NURSING RESEARCH

Generating and Assessing Evidence for Nursing Practice

TENTH EDITION

Denise F. Polit

Cheryl Tatano Beck

The perfect complement to the 10th edition of *Nursing Research: Generating and Assessing Evidence for Nursing Practice,* this knowledge builder strengthens the textbook in important ways. It reinforces the acquisition of basic research skills through systematic learning exercises, with an emphasis on careful reading and critiquing of actual studies—fundamental to designing and planning one's own study.

The Resource Manual includes:

- Full research reports and a grant application in the appendices, which represent a rich array of research endeavors, including quantitative and qualitative studies, an evidence-based practice project report, an instrument development paper, a meta-analysis, and a metasynthesis
- Full critiques of two of the research reports that serve as models for a comprehensive research critique
- A successful grant application that was funded by the National Institute of Nursing Research, together with the Study Section's summary sheet

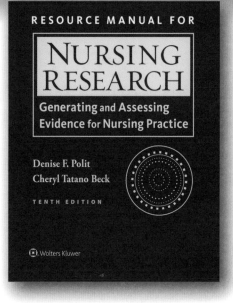

The Resource Manual also includes the invaluable Toolkit, online on thePoint®, which offers important research resources to beginning and advanced researchers. The refined and easily adaptable research tools address a broad range of research situations, are available as editable Word files, and are offered to meet your specific needs.

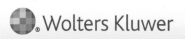 Wolters Kluwer

thePoint®

ISBN: 978-1-4963-1335-5

Quick Guide to an Evidence Hierarchy of Designs
for Cause-Probing Questions

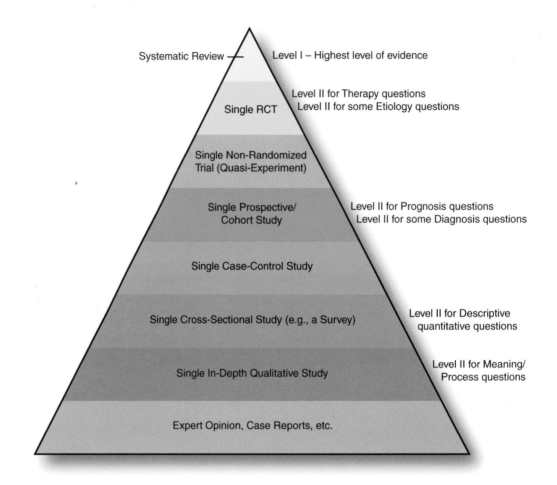

Systematic Review —— Level I – Highest level of evidence

Level II for Therapy questions
Level II for some Etiology questions

Single RCT

Single Non-Randomized
Trial (Quasi-Experiment)

Single Prospective/
Cohort Study

Level II for Prognosis questions
Level II for some Diagnosis questions

Single Case-Control Study

Single Cross-Sectional Study (e.g., a Survey)

Level II for Descriptive
quantitative questions

Single In-Depth Qualitative Study

Level II for Meaning/
Process questions

Expert Opinion, Case Reports, etc.

Quick Guide to Bivariate Statistical Tests

Level of measurement of dependent variable	Group Comparisons: Number of groups (the independent variable)				Correlational analyses (To examine relationship strength)
	2 Groups		3+ Groups		
	Independent Groups Tests	Dependent Groups Tests	Independent Groups Tests	Dependent Groups Tests	
Nominal (Categorical)	χ^2 p. 392 (or Fisher's exact test) p. 393	McNemar"s test p. 393	χ^2 p. 392	Cochran's Q	Phi coefficient (dichotomous) or Cramér's V (not restricted to dichotomous) p. 394
Ordinal (Rank)	Mann-Whitney Test p. 387	Wilcoxon signed ranks test p. 387	Kruskal-Wallis H test p. 391	Friedman's test p. 391	Spearman's rho (or Kendall's tau) pp. 393–394
Interval or Ratio (Continuous)*	Independent group t test pp. 385–386	Paired t test p. 387	ANOVA pp. 388–389	RM-ANOVA pp. 390–391	Pearson's r p. 393
	Multifactor ANOVA for 2+ independent variables p. 389				
	RM-ANOVA for 2+ groups x 2+ measurements over time p. 415				

*For distributions that are markedly nonnormal or samples that are small, the nonparametric tests in the row above may be needed.

NURSING RESEARCH
Generating and Assessing Evidence for Nursing Practice

Tenth Edition

Denise F. Polit, PhD, FAAN
President
Humanalysis, Inc.
Saratoga Springs, New York, *and*
Professor
Griffith University School of Nursing
Brisbane, Australia
(www.denisepolit.com)

Cheryl Tatano Beck, DNSc, CNM, FAAN
Distinguished Professor
School of Nursing
University of Connecticut
Storrs, Connecticut

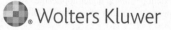 Wolters Kluwer

Philadelphia • Baltimore • New York • London
Buenos Aires • Hong Kong • Sydney • Tokyo

Acquisitions Editor: Christina Burns
Product Development Editor: Katherine Burland
Editorial Assistant: Cassie Berube
Marketing Manager: Dean Karampelas
Production Project Manager: Cynthia Rudy
Design Coordinator: Joan Wendt
Manufacturing Coordinator: Karin Duffield
Prepress Vendor: Absolute Service, Inc.

Tenth edition

9 8 7 6 5 4 3 2 1

Printed in China

Library of Congress Cataloging-in-Publication Data

Polit, Denise F., author.
  Nursing research : generating and assessing evidence for nursing practice / Denise F. Polit, Cheryl Tatano Beck. — Tenth edition.
    p. ; cm.
Includes bibliographical references and index.
ISBN 978-1-4963-0023-2
I. Beck, Cheryl Tatano, author. II. Title.
[DNLM: 1. Nursing Research—methods. WY 20.5]
RT81.5
610.73072—dc23
                                                                                                    2015033543

CCS1215

TO

Our Beloved Family: Our Husbands, Our Children (Spouses/Fiancés), and Our Grandchildren

Husbands: Alan Janosy and Chuck Beck

Children: Alex (Maryanna), Alaine (Jeff), Lauren (Vadim), and Norah (Chris); and Curt and Lisa

Grandchildren: Cormac, Julia, Maren, and Ronan

Acknowledgments

This 10th edition, like the previous nine editions, depended on the contribution of dozens of people. Many faculty and students who used the text have made invaluable suggestions for its improvement, and to all of you we are very grateful. In addition to all those who assisted us during the past 35 years with the earlier editions, the following individuals deserve special mention.

We would like to acknowledge the comments of reviewers of the previous edition of this book, anonymous to us initially, whose feedback influenced our revisions. Faculty at Griffith University in Australia made useful suggestions and also inspired the inclusion of some new content. Valori Banfi, reference librarian at the University of Connecticut, provided ongoing assistance. Dr. Deborah Dillon McDonald was extraordinarily generous in giving us access to her NINR grant application and related material for the *Resource Manual*.

We also extend our thanks to those who helped to turn the manuscript into a finished product. The staff at Wolters Kluwer has been of great assistance to us over the years. We are indebted to Christina Burns, Kate Burland, Cynthia Rudy, and all the others behind the scenes for their fine contributions.

Finally, we thank our family and friends. Our husbands Alan and Chuck have become accustomed to our demanding schedules, but we recognize that their support involves a lot of patience and many sacrifices.

Reviewers

Ellise D. Adams, PhD, CNM
Associate Professor
The University of Alabama in Huntsville
Huntsville, Alabama

Jennifer Bellot, PhD, RN, MHSA
Associate Professor and Director, DNP Program
Thomas Jefferson University
Philadelphia, Pennsylvania

Kathleen D. Black, PhD, RNC
Assistant Professor, Jefferson College of Nursing
Thomas Jefferson University
Philadelphia, Pennsylvania

Dee Campbell, PhD, APRN, NE-BC, CNL
Professor, Graduate Department
Felician College, School of Nursing
Lodi, New Jersey

Patricia Cannistraci, DNS, RN, CNE
Assistant Dean
Excelsior College
Albany, New York

Julie L. Daniels, DNP, CNM
Assistant Professor
Frontier Nursing University
Hyden, Kentucky

Rebecca Fountain, PhD, RN
Associate Professor
University of Texas at Tyler
Tyler, Texas

Teresa S. Johnson, PhD, RN
Associate Professor, College of Nursing
University of Wisconsin—Milwaukee
Milwaukee, Wisconsin

Jacqueline Jones, PhD, RN, FAAN
Associate Professor, College of Nursing
University of Colorado, Anschutz Medical Campus
Aurora, Colorado

Mary Lopez, PhD, RN
Associate Dean, Research
Western University of Health Sciences
Pomona, California

Audra Malone, DNP, FNP-BC
Assistant Professor
Frontier Nursing University
Hyden, Kentucky

Sharon R. Rainer, PhD, CRNP
Assistant Professor, Jefferson College of Nursing
Thomas Jefferson University
Philadelphia, Pennsylvania

Maria A. Revell, PhD, RN
Professor of Nursing
Middle Tennessee State University
Murfreesboro, Tennessee

Stephanie Vaughn, PhD, RN, CRRN
Interim Director, School of Nursing
California State University, Fullerton
Fullerton, California

Preface

Research methodology is not a static enterprise. Even after writing nine editions of this book, we continue to draw inspiration and new material from groundbreaking advances in research methods and in nurse researchers' use of those methods. It is exciting and uplifting to share many of those advances in this new edition. We expect that many of the new methodologic and technologic advances will be translated into powerful evidence for nursing practice. Five years ago, we considered the ninth edition as a watershed edition of a classic textbook. We are persuaded, however, that this 10th edition is even better. We have retained many features that made this book a classic textbook and resource, including its focus on research as a support for evidence-based nursing, but have introduced important innovations that will help to shape the future of nursing research.

NEW TO THIS EDITION

New Chapters

We have added two new chapters on "cutting-edge" topics that are not well covered in any major research methods textbook, regardless of discipline. The first is a chapter on an issue of critical importance to health professionals and yet inadequately addressed in the nursing literature: the clinical significance of research findings. In Chapter 20, we discuss various conceptualizations of clinical significance and present methods of operationalizing those conceptualizations so that clinical significance can be assessed at both the individual and group level. We believe that this is a "must-read" chapter for nurses whose research is designed to inform clinical practice. The second new chapter in this edition concerns the design and conduct of pilot studies. In recent years, experts have written at length about the poor quality of many pilot studies. Chapter 28 provides guidance on how to develop pilot study objectives and draw conclusions about the appropriate next step—that is, whether to proceed to a full-scale study, make major revisions, or abandon the project. This chapter is included in Part 5 of this book, which is devoted to mixed methods research, because pilots can benefit from both qualitative and quantitative evidence.

New Content

Throughout the book, we have included material on methodologic innovations that have arisen in nursing, medicine, and the social sciences during the past 4 to 5 years. The many additions and changes are too numerous to describe here, but a few deserve special mention. In particular, we have totally revised the chapters on measurement (Chapter 14) and scale development (Chapter 15) to reflect emerging ideas about key measurement properties and the assessment of newly developed instruments.

The inclusion of two new chapters made it challenging to keep the textbook to a manageable length. Our solution was to move some content in the ninth edition to supplements that are available online. In fact, every chapter has an online supplement, which gave us the opportunity to add a considerable amount of new content. For example, one supplement is devoted to evidence-based methods to recruit and retain study participants. Other supplements include a description of various randomization methods, an overview of item response theory, guidance on wording proposals to conduct pilot studies, and a discussion of quality improvement studies. Following is a complete list of the supplements for the 31 chapters of this textbook:

1. The History of Nursing Research
2. Evaluating Clinical Practice Guidelines— AGREE II
3. Deductive and Inductive Reasoning
4. Complex Relationships and Hypotheses
5. Literature Review Matrices
6. Prominent Conceptual Models of Nursing Used by Nurse Researchers, and a Guide to Middle-Range Theories
7. Historical Background on Unethical Research Conduct
8. Research Control
9. Randomization Strategies
10. The RE-AIM Framework
11. Other Specific Types of Research
12. Sample Recruitment and Retention
13. Other Types of Structured Self-Reports
14. Cross-Cultural Validity and the Adaptation/ Translation of Measures
15. Overview of Item Response Theory
16. SPSS Analysis of Descriptive Statistics
17. SPSS Analysis of Inferential Statistics
18. SPSS Analysis and Multivariate Statistics
19. Some Preliminary Steps in Quantitative Analysis Using SPSS
20. Clinical Significance Assessment with the Jacobson-Truax Approach
21. Historical Nursing Research
22. Generalizability and Qualitative Research
23. Additional Types of Unstructured Self-Reports
24. Transcribing Qualitative Data
25. Whittemore and Colleagues' Framework of Quality Criteria in Qualitative Research
26. Converting Quantitative and Qualitative Data
27. Complex Intervention Development: Exploratory Questions
28. Examples of Various Pilot Study Objectives
29. Publication Bias in Meta-Analyses
30. Tips for Publishing Reports on Pilot Intervention Studies
31. Proposals for Pilot Intervention Studies

Another new feature of this edition concerns our interest in readers' access to references we cited. To the extent possible, the studies we have chosen as examples of particular research methods are published as open-access articles. These studies are identified with an asterisk in the reference list at the end of each chapter, and a link to the article is included in the Toolkit section of the *Resource Manual*. We hope that these revisions will help users of this book to maximize their learning experience.

ORGANIZATION OF THE TEXT

The content of this edition is organized into six main parts.

- **Part I—Foundations of Nursing Research and Evidence-Based Practice** introduces fundamental concepts in nursing research. Chapter 1 briefly summarizes the history and future of nursing research, discusses the philosophical underpinnings of qualitative research versus quantitative research, and describes major purposes of nursing research. Chapter 2 offers guidance on utilizing research to build an evidence-based practice. Chapter 3 introduces readers to key research terms and presents an overview of steps in the research process for both qualitative and quantitative studies.

- **Part II—Conceptualizing and Planning a Study to Generate Evidence** further sets the stage for learning about the research process by discussing issues relating to a study's conceptualization: the formulation of research questions and hypotheses (Chapter 4), the review of relevant research (Chapter 5), the development of theoretical and conceptual contexts (Chapter 6), and the fostering of ethically sound approaches in doing research (Chapter 7). Chapter 8 provides an overview of important issues that researchers must attend to during the planning of any type of study.

- **Part III—Designing and Conducting Quantitative Studies to Generate Evidence** presents material on undertaking quantitative nursing studies. Chapter 9 describes fundamental principles and applications of quantitative research design, and Chapter 10 focuses on methods to enhance the rigor of a quantitative study, including mechanisms of research control. Chapter 11 examines research with different and distinct purposes, including surveys, outcomes research, and evaluations. Chapter 12 presents strategies for sampling study participants in quantitative research. Chapter 13 describes using structured data collection methods that yield quantitative information. Chapter 14 discusses the concept of measurement and then focuses on methods of assessing the quality of formal measuring instruments. In this edition, we describe methods to assess the properties of point-in-time measurements (reliability and validity) and longitudinal measurements—change scores (reliability of change scores and responsiveness). Chapter 15 presents material on how to develop high-quality self-report instruments. Chapters 16, 17, and 18 present an overview of univariate, bivariate, and multivariate statistical analyses, respectively. Chapter 19 describes the development of an overall analytic strategy for quantitative studies, including material on handling missing data. Chapter 20, a new chapter, discusses the issue of interpreting results and making inferences about clinical significance.
- **Part IV—Designing and Conducting Qualitative Studies to Generate Evidence** presents material on undertaking qualitative nursing studies. Chapter 21 is devoted to research designs and approaches for qualitative studies, including material on critical theory, feminist, and participatory action research. Chapter 22 discusses strategies for sampling study participants in qualitative inquiries. Chapter 23 describes methods of gathering unstructured self-report and observational data for qualitative studies. Chapter 24 discusses methods of analyzing qualitative data, with specific information on grounded theory, phenomenologic, and ethnographic analyses. Chapter 25 elaborates on methods qualitative researchers can use to enhance (and assess) integrity and quality throughout their inquiries.
- **Part V—Designing and Conducting Mixed Methods Studies to Generate Evidence** presents material on mixed methods nursing studies. Chapter 26 discusses a broad range of issues, including asking mixed methods questions, designing a study to address the questions, sampling participants in mixed methods research, and analyzing and integrating qualitative and quantitative data. Chapter 27 presents innovative information about using mixed methods approaches in the development of nursing interventions. In Chapter 28, a new chapter, we provide guidance for designing and conducting a pilot study and using data from the pilot to draw conclusions about how best to proceed.
- **Part VI—Building an Evidence Base for Nursing Practice** provides additional guidance on linking research and clinical practice. Chapter 29 offers an overview of methods of conducting systematic reviews that support EBP, with an emphasis on meta-analyses, metasyntheses, and mixed studies reviews. Chapter 30 discusses dissemination of evidence—how to prepare a research report (including theses and dissertations) and how to publish research findings. The concluding chapter (Chapter 31) offers suggestions and guidelines on developing research proposals and getting financial support and includes information about applying for NIH grants and interpreting scores from NIH's new scoring system.

KEY FEATURES

This textbook was designed to be helpful to those who are learning how to do research as well as to those who are learning to appraise research reports critically and to use research findings in practice. Many of the features successfully used in previous editions have been retained in this 10th edition. Among the basic principles that helped to shape this and earlier editions of this book are (1) an unswerving conviction that the development of research skills is critical to the nursing profession, (2) a fundamental belief that research is intellectually and professionally rewarding, and (3) a steadfast opinion that learning about research methods need be neither intimidating nor dull. Consistent with these principles, we have tried to present the fundamentals of research methods in a way that both facilitates understanding and arouses curiosity and interest. Key features of our approach include the following:

- **Research Examples.** Each chapter concludes with one or two actual research examples designed to highlight critical points made in the chapter and to sharpen the reader's critical thinking skills. In addition, many research examples are used to illustrate key points in the text and to stimulate ideas for a study. Many of the examples used in this edition are open-access articles that can be used for further learning and classroom discussions.
- **Critiquing Guidelines.** Most chapters include guidelines for conducting a critique of each aspect of a research report. These guidelines provide a list of questions that draw attention to specific aspects of a report that are amenable to appraisal.
- **Clear, "user-friendly" style.** Our writing style is designed to be easily digestible and nonintimidating. Concepts are introduced carefully and systematically, difficult ideas are presented clearly, and readers are assumed to have no prior exposure to technical terms.
- **Specific practical tips on doing research.** This textbook is filled with practical guidance on how to translate the abstract notions of research methods into realistic strategies for conducting research. Every chapter includes several tips for applying the chapter's lessons to real-life situations. These suggestions are in recognition of the fact that there is often a large gap between what gets taught in research methods textbooks and what a researcher needs to know to conduct a study.
- **Aids to student learning.** Several features are used to enhance and reinforce learning and to help focus the student's attention on specific areas of text content, including the following: succinct, bulleted summaries at the end of each chapter; tables and figures that provide examples and graphic materials in support of the text discussion; study suggestions at the end of each chapter; a detailed glossary; and a comprehensive index for accessing information quickly.

TEACHING–LEARNING PACKAGE

Nursing Research: Generating and Assessing Evidence for Nursing Practice, 10th edition, has an ancillary package designed with both students and instructors in mind.

- The *Resource Manual* augments the textbook in important ways. The manual itself provides students with exercises that correspond to each text chapter, with a focus on opportunities to critique actual studies. The appendix includes 12 research journal articles in their entirety, plus a successful grant application for a study funded by the National Institute of Nursing Research. The 12 reports cover a range of nursing research ventures, including qualitative, quantitative, and mixed methods studies, an instrument development study, an evidence-based practice translation project, and two systematic reviews. Full critiques of two of the reports are also included and can serve as models for a comprehensive research critique.
- The Toolkit to the *Resource Manual* is a "must-have" innovation that will save considerable time for both students and seasoned researchers. Included on thePoint, the Toolkit offers dozens of research resources in Word documents that can be downloaded and used directly or adapted. The resources reflect best-practice research material, most of which have been pretested and refined in our own research. The Toolkit originated with our realization that in our technologically advanced environment, it is possible to not only *illustrate* methodologic tools as graphics in the textbook but also to make them directly available for use and adaptation. Thus, we have

included dozens of documents in Word files that can readily be used in research projects, without requiring researchers to "reinvent the wheel" or tediously retype material from this textbook. Examples include informed consent forms, a demographic questionnaire, content validity forms, and a coding sheet for a meta-analysis—to name only a few. The Toolkit also has lists of relevant and useful websites for each chapter, which can be "clicked" on directly without having to retype the URL and risk a typographical error. Links to open-access articles cited in the textbook, as well as other open-access articles relevant to each chapter, are included in the Toolkit.

• **The Instructor's Resources on thePoint** include PowerPoint slides summarizing key points in each chapter, test questions that have been placed into a program that allows instructors to automatically generate a test, and an image bank.

It is our hope that the content, style, and organization of this book continue to meet the needs of a broad spectrum of nursing students and nurse researchers. We also hope that this book will help to foster enthusiasm for the kinds of discoveries that research can produce and for the knowledge that will help support an evidence-based nursing practice.

DENISE F. POLIT, PhD, FAAN

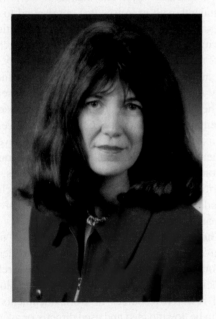

CHERYL TATANO BECK, DNSc, CNM, FAAN

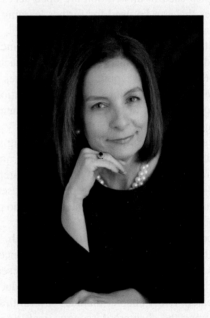

Contents

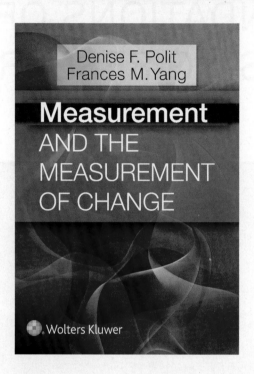

Denise F. Polit
Frances M. Yang

Measurement
AND THE
MEASUREMENT
OF CHANGE

Wolters Kluwer

Check Out the Latest Book Authored by Research Expert Dr. Polit

If you want to make thoughtful but practical decisions about the measurement of health constructs, check out Dr. Polit and Dr. Yang's latest book, a "gentle" introduction to and overview of complex measurement content, called *Measurement and the Measurement of Change*.

This book is for researchers and clinicians from all health disciplines because measurement is vital to high-quality science and to excellence in clinical practice. The text focuses on the measurement of health constructs, particularly those constructs that are not amenable to quantification by means of laboratory analysis or technical instrumentation. These health constructs include a wide range of human attributes, such as quality of life, functional ability, self-efficacy, depression, and pain. Measures of such constructs are proliferating at a rapid rate and often without adequate attention paid to ensuring that standards of scientific rigor are met.

In this book, the authors offer guidance to those who develop new instruments, adapt existing ones, select instruments for use in a clinical trial or in clinical practice, interpret information from measurements and changes in scores, or undertake a systematic review on instruments. This book offers guidance on how to develop new instruments using both "classical" and "modern" approaches from psychometrics as well as methods used in clinimetrics. Much of this book, however, concerns the evaluation of instruments in relation to three key measurement domains: reliability, validity, and responsiveness.

This text was designed to be useful in graduate-level courses on measurement or research methods and will also serve as an important reference and resource for researchers and clinicians.

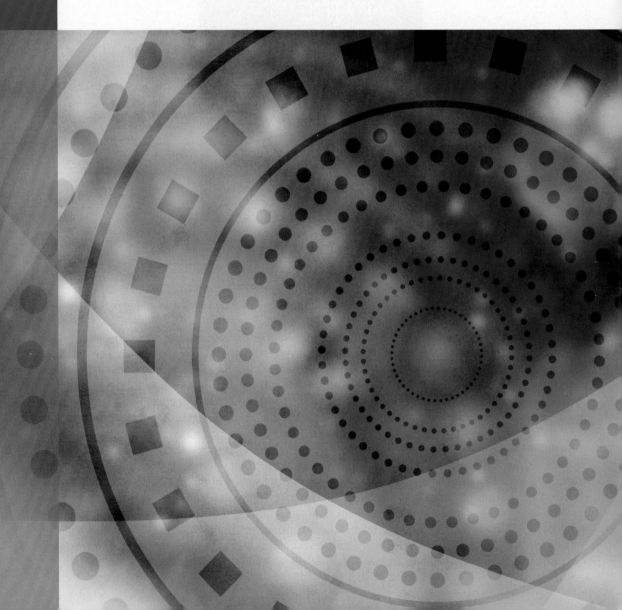

PART 1

FOUNDATIONS OF NURSING RESEARCH

1 | Introduction to Nursing Research in an Evidence-Based Practice Environment

NURSING RESEARCH IN PERSPECTIVE

In all parts of the world, nursing has experienced a profound culture change. Nurses are increasingly expected to understand and conduct research and to base their professional practice on research evidence—that is, to adopt an **evidence-based practice (EBP)**. EBP involves using the best evidence (as well as clinical judgment and patient preferences) in making patient care decisions, and "best evidence" typically comes from research conducted by nurses and other health care professionals.

What Is Nursing Research?

Research is systematic inquiry that uses disciplined methods to answer questions or solve problems. The ultimate goal of research is to develop and expand knowledge.

Nurses are increasingly engaged in disciplined studies that benefit nursing and its clients. **Nursing research** is systematic inquiry designed to generate trustworthy evidence about issues of importance to the nursing profession, including nursing practice, education, administration, and informatics. In this book, we emphasize **clinical nursing research**, that is, research to guide nursing practice and to improve the health and quality of life of nurses' clients.

Nursing research has experienced remarkable growth in the past three decades, providing nurses with a growing evidence base from which

to practice. Yet many questions endure and much remains to be done to incorporate research innovations into nursing practice.

Examples of Nursing Research Questions:

- How effective is pressurized irrigation, compared to a swabbing method, in cleansing wounds, in terms of time to wound healing, pain, patients' satisfaction with comfort, and costs? (Mak et al., 2015)
- What are the experiences of women in Zimbabwe who are living with advanced HIV infection? (Gona & DeMarco, 2015)

The Importance of Research in Nursing

Research findings from rigorous studies provide especially strong evidence for informing nurses' decisions and actions. Nurses are accepting the need to base specific nursing actions on research evidence indicating that the actions are clinically appropriate, cost-effective, and result in positive outcomes for clients.

In the United States, research plays an important role in nursing in terms of credentialing and status. The American Nurses Credentialing Center (ANCC)—an arm of the American Nurses Association and the largest and most prestigious credentialing organization in the United States—developed a Magnet Recognition Program to acknowledge health care organizations that provide high-quality nursing care. As Reigle and her colleagues (2008) noted, "the road to Magnet Recognition is paved with EBP" (p. 102) and the 2014 Magnet application manual incorporated revisions that strengthened evidence-based requirements (Drenkard, 2013). The good news is that there is growing confirmation that the focus on research and evidence-based practice may have important payoffs. For example, McHugh and co-researchers (2013) found that Magnet hospitals have lower risk-adjusted mortality and failure to rescue than non-Magnet hospitals, even when differences among the hospitals in nursing credentials and patient characteristics are taken into account.

Changes to nursing practice now occur regularly because of EBP efforts. Practice changes often are local initiatives that are not publicized, but broader clinical changes are also occurring based on accumulating research evidence about beneficial practice innovations.

Example of Evidence-Based Practice: Numerous clinical practice changes reflect the impact of research. For example, "kangaroo care" (the holding of diaper-clad infants skin to skin by parents) is now practiced in many neonatal intensive care units (NICUs), but this is a relatively new trend. As recently as the 1990s, only a minority of NICUs offered kangaroo care options. Expanded adoption of this practice reflects mounting evidence that early skin-to-skin contact has benefits without negative side effects (e.g., Ludington-Hoe, 2011; Moore et al., 2012). Some of that evidence came from rigorous studies conducted by nurse researchers in several countries (e.g., Chwo et al., 2002; Cong et al., 2009; Cong et al., 2011; Hake-Brooks & Anderson, 2008). Nurses continue to study the potential benefits of kangaroo care in important clinical trials (e.g., Campbell-Yeo et al., 2013).

The Consumer–Producer Continuum in Nursing Research

In our current environment, all nurses are likely to engage in activities along a continuum of research participation. At one end of the continuum are *consumers of nursing research*, who read research reports or research summaries to keep up-to-date on findings that might affect their practice. EBP depends on well-informed nursing research consumers.

At the other end of the continuum are the *producers of nursing research*: nurses who design and

conduct research. At one time, most nurse researchers were academics who taught in schools of nursing, but research is increasingly being conducted by nurses in health care settings who want to find solutions to recurring problems in patient care.

Between these end points on the continuum lie a variety of research activities that are undertaken by nurses. Even if you never personally undertake a study, you may (1) contribute to an idea or a plan for a clinical study; (2) gather data for a study; (3) advise clients about participating in research; (4) solve a clinical problem by searching for research evidence; or (5) discuss the implications of a new study in a **journal club** in your practice setting, which involves meetings (in groups or online) to discuss research articles. In all possible research-related activities, nurses who have some research skills are better able than those without them to make a contribution to nursing and to EBP. An understanding of nursing research can improve the depth and breadth of *every* nurse's professional practice.

Nursing Research in Historical Perspective

Table 1.1 summarizes some of the key events in the historical evolution of nursing research. (An expanded summary of the history of nursing research appears in the Supplement to this chapter on thePoint®).

Most people would agree that research in nursing began with Florence Nightingale in the 1850s. Her most well-known research contribution involved an analysis of factors affecting soldier mortality and morbidity during the Crimean War. Based on skillful analyses, she was successful in effecting changes in nursing care and, more generally, in public health. After Nightingale's work, research was absent from the nursing literature until the early 1900s, but most early studies concerned nurses' education rather than clinical issues.

In the 1950s, research by nurses began to accelerate. For example, a nursing research center was established at the Walter Reed Army Institute of Research. Also, the American Nurses Foundation, which is devoted to the promotion of nursing research, was founded. The surge in the number of studies conducted in the 1950s created the need for

TABLE 1.1 • Historical Landmarks in Nursing Research

YEAR	EVENT
1859	Nightingale's *Notes on Nursing* is published.
1900	*American Journal of Nursing* begins publication.
1923	Columbia University establishes first doctoral program for nurses.
	Goldmark Report with recommendations for nursing education is published.
1936	Sigma Theta Tau awards first nursing research grant in the United States.
1948	Brown publishes report on inadequacies of nursing education.
1952	The journal *Nursing Research* begins publication.
1955	Inception of the American Nurses Foundation to sponsor nursing research.
1957	Establishment of nursing research center at Walter Reed Army Institute of Research.
1963	*International Journal of Nursing Studies* begins publication.
1965	American Nurses Association (ANA) sponsors nursing research conferences.
1969	*Canadian Journal of Nursing Research* begins publication.
1972	ANA establishes a Commission on Research and Council of Nurse Researchers.
1976	Stetler and Marram publish guidelines on assessing research for use in practice.
	Journal of Advanced Nursing begins publication.
1982	Conduct and Utilization of Research in Nursing (CURN) project publishes report.
1983	*Annual Review of Nursing Research* begins publication.
1985	ANA Cabinet on Nursing Research establishes research priorities.
1986	National Center for Nursing Research (NCNR) is established within U.S. National Institutes of Health.
1988	Conference on Research Priorities is convened by NCNR.
1989	U.S. Agency for Health Care Policy and Research (AHCPR) is established.
1993	NCNR becomes a full institute, the National Institute of Nursing Research (NINR).
	The Cochrane Collaboration is established.
	Magnet Recognition Program makes first awards.
1995	Joanna Briggs Institute, an international EBP collaborative, is established in Australia.
1997	Canadian Health Services Research Foundation is established with federal funding.
1999	AHCPR is renamed Agency for Healthcare Research and Quality (AHRQ).
2000	NINR's annual funding exceeds $100 million.
	The Canadian Institute of Health Research is launched.
	Council for the Advancement of Nursing Science (CANS) is established.
2006	NINR issues strategic plan for 2006–2010.
2011	NINR celebrates 25th anniversary and issues a new strategic plan.
2014	NINR budget exceeds $140 million.

a new journal; *Nursing Research* came into being in 1952. As shown in Table 1.1, dissemination opportunities in professional journals grew steadily thereafter.

In the 1960s, nursing leaders expressed concern about the shortage of research on practice issues. Professional nursing organizations, such as the Western Interstate Council for Higher Education in Nursing, established research priorities, and practice-oriented research on various clinical topics began to emerge in the literature.

During the 1970s, improvements in client care became a more visible research priority and nurses also began to pay attention to the clinical utilization of research findings. Guidance on assessing research for application in practice settings became available. Several journals that focus on nursing research were established in the 1970s, including *Advances* in *Nursing Science, Research in Nursing & Health*, and the *Western Journal of Nursing Research*. Nursing research also expanded internationally. For example, the Workgroup of European Nurse Researchers was established in 1978 to develop greater communication and opportunities for partnerships among 25 European National Nurses Associations.

Nursing research continued to expand in the 1980s. In the United States, the National Center for Nursing Research (NCNR) at the National Institutes of Health (NIH) was established in 1986. Several forces outside of nursing also helped to shape the nursing research landscape. A group from the McMaster Medical School in Canada designed a clinical learning strategy that was called evidence-based medicine (EBM). EBM, which promulgated the view that research findings were far superior to the opinions of authorities as a basis for clinical decisions, constituted a profound shift for medical education and practice, and has had a major effect on all health care professions.

Nursing research was strengthened and given more visibility when NCNR was promoted to full institute status within the NIH. In 1993, the *National Institute of Nursing Research* (NINR) was established, helping to put nursing research more into the mainstream of health research. Funding opportunities for nursing research expanded in other countries as well.

Current and Future Directions for Nursing Research

Nursing research continues to develop at a rapid pace and will undoubtedly flourish in the 21st century. Funding continues to grow. For example, NINR funding in fiscal year 2014 was more than $140 million compared to $70 million in 1999—and the competition for available funding is increasingly vigorous as more nurses seek support for testing innovative ideas for practice improvements.

Broadly speaking, the priority for future nursing research will be the promotion of excellence in nursing science. Toward this end, nurse researchers and practicing nurses will be sharpening their research skills and using those skills to address emerging issues of importance to the profession

and its clientele. Among the trends we foresee for the early 21st century are the following:

- *Continued focus on EBP*. Encouragement for nurses to engage in evidence-based patient care is sure to continue. In turn, improvements will be needed both in the quality of studies and in nurses' skills in locating, understanding, critiquing, and using relevant study results. Relatedly, there is an emerging interest in **translational research**—research on how findings from studies can best be translated into practice. Translation potential will require researchers to think more strategically about long-term feasibility, *scalability*, and sustainability when they test solutions to problems.
- *Development of a stronger evidence base through confirmatory strategies*. Practicing nurses are unlikely to adopt an innovation based on weakly designed or isolated studies. Strong research designs are essential, and confirmation is usually needed through the **replication** (i.e., the repeating) of studies with different clients, in different clinical settings, and at different times to ensure that the findings are robust.
- *Greater emphasis on systematic reviews*. **Systematic reviews** are a cornerstone of EBP and will take on increased importance in all health disciplines. Systematic reviews rigorously integrate research information on a topic so that conclusions about the state of evidence can be reached. Best practice clinical guidelines typically rely on such systematic reviews.
- *Innovation*. There is currently a major push for creative and innovative solutions to recurring practice problems. "Innovation" has become an important buzzword throughout NIH and in nursing associations. For example, the 2013 annual conference of the Council for the Advancement of Nursing Science was "Innovative Approaches to Symptom Science." Innovative interventions—and new methods for studying nursing questions—are sure to be part of the future research landscape in nursing.
- *Expanded local research in health care settings*. Small studies designed to solve local problems will likely increase. This trend will be reinforced as more hospitals apply for (and are

recertified for) Magnet status in the United States and in other countries. Mechanisms will need to be developed to ensure that evidence from these small projects becomes available to others facing similar problems, such as communication within and between regional nursing research alliances.

• *Strengthening of interdisciplinary collaboration.* Collaboration of nurses with researchers in related fields is likely to expand in the 21st century as researchers address fundamental health care problems. In turn, such collaborative efforts could lead to nurse researchers playing a more prominent role in national and international health care policies. One of four major recommendations in a 2010 report on the future of nursing by the Institute of Medicine was that nurses should be full partners with physicians and other health care professionals in redesigning health care.

• *Expanded dissemination of research findings.* The Internet and other electronic communication have a big impact on disseminating research information, which in turn helps to promote EBP. Through technologic advances, information about innovations can be communicated more widely and more quickly than ever before.

• *Increased focus on cultural issues and health disparities.* The issue of health disparities has emerged as a central concern in nursing and other health disciplines; this in turn has raised consciousness about the cultural sensitivity of health interventions and the cultural competence of health care workers. There is growing awareness that research must be sensitive to the health beliefs, behaviors, and values of culturally and linguistically diverse populations.

• *Clinical significance and patient input.* Research findings increasingly must meet the test of being clinically significant, and patients have taken center stage in efforts to define clinical significance. A major challenge in the years ahead will involve getting both research evidence and patient preferences into clinical decisions, and designing research to study the process and the outcomes.

Broad research priorities for the future have been articulated by many nursing organizations, including NINR and Sigma Theta Tau International.

Expert panels and research working groups help NINR to identify gaps in current knowledge that require research. The primary areas of research funded by NINR in 2014 were health promotion/disease prevention, eliminating health disparities, caregiving, symptom management, and self-management. Research priorities that have been expressed by Sigma Theta Tau International include advancing healthy communities through health promotion; preventing disease and recognizing social, economic, and political determinants; implementation of evidence-based practice; targeting the needs of vulnerable populations such as the poor and chronically ill; and developing nurses' capacity for research. Priorities also have been developed for several nursing specialties and for nurses in several countries—for example, Ireland (Brenner et al., 2014; Drennan et al., 2007), Sweden (Bäck-Pettersson et al., 2008), Australia (Wynaden et al., 2014), and Korea (Kim et al., 2002).

SOURCES OF EVIDENCE FOR NURSING PRACTICE

Nurses make clinical decisions based on knowledge from many sources, including coursework, textbooks, and their own clinical experience. Because evidence is constantly evolving, learning about best practice nursing perseveres throughout a nurse's career.

Some of what nurses learn is based on systematic research, but much of it is not. What *are* the sources of evidence for nursing practice? Where does knowledge for practice come from? Until fairly recently, knowledge primarily was handed down from one generation to the next based on experience, trial and error, tradition, and expert opinion. Information sources for clinical practice vary in dependability, giving rise to what is called an *evidence hierarchy*, which acknowledges that certain types of evidence are better than others. A brief discussion of some alternative sources of evidence shows how research-based information is different.

Tradition and Authority

Decisions are sometimes based on custom or tradition. Certain "truths" are accepted as given, and such "knowledge" is so much a part of a common heritage that few seek verification. Tradition facilitates communication by providing a common foundation of accepted truth, but many traditions have never been evaluated for their validity. There is concern that some nursing interventions are based on tradition, custom, and "unit culture" rather than on sound evidence. Indeed, a recent analysis suggests that some "sacred cows" (ineffective traditional habits) persist even in a health care center recognized as a leader in evidence-based practice (Hanrahan et al., 2015).

Another common source of information is an authority, a person with specialized expertise. We often make decisions about problems with which we have little experience; it seems natural to place our trust in the judgment of people with specialized training or experience. As a source of evidence, however, authority has shortcomings. Authorities are not infallible, particularly if their expertise is based primarily on personal experience; yet, like tradition, their knowledge often goes unchallenged.

Example of "Myths" in Nursing Textbooks:
A study suggests that even nursing textbooks may contain "myths." In their analysis of 23 widely used undergraduate psychiatric nursing textbooks, Holman and colleagues (2010) found that all books contained at least one unsupported assumption (myth) about loss and grief—that is, assumptions not supported by research evidence. Moreover, many evidence-based findings about grief and loss failed to be included in the textbooks.

Clinical Experience, Trial and Error, and Intuition

Clinical experience is a familiar, functional source of knowledge. The ability to generalize, to recognize regularities, and to make predictions is an important characteristic of the human mind. Nevertheless, personal experience is limited as a knowledge source because each nurse's experience is too narrow to be generally useful. A second limitation is that the same objective event is often experienced and perceived differently by two nurses.

A related method is trial and error in which alternatives are tried successively until a solution to a problem is found. We likely have all used this method in our professional work. For example, many patients dislike the taste of potassium chloride solution. Nurses try to disguise the taste of the medication in various ways until one method meets with the approval of the patient. Trial and error may offer a practical means of securing knowledge, but the method tends to be haphazard and solutions may be idiosyncratic.

Intuition is a knowledge source that cannot be explained based on reasoning or prior instruction. Although intuition and hunches undoubtedly play a role in nursing—as they do in the conduct of research—it is difficult to develop nursing policies and practices based on intuition.

Logical Reasoning

Solutions to some problems are developed by logical thought processes. As a problem-solving method, logical reasoning combines experience, intellectual faculties, and formal systems of thought. **Inductive reasoning** involves developing generalizations from specific observations. For example, a nurse may observe the anxious behavior of (specific) hospitalized children and conclude that (in general) children's separation from their parents is stressful. **Deductive reasoning** involves developing specific predictions from general principles. For example, if we assume that separation anxiety occurs in hospitalized children (in general), then we might predict that (specific) children in a hospital whose parents do not room-in will manifest symptoms of stress. Both systems of reasoning are useful for understanding and organizing phenomena, and both play a role in research. Logical reasoning in and of itself, however, is limited because the validity of reasoning depends on the accuracy of the premises with which one starts.

Assembled Information

In making clinical decisions, health care professionals rely on information that has been assembled for a variety of purposes. For example, local, national, and international *benchmarking data* provide information on such issues as infection rates or the rates of using various procedures (e.g., cesarean births) and can facilitate evaluations of clinical practices. *Cost data*—information on the costs associated with certain procedures, policies, or practices—are sometimes used as a factor in clinical decision making. *Quality improvement and risk data*, such as medication error reports, can be used to assess the need for practice changes. Such sources are useful, but they do not provide a good mechanism for determining whether improvements in patient outcomes result from their use.

Disciplined Research

Research conducted in a disciplined framework is the most sophisticated method of acquiring knowledge. Nursing research combines logical reasoning with other features to create evidence that, although fallible, tends to yield the most reliable evidence. Carefully synthesized findings from rigorous research are at the pinnacle of most evidence hierarchies. The current emphasis on EBP requires nurses to base their clinical practice to the greatest extent possible on rigorous research-based findings rather than on tradition, authority, intuition, or personal experience—although nursing will always remain a rich blend of art and science.

PARADIGMS AND METHODS FOR NURSING RESEARCH

A **paradigm** is a worldview, a general perspective on the complexities of the world. Paradigms for human inquiry are often characterized in terms of the ways in which they respond to basic philosophical questions, such as, What is the nature of reality? (ontologic) and What is the relationship between the inquirer and those being studied? (epistemologic).

Disciplined inquiry in nursing has been conducted mainly within two broad paradigms, *positivism* and *constructivism*. This section describes these two paradigms and outlines the research methods associated with them. In later chapters, we describe the *transformative paradigm* that involves *critical theory research* (Chapter 21), and a *pragmatism paradigm* that involves *mixed methods research* (Chapter 26).

The Positivist Paradigm

The paradigm that dominated nursing research for decades is known as **positivism** (also called *logical positivism*). Positivism is rooted in 19th century thought, guided by such philosophers as Mill, Newton, and Locke. Positivism reflects a broader cultural phenomenon that, in the humanities, is referred to as *modernism*, which emphasizes the rational and the scientific.

As shown in Table 1.2, a fundamental assumption of positivists is that there is a reality *out there* that can be studied and known (an **assumption** is a basic principle that is believed to be true without proof or verification). Adherents of positivism assume that nature is basically ordered and regular and that reality exists independent of human observation. In other words, the world is assumed not to be merely a creation of the human mind. The related assumption of **determinism** refers to the positivists' belief that phenomena are not haphazard but rather have antecedent causes. If a person has a cerebrovascular accident, the researcher in a positivist tradition assumes that there must be one or more reasons that can be potentially identified. Within the positivist paradigm, much research activity is directed at understanding the underlying causes of phenomena.

Positivists value objectivity and attempt to hold personal beliefs and biases in check to avoid contaminating the phenomena under study. The positivists' scientific approach involves using orderly, disciplined procedures with tight controls of the research situation to test hunches about the phenomena being studied.

Strict positivist thinking has been challenged, and few researchers adhere to the tenets of pure positivism. In the **postpositivist paradigm**, there is still a belief in reality and a desire to understand it, but postpositivists recognize the impossibility of total objectivity. They do, however, see objectivity as a goal and strive to be as neutral as possible. Postpositivists also appreciate the impediments to knowing reality with certainty and therefore seek *probabilistic* evidence—that is, learning what the true state of a phenomenon *probably* is, with a high degree of likelihood. This modified positivist

TABLE 1.2 • Major Assumptions of the Positivist and Constructivist Paradigms

TYPE OF QUESTION	POSITIVIST PARADIGM ASSUMPTION	CONSTRUCTIVIST PARADIGM ASSUMPTION
Ontologic: What is the nature of reality?	Reality exists; there is a real world driven by real natural causes and subsequent effects	Reality is multiple and subjective, mentally constructed by individuals; simultaneous shaping, not cause and effect
Epistemologic: How is the inquirer related to those being researched?	The inquirer is independent from those being researched; findings are not influenced by the researcher	The inquirer interacts with those being researched; findings are the creation of the interactive process
Axiologic: What is the role of values in the inquiry?	Values and biases are to be held in check; objectivity is sought	Subjectivity and values are inevitable and desirable
Methodologic: How is evidence best obtained?	Deductive processes → hypothesis testing	Inductive processes → hypothesis generation
	Emphasis on discrete, specific concepts	Emphasis on entirety of some phenomenon, holistic
	Focus on the objective and quantifiable	Focus on the subjective and nonquantifiable
	Corroboration of researchers' predictions	Emerging insight grounded in participants' experiences
	Outsider knowledge—researcher is external, separate	Insider knowledge—researcher is internal, part of process
	Fixed, prespecified design	Flexible, emergent design
	Controls over context	Context-bound, contextualized
	Large, representative samples	Small, information-rich samples
	Measured (quantitative) information	Narrative (unstructured) information
	Statistical analysis	Qualitative analysis
	Seeks generalizations	Seeks in-depth understanding

position remains a dominant force in nursing research. For the sake of simplicity, we refer to it as positivism.

The Constructivist Paradigm

The **constructivist paradigm** (often called the *naturalistic paradigm*) began as a countermovement to positivism with writers such as Weber and Kant. Just as positivism reflects the cultural phenomenon

of modernism that burgeoned after the industrial revolution, naturalism is an outgrowth of the cultural transformation called *postmodernism*. Postmodern thinking emphasizes the value of *deconstruction*—taking apart old ideas and structures—and *reconstruction*—putting ideas and structures together in new ways. The constructivist paradigm represents a major alternative system for conducting disciplined research in nursing. Table 1.2

compares the major assumptions of the positivist and constructivist paradigms.

For the naturalistic inquirer, reality is not a fixed entity but rather is a construction of the individuals participating in the research; reality exists within a context, and many constructions are possible. Naturalists thus take the position of relativism: If there are multiple interpretations of reality that exist in people's minds, then there is no process by which the ultimate truth or falsity of the constructions can be determined.

The constructivist paradigm assumes that knowledge is maximized when the distance between the inquirer and those under study is minimized. The voices and interpretations of study participants are crucial to understanding the phenomenon of interest, and subjective interactions are the primary way to access them. Findings from a constructivist inquiry are the product of the interaction between the inquirer and the participants.

Paradigms and Methods: Quantitative and Qualitative Research

Research methods are the techniques researchers use to structure a study and to gather and analyze information relevant to the research question. The two alternative paradigms correspond to different methods for developing evidence. A key methodologic distinction is between **quantitative research**, which is most closely allied with positivism, and **qualitative research**, which is associated with constructivist inquiry—although positivists sometimes undertake qualitative studies, and constructivist researchers sometimes collect quantitative information. This section provides an overview of the methods associated with the two paradigms.

The Scientific Method and Quantitative Research

The traditional, positivist **scientific method** refers to a set of orderly, disciplined procedures used to acquire information. Quantitative researchers use deductive reasoning to generate predictions that are tested in the real world. They typically move in a systematic fashion from the definition of a problem and the selection of concepts on which to focus to the solution of the problem. By **systematic**, we mean that the investigator progresses logically

through a series of steps, according to a specified plan of action.

Quantitative researchers use various control strategies. **Control** involves imposing conditions on the research situation so that biases are minimized and precision and validity are maximized. Control mechanisms are discussed at length in this book.

Quantitative researchers gather **empirical evidence**—evidence that is rooted in objective reality and gathered through the senses. Empirical evidence, then, consists of observations gathered through sight, hearing, taste, touch, or smell. Observations of the presence or absence of skin inflammation, patients' anxiety level, or infant birth weight are all examples of empirical observations. The requirement to use empirical evidence means that findings are grounded in reality rather than in researchers' personal beliefs.

Evidence for a study in the positivist paradigm is gathered according to an established plan, using structured methods to collect needed information. Usually (but not always) the information gathered is **quantitative**—that is, numeric information that is obtained from a formal measurement and is analyzed statistically.

A traditional scientific study strives to go beyond the specifics of a research situation. For example, quantitative researchers are typically not as interested in understanding why a *particular* person has a stroke as in understanding what factors influence its occurrence in people generally. The degree to which research findings can be generalized to individuals other than those who participated in the study is called the study's **generalizability**.

The scientific method has enjoyed considerable stature as a method of inquiry and has been used productively by nurse researchers studying a range of nursing problems. This is not to say, however, that this approach can solve all nursing problems. One important limitation—common to both quantitative and qualitative research—is that research cannot be used to answer moral or ethical questions. Many persistent, intriguing questions about human beings fall into this area—questions such as whether euthanasia should be practiced or abortion should be legal.

The traditional research approach also must contend with problems of *measurement*. To study a phenomenon, quantitative researchers attempt to measure it by attaching numeric values that express quantity. For example, if the phenomenon of interest is patient stress, researchers would want to assess if patients' stress is high or low, or higher under certain conditions or for some people. Physiologic phenomena such as blood pressure and temperature can be measured with great accuracy and precision, but the same cannot be said of most psychological phenomena, such as stress or resilience.

Another issue is that nursing research focuses on humans, who are inherently complex and diverse. Traditional quantitative methods typically concentrate on a relatively small portion of the human experience (e.g., weight gain, depression) in a single study. Complexities tend to be controlled and, if possible, eliminated, rather than studied directly, and this narrowness of focus can sometimes obscure insights. Finally, quantitative research within the positivist paradigm has been accused of an inflexibility of vision that does not capture the full breadth of human experience.

Constructivist Methods and Qualitative Research

Researchers in constructivist traditions emphasize the inherent complexity of humans, their ability to shape and create their own experiences, and the idea that truth is a composite of realities. Consequently, constructivist studies are heavily focused on understanding the human experience as it is lived, usually through the careful collection and analysis of **qualitative** materials that are narrative and subjective.

Researchers who reject the traditional scientific method believe that it is overly *reductionist*—that is, it reduces human experience to the few concepts under investigation, and those concepts are defined in advance by the researcher rather than emerging from the experiences of those under study. Constructivist researchers tend to emphasize the dynamic, holistic, and individual aspects of human life and attempt to capture those aspects in their entirety, within the context of those who are experiencing them.

Flexible, evolving procedures are used to capitalize on findings that emerge in the course of the study. Constructivist inquiry usually takes place in the **field** (i.e., in naturalistic settings), often over an extended time period. In constructivist research, the collection of information and its analysis typically progress concurrently; as researchers sift through information, insights are gained, new questions emerge, and further evidence is sought to amplify or confirm the insights. Through an inductive process, researchers integrate information to develop a theory or description that helps illuminate the phenomenon under observation.

Constructivist studies yield rich, in-depth information that can elucidate varied dimensions of a complicated phenomenon. Findings from in-depth qualitative research are typically grounded in the real-life experiences of people with first-hand knowledge of a phenomenon. Nevertheless, the approach has several limitations. Human beings are used directly as the instrument through which information is gathered, and humans are extremely intelligent and sensitive—but fallible—tools. The subjectivity that enriches the analytic insights of skillful researchers can yield trivial and obvious "findings" among less competent ones.

Another potential limitation involves the subjectivity of constructivist inquiry, which sometimes raises concerns about the idiosyncratic nature of the conclusions. Would two constructivist researchers studying the same phenomenon in similar settings arrive at similar conclusions? The situation is further complicated by the fact that most constructivist studies involve a small group of participants. Thus, the generalizability of findings from constructivist inquiries is an issue of potential concern.

Multiple Paradigms and Nursing Research

Paradigms should be viewed as lenses that help to sharpen our focus on a phenomenon, not as blinders that limit intellectual curiosity. The emergence of alternative paradigms for studying nursing problems is, in our view, a healthy and desirable path that can maximize the breadth of evidence for practice. Although researchers' worldview may be paradigmatic, knowledge itself is not. Nursing knowledge would be thin if there were not a rich array of methods available within the two paradigms—methods that are often complementary in their strengths and limitations. We believe that intellectual pluralism is advantageous.

We have emphasized differences between the two paradigms and associated methods so that distinctions would be easy to understand—although for many of the issues included in Table 1.2, differences are more on a continuum than they are a dichotomy. Subsequent chapters of this book elaborate further on differences in terminology, methods, and research products. It is equally important, however, to note that the two main paradigms have many features in common, only some of which are mentioned here:

- *Ultimate goals.* The ultimate aim of disciplined research, regardless of the underlying paradigm, is to gain understanding about phenomena. Both quantitative and qualitative researchers seek to capture the truth with regard to an aspect of the world in which they are interested, and both groups can make meaningful—and mutually beneficial—contributions to evidence for nursing practice.
- *External evidence.* Although the word *empiricism* has come to be allied with the classic scientific method, researchers in both traditions gather and analyze evidence empirically, that is, through their senses. Neither qualitative nor quantitative researchers are armchair analysts, depending on their own beliefs and worldviews to generate knowledge.
- *Reliance on human cooperation.* Because evidence for nursing research comes primarily from humans, human cooperation is essential. To understand people's characteristics and experiences, researchers must persuade them to participate in the investigation *and* to speak and act candidly.
- *Ethical constraints.* Research with human beings is guided by ethical principles that sometimes interfere with research goals. As we discuss in Chapter 7, ethical dilemmas often confront researchers, regardless of paradigms or methods.
- *Fallibility of disciplined research.* Virtually all studies have some limitations. Every research question can be addressed in many ways, and inevitably, there are trade-offs. The fallibility of any single study makes it important to understand and critique researchers' methodologic decisions when evaluating evidence quality.

Thus, despite philosophic and methodologic differences, researchers using traditional scientific methods or constructivist methods share overall goals and face many similar challenges. The selection of an appropriate method depends on researchers' personal philosophy and also on the research question. If a researcher asks, "What are the effects of cryotherapy on nausea and oral mucositis in patients undergoing chemotherapy?" the researcher needs to examine the effects through the careful measurement of patient outcomes. On the other hand, if a researcher asks, "What is the process by which parents learn to cope with the death of a child?" the researcher would be hard pressed to quantify such a process. Personal worldviews of researchers help to shape their questions.

In reading about the alternative paradigms for nursing research, you likely were more attracted to one of the two paradigms. It is important, however, to learn about both approaches to disciplined inquiry and to recognize their respective strengths and limitations. In this textbook, we describe methods associated with both qualitative and quantitative research in an effort to assist you in becoming *methodologically bilingual*. This is especially important because large numbers of nurse researchers are now undertaking *mixed methods* research that involves gathering and analyzing both qualitative and quantitative data (Chapters 26–28).

THE PURPOSES OF NURSING RESEARCH

The general purpose of nursing research is to answer questions or solve problems of relevance to nursing. Specific purposes can be classified in various ways. We describe three such classifications—not because it is important for you to categorize a study as having one purpose or the other but rather because this will help us to illustrate the broad range of questions that have intrigued nurses and to further show differences between qualitative and quantitative inquiry.

Applied and Basic Research

Sometimes a distinction is made between basic and applied research. As traditionally defined, **basic**

research is undertaken to enhance the base of knowledge or to formulate or refine a theory. For example, a researcher may perform an in-depth study to better understand normal grieving processes, without having *explicit* nursing applications in mind. Some types of basic research are called *bench research*, which is usually performed in a laboratory and focuses on the molecular and cellular mechanisms that underlie disease.

Example of Basic Nursing Research: Kishi and a multidisciplinary team of researchers (2015) studied the effect of hypo-osmotic shock of epidermal cells on skin inflammation in a rat model, in an effort to understand the physiologic mechanism underlying aquagenic pruritus (disrupted skin barrier function) in the elderly.

Applied research seeks solutions to existing problems and tends to be of greater immediate utility for EBP. Basic research is appropriate for discovering general principles of human behavior and biophysiologic processes; applied research is designed to indicate how these principles can be used to solve problems in nursing practice. In nursing, the findings from applied research may pose questions for basic research, and the results of basic research often suggest clinical applications.

Example of Applied Nursing Research: S. Martin and colleagues (2014) studied whether positive therapeutic suggestions given via headphones to children emerging from anesthesia after a tonsillectomy would help to lower the children's pain.

Research to Achieve Varying Levels of Explanation

Another way to classify research purposes concerns the extent to which studies provide explanatory information. Although specific study goals can range along an explanatory continuum, a fundamental distinction (relevant especially in quantitative research) is between studies whose primary intent is to *describe* phenomena, and those that are **cause-probing**—that is, designed to illuminate the underlying causes of phenomena.

Within a descriptive/explanatory framework, the specific purposes of nursing research include identification, description, exploration, prediction/control, and explanation. For each purpose, various types of question are addressed—some more amenable to qualitative than to quantitative inquiry and vice versa.

Identification and Description

Qualitative researchers sometimes study phenomena about which little is known. In some cases, so little is known that the phenomenon has yet to be clearly identified or named or has been inadequately defined. The in-depth, probing nature of qualitative research is well suited to the task of answering such questions as, "What *is* this phenomenon?" and "What is its name?" (Table 1.3). In quantitative research, by contrast, researchers begin with a phenomenon that has been previously studied or defined—sometimes in a qualitative study. Thus, in quantitative research, identification typically precedes the inquiry.

Qualitative Example of Identification: Wojnar and Katzenmeyer (2013) studied the experiences of preconception, pregnancy, and new motherhood for lesbian nonbiologic mothers. They identified, through in-depth interviews with 24 women, a unique description of a pervasive feeling they called *otherness*.

Description is another important research purpose. Examples of phenomena that nurse researchers have described include patients' pain, confusion, and coping. Quantitative description focuses on the incidence, size, and measurable attributes of phenomena. Qualitative researchers, by contrast, describe the dimensions and meanings of phenomena. Table 1.3 shows descriptive questions posed by quantitative and qualitative researchers.

Quantitative Example of Description: Palese and colleagues (2015) conducted a study to describe the average healing time of stage II pressure ulcers. They found that it took approximately 23 days to achieve complete reepithelialization.

Qualitative Example of Description: Archibald and colleagues (2015) undertook an in-depth study to describe the information needs of parents of children with asthma.

TABLE 1.3 • Research Purposes and Types of Research Questions

PURPOSE	TYPES OF QUESTIONS: QUANTITATIVE RESEARCH	TYPES OF QUESTIONS: QUALITATIVE RESEARCH
Identification		What is this phenomenon? What is its name?
Description	How prevalent is the phenomenon? How often does the phenomenon occur?	What are the dimensions or characteristics of the phenomenon? What is important about the phenomenon?
Exploration	What factors are related to the phenomenon? What are the antecedents of the phenomenon?	What is the full nature of the phenomenon? What is really going on here? How is the phenomenon experienced? What is the process by which the phenomenon evolves?
Explanation	What is the underlying cause of the phenomenon? Does the theory explain the phenomenon?	How does the phenomenon work? What does the phenomenon mean? How did the phenomenon occur?
Prediction	What will happen if we alter a phenomenon or introduce an intervention? If phenomenon X occurs, will phenomenon Y follow?	
Control	Can the occurrence of the phenomenon be prevented or controlled?	

Exploration

Exploratory research begins with a phenomenon of interest, but rather than simply observing and describing it, exploratory research investigates the full nature of the phenomenon, the manner in which it is manifested, and the other factors to which it is related. For example, a *descriptive* quantitative study of patients' preoperative stress might document the degree of stress patients feel before surgery and the percentage of patients who are stressed. An *exploratory* study might ask: What factors diminish or increase a patient's stress? Are nurses' behaviors related to a patient's stress level? Qualitative methods are especially useful for exploring the full nature of a little-understood phenomenon. Exploratory qualitative research is designed to shed light on the various ways in which a phenomenon is manifested and on underlying processes.

Quantitative Example of Exploration: Lee and colleagues (2014) explored the association between physical activity in older adults and their level of depressive symptoms.

Qualitative Example of Exploration: Based on in-depth interviews with adults living on a reservation in the United States, D. Martin and Yurkovich (2014) explored American Indians' perception of a healthy family.

Explanation

The goals of explanatory research are to understand the underpinnings of natural phenomena and to explain systematic relationships among them. Explanatory research is often linked to **theories**, which are a method of integrating ideas about phenomena and their interrelationships. Whereas descriptive research provides new information and exploratory research provides promising insights, explanatory research attempts to offer understanding of the underlying causes or full nature of a phenomenon. In quantitative research, theories or prior findings are used deductively to generate hypothesized explanations that are then tested. In qualitative studies, researchers search for explanations about how or why a phenomenon exists or what a phenomenon means as a basis for *developing* a theory that is grounded in rich, in-depth evidence.

Quantitative Example of Explanation: Golfenshtein and Drach-Zahavy (2015) tested a theoretical model (attribution theory) to understand the role of patients' attributions in nurses' regulation of emotions in pediatric hospital wards.

Qualitative Example of Explanation: Smith-Young and colleagues (2014) conducted an in-depth study to develop a theoretical understanding of the process of managing work-related musculoskeletal disorders while remaining at the workplace. They called this process *constant negotiation*.

Prediction and Control

Many phenomena defy explanation. Yet it is frequently possible to make predictions and to control phenomena based on research findings, even in the absence of complete understanding. For example, research has shown that the incidence of Down syndrome in infants increases with the age of the mother. We can predict that a woman aged 40 years is at higher risk of bearing a child with Down syndrome than is a woman aged 25 years. We can partially control the outcome by educating women about the risks and offering amniocentesis to women older than 35 years of age. The ability to predict and control in this example does not depend on an explanation of *why* older women are at a higher risk of having an abnormal child. In many quantitative studies, prediction and control are key objectives. Although explanatory studies are powerful in an EBP environment, studies whose purpose is prediction and control are also critical in helping clinicians make decisions.

Quantitative Example of Prediction: Dang (2014) studied factors that predicted resilience among homeless youth with histories of maltreatment. Social connectedness and self-esteem were predictive of better mental health.

Research Purposes Linked to Evidence-Based Practice

The purpose of most nursing studies can be categorized on a descriptive–explanatory dimension as just described, but some studies do not fall into such a system. For example, a study to develop and rigorously test a new method of measuring patient outcomes cannot easily be classified on this continuum.

In both nursing and medicine, several books have been written to facilitate evidence-based practice, and these books categorize studies in terms of the types of information needed by clinicians (DiCenso et al., 2005; Guyatt et al., 2008; Melnyk & Fineout-Overholt, 2011). These writers focus on several types of clinical concerns: treatment, therapy, or intervention; diagnosis and assessment; prognosis; prevention of harm; etiology; and meaning. Not all nursing studies have one of these purposes, but most of them do.

Treatment, Therapy, or Intervention

Nurse researchers undertake studies designed to help nurses make evidence-based treatment decisions about how to *prevent* a health problem or how to *manage* an existing problem. Such studies range from evaluations of highly specific treatments or therapies (e.g., comparing two types of cooling blankets for febrile patients) to complex multisession interventions designed to effect major behavioral changes (e.g., nurse-led smoking cessation interventions). Such **intervention research** plays a critical role in EBP.

Example of a Study Aimed at Treatment/Therapy: Ling and co-researchers (2014) tested the effectiveness of a school-based healthy lifestyle intervention designed to prevent childhood obesity in four rural elementary schools.

Diagnosis and Assessment

A burgeoning number of nursing studies concern the rigorous development and evaluation of formal instruments to screen, diagnose, and assess patients and to measure important clinical outcomes. High-quality instruments with documented accuracy are essential both for clinical practice and for further research.

Example of a Study Aimed at Diagnosis/Assessment: Pasek and colleagues (2015) developed a prototype of an electronic headache pain diary for children and evaluated the clinical feasibility of the diary for assessing and documenting concussion headache.

Prognosis

Studies of prognosis examine outcomes associated with a disease or health problem, estimate the probability they will occur, and predict the types of people for whom the outcomes are most likely. Such studies facilitate the development of long-term care plans for patients. They provide valuable information for guiding patients to make lifestyle choices or to be vigilant for key symptoms. Prognostic studies can also play a role in resource allocation decisions.

Example of a Study Aimed at Prognosis: Storey and Von Ah (2015) studied the prevalence and impact of hyperglycemia on hospitalized leukemia patients, in terms of such outcomes as neutropenia, infection, and length of hospital stay.

Prevention of Harm and Etiology (Causation)

Nurses frequently encounter patients who face potentially harmful exposures as a result of environmental agents or because of personal behaviors or characteristics. Providing useful information to patients about such harms and how best to avoid them depends on the availability of accurate evidence about health risks. Moreover, it can be difficult to prevent harms if we do not know what causes them. For example, there would be no smoking cessation programs if research had not provided firm evidence that smoking cigarettes causes or contributes to a wide range of health problems. Thus, identifying factors that affect or cause illness, mortality, or morbidity is an important purpose of many nursing studies.

Example of a Study Aimed at Identifying and Preventing Harms: Hagerty and colleagues (2015) undertook a study to identify risk factors for catheter-associated urinary tract infections in critically ill patients with subarachnoid hemorrhage. The risk factors examined included patients' blood sugar levels, patient age, and levels of anemia requiring transfusion.

Meaning and Processes

Designing effective interventions, motivating people to comply with treatments and health promotion activities, and providing sensitive advice to patients are among the many health care activities that can greatly benefit from understanding the clients' perspectives. Research that provides evidence about what health and illness mean to clients, what barriers they face to positive health practices, and what processes they experience in a transition through a health care crisis are important to evidence-based nursing practice.

Example of a Study Aimed at Studying Meaning: Carlsson and Persson (2015) studied what it means to live with intestinal failure caused by Crohn disease and the influence it has on daily life.

TIP: Several of these EBP-related purposes (except diagnosis and meaning) fundamentally call for cause-probing research. For example, research on interventions focuses on whether an intervention causes improvements in key outcomes. Prognosis research asks if a disease or health condition causes subsequent adverse outcomes, and etiology research seeks explanations about the underlying causes of health problems.

> **BOX 1.1** Questions for a Preliminary Overview of a Research Report
>
> 1. How relevant is the research problem in this report to the actual practice of nursing? Does the study focus on a topic that is a priority area for nursing research?
> 2. Is the research quantitative or qualitative?
> 3. What is the underlying purpose (or purposes) of the study—identification, description, exploration, explanation, or prediction and control? Does the purpose correspond to an EBP focus such as treatment, diagnosis, prognosis, harm/etiology, or meaning?
> 4. Is this study fundamentally cause-probing?
> 5. What might be some clinical implications of this research? To what type of people and settings is the research most relevant? If the findings are accurate, how might I use the results of this study?

ASSISTANCE FOR USERS OF NURSING RESEARCH

This book is designed primarily to help you develop skills for conducting research, but in an environment that stresses EBP, it is extremely important to hone your skills in reading, evaluating, and using nursing studies. We provide specific guidance to consumers in most chapters by including guidelines for critiquing aspects of a study covered in the chapter. The questions in Box 1.1 are designed to assist you in using the information in this chapter in an overall preliminary assessment of a research report.

➔ **TIP:** The *Resource Manual* that accompanies this book offers particularly rich opportunities to practice your critiquing skills. The Toolkit on thePoint with the *Resource Manual* includes Box 1.1 as a Word document, which will allow you to adapt these questions, if desired, and to answer them directly into a Word document without having to retype the questions.

RESEARCH EXAMPLES

Each chapter of this book presents brief descriptions of studies conducted by nurse researchers, focusing on aspects emphasized in the chapter. Reading the full journal articles would prove useful for learning more about the studies, their methods, and the findings.

Research Example of a Quantitative Study

Study: The effects of a community-based, culturally tailored diabetes prevention intervention for high-risk adults of Mexican descent (Vincent et al., 2014)

Study Purpose: The purpose of the study was to evaluate the effectiveness of a 5-month nurse-coached diabetes prevention program (*Un Estilo de Vida Saludable* or EVS) for overweight Mexican American adults.

Study Methods: A total of 58 Spanish-speaking adults of Mexican descent were recruited to participate in the study. Some of the participants, at random, were in a group that received the EVS intervention, while others in a control group did not receive it. The EVS intervention used content from a previously tested diabetes prevention program, but the researchers created a community-based, culturally tailored intervention for their population. The intervention, which was offered in community rooms of churches, consisted of an intensive phase of eight weekly 2-hour sessions, followed by a maintenance phase of 1-hour sessions for the final 3 months. Those in the group not receiving the intervention received educational sessions broadly aimed at health promotion in general. The researchers compared the two groups with regard to several important outcomes, such as weight loss, waist circumference, body mass index, and self-efficacy. Outcome information was gathered three times—at the outset of the study (prior to the intervention), 8 weeks later, and then after the program ended.

Key Findings: The analysis suggested that those in the intervention group had several better outcomes, such as greater weight loss, smaller waist circumference, and lower body mass index, than those in the control group.

Conclusions: Vincent and her colleagues (2014) concluded that implementing the culturally tailored program was feasible, was well-received among participants (e.g., high rates of program retention), and was effective in decreasing risk factors for type 2 diabetes.

Research Example of a Qualitative Study

Study: Silent, invisible, and unacknowledged: Experiences of young caregivers of single parents diagnosed with multiple sclerosis (Bjorgvinsdottir & Halldorsdottir, 2014)

Study Purpose: The purpose of this study was to study the personal experience of being a young caregiver of a chronically ill parent diagnosed with multiple sclerosis (MS).

Study Methods: Young adults in Iceland whose parents were diagnosed with MS were recruited through the Icelandic National Multiple Sclerosis Society, and 11 agreed to be included in the study. Participants were interviewed in their own homes or in the home of the lead researcher, whichever they preferred. In-depth questioning was used to probe the experiences of the participants. The main interview question was: "Can you tell me about your personal experience being a young caregiver of a chronically ill parent with MS?" Several participants were interviewed twice to ensure rich and deep descriptions for a total of 21 interviews.

Key Findings: The young caregivers felt that they were invisible and unacknowledged as caregivers and received limited support and assistance from professionals. Their responsibilities led to severe personal restrictions and they felt they had lived without a true childhood because they were left to manage adult-like responsibilities at a young age. Their role as caregiver was demanding and stressful, and they felt unsupported and abandoned.

Conclusions: The researchers concluded that health professionals should be more vigilant about the needs for support and guidance for children and adolescents caring for chronically ill parents.

SUMMARY POINTS

- **Nursing research** is systematic inquiry to develop knowledge about issues of importance to nurses. Nurses are adopting an **evidence-based practice (EBP)** that incorporates research findings into their clinical decisions.

- Nurses can participate in a range of research-related activities that span a continuum from being *consumers of research* (those who read and evaluate studies) and *producers of research* (those who design and undertake studies).

- Nursing research began with Florence Nightingale but developed slowly until its rapid acceleration in the 1950s. Since the 1970s, nursing research has focused on problems relating to clinical practice.

- The **National Institute of Nursing Research** (NINR), established at the U.S. National Institutes of Health in 1993, affirms the stature of nursing research in the United States.

- Contemporary emphases in nursing research include EBP projects, **replications** of research, research integration through systematic reviews, multisite and interdisciplinary studies, expanded dissemination efforts, and increased focus on health disparities.

- Disciplined research is a better evidence source for nursing practice than other sources, such as tradition, authority, personal experience, trial and error, intuition, and logical reasoning.

- Nursing research is conducted mainly within one of two broad **paradigms**—worldviews with underlying **assumptions** about reality: the positivist paradigm and the constructivist paradigm.

- In the **positivist paradigm**, it is assumed that there is an objective reality and that natural phenomena are regular and orderly. The related assumption of **determinism** is the belief that phenomenas result from prior causes and are not haphazard.

- In the **constructivist (naturalistic) paradigm**, it is assumed that reality is not *fixed* but is rather a construction of human minds; thus, "truth" is a composite of multiple constructions of reality.

- The positivist paradigm is associated with **quantitative research**—the collection and analysis of numeric information. Quantitative research is typically conducted within the traditional **scientific method**, which is a systematic, controlled process. Quantitative researchers gather and analyze **empirical evidence** (evidence collected through the human senses) and strive for **generalizability** of their findings beyond the study setting.

- Researchers within the constructivist paradigm emphasize understanding the human experience as it is lived through the collection and analysis of subjective, narrative materials using flexible procedures that evolve in the **field**; this paradigm is associated with **qualitative research**.
- **Basic research** is designed to extend the knowledge base for the sake of knowledge itself. **Applied research** focuses on discovering solutions to immediate problems.
- A fundamental distinction, especially relevant in quantitative research, is between studies whose primary intent is to *describe* phenomena and those that are **cause-probing**—that is, designed to illuminate underlying causes of phenomena. Specific purposes on the description/explanation continuum include identification, description, exploration, prediction/control, and explanation.
- Many nursing studies can also be classified in terms of a key EBP aim: treatment/therapy/intervention; diagnosis and assessment; prognosis; harm and etiology; and meaning and process.

STUDY ACTIVITIES

Chapter 1 of the *Resource Manual for Nursing Research: Generating and Assessing Evidence for Nursing Practice, 10th edition*, offers study suggestions for reinforcing concepts presented in this chapter. In addition, the following questions can be addressed in classroom or online discussions:

1. Is your worldview closer to the positivist or the constructivist paradigm? Explore the aspects of the two paradigms that are especially consistent with your worldview.
2. Answer the questions in Box 1.1 about the Vincent et al. (2014) study described at the end of this chapter. Could this study have been undertaken as a qualitative study? Why or why not?

3. Answer the questions in Box 1.1 about the Bjorgvinsdottir and Halldorsdottir (2014) study described at the end of this chapter. Could this study have been undertaken as a quantitative study? Why or why not?

STUDIES CITED IN CHAPTER 1

Archibald, M. M., Caine, V., Ali, S., Hartling, L., & Scott, S. (2015). What is left unsaid: An interpretive description of the information needs of parents of children with asthma. *Research in Nursing & Health, 38,* 19–28.

Bäck-Pettersson, S., Hermansson, E., Sernert, N., & Bjökelund, C. (2008). Research priorities in nursing—A Delphi study among Swedish nurses. *Journal of Clinical Nursing, 17,* 2221–2231.

Bjorgvinsdottir, K., & Halldorsdottir, S. (2014). Silent, invisible and unacknowledged: Experiences of young caregivers of single parents diagnosed with multiple sclerosis. *Scandinavian Journal of the Caring Sciences, 28,* 38–48.

Brenner, M., Hilliard, C., Regan, G., Coughlan, B., Hayden, S., Drennan, J., & Kelleher, D. (2014). Research priorities for children's nursing in Ireland. *Journal of Pediatric Nursing, 29,* 301–308.

*Campbell-Yeo, M., Johnston, C., Benoit, B., Latimer, M., Vincer, M., Walker, C., . . . Caddell, K. (2013). Trial of repeated analgesia with kangaroo mother care (TRAKC trial). *BMC Pediatrics, 13,* 182.

Carlsson, E., & Persson, E. (2015). Living with intestinal failure by Crohn disease: Not letting the disease conquer life. *Gastroenterology Nursing, 38,* 12–20.

Chwo, M. J., Anderson, G. C., Good, M., Dowling, D. A., Shiau, S. H., & Chu, D. M. (2002). A randomized controlled trial of early kangaroo care for preterm infants: Effects on temperature, weight, behavior, and acuity. *Journal of Nursing Research, 10,* 129–142.

*Cong, X., Ludington-Hoe, S., McCain, G., & Fu, P. (2009). Kangaroo care modifies preterm infant heart rate variability in response to heel stick pain. *Early Human Development, 85,* 561–567.

Cong, X., Ludington-Hoe, S., & Walsh, S. (2011). Randomized crossover trial of kangaroo care to reduce behavioral pain responses in preterm infants. *Biological Research for Nursing, 13,* 204–216.

Dang, M. T. (2014). Social connectedness and self-esteem: Predictors of resilience in mental health among maltreated homeless youth. *Issues in Mental Health Nursing, 35,* 212–219.

DiCenso, A., Guyatt, G., & Ciliska, D. (2005). *Evidence-based nursing: A guide to clinical practice.* St. Louis, MO: Elsevier Mosby.

Drenkard, K. (2013). Change is good: Introducing the 2014 Magnet Application Manual. *Journal of Nursing Administration, 43*, 489–490.

Drennan, J., Meehan, T., Kemple, M., Johnson, M., Treacy, M., & Butler, M. (2007). Nursing research priorities for Ireland. *Journal of Nursing Scholarship, 39*, 298–305.

Golfenshtein, N., & Drach-Zahavy, A. (2015). An attribution theory perspective on emotional labour in nurse-patient encounters: A nested cross-sectional study in paediatric settings. *Journal of Advanced Nursing, 71*(5), 1123–1134.

Gona, C., & DeMarco, R. (2015). The context and experience of becoming HIV infected for Zimbabwean women: Unheard voices revealed. *Journal of the Association of Nurses in AIDS Care, 26*, 57–68.

Guyatt, G., Rennie, D., Meade, M., & Cook, D. (2008). *Users' guide to the medical literature: Essentials of evidence-based clinical practice* (2nd ed.). New York: McGraw Hill.

Hagerty, T., Kertesz, L., Schmidt, J., Agarwal, S., Claassen, J., Mayer, S., . . . Shang, K. (2015). Risk factors for catheter-associated urinary tract infections in critically ill patients with subarachnoid hemorrhage. *Journal of Neuroscience Nursing, 47*, 51–54.

Hake-Brooks, S., & Anderson, G. (2008). Kangaroo care and breastfeeding of mother-preterm dyads 0–18 months: A randomized controlled trial. *Neonatal Network, 27*, 151–159.

Hanrahan, K., Wagner, M., Matthews, G., Stewart, S., Dawson, C., Greiner, J., . . . Williamson, A. (2015). Sacred cows gone to pasture: A systematic evaluation and integration of evidence-based practice. *Worldview on Evidence-Based Nursing, 12*, 3–11.

Holman, E., Perisho, J., Edwards, A., & Mlakar, N. (2010). The myths of coping with loss in undergraduate psychiatric nursing books. *Research in Nursing & Health, 33*, 486–499.

*Institute of Medicine. (2010). *The future of nursing: Leading change, advancing health.* Washington, DC: The National Academies Press.

Kim, M. J., Oh, E. G., Kim, C. J., Yoo, J. S., & Ko, I. S. (2002). Priorities for nursing research in Korea. *Journal of Nursing Scholarship, 34*, 307–312.

Kishi, C., Minematsu, T., Huang, L., Mugita, Y., Kitamura, A., Nakagami, G., . . . Sanada, H. (2015). Hypo-osmotic shock-induced subclinical inflammation of skin in a rat model of disrupted skin barrier function. *Biological Research for Nursing, 17*, 135–141.

Lee, H., Lee, J., Brar, J., Rush, E., & Jolley, C. (2014). Physical activity and depressive symptoms in older adults. *Geriatric Nursing, 35*, 37–41.

Ling, J., King, K., Speck, B., Kim, S., & Wu, D. (2014). Preliminary assessment of a school-based healthy lifestyle intervention among rural elementary school children. *Journal of School Health, 84*, 247–255.

Ludington-Hoe, S. M. (2011). Thirty years of kangaroo care science and practice. *Neonatal Network, 30*, 357–362.

Mak, S., Lee, M., Cheung, J., Choi, K., Chung, T., Wong, T., . . . & Lee, D. (2015). Pressurised irrigation versus swabbing method

in cleansing wounds healed by secondary intention: A randomized controlled trial with cost effectiveness analysis. *International Journal of Nursing Studies, 52*, 88–101.

Martin, D., & Yurkovich, E. (2014). "Close knit" defines a healthy native American Indian family. *Journal of Family Nursing, 20*, 51–72.

Martin, S., Smith, A., Newcomb, P., & Miller, J. (2014). Effects of therapeutic suggestion under anesthesia on outcomes in children post-tonsillectomy. *Journal of Perianesthesia Nursing, 29*, 94–106.

*McHugh, M. D., Kelly, L. A., Smith, H. L., Wu, E. S., Vanak, J., & Aiken, L. H. (2013). Lower mortality in Magnet hospitals. *Medical Care, 51*, 382–388.

Melnyk, B. M., & Fineout-Overholt, E. (2011). *Evidence-based practice in nursing and healthcare: A guide to best practice* (2nd ed.). Philadelphia: Lippincott Williams & Wilkins.

*Moore, E., Anderson, G., Bergman, N., & Dowswell, T. (2012). Early skin-to-skin contact for mothers and their health newborn infants. *Cochrane Database of Systematic Reviews, (3)*, CD0003519.

Palese, A., Luisa, S., Ilenia, P., Laquintana, D., Stinco, G., & DeLiulio, P. (2015). What is the healing time of stage II pressure ulcers? Findings from a secondary analysis. *Advances in Skin and Would Care, 28*, 79–75.

Pasek, T., Locasto, L., Reichard, J., Fazio Sumrok, V., Johnson, E., & Kontos, A. (2015). The headache electronic diary for children with concussion. *Clinical Nurse Specialist, 29*, 80–88.

Reigle, B. S., Stevens, K., Belcher, J., Huth, M., McGuire, E., Mals, D., & Volz, T. (2008). Evidence-based practice and the road to Magnet status. *The Journal of Nursing Administration, 38*, 97–102.

Smith-Young, J., Solberg, S., & Gaudine, A. (2014). Constant negotiating: Managing work-related musculoskeletal disorders while remaining in the workplace. *Qualitative Health Research, 24*, 217–231.

Storey, S., & Von Ah, D. (2015). Prevalence and impact of hyperglycemia on hospitalized leukemia patients. *European Journal of Oncology Nursing, 19*, 13–17.

Vincent, D., McEwen, M., Hepworth, J., & Stump, C. (2014). The effects of a community-based, culturally tailored diabetes prevention intervention for high-risk adults of Mexican descent. *The Diabetes Educator, 40*, 202–213.

Wojnar, D. M., & Katzenmeyer, A. (2013). Experiences of preconception, pregnancy, and new motherhood for lesbian nonbiological mothers. *Journal of Obstetric, Gynecologic, and Neonatal Nursing, 43*, 50–60.

Wynaden, D., Heslop, K., Omari, O., Nelson, D., Osmond, B., Taylor, M., & Gee, T. (2014). Identifying mental health nursing priorities: A Delphi study. *Contemporary Nurse, 47*, 16–26.

A link to this open-access journal article is provided in the Toolkit for this chapter in the accompanying Resource Manual.

Evidence-Based Nursing: Translating Research Evidence into Practice

2

This book will help you to develop the skills you need to generate and evaluate research evidence for nursing practice. Before we delve into the "how-tos" of research, we discuss key aspects of evidence-based practice (EBP) to clarify the key role that research plays in nursing.

BACKGROUND OF EVIDENCE-BASED NURSING PRACTICE

This section provides a context for understanding evidence-based nursing practice and two closely related concepts, research utilization and knowledge translation.

Definition of Evidence-Based Practice

Pioneer David Sackett defined evidence as "the integration of best research evidence with clinical expertise and patient values" (Sackett et al., 2000, p. 1). Scott and McSherry (2009), in their review of evidence-based nursing concepts, identified 13 overlapping but distinct definitions of evidence-based nursing and EBP. The definition proposed by Sigma Theta Tau International (2008) is as follows: "The process of shared decision-making between practitioner, patient, and others significant to them based on research evidence, the patient's experiences and preferences, clinical expertise or know-how, and other available robust sources of information" (p. 57). A key ingredient in EBP is the effort to personalize "best evidence" to a specific patient's needs within a particular clinical context.

A basic feature of EBP as a clinical problem-solving strategy is that it de-emphasizes decisions based on custom, authority, or ritual. The emphasis is on identifying the best available research evidence and *integrating* it with other factors. In many areas of clinical decision making, research has demonstrated that "tried and true" practices taught in basic nursing education are not always best. For example, although many nurses not so long ago were taught to place infants in the prone sleeping position to prevent aspiration, there is strong evidence that the supine (back) sleeping position decreases the risk of sudden infant death syndrome (SIDS).

> **TIP:** The consequences of *not* using research evidence can be devastating. For example, from 1956 through the 1980s, Dr. Benjamin Spock published several editions of a top-selling book, *Baby and Child Care*, which advised putting babies on their stomachs to sleep. In their systematic review of evidence, Gilbert and colleagues (2005) wrote, "Advice to put infants to sleep on the front for nearly half a century was contrary to evidence from 1970 that this was likely to be harmful" (p. 874). They estimated that if medical advice had been guided by research evidence, over 60,000 infant deaths might have been prevented.

Because research evidence can provide valuable insights about human health and illness, nurses must be lifelong learners who have the skills to search for, understand, and evaluate new information about patient care—as well as the capacity to adapt to change.

Research Utilization

Research utilization (RU) is the use of findings from a study or set of studies in a practical application that is unrelated to the original research. In RU, the emphasis is on translating new knowledge into real-world applications. EBP is a broader concept than RU because it integrates research findings with other factors, as just noted. Also, whereas RU begins with the research itself (How can I put this new knowledge to good use in my clinical setting?), the start point in EBP is a clinical question (What does the evidence say is the best approach to solving this clinical problem?).

➔ TIP: Theorists who have studied the *diffusion* of ideas recognize a continuum of knowledge utilization. At one end of the continuum are identifiable attempts to base specific actions on research findings (e.g., placing infants in supine instead of prone sleeping position). Research findings can also be used in a less focused manner—in a way that reflects awareness or enlightenment. Thus, a qualitative study might provide a rich description of *courage* among individuals with long-term health problems as a process that includes efforts to develop problem-solving skills. The study may make nurses more observant and sensitive in working with patients with long-term illnesses, but it may not lead to formal changes in clinical actions.

During the 1980s, *research utilization* emerged as an important buzzword. In education, nursing schools began to include courses on research methods so that students would become skillful research consumers. In research, there was a shift in focus toward clinical nursing problems. Yet, concerns about the limited use of research evidence in the delivery of nursing care continued to mount.

The need to reduce the gap between research and practice led to formal RU projects, including the groundbreaking *Conduct and Utilization of Research in Nursing (CURN) Project*, a 5-year project undertaken by the Michigan Nurses Association in the 1970s. CURN's objectives were to increase the use of research findings in nurses' daily practice by disseminating current findings and facilitating organizational changes needed to implement innovations (Horsley et al., 1978). The CURN project team concluded that RU by practicing nurses was feasible but only if the research is relevant to practice and if the results are broadly disseminated.

During the 1980s and 1990s, RU projects were undertaken by numerous hospitals and organizations. These projects were institutional attempts to implement changes in nursing practice based on research findings. During the 1990s, however, the call for research utilization began to be superseded by the push for EBP.

The Evidence-Based Practice Movement

The Cochrane Collaboration was an early contributor to the EBP movement. The collaboration was founded in the United Kingdom based on the work of British epidemiologist Archie Cochrane. Cochrane published an influential book in the 1970s that drew attention to the dearth of solid evidence about the effects of health care. He called for efforts to make research summaries of clinical trials available to health care providers. This eventually led to the development of the Cochrane Center in Oxford in 1993, and an international partnership called the Cochrane Collaboration, with centers established in locations throughout the world. Its aim is to help providers make good decisions about health care by preparing and disseminating systematic reviews of the effects of health care interventions.

At about the same time, a group from McMaster Medical School in Canada (including Dr. David Sackett) developed a clinical learning strategy they called *evidence-based medicine*. The evidence-based medicine movement has shifted to a broader conception of using best evidence by all health care practitioners (not just physicians) in a multidisciplinary team. EBP is considered a major shift for health care education and practice. In the EBP environment, a skillful clinician can no longer rely on a repository of memorized information but rather must be adept in accessing, evaluating, and using new evidence.

The EBP movement has advocates and critics. Supporters argue that EBP is a rational approach to providing the best possible care with the most cost-effective use of resources. Advocates also note that EBP provides a framework for self-directed lifelong learning that is essential in an era of rapid clinical advances and the information explosion. Critics worry that the advantages of EBP are exaggerated and that individual clinical judgments and patient inputs are being devalued. They are also concerned that insufficient attention is being paid to the role of qualitative research. Although there is a need for close scrutiny of how the EBP journey unfolds, an EBP path is the one that health care professions will almost surely follow in the years ahead.

> **TIP:** A debate has emerged concerning whether the term "evidence-based practice" should be replaced with *evidence-informed practice* (EIP). Those who advocate for a different term have argued that the word "based" suggests a stance in which patient values and preferences are not sufficiently considered in EBP clinical decisions (e.g., Glasziou, 2005). Yet, as noted by Melnyk (2014), all current models of EBP incorporate clinicians' expertise and patients' preferences. She argued that "changing terms now . . . will only create confusion at a critical time where progress is being made in accelerating EBP" (p. 348). We concur and we use EBP throughout this book.

Knowledge Translation

Research utilization and EBP involve activities that can be undertaken at the level of individual nurses or at a higher organizational level (e.g., by nurse administrators), as we describe later in this chapter. In the early part of this century, a related movement emerged that mainly concerns system-level efforts to bridge the gap between knowledge generation and use. **Knowledge translation (KT)** is a term that is often associated with efforts to enhance systematic change in clinical practice.

It appears that the term was coined by the Canadian Institutes of Health Research (CIHR) in 2000. CIHR defined KT as "the exchange, synthesis, and ethically-sound application of knowledge—within a complex system of interactions among researchers and users—to accelerate the capture of the benefits of research for Canadians through improved health, more effective services and products, and a strengthened health care system" (CIHR, 2004, p. 4).

Several other definitions of KT have been proposed. For example, the World Health Organization (WHO) (2005) adapted the CIHR's definition and defined KT as "the synthesis, exchange and application of knowledge by relevant stakeholders to accelerate the benefits of global and local innovation in strengthening health systems and improving people's health." Institutional projects aimed at KT often use methods and models that are similar to institutional EBP projects.

> **TIP: Translation science** (or **implementation science**) has emerged as a discipline devoted to developing methods to promote knowledge translation. In nursing, the need for translational research was an important impetus for the development of the Doctor of Nursing Practice degree. Several journals have emerged that are devoted to this field (e.g., the journal *Implementation Science*).

EVIDENCE-BASED PRACTICE IN NURSING

Before describing procedures relating to EBP in nursing, we briefly discuss some important issues, including the nature of "evidence" and challenges to pursuing EBP, and resources available to address some of those challenges.

Types of Evidence and Evidence Hierarchies

There is no consensus about the definition of *evidence* nor about what constitutes usable evidence for EBP, but most commentators agree that findings from rigorous research are paramount. Debate continues, however, about what constitutes *rigorous* research and what qualifies as *best* evidence.

At the outset of the EBP movement, there was a strong bias toward reliance on information from studies called *randomized controlled trials* (RCTs). This bias stemmed from the fact that the Cochrane Collaboration initially focused on the effectiveness of therapies rather on other types of health care questions. RCTs are, in fact, very well suited for drawing conclusions about the effects of health care interventions (Chapter 9). The bias in ranking sources of evidence in terms of questions about effective treatments led to some resistance to EBP by nurses who felt that evidence from qualitative and non-RCT studies would be ignored.

Positions about the contribution of various types of evidence are less rigid than previously. Nevertheless, many published **evidence hierarchies** rank evidence sources according to the strength of the evidence they provide, and in most cases, RCTs are near the top of these hierarchies. We offer a modified evidence hierarchy that looks similar to others, but ours illustrates that the ranking of evidence-producing strategies depends on the type of question being asked.

Figure 2.1 shows that **systematic reviews** are at the pinnacle of the hierarchy (Level I), regardless of the type of question, because the strongest evidence comes from careful syntheses of multiple studies. The next highest level (Level II) depends on the nature of inquiry. For Therapy questions regarding the efficacy of an intervention (What works best

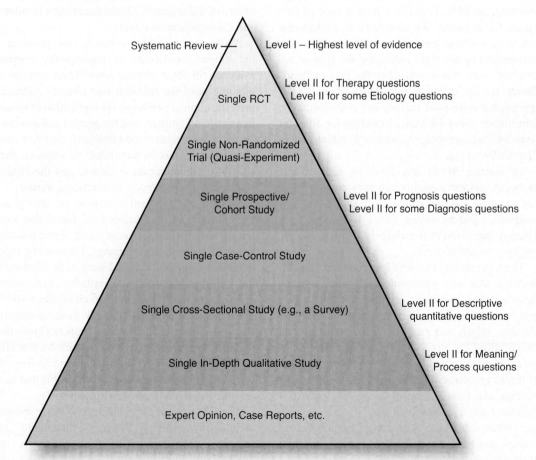

FIGURE 2.1 Evidence hierarchy: levels of evidence.

for improving health outcomes?), individual RCTs constitute Level II evidence (systematic reviews of multiple RCTs are Level I). Going down the "rungs" of the evidence hierarchy for Therapy questions results in less reliable evidence—for example, Level III evidence comes from a type of study called quasi-experimental. In-depth qualitative studies are near the bottom, in terms of evidence regarding intervention effectiveness. (Terms in Figure 2.1 will be discussed in later chapters.)

For a Prognosis question, by contrast, Level II evidence comes from a single prospective cohort study, and Level III is from a type of study called case control (Level I evidence is from a systematic review of cohort studies). Thus, contrary to what is often implied in discussions of evidence hierarchies, there really are multiple hierarchies. If one is interested in best evidence for questions about Meaning, an RCT would be a poor source of evidence, for example. We have tried to portray the notion of multiple hierarchies in Figure 2.1, with information on the right indicating the type of *individual study* that would offer the best evidence (Level II) for different questions. In all cases, appropriate systematic reviews are at the pinnacle. Information about different hierarchies for different types of cause-probing questions is addressed in Chapter 9.

Of course, *within* any level in an evidence hierarchy, evidence quality can vary considerably. For example, an individual RCT could be well designed, yielding strong Level II evidence for Therapy questions, or it could be so flawed that the evidence would be weak.

Thus, in nursing, *best evidence* refers to research findings that are methodologically appropriate, rigorous, and clinically relevant for answering persistent questions—questions not only about the efficacy, safety, and cost-effectiveness of nursing interventions but also about the reliability of nursing assessment tests, the causes and consequences of health problems, and the meaning and nature of patients' experiences. Confidence in the evidence is enhanced when the research methods are compelling, when there have been multiple confirmatory studies, and when the evidence has been carefully evaluated and synthesized.

Of course, there continue to be clinical practice questions for which there is relatively little research evidence. In such situations, nursing practice must rely on other sources—for example, pathophysiologic data, chart review, quality improvement data, and clinical expertise. As Sackett and colleagues (2000) have noted, one benefit of the EBP movement is that a new research agenda can emerge when clinical questions arise for which there is no satisfactory evidence.

Evidence-Based Practice Challenges

Nurses have completed many studies about the use of research in practice, including research on barriers to EBP. Studies on EBP barriers, conducted in several countries, have yielded similar results about constraints on clinical nurses. Most barriers fall into one of three categories: (1) quality and nature of the research, (2) characteristics of nurses, and (3) organizational factors.

With regard to the research, one problem is the limited availability of high-quality research evidence for some practice areas. There remains an ongoing need for research that directly addresses pressing clinical problems, for replication of studies in a range of settings, and for greater collaboration between researchers and clinicians. Another issue is that nurse researchers need to improve their ability to communicate evidence, and the clinical implications of evidence, to practicing nurses.

Nurses' attitudes and education are also potential barriers to EBP. Studies have found that some nurses do not value or know much about research, and others simply resist change. Fortunately, many nurses do value research and want to be involved in research-related activities. Nevertheless, many nurses do not know how to access research evidence and do not possess the skills to critically evaluate research findings—and even those who do may not know how to effectively incorporate research evidence into clinical decision making. Among nurses in non-English-speaking countries, another impediment is that most research evidence is reported in English.

Finally, many of the challenges to using research in practice are organizational. "Unit culture" can undermine research use, and administrative and other organizational barriers also play a major role.

Although many organizations support the idea of EBP in theory, they do not always provide the necessary supports in terms of staff release time and availability of resources. Nurses' time constraints are a crucial deterrent to the use of evidence at the bedside. Strong leadership in health care organizations is essential to making evidence-based practice happen.

RESOURCES FOR EVIDENCE-BASED PRACTICE IN NURSING

The translation of research evidence into nursing practice is an ongoing challenge, but resources to support EBP are increasingly available. We urge you to explore other ideas with your health information librarian because the list of resources is growing as we write.

Preappraised Evidence

Research evidence comes in various forms, the most basic of which is in individual studies. **Primary studies** published in professional journals are not preappraised for quality or use in practice. Chapter 5 discusses how to access primary studies for a literature review.

Preprocessed (preappraised) evidence is evidence that has been selected from primary studies and evaluated for use by clinicians. DiCenso and colleagues (2005) have described a hierarchy of preprocessed evidence. On the first rung above primary studies are synopses of single studies, followed by systematic reviews, and then synopses of systematic reviews. Clinical practice guidelines are at the top of the hierarchy. At each successive step in the hierarchy, the ease in applying the evidence to clinical practice increases. We describe several types of preappraised evidence sources in this section.

Systematic Reviews

Evidence-based practice relies on meticulous integration of research evidence on a topic. Systematic reviews are a pivotal component of EBP: Their "bottom line" is a summary of what the best evidence is at the time the review was written. A systematic review is not just a literature review, such as ones we describe in Chapter 5. A systematic review

is in itself a methodical, scholarly inquiry that follows many of the same steps as those for primary studies. Chapter 29 offers guidance on conducting and critiquing systematic reviews.

Systematic reviews can take various forms. A type of systematic review called a meta-analysis has emerged as an important EBP tool. **Meta-analysis** is a method of integrating quantitative findings statistically. In essence, meta-analysis treats the findings from a study as one piece of information. The findings from multiple studies on the same topic are combined and analyzed statistically. Instead of individual people being the **unit of analysis** (the basic entity of the analysis), individual studies are the unit of analysis in a meta-analysis. Meta-analysis is a convenient, objective method of integrating a body of findings and of observing patterns that might otherwise have gone undetected.

Example of a Meta-Analysis: Du and colleagues (2015) conducted a meta-analysis of the effectiveness of Tai Chi exercise for improving sleep quality in older people. The researchers integrated evidence from five clinical trials. The evidence from these studies suggests that Tai Chi could be an effective alternative and complementary approach to existing therapies for older people with sleep disorders, but the researchers concluded that better confirmatory evidence is needed.

Integrative reviews of qualitative studies often take the form of metasyntheses, which are rich resources for EBP (Beck, 2009). A **metasynthesis**, which involves integrating qualitative research findings on a topic, is distinct from a quantitative meta-analysis: A metasynthesis is less about reducing information and more about amplifying and interpreting it. Strategies are also being developed in the area of **mixed methods synthesis**, which are efforts to integrate and synthesize both quantitative and qualitative evidence (Sandelowski et al., 2013; Thorne, 2009).

Example of a Metasynthesis: Tao and colleagues (2014) did a metasynthesis of 16 studies of the experiences of individuals living with a stoma. They identified three themes concerning patients' personal awareness and behavioral choices on having a stoma: altered self, restricted life, and overcoming restrictions.

Some systematic reviews are published in professional journals that can be accessed using standard literature search procedures; others are available in dedicated databases. In particular, the Cochrane Database of Systematic Reviews contains thousands of systematic reviews (mostly meta-analyses) relating to health care interventions. Cochrane reviews are done with great rigor and have the advantage of being checked and updated regularly.

Example of Cochrane Review: Gillespie and colleagues (2014) conducted a Cochrane review that summarized evidence on the effects of repositioning on the prevention of pressure ulcers in adult patients. The team found evidence from only four studies and concluded that there remains a need for further high-quality research to "assess the effects of position and optimal frequency of repositioning on pressure ulcer incidence" (p. 1).

Many other resources are available for locating systematic reviews as well as synopses of such reviews. Here is information about a few of them:

- The Agency for Healthcare Research and Quality (AHRQ) awarded contracts to establish Evidence-Based Practice Centers that issue *evidence reports* (www.ahrq.gov).
- The Centre for Reviews and Dissemination at the University of York (England) produces useful systematic reviews (http://www.york.ac.uk/inst/crd/index.htm).
- The Joanna Briggs Collaboration, centered in Australia with affiliates worldwide, is another useful source for systematic reviews in nursing and other health fields (http://joannabriggs.org/).
- The Campbell Collaboration includes reviews of interventions that are socially or behaviorally oriented (www.campbellcollaboration.org).

TIP: Websites cited in this chapter, plus additional websites with useful content relating to EBP, are listed in the Toolkit with the accompanying *Resource Manual*. This will allow you to simply use the "Control/Click" feature to go directly to the website, without having to type in the URL and risk a typographical error.

Clinical Practice Guidelines and Care Bundles

Evidence-based **clinical practice guidelines**, like systematic reviews, represent an effort to distill a large body of evidence into a manageable form, but guidelines differ in a number of respects. First, clinical practice guidelines, which are usually based on systematic reviews, give specific recommendations for evidence-based decision making. Their intent is to influence what clinicians do. Second, guidelines attempt to address all of the issues relevant to a clinical decision, including the balancing of benefits and risks. Third, systematic reviews are evidence-driven—that is, they are undertaken when a body of evidence has been produced and needs to be synthesized. Guidelines, by contrast, are "necessity-driven" (Sackett et al., 2000), meaning that guidelines are developed to guide clinical practice—even when available evidence is limited or of unexceptional quality. Fourth, systematic reviews are done by researchers, but guideline development typically involves the consensus of a group of researchers, experts, and clinicians. For this reason, guidelines based on the same evidence may result in different recommendations that take into account contextual factors—for example, guidelines appropriate in the United States may be unsuitable in India.

Also, organizations are developing and adopting **care bundles**—a concept developed by the Institute for Healthcare Improvement—that encompass a set of interventions to treat or prevent a specific cluster of symptoms (www.ihi.org). There is growing evidence that a combination or bundle of strategies produces better outcomes than a single intervention.

Example of a Care Bundle Project: Bates and colleagues (2014) explored the effect of implementing a set of interventions in incremental bundles to patients discharged after coronary artery bypass surgery. Patients who received the bundled interventions had a substantially lower rate of 30-day hospital readmissions than patients discharged prior to implementing the bundles.

Guidelines and bundles are available for many diagnostic and therapeutic decisions. Typically, they define a minimum set of services and actions appropriate for certain clinical conditions. Most guidelines allow for a flexible approach in their application to individual patients who fall outside the scope of their guideline (e.g., those with significant comorbidities).

It can be challenging to find clinical practice guidelines because there is no single guideline repository. One useful approach is to search for guidelines in comprehensive guideline databases, or through specialty organizations that have sponsored guideline development (e.g., the Association of Women's Health, Obstetric and Neonatal Nurses or AWHONN). It would be impossible to list all possible sources, but a few deserve special mention.

- In the United States, nursing and other health care guidelines are maintained by the National Guideline Clearinghouse (www.guideline.gov).
- In Canada, information about clinical practice guidelines can be found through the Registered Nurses' Association of Ontario (RNAO) (www.rnao.org/bestpractices).
- In the United Kingdom, two sources for clinical guidelines are the Translating Research Into Practice (TRIP) database (http://www.tripdatabase.com) and the National Institute for Health and Care Excellence (www.nice.org.uk).
- Another resource is the EBM-Guidelines, which offer recommendations relative to primary care in several languages (www.ebm-guidelines.com).
- The Guidelines International Network makes available guidelines from around the world (www.g-i-n.net).

In addition to looking for guidelines in national clearinghouses and in the websites of professional organizations, you can search bibliographic databases such as MEDLINE or EMBASE. Search terms such as the following can be used: *practice guideline, clinical practice guideline, best practice guideline, evidence-based guideline, standards,* and *consensus statement.* Be aware, though, that a standard search for guidelines in bibliographic databases will yield many references—but often a frustrating mixture of citations to not only the actual guidelines but also to commentaries, anecdotes, case studies, and so on.

Example of a Nursing Clinical Practice Guideline: In 2013, the Registered Nurses' Association of Ontario (RNAO) published the second edition of a best practice guideline called *Assessment and Management of Foot Ulcers for People with Diabetes.* The guideline provides "direction to all nurses and the interprofessional team who provide care in all health care settings to people with type 1 and/or type 2 diabetes and who have established diabetic foot ulcers" (www.rnao.org).

There are many topics for which practice guidelines have not yet been developed, but the opposite problem is also true: The dramatic increase in the number of guidelines means that there are sometimes multiple guidelines on the same topic. Worse yet, because of variation in the rigor of guideline development and in interpreting the evidence, different guidelines sometimes offer different and even conflicting recommendations. Thus, those who wish to adopt clinical practice guidelines are urged to critically appraise them to identify ones that are based on the strongest and most up-to-date evidence, have been meticulously developed, are user-friendly, and are appropriate for local use. We offer some assistance with these tasks later in this chapter.

Clinical Decision Support Tools

Clinical decision support tools are designed to help nurses and other health care professionals to organize information, guide their assessments, and apply appropriate interventions. Among such decision support tools are **clinical decision rules**, which synthesize the best available evidence into convenient guides for practice (Shapiro, 2005). Such decision rules, by standardizing aspects of patient assessments and prescribing specific evidence-based actions, can minimize clinical uncertainty and reduce variations in practice at the bedside.

It has been argued that, to be useful, decision support tools must offer speedy guidance in real time. Technologic advances are making such point-of-care decision-making assistance possible. Computerized decisional support (on computers, tablets, and smart phones) is now available for various clinical settings and specific clinical problems (e.g., Doran, 2009; Doran et al., 2010); DiPietro and colleagues (2012) offer advice on how to make such support useful for point-of-care decisions.

Other Preappraised Evidence

Several other types of preprocessed evidence are useful for EBP. These include the following:

- Synopses of systematic reviews and of single studies are available in evidence-based abstract journals such as *Clinical Evidence* (www.clinical evidence.com) and *Evidence-Based Nursing* (www.evidencebasednursing.com). *Evidence-Based Nursing* presents critical summaries of studies and systematic reviews from more than 150 journals.
- An "evidence digest" feature appears in each issue of *Worldviews on Evidence-Based Nursing*. These digests offer concise summaries of clinically important studies, along with practice implications.
- AHRQ launched its Health Care Innovations Exchange program in 2008, which offers a repository of hundreds of effective health care innovations (www.innovations.ahrq.gov).
- The American Association of Critical-Care Nurses regularly publishes "practice alerts," which are evidence-based recommendations for practice changes (www.aacn.org).

Models for Evidence-Based Practice

Several models of EBP have been developed and are important resources for designing and implementing EBP projects in practice settings. Some models focus on the use of research from the perspective of individual clinicians (e.g., the Stetler Model), but most focus on institutional EBP efforts (e.g., the Iowa Model). Another way to categorize existing models is to distinguish models that are process-oriented models (e.g., the Iowa Model) and models that are explicitly mentor models, such as the Clinical Nurse Scholar model and the ARCC model. Some of these models (e.g., the Ottawa Model of Research Use) have played a prominent role in KT efforts.

The many worthy EBP models are too numerous to list comprehensively, but a few are shown in Box 2.1. For those wishing to follow a formal EBP model, the cited references should be consulted. Gawlinski and Rutledge (2008) and Schaffer and colleagues (2013) offer further descriptions of EBP models and identify features to consider in selecting one to plan an EBP project.

Although each model offers different perspectives on how to translate research findings into practice, several of the steps and procedures are similar across the models. In nursing, the most prominent of these models have been the nurse-developed **PARIHS Model**, the **Stetler Model**, and the **Iowa Model**.

BOX 2.1 Selected Models for Evidence-Based Practice

- ACE Star Model of Knowledge Transformation (Kring, 2008)
- Advancing Research and Clinical Practice Through Close Collaboration (ARCC) Model (Melnyk & Fineout-Overholt, 2015)
- Diffusion of Innovations Theory (Rogers, 1995)
- Framework for Adopting an Evidence-Based Innovation (DiCenso et al., 2005)
- Iowa Model of Evidence-Based Practice to Promote Quality Care (Titler, 2010; Titler et al., 2001)
- Johns Hopkins Nursing Evidence-Based Practice Model (Newhouse et al., 2005)
- Model for Change to Evidence-Based Practice (Rosswurm & Larabee, 1999)
- Ottawa Model of Research Use (Logan & Graham, 1998)
- Promoting Action on Research Implementation in Health Services (PARIHS) Model, (Rycroft-Malone, 2010; Rycroft-Malone et al., 2002)
- Stetler Model of Research Utilization (Stetler, 2001, 2010)

We provide an overview of key activities and issues in EBP initiatives, based on a distillation of common elements from EBP models, in a subsequent section of this chapter. We rely especially heavily on the Iowa Model, a diagram for which is shown in Figure 2.2.

Example of Using an Evidence-Based Practice Model: C. G. Brown (2014) described how the Iowa Model was used to identify evidence-based strategies to reduce patient falls in an oncology unit. An interdisciplinary team worked to develop and implement a practice change and to evaluate effects on decreasing patient falls.

EVIDENCE-BASED PRACTICE IN INDIVIDUAL NURSING PRACTICE

This section and the following one, which are based on the various models of EBP, provide an overview of how research can be put to use in clinical settings. More extensive guidance is available in textbooks devoted to evidence-based nursing (e.g., S. J. Brown, 2013; Craig & Smyth, 2012; DiCenso et al., 2005; Melnyk & Fineout-Overholt, 2015; Schmidt & Brown, 2011). We first discuss strategies and steps for individual clinicians and then describe activities used by teams of nurses.

Clinical Scenarios and the Need for Evidence

Individual nurses make many decisions and are called upon to provide health care advice, and so they have ample opportunity to put research into practice. Here are four clinical scenarios that provide examples of such opportunities:

• Clinical Scenario 1. You work on an intensive care unit and notice that *Clostridium difficile* infection has become more prevalent among surgical patients in your hospital. You want to know if there is a reliable screening tool for assessing the risk of infection so that preventive measures could be initiated in a more timely and effective manner.
• Clinical Scenario 2. You work in an allergy clinic and notice how difficult it is for many children to undergo allergy scratch tests. You wonder if an interactive distraction intervention would help reduce children's anxiety when they are being tested for allergens.
• Clinical Scenario 3. You work in a rehabilitation hospital and one of your elderly patients, who had total hip replacement, tells you she is planning a long airplane trip to visit her daughter after rehabilitation treatments are completed. You know that a long plane ride will increase her risk of deep vein thrombosis and wonder if compression stockings are an effective in-flight treatment. You decide to look for the best possible evidence to answer this question.
• Clinical Scenario 4. You are caring for a hospitalized cardiac patient who tells you that he has sleep apnea. He confides in you that he is reluctant to undergo continuous positive airway pressure (CPAP) treatment because he worries it will hinder intimacy with his wife. You wonder if there is any evidence about what it is like to undergo CPAP treatment so that you can better understand how to address your patient's concerns.

In these and thousands of other clinical situations, research evidence can be put to good use to improve the quality of nursing care. Some situations might lead to unit-wide or institution-wide scrutiny of current practices, but in other situations, individual nurses can personally investigate the evidence to help them address specific problems.

For individual-level EBP efforts, the major steps in EBP include the following:

1. Asking clinical questions that can be answered with research evidence
2. Searching for and retrieving relevant evidence
3. Appraising the evidence
4. Integrating the evidence with your own clinical expertise, patient preferences, and local context
5. Assessing the effectiveness of the decision, intervention, or advice

Asking Well-Worded Clinical Questions

A crucial first step in EBP involves converting information needs into well-worded clinical questions that can be answered with research evidence. Some EBP writers distinguish between background

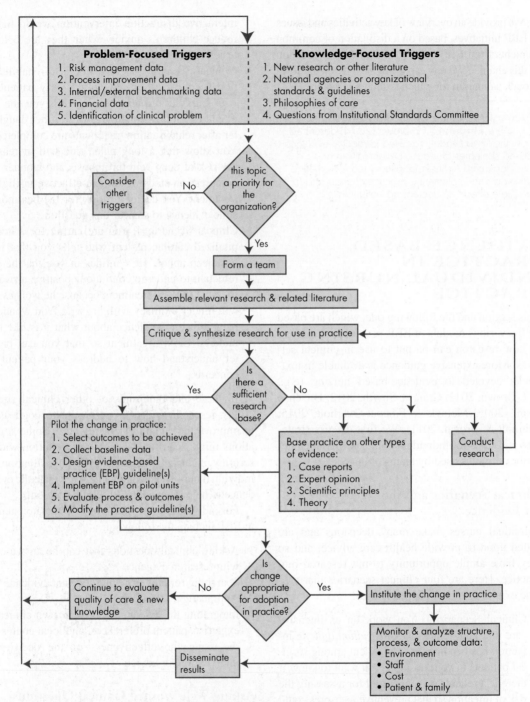

FIGURE 2.2 Iowa Model of Evidence-Based Practice to Promote Quality Care. (Adapted from Titler, M. G., Kleiber, C., Steelman, V., Rakel, B., Budreau, G., Everett, L., . . . Goode, C. [2001]. The Iowa model of evidence-based practice to promote quality care. *Critical Care Nursing Clinics of North America*, *13*, 497–509. Reprinted with permission.)

and foreground questions. *Background questions* are general, foundational questions about a clinical issue, for example: What is cancer cachexia (progressive body wasting), and what is its pathophysiology? Answers to such background questions are typically found in textbooks. *Foreground questions*, by contrast, are those that can be answered based on current best research evidence on diagnosing, assessing, or treating patients, or on understanding the meaning or prognosis of their health problems. For example, we may wonder, is a fish oil–enhanced nutritional supplement effective in stabilizing weight in patients with advanced cancer? The answer to such a question may offer guidance on how best to address the needs of patients with cachexia.

Most guidelines for EBP use the acronyms PIO or PICO to help practitioners develop well-worded questions that facilitate a search for evidence. In the most basic PIO form, the clinical question is worded to identify three components:

1. P: the *population* or *patients* (What are the characteristics of the patients or people?)
2. I: the *intervention*, *influence*, or *exposure* (What are the interventions or therapies of interest? or, What are the potentially harmful influences/exposures of concern?)
3. O: the *outcomes* (What are the outcomes or consequences in which we are interested?)

Applying this scheme to our question about cachexia, our *population* (P) is cancer patients with cachexia; the *intervention* (I) is fish oil–enhanced nutritional supplements; and the *outcome* (O) is weight stabilization. As another example, in the second clinical scenario about scratch tests cited earlier, the population (P) is children being tested for allergies; the intervention is interactive distraction (I); and the outcome is anxiety levels (O).

For questions that can best be answered with qualitative information (e.g., about the meaning of an experience or health problem), two components are most relevant:

1. the *population* (What are the characteristics of the patients or clients?); and
2. the *situation* (What conditions, experiences, or circumstances are we interested in understanding?).

For example, suppose our question was, What is it like to suffer from cachexia? In this case, the question calls for rich qualitative information; the *population* is patients with advanced cancer and the *situation* is the experience of cachexia.

In addition to the basic PIO components, other components are sometimes important in an evidence search. In particular, a comparison (C) component may be needed, when the intervention or influence of interest is contrasted with a specific alternative. For example, we might be interested in learning whether fish oil–enhanced supplements (I) are better than melatonin (C) in stabilizing weight (O) in cancer patients (P). When a *specific* comparison is of interest, a PICO question is required, but if we were interested in uncovering evidence about *all* alternatives to the intervention of primary interest, then PIO components are sufficient. (By contrast, when asking questions to undertake an actual *study*, the "C" must always be specified).

TIP: Other components may be relevant, such as a time frame in which an intervention might be appropriate (adding a "T" for PICOT questions) or a setting (adding an "S" for PICOS questions).

Table 2.1 offers question templates for asking well-framed clinical questions in selected circumstances. The right hand column includes questions with an explicit comparison (PICO questions), while the middle column does not. The questions are categorized in a manner similar to that discussed in Chapter 1 (EBP purposes), as featured in Table 1.3. One exception is that we have added description as a question type. Note that although there are some differences in components across question types, there is always a P component.

TIP: The Toolkit section of Chapter 2 in the accompanying *Resource Manual* includes Table 2.1 in a Word file that can be adapted for your use, so that the template questions can be readily "filled in." Additional EBP resources from this chapter are also in the Toolkit.

TABLE 2.1 • Question Templates for Selected Clinical Foreground Questions: PIO and PICO

TYPE OF QUESTION	QUESTION TEMPLATE FOR QUESTIONS *WITHOUT* AN EXPLICIT COMPARISON	QUESTION TEMPLATE FOR QUESTIONS *WITH* AN EXPLICIT COMPARISON (PICO)
Treatment/ Intervention	In _____ (population), what is the effect of _____ (intervention) on _____ (outcome)?	In _____ (population), what is the effect of _____ (intervention), in comparison to _____ (comparative/ alternative intervention), on _____ (outcome)?
Diagnosis/ assessment	For _____ (population), does _____ (tool/procedure) yield accurate and appropriate diagnostic/assessment information about _____ (outcome)?	For _____ (population), does _____ (tool/procedure) yield more accurate or more appropriate diagnostic/assessment information than _____ (comparative tool/procedure) about _____ (outcome)?
Prognosis	For _____ (population), does _____ (disease or condition) increase the risk of or influence _____ (outcome)?	For _____ (population), does _____ (disease or condition), relative to _____ (comparative disease or condition) increase the risk of or influence _____ (outcome)?
Causation/ Etiology/ Harm	Does _____ (exposure or characteristic) increase the risk of _____ (outcome) in _____ (population)?	Does _____ (exposure or characteristic) increase the risk of _____ (outcome) compared to _____ (comparative exposure or condition) in _____ (population)?
Meaning or Process	What is it like for _____ (population) to experience _____ (condition, illness, circumstance)? OR What is the process by which _____ (population) cope with, adapt to, or live with _____ (condition, illness, circumstance)?	(Explicit comparisons not typical in these types of question)

Finding Research Evidence

By asking clinical questions in the forms suggested, you should be able to more effectively search the research literature for the information you need. Using the templates in Table 2.1, the information inserted into the blanks constitutes *keywords* for undertaking an electronic search.

For an individual EBP endeavor, the best place to begin is to search for evidence in a systematic review or other preappraised source because this leads to a quicker answer—and potentially a superior answer as well if your methodologic skills are limited. Researchers who prepare reviews and clinical guidelines usually have strong research skills and use exemplary standards in evaluating the evidence. Moreover, preappraised evidence is usually developed by teams of researchers, which means that the conclusions are cross-validated. Thus, when preprocessed evidence is available to answer a clinical question, you may not need to look any farther, unless the review is not recent. When preprocessed evidence cannot be located or is old, you will need to look for best evidence in primary studies, using strategies we describe in Chapter 5.

 TIP: In Chapter 5, we provide guidance on using the free Internet resource, PubMed, for searching the bibliographic database MEDLINE. Of special interest to those engaged in an EBP search, PubMed offers a special tool for those seeking evidence for clinical decisions. The "Clinical Queries" link appears under the heading "PubMed Tools" on the PubMed Home Page. In another important database, CINAHL, it is now also possible to delimit a search with a "Clinical Queries" or "Evidence-Based Practice" limiter.

Appraising the Evidence

After locating relevant evidence, it should be appraised before taking clinical action. Critical appraisal for EBP may involve several types of assessments (Box 2.2).

The thoroughness of your appraisal depends on several factors, the most important of which is the nature of the clinical action for which evidence is being sought. Some actions have implications for patient safety, while others are more relevant to patient satisfaction. Using best evidence to guide nursing practice is important for a wide range of outcomes, but appraisal standards would be especially strict for evidence that could affect patient safety and morbidity.

Evidence Quality

The first appraisal issue is the extent to which the findings are valid. That is, were the study methods sufficiently rigorous that the evidence is credible? We offer guidance on critiquing studies and evaluating the strength of evidence from primary studies throughout this book. If there are several primary studies and no existing systematic review, you would need to draw conclusions about the body of evidence taken as a whole. There are several methods for "grading" the quality of a body of evidence, as we discuss in Chapter 27. Clearly, you would need to put most weight on the most rigorous studies. Preappraised evidence is already screened and evaluated, but you may still need to judge its integrity.

Magnitude of Effects

You also need to assess what the results actually *are* and whether they are clinically important. This criterion considers not whether the results are valid but what they are and how powerful are the effects.

BOX 2.2   Questions for Appraising the Evidence

What is the quality of the evidence—that is, how rigorous and reliable is it?
What *is* the evidence—what is the magnitude of effects?
How precise is the estimate of effects?
What evidence is there of any side effect or side benefits?
What is the financial cost of applying (and not applying) the evidence?
Is the evidence relevant to my particular clinical situation?

For example, consider clinical scenario number 3 cited earlier, which corresponds to the following clinical question: Does the use of compression stockings (I) lower the risk of flight-related deep vein thrombosis (O) for high-risk patients (P)? In our search, we find a relevant systematic review in the nursing literature—a meta-analysis of nine randomized controlled trials (Hsieh & Lee, 2005)—and another in the Cochrane database (Clarke et al., 2006). The conclusion of these reviews, based on reliable evidence, is that compression stockings are effective and the magnitude of the effect, in terms of risk reduction, is fairly substantial. Thus, advice about the use of compression stockings may be appropriate, pending an appraisal of other factors.

Determining the magnitude of the effect for quantitative findings is especially important when an intervention is costly or when there are potentially negative side effects. If, for example, there is good evidence that an intervention is only marginally effective in improving a health problem, it is important to consider other factors (e.g., evidence of effects on quality of life).

There are various ways to quantify the magnitude of effects, many of which are described later in this book. An index known as the *effect size*, for example, can provide estimates of the magnitude of effects for outcomes for which average values can be computed (e.g., average body temperature). When outcomes can be dichotomized (e.g., occurrence versus nonoccurrence of a health problem), estimates of magnitude of the effect can be calculated as *absolute risk reduction (ARR)* or *relative risk reduction (RRR)*. For example, if the RRR for the use of compression stockings was 50%, this would mean that this intervention reduced the risk of deep vein thrombosis by 50%, relative to what would occur in its absence. We describe methods of calculating these and other related indexes in Chapter 16.

The magnitude of effects also has a bearing on *clinical significance*. We discuss how to assess whether the findings from a study are clinically significant in Chapter 20.

Precision of Estimates

Another consideration, relevant with quantitative evidence, is how precise the estimate of effect is. This level of appraisal requires some statistical sophistication and so we postpone our discussion of *confidence intervals* to Chapter 17. Suffice it to say that research results provide only an estimate of effects and it is useful to understand not only the exact estimate but also the range within which the actual effect probably lies.

Peripheral Effects

If the evidence is judged to be valid and the magnitude of effects supports further consideration, supplementary information may still be important in guiding decisions. One issue concerns peripheral benefits and costs, evidence for which may emerge during your search. In framing your clinical question, you would have identified the key outcomes in which you were interested—for example, weight stabilization or weight gain for interventions to address cancer cachexia. Primary research on this topic, however, may have involved an examination of other outcomes that could be taken into account—for example, effects on quality of life, side effects, satisfaction, and so on.

Financial Issues

Another issue concerns the financial cost of using the evidence. In some cases, costs may be small or nonexistent. For example, in clinical scenario 4, where the question concerned the experience of CPAP treatment, nursing action would be cost neutral because the evidence would be used to provide information and reassurance to the patient. Some interventions, however, are costly and so the amount of resources needed to put best evidence into practice would need to be factored into any decision. Of course, while the cost of a clinical decision needs to be considered, the cost of *not* taking action is equally important.

Clinical Relevance

Finally, it is important to appraise the evidence in terms of its relevance for the clinical situation at hand—that is, for *your* patient in a specific clinical setting. Best practice evidence can most readily be applied to an individual patient in your care if he or she is similar to people in the study or studies under review. Would your patient have qualified for participation in the study—or is there some factor such as age, illness severity, or comorbidity that would have excluded him or her? DiCenso and colleagues

(2005), who advised clinicians to ask whether there is some compelling reason to conclude that the results may *not* be applicable in their clinical situation, have written some useful tips on applying research results to individual patients.

Actions Based on Evidence Appraisals

Appraisals of the evidence may lead you to different courses of action. You may reach this point and conclude that the evidence is not sufficiently sound, or that the likely effect is too small, or that the cost of applying the evidence is too high. The integration of appraisal information may suggest that "usual care" is the best strategy—or it may suggest the need for a new EBP inquiry. For instance, in the example about cachexia, you likely would have learned that recent best evidence suggests that fish oil–enhanced nutritional supplements may be an ineffective treatment (Ries et al., 2012). However, during your search you may have come across a Cochrane review that concluded that megestrol acetate improves appetite and weight gain in patients with cancer (Ruiz Garcia et al., 2013). This may lead to a new evidence inquiry and to discussions with other members of your health care team about nutrition protocols for your clinical setting. If, however, the initial appraisal of evidence suggests a promising clinical action, then you can proceed to the next step.

Integrating Evidence

As the definition for EBP implies, research evidence needs to be integrated with other types of information, including your own clinical expertise and knowledge of your clinical setting. You may be aware of factors that would make implementation of the evidence, no matter how sound or promising, inadvisable.

Patient preferences and values are also important. A discussion with the patient may reveal negative attitudes toward a potentially beneficial course of action, contraindications (e.g., comorbidities), or possible impediments (e.g., lack of health insurance).

One final issue is the importance of integrating evidence from qualitative research, which can provide rich insights about how patients experience a problem, or about barriers to complying with a treatment. A new intervention with strong potential benefits may fail to achieve desired outcomes if it is not implemented with sensitivity and understanding of the patients' perspectives. As Morse (2005) has so aptly noted, evidence from a clinical trial may tell you whether a pill is effective, but qualitative research can help you understand why patients may not swallow the pill.

Implementing the Evidence and Evaluating Outcomes

After the first four steps of the EBP process have been completed, you can use the resulting information to make an evidence-based decision or provide research-informed advice. Although the steps in the process, as just described, may seem complicated, in reality, the process can be efficient—*if* there is an adequate evidence base and especially if it has been skillfully preprocessed. EBP is most challenging when findings from research are contradictory, inconclusive, or "thin"—that is to say, when better quality evidence is needed.

One last step in an individual EBP effort concerns evaluation. Part of the evaluation involves assessing whether your action achieved the desired outcome. Another part concerns an evaluation of how well you are performing EBP. Sackett and colleagues (2000) offer self-evaluation questions that relate to the five EBP steps, such as asking answerable questions (Am I asking any clinical questions at all? Am I asking well-formulated question?) and finding external evidence (Do I know the best sources of current evidence? Am I becoming more efficient in my searching?). A self-appraisal may lead you to conclude that at least some of the clinical questions in which you are interested are best addressed as a group effort.

EVIDENCE-BASED PRACTICE IN AN ORGANIZATIONAL CONTEXT

Most nurses practice in organizations, such as hospitals or long-term care settings. For some clinical scenarios that trigger an EBP effort, individual nurses may have sufficient autonomy that they can implement research-informed actions on their own (e.g., answering patients' questions about experiences with CPAP). In many situations, however, decisions are best made among a team of nurses working together to solve a common clinical problem. This section describes some additional considerations that are relevant to institutional efforts at EBP—efforts designed to result in a formal policy or protocol affecting the practice of many nurses.

Many of the steps in organizational EBP projects are similar to the ones described in the previous section. For example, asking questions and gathering and appraising evidence are key activities in both. However, there are additional issues of relevance at the organizational level.

Selecting a Problem for an Organizational Evidence-Based Practice Project

An institutional EBP effort can emerge in response to clinical scenarios such as those presented earlier but can also arise in other contexts such as quality improvement efforts. Some EBP projects are "bottoms-up" efforts that originate in discussions among clinicians who develop ideas for problem-solving innovations. Others are "top-down" efforts in which administrators take steps to stimulate creative thought and the use of research evidence. This latter approach often occurs as part of the Magnet recognition process.

Several EBP models distinguish two types of "triggers" for an EBP project—(1) *problem-focused triggers*—a clinical practice problem in need of solution, or (2) *knowledge-focused triggers*—readings in the research literature. Problem-focused triggers may arise in the normal course of clinical practice, as in the clinical scenarios described earlier. A problem-focused approach is likely to have staff support if the problem is widespread.

A second catalyst, knowledge-focused triggers, is research evidence itself. Sometimes this catalyst is a new clinical guideline, and in other cases, the impetus emerges from discussions in a journal club. For EBP projects with knowledge-focused triggers, an assessment of clinical relevance might be needed—that is, will a problem of significance to nurses in that setting be solved by introducing an innovation? Titler and Everett (2001) offered suggestions for selecting interventions, using concepts from Rogers's (1995) influential **Diffusion of Innovations Theory**.

With both types of triggers, consensus about the problem's importance and the need for improving practice is crucial. In the Iowa Model (Figure 2.2), the first decision point involves determining whether the topic is a priority for the organization considering practice changes. Titler and colleagues (2001) advised that, when finalizing a topic, the following issues be taken into account: the topic's fit with the organization's strategic plan, the magnitude of the problem, the number of people invested in the problem, support of nurse leaders and of those in other disciplines, costs, and possible barriers to change.

Addressing Practical Issues in Organizational Evidence-Based Practice Efforts

The most pervasive barriers to EBP are organizational, and so one upfront issue is that nurse administrators need to create structures and processes that facilitate research translation. Nursing leaders can support EBP as an approach to clinical decision making in many ways, including providing nurses with sufficient time away from their daily clinical responsibilities to undertake EBP activities, making available financial and material resources, and developing collaborations with mentors who can provide guidance and direction in the search for and appraisal of evidence.

In an organizational EBP project, some practical matters should be resolved even before a search for evidence begins. One issue concerns the team itself. A motivated and inspiring team leader is essential. The recruitment and development of EBP team members often requires an interdisciplinary perspective. Identifying tasks to be undertaken, developing a realistic timetable and budget, assigning members to tasks, and scheduling meetings are necessary to ensure that the effort will progress. Finally, it is wise for the team to solicit the support of stakeholders who might influence project activities and the eventual implementation of EBP changes.

Finding and Appraising Evidence for Organizational Evidence-Based Practice

For an organizational EBP effort, the best possible scenario involves identifying an appropriate clinical practice guideline, care bundle, or other decision support tool that has been based on rigorous research evidence. For some problem areas, however, clinical guidelines will need to be *developed* based on the evidence and not just implemented or adapted for use.

If a relevant guideline is identified, it should be carefully appraised. Several guideline appraisal instruments are available, but the one that has gained the broadest support is the Appraisal of Guidelines Research and Evaluation (AGREE) Instrument, now in its second version (Brouwers et al., 2010). This tool has been translated into many languages and has been endorsed by the World Health Organization. The AGREE II instrument consists of ratings of quality on a 7-point scale (from strongly agree to strongly disagree) for 23 quality dimensions organized in six domains: scope and purpose, stakeholder involvement, rigor of development, clarity and presentation, applicability, and editorial independence (plus two global assessment ratings). As examples, one of the statements in the Scope and Purpose domain is: "The population (patients, public, etc.) to whom the guideline is meant to apply is specifically described"; one of the statements in the Rigor of Development domain is: "The guideline has been externally reviewed by experts prior to its publication." The AGREE instrument should be applied to the guideline under consideration by a team of two to four appraisers. The Supplement to this chapter briefly discusses aspects of the AGREE II instrument. Another shorter and simpler tool for evaluating guideline quality is called the iCAHE Guideline Quality Check List (Grimmer et al., 2014).

One final issue is that guidelines change more slowly than the evidence. If a high-quality guideline is not recent, it is advisable to determine whether more up-to-date evidence would alter (or strengthen) the guideline's recommendations. It has been recommended that, to avoid obsolescence, guidelines should be reassessed every 3 years.

Making Decisions Based on Evidence Appraisals

In the Iowa Model, the synthesis and appraisal of research evidence provides the basis for a second major decision. The crux of the decision concerns whether the evidence is sufficient to justify an EBP change—for example, whether an existing clinical practice guideline is of sufficiently high quality that it can be used or adapted locally or whether (in the absence of a guideline) research evidence is sufficiently rigorous to recommend a practice innovation.

Coming to conclusions about the adequacy of research evidence can result in several possible outcomes leading to different paths. If the research base is weak, the team could either abandon the EBP project, or they could assemble other types of evidence (e.g., through consultation with experts or surveys of clients) and assess whether these sources suggests a practice change. Another possibility is to pursue an original clinical study to address the question directly. This course of action may be impractical and would result in years of delay before conclusions could be drawn. If, on the other hand, there is a solid evidence base or a high-quality clinical practice guideline, then the team could develop plans for moving forward with implementing a practice innovation.

Assessing Implementation Potential

In some EBP models, the next step is the development and testing of the innovation, followed by an assessment of organizational "fit." Other models recommend early steps to assess the appropriateness of the innovation within the organizational context. In some cases, such an assessment may be warranted even before searching for and appraising evidence. We think an early assessment of the **implementation potential** (or, *environmental readiness*) of a clinical innovation is often sensible, although some situations have little need for a formal assessment.

In determining the implementation potential of an innovation in a particular setting, several issues should be considered, particularly the transferability of the innovation, the feasibility of implementing it, and its cost–benefit ratio.

• *Transferability.* Transferability concerns whether it makes sense to implement the innovation in your practice setting. If some aspects of the setting are fundamentally incongruent with the innovation—in terms of its philosophy, types of client served, staff, or administrative structure—then it might not make sense to try to adopt the innovation, even if there is evidence of clinical effectiveness in other contexts. One possibility, however, is that some organizational changes could be made to make the "fit" better.

• *Feasibility.* Feasibility questions address practical concerns about the availability of staff and resources, the organizational climate, the need for and accessibility of external assistance, and the potential for clinical evaluation. An important issue is whether nurses will have, or share, control over the innovation. If nurses will not have control over a new procedure, the interdependent nature of the project should be identified early so that the EBP team will have needed interdisciplinary representatives.

• *Cost–benefit ratio.* A critical part of a decision to proceed with an EBP project is a careful assessment of costs and benefits of the change. The cost–benefit assessment should encompass likely costs and benefits to various groups (e.g., clients, nurses, the overall organization). If the degree of risk in introducing an innovation is high, then potential benefits must be great and the evidence must be very sound. A cost–benefit assessment should consider the opposite side of the coin as well: the costs and benefits of *not* instituting an innovation. The status quo bears its own risks and failure to change—especially when such change is based on firm evidence—can be costly to clients, to organizations, and to the entire nursing community.

➔ **TIP:** The Toolkit for Chapter 2 in the *Resource Manual* has a worksheet with a series of questions for assessing the implementation potential of a potential innovation.

If the implementation assessment suggests that there might be problems in testing the innovation in that particular practice setting, then the team can either begin the process anew with a different innovation or pursue a plan to improve the implementation potential (e.g., seeking external resources if costs were the inhibiting factor).

➔ **TIP:** Documentation of all steps in the EBP process, including the implementation potential of an innovation, is highly recommended. Committing ideas to writing is useful because it can help to resolve ambiguities, can serve as a problem-solving tool if problems emerge, and can be used to persuade others of the value of the project. All aspects of the EBP project should be transparent.

Developing Evidence-Based Protocols

If the implementation criteria are met and the evidence is adequate, the team can prepare an action plan to move the effort forward, which includes laying out strategies for designing and piloting the new clinical practice. In most cases, a key activity will involve developing a local evidence-based clinical practice protocol or guideline or adapting an existing one.

If a relevant clinical practice guideline has been judged to be of sufficiently high quality, the EBP team needs to decide whether to (1) adopt it in its entirety, (2) adopt only certain recommendations, while disregarding others (e.g., recommendations for which the evidence is less sound), or (3) make adaptations deemed necessary based on local circumstances. The risk in modifying guidelines is that the adaptation will not adequately incorporate the research evidence.

If there is no existing clinical practice guideline, or if existing guidelines are weak, the team will need to develop its own protocol or guideline reflecting the accumulated research evidence. Strategies for developing clinical practice guidelines are suggested in most textbooks on EBP and in several handbooks (Ansari & Rashidian, 2012; Turner et al., 2008). Whether a guideline is developed "from scratch" or adapted from an existing one, independent peer review is advisable to ensure that the guidelines are clear, comprehensive, and congruent with best existing evidence.

➔ **TIP:** Guidelines should be user-friendly. Visual devices such as flowcharts and decision trees are often useful.

Implementing and Evaluating the Innovation

Once an EBP protocol has been developed, the next step is to **pilot test** it (give it a trial run) in a clinical setting and to evaluate the outcome. Building on the Iowa Model, this phase of the project likely would involve the following activities:

1. Developing an evaluation plan (e.g., identifying outcomes to be achieved, deciding how many clients to involve, settling on when and how often to collect outcome information)
2. Collecting information on the outcomes for clients prior to implementing the innovation to develop a comparison against which the outcomes of the innovation can be assessed
3. Training staff in the use of the new protocol and, if necessary, "marketing" the innovation to users so that it is given a fair test
4. Trying the protocol out on one or more units or with a group of clients
5. Evaluating the pilot project, in terms of both process (e.g., How was the innovation received, what implementation problems were encountered?) and outcomes (e.g., How were outcomes affected, what were the costs?)

TIP: The Registered Nurses' Association of Ontario or RNAO (2012) has developed a toolkit to facilitate the implementation of clinical practice guidelines. The toolkit (second edition) is available at http://rnao.ca/bpg/resources/toolkit-implementation-best-practice-guidelines-second-edition.

A variety of research strategies and designs can be used to evaluate the innovation (see Chapter 11). In most cases, an informal evaluation will be adequate, for example, comparing outcome information from hospital records before and after the innovation and gathering information about patient and staff satisfaction. Qualitative information can also contribute to the evaluation: Qualitative data can uncover subtleties about the implementation process and help to explain findings.

Evaluation information should be gathered over a sufficiently long period (6 to 12 months) to allow for a true test of a "mature" innovation. An even longer time frame is useful for learning about the *sustainability* of an innovation. The end result is a decision about whether to adopt the innovation, to modify it for ongoing use, or to revert to prior practices. Another advisable step is to disseminate the results so that other nurses and nursing administrators can benefit. Finally, the EBP team should develop a plan for when the new protocol will be reviewed and, if necessary, updated based on new research evidence or ongoing feedback about outcomes.

TIP: Every nurse can play a role in using research evidence. Here are some strategies:

- *Read widely and critically.* Professionally accountable nurses keep abreast of important developments and read journals relating to their specialty, including research reports in them.
- *Attend professional conferences.* Nursing conferences include presentations of studies with clinical relevance. Conference attendees have opportunities to meet researchers and to explore practice implications.
- *Insist on evidence that a procedure is effective.* Every time nurses or nursing students are told about a standard nursing procedure, they have a right to ask: Why? Nurses need to develop expectations that the clinical decisions they make are based on sound, evidence-based rationales.
- *Become involved in a journal club.* Many organizations that employ nurses sponsor journal clubs that review studies with potential relevance to practice. The traditional approach for a journal club (nurses coming together as a group to discuss and critique an article) is in some settings being replaced with online journal clubs that acknowledge time constraints and the inability of nurses from all shifts to come together at one time.
- *Pursue and participate in EBP projects.* Several studies have found that nurses who are involved in research activities (e.g., an EBP project or data collection activities) develop more positive attitudes toward research and better research skills.

●●●●●●●●●●●●●●●●●●●●●●●

RESEARCH EXAMPLE

Thousands of EBP projects are underway in practice settings. Many that have been described in the nursing literature offer useful information about planning and implementing such an endeavor. One is described here, and another full article is included in the *Resource Manual*.

Study: Implementing skin-to-skin contact at birth using the Iowa Model (Haxton et al., 2012).

Purpose: An evidence-based practice implementation project was undertaken at a Midwestern academic medical center. The focus of the project was to promote early skin-to-skin contact (SSC) as a best practice for healthy term newborns.

Framework: The project used the Iowa Model as its guiding framework. The EBP team identified early SSC as having a knowledge-focused trigger: New guidelines supporting SSC had recently been published, and yet many nurses in the medical center did not routinely engage in the practice.

Early Iowa Model Steps: After conducting a small study in which 30 mothers of health newborns were interviewed, the project leaders decided to focus on "improving staff knowledge and philosophy of care related to SSC" (p. 224). They addressed the issue of organizational priorities by making a presentation of evidence on the benefits of SSC to the hospital's Best Practice Committee. The Committee and the leadership within the hospital's Birth Center gave their enthusiastic support for the project. Next, a project team was organized. The team consisted of nurses, physicians, nursing assistants, and lactation consultants, under the leadership of the Birth Center's Clinical Nurse Specialist. Nurses from all shifts joined the team. Members of the team participated in a group approach to assembling, reviewing, and critiquing the evidence.

Protocol Development: The team discovered that implementing early SSC was in conflict with standard practices at the Birth Center, which involved having a second nurse in the patient's room to accept the newborn from the physician or midwife, complete a series of common measurements and interventions, wrap the newborn in a blanket, and then hand the infant to the mother. After reviewing evidence that delaying common newborn interventions would not put the baby at risk, the team concluded that if a newborn was stable and the mother expressed a desire to perform SSC, then the second nurse could be dismissed earlier. Subsequently, the team "negotiated a detailed step-by-step protocol for early SSC intervention after vaginal birth" (p. 226). Educational material for mothers was developed. The electronic medical record also had to be modified.

Evaluation: The protocol was then pilot tested, beginning with the development and implementation of four training sessions for the labor and delivery nursing staff. Once training was complete, several evaluation activities were undertaken. For example, the team first examined whether SSC was actually being offered and delivered. In the pilot study, several outcomes were assessed such as the rate of breastfeeding initiation and maternal satisfaction. The evaluation involved examination of charts before and after implementing the protocol and interviews with staff and mothers.

Findings and Conclusions: Based on chart review in the four quarters before and after initiating the pilot, the researchers found that the rate of breastfeeding initiation increased from around 74% to 84%. Most mothers who were interviewed acknowledged that their nurse had explained SSC and its benefits to them, and most made positive comments about the SSC experience. Nurses anecdotally reported that the protocol did not increase their workload and did not result in delays in transferring mothers to the postpartum unit. The authors of the article acknowledged that the project was challenging and many barriers were encountered, but they emphasized that they were able to overcome the challenges and were encouraged by the preliminary results from the pilot.

●●●●●●●●●●●●●●●●●●●●●●●

SUMMARY POINTS

- **Evidence-based practice (EBP)** is the conscientious integration of current best evidence with clinical expertise and patient preferences in making clinical decisions; it is a clinical problem-solving strategy that de-emphasizes decision making based on custom.

- **Research utilization (RU)** and EBP are overlapping concepts that concern efforts to use research as a basis for clinical decisions, but RU *starts* with a research-based innovation that gets evaluated for possible use in practice.

- **Knowledge translation (KT)** is a term used primarily about system-wide efforts to enhance systematic change in clinical practice or policies.

- Two underpinnings of the EBP movement are the **Cochrane Collaboration** (which is based on the work of British epidemiologist Archie Cochrane) and the clinical learning strategy called *evidence-based medicine* developed at the McMaster Medical School.

- EBP typically involves weighing various types of evidence in an effort to determine *best evidence*. Often, an **evidence hierarchy** is used to grade study findings according to the strength of evidence provided, but different hierarchies are appropriate for different types of questions. In all evidence hierarchies, however, systematic reviews are at the pinnacle.

- Resources to support EBP are growing at a phenomenal pace. Among the resources are systematic reviews (and electronic databases that make them easy to locate); evidence-based clinical practice guidelines, care bundles, and other decision support tools; a wealth of other preappraised evidence that makes it possible to practice EBP efficiently; and models of EBP that provide a framework for planning and undertaking EBP projects.

- **Systematic reviews** are rigorous integrations of research evidence from multiple studies on a topic. Systematic reviews can involve either qualitative, narrative approaches to integration (including **metasynthesis** of qualitative studies), or quantitative methods (**meta-analysis**) that integrate findings statistically.

- Evidence-based **clinical practice guidelines** combine a synthesis and appraisal of research evidence with specific recommendations for clinical decision making. Clinical practice guidelines should be carefully and systematically appraised, for example, using the Appraisal of Guidelines Research and Evaluation (*AGREE II*) Instrument.

- Many models of EBP have been developed, including models that provide a framework for individual clinicians (e.g., the **Stetler Model**) and others for organizations or teams of clinicians (e.g., the **Iowa Model** of Evidence-Based Practice to Promote Quality Care, Promoting Action on Research Implementation in Health Services or **PARIHS Model**).

- Individual nurses can put research into practice, using five basic steps: (1) framing an answerable clinical question, (2) searching for relevant research evidence, (3) appraising and synthesizing the evidence, (4) integrating evidence with other factors, and (5) assessing effectiveness.

- One scheme for asking well-worded clinical questions involves four primary components, an acronym for which is **PICO**: Population (P), Intervention or influence (I), Comparison (C), and Outcome (O). When there is no explicit comparison, the acronym is PIO.

- An appraisal of the evidence involves such considerations as the validity of study findings, their clinical importance, the precision of estimates of effects, associated costs and risks, and utility in a particular clinical situation.

- EBP in an organizational context involves many of the same steps as an individual EBP effort but tends to be more formalized and must take organizational and interpersonal factors into account. "Triggers" for an organizational project include both pressing clinical problems and existing knowledge.

- Team-based or organizational EBP projects typically involve the development or adaptation of clinical protocols. Before these products can be tested, there should be an assessment of the **implementation potential** of the innovation, which includes the dimensions of transferability of findings, feasibility of using the findings in the new setting, and the cost–benefit ratio of a new practice.

- Once an evidence-based protocol or guideline has been developed and deemed worthy of implementation, the team can move forward with a **pilot test** of the innovation and an assessment of the outcomes prior to widespread adoption.

STUDY ACTIVITIES

Chapter 2 of the *Resource Manual for Nursing Research: Generating and Assessing Evidence for Nursing Practice, 10th edition*, offers study suggestions for reinforcing concepts presented in this chapter. In addition, the following questions can be addressed in classroom or online discussions:

1. Think about your own clinical situation and identify a problem area. Now pose a well-worded clinical question using the templates in Table 2.1. Identify the various components of the question—that is, population, intervention or issue, comparison, and outcome.
2. Discuss the overall approach used in the example featured at the end of this chapter (Haxton et al., 2012).

STUDIES CITED IN CHAPTER 2

*Ansari, S., & Rashidian, A., (2012). Guidelines for guidelines: Are they up to the task? A comparative assessment of clinical practice guideline development handbooks. *PloS One, 7*, e49864.

Bates, O. L., O'Connor, N., Dunn, D., & Hasenau, S. (2014). Applying SRAAT interventions in incremental bundles: Improving post-CABG surgical patient care. *Worldviews on Evidence-Based Nursing, 11*, 89–97.

Beck, C. (2009). Metasynthesis: A goldmine for evidence-based practice. *AORN Journal, 90*, 701–702.

*Brouwers, M., Kho, M., Browman, G., Burgers, J., Cluzeau, F., Feder, G., . . . Zitzelsberger, L. (2010). AGREE II: Advancing guideline development, reporting and evaluation in health care. *Canadian Medical Association Journal, 182*, E839–E842.

Brown, C. G. (2014). The Iowa model of evidence-based practice to promote quality care: An illustrated example in oncology nursing. *Clinical Journal of Oncology Nursing, 18*, 157–159.

Brown, S. J. (2013). *Evidence-based nursing: The research-practice connection* (3rd ed.). Boston: Jones and Bartlett.

Canadian Institutes of Health Research. (2004). *Knowledge translation strategy 2004–2009: Innovation in action.* Ottawa, Canada: Author.

Clarke, M., Hopewell, S., Juszczak, E., Eisinga, A., & Kjeldstrom, M. (2006). Compression stockings for preventing deep vein thrombosis in airline passengers. *Cochrane Database of Systematic Reviews,* (2), CD004002.

Craig, J., & Smyth, R. (2012). *The evidence-based practice manual for nurses* (3rd ed.). Edinburgh, Scotland: Churchill Livingstone Elsevier.

DiCenso, A., Guyatt, G., & Ciliska, D. (2005). *Evidence-based nursing: A guide to clinical practice.* St. Louis, MO: Elsevier Mosby.

DiPietro, T., Nhuyen, H., & Doran, D. (2012). Usability evaluation: Results from "evaluation of mobile information technology to improve nurses' access to and use of research evidence." *Computers, Informatics, Nursing, 30*, 440–448.

Doran, D. (2009). The emerging role of PDAs in information use and clinical decision making. *Evidence-Based Nursing, 12*, 35–38.

Doran, D., Haynes, R., Kushniruk, A., Straus, S., Grimshaw, J., Hall, L., . . . Jedras, D. (2010). Supporting evidence-based practice for nurses through information technologies. *Worldviews on Evidence-Based Nursing, 7*, 4–15.

Du, S., Dong, J., Zhang, H., Jin, S., Xu, G., Liu, Z., . . . Sun, Z. (2015). Tai chi exercise for self-rated sleep quality in older people: A systematic review and meta-analysis. *International Journal of Nursing Studies, 52*, 368–379.

Gawlinski, A., & Rutledge, D. (2008). Selecting a model for evidence-based practice changes. *AACN Advanced Critical Care, 19*, 291–300.

*Gilbert, R., Salanti, G., Harden, M., & See, S. (2005). Infant sleeping position and the sudden infant death syndrome: Systematic review of observational studies and historical review of recommendations from 1940 to 2002. *International Journal of Epidemiology, 34*, 874–887.

Gillespie, B., Chaboyer, W., McInnes, E., Kent, B., Whitty, J., & Thalib, L. (2014). Repositioning for pressure ulcer prevention in adults. *Cochrane Database of Systematic Reviews,* (4), CD009958.

Glasziou, P. (2005). Evidence-based medicine: Does it make a difference? Make it evidence informed with a little wisdom. *British Medical Journal, 330*(7482), 92.

*Grimmer, K., Dizon, J., Milanese, S., King, E., Beaton, K., Thorpe, O., . . . Kumar, S. (2014). Efficient clinical evaluation of guideline quality: Development and testing of a new tool. *BMC Medical Research Methodology, 14*, 63.

Haxton, D., Doering, J., Gingras, L., & Kelly, L. (2012). Implementing skin-to-skin contact at birth using the Iowa Model. *Nursing for Women's Health, 16*, 221–230.

Horsley, J. A., Crane, J., & Bingle, J. D. (1978). Research utilization as an organizational process. *Journal of Nursing Administration, 8*, 4–6.

Hsieh, H. F., & Lee, F. P. (2005). Graduated compression stockings as prophylaxis for flight-related venous thrombosis: Systematic literature review. *Journal of Advanced Nursing, 51*, 83–98.

Kring, D. L. (2008). Clinical nurse specialist practice domains and evidence-based practice competencies: A matrix of influence. *Clinical Nurse Specialist, 22*, 179–183.

Logan, J., & Graham, I. (1998). Toward a comprehensive interdisciplinary model of health care research use. *Science Communication, 20*, 227–246.

Melnyk, B. M. (2014). Evidence-based practice versus evidence-informed practice: A debate that could stall forward momentum in improving healthcare quality, safety, patient outcomes, and costs. *Worldviews on Evidence-Based Nursing*, *11*, 347–349.

Melnyk, B. M., & Fineout-Overholt, E. (2015). *Evidence-based practice in nursing and healthcare* (3rd ed.). Philadelphia: Lippincott Williams & Wilkins.

Morse, J. M. (2005). Beyond the clinical trial: Expanding criteria for evidence. *Qualitative Health Research*, *15*, 3–4.

Newhouse, R., Dearholt, S., Poe, S., Pugh, L. C., & White, K. M. (2005). Evidence-based practice: A practical approach to implementation. *Journal of Nursing Administration*, *35*, 35–40.

Registered Nurses' Association of Ontario. (2012). *Toolkit: Implementation of best practice guidelines* (2nd ed.). Retrieved from http://rnao.ca/bpg/resources/toolkit-implementation-best-practice-guidelines-second-edition

Registered Nurses' Association of Ontario. (2013). *Assessment and management of foot ulcers for people with diabetes* (2nd ed.). Retrieved from http://rnao.ca/bpg/guidelines/assessment-and-management-foot-ulcers-people-diabetes-second-edition

Ries, A., Trottenberg, P., Elsner, F., Stiel, S., Haugen, D., Kaasa, S., & Radbruch, L. (2012). A systematic review on the role of fish oil for the treatment of cachexia in advanced cancer. *Palliative Medicine*, *26*, 294–304.

Rogers, E. M. (1995). *Diffusion of innovations* (4th ed.). New York: Free Press.

Rosswurm, M. A., & Larrabee, J. H. (1999). A model for change to evidence-based practice. *Image: The Journal of Nursing Scholarship*, *31*, 317–322.

Ruiz Garcia, V., López-Briz, E., Carbonell Sanchis, R., Gonzalvez Perales, J., & Bort-Marti, S. (2013). Megestrol acetate for treatment of anorexia-cachexia syndrome. *Cochrane Database of Systematic Reviews*, (3), CD004310.

Rycroft-Malone, J. (2010). Promoting Action on Research Implementation in Health Services (PARIHS). In J. Rycroft-Malone & T. Bucknall (Eds.), *Models and frameworks for implementing evidence-based practice: Linking evidence to action* (pp. 109–133). Malden, MA: Wiley-Blackwell.

*Rycroft-Malone, J., Kitson, A., Harvey, G., McCormack, B., Seers, K., Titchen, A., & Estabrooks, C. (2002). Ingredients for change: Revisiting a conceptual framework. *Quality and Safety in Health Care*, *11*, 174–180.

Sackett, D. L., Straus, S. E., Richardson, W. S., Rosenberg, W., & Haynes, R. B. (2000). *Evidence-based medicine: How to practice and teach EBM* (2nd ed.). Edinburgh, Scotland: Churchill Livingstone.

Sandelowski, M., Voils, C. I., Crandell, J. L., & Leeman, J. (2013). Synthesizing qualitative and quantitative research findings. In C. T. Beck (Ed.), *Routledge international handbook of qualitative nursing research* (pp. 347–356). New York: Routledge.

Schaffer, M. A., Sandau, K., & Diedrick, L. (2013). Evidence-based practice models for organizational change: Overview and practical applications. *Journal of Advanced Nursing*, *69*, 1197–1209.

Schmidt, N. A., & Brown, J. M. (2011). *Evidence-based practice for nurses: Appraisal and application of research* (2nd ed.). Sudbury, MA: Jones & Bartlett.

Scott, K., & McSherry, R. (2009). Evidence-based nursing: Clarifying the concepts for nurses in practice. *Journal of Clinical Nursing*, *18*, 1085–1095.

Shapiro, S. E. (2005). Evaluating clinical decision rules. *Western Journal of Nursing Research*, *27*, 655–664.

Sigma Theta Tau International. (2008). Sigma Theta Tau International position statement on evidence-based practice, February 2007 summary. *Worldviews of Evidence-Based Nursing*, *5*, 57–59.

Stetler, C. B. (2001). Updating the Stetler model of research utilization to facilitate evidence-based practice. *Nursing Outlook*, *49*, 272–279.

Stetler, C. B. (2010). Stetler model. In J. Rycroft-Malone & T. Bucknall (Eds.), *Models and frameworks for implementing evidence-based practice: Linking evidence to action* (pp. 51–77). Malden, MA: Wiley-Blackwell.

Tao, H., Songwathana, P., Isaralali, S., & Zhang, Y. (2014). Personal awareness and behavioural choices on having a stoma: A qualitative metasynthesis. *Journal of Clinical Nursing*, *23*, 1186–1200.

Thorne, S. (2009). The role of qualitative research within an evidence-based context: Can metasynthesis be the answer? *International Journal of Nursing Studies*, *46*, 569–575.

Titler, M. (2010). Iowa model of evidence-based practice. In J. Rycroft-Malone & T. Bucknall (Eds.), *Models and frameworks for implementing evidence-based practice: Linking evidence to action* (pp. 169–182). Malden, MA: Wiley-Blackwell.

Titler, M. G., & Everett, L. Q. (2001). Translating research into practice. Considerations for critical care investigators. *Critical Care Nursing Clinics of North America*, *13*, 587–604.

Titler, M. G., Kleiber, C., Steelman, V., Rakel, B., Budreau, G., Everett, L., . . . Goode, C. (2001). The Iowa model of evidence-based practice to promote quality care. *Critical Care Nursing Clinics of North America*, *13*, 497–509.

*Turner, T., Misso, M., Harris, C., & Green, S. (2008). Development of evidence-based clinical practice guidelines (CPGs): Comparing approaches. *Implementation Science*, *3*, 45.

*World Health Organization. (2005). *Bridging the "Know-Do" gap: Meeting on knowledge translation in global health.* Retrieved from http://www.who.int/kms/WHO_EIP_KMS_2006_2.pdf

***A link to this open-access journal article is provided in the Toolkit for this chapter in the accompanying Resource Manual.*

Key Concepts and Steps in Qualitative and Quantitative Research

3

This chapter covers a lot of ground—but, for many of you, it is familiar ground. For those who have taken an earlier research course, this chapter provides a review of key terms and steps in the research process. For those without previous exposure to research methods, this chapter offers basic grounding in research terminology.

Research, like any discipline, has its own language—its own *jargon*. Some terms are used by both qualitative and quantitative researchers, but others are used mainly by one or the other group. To make matters more complex, some nursing research jargon has its roots in the social sciences, but sometimes different terms for the same concepts are used in medical research; we cover both.

FUNDAMENTAL RESEARCH TERMS AND CONCEPTS

When researchers address a problem—regardless of the underlying paradigm—they undertake a **study** (or an **investigation**). Studies involve people working together in different roles.

The Faces and Places of Research

Studies with humans involve two sets of people: those who do the research and those who provide the information. In a quantitative study, the people being studied are called **subjects** or **study participants** (Table 3.1). In a qualitative study, those cooperating in the study are called study par-

ticipants, **informants**, or **key informants**. Collectively, study participants comprise the **sample**.

The person who conducts a study is the **researcher** or **investigator**. When a study is done by a team, the person directing the study is the **principal investigator (PI)**. In large-scale projects, dozens of individuals may be involved in planning, managing, and conducting the study. The following examples of staffing configurations span the continuum from an extremely large project to a more modest one.

Examples of Staffing on a Quantitative Study: The first author of this book was involved in a multicomponent, interdisciplinary study of poor women living in four major U.S. cities. As part of the study, she and two colleagues prepared a report documenting the health problems of 4,000 welfare mothers who were interviewed twice over a 3-year period (Polit et al., 2001). The project was staffed by over 100 people, including lead investigators of six project components (Polit was one), over 50 interviewers, and dozens of research assistants, computer programmers, and other support staff. Several health consultants, including a prominent nurse researcher (Linda Aiken), served as reviewers.

Examples of Staffing on a Qualitative Study: Beck (2009) conducted a qualitative study focusing on the experiences of mothers caring for their children with a brachial plexus injury. The team consisted Beck as the PI (who gathered and analyzed all the data), members of the United Brachial Plexus Executive Board (who helped to recruit

TABLE 3.1 • Key Terms in Quantitative and Qualitative Research

CONCEPT	QUANTITATIVE TERM	QUALITATIVE TERM
Person contributing information	Subject Study participant —	— Study participant Informant, key informant
Person undertaking the study	Researcher Investigator	Researcher Investigator
That which is being investigated	— Concepts Constructs Variables	Phenomena Concepts — —
System of organizing concepts	Theory, theoretical framework Conceptual framework, conceptual model	Theory Conceptual framework, sensitizing framework
Information gathered	Data (numerical values)	Data (narrative descriptions)
Connections between concepts	Relationships (cause-and-effect, associative)	Patterns of association
Logical reasoning processes	Deductive reasoning	Inductive reasoning

mothers for the study), a transcriber (who listened to the tape-recorded interviews and typed them up verbatim), and an undergraduate nursing student (who checked the accuracy of the interview transcripts against the tape-recorded interviews).

Research can be undertaken in a variety of *settings* (the specific places where information is gathered) and in one or more *sites*. Some studies take place in *naturalistic settings* in the field, such as in people's homes, but some studies are done in controlled laboratory or clinical settings. Qualitative researchers are especially likely to engage in **fieldwork** in natural settings because they are interested in the contexts of people's experiences. The *site* is the overall location for the research—it could be an entire community (e.g., a Haitian neighborhood in Miami) or an institution (e.g., a hospital in Toronto). Researchers sometimes engage in **multisite studies** because the use of multiple sites offers a larger or more diverse sample of participants.

The Building Blocks of Research

Phenomena, Concepts, and Constructs

Research involves abstractions. For example, *pain*, *quality of life*, and *resilience* are abstractions of particular aspects of human behavior and characteristics. These abstractions are called **concepts** or, in qualitative studies, **phenomena**.

Researchers also use the term **construct**. Like a concept, a construct is an abstraction inferred from situations or behaviors. Kerlinger and Lee (2000) distinguish concepts from constructs by noting that constructs are abstractions that are deliberately invented (constructed) by researchers. For example, *self-care* in Orem's model of health maintenance is a construct. The terms *construct* and *concept* are sometimes used interchangeably but, by convention, a construct typically refers to a more complex abstraction than a concept.

Theories and Conceptual Models

A **theory** is a systematic, abstract explanation of some aspect of reality. Theories, which knit concepts together into a coherent system, play a role in both qualitative and quantitative research.

Quantitative researchers may start with a theory, *framework*, or *conceptual model* (distinctions are discussed in Chapter 6). Based on theory, researchers predict how phenomena will behave in the real world *if the theory is true*—researchers use *deductive reasoning* to go from a theory to specific hypotheses. Predictions deduced from theory are tested through research, and results are used to support, reject, or modify the theory.

In qualitative research, theories may be used in various ways. Sometimes conceptual or **sensitizing frameworks**, derived from qualitative research traditions we describe later in this chapter, offer an orienting worldview. In such studies, the framework helps to guide the inquiry and to interpret research evidence. In other qualitative studies, theory is the *product* of the research: The investigators use information from participants *inductively* to develop a theory rooted in the participants' experiences.

S Deductive and inductive logical reasoning processes are described more fully on the Supplement to this chapter on thePoint®.

Variables

In quantitative studies, concepts often are called **variables**. A variable, as the name implies, is something that varies. Weight, fatigue, and anxiety are variables—each varies from one person to another. In fact, most aspects of humans are variables. If everyone weighed 150 pounds, weight would not be a variable, it would be a *constant*. It is precisely because people and conditions *do* vary that most research is conducted. Quantitative researchers seek to understand how or why things vary and to learn if differences in one variable are related to differences in another. For example, lung cancer research is concerned with the variable of lung cancer, which is a variable because not everyone has this disease. Researchers have studied factors that might be linked to

lung cancer, such as cigarette smoking. Smoking is also a variable because not everyone smokes. A variable, then, is any quality of a person, group, or situation that varies or takes on different values. Variables are the building blocks of quantitative studies.

When an attribute is highly varied in the group under study, the group is **heterogeneous** with respect to that variable. If the amount of variability is limited, the group is **homogeneous**. For example, for the variable height, a sample of 2-year-old children would be more homogeneous than a sample of 21-year-olds.

Variables may be inherent characteristics of people, such as their age, blood type, or weight. Sometimes, however, researchers *create* a variable. For example, if a researcher tests the effectiveness of patient-controlled analgesia as opposed to intramuscular analgesia in relieving pain after surgery, some patients would be given patient-controlled analgesia and others would receive intramuscular analgesia. In the context of this study, method of pain management is a variable because different patients get different analgesic methods.

Continuous, Discrete, and Categorical Variables. Some variables take on a wide range of values. A person's age, for instance, can take on values from zero to more than 100, and the values are not restricted to whole numbers. **Continuous variables** have values along a continuum and, in theory, can assume an infinite number of values between two points. Consider the continuous variable *weight*: between 1 and 2 pounds, the number of values is limitless: 1.05, 1.8, 1.333, and so on.

By contrast, a **discrete variable** has a finite number of values between any two points, representing discrete quantities. For example, if people were asked how many children they had, they might answer 0, 1, 2, 3, or more. The value for number of children is discrete, because a number such as 1.5 is not meaningful. Between 1 and 3, the only possible value is 2.

Other variables take on a small range of values that do not represent a *quantity*. Blood type, for example, has four values—A, B, AB, and O. Variables that take on a handful of discrete nonquantitative values are **categorical variables**. When categorical variables take on only two values, they are **dichotomous variables**. Gender, for example, is dichotomous: male and female.

Dependent and Independent Variables. Many studies seek to unravel and understand causes of phenomena. Does a nursing intervention *cause* improvements in patient outcomes? Does smoking *cause* lung cancer? The presumed cause is the **independent variable**, and the presumed effect is the **dependent variable** (or, the **outcome variable**). In terms of the PICO scheme discussed in Chapter 2, the dependent variable corresponds to the "O" (outcome). The independent variable corresponds to the "I" (the intervention, influence, or exposure) *plus* the "C" (the comparison). In searching for existing evidence, you might want to learn about the effects of an intervention or influence (I), compared to *any* alternative, on an outcome (O) of interest. In a study, however, researchers must always specify the comparator (the "C").

Variation in the dependent variable is presumed to *depend on* variation in the independent variable. For example, researchers study the extent to which lung cancer (the dependent variable) depends on smoking (the independent variable). Or, investigators might study the extent to which patients' pain (the dependent variable) depends on different nursing actions (the independent variable). The dependent variable is the outcome that researchers want to understand, explain, or predict.

The terms *independent variable* and *dependent variable* can also be used to indicate *direction of influence* rather than a cause and effect. For example, suppose a researcher studied the mental health of the spousal caregivers of patients with Alzheimer's disease and found lower depression for wives than for husbands. We could not conclude that depression was *caused* by gender. Yet the direction of influence clearly runs from gender to depression: A patient's level of depression does not influence their gender. Although it may not make sense to infer a cause-and-effect connection, it is appropriate to consider depression as the outcome variable and gender as an independent variable.

Most outcomes have multiple causes or influences. If we were studying factors that influence people's body mass index (the dependent variable), we might consider height, physical activity, and diet as independent variables. Two or more *dependent* variables also may be of interest. For example, a researcher may compare the effects of two methods of nursing care for children with cystic fibrosis. Several dependent variables could be used to assess treatment effectiveness, such as length of hospital stay, number of recurrent respiratory infections, and so on. It is common to design studies with multiple independent and dependent variables.

Variables are not *inherently* dependent or independent. A dependent variable in one study could be an independent variable in another. For example, a study might examine the effect of an exercise intervention (the independent variable) on osteoporosis (the dependent variable) to answer a Therapy question. Another study might investigate the effect of osteoporosis (the independent variable) on bone fracture incidence (the dependent variable) to address a Prognosis question. In short, whether a variable is independent or dependent is a function of the role that it plays in a particular study.

Example of Independent and Dependent Variables: *Research question (Etiology/Harm question)*: Are interruptions during patient medication rounds in a mental health hospital associated with higher rates of nurses' medication-administration errors? (Cottney & Innes, 2015)
Independent variable: Interruptions during medication rounds
Dependent variable: Medication administration errors

Conceptual and Operational Definitions

Concepts are abstractions of observable phenomena, and researchers' worldviews shape how those concepts are defined. A **conceptual definition** presents the abstract or theoretical meaning of concepts under study. Even seemingly straightforward terms need to be conceptually defined. The classic example is the concept of *caring*. Morse and colleagues (1990) examined how researchers and theorists defined *caring* and identified five classes of conceptual definition: as a human trait, a moral imperative, an affect, an interpersonal relationship, and a therapeutic intervention. Researchers undertaking studies of caring need to clarify which conceptual definition they have adopted.

In qualitative studies, conceptual definitions of key phenomena may be a major end product, reflecting an intent to have the meaning of concepts defined by those being studied. In quantitative studies, however, researchers must define concepts at the outset because they must decide how the variables will be observed and measured. An **operational definition** of a concept specifies what the researchers must do to measure the concept and collect needed information.

Variables differ in the ease with which they can be operationalized. The variable weight, for example, is easy to define and measure. We might operationally define weight as the amount that an object weighs, to the nearest half pound. This definition designates that weight will be measured using one system (pounds) rather than another (grams). We could also specify that weight will be measured using a digital scale with participants fully undressed after 10 hours of fasting. This operational definition clarifies what we mean by the variable *weight*.

Few variables are operationalized as easily as weight. Most variables can be measured in different ways, and researchers must choose the one that best captures the variables as they conceptualize them. Take, for example, *anxiety*, which can be defined in terms of both physiologic and psychological functioning. For researchers choosing to emphasize physiologic aspects, the operational definition might involve a measure such as pulse rate. If researchers conceptualize anxiety as a psychological state, the operational definition might be scores on a paper-and-pencil test such as the State Anxiety Scale. Readers of research articles may not agree with how variables were conceptualized and measured, but definitional precision is important for communicating exactly what concepts mean within the study.

➔ TIP: Operationalizing a concept is often a two-part process that involves deciding (1) how to accurately measure the variable and (2) how to represent it in an analysis. For example, a person's age might be obtained by asking them to report their birthdate but operationalized in an analysis in relation to a threshold (e.g., under 65 versus 65 or older).

Example of Conceptual and Operational Definitions: Fogg and colleagues (2011) developed a scale to measure people's beliefs and intentions about HIV screening. The scale relied on constructs from a theory called the Theory of Planned Behavior (see Chapter 6). The researchers provided examples of both conceptual and operational definitions of key constructs. For example, "subjective norm" was conceptually defined as "the overall perception of social pressure to perform or not perform the behavior" and a scale item used to measure this construct in the context of HIV screening was "The people in my life whose opinions I value are regularly tested for HIV" (p. 76).

Data

Research **data** (singular, datum) are the pieces of information obtained in a study. In quantitative studies, researchers identify and define their variables and then collect relevant data from study participants. Quantitative researchers collect primarily **quantitative data**—data in numeric form. For example, suppose we conducted a quantitative study in which a key variable was depression. We might ask, "Thinking about the past week, how depressed would you say you have been on a scale from 0 to 10, where 0 means 'not at all' and 10 means 'the most possible'?" Box 3.1 presents quantitative data for three fictitious people. Subjects provided a number along the 0 to 10 continuum representing their degree of depression—*9* for subject 1 (a high level of depression), *0* for subject 2 (no depression), and *4* for subject 3 (little depression). The numeric values for all people, collectively, would comprise the data on depression.

In qualitative studies, researchers collect **qualitative data**, that is, narrative descriptions. Narrative information can be obtained by having conversations with participants, by making detailed notes about how people behave in naturalistic settings, or by obtaining narrative records, such as diaries. Suppose we were studying depression qualitatively. Box 3.2 presents qualitative data for three people responding conversationally to the question, "Tell me about how you've been feeling lately—have you felt sad or depressed at all, or have you generally been in good spirits?" The data consist of rich narrative descriptions of participant's emotional state.

Relationships

Researchers are rarely interested in isolated concepts, except in descriptive studies. For example,

> ## BOX 3.1 Example of Quantitative Data
>
> **Question:** Thinking about the past week, how depressed would you say you have been on a scale from 0 to 10, where 0 means "not at all" and 10 means "the most possible"?
>
> **Data:** 9 (Subject 1)
> 0 (Subject 2)
> 4 (Subject 3)

a researcher might describe the percentage of patients receiving intravenous (IV) therapy who experience IV infiltration. In this example, the variable is IV infiltration versus no infiltration. Usually, however, researchers study phenomena in relation to other phenomena—that is, they focus on relationships. A **relationship** is a bond or a connection between phenomena. For example, researchers repeatedly have found a *relationship* between cigarette smoking and lung cancer. Both qualitative and quantitative studies examine relationships but in different ways.

In quantitative studies, researchers examine the relationship between the independent and dependent variables. Researchers ask whether variation in the dependent variable (the outcome) is systematically related to variation in the independent variable. Relationships are usually expressed in quantitative terms, such as *more than*, *less than*, and so on. For example, let us consider a person's

weight as our dependent variable. What variables are related to (associated with) body weight? Some possibilities are height, caloric intake, and exercise. For each independent variable, we can make a prediction about its relationship to the outcome variable:

Height: Taller people will weigh more than shorter people.
Caloric intake: People with higher caloric intake will be heavier than those with lower caloric intake.
Exercise: The lower the amount of exercise, the greater will be the person's weight.

Each statement expresses a predicted relationship between weight (the dependent variable) and a measurable independent variable. Terms such as *more than* and *heavier than* imply that as we observe a change in one variable, we are likely to observe a change in weight. If Alex is taller than

> ## BOX 3.2 Example of Qualitative Data
>
> **Question:** Tell me about how you've been feeling lately—have you felt sad or depressed at all, or have you generally been in good spirits?
>
> **Data:** "Well, actually, I've been pretty depressed lately, to tell you the truth. I wake up each morning and I can't seem to think of anything to look forward to. I mope around the house all day, kind of in despair. I just can't seem to shake the blues, and I've begun to think I need to go see a shrink." (Participant 1)
>
> "I can't remember ever feeling better in my life. I just got promoted to a new job that makes me feel like I can really get ahead in my company. And I've just gotten engaged to a really great guy who is very special." (Participant 2)
>
> "I've had a few ups and downs the past week, but basically things are on a pretty even keel. I don't have too many complaints." (Participant 3)

Tom, we would predict (in the absence of any other information) that Alex is heavier than Tom.

Quantitative studies can address one or more of the following questions about relationships:

- Does a relationship between variables *exist*? (e.g., Is cigarette smoking related to lung cancer?)
- What is the *direction* of the relationship between variables? (e.g., Are people who smoke *more* likely or *less* likely to get lung cancer than those who do not?)
- How *strong* is the relationship between the variables? (e.g., How much higher is the risk that smokers will develop lung cancer?)
- What is the *nature* of the relationship between variables? (e.g., Does smoking *cause* lung cancer? Does some other factor *cause* both smoking and lung cancer?)

As the last question suggests, variables can be related to one another in different ways. One type of relationship is called a **cause-and-effect** (or **causal**) **relationship**. Within the positivist paradigm, natural phenomena are assumed not to be haphazard; they have antecedent causes that are presumably discoverable. In our example about a person's weight, we might speculate that there is a causal relationship between caloric intake and weight: Consuming more calories causes weight gain. As noted in Chapter 1, many quantitative studies are *cause-probing*—they seek to illuminate the causes of phenomena.

Example of a Study of Causal Relationships: Townsend-Gervis and colleagues (2014) studied whether interdisciplinary rounds and a structured communication protocol had an impact on patient satisfaction, patient readmission, and Foley catheter removal compliance.

As noted earlier, not all relationships between variables can be interpreted as causal ones. There is a relationship, for example, between a person's pulmonary artery and tympanic temperatures: People with high readings on one tend to have high readings on the other. We cannot say, however, that pulmonary artery temperature *caused* tympanic temperature nor that tympanic temperature *caused* pulmonary artery temperature. This type of relationship is called a **functional** (or an **associative**) **relationship** rather than as a causal relationship.

Example of a Study of Associative Relationships: Hsieh and colleagues (2014) examined the relationship between physical activity, body mass index, and cardiorespiratory fitness among Taiwanese school children.

Qualitative researchers are not concerned with quantifying relationships nor in testing causal relationships. Qualitative researchers seek patterns of association as a way to illuminate the underlying meaning and dimensionality of phenomena. Patterns of interconnected themes and processes are identified as a means of understanding the whole.

Example of a Qualitative Study of Patterns: Martsolf and colleagues (2012) investigated patterns of dating violence in 88 young adults aged 18 to 21 who had experienced violent dating relationships as teenagers. Analysis of the in-depth interviews revealed four patterns of adolescent dating violence based on the number of violent relationships in which each teen had been involved.

MAJOR CLASSES OF QUANTITATIVE AND QUALITATIVE RESEARCH

Researchers usually work within a paradigm that is consistent with their worldview and that gives rise to questions that excite their curiosity. The maturity of the focal concept also may lead to one or the other paradigm: When little is known about a topic, a qualitative approach is often more fruitful than a quantitative one. In this section, we briefly describe broad categories of quantitative and qualitative research.

Quantitative Research: Experimental and Nonexperimental Studies

A basic distinction in quantitative studies is between experimental and nonexperimental research. In **experimental research**, researchers actively introduce an intervention or treatment—most often, to address Therapy questions. In **nonexperimental research**, researchers are bystanders—they collect data without intervening (most often, to address Etiology, Prognosis, or Diagnosis questions). For example, if a researcher gave bran flakes to one group of people and prune juice to another to evaluate which method facilitated elimination more effectively, the study would be experimental because the researcher intervened in the normal course of things. If, on the other hand, a researcher compared elimination patterns of two groups whose regular eating patterns differed, the study would be nonexperimental because there is no intervention. In medical research, an experimental study usually is called a **clinical trial**, and a nonexperimental inquiry is called an **observational study**. As we discuss in Chapter 9, a *randomized controlled trial* or RCT is a particular type of clinical trial.

→ **TIP:** On the evidence hierarchy shown in Figure 2.1, the two rungs below systematic reviews (RCTs and quasi-experiments) involve interventions and are experimental. The four rungs below that are nonexperimental.

Experimental studies are explicitly cause-probing—they test whether an intervention *caused* changes in the dependent variable. Sometimes nonexperimental studies also explore causal relationships, but the resulting evidence is usually less conclusive. Experimental studies offer the possibility of greater control over confounding influences than nonexperimental studies, and so causal inferences are more plausible.

Example of Experimental Research: Williams and colleagues (2014) tested the effect of an intervention called Reasoning Exercises in Assisted Living on residents' problem solving and reasoning. Some study participants received the cognitive training intervention, and others did not.

In this example, the researchers intervened by giving some patients the special intervention but not giving it to others. In other words, the researcher *controlled* the independent variable, which in this case was receipt or nonreceipt of the cognitive training intervention.

Example of Nonexperimental Research: Huang and colleagues (2014) studied factors that predicted fatigue severity in Taiwanese women with breast cancer 1 year after surgery. They found, for example, that women who were married and who had poorer functional performance at diagnosis had higher levels of fatigue.

In this nonexperimental study to address a Prognosis question, the researchers did not intervene in any way. Their intent was to explore existing relationships rather than to test a potential solution to a problem.

Qualitative Research: Disciplinary Traditions

The majority of qualitative studies can best be described as **qualitative descriptive research**. Many qualitative studies, however, are rooted in research traditions that originated in anthropology, sociology, and psychology. Three such traditions that are prominent in qualitative nursing research are briefly described here. Chapter 21 provides a fuller discussion of these traditions and the methods associated with them.

Grounded theory research, with roots in sociology, seeks to describe and understand the key social psychological processes that occur in social settings. Most grounded theory studies focus on a developing social experience—the social and psychological processes that characterize an event or episode. A major component of grounded theory is the discovery of not only the basic social psychological problem but also a *core variable* that is central in explaining what is going on in that social scene. Grounded theory researchers strive to generate explanations of phenomena that are grounded in reality. Grounded theory was developed in the 1960s by two sociologists, Glaser and Strauss (1967).

Example of a Grounded Theory Study: Ramirez and Badger (2014) conducted a grounded theory study to explore the social psychological processes of men who suffer from depression. They uncovered six stages through which men navigated in their experiences with depression.

Phenomenology, rooted in a philosophical tradition developed by Husserl and Heidegger, is concerned with the lived experiences of humans. Phenomenology is an approach to thinking about what life experiences of people are like and what they mean. The phenomenologic researcher asks the questions: What is the *essence* of this phenomenon as experienced by these people? Or, What is the meaning of the phenomenon to those who experience it?

Example of a Phenomenologic Study: Ekwall and co-researchers (2014) conducted in-depth interviews to explore the lived experience of having recurring ovarian cancer.

Ethnography, the primary research tradition in anthropology, provides a framework for studying the patterns, lifeways, and experiences of a defined cultural group in a holistic manner. Ethnographers typically engage in extensive fieldwork, often participating in the life of the culture under study. Ethnographic research can be concerned with broadly defined cultures (e.g., Hmong refugee communities) but sometimes focuses on more narrowly defined cultures (e.g., the culture of an intensive care unit). Ethnographers strive to learn from members of a cultural group, to understand their worldview, and to describe their customs and norms.

Example of an Ethnographic Study: Broadbent and colleagues (2014) conducted ethnographic fieldwork to investigate the emergency department triage environment and its effect on triage practices for clients with a mental illness.

MAJOR STEPS IN A QUANTITATIVE STUDY

In quantitative studies, researchers move from the beginning of a study (posing a question) to the end point (obtaining an answer) in a reasonably linear sequence of steps that is broadly similar across studies. In some studies, the steps overlap; in others, some steps are unnecessary. Still, a general flow of activities is typical in a quantitative study (see Figure 3.1). This section describes that flow, and the next section describes how qualitative studies differ.

Phase 1: The Conceptual Phase

Early steps in a quantitative study typically have a strong conceptual element. These activities include reading, conceptualizing, theorizing, and reviewing ideas with colleagues or advisers. During this phase, researchers call on such skills as creativity, deductive reasoning, and a firm grounding in previous research on a topic of interest.

Step 1: Formulating and Delimiting the Problem

Quantitative researchers begin by identifying an interesting, significant research problem and formulating **research questions**. Good research requires starting with good questions. In developing research questions, nurse researchers must attend to substantive issues (What kind of new evidence is needed?), theoretical issues (Is there a conceptual context for understanding this problem?), clinical issues (How could evidence from this study be used in clinical practice?), methodologic issues (How can this question best be studied to yield high-quality evidence?), and ethical issues (Can this question be rigorously addressed in an ethical manner?)

> ⇨ **TIP:** A critical ingredient in developing good research questions is personal interest. Begin with topics that fascinate you or about which you have a passionate interest or curiosity.

Step 2: Reviewing the Related Literature

Quantitative research is conducted in a context of previous knowledge. Quantitative researchers typically strive to understand what is already known about a topic by undertaking a literature review. A thorough **literature review** provides a foundation on which to base new evidence and usually is conducted before data are collected. For clinical problems, it may also be necessary to learn the "status quo" of current procedures and to review existing practice guidelines.

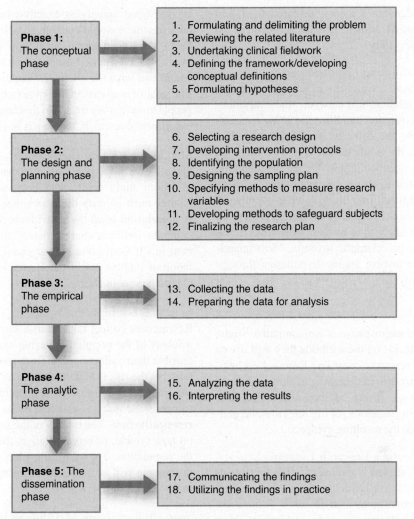

Phase 1:
The conceptual phase

1. Formulating and delimiting the problem
2. Reviewing the related literature
3. Undertaking clinical fieldwork
4. Defining the framework/developing conceptual definitions
5. Formulating hypotheses

Phase 2:
The design and planning phase

6. Selecting a research design
7. Developing intervention protocols
8. Identifying the population
9. Designing the sampling plan
10. Specifying methods to measure research variables
11. Developing methods to safeguard subjects
12. Finalizing the research plan

Phase 3:
The empirical phase

13. Collecting the data
14. Preparing the data for analysis

Phase 4:
The analytic phase

15. Analyzing the data
16. Interpreting the results

Phase 5: The dissemination phase

17. Communicating the findings
18. Utilizing the findings in practice

FIGURE 3.1 Flow of steps in a quantitative study.

Step 3: Undertaking Clinical Fieldwork

Unless the research problem originated in a clinical setting, researchers embarking on a clinical nursing study benefit from spending time in relevant clinical settings, discussing the problem with clinicians and administrators, and observing current practices. Clinical fieldwork can provide perspectives on recent clinical trends, current diagnostic procedures, and relevant health care delivery models; it can also help researchers better understand clients and the settings in which care is provided. Such fieldwork can also be valuable in gaining access to an appropriate site or in developing research

strategies. For example, in the course of clinical fieldwork, researchers might discover the need for research assistants who are bilingual.

Step 4: Defining the Framework and Developing Conceptual Definitions

Theory is the ultimate aim of science: It transcends the specifics of a particular time, place, and group and aims to identify regularities in the relationships among variables. When quantitative research is performed within the context of a theoretical framework, the findings often have broader significance and utility. Even when the research question is not embedded in a theory, researchers should have a conceptual rationale and a clear vision of the concepts under study.

Step 5: Formulating Hypotheses

Hypotheses state researcher's expectations (predictions) about relationships between study variables. The research question identifies the study concepts and asks how the concepts might be related; a hypothesis is the predicted answer. For example, the research question might be: Is preeclamptic toxemia related to stress during pregnancy? This might be translated into the following hypothesis: Women with high levels of stress during pregnancy will be more likely than women with lower stress to experience preeclamptic toxemia. Most quantitative studies involve testing hypotheses through statistical analysis.

Phase 2: The Design and Planning Phase

In the second major phase of a quantitative study, researchers decide on the methods they will use to address the research question. Researchers usually have flexibility in designing a study and make many decisions. These methodologic decisions have crucial implications for the integrity and generalizability of the resulting evidence.

Step 6: Selecting a Research Design

The **research design** is the overall plan for obtaining answers to the research questions. Many experimental and nonexperimental research designs are available. In designing the study, researchers select a specific design and identify strategies to minimize bias. Research designs indicate how often data will be collected, what types of comparisons will be made, and where the study will take place. The research design is the architectural backbone of the study.

Step 7: Developing Protocols for the Intervention

In experimental research, researchers create an intervention (the independent variable), and so they need to develop its specifications. For example, if we were interested in testing the effect of biofeedback on hypertension, the independent variable would be exposure to biofeedback compared with either an alternative treatment (e.g., relaxation) or no treatment. An **intervention protocol** for the study must

be developed, specifying exactly what the biofeedback treatment would entail (e.g., what type of feedback, who would administer it, how frequently and over how long a period the treatment would last, and so on) *and* what the alternative condition would be. The goal of well-articulated protocols is to have all people in each group treated in the same way. (In nonexperimental research, this step is not necessary.)

Step 8: Identifying the Population

Quantitative researchers need to clarify the group to whom study results can be generalized—that is, they must identify the population to be studied. A **population** is *all* the individuals or objects with common, defining characteristics (the "P" component in PICO questions). For example, the population of interest might be all patients undergoing chemotherapy in Dallas.

Step 9: Designing the Sampling Plan

Researchers collect data from a sample, which is a subset of the population. Using samples is more feasible than collecting data from an entire population, but the risk is that the sample might not reflect the population's traits. In a quantitative study, a sample's adequacy is assessed by its size and **representativeness**. The quality of the sample depends on how typical, or representative, the sample is of the population. The **sampling plan** specifies how the sample will be selected and recruited and how many subjects there will be.

Step 10: Specifying Methods to Measure Research Variables

Quantitative researchers must develop or borrow methods to measure their research variables. The primary methods of data collection are *self-reports* (e.g., interviews), *observations* (e.g., observing the sleep–wake state of infants), and *biophysiologic measurements*. Self-reported data from patients is the largest class of data collection methods and is often referred to as **patient-reported outcomes (PROs)**. The task of measuring research variables and developing a **data collection plan** is complex and challenging.

Step 11: Developing Methods to Safeguard Human/Animal Rights

Most nursing research involves humans, and so procedures need to be developed to ensure that the

The Abstract

The **abstract** is a brief description of the study placed at the beginning of the article. The abstract answers, in about 250 words, the following: What were the research questions? What methods did the researcher use to address the questions? What did the researcher find? What are the implications for practice? Readers review abstracts to assess whether the entire report is of interest. Some journals have moved from traditional abstracts—single paragraphs summarizing the study's main features—to longer, structured abstracts with specific headings. For example, in *Nursing Research,* the abstracts are organized under the following headings: Background, Objectives, Method, Results, and Conclusions.

The Introduction

The introduction communicates the research problem and its context. The introduction, which often is not be specifically labeled "Introduction," follows immediately after the abstract. This section typically describes (1) the central phenomena, concepts, or variables under study; (2) the population of interest; (3) the current state of evidence, based on a literature review; (4) the theoretical framework; (5) the study purpose, research questions, or hypotheses to be tested; and (6) the study's significance. Thus, the introduction sets the stage for a description of what the researcher did and what was learned. The introduction corresponds roughly to the conceptual phase (Phase 1) of a study.

The Method Section

The method section describes the methods used to answer the research questions. This section lays out methodologic decisions made in the design and planning phase (Phase 2) and may offer rationales for those decisions. In a quantitative study, the method section usually describes (1) the research design, (2) the sampling plan for selecting participants from the population of interest, (3) methods of data collection and specific instruments used, (4) study procedures (including ethical safeguards), and (5) analytic procedures and methods.

Qualitative researchers discuss many of the same issues but with different emphases. For example, a qualitative study often provides more information about the research setting and the study context and less information on sampling. Also, because formal instruments are not used to collect qualitative data, there is less discussion about data collection methods, but there may be more information on data collection procedures. Increasingly, reports of qualitative studies are including descriptions of the researchers' efforts to enhance the trustworthiness of the study.

The Results Section

The results section presents the **findings** (results) from the data analyses. The text summarizes key findings, and (in quantitative reports) tables provide greater detail. Virtually all results sections contain a description of the participants (e.g., their average age, percent male/female).

In quantitative studies, the results section provides information about **statistical tests**, which are used to test hypotheses and evaluate the believability of the findings. For example, if the percentage of smokers who smoke two packs or more daily is computed to be 40%, how *probable* is it that the percentage is accurate? If the researcher finds that the average number of cigarettes smoked weekly is lower for those in an intervention group than for those not getting the intervention, how *probable* is it that the intervention effect is *real*? Is the effect of the intervention on smoking likely to be replicated with a new sample of smokers—or does the result reflect a peculiarity of the sample? Statistical tests help to answer such questions. Researchers typically report:

- *The names of statistical tests used.* Different tests are appropriate for different situations but are based on common principles. You do not have to know the names of all statistical tests—there are dozens of them—to comprehend the findings.
- *The value of the calculated statistic.* Computers are used to calculate a numeric value for the particular statistical test used. The value allows researchers to draw conclusions about the meaning of the results. The *actual* numeric value of the statistic, however, is not inherently meaningful and need not concern you.

- *The significance.* A critical piece of information-tion is whether the value of the statistic was significant (not to be confused with important or clinically relevant). When researchers say that results are **statistically significant**, it means the findings are probably reliable and replicable with a new sample. Research reports indicate the **level of significance**, which is an index of how probable it is that the findings are reliable. For example, if a report says that a finding was significant at the .05 level, this means that only 5 times out of 100 $(5 \div 100 = .05)$ would the result be spurious. In other words, 95 times out of 100, similar results would be obtained with a new sample. Readers can have a high degree of confidence—but not total assurance—that the evidence is reliable.

> **Example from the Results Section of a Quantitative Study:** Edwards and colleagues (2014) evaluated whether the introduction of an aquarium into dementia units would result in improved resident behavior and increased staff satisfaction. Here is what they reported: "Residents' behavior improved along four domains: uncooperative, irrational, sleep, and inappropriate behaviors. The overall residents' behavior score was significantly improved after an aquarium was introduced, $F = 15.60$, $p < .001$" (p. 1309).

In this study, Edwards et al. found improvement over time (from an initial measurement to a second measurement after aquariums were introduced) in various realms of behavior among dementia unit residents. This finding is highly reliable: Less than one time in 1,000 $(p < .001)$ would changes as great as those observed have occurred as a fluke. To understand this finding, you do not have to understand what an *F* statistic is nor do you need to worry about the actual value of the statistic, 15.60.

Results sections of qualitative reports often have several subsections, the headings of which correspond to the themes, processes, or categories identified in the data. Excerpts from the raw data are presented to support and provide a rich description of the thematic analysis. The results section of qualitative studies may also present the researcher's emerging theory about the phenomenon under study.

The Discussion Section

In the discussion section, researchers draw conclusions about what the results mean and how the evidence can be used in practice. The discussion in both qualitative and quantitative reports may include the following elements: (1) an interpretation of the results and their clinical significance, (2) implications for clinical practice and for future and research, and (3) study limitations and ramifications for the integrity of the results. Researchers are in the best position to point out sample deficiencies, design problems, weaknesses in data collection, and so forth. A discussion section that presents these limitations demonstrates to readers that the author was aware of these limitations and probably took them into account in interpreting the findings.

The Style of Research Journal Articles

Research reports tell a story. However, the style in which many research journal articles are written—especially reports of quantitative studies—makes it difficult for many readers to figure out the story or become intrigued by it. To unaccustomed audiences, research reports may seem stuffy, pedantic, and bewildering. Four factors contribute to this impression:

1. *Compactness.* Journal space is limited, so authors compress a lot of information into a short space. Interesting, personalized aspects of the study are not reported. In qualitative studies, only a handful of supporting quotes can be included.
2. *Jargon.* The authors of research reports use terms that may seem esoteric.
3. *Objectivity.* Quantitative researchers tell their stories objectively, often in a way that makes them sound impersonal. For example, most quantitative reports are written in the passive voice (i.e., personal pronouns are avoided), which tends to make a report less inviting and lively than use of the active voice. Qualitative reports, by contrast, are more subjective and personal and written in a more conversational style.
4. *Statistical information.* Quantitative reports summarize the results of statistical analyses. Numbers and statistical symbols can intimidate readers who do not have statistical training.

BOX 3.3 Additional Questions for a Preliminary Review of a Study

1. What is the study all about? What are the main phenomena, concepts, or constructs under investigation?
2. If the study is quantitative, what are the independent and dependent variables?
3. Do the researchers examine relationships or patterns of association among variables or concepts? Does the report imply the possibility of a causal relationship?
4. Are key concepts clearly defined, both conceptually and operationally?
5. What type of study does it appear to be, in terms of types described in this chapter: Quantitative— experimental? nonexperimental? Qualitative—descriptive? grounded theory? phenomenologic? ethnographic?
6. Does the report provide any information to suggest how long the study took to complete?
7. Does the format of the report conform to the traditional IMRAD format? If not, in what ways does it differ?

In this textbook, we try to assist you in dealing with these issues and also strive to encourage you to tell *your* research stories in a manner that makes them accessible to practicing nurses.

Tips on Reading Research Reports

As you progress through this textbook, you will acquire skills for evaluating various aspects of research reports critically. Some preliminary hints on digesting research reports follow.

- Grow accustomed to the style of research articles by reading them frequently, even though you may not yet understand all the technical points.
- Read from an article that has been copied (or downloaded and printed) so that you can highlight portions and write marginal notes.
- Read articles slowly. Skim the article first to get major points and then read it more carefully a second time.
- On the second reading of a journal article, train yourself to be an *active* reader. Reading actively means that you constantly monitor yourself to assess your understanding of what you are reading. If you have problems, go back and reread difficult passages or make notes so that you can ask someone for clarification. In most cases, that "someone" will be your research instructor but also consider contacting researchers themselves via e-mail.
- Keep this textbook with you as a reference while you are reading articles, so that you can look up unfamiliar terms in the glossary or index.

- Try not to get scared away by statistical information. Try to grasp the gist of the story without letting numbers frustrate you.
- Until you become accustomed to research journal articles, you may want to "translate" them by expanding compact paragraphs into looser constructions, by translating jargon into familiar terms, by recasting the report into an active voice, and by summarizing findings with words rather than numbers. (Chapter 3 in the accompanying *Resource Manual* has an example of such a translation.)

GENERAL QUESTIONS IN REVIEWING A RESEARCH STUDY

Most chapters of this book contain guidelines to help you evaluate different aspects of a research report critically, focusing primarily on the researchers' methodologic decisions. Box 3.3 presents some further suggestions for performing a preliminary overview of a research report, drawing on concepts explained in this chapter. These guidelines supplement those presented in Box 1.1, Chapter 1.

RESEARCH EXAMPLES

In this section, we illustrate the progression of activities and discuss the time schedule of two studies (one quantitative and the other qualitative) conducted by the second author of this book.

Project Schedule for a Quantitative Study

Study: Postpartum depressive symptomatology: Results from a 2-stage U.S. national survey (Beck et al., 2011)

Study Purpose: Beck and colleagues undertook a study to estimate the prevalence of mothers with elevated postpartum depressive symptom levels in the United States and the factors that contributed to variability in symptom levels.

Study Methods: This study required a little less than 3 years to complete. Key activities and methodologic decisions included the following:

Phase 1. Conceptual Phase:
1 Month

Beck had been a member of the Listening to Mothers II National Advisory Council. The data for their national survey (the Childbirth Connection: Listening to Mothers II U.S. National Survey) had already been collected when Beck was approached to analyze the variables in the survey relating to postpartum depressive (PPD) symptoms. The first phase took only 1 month because data collection was already completed and Beck, a world expert on PPD, just needed to update a review of the literature.

Phase 2. Design and Planning Phase:
3 Months

The design phase entailed identifying which of the hundreds of variables on the national survey the researchers would focus on in their analysis. Also, their research questions were formalized during this phase. Approval from a human subjects committee also was obtained during this phase.

Phase 3. Empirical Phase:
0 Month

In this study, the data from nearly 1,000 postpartum women had already been collected.

Phase 4. Analytic Phase:
12 Months

Statistical analyses were performed to (1) estimate the percentage of new mothers experiencing elevated postpartum depressive symptom levels and (2) to identify which demographic, antepartum, intrapartum, and postpartum variables were significantly related to these elevated symptom levels.

Phase 5. Dissemination Phase:
18 Months

The researchers prepared and submitted their report to the *Journal of Midwifery & Women's Health* for possible publication. It was accepted within 5 months and was "in press" (awaiting publication) another 4 months before being published. The article received the *Journal of Midwifery & Women's Health* 2012 Best Research Article Award.

Project Schedule for a Qualitative Study

Study: Subsequent childbirth after a previous traumatic birth (Beck & Watson, 2010)

Study Purpose: The purpose of this study was to describe the meaning of women's experiences of a subsequent childbirth after a previous traumatic birth.

Study Methods: The total time required to complete this study was a little more than 4 years. Beck and Watson's key activities included the following:

Phase 1. Conceptual Phase:
2 Months

Beck had previously studied traumatic childbirth, and one of the mothers in the initial study inspired an interest in what happened to these mothers in a subsequent pregnancy and childbirth. During this phase, Beck reviewed the literature on subsequent childbirth following birth trauma.

Phase 2. Design and Planning Phase:
5 Months

Beck and Watson chose a descriptive phenomenologic design for this study. Once their proposal was finalized, it was submitted to the university's committee for reviewing ethical research conduct for approval.

Phase 3. Empirical/Analytic Phases:
26 Months

A recruitment notice was placed on the website of Trauma and Birth Stress, a charitable Trust located in New Zealand. Thirty-five women sent their stories of their subsequent childbirth after a previous traumatic birth to Beck via the Internet. Analysis of the mothers' stories took an additional 5 months. Four themes emerged from the data analysis: (1) riding the turbulent wave of panic during pregnancy, (2) strategizing: attempts to reclaim their body and complete the journey to motherhood, (3) bringing reverence to the birthing process and empowering women, and (4) still elusive: the longed-for healing birth experience.

Phase 4: Dissemination Phase: 17 Months

It took 6 months to prepare the manuscript for this study. It was submitted to the journal *Nursing Research* on August 17, 2009. On October 13, 2009, Beck and Watson received a letter from the journal's editor indicating that the reviewers recommended they revise and resubmit the paper. On December 18, 2009, Beck and Watson submitted a revised manuscript that incorporated the reviewers' recommendations. On January 27, 2010, Beck and Watson were notified that their manuscript had been accepted for publication and the article was published in the July/August 2010 issue. Beck has also presented the findings at national conferences.

SUMMARY POINTS

- The people who provide information to the **researchers** (investigators) in a study are called **subjects** or **study participants** (in quantitative research) or study participants or **informants** in qualitative research; collectively, the participants comprise the **sample**.
- The *site* is the overall location for the research; researchers sometimes engage in **multisite studies**. *Settings* are the more specific places where data collection occurs. Settings can range from totally naturalistic environments to formal laboratories.
- Researchers investigate **concepts** (or **constructs**) and **phenomena**, which are abstractions or mental representations inferred from behavior or characteristics.
- Concepts are the building blocks of **theories**, which are systematic explanations of some aspect of the real world.
- In quantitative studies, concepts are called *variables*. A **variable** is a characteristic or quality that takes on different values (i.e., varies from one person to another). Groups that are varied with respect to an attribute are **heterogeneous**; groups with limited variability are **homogeneous**.
- **Continuous variables** can take on an infinite range of values along a continuum (e.g., weight). **Discrete variables** have a finite number of values between two points (e.g., number of children).

- **Categorical variables** have distinct categories that do not represent a quantity (e.g., blood type).
- The **dependent** (or **outcome**) **variable** is the behavior or characteristic the researcher is interested in explaining, predicting, or affecting (the "O" in the PICO scheme). The **independent variable** is the presumed cause of, antecedent to, or influence on the dependent variable. The independent variable corresponds to the "I" and the "C" components in the PICO scheme.
- A **conceptual definition** describes the abstract or theoretical meaning of a concept being studied. An **operational definition** specifies how the variable will be measured.
- **Data**—information collected during a study—may take the form of narrative information (**qualitative data**) or numeric values (**quantitative data**).
- A **relationship** is a bond or connection between two variables. Quantitative researchers examine the relationship between the independent variable and dependent variable.
- When the independent variable causes the dependent variable, the relationship is a **cause-and-effect** (or **causal**) **relationship**. In an **associative** (*functional*) **relationship**, variables are related in a noncausal way.
- A key distinction in quantitative studies is between **experimental research**, in which researchers intervene, and **nonexperimental** (or **observational) research**, in which researchers make observations of existing phenomena without intervening.
- Qualitative research sometimes is rooted in research traditions that originate in other disciplines. Three such traditions are grounded theory, phenomenology, and ethnography.
- **Grounded theory** seeks to describe and understand key social psychological processes that occur in social settings.
- **Phenomenology** focuses on the lived experiences of humans and is an approach to learning what the life experiences of people are like and what they mean.
- **Ethnography** provides a framework for studying the meanings, patterns, and lifeways of a culture in a holistic fashion.

- Quantitative researchers usually progress in a fairly linear fashion from asking research questions to answering them. The main phases in a quantitative study are the conceptual, planning, empirical, analytic, and dissemination phases.
- The *conceptual phase* involves (1) defining the problem to be studied, (2) doing a **literature review**, (3) engaging in **clinical fieldwork** for clinical studies, (4) developing a framework and conceptual definitions, and (5) formulating **hypotheses** to be tested.
- The *planning phase* entails (6) selecting a **research design**, (7) developing **intervention protocols** if the study is experimental, (8) specifying the **population**, (9) developing a **sampling plan**, (10) specifying methods to measure research variables, (11) developing strategies to safeguard the rights of participants, and (12) finalizing the research plan (e.g., *pretesting* instruments).
- The *empirical phase* involves (13) collecting data and (14) preparing data for analysis.
- The *analytic phase* involves (15) analyzing data through **statistical analysis** and (16) interpreting the results.
- The *dissemination phase* entails (17) communicating the findings in a **research report** and (18) promoting the use of the study evidence in nursing practice.
- The flow of activities in a qualitative study is more flexible and less linear. Qualitative studies typically involve an **emergent design** that evolves during data collection.
- Qualitative researchers begin with a broad question regarding a phenomenon, often focusing on a little-studied aspect. In the early phase of a qualitative study, researchers select a site and seek to **gain entrée** into it, which typically involves enlisting the cooperation of **gatekeepers**.
- Once in the field, researchers select informants, collect data, and then analyze and interpret them in an iterative fashion. Knowledge gained during data collection helps in to shape the design of the study.
- Early analysis in qualitative research leads to refinements in sampling and data collection, until **saturation** (redundancy of information) is achieved.

- Both qualitative and quantitative researchers disseminate their findings, often in **journal articles** that concisely communicate what the researchers did and what they found.
- Journal articles typically consist of an **abstract** (a brief synopsis) and four major sections in an **IMRAD format**: an **I**ntroduction (explanation of the study problem and its context), **M**ethod section (the strategies used to address the problem), **R**esults section (study findings), **and D**iscussion (interpretation of the findings).
- Research reports can be difficult to read because they are dense and contain a lot of jargon. Quantitative research reports may be intimidating at first because, compared to qualitative reports, they are more impersonal and include statistical information.
- **Statistical tests** are procedures for testing research hypotheses and evaluating the believability of the findings. Findings that are **statistically significant** are ones that have a high probability of being "real."

STUDY ACTIVITIES

Chapter 3 of the *Resource Manual for Nursing Research: Generating and Assessing Evidence for Nursing Practice, 10th edition*, offers study suggestions for reinforcing concepts presented in this chapter. In addition, the following questions can be addressed in classroom or online discussions:

1. Suggest ways of conceptually and operationally defining the following concepts: nursing competency, aggressive behavior, pain, and body image.
2. Name three continuous, three discrete, and three categorical variables; identify which, if any, are dichotomous.
3. In the following research problems, identify the independent and dependent variables:
   a. Does screening for intimate partner violence among pregnant women improve birth and delivery outcomes?
   b. Do elderly patients have lower pain thresholds than younger patients?

c. Are the sleeping patterns of infants affected by different forms of stimulation?

d. Can home visits by nurses to released psychiatric patients reduce readmission rates?

oooooooooooooooooooooooooooooooo

STUDIES CITED IN CHAPTER 3

Beck, C. T. (2009). The arm: There is no escaping the reality for mothers of children with obstetric brachial plexus injuries. *Nursing Research, 58,* 237–245.

Beck, C. T., Gable, R. K., Sakala, C., & Declercq, E. R. (2011). Postpartum depressive symptomatology: Results from a two-stage U.S. national survey. *Journal of Midwifery & Women's Health, 56,* 427–435.

Beck, C. T., & Watson, S. (2010). Subsequent childbirth after a previous traumatic birth. *Nursing Research, 59,* 241–249.

Broadbent, M., Moxham, L., & Dwyer, T. (2014). Implications of the emergency department triage environment on triage practice for clients with a mental illness at triage in an Australian context. *Australasian Emergency Nursing Journal, 17,* 23–29.

Cottney, A., & Innes, J. (2015). Medication-administration errors in an urban mental health hospital: A direct observation study. *International Journal of Mental Health Nursing, 24,* 65–74.

Edwards, N. E., Beck, A., & Lim, E. (2014). Influence of aquariums on resident behavior and staff satisfaction in dementia units. *Western Journal of Nursing Research, 36,* 1309–1322.

Ekwall, E., Ternestedt, B., Sorbe, B., & Sunvisson, H. (2014). Lived experiences of women with recurring ovarian cancer. *European Journal of Oncology Nursing, 18,* 104–109.

Fogg, C., Mawn, B., & Porell, F. (2011). Development of the Fogg Intent-to-Screen for HIV (ITS HIV) questionnaire. *Research in Nursing & Health, 34,* 73–84.

*Gitsels-van der Wal, J. T., Martin, L., Manniën, J., Verhoeven, P., Hutton, E., & Reinders, H. (2015). A qualitative study on how Muslim women of Moroccan descent approach antenatal anomaly screening. *Midwifery, 31,* e43–e49.

Glaser, B. G., & Strauss, A. L. (1967). *The discovery of grounded theory: Strategies for qualitative research.* Chicago: Aldine.

*Hsieh, P. L., Chen, M., Huang, C., Chen, W., Li, C., & Chang, L. (2014). Physical activity, body mass index, and cardiorespiratory fitness among school children in Taiwan. *International Journal of Environmental Research and Public Health, 11,* 7275–7285.

Huang, H. P., Chen, M., Liang, J., & Miaskowski, C. (2014). Changes in and predictors of severity of fatigue in women with breast cancer: A longitudinal study. *International Journal of Nursing Studies, 51,* 582–592.

Kerlinger, F. N., & Lee, H. B. (2000). *Foundations of behavioral research* (4th ed.). Orlando, FL: Harcourt College.

Martsolf, D. S., Draucker, C., Stephenson, P., Cook, C., & Heckman, T. (2012). Patterns of dating violence across adolescence. *Qualitative Health Research, 22,* 1271–1283.

Morse, J. M., Solberg, S. M., Neander, W. L., Bottorff, J. L., & Johnson, J. L. (1990). Concepts of caring and caring as a concept. *Advances in Nursing Science, 13,* 1–14.

Polit, D. F., London, A., & Martinez, J. (2001). *The health of poor urban women.* New York: Manpower Demonstration Research Corporation. Retrieved from htpp://www.mdrc.org

Ramirez, J., & Badger, T. (2014). Men navigating inward and outward through depression. *Archives of Psychiatric Nursing, 28,* 21–28.

Townsend-Gervis, M., Cornell, P., & Vardaman, J. (2014). Interdisciplinary rounds and structured communication reduce re-admissions and improve some patient outcomes. *Western Journal of Nursing Research, 36,* 917–928.

*Williams, K., Herman, R., & Bontempo, D. (2014). Reasoning exercises in assisted living: A cluster randomized trial to improve reasoning and everyday problem solving. *Clinical Interventions in Aging, 9,* 981–996.

***A link to this open-access journal article is provided in the Toolkit for this chapter in the accompanying* Resource Manual.** ⊗

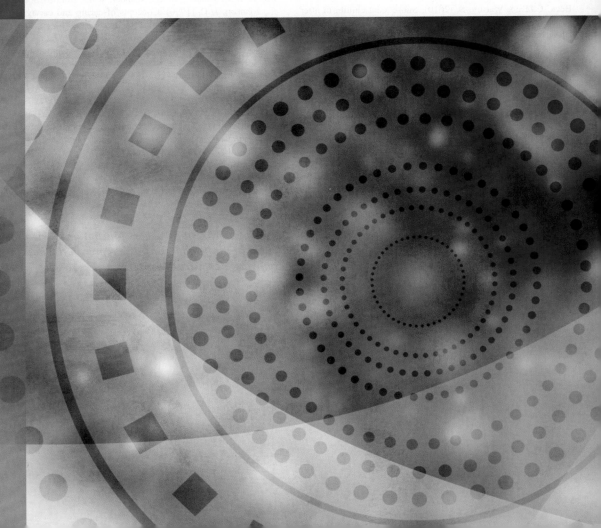

PART 2

CONCEPTUALIZING AND PLANNING A STUDY TO GENERATE EVIDENCE FOR NURSING

4 | Research Problems, Research Questions, and Hypotheses

OVERVIEW OF RESEARCH PROBLEMS

Studies begin, much like an EBP effort, with a problem that need to be solved or a question that needs to be answered. This chapter discusses the development of research problems. We begin by clarifying some relevant terms.

Basic Terminology

At a general level, a researcher selects a **topic** or a phenomenon on which to focus. Examples of research topics are claustrophobia during MRI tests, pain management for sickle cell disease, and nutrition during pregnancy. Within broad topic areas are many potential research problems. In this section, we illustrate various terms using the topic *side effects of chemotherapy*.

A **research problem** is an enigmatic or troubling condition. Researchers identify a research problem within a topic of interest. The purpose of research is to "solve" the problem—or to contribute to its solution—by generating relevant evidence. Researchers articulate the problem in a **problem statement** and explain the need for a study by developing an *argument*. Table 4.1 presents a simplified problem statement related to the topic of side effects of chemotherapy.

Research questions are the specific queries researchers want to answer in addressing the problem. Research questions guide the types of data to collect in a study. Researchers who make predictions about answers to research questions pose **hypotheses** that can be tested.

Many reports include a **statement of purpose** (or purpose statement), which summarizes the study goals. Researchers might also identify several **research aims** or **objectives**—the specific accomplishments they hope to achieve by conducting the study. The objectives include answering research questions or testing research hypotheses but may also encompass broader aims (e.g., developing an effective intervention).

These terms are not always consistently defined in research methods textbooks, and differences among them are often subtle. Table 4.1 illustrates the terms as we define them.

Research Problems and Paradigms

Some research problems are better suited to qualitative versus quantitative methods. Quantitative studies usually focus on concepts that are fairly well developed, about which there is existing evidence, and for which reliable methods of measurement have been (or can be) developed. For example, a quantitative study might be undertaken to explore whether older people with chronic illness who continue working are less (or more) depressed than those who retire. There are relatively good measures of depression that would yield quantitative information about the level of

TABLE 4.1 • Example of Terms Relating to Research Problems

TERM	EXAMPLE
Topic/focus	Side effects of chemotherapy
Research problem (Problem statement)	Nausea and vomiting are common side effects among patients on chemotherapy, and interventions to date have been only moderately successful in reducing these effects. New interventions that can reduce or prevent these side effects need to be identified.
Statement of purpose	The purpose of the study is to test an intervention to reduce chemotherapy-induced side effects—specifically, to compare the effectiveness of patient-controlled and nurse-administered antiemetic therapy for controlling nausea and vomiting in patients on chemotherapy.
Research question	What is the relative effectiveness of patient-controlled antiemetic therapy versus nurse-controlled antiemetic therapy with regard to (a) medication consumption and (b) control of nausea and vomiting in patients on chemotherapy?
Hypotheses	Subjects receiving antiemetic therapy by a patient-controlled pump will (1) be less nauseous, (2) vomit less, and (3) consume less medication than subjects receiving the therapy by nurse administration.
Aims/objectives	This study has as its aim the following objectives: (1) to develop and implement two alternative procedures for administering antiemetic therapy for patients receiving moderate emetogenic chemotherapy (patient controlled versus nurse controlled), (2) to test three hypotheses concerning the relative effectiveness of the alternative procedures on medication consumption and control of side effects, and (3) to use the findings to develop recommendations for possible changes to clinical procedures.

depression in a sample of employed and retired chronically ill seniors.

Qualitative studies are often undertaken because a researcher wants to develop a rich and context-bound understanding of a poorly understood phenomenon. Researchers sometimes initiate qualitative studies to heighten awareness and create a dialogue about a phenomenon. Qualitative methods would not be well suited to comparing levels of depression among employed and retired seniors, but they would be ideal for exploring, for example, the meaning or experience of depression among chronically ill retirees. Thus, the nature of the research question is linked to paradigms and to research traditions within paradigms.

Sources of Research Problems

Where do ideas for research problems come from? At a basic level, research topics originate with researchers' interests. Because research is a time-consuming enterprise, curiosity about and interest in a topic are essential. Research reports rarely indicate the source of researchers' inspiration, but a variety of explicit sources can fuel their interest, including the following:

* *Clinical experience.* Nurses' everyday clinical experience is a rich source of ideas for research topics. Immediate problems that need a solution—analogous to problem-focused triggers discussed in Chapter 2—may generate enthusiasm, and they have high potential for clinical relevance.

- *Quality improvement efforts*. Important clinical questions sometimes emerge in the context of findings from quality improvement studies. Personal involvement on a quality improvement team can sometimes lead to ideas for a study.
- *Nursing literature*. Ideas for studies often come from reading the nursing literature. Research articles may suggest problems indirectly by stimulating the reader's curiosity and directly by noting needed research. Familiarity with existing research or with emerging clinical issues is an important route to developing a research topic.
- *Social issues*. Topics are sometimes suggested by global social or political issues of relevance to the health care community. For example, the feminist movement raised questions about such topics as gender equity in health care. Public awareness about health disparities has led to research on health care access and culturally sensitive interventions.
- *Theories*. Theories from nursing and other disciplines sometimes suggest a research problem. Researchers ask, "If this theory is correct, what would I predict about people's behaviors, states, or feelings?" The predictions can then be tested through research.
- *Ideas from external sources*. External sources and direct suggestions can sometimes provide the impetus for a research idea. For example, ideas for studies may emerge by reviewing a funding agency's research priorities or from brainstorming with other nurses.

Additionally, researchers who have developed a *program of research* on a topic area may get inspiration for "next steps" from their own findings or from a discussion of those findings with others.

Example of a Problem Source in a Program of Research: Beck, one of this book's authors, has developed a strong research program on postpartum depression (PPD). Beck was approached by Dr. Carol Lammi-Keefe, a professor in nutritional sciences, and her PhD student, Michelle Judge, who had been researching the effect of DHA (docosahexaenoic acid, a fat found in cold-water fish) on fetal brain development. The literature suggested that DHA might play a role in reducing the severity of PPD and so these researchers collaborated in a project to test the effectiveness of dietary supplements of DHA on the incidence and severity of PPD. The results of their study indicated that women in the DHA experimental group had fewer symptoms of postpartum depression compared to women who did not receive the DHA intervention (Judge et al., 2014).

TIP: Personal experiences in clinical settings are a provocative source of research ideas and questions. Here are some hints:

- Watch for a recurring problem and see if you can discern a pattern in situations that lead to the problem.

Example: Why do many patients complain of being tired after being transferred from a coronary care unit to a progressive care unit?

- Think about aspects of your work that are frustrating or do not result in the intended outcome—then try to identify factors contributing to the problem that could be changed.

Example: Why is suppertime so frustrating in a nursing home?

- Critically examine your own clinical decisions. Are they based on tradition, or are they based on systematic evidence that supports their efficacy?

Example: What would happen if you used the return of flatus to assess the return of GI motility after abdominal surgery rather than listening to bowel sounds?

DEVELOPING AND REFINING RESEARCH PROBLEMS

Unless a research problem is based on an explicit suggestion, actual procedures for developing one are difficult to describe. The process is rarely a smooth and orderly one; there are likely to be false starts, inspirations, and setbacks. The few suggestions offered here are not intended to imply that there are techniques for making this first step easy but rather to encourage you to persevere in the absence of instant success.

Selecting a Topic

Developing a research problem is a creative process. In the early stages of initiating research ideas, try not to be too self-critical. It is better to relax and jot down topics of interest as they come to mind. It does not matter if the ideas are abstract or concrete, broad or specific, technical or colloquial—the important point is to put ideas on paper.

After this first step, ideas can be sorted in terms of interest, knowledge about the topics, and the perceived feasibility of turning the topics into a study. When the most fruitful idea has been selected, the list should not be discarded; it may be necessary to return to it.

TIP: The process of selecting and refining a research problem usually takes longer than you might think. The process involves starting with some preliminary ideas, having discussions with colleagues and advisers, perusing the research literature, looking at what is happening in clinical settings, and a lot of reflection.

Narrowing the Topic

Once you have identified a topic of interest, you can begin to ask some broad questions that can lead you to a researchable problem. Examples of question stems that might help to focus an inquiry include the following:

- What is going on with . . . ?
- What is the process by which . . . ?
- What is the meaning of . . . ?
- What is the extent of . . . ?
- What influences or causes . . . ?
- What differences exist between . . . ?
- What are the consequences of . . . ?
- What factors contribute to . . . ?

Again, early criticism of ideas can be counterproductive. Try not to jump to the conclusion that an idea sounds trivial or uninspired without giving it more careful consideration or exploring it with others. Another potential danger is that new researchers sometimes develop problems that are too broad in scope or too complex for their level

of methodologic expertise. The transformation of a general topic into a workable problem typically is accomplished in uneven steps. Each step should result in progress toward the goals of narrowing the scope of the problem and sharpening the concepts.

As researchers move from general topics to more specific ideas, several possible research problems may emerge. Consider the following example. Suppose you were working on a medical unit and were puzzled by that fact that some patients always complained about having to wait for pain medication when certain nurses were assigned to them. The general problem is discrepancy in patient complaints regarding pain medications. You might ask: What accounts for the discrepancy? How can I improve the situation? These are not research questions, but they may lead you to ask such questions as the following: How do the two groups of nurses differ? or What characteristics do the complaining patients share? At this point, you may observe that the ethnic background of the patients and nurses could be relevant. This may lead you to search the literature for studies about ethnicity in relation to nursing care, or it may provoke you to discuss the observations with others. These efforts may result in several research questions, such as the following:

- What is the nature of patient complaints among patients of different ethnic backgrounds?
- Is the ethnic background of nurses related to the frequency with which they dispense pain medication?
- Does the number of patient complaints increase when patients are of dissimilar ethnic backgrounds as opposed to when they are of the same ethnic background as nurses?
- Do nurses' dispensing behaviors change as a function of the similarity between their own ethnic background and that of patients?

These questions stem from the same problem, yet each would be studied differently. Some suggest a qualitative approach and others suggest a quantitative one. A quantitative researcher might be curious about ethnic differences in nurses' dispensing behaviors. Both ethnicity and nurses' dispensing behaviors are variables that can be measured reliably.

A qualitative researcher would likely be more interested in understanding the *essence* of patients' complaints, their *experience* of frustration, or the *process* by which the problem got resolved. These are aspects of the research problem that would be difficult to quantify.

Researchers choose a problem to study based on several factors, including its inherent interest and its compatibility with a paradigm of preference. In addition, tentative problems vary in their feasibility and worth. A critical evaluation of ideas is appropriate at this point.

Evaluating Research Problems

Although there are no rules for selecting a research problem, four important considerations to keep in mind are the problem's significance, researchability, feasibility, and interest to you.

Significance of the Problem

A crucial factor in selecting a problem is its significance to nursing. Evidence from the study should have potential to contribute meaningfully to nursing practice: The new study should be the right "next step." The right next step could be an original study, but it could also be a replication to answer previously asked questions with greater rigor or with a different population.

In evaluating the significance of an idea, you can ask the following kinds of questions: Is the problem important to nursing and its clients? Will patient care benefit from the evidence? Will the findings challenge (or lend support to) existing practices? If the answer to all these questions is "no," then the problem should be abandoned.

Researchability of the Problem

Not all problems are amenable to research inquiry. Questions of a moral or ethical nature, although provocative, cannot be researched. For example, should assisted suicide be legalized? There are no *right* or *wrong* answers to this question, only points of view. To be sure, it is possible to ask related questions that could be researched, such as the following: What are terminally ill patients' attitudes toward assisted suicide? What moral dilemmas are perceived by nurses who might be involved in assisted suicide? Do patients living with high levels of pain hold more favorable attitudes toward assisted suicide than those with less pain? The findings from studies addressing such questions would have no bearing on whether assisted suicide should be legalized, but they could be useful in developing a better understanding of the issues.

Feasibility of the Problem

A third consideration concerns feasibility, which encompasses several issues. Not all of the following factors are universally relevant, but they should be kept in mind in making a decision.

Time. Most studies have deadlines or goals for completion, so the problem must be one that can be studied in the allotted time. The scope of the problem should be scaled to ensure sufficient time for the steps reviewed in Chapter 3. It is prudent to be conservative in estimating time for various tasks because research activities often require more time than anticipated.

Researcher Experience. The problem should relate to a topic about which you have some prior knowledge or experience. The issue of research expertise also should be considered. Beginning researchers should avoid research problems that might require the development of sophisticated measuring instruments or that demand complex analyses.

Availability of Study Participants. In any study involving humans, researchers need to consider whether people with the desired characteristics will be available and willing to cooperate. Securing people's cooperation is often challenging. Some people may not have the time or interest, and others may not feel well enough to participate. Researchers may need to put considerable effort into recruiting participants or may need to offer a monetary incentive.

Cooperation of Others. As noted in Chapter 3, it may be necessary to gain entrée into an appropriate community or setting and to develop the trust of gatekeepers. In institutional settings (e.g., hospitals), access to clients, personnel, or records require authorization.

Ethical Considerations. A research problem may be unfeasible if the study would pose unfair or unethical demands on participants. An overview of ethical issues in research is presented in Chapter 7 and should be reviewed when considering the study's feasibility.

Facilities and Equipment. All studies have resource requirements, although needs are sometimes modest. It is prudent to consider what facilities and equipment will be needed and whether they will be available before embarking on a study.

Money. Monetary needs for studies vary widely, ranging from $100 or less for small student projects to hundreds of thousands of dollars for large-scale research. If you are on a limited budget, you should think carefully about projected expenses before selecting a problem. Major categories of research-related expenditures include the following:

- Personnel costs—payments to individuals to help with the study (e.g., for conducting interviews, coding, data entry, transcribing)
- Participant costs—payments to participants as an incentive for their cooperation or to offset their expenses (e.g., parking or baby-sitting costs)
- Supplies—paper, envelopes, computer disks, postage, and so forth
- Printing and duplication—costs for reproducing forms, questionnaires, and so on
- Equipment—laboratory apparatus, computers and software, audio or video recorders, calculators, and the like
- Laboratory fees for the analysis of biophysiologic data
- Transportation costs (e.g., travel to participants' homes)

Researcher Interest

Even if a tentative problem is researchable, significant, and feasible, there is one more criterion: your own interest in the problem. Genuine curiosity about a research problem is an important prerequisite to a successful study. A lot of time and energy are expended in a study; there is little sense devoting these resources to a project about which you are not enthusiastic.

➲ TIP: New researchers often seek suggestions about a topic area, and such assistance may be helpful in getting started. Nevertheless, it is unwise to be talked into a topic toward which you are not personally inclined. If you do not find a problem interesting in the beginning phase of a study, then you are likely to regret your choice later.

COMMUNICATING RESEARCH PROBLEMS AND QUESTIONS

Every study needs a problem statement—an articulation of what is problematic and is the impetus for the research. Most research reports also present either a statement of purpose, research questions, or hypotheses, and often combinations of these elements are included.

Many people do not really understand problem statements and may have trouble identifying them in a research article—not to mention developing one. A problem statement often begins with the very first sentence after the abstract. Specific research questions, purposes, or hypotheses appear later in the introduction. Typically, however, researchers *begin* their inquiry with a research question and *then* develop an argument in their problem statement to present the rationale for the new research. This section describes the wording of statements of purpose and research questions, followed by a discussion of problem statements.

Statements of Purpose

Many researchers articulate their research goals as a statement of purpose, worded declaratively. It is usually easy to identify a purpose statement because the word *purpose* is explicitly stated: "The purpose of this study was . . . "—although sometimes the words *aim*, *goal*, *intent*, or *objective* are used instead, as in "The aim of this study was . . . "

In a quantitative study, a statement of purpose identifies the key study variables and their possible interrelationships as well as the population of interest (i.e., all the PICO elements).

Example of a Statement of Purpose from a Quantitative Study: "Purpose/Objectives: To examine the association of the serotonin transport gene and postdischarge nausea and vomiting (PNDV) in women following breast cancer surgery" (Wesmiller et al., 2014, p. 195).

This purpose statement identifies the population—women who had breast cancer surgery. The aim is to examine the relationship between the women's serotonin transport gene, which is the independent variable, and postdischarge nausea and vomiting, which are the dependent variables.

In qualitative studies, the statement of purpose indicates the key concept or phenomenon and the group, community, or setting under study.

Example of a Statement of Purpose from a Qualitative Study: "The aim of this qualitative study was to describe the lived experience of chronic venous insufficiency (CVI) sufferers and to explore how this chronic disease affected their health-related quality of life" (Wellborn & Moceri, 2014, p. 122).

This statement indicates that the central phenomenon in this study was the experience of living with chronic venous insufficiency, with emphasis on the disease's impact on quality of life, and that the group under study was patients suffering from CVI.

The statement of purpose communicates more than just the nature of the problem. Researchers' selection of verbs in a purpose statement suggests how they sought to solve the problem or the state of knowledge on the topic. A study whose purpose is to *explore* or *describe* a phenomenon is likely an investigation of a little-researched topic, sometimes involving a qualitative approach. A purpose statement for a qualitative study may also use verbs such as *understand*, *discover*, *develop*, or *generate*. Statements of purpose in qualitative studies may "encode" the tradition of inquiry, not only through the researcher's choice of verbs but also through the use of "buzzwords" associated with those traditions, as follows:

- *Grounded theory*: processes, social structures, social interactions

- *Phenomenologic studies*: experience, lived experience, meaning, essence
- *Ethnographic studies*: culture, roles, lifeways, cultural behavior

Quantitative researchers also suggest the nature of the inquiry through their selection of verbs. A statement indicating that the study's purpose is to *test* or *evaluate* something (e.g., an intervention) suggests an experimental design. A study whose purpose is to *examine* or *explore* the relationship between two variables likely involves a nonexperimental design. In some cases, the verb is ambiguous: A purpose statement indicating that the researcher's intent is to *compare* could be referring to a comparison of alternative treatments (using an experimental approach) or a comparison of preexisting groups (using a nonexperimental approach). In any event, verbs such as *test*, *evaluate*, and *compare* suggest an existing knowledge base and quantifiable variables.

The verbs in a purpose statement should connote objectivity. A statement of purpose indicating that the study goal was to *prove*, *demonstrate*, or *show* something suggests a bias. The word *determine* should usually be avoided as well because research methods almost never provide definitive answers to research questions.

➔ **TIP:** In wording your statement of purpose, it may be useful to look at published research articles for models. Unfortunately, some reports fail to state unambiguously the study purpose, leaving readers to infer the purpose from such sources as the title of the report. In other reports, the purpose is clearly stated but may be difficult to find. Researchers most often state their purpose toward the end of the report's introduction.

Research Questions

Research questions are sometimes direct rewordings of purpose statements, phrased interrogatively rather than declaratively, as in the following example:

- *Purpose*: The purpose of this study was to assess the relationship between the functional dependence level of renal transplant recipients and their rate of recovery.

• *Question*: What is the relationship between the functional dependence level (I) of renal transplant recipients (P) and their rate of recovery (O)?

Questions have the advantage of simplicity and directness—they invite an answer and help to focus attention on the kinds of data needed to provide that answer. Some research reports thus omit a statement of purpose and state only research questions. Other researchers use a set of research questions to clarify or lend greater specificity to a global purpose statement.

Research Questions in Quantitative Studies

In Chapter 2, we discussed the framing of clinical foreground questions to guide an EBP inquiry. Many of the EBP question templates in Table 2.1 could yield questions to guide a study as well, but *researchers* tend to conceptualize their questions in terms of their *variables*. Take, for example, the first question in Table 2.1, which states, "In (population), what is the effect of (intervention) on (outcome)?" A researcher would likely think of the question in these terms: "In (population), what is the effect of (independent variable) on (dependent variable)?" Thinking in terms of variables is advantageous because researchers must decide how to operationalize their variables. Thus, in quantitative studies, research questions identify the population (P) under study, the key study variables (I, C, and O components), and possible relationships among the variables. The variables are all quantifiable concepts.

Most research questions concern relationships, and so many quantitative research questions could be articulated using a general question template: "In (population), what is the relationship between (independent variable or IV) and (dependent variable or DV)?" Examples of variations include the following:

• *Treatment, intervention*: In (population), what is the effect of (IV: intervention versus an alternative) on (DV)?
• *Prognosis*: In (population), does (IV: disease or illness versus its absence) affect or increase the risk of (DV: adverse consequences)?
• *Etiology/harm*: In (population), does (IV: exposure versus nonexposure) cause or increase the risk of (DV: disease, health problem)?

As noted in Chapter 2, there is an important distinction between clinical foreground questions for an EBP-focused search and a question for a study. As shown in Table 2.1, sometimes clinicians ask questions about explicit comparisons (e.g., they want to compare intervention A to intervention B) and sometimes they do not (e.g., they want to learn the effects of intervention A, compared to any other intervention or to the absence of an intervention). In a research question, there must *always* be a designated comparison, because the independent variable must be operationally defined; this definition would articulate exactly what is being studied.

→ TIP: Research questions are sometimes more complex than clinical foreground questions for EBP. They may include, in addition to the independent and dependent variable, elements called moderator variables or mediating variables. A **moderator variable** is a variable that influences the strength or direction of a relationship between two variables (e.g., a person's age might moderate the effect of exercise on physical function). A **mediating variable** is one that acts like a "go between" in a link between two variables (e.g., a smoking cessation intervention may affect smoking behavior through the intervention's effect on motivation). The supplementary material for this chapter on thePoint® describes the role these variables play in complex research questions and complex hypotheses.

Some research questions are primarily descriptive. As examples, here are some descriptive questions that could be answered in a study on nurses' use of humor:

• What is the frequency with which nurses use humor as a complementary therapy with hospitalized cancer patients?
• What are the reactions of hospitalized cancer patients to nurses' use of humor?
• What are the characteristics of nurses who use humor as a complementary therapy with hospitalized cancer patients?
• Is my *Use of Humor Scale* a reliable and valid measure of nurses' use of humor with patients in clinical settings?

Answers to such questions might, if addressed in a methodologically sound study, be useful in developing strategies for reducing stress in patients with cancer.

Example of a Research Question from a Quantitative Study: Schmidt and colleagues (2014) studied older adults' performance in technology-based tasks. One of their research questions was: *Do older participants without cognitive impairment and those with mild cognitive impairment differ in their ability to use technology?*

➔ **TIP:** The Toolkit section of Chapter 4 of the accompanying *Resource Manual* includes question templates in a Word document that can be "filled in" to generate many types of research questions for both qualitative and quantitative studies.

Research Questions in Qualitative Studies

Research questions for qualitative studies state the phenomenon of interest and the group or population of interest. Researchers in the various qualitative traditions vary in their conceptualization of what types of questions are important. Grounded theory researchers are likely to ask *process* questions, phenomenologists tend to ask *meaning* questions, and ethnographers generally ask *descriptive* questions about cultures. The terms associated with the various traditions, discussed previously in connection with purpose statements, are likely to be incorporated into the research questions.

Example of a Research Question from a Phenomenologic Study: What is the lived experience of mothers of children with a rare disease in using online health communications to manage their chronic sorrow? (Glenn, 2015)

Not all qualitative studies are rooted in a specific research tradition. Many researchers use qualitative methods to describe or explore phenomena without focusing on cultures, meaning, or social processes.

Example of a Research Question from a Descriptive Qualitative Study: In their descriptive qualitative study, Oliveira and colleagues (2015) explored the role of smoking in the lives of patients hospitalized in a Brazilian psychiatric ward.

In qualitative studies, research questions may evolve over the course of the study. Researchers begin with a *focus* that defines the broad boundaries of the study, but the boundaries are not cast in stone. The boundaries "can be altered and, in the typical naturalistic inquiry, will be" (Lincoln & Guba, 1985, p. 228). The naturalist begins with a research question that provides a general starting point but does not prohibit discovery. Qualitative researchers are sufficiently flexible that questions can be modified as new information makes it relevant to do so.

Problem Statements

Problem statements express the dilemma or troubling situation that needs investigation and that provide a rationale for a new inquiry. A good problem is a well-structured formulation of what is problematic, what "needs fixing," or what is poorly understood. Problem statements, especially for quantitative studies, often have most of the following six components:

1. *Problem identification*: What is wrong with the current situation?
2. *Background*: What is the context of the problem that readers need to understand?
3. *Scope of the problem*: How big a problem is it, how many people are affected?
4. *Consequences of the problem*: What are the costs of *not* fixing the problem?
5. *Knowledge gaps*: What information about the problem is lacking?
6. *Proposed solution*: What is the basis for believing that the proposed study would contribute to the solution of the problem?

➔ **TIP:** The Toolkit section of Chapter 4 of the accompanying *Resource Manual* includes these questions in a Word document that can be "filled in" and reorganized as needed, as an aid to developing a problem statement.

BOX 4.1 Draft Problem Statement on Humor and Stress

A diagnosis of cancer is associated with high levels of stress. Sizeable numbers of patients who receive a cancer diagnosis describe feelings of uncertainty, fear, anger, and loss of control. Interpersonal relationships, psychological functioning, and role performance have all been found to suffer following cancer diagnosis and treatment.

A variety of alternative/complementary therapies have been developed in an effort to decrease the harmful effects of stress on psychological and physiologic functioning, and resources devoted to these therapies (money and staff) have increased in recent years. However, many of these therapies have not been carefully evaluated to determine their efficacy, safety, or cost-effectiveness. For example, the use of humor has been recommended as a therapeutic device to improve quality of life, decrease stress, and perhaps improve immune functioning, but the evidence to support this claim is scant.

Suppose our topic was humor as a complementary therapy for reducing stress in hospitalized patients with cancer. Our research question is, "What is the effect of nurses' use of humor on stress and natural killer cell activity in hospitalized cancer patients?" Box 4.1 presents a rough draft of a problem statement for such a study. This problem statement is a reasonable first draft. The draft has several, but not all, of the six components.

Box 4.2 illustrates how the problem statement could be strengthened by adding information about scope (component 3), long-term consequences (component 4), and possible solutions (component 6).

This second draft builds a more compelling argument for new research: Millions of people are affected by cancer, and the disease has adverse consequences not only for those diagnosed and their families but also for society. The revised problem statement also suggests a basis for the new study by describing a solution on which the new study might build.

As this example suggests, the problem statement is usually interwoven with supportive evidence from the research literature. In many research articles, it is difficult to disentangle the problem statement from the literature review, unless there is a subsection specifically labeled "Literature Review."

BOX 4.2 Some Possible Improvements to Problem Statement on Humor and Stress

Each year, more than 1 million people are diagnosed with cancer, which remains one of the top causes of death among both men and women (reference citations). Numerous studies have documented that a diagnosis of cancer is associated with high levels of stress. Sizeable numbers of patients who receive a cancer diagnosis describe feelings of uncertainty, fear, anger, and loss of control (citations). Interpersonal relationships, psychological functioning, and role performance have all been found to suffer following cancer diagnosis and treatment (citations). These stressful outcomes can, in turn, adversely affect health, long-term prognosis, and medical costs among cancer survivors (citations).

A variety of alternative/complementary therapies have been developed in an effort to decrease the harmful effects of stress on psychological and physiologic functioning, and resources devoted to these therapies (money and staff) have increased in recent years (citations). However, many of these therapies have not been carefully evaluated to determine their efficacy, safety, or cost-effectiveness. For example, the use of humor has been recommended as a therapeutic device to improve quality of life, decrease stress, and perhaps improve immune functioning (citations), but the evidence to support this claim is scant. Preliminary findings from a recent small-scale endocrinology study with a healthy sample exposed to a humorous intervention (citation), holds promise for further inquiry with immunocompromised populations.

Problem statements for a qualitative study similarly express the nature of the problem, its context, its scope, and information needed to address it.

Example of a Problem Statement from a Qualitative Study: "Although we know that partners of men with prostate cancer experience significant distress, we know little about how they manage their distress, what parts of their cancer experiences cause them the most distress, or how they conceptualize caring for their recovering partner . . . Without a better understanding of the experiences and needs of partners of men with prostate cancer, we cannot truly treat prostate cancer as the couple's disease that we now understand it to be." The researchers used a qualitative design to "describe the experiences of low-income Latinas longitudinally as their husbands recovered from radical prostatectomy for prostate cancer" (Williams et al., 2014, p. 307).

Qualitative studies embedded in a particular research tradition usually incorporate terms and concepts in their problem statements that foreshadow the tradition. For example, the problem statement in a grounded theory study might refer to the need to generate a theory relating to social processes. A problem statement for a phenomenologic study might note the need to gain insight into people's experiences or the meanings they attribute to those experiences. And an ethnographer might indicate the need to understand how cultural forces affect people's behavior.

RESEARCH HYPOTHESES

A hypothesis is a prediction, almost always a prediction about the relationship between variables.* In qualitative studies, researchers do not have an *a priori* hypothesis, in part because there is too little known to justify a prediction, and in part because qualitative researchers want the inquiry to be guided by participants' viewpoints rather than by their own hunches. Thus, our discussion here focuses on hypotheses in quantitative research.

_____
*Although this does not occur with great frequency, it is possible to make a hypothesis about a specific value. For example, we might hypothesize that the rate of medication compliance in a specific population is 60%.

Function of Hypotheses in Quantitative Research

Research questions, as we have seen, are usually queries about relationships between variables. Hypotheses are predicted answers to these queries. For instance, the research question might ask: Does sexual abuse in childhood (I) affect the development of irritable bowel syndrome (O) in women (P)? The researcher might predict the following: Women who were sexually abused in childhood have a higher incidence of irritable bowel syndrome than women who were not.

Hypotheses sometimes follow from a theory. Scientists reason from theories to hypotheses and test those hypotheses in the real world. Take, as an example, the theory of reinforcement, which maintains that behavior that is positively reinforced (rewarded) tends to be learned or repeated. Predictions based on this theory could be tested. For example, we could test the following hypothesis: Pediatric patients who are given a reward (e.g., a balloon or permission to watch television) when they cooperate during nursing procedures tend to be more cooperative during those procedures than nonrewarded peers. This hypothesis can be put to a test, and the theory gains credibility if it is supported with real data.

Even in the absence of a theory, well-conceived hypotheses offer direction and suggest explanations. For example, suppose we hypothesized that the incidence of bradycardia in extremely low birth weight infants undergoing intubation and ventilation would be lower using the closed tracheal suction system (CTSS) than using the partially ventilated endotracheal suction method (PVETS). We could justify our speculation based on earlier studies or clinical observations, or both. *The development of predictions forces researchers to think logically and to tie together earlier research findings.*

Now let us suppose the preceding hypothesis is not confirmed: We find that rates of bradycardia are similar for both the PVETS and CTSS methods. *The failure of data to support a prediction forces researchers to analyze theory or previous research critically, to consider study limitations, and to explore alternative explanations for the findings.* The use of hypotheses tends to induce critical thinking and encourages careful interpretation of the evidence.

To illustrate further the utility of hypotheses, suppose we conducted the study guided only by the research question, Is there a relationship between suction method and incidence of bradycardia? The investigator without a hypothesis is apparently prepared to accept any results. The problem is that it is almost always possible to explain something superficially after the fact, no matter what the findings are. Hypotheses reduce the risk that spurious results will be misconstrued.

Characteristics of Testable Hypotheses

Testable hypotheses state the expected relationship between the independent variable (the presumed cause or antecedent) and the dependent variable (the presumed effect or outcome) within a population.[†]

> **Example of a Research Hypothesis:** Leutwyler and co-researchers (2014) hypothesized that, in a sample of older adults with schizophrenia, more severe neurocognitive deficits are associated with lower levels of physical activity.

In this example, the population is older adults with schizophrenia, the independent variable is severity of neurocognitive deficits, and the dependent variable is amount of physical activity. The hypothesis predicts that these two variables are related within the population—greater physical activity is predicted among patients with less severe neurocognitive deficits.

Hypotheses that do not make a relational statement are difficult to test. Take the following example: *Pregnant women who receive prenatal instruction about postpartum experiences are not likely to experience postpartum depression.* This statement expresses no anticipated relationship—there is only one variable (postpartum depression), and a relationship requires at least two variables.

The problem is that without a prediction about an anticipated relationship, the hypothesis cannot readily be tested using standard statistical procedures. In our example, how would we know whether the hypothesis was supported—what standard could be used to decide whether to accept or reject it? To illustrate this concretely, suppose we asked a group of mothers who had been given instruction on postpartum experiences the following question 1 month after delivery: On the whole, how depressed have you been since you gave birth? Would you say (1) extremely depressed, (2) moderately depressed, (3) a little depressed, or (4) not at all depressed?

Based on responses to this question, how could we compare the actual outcome with the predicted outcome? Would *all* the women have to say they were "not at all depressed?" Would the prediction be supported if 51% of the women said they were "not at all depressed" *or* "a little depressed?" It is difficult to test the accuracy of the prediction.

A test is simple, however, if we modify the prediction as follows: Pregnant women who receive prenatal instruction are less likely to experience postpartum depression than those with no prenatal instruction. Here, the outcome variable (O) is the women's depression, and the independent variable is receipt (I) versus nonreceipt (C) of prenatal instruction. The relational aspect of the prediction is embodied in the phrase *less than*. If a hypothesis lacks a phrase such as *more than, less than, greater than, different from, related to, associated with*, or something similar, it is probably not amenable to statistical testing. To test this revised hypothesis, we could ask two groups of women with different prenatal instruction experiences to respond to the question on depression and then compare the groups' responses. The absolute degree of depression of either group would not be at issue.

Hypotheses should be based on justifiable rationales. Hypotheses often follow from previous research findings or are deduced from a theory. When a new area is being investigated, the researcher may have to turn to logical reasoning or clinical experience to justify predictions.

The Derivation of Hypotheses

Many students ask, How do I go about developing hypotheses? Two basic processes—induction and deduction—are the intellectual machinery involved in deriving hypotheses. (The Supplement to Chapter 3 (S) on thePoint® described induction and deduction).

[†]It is possible to test hypotheses about the value of a single variable, but this happens rarely. See Chapter 17 for an example.

An **inductive hypothesis** is inferred from observations. Researchers observe certain patterns or associations among phenomena and then make predictions based on the observations. An important source for inductive hypotheses is clinical experiences. For example, a nurse might notice that presurgical patients who ask a lot of questions about pain have a more difficult time than other patients in learning postoperative procedures. The nurse could formulate a hypothesis, such as: Patients who are stressed by fear of pain have more difficulty in deep breathing and coughing after surgery than patients who are not stressed. Qualitative studies are an important source of inspiration for inductive hypotheses.

Example of Deriving an Inductive Hypothesis: Beck and colleagues (2013) studied women's experiences of eye movement desensitization reprocessing (EMDR) therapy for their posttraumatic stress symptoms following birth trauma. One of their findings was that women who had experienced both EMDR and cognitive therapy said that EMDR therapy gave them symptom relief much faster than cognitive therapy. A hypothesis that can be derived from this qualitative finding might be as follows: Women who undergo EMDR therapy for their posttraumatic stress symptoms due to traumatic childbirth have faster relief of their symptoms than women who have cognitive therapy.

Inductive hypotheses begin with specific observations and move toward generalizations. **Deductive hypotheses** have theories as a starting point, as in our earlier example about reinforcement theory. Researchers deduce that if the theory is true, then certain outcomes can be expected. If hypotheses are supported, then the theory is strengthened. The advancement of nursing knowledge depends on both inductive and deductive hypotheses. Researchers need to be organizers of concepts (think inductively), logicians (think deductively), and critics and skeptics of resulting formulations, constantly demanding evidence.

Wording of Hypotheses

A good hypothesis is worded clearly and concisely and in the present tense. Researchers make predictions about relationships that exist in the population and not just about a relationship that will be revealed in a particular sample. There are various types of hypotheses.

Directional versus Nondirectional Hypotheses
Hypotheses can be stated in a number of ways, as in the following example:

1. Older patients are more likely to fall than younger patients.
2. There is a relationship between the age of a patient and the risk of falling.
3. The older the patient, the greater the risk that he or she will fall.
4. Older patients differ from younger ones with respect to their risk of falling.
5. Younger patients tend to be less at risk of a fall than older patients.
6. The risk of falling increases with the age of the patient.

In each example, the hypothesis indicates the population (patients), the independent variable (patients' age), the dependent variable (a fall), and the anticipated relationship between them.

Hypotheses can be either directional or nondirectional. A **directional hypothesis** is one that specifies not only the existence but also the expected direction of the relationship between variables. In our example, versions 1, 3, 5, and 6 are directional hypotheses because there is an explicit prediction that older patients are more likely to fall than younger ones. A **nondirectional hypothesis** does not state the direction of the relationship, as illustrated by versions 2 and 4. These hypotheses predict that a patient's age and risk of falling are related, but they do not stipulate whether the researcher thinks that *older* patients or *younger* ones are at greater risk.

Hypotheses derived from theory are almost always directional because theories provide a rationale for expecting variables to be related in a certain way. Existing studies also offer a basis for directional hypotheses. When there is no theory or related research, when findings of prior studies are contradictory, or when researchers' own experience leads to ambivalence, nondirectional hypotheses may be appropriate. Some people argue, in fact, that nondirectional hypotheses are preferable because they connote impartiality. Directional hypotheses, it is said, imply that researchers are intellectually committed to certain outcomes, and such a commitment might lead to bias. Yet, researchers typically *do* have hunches about outcomes, whether they state them explicitly or not. We prefer directional hypotheses when there is a reasonable basis for them, because they clarify the study's framework and demonstrate that researchers have thought critically about the study variables.

→ **TIP:** Hypotheses can be either *simple hypotheses* (ones with one independent variable and one dependent variable) or *complex* (ones with three or more variables—i.e., multiple independent or dependent variables). Supplementary information about complex relationships and hypotheses is available on thePoint®. ⑤

Research versus Null Hypotheses

Hypotheses can be described as either research hypotheses or null hypotheses. **Research hypotheses** (also called *substantive* or *scientific* hypotheses) are statements of expected relationships between variables. All hypotheses presented thus far are research hypotheses that state actual predictions.

Statistical inference uses a logic that may be confusing. This logic requires that hypotheses be expressed as an expected *absence* of a relationship. **Null hypotheses** (or *statistical hypotheses*) state that there is no relationship between the independent and dependent variables. The null form of the hypothesis used in our example might be: "Patients' age is unrelated to their risk of falling" or "Older patients are just as likely as younger patients to fall." The null hypothesis might be compared with the assumption of innocence of an accused criminal in English-based systems of justice: The variables are assumed to be "innocent" of any relationship until they can be shown "guilty" through appropriate statistical procedures. The null hypothesis represents the formal statement of this assumption of innocence.

Research articles typically state research rather than null hypotheses. Indeed, you should avoid stating hypotheses in null form in a proposal or a report because this gives an amateurish impression. In statistical testing, underlying null hypotheses are assumed without being stated. If the researcher's *actual* research hypothesis is that no relationship among variables exists, complex procedures are needed to test it.

Hypothesis Testing and Proof

Researchers seek evidence through statistical analysis that their research hypotheses have a high probability of being correct. However, hypotheses are never *proved* through hypothesis testing; rather, they are *accepted* or *supported*. Findings are always tentative. If the same results are replicated in numerous studies, then greater confidence can be placed in the conclusions. Hypotheses come to be increasingly supported with evidence from multiple studies.

Let us look at why this is so. Suppose we hypothesized that height and weight are related. We predict that, on average, tall people weigh more than short people. We then obtain height and weight measurements from a sample and analyze the data. Now suppose we happened by chance to get a sample that consisted of short, heavy people and tall, thin people. Our results might indicate that there is no relationship between height and weight. Would we be justified in stating that this study *proved* that height and weight are unrelated?

As another example, suppose we hypothesized that tall nurses are more effective than short ones. In reality, we would expect no relationship between height and a nurse's job performance. Now suppose that, by chance again, we drew a sample in which tall nurses received better job evaluations than short ones. Could we say that we *proved* that height is related to a nurse's performance? These two examples illustrate the difficulty of using observations from a sample to come to definitive conclusions about a population. Issues such as the accuracy of the measures, the effects of uncontrolled variables, and idiosyncrasies of the sample prevent researchers from concluding with finality that hypotheses are proved.

TIP: If a researcher uses any statistical tests (as is true in most quantitative studies), it means that there were underlying hypotheses—regardless of whether the researcher explicitly stated them—because statistical tests are designed to test hypotheses. In planning a quantitative study of your own, do not be afraid to make predictions—that is, to state hypotheses.

CRITIQUING RESEARCH PROBLEMS, RESEARCH QUESTIONS, AND HYPOTHESES

In critiquing research articles, you need to evaluate whether researchers have adequately communicated their problem. The problem statement, purpose, research questions, and hypotheses set the stage for a description of what the researchers did and what they learned. Ideally, you would not have to dig deeply to decipher the research problem or the questions.

A critique of the research problem is multidimensional. Substantively, you need to consider whether the problem has significance for nursing. Studies that build in a meaningful way on existing knowledge are well-poised to contribute to evidence-based nursing practice. Researchers who develop a systematic *program of research*, building on their own earlier findings, are especially likely to make important contributions (Conn, 2004). For example, Beck's series of studies relating to postpartum depression have influenced women's health care worldwide. Also, research problems stemming from established research priorities (Chapter 1) have a high likelihood of yielding important new evidence for nurses because they reflect expert opinion about areas of needed research.

Another dimension in critiquing the research problem is methodologic—in particular, whether the research problem is compatible with the chosen research paradigm and its associated methods. You should also evaluate whether the statement of purpose or research questions have been properly worded and lend themselves to empirical inquiry.

In a quantitative study, if the research article does not contain explicit hypotheses, you need to consider whether their absence is justified. If there are hypotheses, you should evaluate whether they are logically connected to the problem and are consistent with existing evidence or relevant theory. The wording of hypotheses should also be assessed. To be testable, the hypothesis should contain a prediction about the relationship between two or more measurable variables. Specific guidelines for critiquing research problems, research questions, and hypotheses are presented in Box 4.3.

RESEARCH EXAMPLES

This section describes how the research problem and research questions were communicated in two nursing studies, one quantitative and one qualitative.

Research Example of a Quantitative Study

Study: Night and day in the VA: Associations between night shift staffing, nurse workforce characteristics, and length of stay (de Cordova et al., 2014)

Problem Statement: "Although the intensity of nursing work may differ at certain hours during the day, nurses are essential in ensuring patient safety at all hours. Patient outcomes are worse when critical events occur at times other than on weekdays from 9 a.m. to 5 p.m. In a comprehensive systematic review of patient and employee outcomes on off-shifts (i.e., nights and weekends), we also found that both patient and employee outcomes were worse on off-shifts than on more regular hours. Although evidence suggests that patients admitted to hospitals on off-shifts have worse outcomes than those admitted during the day, there is a paucity of evidence on the staffing and workforce characteristics on off-shifts that might explain these worse outcomes" (p. 90). (Citations were omitted to streamline the presentation).

Statement of Purpose: "The aim of this study was to examine the association between night nurse staffing and workforce characteristics and the length of stay (LOS) in 138 Veteran Affairs (VA) hospitals . . . " (p. 90).

Research Question: The authors posed this research question: "What is the relationship between LOS and

BOX 4.3 Guidelines for Critiquing Research Problems, Research Questions, and Hypotheses

1. What is the research problem? Is the problem statement easy to locate and is it clearly stated? Does the problem statement build a cogent and persuasive argument for the new study?
2. Does the problem have significance for nursing? How might the research contribute to nursing practice, administration, education, or policy?
3. Is there a good fit between the research problem and the paradigm in which the research was conducted? Is there a good fit between the problem and the qualitative research tradition (if applicable)?
4. Does the report formally present a statement of purpose, research question, and/or hypotheses? Is this information communicated clearly and concisely, and is it placed in a logical and useful location?
5. Are purpose statements or questions worded appropriately? For example, are key concepts/variables identified, and is the population of interest specified? Are verbs used appropriately to suggest the nature of the inquiry and/or the research tradition?
6. If hypotheses were not formally stated, is their absence justified? Are statistical tests used in analyzing the data despite the absence of stated hypotheses?
7. Do hypotheses (if any) flow from a theory or previous research? Is there a justifiable basis for the predictions?
8. Are hypotheses (if any) properly worded—do they state a predicted relationship between two or more variables? Are they directional or nondirectional, and is there a rationale for how they were stated? Are they presented as research or as null hypotheses?

RN staffing levels, skill mix, and experience on the night shift?" (p. 91).

Hypotheses: The researchers hypothesized that "1) RN staffing at night is negatively related to LOS; 2) RN skill mix at night is negatively related to LOS; and 3) RN experience at night is negatively related to LOS" (p. 91).

Study Methods: The study was conducted using data from acute care units in 138 veterans affairs hospitals in the United States, collected over the 2002-2006 period. Patient and nurse data were drawn from the hospitals' administrative and electronic data sources.

Key Findings: In these VA acute care units, there were fewer nurses and a less well-educated workforce at night. The researchers also found that higher night staffing and a higher skill mix were associated with reduced patient length of stay in the hospitals.

Research Example of a Qualitative Study

Study: Conceptions of diabetes and diabetes care in young people with minority backgrounds (Boman et al., 2015)

Problem Statement: "People with type 1 diabetes (T1DM) who fail to take sufficiently good care of their health with regard to their disease can in the

long term suffer severe medical complications that can gravely impair quality and length of life . . . Successful prevention of future medical complications requires self-care in terms of strict and repeated metabolic control of blood glucose levels throughout the day, achieved by taking blood tests and balancing physical activity, food intake, and insulin injections. Teenagers, whom researchers have identified as the least successful group regarding diabetic metabolic control, are a vulnerable group of patients . . . [Research has] shown that belonging to a minority ethnic group might contribute to poor metabolic diabetes control among young people and thus to poor long-term quality of life" (p. 5) (Excerpt; citations omitted to streamline presentation).

Statement of Purpose: "The aim of this study was to gain in-depth knowledge on the experience of adolescents with T1DM and a non-Swedish background regarding factors that might influence their ability to take care of themselves" (p. 5).

Research Questions: "Which factors are important for the adolescents to consistently take responsibility for self-care, and which factors might counteract taking such responsibility? Which factors related to the pediatric diabetes care unit are important motivators or demotivators for the adolescents? What types of support for self-care are available to the adolescents in their social context, and what types of support do they wish for? How do the adolescents perceive their ability to influence their health situation?" (p. 6).

Method: Twelve adolescents who were first- or second-generation immigrants who were treated for T1DM in a Swedish hospital agreed to participate in the study. A trained interviewer conducted in-depth interviews with the adolescents, mostly in their homes. The interviews were recorded and subsequently transcribed for analysis.

Key Findings: The results indicated resources as well as constraints in the adolescents' social context as well as in the health care organization where they received treatment. The results strongly indicated that the focus predominantly on Hb1Ac levels permeated the adolescents' experiences before, during, and after their clinic visits.

SUMMARY POINTS

- A **research problem** is a perplexing or enigmatic situation that a researcher wants to address through disciplined inquiry. Researchers usually identify a broad **topic**, narrow the problem scope, and identify questions consistent with a paradigm of choice.
- Common sources of ideas for nursing research problems are clinical experience, relevant literature, quality improvement initiatives, social issues, theory, and external suggestions.
- Key criteria in assessing a research problem are that the problem should be clinically significant, researchable, feasible, and of personal interest.
- Feasibility involves the issues of time, researcher skills, cooperation of participants and other people, availability of facilities and equipment, and ethical considerations.
- Researchers communicate their aims as problem statements, statements of purpose, research questions, or hypotheses.
- **Problem statements**, which articulate the nature, context, and significance of a problem, include several components organized to form an *argument* for a new study: problem identifica-

tion; the background, scope, and consequences of the problem; knowledge gaps; and possible solutions to the problem.
- A **statement of purpose**, which summarizes the overall study goal, identifies key concepts (variables) and the population. Purpose statements often communicate, through the use of verbs and other key terms, the underlying research tradition of qualitative studies, or whether study is experimental or nonexperimental in quantitative ones.
- A **research question** is the specific query researchers want to answer in addressing the research problem. In quantitative studies, research questions usually concern the existence, nature, strength, and direction of relationships.
- In quantitative studies, a **hypothesis** is a statement of predicted relationships between two or more variables.
- **Directional hypotheses** predict the direction of a relationship; **nondirectional hypotheses** predict the existence of relationships, not their direction.
- **Research hypotheses** predict the existence of relationships; **null hypotheses**, which express the absence of a relationship, are the hypotheses subjected to statistical testing.
- Hypotheses are never proved or disproved in an ultimate sense—they are accepted or rejected and supported or not supported by the data.

STUDY ACTIVITIES

Chapter 4 of the *Resource Manual for Nursing Research: Generating and Assessing Evidence for Nursing Practice, 10th edition*, offers study suggestions for reinforcing concepts presented in this chapter. In addition, the following questions can be addressed in classroom or online discussions:

1. Think of a frustrating experience you have had as a nursing student or as a practicing nurse. Identify the problem area. Ask yourself a series of questions until you have one that you think is researchable. Evaluate the problem in terms of the evaluation criteria discussed in this chapter.

2. To the extent possible, use the critiquing questions in Box 4.3 to appraise the research problems for the two studies used as research examples at the end of this chapter.

STUDIES CITED IN CHAPTER 4

Beck, C. T., Driscoll, J. W., & Watson, S. (2013). *Traumatic childbirth*. New York: Routledge.

Boman, A., Bohlin, M., Eklör, M., Forsander, G., & Törner, M. (2015). Conceptions of diabetes and diabetes care in young people with minority backgrounds. *Qualitative Health Research, 25*, 5–15.

Conn, V. (2004). Building a research trajectory. *Western Journal of Nursing Research, 26*, 592–594.

de Cordova, P. B., Phibbs, C., Schmitt, S., & Stone, P. (2014). Night and day in the VA: Associations between night shift staffing, nurse workforce characteristics, and length of stay. *Research in Nursing & Health, 37*, 90–97.

Glenn, A. D. (2015). Using online health communication to manage chronic sorrow: Mothers of children with rare diseases speak. *Journal of Pediatric Nursing, 30*, 17–24.

Judge, M. P., Beck, C. T., Durham, H., McKelvey, M., & Lammi-Keefe, C. (2014). Pilot trial evaluating maternal docosahexaenoic acid consumption during pregnancy: Decreased postpartum depressive symptomatology. *International Journal of Nursing Sciences, 1*, 339–345.

Leutwyler, H., Hubbard, E., Jeste, D., Miller, B., & Vinogradov, S. (2014). Association between schizophrenia symptoms and neurocognition with physical activity in older adults with schizophrenia. *Biological Research for Nursing, 16*, 23–30.

Lincoln, Y. S., & Guba, E. G. (1985). *Naturalistic inquiry*. Newbury Park, CA: Sage.

Oliveira, R., Siqueira-Junior, A., & Furegato, A. (2015). The meaning of smoking for patients with mental disorder. *Issues in Mental Health Nursing, 36*, 127–134.

Schmidt, L. I., Wahl, H., & Piclschke, H. (2014). Older adults' performance in technology-based tasks: Cognitive ability and beyond. *Journal of Gerontological Nursing, 40*, 18–24.

Wellborn, J., & Moceri, J. T. (2014). The lived experience of persons with chronic venous insufficiency and lower extremity ulcers. *Journal of Wound, Ostomy, & Continence Nursing, 41*, 122–126.

*Wesmiller, S. W., Bender, C., Serieka, S., Ahrendt, G., Bonaventura, M., Bovbjerg, D., & Conley, Y. (2014). Association between serotonin transport polymorphisms and postdischarge nausea and vomiting in women following breast cancer surgery. *Oncology Nursing Forum, 41*, 195–202.

Williams, K. C., Hicks, E. M., Chang, N., Connor, S. E., & Maliski, S. L. (2014). Purposeful normalization when caring for husbands recovering from prostate cancer. *Qualitative Health Research, 24*, 306–316.

A link to this open-access journal article is provided in the Toolkit for this chapter in the accompanying Resource Manual. ✖

5 | Literature Reviews: Finding and Critiquing Evidence

Researchers typically undertake a thorough **literature review** as an early step in a study. This chapter describes activities associated with literature reviews, including locating and critiquing studies. Many activities overlap with early steps in an EBP project, as described in Chapter 2.

GETTING STARTED ON A LITERATURE REVIEW

Before discussing the steps involved in doing a research-based literature review, we briefly discuss some general issues. The first concerns the viewpoint of qualitative researchers.

Literature Reviews in Qualitative Research Traditions

Qualitative researchers have varying opinions about reviewing the literature before doing a new study. Some of the differences reflect viewpoints associated with qualitative research traditions.

Grounded theory researchers often collect their data before reviewing the literature. The grounded theory takes shape as data are analyzed. Researchers then turn to the literature when the theory is sufficiently developed, seeking to relate the theory to prior findings. Glaser (1978) warned, "It's hard enough to generate one's own ideas without the 'rich' detailment provided by literature in the same field" (p. 31). Thus, grounded theory researchers may defer a literature review, but then they

consider how previous research fits with or extends the emerging theory.

Phenomenologists often undertake a search for relevant materials at the outset of a study. In reviewing the literature, phenomenologic researchers look for experiential descriptions of the phenomenon being studied (Munhall, 2012). The purpose is to expand the researcher's understanding of the phenomenon from multiple perspectives, and this may include an examination of artistic sources in which the phenomenon is described (e.g., in novels or poetry).

Even though "ethnography starts with a conscious attitude of almost complete ignorance" (Spradley, 1979, p. 4), literature relating to the cultural problem to be studied is often reviewed before data collection. A second, more thorough literature review is often done during data analysis and interpretation so that findings can be compared with previous findings.

Regardless of tradition, if funding is sought for a qualitative project, an up-front literature review is usually necessary. Proposal reviewers need to understand the context for a proposed study when deciding whether it should be funded.

Purposes and Scope of Research Literature Reviews

Written literature reviews are undertaken for many reasons. The length of the product depends on its purpose but, regardless of length, a good review requires thorough familiarity with available evidence. As Garrard (2014) advised, you must strive to *own* the literature on a topic to be confident of preparing a state-of-the-art review. Major types of written research review include the following:

- *A review embedded in a research report*. Literature reviews in the introduction to a report provide readers with an overview of existing evidence and contribute to the argument for a new study. These reviews are usually only two to three double-spaced pages, and so only key studies can be cited. The emphasis is on summarizing an overall body of evidence.
- *A review in a proposal*. A literature review in a proposal provides context and confirms the need for new research. The length of such reviews is specified in proposal guidelines but is often just a few pages. This means that the review must reflect expertise on the topic in a succinct fashion.
- *A review in a thesis or dissertation*. Dissertations in the traditional format (see Chapter 30) often include a thorough, critical literature review. An entire chapter may be devoted to the review, and such chapters are often 15-30 pages long. These reviews typically include an evaluation of the overall body of literature as well as critiques of key individual studies.
- *Free-standing literature reviews*. Nurses also prepare reviews that critically appraise and summarize a body of research, sometimes for a course or for an EBP project. Researchers who are experts in a field also may do reviews that are published in journals. Free-standing reviews are usually 15 to 25 pages long.

By doing a thorough review, researchers can determine how best to make a contribution to existing evidence—for example, whether there are gaps or inconsistencies in a body of research or whether a replication with a new population is the right next step. A literature review also facilitates researchers' interpretations of their findings after their data are analyzed.

Types of Information for a Research Review

Written materials vary in their quality and the kind of information they contain. In performing a literature review, you will have to decide what to read and what to include in a written review.

The most important type of information for a research review is findings from prior studies. You should rely mostly on **primary source** research reports, which are descriptions of studies written by the researchers who conducted them.

Secondary sources are descriptions of studies prepared by someone other than the original researcher. Literature reviews, for example, are secondary sources.* If reviews are recent, they are a good place to start because they provide an overview of the topic and a valuable bibliography. Secondary sources are not substitutes for primary sources because they typically fail to provide much detail about studies and are seldom completely objective.

➔ **TIP:** For an EBP project, a recent, high-quality review may be sufficient to provide needed information about existing evidence, although it is wise to search for recent studies not covered by the review.

In addition to research reports, your search may yield nonresearch references, such as case reports, anecdotes, editorials, or clinical descriptions. Nonresearch materials may broaden understanding of a problem, demonstrate a need for research, or describe aspects of clinical practice. These writings may help in formulating research ideas, but they usually have limited utility in written research reviews because they do not address the central question: What is the current state of *evidence* on this research problem?

Major Steps and Strategies in Doing a Literature Review

Conducting a literature review is a little like doing a full study, in the sense that reviewers start with a question, formulate and implement a plan for gathering information, and then analyze and interpret information. The "findings" are then summarized in a written product.

---

*Garrard (2014) calls systematic reviews and clinical practice guidelines *tertiary sources*.

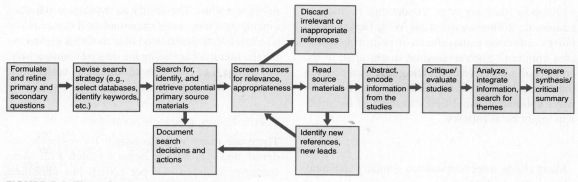

FIGURE 5.1 Flow of tasks in a literature review.

Figure 5.1 outlines the literature review process. As the figure shows, there are several potential feedback loops, with opportunities to retrace earlier steps in search of more information. This chapter discusses each step, but some steps are elaborated in Chapter 29 in our discussion of systematic reviews.

Conducting a high-quality literature review is more than a mechanical exercise—it is an art and a science. Several qualities characterize a high-quality review. First, the review must be comprehensive, thorough, and up-to-date. To "own" the literature (Garrard, 2014), you must be determined to become an expert on your topic, which means that you need to be diligent in hunting down leads for possible sources of evidence.

> ⮞ **TIP:** Locating all relevant information on a research question is like being a detective. The literature retrieval tools we discuss in this chapter are essential aids, but there inevitably needs to be some digging for the clues to evidence on a topic. Be prepared for sleuthing.

Second, a high-quality review is systematic. Decision rules should be clear, and criteria for including or excluding a study need to be explicit. This is because a third characteristic of a good review is that it is reproducible, which means that another diligent reviewer would be able to apply the same decision rules and criteria and come to similar conclusions about the evidence.

Another desirable attribute of a literature review is the absence of bias. This is more easily achieved

when systematic rules for evaluating information are followed or when a team of researchers participates in the review. Finally, reviewers should strive for a review that is insightful and that is more than "the sum of its parts." Reviewers can contribute to knowledge through an astute synthesis of the evidence.

We recommend thinking of doing a literature review as similar to doing a qualitative study. This means having a flexible approach to "data collection" and thinking creatively about ideas for new sources of information. It means pursuing leads until "saturation" is achieved—that is, until your search strategies yield redundant information about studies to include. And it also means that the analysis of your "data" will typically involve a search for important themes.

Primary and Secondary Questions for a Review

For free-standing literature reviews and EBP projects, reviewers may summarize evidence about a single focused question such as those described in Chapter 2. For those who are undertaking a literature review as part of a new study, the *primary question* for the literature review is the same as the actual research question for the new study. The researcher wants to know: What is the current state of knowledge on the question that I will be addressing in *my* study?

If you are doing a review for a new study, you inevitably will need to search for existing evidence on several *secondary questions* because you will need to develop an argument for the new study in the problem statement. An example will clarify this point.

Suppose that we were conducting a study to address the following question: What factors affect nurses' effective management of pain in hospitalized children? Such a question might arise in the context of a perceived problem, such as a concern that nurses' treatment of children's pain is not always optimal. A simplified statement of the problem might be as follows:

• • •

Many children are hospitalized annually and many hospitalized children experience high levels of pain. Although effective analgesic and nonpharmacologic methods of controlling children's pain exist, and although there are reliable methods of assessing children's pain, it has been found that nurses do not always manage children's pain adeptly. *What factors associated with the nurses or their practice settings are associated with effective management of hospitalized children's pain?*

This rudimentary problem statement suggests a number of *secondary questions* for which evidence from the literature will need to be located and evaluated. Examples of such secondary questions include the following:

- What types and levels of pain do hospitalized children experience?
- How can pain in hospitalized children be reliably assessed and what are effective treatments?
- How knowledgeable are nurses about pain assessment and pain management strategies for children?
- What are the barriers to effective pain management for hospitalized children?

Thus, a literature review tends to be a multipronged task when it is done as part of a new study. It is important to keep in mind all questions for which information from the research literature needs to be retrieved.

LOCATING RELEVANT LITERATURE FOR A RESEARCH REVIEW

As shown in Figure 5.1, an early step in a literature review is devising a strategy to locate relevant studies. The ability to locate research documents on a topic is an important skill that requires adaptability. Sophisticated new methods of searching the literature are being introduced continuously. We urge you to consult with librarians, colleagues, or faculty for suggestions.

Formulating a Search Strategy

There are many ways to search for research evidence, and it is wise to begin a search with some strategies in mind. Cooper (2010) has identified several approaches, one of which we describe in some detail in this chapter: searching for references in bibliographic databases. Another approach, called the *ancestry approach*, involves using references cited in relevant studies to track down earlier research on the same topic (the "ancestors"). A third method, the *descendancy approach*, is to find a pivotal early study and to search forward in citation indexes to find more recent studies ("descendants") that cited the key study. Other strategies exist for tracking down what is called the *grey literature*, which refers to studies with more limited distribution, such as conference papers, unpublished reports, and so on. We describe these strategies in Chapter 29 on systematic reviews. If your intent is to "own" the literature, then you will likely want to adopt all of these strategies, but in many cases, the first two or three might suffice.

> **TIP:** You may be tempted to begin a literature search through an Internet search engine, such as Yahoo, Google, or Bing. Such a search is likely to yield a lot of "hits" on your topic but is unlikely to give you full bibliographic information on *research* literature on your topic. However, such searches can provide useful leads for *search terms* as well as basic background information relating to secondary questions.

Search plans also involve decisions about delimiting the search. These decisions need to be explicit to ensure reproducibility. If you are not multilingual, you may need to constrain your search to studies written in your own language. You may also want to limit your search to studies conducted within a certain time frame (e.g., within the past 15 years). You may want to exclude studies with certain types of participants. For instance, in our example of a literature search about factors affecting nurses' management of children's pain, we might want to exclude studies in which the children were neonates.

> **➲ TIP:** Constraining your search might help you to avoid irrelevant material, but be cautious about putting too many restrictions on your search, especially initially. You can always make decisions to exclude studies at a later point, provided you have clear criteria and a rationale. Be sure not to limit your search to very recent studies or to studies exclusively in the nursing literature.

Searching Bibliographic Databases

Reviewers typically begin by searching bibliographic databases that can be accessed by computer. The databases contain entries for thousands of journal articles, and in most databases, the articles are coded to facilitate retrieval. For example, articles may be coded for language used (e.g., English), subject matter (e.g., pain), type of journal (e.g., nursing), and so on. Some databases can be accessed free of charge (e.g., PubMed, Google Scholar), whereas others are sold commercially—but are often available through hospital or university libraries. Most programs are user-friendly, offering menu-driven systems with on-screen support so that retrieval can proceed with minimal instruction.

Getting Started with a Bibliographic Database

Before searching an electronic database, you should become familiar with the features of the software you are using to access the database. The software gives you options for limiting your search, for combining the results of two searches, for saving your search, and so on. Most programs have tutorials that can improve the efficiency and effectiveness of your search. In many cases, a "Help" button provides a lot of information.

Most bibliographic software has mapping capabilities. *Mapping* is a feature that allows you to search for topics using your own **keywords** rather than needing to enter a term that is exactly the same

as a **subject heading** (subject codes) in the controlled vocabulary of the database. The software translates ("maps") the keywords you enter into the most plausible subject heading. In addition to mapping your term onto subject heading codes, most programs will also search in the *text fields* of records (e.g., the title and abstract) for the keywords you enter.

> **➲ TIP:** The keywords are often the major independent or dependent variables. If you have used the question templates in Table 2.1, the words you entered in the blanks would be keywords.

Even when there are mapping capabilities, you should learn the relevant subject headings of the database you are using because keyword searches and subject heading searches yield overlapping but nonidentical results. Subject headings for databases can be located in the database's thesaurus or other reference tools.

> **➲ TIP:** To identify all major research reports on a topic, you need to be flexible and to think broadly about keywords that could be related to your topic. For example, if you are interested in anorexia nervosa, you might search *anorexia*, *eating disorder*, and *weight loss*, and perhaps *appetite*, *eating behavior*, *food habits*, *bulimia*, and *body weight change*.

General Database Search Features

Some features of an electronic search are similar across databases. One feature is that you usually can use **Boolean operators** to expand or delimit a search. Three widely used Boolean operators are AND, OR, and NOT (in all caps). The operator *AND* delimits a search. If we searched for *pain AND children*, the software would retrieve only records that have both terms. The operator *OR* expands the search: *pain OR children* could be used in a search to retrieve records with either term. Finally, *NOT* narrows a search: *pain NOT children* would retrieve all records with pain that did not include the term children.

Wildcard and truncation symbols are other useful tools for searching databases. These symbols vary from one database to another, but their function is to expand the search. A **truncation symbol** (often an asterisk, *) expands a search term to include all forms of a root word. For example, a search for *child** would instruct the computer to search for any word that begins with "child" such as children, childhood, or childrearing. **Wildcard symbols** (often a question mark or asterisk) inserted into the middle of a search term permits a search for alternative spellings. For example, a search for *behavio?r* would retrieve records with either *behavior* or *behaviour*. For each database, it is important to learn what these special symbols are and how they work. For example, many databases require at least three letters at the beginning of a search term before a wildcard or truncation symbol can be used (e.g., ca* would not be allowed). Moreover, not every database allows wildcard codes in the middle of a search term.

Another important thing to know is that use of special symbols may turn off a software's mapping feature. For example, a search for *child** would retrieve records in which any form of "child" appeared in text fields, but it would not map any of these concepts onto the database's subject headings.

Sometimes it is important to keep words together in a search, as in a search for records with *blood pressure*. Some bibliometric software would treat this as *blood AND pressure* and would search for records with both terms somewhere in text fields, even if they are not contiguous. Quotation marks often can be used to ensure that the words are searched in combination, as in "*blood pressure.*" Also, in most databases, it is possible to undertake either a *subject search*, looking for references on a topic of interest, or an *author search*, looking for papers by a particular researcher.

Key Electronic Databases for Nurse Researchers

Two especially useful electronic databases for nurse researchers are CINAHL (**C**umulative **I**ndex to **N**ursing and **A**llied **H**ealth **L**iterature) and MEDLINE (**Med**ical Literature On-**Line**), which we discuss in the next sections. We also briefly discuss Google Scholar. Other potentially useful bibliographic databases or search engines for nurses include the following:

- British Nursing Index
- Cochrane Database of Systematic Reviews
- EMBASE (the **E**xcerpta **M**edica data**base**)
- HaPI (**H**ealth **a**nd **P**sychosocial **I**nstruments database)
- Health Source: Nursing/Academic Edition
- ISI Web of Knowledge
- PsycINFO (**Psyc**hology **Info**rmation)
- Scopus

Note that a search strategy that works well in one database does not always produce good results in another. Thus, it is important to explore strategies in each database and to understand how each database is structured—for example, what subject headings are used and how they are organized in a hierarchy. Each database and software program also has certain peculiarities. For example, using PubMed (to be discussed later) to search the MEDLINE database, you might restrict your search to nursing journals. However, if you did this you would be excluding studies in several journals in which nurses often publish, such as *Birth* and *Qualitative Health Research* because these journals are not currently coded for the nursing subset of PubMed.

TIP: In the following sections, we provide specific information about using CINAHL and MEDLINE via PubMed. Note, however, that databases and the software through which they are accessed change periodically, and so our instructions may not be current.

Cumulative Index to Nursing and Allied Health Literature

CINAHL is an important electronic database: It covers references to virtually all English-language nursing and allied health journals and also includes books, dissertations, and selected conference proceedings in nursing and allied health fields. There are several versions of the CINAHL database (e.g., CINAHL, CINAHL Plus, CINAHL Complete), each with somewhat different features relating to full text availability and journal coverage. All are offered through EBSCOhost.

The basic CINAHL database indexes material from more than 3,000 journals dating from 1981 and contains about 3 million records. In addition to providing bibliographic information for references (i.e., author, title, journal, year of publication, volume, and page numbers), CINAHL provides abstracts of most citations. Supplementary information, such as names of data collection instruments, is available for many records, and links to the actual article are often provided. We illustrate features of CINAHL, but note that some features may be different at your institution.

At the outset, you might begin with a "basic search" by simply entering keywords or phrases relevant to your primary question. In the basic search screen, you could limit your search in a number of ways, for example, by limiting the records retrieved to those with certain features (e.g., only ones with abstracts or only those in journals with peer review), to specific publication dates (e.g., only those from 2005 to the present), or to those coded as being in a particular journal subset (e.g., nursing). The basic search screen also allows you to expand your search by clicking an option labeled "Apply related words."

As an example, suppose we were interested in recent research on nurses' pain management for children. If we searched for *pain*, we would get nearly 160,000 records. Searching for *pain AND child* AND nurs** would bring the number down to about 2,600. (In CINAHL, an asterisk is the truncation symbol and a question mark is the wildcard.) We could pare the number down to about 500 by limiting the search to articles with abstracts published in nursing journals after 2004.

The advanced search mode in CINAHL permits even more fine-tuning. For example, we could stipulate that we wanted only research articles published in English. These restrictions, which take only seconds to execute, would get us down to a more manageable number of records (300) that could be reviewed for relevance. The advanced search mode offers many additional options that should be more fully explored.

The full records for the 300 references would then be displayed on the monitor in a Results List. The Results List has sidebar options that allow you to narrow your search even farther, if desired. From the Results List, we could place promising references

into a folder for later scrutiny, or we could immediately retrieve and print full bibliographic information for records of interest. An example of an abridged CINAHL record entry for a study identified through the search on children's pain is presented in Figure 5.2. The record begins with the article title, the authors' names and affiliation, and source. The source indicates the following:

- Name of the journal (*Journal for Specialists in Pediatric Nursing*)
- Year and month of publication (2013 Jul)
- Volume (18)
- Issue (3)
- Page numbers (189–201)
- Number of cited references (57)

The record also shows the major and minor CINAHL subject headings that were coded for this study. Any of these headings could have been used to retrieve this reference. Note that the subject headings include substantive codes such as *Postoperative Pain*, and also methodologic codes (e.g., *Content Analysis*) and person characteristic codes (e.g., *Child*). Next, the abstract for the study is shown. Based on the abstract, we would decide whether this reference was pertinent. Additional information on the record includes the journal subset, special interest category, and instrumentation. Each entry also shows an accession number that is the unique identifier for each record in the CINAHL database as well as other identifying numbers.

An important feature of CINAHL and other databases is that it allows you to find other relevant references once a good one has been found. In Figure 5.2, you can see that the record offers many embedded links on which you can click. For example, you could click on any of the authors' names to see if they published other related articles. You could also click on subject headings to track down other leads. There is also a link in each record called *Cited References*. By clicking this link, the entire reference list for the record (i.e., all the references cited in the article) would be retrieved, and you could then examine any of the citations. There is also a sidebar link in each record called *Times Cited in this Database*, which would retrieve records for articles that had cited this paper (for a descendancy search), and another link for *Find Similar Results*

Title:	Pediatric nurses' postoperative pain management practices: An observational study.
Authors:	Twycross, Alison; Finley, G. Allen; Latimer, Margot
Affiliation:	Children's Nursing, Faculty of Health, Social Care and Education, Kingston University St George's University of London
Source:	Journal for Specialists in Pediatric Nursing (J SPEC PEDIATR NURS), 2013 Jul; 18(3): 189–201. (57 ref)
Publication Type:	journal article – **research**, tables/charts
Language:	English
Major Subjects:	Postoperative Pain – Nursing – In Infancy and Childhood; Postoperative Pain – Drug Therapy – In Infancy and Childhood; Pediatric Nursing; Nursing Practice; Postoperative Care
Minor Subjects:	Pain Measurement; Surgical Patients; Hospitals, Pediatric; Canada; Participant Observation; Infant, Newborn; Infant; Child, Preschool; Child; Adolescence; Purposive Sample; Field Notes; Registered Nurses; Content Analysis; Thematic Analysis; Clinical Assessment Tools; Scales; Summated Rating Scaling; Nursing Assessment; Nursing Interventions; Analgesics – Administration and Dosage; Cryotherapy; Communication; Parents; Documentation; Pediatric Units; Inpatients; Human; Descriptive Statistics; Patient Satisfaction
Abstract:	Purpose This study was an in-depth examination of pediatric postoperative **pain** care. Design and Methods Participant observational data were collected on the care of 10 **children**. Particular attention was paid to actions when **pain** scores were ≥5 and to the relationship between **pain** scores and medications administered. Results A pattern of care emerged of giving **pain** medications regularly even if they were prescribed pro re nata. Actions when **pain** scores were ≥5 varied. Recorded **pain** scores rarely guided treatment choices. Practice Implications: The use of **pain** scores to guide treatment choices needs further debate. Future **research** should explore the implications of divorcing treatment from **pain** scores on **children's pain** experience.
Journal Subset:	Core nursing; Nursing; Peer reviewed; USA
Special Interest:	Pain and Pain Management; Pediatric Care; Perioperative Care
Instrumentation:	FACES pain scale (FPS)
MEDLINE info:	*PMID: 23822843 NLM UID*: 101142025
Accession No.	2012170940

FIGURE 5.2 Example of a record from a CINAHL search.

that suggests other relevant references. A useful tool in CINAHL appears in the right-hand sidebar: When you click on the *Cite* link, you can retrieve the article's citation format for the American Medical Association or the American Psychological Association, and this information can be exported (e.g., to EndNote or ProCite).

In CINAHL, you can also explore the structure of the database's thesaurus to get additional leads for searching. The toolbar at the top of the screen has a tab called *CINAHL Headings*. When you click on this tab, you can enter a term of interest in the *Browse* field and select one of three options: *Term Begins With*, *Term Contains*, or *Relevance Ranked* (which is the default). For example, if we entered *pain* and then clicked on Browse, we would be shown the 16 major subject headings relating to

pain, and most have several subheadings as well. We could then search the database for any of the listed subject headings.

> **TIP:** Note that the keywords we used to illustrate the search would not be adequate for a comprehensive retrieval of studies relevant to the research problem we identified earlier. For example, we would want to search for such additional terms (e.g., *pediatric*).

The MEDLINE Database
The MEDLINE database was developed by the U.S. National Library of Medicine (NLM) and is widely recognized as the premier source for bibliographic coverage of the biomedical literature.

MEDLINE covers about 5,600 medical, nursing, and health journals published in about 70 countries and contains more than 23 million records dating back to the mid-1940s. In 1999, abstracts of reviews from the Cochrane Collaboration became available through MEDLINE.

The MEDLINE database can be accessed through a commercial vendor, but it can be accessed for free through the PubMed website (http://www.ncbi.nlm.nih.gov/PubMed). This means that anyone, anywhere in the world with Internet access can search for journal articles, and thus, PubMed is a lifelong resource regardless of your institutional affiliation. PubMed has an excellent tutorial.

On the Home page of PubMed, you can launch a basic search that looks for your keyword in text fields of the record. As you begin to enter your keyword in the search box, automatic suggestions will display, and you can click on the one that is the best match.

MEDLINE uses a controlled vocabulary called MeSH (Medical Subject Headings) to index articles. MeSH provides a consistent way to retrieve information that may use different terms for the same concepts. You can learn about relevant MeSH terms by clicking on the "MeSH database" link on the Home page (under *More Resources*). If, for example, we searched the MeSH database for "pain," we would find that Pain is a MeSH subject heading (a definition is provided) and there are 60 additional related categories—for example, "Pain measurement" and "Headache." Each category has numerous subheadings, such as "Complications" and "Etiology."

If you begin using your own keyword in a basic search, you can see how your term mapped onto MeSH terms by scrolling down and looking in the right hand panel for a section labeled *Search Details*. For example, if we entered the keyword "children" in the search field of the initial screen, Search Details would show us that PubMed searched for all references that have "child" or "children" in text fields of the database record, *and* it also searched for all references that had been coded "child" as a subject heading, because "child" is a MeSH subject heading.

If we did a PubMed search of MEDLINE similar to the one we described earlier for CINAHL, we would find that a simple search for *pain* would yield about 565,000 records, and *pain AND child**

AND nurs* would yield about 3,900. We can place restrictions on the search using filters that appear in the left sidebar. If we limited our search to entries with abstracts, written in English, published in 2005 or later, and coded in the Nursing subset, the search would yield about 750 citations. This PubMed search yielded more references than the CINAHL search, but we were not able to limit the search to research reports: PubMed does not have a generic category that distinguishes all research articles from nonresearch articles.

Figure 5.3 shows the full citation for the same study we located earlier in CINAHL. Beneath the abstract, when you click on "MeSH Terms," the display presents the MeSH terms that were used for this particular study. (Those marked with an asterisk indicates that the MeSH subject heading is a major focus of the article.) As you can see, the MeSH terms are different than the subject headings for the same article in CINAHL. As with CINAHL, you can click on highlighted record entries (author names and MeSH terms) for possible leads.

In the right panel of the screen for PubMed records, there is a list of *Related Citations*, which is a useful feature once you have found a study that is a good exemplar of evidence for what you are looking. Further down in the right panel, PubMed provides a list of any articles in the MEDLINE database that had cited this study, which is useful for a descendancy search.

An interesting feature of MEDLINE is that it provides access to new research by including citations to forthcoming articles in many journals. The records for these not-yet-published articles have the tag "Epub ahead of print."

⮕ **TIP:** Searching for qualitative studies can pose special challenges. Wilczynski and colleagues (2007) described optimal search strategies for qualitative studies in the CINAHL database. Flemming and Briggs (2006) compared three alternative strategies for finding qualitative research. Finfgeld-Connett and Johnson (2013) offered search strategies for qualitative systematic reviews.

J Spec Pediatr Nurs. 2013 Jul;18(3):189–201. doi: 10.1111/jspn.12026. Epub 2013 Mar 24.

Pediatric nurses' postoperative pain management practices: an observational study.

Twycross A[1], Finley GA, Latimer M.

Author information: [1]Faculty of Health, Social Care and Education, St George's University of London, London, United Kingdom. a.twycross@sgul.kingston.ac.uk

Abstract:
PURPOSE: This study was an in-depth examination of pediatric postoperative pain care.
DESIGN AND METHODS: Participant observational data were collected on the care of 10 children. Particular attention was paid to actions when pain scores were ≥5 and to the relationship between pain scores and medications administered.
RESULTS: A pattern of care emerged of giving pain medications regularly even if they were prescribed pro re nata. Actions when pain scores were ≥5 varied. Recorded pain scores rarely guided treatment choices.
PRACTICE IMPLICATIONS: The use of pain scores to guide treatment choices needs further debate. Future research should explore the implications of divorcing treatment from pain scores on children's pain experience. © 2013, Wiley Periodicals, Inc.
KEYWORDS: Pain assessment, pediatric pain, postoperative pain

Comment in Our incredible failure to incorporate evidence about pediatric pain management into clinical practice. [J Spec Pediatr Nurs. 2013]

PMID: 23822843 [PubMed - indexed for MEDLINE]

Publication Types, MeSH Terms, Substances
Publication Types Research Support, Non–U.S. Gov't

MeSH Terms
- Adolescent
- Analgesics/therapeutic use*
- Child
- Child, Hospitalized
- Child, Preschool
- Female
- Humans
- Infant
- Infant, Newborn
- Male
- Pain Measurement/nursing*
- Pain, Postoperative/drug therapy*
- Pain, Postoperative/nursing*
- Pediatric Nursing/methods*

Substances Analgesics

FIGURE 5.3 Example of a record from a PubMed search.

Google Scholar

Google Scholar (GS) has become an increasingly popular bibliographic search engine that was launched in 2004. Google Scholar includes articles in journals from scholarly publishers in all disciplines and also includes scholarly books, technical reports, and other documents. A powerful advantage of GS is that it is accessible free of charge over the Internet. Like other bibliographic search engines, GS allows users to search by topic, by a title, and by author, and uses Boolean operators and other search conventions. Also like PubMed and CINAHL, GS has a *Cited By* feature for a descendancy search and a *Related Articles* feature to locate other sources with relevant content to an identified article. Because of its expanded coverage of material, GS can provide greater access to free full-text publications.

Unlike other scholarly databases, GS does not allow users to order retrieved references by publication date. The reference list ordering in GS is determined by an algorithm that puts most weight on the number of times a reference has been cited—and this in turn means that older references are usually earlier on the list. Another disadvantage of GS is that the ability to impose search limits and search filters is limited.

In the field of medicine, GS has generated considerable controversy, with some arguing that it is of similar utility and quality to popular medical databases (Gehanno et al., 2013), and others urging caution in depending primarily on GS (e.g., Boeker et al., 2013; Bramer et al., 2013). Some have found that for quick clinical searches, GS returns more citations than PubMed (Shariff et al., 2013). The capabilities and features of Google Scholar may improve in the years ahead, but at the moment, it may be risky to depend on GS exclusively. For a full literature review, we think it is best to combine searches using GS with searches of other databases.

Screening and Gathering References

References that have been identified through a literature search need to be screened. By perusing the abstract, one can usually come to some conclusions about its relevance for a review. When there is no abstract, article titles may be insufficiently informative—it may be necessary to screen the full article. During the screening, keep in mind that some articles judged to be not relevant for your primary question may be useful for a secondary question.

The next step is to retrieve the references that you think may have potential value for your review. If you are affiliated with a large institution, you may have online access to most full-text articles. If you are not so fortunate, more effort will be required to obtain the articles. One possibility is to copy the article from a hard copy of a journal in a library, and another is to request a copy through an interlibrary loan.

The **open-access journal** movement is gaining momentum in health care publishing. Open-access journals provide articles free of charge online.

Some journals have a hybrid format in which most articles are not open-access, but individual articles can be designated as open-access (usually through the payment of a fee by authors or their institutions). Bibliographic databases indicate which articles can be accessed, and this can be accomplished simply by clicking on a link. (In PubMed, the link to click on states "Free Article.")

TIP: We provide links to open-access articles with content relevant to each chapter of this book in the Toolkit section of the accompanying *Resource Manual.*

When an article is not freely available online, you may be able to access it by communicating with the lead author. Bibliographic databases often provide an e-mail address for the lead author and their institutional affiliation. Another alternative is to go to websites such as *ResearchGate* (www.researchgate.net) and do a search for a particular author. Authors sometimes upload articles onto their profile for access by others. If an article has not been uploaded, ResearchGate provides a mechanism for you to send the author a message.

Most articles for your review will likely be retrieved electronically. It is a good idea to put all articles into a designated document folder and to give each article file a name that makes it easy to find. For example, for the article shown in Figures 5.2 and 5.3, the file name could be Twycross_2013_JSPN.pdf. This file name indicates the first author, year of publication, and an acronym for the journal. This system would result in a document folder with articles listed alphabetically by the first authors' last names. For simple reviews, reading each article on a computer screen may suffice, but for more complex reviews that involve a coding scheme, printing a copy of the article is usually useful.

Documentation in Literature Retrieval

If your goal is to "own" the literature, you will be using a variety of databases, keywords, subject headings, and strategies in an effort to pursue all leads. As you meander through the complex world of research information, you will likely lose track of your efforts if you do not document your actions from the outset.

It is highly advisable to use a notebook (or a spreadsheet) to record your search strategies and search results. You should make note of information such as databases searched; limits put on your search; specific keywords, subject headings, or authors used to direct the search; studies used to inaugurate a "Related Articles" or "descendancy" search; websites visited; links pursued; authors contacted to request further information or copies of articles not readily available; and any other information that would help you keep track of what you have done. Part of your strategy usually can be documented by printing your search history from bibliographic databases.

By documenting your actions, you will be able to conduct a more efficient search—that is, you will not inadvertently duplicate a strategy you have already pursued. Documentation will also help you to assess what else needs to be tried—where to go next in your search. Finally, documenting your efforts is a step in ensuring that your literature review is reproducible.

➔ **TIP:** The Toolkit section of the accompanying *Resource Manual* offers a template for documenting certain types of information during a literature search. The template, as a Word document, can easily be augmented and adapted.

ABSTRACTING AND RECORDING INFORMATION

Tracking down relevant research on a topic is only the beginning of doing a literature review. Once you have a set of useful articles, you need to develop a strategy for making sense of the information in them. If a literature review is fairly simple, it may be sufficient to jot down notes about key features of the studies under review and to use these notes as the basis for your analysis. However, literature reviews are often complex—for example, there may be dozens of studies, or study findings may vary. In such situations, it is useful to adopt a system of recording

key information about each study. One mechanism for doing this is to use a formal protocol and another is to create matrices. First, though, we discuss the advantages of developing a coding scheme.

Coding the Studies

Reviewers who undertake systematic reviews usually develop coding systems to support statistical analyses. Coding may not be necessary in less formal reviews, but we do think that coding can be useful, and so we offer some a few suggestions and an example.

To develop a coding scheme, you need to read a subset of studies and look for opportunities to categorize information. One approach is to code the findings for key variables or themes. Let us take the example we have used in this chapter, the relationship between factors affecting nurses' management of children's pain (independent variables) on the one hand and nurses' actual pain management behaviors (dependent variables) on the other. By perusing the articles we retrieved, we find that several factors have been studied—for example, nurses' knowledge about children's pain management, their attitudes about pain, organizational factors, and so on. We can assign codes to each factor. With regard to the dependent variable, we find that some studies have focused on nurses' pain assessment, whereas others have studied nurses' use of analgesia, and so on. These different outcomes can also be coded. An example of a simple coding scheme is presented in Box 5.1.

The codes can then be applied to each study. You can record these codes in a protocol or on a matrix (which we discuss next), but it is useful to note the codes in the margins of the articles themselves, so you can easily find the information. Figure 5.4, which presents an excerpt from the results section of a study by Twycross and Collins (2013), shows marginal coding of key variables.

Coding can be a useful organizational tool even when a review is focused. For example, if our research question was about nurses' use of nonpharmacologic methods of pain treatment (i.e., not about use of analgesics or pain assessment), the outcome categories might be specific nonpharmacologic approaches, such as distraction, guided imagery, massage, and so on. The point is to organize

---

BOX 5.1 Substantive Codes for a Review on Factors Affecting Nurses' Management of Children's Pain

CODES FOR FACTORS AFFECTING NURSES' PAIN MANAGEMENT BEHAVIOR
1. Nurses' pain knowledge/years of nursing experience
2. Nurses' pain attitudes and perceptions
3. Demographic nurse factors (e.g., age, education, number of own children)
4. Other nurse factors (e.g., self-efficacy, personal experience with pain)
5. Organizational factors (e.g., nurses' workload, organizational culture)
6. Specific interventions to improve nurses' pain management behavior
7. Other factors (e.g., physician factors, parental complaints)

CODES FOR NURSES' PAIN MANAGEMENT BEHAVIOR
A. Nurses' assessment of children's pain
B. Nurses' use of pain reducing strategies/ability to overcome barriers
   a. Use of analgesics
   b. Use of nonpharmacologic methods
C. Provision of information to parents about managing their child's pain

---

information in a way that facilitates retrieval and analysis. Further guidance on coding is offered in the Supplement to this chapter.

Literature Review Protocols

One method of organizing information from research articles is to complete a formal protocol for each relevant reference, either in writing or in a word processing file. Protocols are a means of summarizing key aspects of a study systematically, including the full citation, theoretical foundations, methodologic features, findings, and conclusions. Evaluative information (e.g., your assessment of the study's strengths and weaknesses) can be noted. The study abstract can be attached to the protocol (e.g., copied and pasted from the bibliographic database onto the back of the protocol) for easy review.

There is no fixed format for such a protocol—you must decide what elements are important to record *consistently* across studies to help you organize and analyze information. Figure 5.5 provides an example that can be adapted to fit your needs. (Although many terms on this protocol may not be familiar to you yet, you will learn about them in later chapters.) If you developed a coding scheme, you can use the codes to record information about study variables rather than writing out their names. By using codes, it is easier to retrieve all the articles with a certain code—for example, all articles about

---

More than one-half of the parents remembered their child having a pain history taken on admission, with just over one-half indicating that their child had used a pain assessment tool. Nonpharmacologic methods of pain relief were recommended to only 19% of children. Most parents felt that they and their child were asked about pain and had ways of relieving pain discussed with them the right amount of time.   *A*
    B.b
    C

Excerpt from Twycross & Collins (2013), p. e210.
*Codes in margin are shown in Box 5.1.

FIGURE 5.4 Coded excerpt from the results section of a research article: nurses' management of children's pain example.

Citation	Authors: _____ Title: _____ Journal: _____ Year: _____ Volume: _____ Issue: _____ Pages: _____
Type of Study:	☐ Quantitative ☐ Qualitative ☐ Mixed Method
Location/setting:	_____ ☐ Multi-site
Key Concepts/ Variables (or Codes):	Concepts: _____ Intervention/Independent Variable(s): _____ Dependent Variable(s): _____ Controlled Variable(s): _____
Framework/Theory:	_____
Quant. Design:	☐ Experimental ☐ Quasi-experimental ☐ Nonexperimental Specific Design: _____ Blinding? ☐ None ☐ Yes: Who? _____ Description of Intervention: _____ _____ _____ Comparison group(s): _____ ☐ Cross-sectional ☐ Longitudinal/prospective No. of data collection points: ___ Rate of refusal/nonparticipation: _____ % Rate of attrition: _____ %
Qual. Tradition:	☐ Grounded theory ☐ Phenomenology ☐ Ethnography ☐ Descriptive ☐ Other: _____
Sample:	Size: _____ Sampling method: _____ Sample characteristics: _____
Data Sources:	Type: ☐ Self-report ☐ Observational ☐ Biophysiologic ☐ Other_____ Description of measures: _____ _____ Data Quality: _____
Statistical Tests:	Bivariate (e.g., *t*-test, ANOVA, Pearson's *r*): _____ Multivariate (e.g., multiple regression, logistic regression): _____
Findings/Themes/ Effect Sizes	_____ _____ _____ _____
Conclusions:	_____ _____
Strengths:	_____ _____
Weaknesses:	_____ _____

FIGURE 5.5 Example of a literature review protocol.

nurses' pain knowledge or experience. Once you have developed a draft protocol, you should pilot test it with several studies to make sure it is sufficiently comprehensive.

Literature Review Matrices

For traditional narrative reviews of the literature, we prefer using two-dimensional matrices to organize information because matrices directly support a thematic analysis of the retrieved evidence. In a matrix, reviewers put each study on a row and all other pertinent information—about methods, results, and so on—into the columns. The Supplement to this chapter on thePoint® provides guidance about the use of literature review matrices together with examples. 🅢

CRITIQUING STUDIES AND EVALUATING THE EVIDENCE

In drawing conclusions about a body of research, reviewers must record not only factual information about studies—methodologic features and findings—but must also make judgments about the worth of the evidence. This section discusses issues relating to research critiques.

Research Critiques of Individual Studies

A research **critique** is an appraisal of the strengths and weaknesses of a study. A good critique identifies areas of adequacy and inadequacy in an unbiased manner. Although this chapter emphasizes the evaluation of a body of research evidence for a literature review, we pause to offer advice about other types of critiques.

Many critiques focus on a single study. For example, most journals that publish research articles have a policy of soliciting critiques by two or more **peer reviewers** who prepare written critiques and make recommendations about whether or not to publish a manuscript. Peer reviewers' critiques typically are brief and focus on key substantive and methodologic issues. Note that peer-reviewed journals are held in higher esteem than journals that publish without peer review.

Students taking a research course may be asked to critique a study to document their mastery of

methodologic concepts. Such critiques usually are expected to be comprehensive, encompassing various dimensions of a report, including substantive and theoretical aspects, ethical issues, methodologic decisions, interpretation, and the report's presentation. The purpose of such a thorough critique is to cultivate critical thinking, to induce students to apply new research skills, and to prepare students for a professional nursing career in which evaluating research may play a role.

We provide support for comprehensive critiques of individual studies in several ways. First, critiquing suggestions corresponding to chapter content are included at the end of most chapters. We also offer key critiquing questions for quantitative and qualitative reports here in this chapter, in Boxes 5.2 ✖ and 5.3 ✖, respectively. Finally, it can be illuminating to have a good model, and so Appendix H and I of the accompanying *Resource Manual* include comprehensive research critiques of a quantitative and a mixed methods study.

➲ **TIP:** For mixed methods studies that include both quantitative and qualitative components, questions from Boxes 5.2 *and* 5.3 can be used. Additional critiquing guidelines for mixed methods studies are offered in Chapter 26.

The questions in Boxes 5.2 and 5.3 are organized according to the structure of most research articles—Abstract, Introduction, Method, Results, and Discussion. The second column lists key critiquing questions, and the third column cross-references the detailed guidelines in other chapters. Many critiquing questions are likely too difficult for you to answer at this point, but your methodologic and critiquing skills will develop as you progress through this book.

A few comments about these guidelines are in order. First, the questions call for a yes or no answer (although for some, the answer may be "Yes, *but* . . . "). In all cases, the desirable answer is "yes." That is, a "no" suggests a possible limitation and a "yes" suggests a strength. Therefore, the more "yeses" a study gets, the stronger it is likely to be. These guidelines can thus cumulatively suggest

BOX 5.2 Guide to an Overall Critique of a Quantitative Research Report

Aspect of the Report	Critiquing Questions	Detailed Critiquing Guidelines
Title	• Is the title a good one, succinctly suggesting key variables and the study population?	
Abstract	• Did the abstract clearly and concisely summarize the main features of the report (problem, methods, results, conclusions)?	
Introduction		
Statement of the problem	• Was the problem stated unambiguously, and was it easy to identify? • Is the problem significant for nursing? • Did the problem statement build a persuasive argument for the new study? • Was there a good match between the research problem and the methods used—that is, was a quantitative approach appropriate?	Box 4.3, page 84
Hypotheses or research questions	• Were research questions and/or hypotheses explicitly stated? If not, was their absence justified? • Were questions and hypotheses appropriately worded, with clear specification of key variables and the study population? • Were the questions/hypotheses consistent with existing knowledge?	Box 4.3, page 84
Literature review	• Was the literature review up-to-date and based mainly on primary sources? • Did the review provide a state-of-the-art synthesis of evidence on the problem? • Did the literature review provide a strong basis for the new study?	Box 5.4, page 113
Conceptual/theoretical framework	• Were key concepts adequately defined conceptually? • Was a conceptual/theoretical framework articulated—and, if so, was it appropriate? If not, is the absence of a framework justified? • Were the questions/hypotheses consistent with the framework?	Box 6.2, page 132
Method		
Protection of human rights	• Were appropriate procedures used to safeguard the rights of study participants? • Was the study externally reviewed by an IRB/ethics review board? • Was the study designed to minimize risks and maximize benefits to participants?	Box 7.3, page 154

BOX 5.2 Guide to an Overall Critique of a Quantitative Research Report (continued)

Aspect of the Report	Critiquing Questions	Detailed Critiquing Guidelines
Research design	• Was the most rigorous design used, given the study purpose? • Were appropriate comparisons made to enhance interpretability of the findings? • Was the number of data collection points appropriate? • Did the design minimize biases and threats to the internal, construct, and external validity of the study (e.g., was blinding used, was attrition minimized)?	Box 9.1, page 210; Box 10.1, page 232
Population and sample	• Was the population identified? Was the sample described in sufficient detail? • Was the best possible sampling design used to enhance the sample's representativeness? Were sampling biases minimized? • Was the sample size adequate? Was the sample size based on a power analysis?	Box 12.1, page 263
Data collection and measurement	• Were the operational and conceptual definitions congruent? • Were key variables measured using an appropriate method (e.g., interviews, observations, and so on)? • Were specific instruments adequately described and were they good choices, given the study population and the variables being studied? • Did the report provide evidence that the data collection methods yielded data that were reliable, valid, and responsive?	Box 13.1, page 279; Box 14.1, page 325
Procedures	• If there was an intervention, was it adequately described, and was it rigorously developed and implemented? Did most participants allocated to the intervention group actually receive it? Was there evidence of intervention fidelity? • Were data collected in a manner that minimized bias? Were the staff who collected data appropriately trained?	Box 9.1, page 210; Box 10.1, page 232

(box continues on page 104)

BOX 5.2 Guide to an Overall Critique of a Quantitative Research Report (continued)

Aspect of the Report	Critiquing Questions	Detailed Critiquing Guidelines
Results		
Data analysis	• Were analyses undertaken to address each research question or test each hypothesis? • Were appropriate statistical methods used, given the level of measurement of the variables, number of groups being compared, and assumptions of the tests? • Was a powerful analytic method used? (e.g., did the analysis help to control for confounding variables)? • Were Type I and Type II errors avoided or minimized? • In intervention studies, was an intention-to-treat analysis performed? • Were problems of missing values evaluated and adequately addressed?	Box 16.1, page 371; Box 17.1, page 399
Findings	• Was information about statistical significance presented? Was information about effect size and precision of estimates (confidence intervals) presented? • Were the findings adequately summarized, with good use of tables and figures? • Were findings reported in a manner that facilitates a meta-analysis, and with sufficient information needed for EBP?	Box 17.1, page 399; Box 28.1, page 641
Discussion		
Interpretation of the findings	• Were all major findings interpreted and discussed within the context of prior research and/or the study's conceptual framework? • Were causal inferences, if any, justified? • Was the issue of clinical significance discussed? • Were interpretations well-founded and consistent with the study's limitations? • Did the report address the issue of the generalizability of the findings?	Box 20.1, page 457
Implications/ recommendations	• Did the researchers discuss the implications of the study for clinical practice or further research—and were those implications reasonable and complete?	Box 20.1, page 457

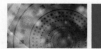

BOX 5.2 Guide to an Overall Critique of a Quantitative Research
Report (continued)

Aspect of the Report	Critiquing Questions	Detailed Critiquing Guidelines
General Issues		
Presentation	• Was the report well-written, organized, and sufficiently detailed for critical analysis? • In intervention studies, was a CONSORT flowchart provided to show the flow of participants in the study? • Was the report written in a manner that makes the findings accessible to practicing nurses?	Box 30.2, page 696
Researcher credibility	• Do the researchers' clinical, substantive, or methodologic qualifications and experience enhance confidence in the findings and their interpretation?	
Summary assessment	• Despite any limitations, do the study findings appear to be valid—do you have confidence in the *truth* value of the results? • Does the study contribute any meaningful evidence that can be used in nursing practice or that is useful to the nursing discipline?	

a global assessment: A report with 25 "yeses" is likely to be superior to one with only 10. Not all "yeses" are equal, however. Some elements are more important in drawing conclusions about study rigor than others. For example, the inadequacy of the article's literature review is less damaging to the worth of the study's *evidence* than the use of a faulty design. In general, questions about methodologic decisions (i.e., the questions under "Method") and about the analysis are especially important in evaluating the quality of the study's evidence.

Although the questions in these boxes elicit yes or no responses, a comprehensive critique would do more than point out what the researchers did and did not do. Each criticism should be explained and justified. For example, if you answered "no" to the question about whether a rigorous design was used, you would need to describe your concerns and suggest a stronger alternative.

Our simplified critiquing guidelines have a number of shortcomings. In particular, they are generic despite the fact that critiquing cannot use a one-size-fits-all list of questions. Some critiquing questions that are relevant to, say, clinical trials do not make sense for all quantitative studies. Thus, you need to use some judgment about whether the guidelines are sufficiently comprehensive for the type of study you are critiquing and perhaps supplement them with some of the critiquing questions from other chapters of this book.

Finally, there are questions in these guidelines for which there are no objective answers. Even experts sometimes disagree about what are the best methodologic strategies for a study. You should not be afraid to express an evaluative opinion—but be sure that your comments have some basis in methodologic principles discussed in this book.

Evaluating a Body of Research

In reviewing the literature, you would not undertake a *comprehensive* critique of each study—but

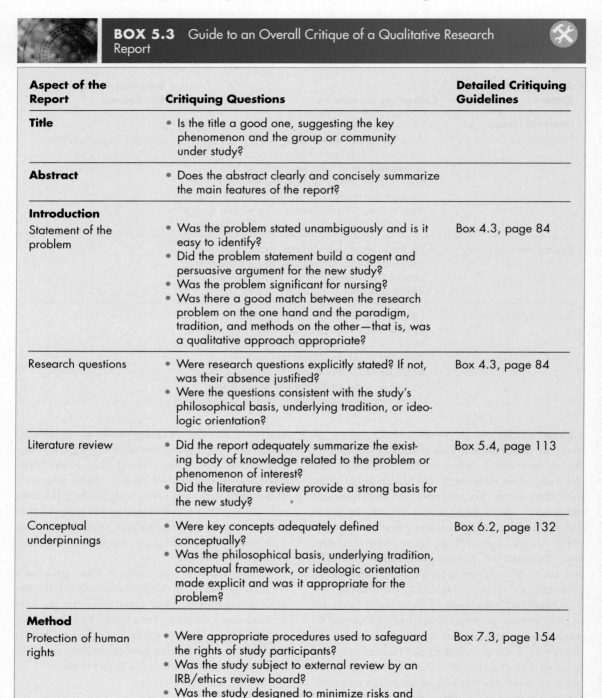

BOX 5.3 Guide to an Overall Critique of a Qualitative Research Report

Aspect of the Report	Critiquing Questions	Detailed Critiquing Guidelines
Title	• Is the title a good one, suggesting the key phenomenon and the group or community under study?	
Abstract	• Does the abstract clearly and concisely summarize the main features of the report?	
Introduction Statement of the problem	• Was the problem stated unambiguously and is it easy to identify? • Did the problem statement build a cogent and persuasive argument for the new study? • Was the problem significant for nursing? • Was there a good match between the research problem on the one hand and the paradigm, tradition, and methods on the other—that is, was a qualitative approach appropriate?	Box 4.3, page 84
Research questions	• Were research questions explicitly stated? If not, was their absence justified? • Were the questions consistent with the study's philosophical basis, underlying tradition, or ideologic orientation?	Box 4.3, page 84
Literature review	• Did the report adequately summarize the existing body of knowledge related to the problem or phenomenon of interest? • Did the literature review provide a strong basis for the new study?	Box 5.4, page 113
Conceptual underpinnings	• Were key concepts adequately defined conceptually? • Was the philosophical basis, underlying tradition, conceptual framework, or ideologic orientation made explicit and was it appropriate for the problem?	Box 6.2, page 132
Method Protection of human rights	• Were appropriate procedures used to safeguard the rights of study participants? • Was the study subject to external review by an IRB/ethics review board? • Was the study designed to minimize risks and maximize benefits to participants?	Box 7.3, page 154

BOX 5.3   Guide to an Overall Critique of a Qualitative Research Report (continued)

Aspect of the Report	Critiquing Questions	Detailed Critiquing Guidelines
Research design and research tradition	• Was the identified research tradition (if any) congruent with the methods used to collect and analyze data? • Was an adequate amount of time spent with study participants? • Did the design unfold during data collection, giving researchers opportunities to capitalize on early understandings? • Was there an adequate number of contacts with study participants?	Box 21.1, page 483
Sample and setting	• Was the group or population of interest adequately described? Were the setting and sample described in sufficient detail? • Was the approach used to recruit participants or gain access to the site productive and appropriate? • Was the best possible method of sampling used to enhance information richness and address the needs of the study? • Was the sample size adequate? Was saturation achieved?	Box 22.1, page 501
Data collection	• Were the methods of gathering data appropriate? Were data gathered through two or more methods to achieve triangulation? • Did the researcher ask the right questions or make the right observations, and were they recorded in an appropriate fashion? • Was a sufficient amount of data gathered? Were the data of sufficient depth and richness?	Box 23.1, page 521
Procedures	• Were data collection and recording procedures adequately described and do they appear appropriate? • Were data collected in a manner that minimized bias? Were the staff who collected data appropriately trained?	Box 23.1, page 521

(box continues on page 108)

BOX 5.3 Guide to an Overall Critique of a Qualitative Research Report (continued)

Aspect of the Report	Critiquing Questions	Detailed Critiquing Guidelines
Enhancement of trustworthiness	• Did the researchers use effective strategies to enhance the trustworthiness/integrity of the study, and was there a good description of those strategies? • Were the methods used to enhance trustworthiness adequate? • Did the researcher document research procedures and decision processes sufficiently that findings are auditable and confirmable? • Was there evidence of researcher reflexivity? • Was there "thick description" of the context, participants, and findings, and was it at a sufficient level to support transferability?	Box 25.1, page 571; Table 25.1, page 562
Results Data analysis	• Were the data management and data analysis methods adequately described? • Was the data analysis strategy compatible with the research tradition and with the nature and type of data gathered? • Did the analysis yield an appropriate "product" (e.g., a theory, taxonomy, thematic pattern)? • Did the analytic procedures suggest the possibility of biases?	Box 24.1, page 532
Findings	• Were the findings effectively summarized, with good use of excerpts and supporting arguments? • Did the themes adequately capture the meaning of the data? Does it appear that the researcher satisfactorily conceptualized the themes or patterns in the data? • Did the analysis yield an insightful, provocative, authentic, and meaningful picture of the phenomenon under investigation?	Box 24.1, page 532
Theoretical integration	• Were the themes or patterns logically connected to each other to form a convincing and integrated whole? • Were figures, maps, or models used effectively to summarize conceptualizations? • If a conceptual framework or ideologic orientation guided the study, were the themes or patterns linked to it in a cogent manner?	Box 24.1 page 532; Box 6.2, page 132

BOX 5.3 Guide to an Overall Critique of a Qualitative Research Report (continued)

Aspect of the Report	Critiquing Questions	Detailed Critiquing Guidelines
Discussion		
Interpretation of the findings	• Were the findings interpreted within an appropriate social or cultural context? • Were major findings interpreted and discussed within the context of prior studies? • Were the interpretations consistent with the study's limitations?	Box 24.1, page 532
Implications/ recommendations	• Did the researchers discuss the implications of the study for clinical practice or further research—and were those implications reasonable and complete?	
General Issues		
Presentation	• Was the report well-written, organized, and sufficiently detailed for critical analysis? • Was the description of the methods, findings, and interpretations sufficiently rich and vivid?	Box 30.2, page 696
Researcher credibility	• Do the researchers' clinical, substantive, or methodologic qualifications and experience enhance confidence in the findings and their interpretation?	
Summary assessment	• Do the study findings appear to be trustworthy—do you have confidence in the *truth* value of the results? • Does the study contribute any meaningful evidence that can be used in nursing practice or that is useful to the nursing discipline?	

you would need to assess the quality of evidence in each study so that you could draw conclusions about the overall body of evidence. Critiques for a literature review tend to focus on the methodologic strengths and weaknesses of key studies, often the ones that are recent.

TIP: In systematic reviews, methodologic quality sometimes plays a role in study selection—that is, investigations judged to be of low quality may be screened out of the review. Using methodologic quality as a screening criterion is controversial, however, as discussed in Chapter 29.

In preparing a literature review for a new primary study, methodologic features of studies under review need to be assessed with an eye to answering a broad question: To what extent do the cumulative findings accurately reflect the *truth* or, conversely, to what extent do methodologic flaws undermine the believability of the evidence? The "truth" is most likely to be revealed when researchers use powerful designs, good sampling plans, strong data collection instruments and procedures, and appropriate analyses.

The use of literature review matrices, as described in the chapter Supplement ⓢ, supports the analysis of multiple studies. For example, if there is a column for sample size in the matrix,

TABLE 5.1 • Thematic Possibilities for a Literature Review

TYPE OF THEME	QUESTIONS FOR THEMATIC ANALYSIS
Substantive	What is the pattern of evidence? How much evidence is there? How consistent is the body of evidence? How powerful are the observed effects? How persuasive is the evidence? What gaps are there in the body of evidence?
Theoretical	What theoretical or conceptual frameworks have been used to address the primary question—or has most research been atheoretical? How congruent are the theoretical frameworks? Do findings vary in relation to differences in frameworks?
Generalizability/ Transferability	To what types of people or settings do the findings apply? Do the findings vary for different types of people (e.g., men versus women) or setting (e.g., urban versus rural)?
Historical	Have there been substantive, theoretical, or methodologic trends over time? Is the evidence getting better? When was most of the research conducted?
Researcher	Who has been doing the research, in terms of discipline, specialty area, nationality, prominence, and so on? Has the research been developed within a systematic program of research?

one could readily see at a glance that, for example, much of the evidence is from studies with a small sample size.

ANALYZING AND SYNTHESIZING INFORMATION

Once all the relevant studies have been retrieved, read, abstracted, and critiqued, the information has to be analyzed and synthesized. As previously noted, doing a literature review is similar to doing a qualitative study, particularly with respect to the analysis of the "data" (i.e., information from the retrieved studies). In both, the focus is on identifying important *themes*.

A thematic analysis essentially involves detecting patterns and regularities as well as inconsistencies and gaps. Several different types of themes can be identified, as described in Table 5.1. The reason we recommend using literature review matrices can be seen by reading the list of possible themes: It is easier to discern patterns by reading down the columns of the matrices than by flipping through

a stack of review protocols or skimming through articles.

Clearly, it is not possible—even in lengthy free-standing reviews—to analyze all the themes in Table 5.1. Reviewers have to make decisions about which patterns to pursue. In preparing a review as part of a new study, you would need to determine which pattern is of greatest relevance for developing an argument and providing a context for the new research.

PREPARING A WRITTEN LITERATURE REVIEW

Writing literature reviews can be challenging, especially when voluminous information must be condensed into a small number of pages, as is typical for a journal article or proposal. We offer a few suggestions, but acknowledge that skills in writing literature reviews develop over time.

Organizing the Review

Organization is crucial in a written review. Having an outline helps to structure the flow of presentation.

If the review is complex, a written outline is recommended. The outline should list the main topics or themes to be discussed and indicate the order of presentation. The important point is to have a plan before starting to write so that the review has a coherent flow. The goal is to structure the review in such a way that the presentation is logical, demonstrates meaningful thematic integration, and leads to a conclusion about the state of evidence on the topic.

Writing a Literature Review

Although it is beyond the scope of this book to offer detailed guidance on writing research reviews, we offer a few comments on their content and style. Additional assistance is provided in books such as the ones by Fink (2014) and Galvan (2012).

Content of the Written Literature Review

A written research review should provide readers with an objective, organized synthesis of evidence on a topic. A review should be neither a series of quotes nor a series of abstracts. The central tasks are to summarize and critically evaluate the overall evidence so as to reveal the current state of knowledge—not simply to describe what researchers have done.

Although key studies may be described in some detail, it is not necessary to provide particulars for every reference, especially when there are page constraints. Studies with comparable findings often are summarized together.

Example of Grouped Studies: Pinto and colleagues (2015) summarized findings from several studies in their introduction to a study of health-related quality of life and psychological well-being in patients with benign prostatic hyperplasia (BPH). Here is one excerpt: "Previous studies have consistently reported on the negative impact of LUTS (lower urinary tract symptoms) on the health-related quality of life (HRQoL) of men with BPH (Garraway & Kirby, 1994; Girman et al., 1994; Sagnier et al., 1995; Peters et al., 1997; Eckhardt et al., 2001; Van Dijk et al., 2009)" (p. 513).

The review should demonstrate that you have considered the cumulative worth of the body of research. The review should be objective to the extent possible. Studies that are at odds with your

hypotheses should not be omitted, and the review should not ignore a study because its findings contradict other studies. Inconsistent results should be analyzed and the supporting evidence evaluated objectively.

A literature review typically concludes with a concise summary of evidence on the topic and gaps in the evidence. If the review is conducted for a new study, this critical summary should demonstrate the need for the research and should clarify the basis for any hypotheses.

TIP: As you progress through this book, you will acquire proficiency in critically evaluating studies. We hope you will understand the *mechanics* of doing a review after reading this chapter, but we do not expect you to be able to write a state-of-the-art review until you have gained more skills in research methods.

Style of a Research Review

Students preparing their first written research review often struggle with stylistic issues. Students sometimes accept research findings uncritically, perhaps reflecting a common misunderstanding about the conclusiveness of research. You should keep in mind that hypotheses cannot be proved or disproved by empirical testing, and no research question can be answered definitely in a single study. The issue is partly semantic: Hypotheses are not proved; they are *supported* by research findings. Research reviews should be written in a style that suggests tentativeness.

TIP: When describing study findings, you can use phrases indicating that results may not be definitive, such as the following:

- Several studies have *found* . . .
- Findings thus far *suggest* . . .
- The data *supported* the hypothesis that . . .
- There *appears* to be good evidence that . . .

A related stylistic problem is the interjection of opinions into the review. The review should include

TABLE 5.2 • Examples of Stylistic Difficulties for Research Literature Reviews

PROBLEMATIC STYLE OR WORDING	IMPROVED STYLE OR WORDING
Women who do not participate in childbirth preparation classes manifest a high degree of anxiety during labor.	*Studies have found that* women who participate in childbirth preparation classes *tend to* manifest less anxiety than those who do not (Franck, 2013; Matthiesen, 2015; Yepsen, 2014).
Studies have proved that doctors and nurses do not fully understand the psychobiologic dynamics of recovery from a myocardial infarction.	Studies by Fortune (2015) and Crampton (2012) *suggest that many* doctors and nurses do not fully understand the psychobiologic dynamics of recovery from a myocardial infarction.
Attitudes cannot be changed quickly.	Attitudes *have been found to be* relatively stable, enduring attributes that do not change quickly (Nicolet, 2013; Brusser & Lace, 2011).
It is known that uncertainty engenders stress.	*According to* Dr. A. Cassard (2015), an international expert on stress and anxiety, uncertainty is a major stressor.

Note. Italicized words in the improved version indicate key alternations. All citations are fictitious.

opinions sparingly and should be explicit about their source. Reviewers' opinions do not belong in a literature review, except for assessments of study quality.

The left-hand column of Table 5.2 presents several examples of stylistic flaws for a review. The right-hand column offers suggested rewordings that are more acceptable for a research literature review. Many alternative wordings are possible.

CRITIQUING RESEARCH LITERATURE REVIEWS

We conclude this chapter with some advice about critiquing a literature review written by another person. It is often difficult to critique a research review because the author is almost invariably more knowledgeable about the topic than the readers. It is thus not usually possible to judge whether the author has included all relevant literature and has adequately summarized evidence on that topic—although you may have suspicions that the review is deficient if none of the citations are to recent papers. Several aspects of a review, however, are

amenable to evaluation by readers who are not experts on the topic. Some suggestions for critiquing written research reviews are presented in Box 5.4. (These questions could be used to review your own literature review as well.) When a review is published as a stand-alone article, it should include information to help readers evaluate the author's search strategies, as we discuss in Chapter 29.

In assessing a literature review, the key question is whether it summarizes the current state of research evidence adequately. If the review is written as part of an original research report, an equally important question is whether the review lays a solid foundation for the new study.

RESEARCH EXAMPLES OF LITERATURE REVIEWS

The best way to learn about the style and organization of a research literature review is to read reviews

> **BOX 5.4** Guidelines for Critiquing Literature Reviews
>
> 1. Is the review thorough—does it include all major studies on the topic? Does it include *recent* research (studies published within previous 2–3 years)? Are studies from other related disciplines included, if appropriate?
> 2. Does the review rely mainly on primary source research articles? Are the articles from peer-reviewed journals?
> 3. Is the review merely a summary of existing work, or does it critically appraise and compare key studies? Does the review identify important gaps in the literature?
> 4. Is the review well organized? Is the development of ideas clear?
> 5. Does the review use appropriate language, suggesting the tentativeness of prior findings? Is the review objective? Does the author paraphrase, or is there an overreliance on quotes from original sources?
> 6. If the review is part of a research report for a new study, does the review support the need for the study?
> 7. If it is a review designed to summarize evidence for clinical practice, does the review draw reasonable conclusions about practice implications?

in nursing journals. We present excerpts from two reviews that were in the introduction to a report for an original study. We urge you to read others on a topic of interest to you.[†]

Literature Review from a Quantitative Research Report

Study: Sleep in persons with frontotemporal dementia and their family caregivers (Merrilees et al., 2014)

Statement of Purpose: The purpose of this study was to characterize sleep (using actigraphy and subjective assessments) in patients with mild to moderate frontotemporal dementia and their family caregivers.

Literature Review (Excerpt): "The neurological deterioration associated with dementia contributes to disturbances in nighttime behavior and sleep. Disrupted nighttime sleep occurs in many types of dementia. In Alzheimer's disease (AD), such disruptions include insomnia, frequent nighttime awakenings, decreased total nighttime sleep, increased daytime sleep, and evening agitation (Dowling et al., 2005). Nighttime sleep disruption is even more common in dementia with Lewy bodies (DLB) compared to AD. Patients with DLB suffer more movement disorders during sleep and more daytime sleepiness (Bliwise et al., 2011). Patients with vascular dementia experience

disruption in sleep–wake cycles and decreased sleep efficiency (Aharon-Peretz et al., 1991). Nighttime sleep disruption is difficult to treat and pharmacological management is associated with negative side effects (McCurry & Ancoli-Israel, 2003).

Much less is known about sleep in frontotemporal dementia (FTD). FTD refers to a range of neurodegenerative disorders characterized by focal atrophy of the frontal and/or anterior temporal lobes of the brain, resulting in profound behavioral, cognitive, and emotional symptoms (Brun, 1987; Neary et al., 1998; Rosen et al., 2005). Two subtypes of FTD include the behavioral variant (bvFTD) and semantic dementia (SD). Sleep disruption, characterized by increased nocturnal activity, decreased morning activity, and excessive daytime sleepiness, have been reported, but not well characterized, in FTD (Anderson, Hatfield, Kipps, Hastings, & Hodges, 2009; Harper et al., 2001; Merrilees, Hubbard, Mastick, Miller, & Dowling, 2009).

Sleep is an important issue for the family members who care for patients with dementia. Approximately two thirds of adult family caregivers complain of disrupted sleep (McCurry et al., 1999; Wilcox & King, 1999). Dementia family caregivers sleep less and have poorer ratings of sleep quality compared to noncaregivers (McKibbin et al., 2005; von Känel et al., 2010). Nighttime behaviors of patients with dementia are often associated with sleep problems in family caregivers (McCurry, Logsdon, Teri, & Vitiello, 2007), and sleep disruption is a major reason why

---

[†]Consult the full research reports for references cited within these excerpted literature reviews.

family members institutionalize their care recipients (Hope, Keene, Gedling, Fairburn, & Jacoby, 1998; Yaffe et al., 2002). Poor sleep quality has been shown to contribute to depression and elevated biomarkers of increased atherosclerotic risk among family caregivers of persons with AD (Rowe, McCrae, Campbell, Benito, & Cheng, 2008; Simpson & Carter, 2013; von Känel et al., 2010), and more research describing the nature of sleep disruptions and their impact on sleep quality in patients with FTD and their caregivers are needed. Caregivers of patients with FTD have not been the focus of sleep research, although a case of a spouse caregiver of a patient with bvFTD whose ratings of emotional distress for the patient's nighttime behavior increased during a 3-year period of caregiving was reported (Merrilees et al., 2009). The purposes of this study were to characterize sleep (using actigraphy and subjective assessments) in patients with mild to moderate bvFTD and SD and their primary family caregivers, and to compare patient and caregiver data" (pp. 129–130).

Literature Review from a Qualitative Research Report

Study: The everyday life of the young child shortly after receiving a cancer diagnosis, from both children's and parent's perspectives (Darcy et al., 2014)

Statement of Purpose: The purpose of this study was to explore young children's and their parents' perceptions of how cancer affects the child's health and everyday life shortly after diagnosis.

Literature Review (Excerpt): "There are very few published studies describing the health and everyday life of children with cancer. Only 1 study has been found in which young children with cancer were asked about their health and quality of life (Hicks et al., 2003). Focus group interviews with 13 children in the 5- to 9-year-old age bracket showed that they were affected by treatment and medication with impacts including tiredness, hair loss, and limited possibilities for activities and relationships.

A recent study offering a perspective on the needs and preferences of children and young people receiving cancer care included 2 children in the group of those younger than 5 years (Gibson et al., 2010). Researchers proposed a model of communication among children, parents, and health professionals suggesting that chil-

dren worry when they are not informed about their condition and treatment. Young children remain in the background and rely on their parents to speak for them, whereas teenagers tend to step into the foreground and speak for themselves, as they progressively gain increased autonomy, responsibility, and independence.

Other studies that are published describing young children's health and everyday life are predominantly proxy studies where staff or parents have described how the child feels (Hedstrom et al., 2003; Bjork et al., 2007; Von Essen et al., 2002). According to parents and staff, the most common sources of distress experienced by the young child include the illness, physical pain due to procedures, tiredness, and emotional difficulties, such as a sense of unfamiliarity with oneself. The primary needs of these children, according to their parents' perceptions, were to have a normal family life and interact with friends.

Observational studies suggest that during hospitalization parents are the most important people in a child's life. Nevertheless, children want to be active participants in their own care, to be kept informed, and to be treated with respect, by health professionals who are nice and approachable (Bjork et al., 2007; Von Essen et al., 2002; Gibson & Hopkins, 2005).

The Convention on the Rights of the Child states that children have the right to be consulted and listened to in matters that affect them (United Nations, 1989). Young children's understanding of illness and health is dependent on their cognitive abilities, previous experiences, and the environment they grow up in. Preschool-aged children strongly associate the concept of health with taking part in what they understand to be daily activities with their family and peers (Almqvist et al., 2006). Young children can offer subjective assessments about their health and should be encouraged to report them, when possible (Chaplin et al., 2008)" (p. 447).

●○●○●○●○●○●○●○●○●○●○●○●○

SUMMARY POINTS

- A research **literature review** is a written summary of evidence on a research problem.
- The major steps in preparing a written research review include formulating a question, devising

a search strategy, conducting a search, retrieving relevant sources, abstracting information, critiquing studies, analyzing aggregated information, and preparing a written synthesis.

- Study findings are the major focus of research reviews. Information in nonresearch references—for example, opinion articles, case reports—may broaden understanding of a research problem but has limited utility in research reviews.
- A **primary source** is the original description of a study prepared by the researcher who conducted it; a **secondary source** is a description of the study by a person unconnected with it. Literature reviews should be based on primary source material.
- Strategies for finding studies on a topic include the use of bibliographic tools but also include the *ancestry approach* (tracking down earlier studies cited in a reference list of a report) and the *descendancy approach* (using a pivotal study to search forward to subsequent studies that cited it).
- An important method for locating references is an electronic search of bibliographic databases. For nurses, the CINAHL and MEDLINE databases are especially useful, and Google Scholar is becoming popular because it is freely available.
- In searching a database, users can perform a **keyword search** that looks for searcher-specified terms in text fields of a database record (or that *maps* keywords onto the database's subject codes) or can search according to **subject heading** codes themselves.
- Access to many journal articles is becoming easier through online resources, especially for articles available in an **open-access** format.
- References must be screened for relevance, and then pertinent information must be abstracted for analysis. Formal review protocols and two-dimensional review matrices facilitate abstraction, as does a good coding scheme.
- A research **critique** is a careful appraisal of a study's strengths and weaknesses. Critiques for a research review tend to focus on the methodologic aspects of a set of studies and

the overall findings. Critiques of individual studies tend to be more comprehensive.

- The analysis of information from a literature search involves the identification of important themes—regularities (and inconsistencies) in the information. Themes can take many forms, including substantive, methodologic, and theoretic themes.
- In preparing a written review, it is important to organize materials logically. The reviewers' role is to describe study findings, the dependability of the evidence, evidence gaps, and (in the context of a new study) contributions that the new study would make.

STUDY ACTIVITIES

Chapter 5 of the *Resource Manual for Nursing Research: Generating and Assessing Evidence for Nursing Practice, 10th edition*, offers study suggestions for reinforcing concepts presented in this chapter. In addition, the following questions can be addressed in classroom or online discussions:

1. Suppose you were planning to study the relationship between chronic transfusion therapy and quality of life in adolescents with sickle cell disease. Identify 5 to 10 keywords that could be used to search for relevant studies and compare them with those found by other students.
2. Suppose you were studying factors affecting the discharge of chronic psychiatric patients. Obtain references for five studies for this topic and compare them with those of other students.

STUDIES CITED IN CHAPTER 5

*Boeker, M., Vach, W., & Motschall, E. (2013). Google Scholar as replacement for systematic literature searches: Good relative recall and precision are not enough. *BMC Medical Research Methodology, 13*, 131.
*Bramer, W. M., Giustini, D., Kramer, B., & Anderson, P. (2013). The comparative recall of Google Scholar versus PubMed in identical searches for biomedical systematic reviews. *Systematic Reviews, 2*, 115.

Cooper, H. (2010). *Research synthesis and meta-analysis* (4th ed.). Thousand Oaks, CA: Sage.

Darcy, L., Knutsson, S., Huus, K., & Enskar, K. (2014). The everyday life of the young child shortly after receiving a cancer diagnosis, from both children's and parent's perspectives. *Cancer Nursing, 37*, 445–456.

*Finfgeld-Connett, D., & Johnson, E. (2013). Literature search strategies for conducting knowledge-building and theory-generating qualitative systematic reviews. *Journal of Advanced Nursing, 69*, 194–204.

Fink, A. (2014). *Conducting research literature reviews: From the Internet to paper.* Thousand Oaks, CA: Sage.

Flemming, K., & Briggs, M. (2006). Electronic searching to locate qualitative research: Evaluation of three strategies. *Journal of Advanced Nursing, 57*, 95–100.

Galvan, J. L. (2012). *Writing literature reviews: A guide for students of the social and behavioral sciences.* Los Angeles, CA: Pyrczak.

Garrard, J. (2014). *Health sciences literature review made easy: The matrix method* (4th ed.). Burlington, MA: Jones & Bartlett.

*Gehanno, J. F., Rollin, L., & Darmon, S. (2013). Is the coverage of Google Scholar enough to be used along for systematic reviews? *BMC Medical Informatics and Decision Making, 13*, 7.

Glaser, B. (1978). *Theoretical sensitivity.* Mill Valley, CA: The Sociology Press.

Merrilees, J., Hubbard, E., Mastick, J., Miller, B., & Dowling, G. (2014). Sleep in persons with frontotemporal dementia and their family caregivers. *Nursing Research, 63*, 129–136.

Munhall, P. L. (2012). *Nursing research: A qualitative perspective* (5th ed.). Sudbury, MA: Jones & Bartlett.

Pinto, J. D., He, H., Chan, S., Toh, P., Esuvaranathan, K., & Wang, W. (2015). Health-related quality of life and psychological well-being in patients with benign prostatic hyperplasia. *Journal of Clinical Nursing, 24*, 511–522.

*Shariff, S. Z., Bejaimal, S., Sontrop, J., Iansavichus, A., Haynes, R. B., Weir, M., & Garg, A. (2013). Retrieving clinical evidence: A comparison of PubMed and Google Scholar for quick clinical searches. *Journal of Medical Internet Research, 15*(8), e164.

Spradley, J. (1979). *The ethnographic interview.* New York: Holt Rinehart & Winston.

Twycross, A., & Collis, S. (2013). How well is acute pain managed? A snapshot in one English hospital. *Pain Management Nursing, 14*, e204–e215.

Wilczynski, N., Marks, S., & Haynes, R. (2007). Search strategies for identifying qualitative studies in CINAHL. *Qualitative Health Research, 17*, 705–710.

A link to this open-access journal article is provided in the Toolkit for this chapter in the accompanying Resource Manual. ✪

6 | Theoretical Frameworks

High-quality studies achieve a high level of *conceptual integration*. This means that the methods are appropriate for the research questions, the questions are consistent with existing evidence, and there is a plausible conceptual rationale for the way things are expected to unfold—including a rationale for hypotheses to be tested or for the design of an intervention.

For example, suppose we hypothesized that a smoking cessation intervention would reduce rates of smoking among patients with cardiovascular disease. Why would we make this prediction? That is, what is our "theory" (our theoretical rationale) about how the intervention might bring about behavior change? Do we predict that the intervention will change patients' knowledge? motivation? sense of control over their decision making? Our view of how the intervention would "work"—what would *mediate* the relationship between intervention receipt and the desired outcome—should guide the design of the intervention and the study.

In designing research, researchers need to have a conceptualization of people's behaviors or characteristics, and how these affect or are affected by interpersonal, environmental, or biologic forces. In high-quality research, a strong, defensible conceptualization is made explicit. This chapter discusses theoretical and conceptual contexts for nursing research problems.

THEORIES, MODELS, AND FRAMEWORKS

Many terms are used in connection with conceptual contexts for research, such as theories, models, frameworks, schemes, and maps. We offer guidance in distinguishing these terms, but note that our definitions are not universal—indeed a confusing aspect of theory-related writings is that there is no consensus about terminology.

Theories

The term *theory* is used in many ways. For example, nursing instructors and students often use the term to refer to classroom content, as opposed to the actual practice of performing nursing actions. In both lay and scientific usage, the term *theory* connotes an *abstraction*.

In research circles, the term theory is used differently by different authors. Classically, **theory** refers to an abstract generalization that explains how phenomena are interrelated. In this definition, a theory embodies at least two concepts that are related in a manner that the theory purports to explain. Traditional theories typically have explanation or prediction as their purpose.

Others, however, use the term *theory* less restrictively to refer to a broad characterization that can thoroughly describe a single phenomenon. Some authors refer to this type of theory as *descriptive theory*, while others have used the term *factor isolating theory*. Broadly speaking, descriptive theories are ones that describe or categorize characteristics of individuals, groups, or situations by abstracting common features observed across multiple manifestations. Descriptive theory plays an important role in qualitative studies. Qualitative researchers often strive to develop conceptualizations of phenomena that are grounded in actual observations. Descriptive theory is sometimes a precursor to predictive and explanatory theories.

Components of a Traditional Theory

Writings on scientific theory include such terms as *proposition*, *premise*, *axiom*, *principle*, and so forth. Here we present a simplified analysis of the components of a theory.

Concepts are the basic building blocks of a theory. Classical theories comprise a set of propositions that indicate relationships among the concepts. Relationships are denoted by such terms as "is associated with," "varies directly with," or "is contingent on." The propositions form a logically interrelated deductive system. This means that the theory provides a mechanism for logically deriving new statements from the original propositions.

Let us illustrate with the **Theory of Planned Behavior** (TPB; Ajzen, 2005), which is related to another theory called the *Theory of Reasoned Action* or *TRA* (Fishbein & Ajzen, 2010). TPB provides a framework for understanding people's behavior and its psychological determinants. A greatly simplified construction of the TPB consists of the following propositions:

1. Behavior that is volitional is determined by people's intention to perform that behavior.
2. Intention to perform or not perform a behavior is determined by three factors:
   - Attitudes toward the behavior (i.e., the overall evaluation of performing the behavior)
   - Subjective norms (i.e., perceived social pressure to perform or not perform the behavior)
   - Perceived behavioral control (i.e., self-efficacy beliefs—the anticipated ease or difficulty of engaging in the behavior)
3. The relative importance of the three factors in influencing intention varies across behaviors and situations.

> **→ TIP:** There are websites devoted to many of the theories and conceptual models mentioned in this chapter, including the TPB. Several specific websites are listed in the "Useful Websites for Chapter 6" table in the Toolkit of the accompanying *Resource Manual* for you to click on directly.

The concepts that form the basis of the TPB include behaviors, intentions, attitudes, subjective norms, and perceived self-control. The theory, which specifies the nature of the relationship among these concepts, provides a framework for generating hypotheses relating to health behaviors. We might hypothesize on the basis of the TPB, for example, that compliance with a medical regimen (the behavior) could be enhanced by influencing people's attitudes toward compliance or by increasing their sense of control. The TPB has been used as the underlying theory for studying a wide range of health decision-making behaviors (e.g., condom use, preventive health screening) as well as in developing health-promoting interventions.

Example Using the TPB: Ben Natan and colleagues (2014) used the Theory of Planned Behavior to study factors affecting Israeli women's decision about donating cord blood.

Levels of Theories

Theories differ in their level of generality and abstraction. The most common labels used in nursing for levels or scope of theory are *grand*, *middle-range*, and *micro* or *practice*.

Grand theories or *macrotheories* purport to describe and explain large segments of the human experience. In nursing, there are several grand theories that offer explanations of the whole of nursing and that address the nature, goals, and mission of nursing practice, as distinct from the discipline of medicine. An example of a nursing theory that has been described as a grand theory is Parse's Human-becoming Paradigm (Parse, 2014).

Theories of relevance to researchers are often more focused than grand theories. **Middle-range theories** attempt to explain such phenomena as decision making, stress, comfort, health promotion, and unpleasant symptoms. In comparison to grand theories, middle-range theories tend to involve fewer concepts or propositions, are more specific, and are more amenable to empirical testing (Peterson & Bredow, 2012). Nurse researchers are increasingly turning to middle-range theories for their conceptual inspiration. There are literally dozens of middle-range theories developed by or used by nurses, several of which we briefly describe in this chapter.

The least abstract level of theory is *practice theory* (sometimes called *micro theory* or *situation-specific theory*). Such theories are highly specific, narrow in scope, and have an action orientation. They are seldom associated with research, and there is ongoing debate about whether they should be called "theory" (Peterson & Bredow, 2012).

Models

Conceptual models, *conceptual frameworks*, or *conceptual schemes* (we use the terms interchangeably) are considered a less formal means of organizing phenomena than theories. Like theories, conceptual models deal with abstractions (concepts) that are assembled by virtue of their relevance to a common theme. What is absent from conceptual models is the deductive system of propositions that assert and explain relationships among concepts. Conceptual models provide a perspective regarding interrelated phenomena but are more loosely structured than theories. A conceptual model broadly presents an understanding of the phenomenon of interest and reflects the assumptions and philosophic views of the model's designer. Conceptual models can serve as springboards for generating hypotheses, but conceptual models in their entirety are not formally "tested."

The term *model* is often used in connection with symbolic representations of a conceptualization. **Schematic models** (or **conceptual maps**) are visual representations of some aspect of reality. Like conceptual models and theories, they use concepts as building blocks but with a minimal use of words. A visual or symbolic representation of a theory or conceptual framework often helps to express abstract ideas in a concise and accessible form.

Schematic models are common in both qualitative and quantitative research. Concepts and the linkages between them are represented through the use of boxes, arrows, or other symbols. As an example, Figure 6.1 shows **Pender's Health Promotion Model**, which is a model for explaining and predicting the health-promotion component of lifestyle (Pender et al., 2015). Such schematic models can be useful in clarifying and succinctly communicating linkages among concepts.

Frameworks

A **framework** is the overall conceptual underpinnings of a study. Not every study is based on a formal theory or conceptual model, but every study has a framework—that is, a conceptual rationale. In a study based on a theory, the framework is a **theoretical framework**; in a study with roots in a conceptual model, the framework is a **conceptual framework** (although the terms conceptual framework and theoretical framework are frequently used interchangeably).

In most nursing studies, the framework is not an explicit theory or conceptual model, and sometimes the underlying conceptual rationale for the inquiry is not explained. Frameworks are often implicit, without being formally acknowledged or described. In studies that fail to articulate a conceptual framework, it may be difficult to figure out what the researchers thought was "going on."

Sometimes researchers fail even to adequately describe key constructs at the conceptual level. The concepts in which researchers are interested are by definition abstractions of observable phenomena, and our worldview, and views on nursing, shape how those concepts are defined and operationalized. Researchers should make clear the conceptual definition of their key variables, thereby providing information about the study's framework.

In most qualitative studies, the frameworks are part of the research tradition in which the study is embedded. For example, ethnographers usually begin their work within a theory of culture. Grounded theory researchers incorporate sociologic principles into their framework and their approach to looking at phenomena. The questions that most qualitative researchers ask and the methods

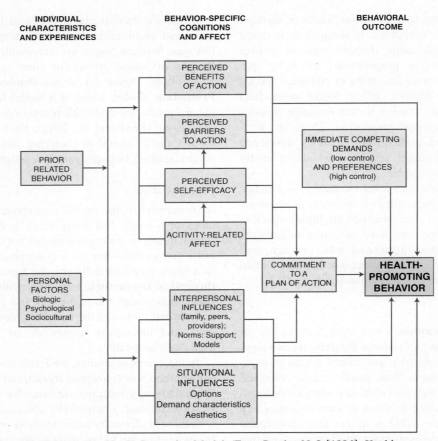

FIGURE 6.1 The Health Promotion Model. (From Pender, N. J. [1996]. *Health promotion diagram*. Retrieved from http://www.nursing.umich.edu/faculty/pender/chart.gif)

they use to address those questions inherently reflect certain theoretical formulations.

In recent years, *concept analysis* has become an important enterprise among students and nurse scholars. Several methods have been proposed for undertaking a concept analysis and clarifying conceptual definitions (e.g., Schwartz-Barcott & Kim, 2000; Walker & Avant, 2010). Efforts to analyze concepts of relevance to nursing practice should facilitate greater conceptual clarity among nurse researchers.

Example of Developing a Conceptual Definition: Ramezani and colleagues (2014) used Walker and Avant's eight-step concept analysis methods to conceptually define *spiritual care in nursing*.

They searched and analyzed national and international databases and found 151 relevant articles and 7 books. They proposed the following definition:

"The attributes of spiritual care are healing presence, therapeutic use of self, intuitive sense, exploration of the spiritual perspective, patient centredness, meaning-centred therapeutic intervention and creation of a spiritually nurturing environment." (p. 211)

THE NATURE OF THEORIES AND CONCEPTUAL MODELS

Theories and conceptual models have much in common, including their origin, general nature, purposes, and role in research. In this section, we examine some characteristics of theories and conceptual models. We use the term *theory* in a broad sense, inclusive of conceptual models.

Origin of Theories and Models

Theories, conceptual frameworks, and models are not *discovered*; they are created and invented. Theory building depends not only on facts and observable evidence but also on the originator's ingenuity in pulling facts together and making sense of them. Theory construction is a creative and intellectual enterprise that can be undertaken by anyone who is insightful, has a firm grounding in existing evidence, and has the ability to knit together evidence into an intelligible pattern.

Tentative Nature of Theories and Models

Theories and conceptual models cannot be proved—they represent a theorist's best effort to describe and explain phenomena. Today's flourishing theory may be discredited or revised tomorrow. This may happen if new evidence or observations undermine a previously accepted theory. Or, a new theory might integrate new observations into an existing theory to yield a more parsimonious or accurate explanation of a phenomenon.

Theories and models that are not congruent with a culture's values also may fall into disfavor over time. For example, certain psychoanalytic and structural social theories, which had broad support for decades, have come to be challenged as a result of changing views about women's roles. Theories are deliberately invented by humans, and so they are not free from human values, which can change over time. Thus, theories and models are never considered final and verified. We have no way of knowing the ultimate accuracy and utility of any theory.

The Role of Theories and Models

Theoretical and conceptual frameworks play interrelated roles in the progress of a science. Theories allow researchers to integrate observations and findings into an orderly scheme. Theories are efficient for drawing together accumulated facts, often from separate investigations. The linkage of findings into a coherent structure can make a body of evidence more accessible and more useful.

In addition to summarizing, theories and models can guide a researcher's understanding of not only the *what* of natural phenomena but also the *why* of their occurrence. Theories often provide a basis for predicting phenomena. Prediction, in turn, has implications for the control of those phenomena. A utilitarian theory has potential to bring about desirable changes in people's behavior or health. Thus, theories are an important resource for developing nursing interventions.

Theories and conceptual models help to stimulate research and the extension of knowledge by providing both direction and impetus. Thus, theories may serve as a springboard for advances in knowledge and the accumulation of evidence for practice.

Relationship between Theory and Research

Theory and research have a reciprocal relationship. Theories are built inductively from observations, and research is an excellent source for those observations. Concepts and relationships that are validated through research become the foundation for theory development. The theory, in turn, must be tested by subjecting deductions from it (hypotheses) to systematic inquiry. Thus, research plays a dual and continuing role in theory building. Theory guides and generates ideas for research; research assesses the worth of the theory and provides a foundation for new theories.

CONCEPTUAL MODELS AND THEORIES USED IN NURSING RESEARCH

Nurse researchers have used nursing and nonnursing frameworks to provide a conceptual context for their studies. This section briefly discusses several frameworks that have been found useful.

Conceptual Models and Theories of Nursing

In the past few decades, several nurses have formulated theories and models of nursing practice. These models constitute formal explanations of what nursing is and what the nursing process entails, according to the model developer's point of view. As Fawcett and DeSanto-Madeya (2013) have noted, four concepts are central to models of nursing: *human beings*, *environment*, *health*, and *nursing*. The various conceptual models, however, define these concepts differently, link them in diverse ways, and emphasize different relationships among them. Moreover, different models portray different processes as being central to nursing.

The conceptual models were not developed primarily as a base for nursing research. Indeed, most models have had more impact on nursing education and clinical practice than on research. Nevertheless, nurse researchers have been inspired by these conceptual frameworks in formulating research questions and hypotheses. Two nursing models that have generated particular interest as a basis for research are described in greater detail.

Roy's Adaptation Model

In **Roy's Adaptation Model**, humans are viewed as biopsychosocial adaptive systems who cope with environmental change through the process of adaptation (Roy & Andrews, 2009). Within the human system, there are four subsystems: physiologic/physical, self-concept/group identity, role function, and interdependence. These subsystems constitute adaptive modes that provide mechanisms for coping with environmental stimuli and change. Health is viewed as both a state and a process of being and becoming integrated and whole that reflects the mutuality of persons and environment. The goal of nursing, according to this model, is to promote client adaptation. Nursing also regulates stimuli affecting adaptation. Nursing interventions usually take the form of increasing, decreasing, modifying, removing, or maintaining internal and external stimuli that affect adaptation. Roy's Adaptation Model has been the basis for several middle-range theories and dozens of studies.

Example Using Roy's Adaptation Model:
Aber and colleagues (2013) studied women's adaptation to motherhood in the first 3 to 6 weeks postpartum, using concepts from Roy's Adaptation Model. The physical, emotional, functional, and social components of adaptation were studied.

Rogers' Science of Unitary Human Beings

The building blocks of **Rogers' Science of Unitary Human Beings** (Rogers, 1990, 1994) are five assumptions relating to human life processes: wholeness (a human as a unified whole, more than the sum of the parts), openness (humans and the environment continuously exchanging matter and energy), unidirectionality (life processes existing along an irreversible space/time continuum), pattern and organization (which identify humans and reflect their wholeness), and sentience and thought (a human as capable of abstraction, imagery, language, and sensation). Four critical elements are basic to Rogers' proposed system: *energy fields*, *open systems*, *pattern*, and *pandimensionality*. The key to Rogers' conceptual framework are her principles of homeodynamics, which represent a way of viewing unitary human beings and provide guidance to nursing practice. The principles include integrality, helicy, and resonancy. *Integrality* concerns the continuous and mutual processes between human and environmental fields—changes in one field will bring about changes in the other. *Helicy* refers to the continuous and innovative diversity of human and environmental field patterns. Finally, *resonancy* describes the continuous change from lower to higher frequency wave patterns in human and environmental energy fields. Rogerian science continues to be developed by theorists and researchers.

Example Using a Rogerian Framework:
Reis and Alligood (2014) explored changes in optimism, power, and well-being among women who participated in a prenatal yoga program, and conceptualized the study from the perspective of Rogers' Science of Unitary Human Beings.

Other Models and Middle-Range Theories Developed by Nurses

In addition to conceptual models that are designed to describe and characterize the nursing process, nurses have developed middle-range theories and models that focus on more specific phenomena of interest to nurses. Examples of middle-range theories that have been used in research include

- Beck's (2012) Theory of Postpartum Depression
- Kolcaba's (2003) Comfort Theory

- Symptom Management Model (Dodd et al., 2001)
- Theory of Transitions (Meleis et al., 2000)
- Peplau's (1997) Theory of Interpersonal Relations
- Pender's Health Promotion Model (Pender et al., 2015)
- Mishel's Uncertainty in Illness Theory (Mishel, 1990)

The latter two are briefly described here.

The Health Promotion Model

Nola Pender's (Pender et al., 2015) Health Promotion Model (HPM) focuses on explaining health-promoting behaviors, using a wellness orientation. According to the model (see Figure 6.1), *health promotion* entails activities directed toward developing resources that maintain or enhance a person's well-being. The model embodies a number of theoretical propositions that can be used in developing interventions and understanding health behaviors. For example, one HPM proposition is that people commit to engaging in behaviors from which they anticipate deriving valued benefits, and another is that perceived competence or self-efficacy relating to a given behavior increases the likelihood of actual performance of the behavior. Greater perceived self-efficacy is viewed as resulting in fewer perceived barriers to a specific health behavior. The model also incorporates interpersonal and situational influences on a person's commitment to health-promoting actions.

Example Using the HPM: Cole and Gaspar (2015) used the Health Promotion Model as their framework for an evidence-based project designed to examine the disease management behaviors of patients with epilepsy and to guide the implementation of a self-management protocol for these patients.

Uncertainty in Illness Theory

Mishel's Uncertainty in Illness Theory (Mishel, 1990) focuses on the concept of uncertainty—the inability of a person to determine the meaning of illness-related events. According to this theory, people develop subjective appraisals to assist them in interpreting the experience of illness and treatment. Uncertainty occurs when people are unable to recognize and categorize stimuli. Uncertainty results in the inability to obtain a clear conception of the situation, but a situation appraised as uncertain will mobilize individuals to use their resources to adapt to the situation. Mishel's theory as originally conceptualized was most relevant to patients in an acute phase of illness or in a downward illness trajectory, but it has been reconceptualized to include constant uncertainty in chronic or recurrent illness. Mishel's conceptualization of uncertainty, and her Uncertainty in Illness Scale, have been used in many nursing studies.

Example Using Uncertainty in Illness Theory: Germino and colleagues (2013) tested whether breast cancer survivors who received an uncertainty management intervention would have less uncertainty, fewer cancer-specific concerns, and better psychological outcomes than women who did not receive the intervention.

Other Models and Theories Used by Nurse Researchers

Many concepts of interest to nurse researchers are not unique to nursing, and so their studies are sometimes linked to frameworks that are not models from the nursing profession. Several of these alternative models have gained special prominence in the development of nursing interventions to promote health-enhancing behaviors. In addition to the previously described Theory of Planned Behavior, four non-nursing models or theories have often been used in nursing studies: Bandura's Social Cognitive Theory, Prochaska's Transtheoretical (Stages of Change) Model, the Health Belief Model, and Lazarus and Folkman's Theory of Stress and Coping.

Bandura's Social Cognitive Theory

Social Cognitive Theory (Bandura, 1997, 2001), which is sometimes called **self-efficacy theory**, offers an explanation of human behavior using the concepts of self-efficacy and outcome expectations. Self-efficacy concerns people's belief in their own capacity to carry out particular behaviors (e.g., smoking cessation). Self-efficacy expectations influences the behaviors a person chooses to perform, the degree of perseverance, and the quality of the performance. Bandura identified four factors that influence a person's cognitive appraisal of self-efficacy: (1) their own mastery experience;

(2) verbal persuasion; (3) vicarious experience; and (4) physiologic and affective cues, such as pain and anxiety. The role of self-efficacy has been studied in relation to numerous health behaviors (e.g., weight control, smoking).

➔ TIP: Bandura's self-efficacy construct is a key mediating variable in several theories discussed in this chapter. Self-efficacy has repeatedly been found to explain a significant amount of variation in people's behaviors *and* to be amenable to change. As a result, self-efficacy enhancement is often a goal in interventions designed to change people's health-related behaviors (Conn et al., 2001).

Example Using Social Cognitive Theory: Guided by Social Cognitive Theory, Chilton and colleagues (2014) examined the effect of a comprehensive wellness intervention on the health behaviors and physical fitness outcomes of adolescent females.

The Transtheoretical (Stages of Change) Model

There are several dimensions in the **Transtheoretical Model** (Prochaska et al., 2002; Prochaska & Velicer, 1997), a model that has been the basis of numerous interventions designed to change people's behavior such as smoking. The core construct around which the other dimensions are organized are the *stages of change*, which conceptualizes a continuum of *motivational readiness* to change problem behavior. The five stages of change are precontemplation, contemplation, preparation, action, and maintenance. Transitions from one stage to the next are affected by processes of change. Studies have shown that successful self-changers use different processes at each particular stage, thus suggesting the desirability of interventions that are individualized to the person's stage of readiness for change. The model also incorporates a series of intervening variables, one of which is self-efficacy.

Example Using the Transtheoretical Model: Lee and colleagues (2015) tested a web-based self-management intervention for breast cancer survivors.

The exercise and diet intervention program incorporated transtheoretical model-based strategies.

The Health Belief Model

The **Health Belief Model** (HBM; Becker, 1976, 1978) has become a popular framework in nursing studies focused on patient compliance and preventive health care practices. The model postulates that health-seeking behavior is influenced by a person's perception of a threat posed by a health problem and the value associated with actions aimed at reducing the threat. The major components of the HBM include perceived susceptibility, perceived severity, perceived benefits and costs, motivation, and enabling or modifying factors. Perceived susceptibility is a person's perception that a health problem is personally relevant or that a diagnosis is accurate. Even when one recognizes personal susceptibility, action will not occur unless the individual perceives the severity to be high enough to have serious implications. Perceived benefits are the patients' beliefs that a given treatment will cure the illness or help prevent it, and perceived barriers include the complexity, duration, and accessibility of the treatment. Motivation is the desire to comply with a treatment. Among the modifying factors that have been identified are personality variables, patient satisfaction, and sociodemographic factors.

Example Using the HBM: Bae and co-researchers (2014) used the Health Belief Model as the framework for studying factors associated with adherence to fecal occult blood testing for colorectal cancer screening in Korean adults.

Lazarus and Folkman's Theory of Stress and Coping

The **Transactional Theory of Stress and Coping** (Lazarus, 2006; Lazarus & Folkman, 1984) is an effort to explain people's methods of dealing with stress—that is, environmental and internal demands that tax or exceed a person's resources and endanger his or her well-being. The model posits that coping strategies are learned, deliberate responses used to adapt to or change stressors. According to this model, a person's perception of mental and physical health is related to the ways he or she evaluates and copes with the stresses of living.

Example Using the Theory of Stress and Coping: Using Lazarus and Folkman's Theory of Stress and Coping as a framework, Knapp and colleagues (2013) tested a "family bundle" designed to improve family members' stress and coping following the patient's admission to a surgical intensive care unit.

➔ **TIP:** Several controversies surround the issue of theoretical frameworks in nursing. One controversy involves the source of theories for nursing research. Some commentators advocate the development of unique nursing theories, claiming that only through such development can knowledge to guide nursing practice be produced. Others argue that well-respected theories from other disciplines, such as physiology or psychology (so-called **borrowed theories**), can be applied to nursing problems. (When the appropriateness of borrowed theories for nursing inquiry is confirmed, the theories are sometimes called **shared theories**.) Nurse researchers are likely to continue on their current path of conducting studies within a multidisciplinary, multitheoretical perspective.

Selecting a Theory or Model for Nursing Research

As we discuss in the next section, theory can be used by qualitative and quantitative researchers in various ways. A task common to many efforts to develop a study with a conceptual context, however, is the identification of an appropriate model or theory—a task made especially daunting because of the burgeoning number available. There are no rules for how this can be done, but there are two places to start—with the theory or model, or with the phenomenon being studied.

Readings in the theoretical literature often give rise to research ideas, so it is useful to become familiar with a variety of grand and middle-range theories. Several nursing theory textbooks provide good overviews of major nurse theorists (e.g., McEwen & Wills, 2011; Alligood, 2014). Resources for learning more about middle-range theories include M. J. Smith and Liehr (2014), Alligood (2014), and Peterson and Bredow (2012).

The Supplement for this chapter on the**Point**® includes a table that lists 10 nursing models that have been used by researchers. The table briefly describes the model's key feature and identifies a study that has claimed the model as its framework. Additionally, the Supplement offers references for about 100 middle-range theories and models that have been used in nursing research, organized in broad domains (e.g., aging, mental health, pain).

If you begin with a particular research problem or topic and are looking for a theory, a good strategy is to examine the conceptual contexts of existing studies on a similar topic. You may find that several different models or theories have been used, and so the next step is to learn as much as possible about the most promising ones so that you can select an appropriate one for your own study.

➔ **TIP:** Although it may be tempting to read about the features of a theory in a secondary source, it is best to consult a primary source and to rely on the most up-to-date reference because models are often revised as research accumulates. However, it is also a good idea to review studies that have used the theory. By reading other studies, you will be better able to judge how much empirical support the theory has received and how key variables were measured.

Many writers have offered advice on how to do an analysis and evaluation of a theory for use in nursing practice and nursing research (e.g., Chinn & Kramer, 2015; Fawcett & DeSanto-Madeya, 2013; Parker & Smith, 2011). Box 6.1 ⊗ presents some basic questions that can be asked in a preliminary assessment of a theory or model.

In addition to evaluating the general integrity of the model or theory, it is important to make sure that there is a proper "fit" between the theory and the research question to be studied. A critical issue is whether the theory has done a good job of explaining, predicting, or describing constructs that

BOX 6.1 Some Questions for a Preliminary Assessment of a Model or Theory

Issue	Questions
Theoretical clarity	• Are key concepts defined and are definitions sufficiently clear? • Do all concepts "fit" within the theory? Are concepts used in the theory in a manner compatible with conceptual definitions? • Are basic assumptions consistent with one another? • Are schematic models compatible with the text? Are schematic models needed but not presented? • Can the theory be followed—is it adequately explained? Are there ambiguities?
Theoretical complexity	• Is the theory sufficiently rich and detailed? • Is the theory overly complex? • Can the theory be used to explain or predict, or only to describe phenomena?
Theoretical grounding	• Are the concepts identifiable in reality? • Is there a research basis for the theory, and is the basis a sound one?
Appropriateness of the theory	• Are the tenets of the theory compatible with nursing's philosophy? • Are the key concepts within the domain of nursing?
Importance of the theory	• Could research based on this theory answer critical questions for nursing? • How will testing the theory contribute to nursing's evidence base?
General issue	• Are there other theories or models that would do a better job of explaining phenomena of interest? • Is the theory compatible with your worldview?

are key to your research problem. A few additional questions include the following:

- Has the theory been applied to similar research questions, and do the findings from prior research lend credibility to the theory's utility for research?
- Are the theoretical constructs in the model or theory readily operationalized? Are there existing instruments of adequate quality?
- Is the theory compatible with your worldview, and with the worldview implicit in the research question?

TIP: If you begin with a research problem and need to identify a suitable framework, it is wise to confer with people who may be familiar with a broad range of theoretical perspectives.

TESTING, USING, AND DEVELOPING A THEORY OR FRAMEWORK

In this section, we elaborate on the manner in which theory and conceptual frameworks are used by qualitative and quantitative researchers. In the discussion, we use the term *theory* broadly to include conceptual models, formal theories, and frameworks.

Theories and Qualitative Research

Theory is almost always present in studies that are embedded in a qualitative research tradition such as ethnography, phenomenology, or grounded theory. These research traditions inherently provide an overarching framework that gives qualitative studies a theoretical grounding. However, different traditions involve theory in different ways.

Sandelowski (1993) made a useful distinction between **substantive theory** (conceptualizations of the target phenomenon under study) and theory that reflects a conceptualization of human inquiry. Some qualitative researchers insist on an atheoretical stance vis-a-vis the phenomenon of interest, with the goal of suspending *a priori* conceptualizations (substantive theories) that might bias their collection and analysis of data. For example, phenomenologists are in general committed to theoretical naiveté and explicitly try to hold preconceived views of the phenomenon in check. Nevertheless, they are guided in their inquiries by a framework or philosophy that focuses their analysis on certain aspects of a person's life. That framework is based on the premise that human experience is an inherent property of the experience itself, not constructed by an outside observer.

Ethnographers typically bring a strong cultural perspective to their studies, and this perspective shapes their initial fieldwork. Fetterman (2010) has observed that most ethnographers adopt one of two cultural theories: **ideational theories**, which suggest that cultural conditions and adaptation stem from mental activity and ideas, or **materialistic theories**, which view material conditions (e.g., resources, money, production) as the source of cultural developments.

The theoretical underpinning of grounded theory is a melding of sociologic formulations. The most prominent theoretical system in grounded theory is **symbolic interaction** (or *interactionism*), which has three underlying premises (Blumer, 1986). First, humans act toward things based on the meanings that the things have for them. Second, the meaning of things arises out of the interaction humans have with other fellow humans. Last, meanings are handled in, and modified through, an interpretive process in dealing with the things humans encounter. Despite having a theoretical umbrella, grounded theory researchers, like phenomenologists, attempt to hold prior substantive theory (existing knowledge and conceptualizations about the phenomenon) in abeyance until their own substantive theory begins to emerge.

Example of a Grounded Theory Study:
Komatsu and colleagues (2014) conducted a grounded theory study based on a symbolic interactionist framework to explore the process of fertility preservation among women with cervical cancer who underwent radical trachelectomy.

Grounded theory methods are designed to facilitate the generation of theory that is *conceptually dense*, that is, with many conceptual patterns and relationships. Grounded theory researchers seek to develop a conceptualization of a phenomenon that is *grounded* in actual observations—that is, to explicate an empirically based conceptualization for integrating and making sense of a process or phenomenon. During the ongoing analysis of data, the researchers move from specific pieces of data to abstract generalizations that synthesize and give structure to the observed phenomenon. The goal is to use the data to provide a description or an explanation of events as they occur—not as they have been conceptualized in existing theories. Once the grounded theory begins to take shape, however, previous literature is used for comparison with the emerging and developing categories of the theory. Sandelowski (1993) has noted that previous substantive theories or conceptualizations, when used in this manner, are essentially data themselves, and can be taken into consideration, along with study data, as part of an inductively driven new conceptualization.

⊙ **TIP:** The use of theory in qualitative studies has been the topic of some debate. Morse (2002) called for qualitative researchers to not be "theory ignorant but theory smart" (p. 296) and to "get over" their theory phobia. She elaborated by noting that qualitative research does not necessarily begin with holding in check all prior knowledge of the phenomenon under study (Morse, 2004). She suggested that if the boundaries of the concept of interest can be identified, a qualitative researcher can use these boundaries as a scaffold to inductively explore the attributes of the concept.

Some qualitative nurse researchers have adopted a perspective known as critical theory as their framework. **Critical theory** is a paradigm that involves a critique of society and societal processes and structures, as we discuss in greater detail in Chapter 21.

Qualitative researchers sometimes use conceptual models of nursing as an interpretive framework rather than as a guide for the conduct of a study. For example, some qualitative nurse researchers acknowledge that the philosophic roots of their studies lie in conceptual models of nursing developed by Newman, Parse, and Rogers.

One final note is that a systematic review of qualitative studies on a specific topic is another strategy leading to theory development. In metasyntheses, qualitative studies on a topic are scrutinized to identify essential elements. The findings from different sources are then used for theory building. We discuss metasyntheses in Chapter 29.

Theories and Models in Quantitative Research

Quantitative researchers, like qualitative researchers, link research to theory or models in several ways. The classic approach is to test hypotheses deduced from an existing theory.

Testing an Existing Theory

Theories sometimes stimulate new studies. For example, a nurse might read about Pender's Health Promotion Model (see Figure 6.1) and, as reading progresses, the following type of reasoning might occur: "If the HPM is valid, then I would expect that patients with osteoporosis who perceived the benefit of a calcium-enriched diet would be more likely to alter their eating patterns than those who perceived no benefits." Such a conjecture can serve as a starting point for testing the model.

In testing a theory or model, quantitative researchers deduce implications (as in the preceding example) and develop hypotheses, which are predictions about the manner in which variables would be interrelated if the theory were valid. The hypotheses are then subjected to testing through systematic data collection and analysis.

The testing process involves a comparison between observed outcomes with those hypothesized. Through this process, a theory is continually subjected to potential disconfirmation. If studies repeatedly fail to disconfirm a theory, it gains support.

Testing continues until pieces of evidence cannot be interpreted within the context of the theory but *can* be explained by a new theory that also accounts for previous findings. Theory-testing studies are most useful when researchers devise logically sound deductions from the theory, design a study that reduces the plausibility of alternative explanations for observed relationships, and use methods that assess the theory's validity under maximally heterogeneous situations so that potentially competing theories can be ruled out.

Researchers sometimes base a new study on a theory in an effort to explain earlier descriptive findings. For example, suppose several researchers had found that nursing home residents demonstrate greater levels of anxiety and noncompliance with nursing staff around bedtime than at other times. These findings shed no light on underlying causes of the problem and so suggest no way to improve it. Several explanations, rooted in models such as Lazarus and Folkman's Theory of Stress and Coping, may be relevant in explaining the residents' behavior. By directly testing the theory in a new study (i.e., deducing hypotheses derived from the theory), a researcher might learn *why* bedtime is a vulnerable period for nursing home residents.

Researchers sometimes combine elements from more than one theory as a basis for generating hypotheses. In doing this, researchers need to be thoroughly knowledgeable about *both* theories to see if there is an adequate conceptual basis for conjoining them. If underlying assumptions or conceptual definitions of key concepts are not compatible, the theories should not be combined (although perhaps elements of the two can be used to create a new conceptual framework with its own assumptions and definitions).

Another strategy that can be used in theory-testing research (but is used infrequently) is to test two competing theories directly—that is, to test alternative explanations of a phenomenon in a single study. There are competing theories for such phenomena as stress, behavior change, and so on, and each competing theory suggests alternative approaches to achieving positive outcomes or avoiding negative ones. Researchers who deliberately test multiple theories with a single sample of participants may be able to make powerful comparisons about the utility of competing explanations, but such a study requires considerable advance planning and the measurement of a wider array of constructs than would otherwise be the case.

Tests of a theory increasingly are taking the form of testing theory-based interventions. If a theory is correct, it has implications for strategies to influence people's health-related attitudes or behavior, and hence their health outcomes. And, if an intervention is developed on the basis of an explicit conceptualization of human behavior and thought, then it likely has a greater chance of being effective than if it is developed in a conceptual vacuum. The role of theory in the development of interventions is discussed at greater length in Chapter 27.

> **Example of a Theory-Based Intervention:**
> D. M. Smith and colleagues (2015) tested the effectiveness of a theory-based (Social Cognitive Theory) lifestyle program for pregnant women whose body mass index exceeded 30.

Using a Model or Theory as an Organizing Structure

Many researchers who cite a theory or model as their framework are not directly testing it but rather using the theory as organizational or interpretive tools. In such studies, researchers begin with a conceptualization of nursing (or stress, health beliefs, and so on) that is consistent with that of a model developer. The researchers *assume* that the model used as a framework is valid and proceed to conceptualize and operationalize constructs with the model in mind. Using models in this fashion can serve a valuable organizing purpose, but such studies do not address the issue of whether the theory itself is sound. Keller and colleagues (2009) have offered some guidelines for assessing fidelity to theory in intervention studies.

→ **TIP:** The Toolkit with the accompanying *Resource Manual* offers some criteria for drawing conclusions about whether researchers were truly testing a theory or using a theory as an organizational or interpretive aid.

We should note that the framework for a quantitative study need not be a formal theory such as those described in the previous section. Sometimes quantitative studies are undertaken to further explicate constructs identified in grounded theory or other qualitative research.

Fitting a Problem to a Theory

Researchers sometimes develop a set of research questions or hypotheses and then subsequently try to devise a theoretical context in which to frame them. Such an approach may in some cases be worthwhile, but we caution that an after-the-fact linkage of theory to a problem does not always enhance a study. An important exception is when the researcher is struggling to make sense of findings and calls on an existing theory to help explain or interpret them.

If it is necessary to find a relevant theory or model after a research problem is selected, the search for such a theory must begin by first conceptualizing the problem on an abstract level. For example, take the following research question: "Do daily telephone conversations between a psychiatric nurse and a patient for 2 weeks after hospital discharge reduce rates of readmission by short-term psychiatric patients?" This is a relatively concrete research problem, but it might profitably be viewed within the context of Orem's Self-Care Deficit Theory, reinforcement theory, a theory of social support, or a theory of crisis resolution. Part of the difficulty in finding a theory is that a single phenomenon of interest can be conceptualized in a number of ways.

Fitting a problem to a theory after-the-fact should be done with circumspection. Although having a theoretical context can enhance the meaningfulness of a study, artificially linking a problem to a theory is not the route to scientific utility nor to enhancing nursing's evidence base. There are many published studies that purport to have a conceptual framework when, in fact, the tenuous *post hoc* linkage is all too evident. If a conceptual model is really linked to a problem, then the design of the study, decisions about what to measure and how to measure it, and the interpretation of the findings *flow* from that conceptualization.

> **TIP:** If you begin with a research question and then subsequently identify a theory or model, be willing to adapt or augment your original research problem as you gain greater understanding of the theory. The linking of theory and research question may involve an iterative approach.

Developing a Framework in a Quantitative Study

Novice researchers may think of themselves as unqualified to develop a conceptual scheme of their own. But theory development depends less on research experience than on powers of observation, grasp of a problem, and knowledge of prior research. There is nothing to prevent a creative and astute person from formulating an original conceptual framework for a study. The framework may not be a full-fledged theory, but it should place the issues of the study into some broader perspective.

The basic intellectual process underlying theory development is induction—that is, reasoning from particular observations and facts to broader generalizations. The inductive process involves integrating what one has experienced or learned into an organized scheme. For quantitative research, the observations used in the inductive process usually are findings from other studies. When patterns of relationships among variables are derived in this

fashion, one has the makings of a theory that can be put to a more rigorous test. The first step in the development of a framework, then, is to formulate a generalized scheme of relevant concepts that is firmly grounded in the research literature.

Let us use as an example a hypothetical study question that we described in Chapter 4, namely, What is the effect of humor on stress in patients with cancer? (See the problem statement in Box 4.2). In undertaking a literature review, we find that researchers and reviewers have suggested a myriad of complex relationships among such concepts as humor, social support, stress, coping, appraisal, immune function, and neuroendocrine function on the one hand and various health outcomes (pain tolerance, mood, depression, health status, and eating and sleeping disturbances) on the other (e.g., Christie & Moore, 2005). While there is a fair amount of research evidence for the existence of these relationships, it is not clear how they all fit together. Without some kind of "map" or conceptualization of what might be going on, it would be difficult to design a strong study—we might, for example, not measure all the key variables or we might not undertake an appropriate analysis. And, if our goal is to design a humor therapy, we might struggle in developing a strong intervention in the absence of a framework.

The conceptual map in Figure 6.2 represents an attempt to put the pieces of the puzzle together

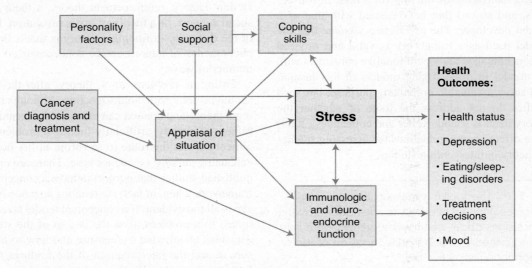

FIGURE 6.2 Conceptual Model of Stress and Health Outcomes in Patients with Cancer.

for a study involving a test of a humor intervention to improve health outcomes for patients with cancer. According to this map, stress is affected by a cancer diagnosis and treatment both directly and indirectly, through the person's appraisal of the situation. That appraisal, in turn, is affected by the patient's coping skills, personality factors, and available social supports (factors which themselves are interrelated). Stress and physiologic function (neuroendocrine and immunologic) have reciprocal relationships.

Note that we have not yet put in a "box" for humor in Figure 6.2. How do we think humor might operate? If we see humor as having primarily a direct effect on physiologic response, we would place humor near the bottom and draw an arrow from the box to immune and neuroendocrine function. But perhaps humor reduces stress because it helps a person cope (i.e., its effects are primarily psychological). Or maybe humor will affect the person's appraisal of the situation. Alternatively, a nurse-initiated humor therapy might have its effect primarily because it is a form of social support. Each conceptualization has a different implication for study design. To give but one example, if the humor therapy is viewed primarily as a form of social support, then we might want to compare our intervention to an alternative intervention that involves the presence of a comforting nurse (another form of social support), without any special effort at including humor.

This type of inductive conceptualization based on existing research is a useful means of providing theoretical grounding for a study. Of course, our research question in this example could have been addressed within the context of an existing conceptualization, such as Lazarus and Folkman's Theory of Stress and Coping or the psychoneuroimmunology (PNI) framework of McCain et al. (2005), but hopefully our example illustrates how developing an original framework can inform researchers' decisions and strengthen the study. Havenga and colleagues (2014) offer additional tips on developing a model.

◆ TIP: We strongly encourage you to draw a conceptual map before launching an investigation based on either a formal theory or your own

inductive conceptualization—even if you do not plan to formally test the entire model or present the model in a report. Such maps are valuable heuristic devices in planning a study.

Example of Developing a New Model:
Hoffman and colleagues (2014) developed a rehabilitation program for lung cancer patients and then pilot tested it. The intervention was based on their own model, which represented a synthesis of two theories, the Theory of Symptom Self-Management and the Transitional Care Model.

CRITIQUING FRAMEWORKS IN RESEARCH REPORTS

It is often challenging to critique the theoretical context of a published research report—or its absence—but we offer a few suggestions.

In a qualitative study in which a grounded theory is developed and presented, you probably will not be given enough information to refute the proposed theory because only evidence supporting it is presented. You can, however, assess whether the theory seems logical, whether the conceptualization is insightful, and whether the evidence in support of it is persuasive. In a phenomenologic study, you should look to see if the researcher addresses the philosophical underpinnings of the study. The researcher should briefly discuss the philosophy of phenomenology upon which the study was based.

Critiquing a theoretical framework in a quantitative report is also difficult, especially because you are not likely to be familiar with a range of relevant theories and models. Some suggestions for evaluating the conceptual basis of a quantitative study are offered in the following discussion and in Box 6.2. ✪

The first task is to determine whether the study does, in fact, have a theoretical or conceptual framework. If there is no mention of a theory, model, or framework, you should consider whether the study's contribution is weakened by the absence of a conceptual context. Nursing has been criticized for producing pieces of isolated research that are difficult to integrate because of the absence of a theoretical foundation, but in some cases, the research may be

BOX 6.2 Guidelines for Critiquing Theoretical and Conceptual Frameworks

1. Did the report describe an explicit theoretical or conceptual framework for the study? If not, does the absence of a framework detract from the usefulness or significance of the research?
2. Did the report adequately describe the major features of the theory or model so that readers could understand the conceptual basis of the study?
3. Is the theory or model appropriate for the research problem? Would a different framework have been more fitting?
4. If there is an intervention, was there a cogent theoretical basis or rationale for the intervention?
5. Was the theory or model used as a basis for generating hypotheses, or was it used as an organizational or interpretive framework? Was this appropriate?
6. Did the research problem and hypotheses (if any) naturally flow from the framework, or did the purported link between the problem and the framework seem contrived? Were deductions from the theory logical?
7. Were concepts adequately defined in a way that is consistent with the theory? If there was an intervention, were intervention components consistent with the theory?
8. Was the framework based on a conceptual model of nursing or on a model developed by nurses? If it was borrowed from another discipline, is there adequate justification for its use?
9. Did the framework guide the study methods? For example, was the appropriate research tradition used if the study was qualitative? If quantitative, did the operational definitions correspond to the conceptual definitions?
10. Did the researcher tie the study findings back to the framework in the Discussion section? Did the findings support or challenge the framework? Were the findings interpreted within the context of the framework?

so pragmatic that it does not really need a theory to enhance its usefulness. If, however, the study involves evaluating a complex intervention or testing hypotheses, the absence of a formally stated theoretical framework or rationale suggests conceptual fuzziness.

If the study does have an explicit framework, you must then ask whether the particular framework is appropriate. You may not be in a position to challenge the researcher's use of a particular theory or to recommend an alternative, but you can evaluate the logic of using that framework and assess whether the link between the problem and the theory is genuine. Does the researcher present a convincing rationale for the framework used? Do the hypotheses flow from the theory? Will the findings contribute to the validation of the theory? Does the researcher interpret the findings within the context of the framework? If the answer to such questions is no, you may have grounds for criticizing the study's framework, even though you may not be able to articulate how the conceptual basis of the study could be improved.

RESEARCH EXAMPLES

Throughout this chapter, we have mentioned studies that were based on various conceptual and theoretical models. This section presents more detailed examples of the linkages between theory and research from the nursing research literature—one from a quantitative study and the other from a qualitative study.

Research Example from a Quantitative Study: Health Promotion Model

Study: The effects of coping skills training among teens with asthma (Srof et al., 2012)

Statement of Purpose: The purpose of the study was to evaluate the effects of a school-based intervention, Coping Skills Training (CST), for teenagers with asthma.

Theoretical Framework: The Health Promotion Model (HPM), shown in Figure 6.1, was the guiding framework for the intervention. The authors noted that within the HPM, various behavior-specific cognitions (e.g., perceived barriers to behavior, perceived self-efficacy) influence health-promoting behavior *and* are modifiable through an intervention. In this study, the overall behavior of interest was asthma self-management. The CST intervention was a five-session small-group strategy designed to promote problem solving, cognitive-behavior modification, and conflict resolution using strategies to improve self-efficacy and reduce perceived barriers. The researchers hypothesized that participation in CST would result in improved outcomes: asthma self-efficacy, asthma-related quality of life, social support, and peak expiratory flow rate (PEFR).

Method: In this pilot study, 39 teenagers with asthma were randomly assigned to one of two groups—one that participated in the intervention and the other that did not. The researchers collected data about the outcomes from all participants at two points in time, before the start of the intervention and 6 weeks later.

Key Findings: Teenagers in the treatment group scored significantly higher at the end of the study on self-efficacy, activity-related quality of life, and social support than those in the control group.

Conclusions: The researchers noted that the self-efficacy and social support effects of the intervention were consistent with the HPM. They recommended that, although the findings were promising, replication of the study and an extension to specifically examine asthma self-management behavior would be useful.

Research Example from a Qualitative Study: A Grounded Theory

Study: Transition from patient to survivor in African American breast cancer survivors (Mollica & Nemeth, 2015)

Statement of Purpose: The purpose of the study was to examine the experience of African American women as they transition between breast cancer patient and breast cancer survivor.

Theoretical Framework: A grounded theory approach was chosen because the researchers noted as a goal "the discovery of theory from data systematically obtained and analyzed" (p. 17). The researchers further noted the use of induction that is inherent in a grounded theory approach: "An open, exploratory approach was used to identify recurrent meaningful concepts through systematic, inductive analysis of content" (p. 17).

Method: Data were collected through interviews with 15 community-based African American women who had completed treatment for primary breast cancer between 6 and 18 months prior to the interviews. Women were recruited from community settings in two American cities, through community and support groups. The women were interviewed by telephone. Each interview, which lasted about 45 minutes, was audiorecorded so that the interviews could be transcribed. The interviewer asked broad questions about the women's experiences following their treatment for breast cancer. Recruitment and interviewing continued until no new information was revealed—that is, until data saturation occurred.

Key Findings: Based on their analysis of the in-depth interviews, the researchers identified four main processes: perseverance through struggles supported by reliance on faith, dealing with persistent physical issues, needing anticipatory guidance after treatment, and finding emotional needs as important as physical ones. A schematic model for the substantive theory is presented in Figure 6.3.

SUMMARY POINTS

- High-quality research requires *conceptual integration*, one aspect of which is having a defensible theoretical rationale for undertaking the study in a given manner or for testing specific hypotheses. Researchers demonstrate their conceptual clarity through the delineation of a theory, model, or framework on which the study is based.

- A **theory** is a broad abstract characterization of phenomena. As classically defined, a theory is an abstract generalization that systematically explains relationships among phenomena. **Descriptive theory** thoroughly describes a phenomenon.

- Concepts are the basic components of a theory. Classically defined theories consist of a set of propositions about the interrelationships among concepts, arranged in a logically interrelated system that permits new statements to be deduced from them.

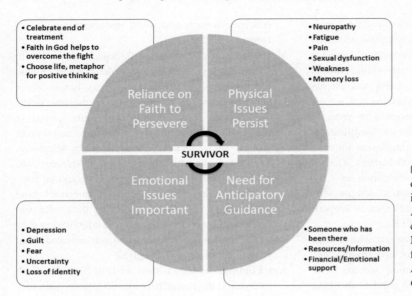

FIGURE 6.3 A grounded theory of the experience of transitioning into survivorship among African American women with breast cancer. (From Mollica, M., & Nemeth, L. [2015]. Transition from patient to survivor in African American breast cancer survivors. *Cancer Nursing*, *38*, 16–22.)

- **Grand theories** (or *macrotheories*) attempt to describe large segments of the human experience. **Middle-range theories** are more specific to certain phenomena and are increasingly important in nursing research.
- Concepts are also the basic elements of **conceptual models**, but concepts are not linked in a logically ordered, deductive system. Conceptual models, like theories, provide context for nursing studies.
- The goal of theories and models in research is to make findings meaningful, to integrate knowledge into coherent systems, to stimulate new research, and to explain phenomena and relationships among them.
- **Schematic models** (or **conceptual maps**) are graphic, theory-driven representations of phenomena and their interrelationships using symbols or diagrams and a minimal use of words.
- A **framework** is the conceptual underpinning of a study, including an overall rationale and conceptual definitions of key concepts. In qualitative studies, the framework often springs from distinct research traditions.
- Several conceptual models and grand theories of nursing have been developed. The concepts central to models of nursing are human beings, environment, health, and nursing. Two major

conceptual models of nursing used by researchers are Roy's Adaptation Model and Rogers' Science of Unitary Human Beings.
- Non-nursing models used by nurse researchers (e.g., Bandura's Social Cognitive Theory) are **borrowed theories**; when the appropriateness of borrowed theories for nursing inquiry is confirmed, the theories become **shared theories**.
- In some qualitative research traditions (e.g., phenomenology), the researcher strives to suspend previously held **substantive theories** of the phenomena under study, but there is a rich theoretical underpinning associated with the tradition itself.
- Some qualitative researchers specifically seek to develop *grounded theories*, data-driven explanations to account for phenomena under study through inductive processes.
- In the classical use of theory, researchers test hypotheses deduced from an existing theory. An emerging trend is the testing of theory-based interventions.
- In both qualitative and quantitative studies, researchers sometimes use a theory or model as an organizing framework or as an interpretive tool.
- Researchers sometimes develop a problem, design a study, and *then* look for a conceptual framework; such an after-the-fact selection of

a framework usually is less compelling than a more systematic application of a particular theory.

- Even in the absence of a formal theory, quantitative researchers can inductively weave together the findings from prior studies into a conceptual scheme that provides methodologic and conceptual direction to the inquiry.

STUDY ACTIVITIES

Chapter 6 of the *Resource Manual for Nursing Research: Generating and Assessing Evidence for Nursing Practice, 10th edition*, offers study suggestions for reinforcing concepts presented in this chapter. In addition, the following questions can be addressed in classroom or online discussions:

1. Select one of the conceptual models or theories described in this chapter. Formulate a research question and one or two hypotheses that could be used empirically to test the utility of the conceptual framework or model in nursing practice.
2. Answer appropriate questions from Box 6.2 regarding the Srof et al. (2012) intervention study for teens with asthma described at the end of the chapter. Also, consider what the implications of the study are in terms of the utility of the HPM.
3. Answer appropriate questions from Box 6.2 regarding Mollica and Nemeth's (2015) grounded theory study of the transition from breast cancer patient to survivor. Also answer these questions: (a) In what way was the use of theory different in this study than in the previous study by Srof and colleagues (2012)? (b) Comment on the utility of the schematic model shown in Figure 6.3.

STUDIES CITED IN CHAPTER 6

Aber, C., Weiss, M., & Fawcett, J. (2013). Contemporary women's adaptation to motherhood: The first 3 to 6 weeks postpartum. *Nursing Science Quarterly, 26,* 344–351.

Ajzen, I. (2005). *Attitudes, personality and behavior* (2nd ed.). New York: McGraw Hill.

Alligood, M. R. (2014). *Nurse theorists and their work.* (8th ed.). St. Louis, MO: Elsevier Mosby.

Bae, N., Park, S., & Lim, S. (2014). Factors associated with adherence to fecal occult blood testing for colorectal cancer screening among adults in the Republic of Korea. *European Journal of Oncology Nursing, 18,* 72–77.

Bandura, A. (1997). *Self-efficacy: The exercise of control.* New York: W. H. Freeman.

Bandura, A. (2001). Social cognitive theory: An agentic perspective. *Annual Review of Psychology, 52,* 1–26.

Beck, C. T. (2012). Exemplar: Teetering on the edge: A second grounded theory modification. In P. L. Munhall (Ed.), *Nursing research: A qualitative perspective* (5th ed., pp. 257–284). Sudbury, MA: Jones & Bartlett.

Becker, M. (1976). *Health belief model and personal health behavior.* Thorofare, NJ: Slack.

Becker, M. (1978). The Health Belief Model and sick role behavior. *Nursing Digest, 6,* 35–40.

Ben Natan, M., Grinberg, K., Galula, S., & Biton, M. (2014). Factors affecting Israeli women's decision whether to donate cord blood. *MCN: The American Journal of Maternal/Child Nursing, 39,* 96–101.

Blumer, H. (1986). *Symbolic interactionism: Perspective and method.* Berkeley, CA: University of California Press.

Chilton, J. M., Haas, B., & Gosselin, K. (2014). The effect of a wellness program on adolescent females. *Western Journal of Nursing Research, 36,* 581–598.

Chinn, P. L., & Kramer, M. K. (2015). *Knowledge development in nursing: Theory and process* (9th ed.). St. Louis, MO: Elsevier Mosby.

Christie, W., & Moore, C. (2005). The impact of humor on patients with cancer. *Clinical Journal of Oncology Nursing, 9,* 211–218.

Cole, K. A., & Gaspar, P. (2015). Implementation of an epilepsy self-management protocol. *Journal of Neuroscience Nursing, 47,* 3–9.

Conn, V. S., Rantz, M. J., Wipke-Tevis, D. D., & Maas, M. L. (2001). Designing effective nursing interventions. *Research in Nursing & Health, 24,* 433–442.

Dodd, M., Janson, S., Facione, N., Fawcett, J., Froelicher, E. S., Humphreys, J., . . . Taylor, D. (2001). Advancing the science of symptom management. *Journal of Advanced Nursing, 33,* 668–676.

Fawcett, J., & DeSanto-Madeya, S. (2013). *Contemporary nursing knowledge: Analysis and evaluation of nursing models and theories* (3rd ed.). Philadelphia: F.A. Davis.

Fetterman, D. M. (2010). *Ethnography: Step by step* (3rd ed.). Thousand Oaks, CA: Sage.

Fishbein, M., & Ajzen, I. (2010). *Predicting and changing behavior: The reasoned action approach.* New York: Psychology Press.

*Germino, B. B., Mishel, M., Crandell, J., Porter, L., Blyler, D., Jenerette, C., & Gil, K. (2013). Outcomes of an uncertainty management intervention in younger African American and Caucasian breast cancer survivors. *Oncology Nursing Forum, 40,* 82–92.

Havenga, Y., Poggenpoel, M., & Myburgh, C. (2014). Developing a model: An illustration. *Nursing Science Quarterly, 27,* 149–156.

*Hoffman, A., Brintnall, R., von Eye, A., Jones, L., Alderlink, G., Patelt, L., & Brown, J. (2014). A rehabilitation program for lung cancer patients during postthoracotomy chemotherapy. *OncoTargets and Therapy*, 7, 415–423.

Keller, C., Fleury, J., Sidano, S., & Ainsworth, B. (2009). Fidelity to theory in PA intervention research. *Western Journal of Nursing Research*, 31, 289–311.

Knapp, S. J., Sole, M. L., & Byers, J. (2013). The EPICS Family Bundle and its effect on stress and coping of families of critically ill trauma patients. *Applied Nursing Research*, 26, 51–57.

Kolcaba, K. (2003). *Comfort theory and practice*. New York: Springer.

Komatsu, H., Yagasaki, K., Shoda, R., Chung, Y., Iwata, T., Sugiyama, J., & Fuji, T. (2014). Repair of threatened feminine identity: Experience of women with cervical cancer undergoing fertility preservation surgery. *Cancer Nursing*, 37, 75–82.

Lazarus, R. (2006). *Stress and emotion: A new synthesis*. New York: Springer.

Lazarus, R., & Folkman, S. (1984). *Stress, appraisal, and coping*. New York: Springer.

Lee, M. K., Yun, Y., Park, H., Lee, E., Jung, K., & Noh, D. (2015). A web-based self-management exercise and diet intervention for breast cancer survivors. *International Journal of Nursing Studies*, 51, 1557–1567.

*McCain, N. L., Gray, D. P., Walter, J. M., & Robins, J. (2005). Implementing a comprehensive approach to the study of health dynamics using the psychoimmunology paradigm. *Advances in Nursing Science*, 28, 320–332.

McEwen, M., & Wills, E. (2011). *Theoretical basis for nursing* (3rd ed.). Philadelphia: Lippincott Williams & Wilkins.

Meleis, A. I., Sawyer, L. M., Im, E., Hilfinger Messias, D., & Schumacher, K. (2000). Experiencing transitions: An emerging middle-range theory. *Advances in Nursing Science*, 23,12–28.

Mishel, M. H. (1990). Reconceptualization of the uncertainty in illness theory. *Image: Journal of Nursing Scholarship*, 22, 256–262.

Mollica, M., & Nemeth, L. (2015). Transition from patient to survivor in African American breast cancer survivors. *Cancer Nursing*, 38, 16–22.

Morse, J. M. (2002). Theory innocent or theory smart? *Qualitative Health Research*, 12, 295–296.

Morse, J. M. (2004). Constructing qualitatively derived theory. *Qualitative Health Research*, 14, 1387–1395.

Parker, M. E., & Smith, M. C. (2011). *Nursing theories and nursing practice* (3rd ed.). Philadelphia: F.A. Davis.

Parse, R. R. (2014). *The humanbecoming paradigm: A transformational worldview*. Pittsburgh, PA: Discovery International.

Pender, N. J., Murdaugh, C., & Parsons, M. A. (2015). *Health promotion in nursing practice* (7th ed.). Upper Saddle River, NJ: Prentice Hall.

Peplau, H. E. (1997). Peplau's theory of interpersonal relations. *Nursing Science Quarterly*, 10, 162–167.

Peterson, S. J., & Bredow, T. S. (2012). *Middle range theories: Applications to nursing research* (3rd ed.). Philadelphia: Lippincott Williams & Wilkins.

Prochaska, J. O., Redding, C. A., & Evers, K. E. (2002). The transtheoretical model and stages of changes. In F. M. Lewis (Ed.), *Health behavior and health education: Theory, research and practice* (pp. 99–120). San Francisco, CA: Jossey Bass.

Prochaska, J. O., & Velicer, W. F. (1997). The transtheoretical model of health behavior change. *American Journal of Health Promotion*, 12, 38–48.

Ramezani, M., Ahmadi, F., Mohammadi, E., & Kazamnejad, A. (2014). Spiritual care in nursing: A concept analysis. *International Nursing Review*, 61, 211–219.

Reis, P. J., & Alligood, M. (2014). Prenatal yoga in late pregnancy and optimism, power, and well-being. *Nursing Science Quarterly*, 27, 30–36.

Rogers, M. E. (1990). Nursing: A science for unitary, irreducible human beings: Update 1990. In E. Barrett (Ed.), *Visions of Rogers' science-based nursing*. New York: National League for Nursing.

Rogers, M. E. (1994). The science of unitary human beings: Current perspectives. *Nursing Science Quarterly*, 7, 33–35.

Roy, C., Sr., & Andrews, H. (2009). *The Roy adaptation model*. (3rd ed.). Upper Saddle River, NJ: Prentice Hall.

Sandelowski, M. (1993). Theory unmasked: The uses and guises of theory in qualitative research. *Research in Nursing & Health*, 16, 213–218.

Schwartz-Barcott, D., & Kim, H. S. (2000). An expansion and elaborating of hybrid model of concept development. In B. L. Rodgers & K. A. Knafl (Eds.), *Concept development in nursing* (pp. 107–133). Philadelphia: Saunders.

Smith, D. M., Taylor, W., Whitworth, M., Roberts, S., Sibley, C., & Lavender, T. (2015). The feasibility phase of a community antenatal lifestyle programme [The Lifestyle Course (TLC)] for women with body mass index (BMI) $\geq$ 30 kg/m^2. *Midwifery*, 31, 280–287.

Smith, M. J., & Liehr, P. (2014). *Middle-range theory for nursing* (3rd ed.). New York: Springer.

Srof, B., Velsor-Friedrich, B., & Penckofer, S. (2012). The effects of coping skills training among teens with asthma. *Western Journal of Nursing Research*, 34, 1043–1061.

Walker, L. O., & Avant, K. C. (2010). *Strategies for theory construction in nursing* (5th ed.). Upper Saddle River, NJ: Prentice Hall.

***A link to this open-access journal article is provided in the Toolkit for this chapter in the accompanying* Resource Manual.** ✪

7 | Ethics in Nursing Research

Researchers who study human beings or animals must deal with ethical issues. Ethical demands can be challenging because ethical requirements sometimes conflict with the desire to produce rigorous evidence. This chapter discusses major ethical principles for conducting research.

ETHICS AND RESEARCH

When humans are used as study participants, care must be exercised to ensure that their rights are protected. The obligation for ethical conduct may strike you as self-evident, but ethical considerations have not always been given adequate attention, as we describe in the Supplement to this chapter on thePoint® regarding historical examples of ethical transgressions. Ⓢ

Codes of Ethics

In recognition that human rights violations have occurred in the name of science, various **codes of ethics** have been developed. The *Nuremberg Code*, developed after Nazi crimes were made public in the Nuremberg trials, was an international effort to establish ethical standards. The *Declaration of Helsinki*, another international set of standards, was adopted in 1964 by the World Medical Association and was most recently revised in 2013.

Most disciplines (e.g., psychology, sociology, medicine) have established their own ethical codes. In nursing, the American Nurses Association (ANA)

issued *Ethical Guidelines in the Conduct, Dissemination, and Implementation of Nursing Research* (Silva, 1995). The ANA, which declared 2015 the Year of Ethics, published a revised *Code of Ethics for Nurses with Interpretive Statements*, a document that covers primarily ethical issues for practicing nurses but that also includes principles that apply to nurse researchers. In Canada, the Canadian Nurses Association published a document entitled *Ethical Research Guidelines for Registered Nurses* in 2002. In Australia, three nursing organizations collaborated to develop the *Code of Ethics for Nurses in Australia* (2008).

Some nurse ethicists have called for an international ethics code for nursing research, but nurses in most countries have developed their own professional codes or follow the codes established by their governments. The International Council of Nurses (ICN), however, has developed the *ICN Code of Ethics for Nurses*, updated in 2012.

➲ **TIP:** In their study of 27 ethical review boards in the United States, Rothstein and Phuong (2007) found nurses to be more sensitive to ethical issues than physicians and other board members.

Government Regulations for Protecting Study Participants

Governments throughout the world fund research and establish rules for adhering to ethical principles. For example, Health Canada specified the

Tri-Council Policy Statement: Ethical Conduct for Research Involving Humans as the guidelines to protect study participants in all types of research, most recently in 2010. In Australia, the National Health and Medical Research Council issued the *National Statement on Ethical Conduct in Research Involving Humans* in 2007.

In the United States, the National Commission for the Protection of Human Subjects of Biomedical and Behavioral Research adopted a code of ethics in 1978. The commission, established by the National Research Act, issued the **Belmont Report**, which provided a model for many disciplinary guidelines. The Belmont Report also served as the basis for regulations affecting research sponsored by the U.S. government, including studies supported by National Institute of Nursing Research (NINR). The U.S. Department of Health and Human Services (DHHS) has issued ethical regulations that have been codified as Title 45 Part 46 of the Code of Federal Regulations (45 CFR 46). These regulations, revised most recently in 2009, are among the most widely used guidelines in the United States for evaluating the ethical aspects of studies.

➔ TIP: Many useful websites are devoted to ethical principles, only some of which are mentioned in this chapter. Several websites are listed in the "Useful Websites for Chapter 7" file in the Toolkit of the accompanying *Resource Manual* for you to click on directly.

Ethical Dilemmas in Conducting Research

Research that violates ethical principles is rarely done to be cruel or insensitive but usually reflects a conviction that knowledge is important and beneficial in the long run. There are situations in which participants' rights and study demands are in direct conflict, posing **ethical dilemmas** for researchers. Here are examples of research problems in which the desire for rigor conflicts with ethical considerations:

1. *Research question*: Does a new medication prolong life in patients with AIDS?
Ethical dilemma: The best way to test the effectiveness of an intervention is to administer the intervention to some participants but withhold it from others to see if differences between the groups emerge. However, if the intervention is untested (e.g., a new drug), the group receiving the intervention may be exposed to potentially hazardous side effects. On the other hand, the group *not* receiving the drug may be denied a beneficial treatment.

2. *Research question*: Are nurses equally empathic in their treatment of male and female patients in the ICU?
Ethical dilemma: Ethics require that participants be aware of their role in a study. Yet if the researcher informs nurse participants that their empathy in treating male and female ICU patients will be scrutinized, will their behavior be "normal"? If the nurses' usual behavior is altered because of the known presence of research observers, then the findings will be inaccurate.

3. *Research question*: What are the coping mechanisms of parents whose children have cancer?
Ethical dilemma: To answer this question, the researcher may need to probe into the psychological state of parents at a vulnerable time; such probing could be painful or traumatic. Yet knowledge of the parents' coping mechanisms might help to design effective interventions for dealing with parents' stress.

4. *Research question*: What is the process by which adult children adapt to the day-to-day stresses of caring for a parent with Alzheimer's disease?
Ethical dilemma: Sometimes, especially in qualitative studies, a researcher may get so close to participants that they become willing to share "secrets" and privileged information. Interviews can become confessions—sometimes of unseemly or illegal behavior. In this example, suppose a woman admitted to physically abusing her mother—how does the researcher respond to that information without undermining a pledge of confidentiality? And, if the researcher divulges the information to authorities, how can a pledge of confidentiality be given in good faith to other participants?

As these examples suggest, researchers are sometimes in a bind. They strive to develop good evidence for practice, using the best methods available, but they must also adhere to rules for protecting human rights. Another dilemma can arise if nurse researchers are confronted with conflict-of-interest situations, in which their expected behavior as researchers conflicts with their expected behavior as nurses (e.g., deviating from a research protocol to give assistance to a patient). It is precisely because of such dilemmas that codes of ethics have been developed to guide researchers' efforts.

ETHICAL PRINCIPLES FOR PROTECTING STUDY PARTICIPANTS

The *Belmont Report* articulated three broad principles on which standards of ethical conduct in research in the United States are based: beneficence, respect for human dignity, and justice. We briefly discuss these principles and then describe procedures researchers adopt to comply with them.

Beneficence

Beneficence imposes a duty on researchers to minimize harm and maximize benefits. Human research should be intended to produce benefits for participants or—a more common situation—for others. This principle covers multiple aspects.

The Right to Freedom from Harm and Discomfort

Researchers have an obligation to avoid, prevent, or minimize harm (*nonmaleficence*) in studies with humans. Participants should not be subjected to unnecessary risks of harm or discomfort, and their participation must be essential to achieving societally important aims that could not otherwise be realized. In research with humans, *harm* and *discomfort* can be physical (e.g., injury, fatigue), emotional (e.g., stress, fear), social (e.g., loss of social support), or financial (e.g., loss of wages). Ethical researchers must use strategies to minimize all types of harms and discomforts, even ones that are temporary.

Research should be conducted only by qualified people, especially if potentially dangerous equipment or specialized procedures are used. Ethical researchers must be prepared to terminate a study if they suspect that continuation would result in injury, death, or undue distress to participants. When a new medical procedure or drug is being tested, prior experimentation with animals or tissue cultures is often advisable. (Guidelines for the ethical treatment of animals are discussed later in this chapter).

Protecting human beings from physical harm may be straightforward, but the psychological consequences of study participation are usually subtle and require sensitivity. For example, participants may be asked questions about their personal views, weaknesses, or fears. Such queries might lead people to reveal highly personal information. The point is not that researchers should refrain from asking questions but that they need to be aware of the intrusion on people's psyches.

The need for sensitivity may be greater in qualitative studies, which often involve in-depth exploration on personal topics. In-depth probing may expose deep-seated fears that study participants had previously repressed. Qualitative researchers, regardless of the underlying research tradition, must be especially vigilant in anticipating complications.

The Right to Protection from Exploitation

Study involvement should not place participants at a disadvantage or expose them to damages. Participants need to be assured that their participation, or information they might provide, will not be used against them. For example, people describing their finances to a researcher should not be exposed to the risk of losing public health care benefits; those divulging illegal drug use should not fear exposure to criminal authorities.

Study participants enter into a special relationship with researchers, and this relationship should never be exploited. Exploitation may be overt and malicious (e.g., sexual exploitation, use of donated blood for a commercial product) but might also be more elusive. For example, suppose people agreed to participate in a study requiring 30 minutes of their time but the time commitment was actually much longer (e.g., 90 minutes). In such a situation, the researcher might be accused of exploiting the researcher–participant relationship.

Because nurse researchers may have a nurse–patient (in addition to a researcher–participant) relationship, special care may be required to avoid exploiting that bond. Patients' consent to participate in a study may result from their understanding of the researcher's role as *nurse*, not as *researcher*.

In qualitative research, psychological distance between researchers and participants often declines as the study progresses. The emergence of a pseudotherapeutic relationship is not uncommon, which can heighten the risk that exploitation could occur inadvertently (Eide & Kahn, 2008). On the other hand, qualitative researchers often are in a better position than quantitative researchers to *do good*, rather than just to avoid doing harm, because of the relationships they often develop with participants. Munhall (2012) has argued that qualitative nurse researchers have the responsibility of ensuring that, if there is a conflict, the clinical and therapeutic imperative of nursing takes precedence over the research imperative of advancing knowledge.

Example of Therapeutic Research Experiences: In their study on secondary traumatic stress among certified nurse-midwives, Beck and colleagues (2015) were told by some participants that it was therapeutic for them to write about traumatic births they had attended. One participant wrote,

"I think it's fascinating how little respect our patients and coworkers give to the traumatic experiences we suffer. It is healing to be able to write out my experiences in this study and actually have researchers interested in studying this topic."

Respect for Human Dignity

Respect for human dignity is the second ethical principle in the *Belmont Report*. This principle includes the right to self-determination and the right to full disclosure.

The Right to Self-Determination

Humans should be treated as autonomous agents, capable of controlling their actions. **Self-determination** means that prospective participants can voluntarily decide whether to take part in a study, without risk of prejudicial treatment. It also means that people have the right to ask questions, to refuse to give information, and to withdraw from the study.

A person's right to self-determination includes freedom from **coercion**, which involves threats of penalty from failing to participate in a study or excessive rewards from agreeing to participate. Protecting

people from coercion requires careful thought when the researcher is in a position of authority or influence over potential participants, as is often the case in a nurse–patient relationship. The issue of coercion may require scrutiny even when there is not a pre-established relationship. For example, a generous monetary incentive (or **stipend**) offered to encourage participation among an economically disadvantaged group (e.g., the homeless) might be considered mildly coercive because such incentives might pressure prospective participants into cooperation.

The Right to Full Disclosure

People's right to make informed, voluntary decisions about study participation requires full disclosure. **Full disclosure** means that the researcher has fully described the study, the person's right to refuse participation, the researcher's responsibilities, and likely risks and benefits. The right to self-determination and the right to full disclosure are the two major elements on which informed consent—discussed later in this chapter—is based.

Full disclosure is not always straightforward because it can create biases and sample recruitment problems. Suppose we were testing the hypothesis that high school students with a high rate of absenteeism are more likely to be substance abusers than students with good attendance. If we approached potential participants and fully explained the study purpose, some students likely would refuse to participate, and nonparticipation would be selective; those least likely to volunteer might well be substance-abusing students—the group of primary interest. Moreover, by knowing the research question, those who *do* participate might not give candid responses. In such a situation, full disclosure could undermine the study.

A technique that is sometimes used in such situations is **covert data collection** (*concealment*), which is the collection of data without participants' knowledge and consent. This might happen, for example, if a researcher wanted to observe people's behavior in real-world settings and worried that doing so openly would affect the behavior of interest. Researchers might choose to obtain the information through concealed methods, such as by videotaping with hidden equipment or observing while pretending to be engaged in other activities.

Covert data collection may in some cases be acceptable if risks are negligible and participants' right to privacy has not been violated. Covert data collection is least likely to be ethically tolerable if the study is focused on sensitive aspects of people's behavior, such as drug use or sexual conduct.

A more controversial technique is the use of **deception**, which involves deliberately withholding information about the study or providing participants with false information. For example, in studying high school students' use of drugs, we might describe the research as a study of students' health practices, which is a mild form of misinformation.

Deception and concealment are problematic ethically because they interfere with people's right to make informed decisions about personal costs and benefits of participation. Some people argue that deception is never justified. Others, however, believe that if the study involves minimal risk to participants and if there are anticipated benefits to society, then deception may be justified to enhance the validity of the findings.

Another issue that has emerged in this era of electronic communication concerns data collection over the Internet. For example, some researchers analyze the content of messages posted to blogs, listservs, or social media sites. The issue is whether such messages can be treated as research data without permission and informed consent. Some researchers believe that messages posted electronically are in the public domain and can be used without consent for research purposes. Others, however, feel that standard ethical rules should apply in cyberspace research and that researchers must carefully protect the rights of those who participate in "virtual" communities. Guidance for the ethical conduct of health research on the Internet has been developed by such writers as Ellett et al. (2004) and Holmes (2009).

Justice

The third broad principle articulated in the *Belmont Report* concerns justice, which includes participants' right to fair treatment and their right to privacy.

The Right to Fair Treatment
One aspect of justice concerns the equitable distribution of benefits and burdens of research. Participant selection should be based on study requirements and not on a group's vulnerability. Participant selection has been a key ethical issue historically, with researchers sometimes selecting groups with lower social standing (e.g., poor people, prisoners) as participants. The principle of justice imposes particular obligations toward individuals who are unable to protect their own interests (e.g., dying patients) to ensure that they are not exploited.

Distributive justice also imposes duties to neither neglect nor discriminate against individuals or groups who may benefit from research. During the 1980s and 1990s, it became evident that women and minorities were being unfairly excluded from many clinical studies in the United States. This led to the promulgation of regulations requiring that researchers who seek funding from the National Institutes of Health (NIH) include women and minorities as participants. The regulations also require researchers to examine whether clinical interventions have differential effects (e.g., whether benefits are different for men than for women), although this provision has had limited adherence (Polit & Beck, 2009, 2013).

The fair treatment principle covers issues other than participant selection. The right to fair treatment means that researchers must treat people who decline to participate (or who withdraw from the study after initial agreement) in a nonprejudicial manner; that they must honor all agreements made with participants (including payment of any promised stipends); that they demonstrate respect for the beliefs, habits, and lifestyles of people from different backgrounds or cultures; that they give participants access to research staff for desired clarification; and that they afford participants courteous and tactful treatment at all times.

The Right to Privacy
Research with humans involves intrusions into personal lives. Researchers should ensure that their research is not more intrusive than it needs to be and that participants' privacy is maintained. Participants have the right to expect that their data will be kept in strictest confidence.

Privacy issues have become especially salient in the U.S. health care community since the passage of the Health Insurance Portability and Accountability Act of 1996 (HIPAA), which articulates federal standards to protect patients' health information. In response to the HIPAA legislation, the U.S. Department of Health and Human Services issued the regulations *Standards for Privacy of Individually Identifiable Health Information*. For most health care providers who transmit health information electronically, compliance with these regulations, known as the Privacy Rule, was required as of April 14, 2003.

TIP: Some information relevant to HIPAA compliance is presented in this chapter, but you should confer with organizations that are involved in your research (if they are covered entities) regarding their practices and policies relating to HIPAA provisions. Websites that provide information about the implications of HIPAA for health research include http://privacyruleandresearch.nih.gov/ and www.hhs.gov/ocr/hipaa/guidelines/research.pdf.

PROCEDURES FOR PROTECTING STUDY PARTICIPANTS

Now that you are familiar with fundamental ethical principles in research, you need to understand procedures that researchers use to adhere to them.

Risk/Benefit Assessments

One strategy that researchers can use to protect participants is to conduct a **risk/benefit assessment**. Such an assessment is designed to evaluate whether the benefits of participating in a study are in line with the costs, be they financial, physical, emotional, or social—that is, whether the *risk/benefit ratio* is acceptable. A summary of risks and benefits should be communicated to recruited individuals so that they can evaluate whether it is in their best interest to participate. Box 7.1 summarizes major costs and benefits of research participation.

TIP: The Toolkit in the accompanying *Resource Manual* includes a Word document with the factors in Box 7.1 arranged in worksheet form for you to complete in doing a risk/benefit assessment. By completing the worksheet, it may be easier for you to envision opportunities for "doing good" and to avoid possibilities of doing harm.

The risk/benefit ratio should take into consideration whether risks to participants are commensurate with benefits to society. A broad guideline is that the degree of risk by participants should never exceed the potential humanitarian benefits of the knowledge to be gained. Thus, the selection of a significant topic that has the potential to improve patient care is the first step in ensuring that research is ethical. Gennaro (2014) has written eloquently about this issue.

All research involves some risks, but risk is sometimes minimal. **Minimal risk** is defined as risks no greater than those ordinarily encountered in daily life or during routine tests or procedures. When the risks are not minimal, researchers must proceed with caution, taking every step possible to diminish risks and maximize benefits. If expected risks to participants outweigh the anticipated benefits of the study, the research should be redesigned.

In quantitative studies, most details of the study usually are spelled out in advance, and so a reasonably accurate risk/benefit ratio assessment can be developed. Qualitative studies, however, usually evolve as data are gathered, and so it may be more difficult to assess all risks at the outset. Qualitative researchers must remain sensitive to potential risks throughout the study.

Example of Ongoing Risk/Benefit Assessment: Carlsson and colleagues (2007) discussed ethical issues relating to the conduct of interviews with people who have brain damage. The researchers noted the need for ongoing vigilance and attention to cues about risks and benefits. For example, one interview had to be interrupted because the participant displayed signs of distress. Afterward, however, the participant expressed gratitude for the opportunity to discuss his experience.

BOX 7.1 Potential Benefits and Risks of Research to Participants

MAJOR POTENTIAL BENEFITS TO PARTICIPANTS

- Access to a potentially beneficial intervention that might otherwise be unavailable
- Comfort in being able to discuss their situation or problem with a friendly, impartial person
- Increased knowledge about themselves or their conditions, either through opportunity for introspection and self-reflection or through direct interaction with researchers
- Escape from normal routine
- Satisfaction that information they provide may help others with similar conditions
- Direct monetary or material gains through stipends or other incentives

MAJOR POTENTIAL RISKS TO PARTICIPANTS

- Physical harm, including unanticipated side effects
- Physical discomfort, fatigue, or boredom
- Emotional distress resulting from self-disclosure, introspection, fear of the unknown, discomfort with strangers, fear of repercussions, anger or embarrassment at the questions being asked
- Social risks, such as the risk of stigma, adverse effects on personal relationships, loss of status
- Loss of privacy
- Loss of time
- Monetary costs (e.g., for transportation, child care, time lost from work)

One potential benefit to participants is monetary. Stipends offered to prospective participants are rarely viewed as an opportunity for financial gain, but there is ample evidence that stipends are useful incentives to participant recruitment and retention (Edwards et al., 2009). Financial incentives are especially effective when the group under study is difficult to recruit, when the study is time-consuming or tedious, or when participants incur study-related costs (e.g., for childcare or transportation). Stipends range from $1 to hundreds of dollars, but many are in the $20 to $30 range.

➔ **TIP:** In evaluating the anticipated risk/benefit ratio of a study design, you might want to consider how comfortable *you* would feel about being a study participant.

Informed Consent and Participant Authorization

A particularly important procedure for safeguarding participants is to obtain their informed con-

sent. **Informed consent** means that participants have adequate information about the research, comprehend that information, and have the ability to consent to or decline participation voluntarily. This section discusses procedures for obtaining informed consent and for complying with HIPAA rules regarding accessing patients' health information.

The Content of Informed Consent

Fully informed consent involves communicating the following pieces of information to participants:

1. *Participant status.* Prospective participants need to understand the distinction between *research* and *treatment*. They should be told which health care activities are routine and which are implemented specifically for the study. They also should be informed that data they provide will be used for research purposes.
2. *Study goals.* The overall goals of the research should be stated in lay rather than technical terms. The use to which the data will be put should be described.

3. *Type of data.* Prospective participants should be told what type of data (e.g., self-report, laboratory tests) will be collected.

4. *Procedures.* Prospective participants should be given a description of the data collection procedures and of procedures to be used in any innovative treatment.

5. *Nature of the commitment.* Participants should be told the expected time commitment at each point of contact and the number of contacts within a given time frame.

6. *Sponsorship.* Information on who is sponsoring or funding the study should be noted; if the research is part of an academic requirement, this information should be shared.

7. *Participant selection.* Prospective participants should be told how they were selected for recruitment and how many people will be participating.

8. *Potential risks.* Foreseeable risks (physical, psychological, social, or economic) or discomforts should be communicated as well as efforts that will be made to minimize risks. The possibility of unforeseeable risks should also be discussed, if appropriate. If injury or damage is possible, treatments that will be made available to participants should be described. When risks are more than minimal, prospective participants should be encouraged to seek advice before consenting.

9. *Potential benefits.* Specific benefits to participants, if any, should be described as well as possible benefits to others.

10. *Alternatives.* If appropriate, participants should be told about alternative procedures or treatments that might be advantageous to them.

11. *Compensation.* If stipends or reimbursements are to be paid (or if treatments are offered without any fee), these arrangements should be discussed.

12. *Confidentiality pledge.* Prospective participants should be assured that their privacy will at all times be protected. If anonymity can be guaranteed, this should be stated.

13. *Voluntary consent.* Researchers should indicate that participation is strictly voluntary and that failure to volunteer will not result in any penalty or loss of benefits.

14. *Right to withdraw and withhold information.* Prospective participants should be told that, after consenting, they have the right to withdraw from the study or to withhold any specific piece of information. Researchers may need to describe circumstances under which researchers would terminate the study.

15. *Contact information.* The researcher should tell participants whom they could contact in the event of further questions, comments, or complaints.

In qualitative studies, especially those requiring repeated contact with participants, it may be difficult to obtain meaningful informed consent at the outset. Qualitative researchers do not always know in advance how the study will evolve. Because the research design emerges during data collection, researchers may not know the exact nature of the data to be collected, what the risks and benefits to participants will be, or how much of a time commitment they will be expected to make. Thus, in a qualitative study, consent is often viewed as an ongoing, transactional process, sometimes called **process consent**. In process consent, the researcher continually renegotiates the consent, allowing participants to play a collaborative role in making decisions about ongoing participation.

Example of Process Consent: Darcy and colleagues (2014) studied the process of striving for an "ordinary, everyday life" among young children with cancer. In-depth interviews were conducted with children and their parents at 6 months and 1 year after diagnosis. Informed consent was obtained from parents, and verbal assent was obtained from children, at the first interview and confirmed at the second interview.

Comprehension of Informed Consent

Consent information is typically presented to prospective participants while they are being recruited, either orally or in writing. Written notices should not, however, take the place of spoken explanations, which provide opportunities for elaboration and for participants to question and "screen" the researchers.

Because informed consent is based on a person's evaluation of the potential risks and benefits of participation, the information must not only be communicated but understood. Researchers may have to play a "teacher" role in communicating consent information. They should be careful to use simple language and to avoid jargon and technical terms whenever possible; they should also avoid language that might unduly influence the person's decision to participate. Written statements should be consistent with the participants' reading levels and educational attainment. For participants from a general population (e.g., patients in a hospital), the statement should be written at about the 7th or 8th grade reading level.

⊃ TIP: Innovations to improve understanding of consent are being developed (e.g., Yates et al., 2009). Nishimura and colleagues (2013) have undertaken a systematic review of 54 of them.

For some studies, especially those involving more than minimal risk, researchers need to ensure that prospective participants understand what participation will entail. In some cases, this might involve testing participants for their comprehension of the informed consent material before deeming them eligible. Such efforts are especially warranted with participants whose native tongue is not English or who have cognitive impairments (Simpson, 2010).

Example of Evaluating Comprehension in Informed Consent: Horgas and colleagues (2008) studied the relationship between pain and functional disability in older adults. Prospective participants had to demonstrate ability to provide informed consent:

"Ability to consent was ascertained by explaining the study to potential participants, who were then asked to describe the study" (p. 344). All written materials for the study, including consent forms, were at the 8th grade reading level and printed in 14-point font.

Documentation of Informed Consent

Researchers usually document informed consent by having participants sign a **consent form**. In the United States, federal regulations for studies funded by the government require written consent of participants except under certain circumstances. When the study does not involve an intervention and data

are collected anonymously—or when existing data from records or specimens are used without linking identifying information to the data—regulations requiring written informed consent do not apply. HIPAA legislation is explicit about the type of information that must be eliminated from patient records for the data to be considered **de-identified**.

The consent form should contain all the information essential to informed consent. Prospective participants (or a legally authorized representative) should have ample time to review the document before signing it. The consent form should also be signed by the researcher, and a copy should be retained by both parties.

An example of a written consent form used in a study of one of the authors is presented in Figure 7.1. The numbers in the margins of this figure correspond to the types of information for informed consent outlined earlier. (The form does not indicate how people were selected; prospective participants were aware of recruitment through a particular support group.)

⊃ TIP: In developing a consent form, the following suggestions might prove helpful:

1. Organize the form coherently so that prospective participants can follow the logic of what is being communicated. If the form is complex, use headings as an organizational aid.
2. Use a large enough font so that the form can be easily read, and use spacing that avoids making the document appear too dense. Make the form attractive and inviting.
3. In general, simplify. Avoid technical terms if possible. If technical terms are needed, include definitions. Some suggestions are offered in the Toolkit.
4. Assess the form's reading level by using a **readability formula** to ensure an appropriate level for the group under study. There are several such formulas, including the Flesch Reading Ease score and Flesch-Kincaid Grade Level score (Flesch, 1948). Microsoft Word provides Flesch readability statistics.
5. Test the form with people similar to those who will be recruited, and ask for feedback.

Informed Consent Form

1 2 3,5 4 12 11 8	I understand that I am being asked to participate in a research study at Saint Francis Hospital and Medical Center. This research study will evaluate: What it is like being a mother of multiples during the first year of the infants' lives. If I agree to participate in the study, I will be interviewed for approximately 30 to 60 minutes about my experience as a mother of multiple infants. The interview will be tape-recorded and take place in a private office at Saint Francis Hospital. No identifying information will be included when the interview is transcribed. I understand I will receive $25.00 for participating in the study. There are no known risks associated with this study.
7	I realize that I may not participate in the study if I am younger than 18 years of age or I cannot speak English.
10	I realize that the knowledge gained from this study may help either me or other mothers of multiple infants in the future.
13 14	I realize that my participation in this study is entirely voluntary, and I may withdraw from the study at any time I wish. If I decide to discontinue my participation in this study, I will continue to be treated in the usual and customary fashion.
12	I understand that all study data will be kept confidential. However, this information may be used in nursing publications or presentations.
8	I understand that if I sustain injuries from my participation in this research project, I will not be automatically compensated by Saint Francis Hospital and Medical Center.
15	If I need to, I can contact Dr. Cheryl Beck, University of Connecticut, School of Nursing, any time during the study.
1,2	The study has been explained to me. I have read and understand this consent form, all of my questions have been answered, and I agree to participate. I understand that I will be given a copy of this signed consent form.

_____   _____

Signature of Participant   Date

_____   _____

Signature of Investigator   Date

FIGURE 7.1 Example of an informed consent form.

In certain circumstances (e.g., with non-English-speaking participants), researchers have the option of presenting the full information orally and then summarizing essential information in a **short form**. If a short form is used, however, the oral presentation must be witnessed by a third party, and the witness's signature must appear on the short consent form. The signature of a third-party witness is also advisable in studies involving more than minimal risk, even when a comprehensive consent form is used.

When the primary means of data collection is through a self-administered questionnaire, some researchers do not obtain written informed consent because they assume **implied consent** (i.e., that the return of the completed questionnaire reflects voluntary consent to participate). This assumption, however, may not always be warranted (e.g., if patients feel that their treatment might be affected by failure to cooperate with the researcher).

➲ **TIP:** The Toolkit in the accompanying *Resource Manual* includes several informed consent forms as Word documents that can be adapted for your use. (Many universities offer templates for consent forms.) The Toolkit also includes several other resources designed to help you with the ethical aspects of a study.

Authorization to Access Private Health Information

Under HIPAA regulations in the United States, a covered entity such as a hospital can disclose individually identifiable health information (IIHI) from its records if the patient signs an authorization. The authorization can be incorporated into the consent form, or it can be a separate document. ✴ Using a separate authorization form may be advantageous to protect the patients' confidentiality because the form does not need to provide detailed information about the study purpose. If the research purpose is not sensitive, or if the entity is already cognizant of the study purpose, an integrated form may suffice.

The authorization, whether obtained separately or as part of the consent form, must include the following: (1) who will receive the information, (2) what type of information will be disclosed, and (3) what further disclosures the researcher anticipates. Patient authorization to access IIHI can be waived only under certain circumstances. Patient authorization usually must be obtained for data that are *created* as part of the research as well as for information already maintained in institutional records (Olsen, 2003).

Confidentiality Procedures

Study participants have the right to expect that data they provide will be kept in strict confidence. Participants' right to privacy is protected through various confidentiality procedures.

Anonymity

Anonymity, the most secure means of protecting confidentiality, occurs when the researcher cannot link participants to their data. For example, if questionnaires were distributed to a group of nursing home residents and were returned without any identifying information, responses would be anonymous. As another example, if a researcher reviewed hospital records from which all identifying

information had been expunged, anonymity would again protect participants' right to privacy. Whenever it is possible to achieve anonymity, researchers should strive to do so.

Example of Anonymity: Johnson and McRee (2015) studied health-risk behavior among high school athletes. The data for the study were collected via questionnaires, completed anonymously by nearly 50,000 student athletes in the state of Minnesota.

Confidentiality in the Absence of Anonymity

When anonymity is not possible, other confidentiality procedures are needed. A promise of **confidentiality** is a pledge that any information participants provide will not be publicly reported in a manner that identifies them and will not be accessible to others. This means that research information should not be shared with strangers nor with people known to participants (e.g., relatives, doctors, other nurses), unless participants give explicit permission to do so.

Researchers can take a number of steps to ensure that a *breach of confidentiality* does not occur, including the following:

- Obtain identifying information (e.g., name, address) from participants only when essential.
- Assign an **identification** (ID) **number** to each participant and attach the ID number rather than other identifiers to the actual data.
- Maintain identifying information in a locked file.
- Restrict access to identifying information to only a few people on a need-to-know basis.
- Enter no identifying information onto computer files.
- Destroy identifying information as quickly as practical.
- Make research personnel sign confidentiality pledges if they have access to data or identifying information. ✴
- Report research information in the aggregate; if information for an individual is reported, disguise the person's identity, such as through the use of a fictitious name.

➜ **TIP:** Researchers who plan to collect data from participants multiple times (or who use multiple forms that need to be linked) do not have to forego anonymity. A technique that has been successful is to have participants themselves generate an ID number. They might be instructed, for example, to use their birth year and the first three letters of their mother's maiden names as their ID code (e.g., 1946CRU). This code would be put on every form so that forms could be linked, but researchers would not know participants' identities.

Qualitative researchers may need to take extra steps to safeguard participants' privacy. Anonymity is rarely possible in qualitative studies because researchers typically become closely involved with participants. Moreover, because of the in-depth nature of qualitative studies, there may be a greater invasion of privacy than is true in quantitative research. Researchers who spend time in the home of a participant may, for example, have difficulty segregating the public behaviors that the participant is willing to share from private behaviors that unfold during data collection. A final issue is adequately disguising participants in reports. Because the number of participants is small, qualitative researchers may need to take extra precautions to safeguard identities. This may mean more than simply using a fictitious name. Qualitative researchers may have to slightly distort identifying information or provide only general descriptions. For example, a 49-year-old antique dealer with ovarian cancer might be described as "a middle-aged cancer patient who worked in sales" to avoid identification that could occur with the more detailed description.

Example of Confidentiality Procedures in a Qualitative Study: Dale and colleagues (2015) explored factors that contribute to poor attendance in cardiac rehabilitation programs among men with coronary heart disease and type 2 diabetes, including factors relating to the men's masculinity and perceptions about gender roles. Potential participants were provided with an informational packet and then informed consent procedures were initiated, including assurances of confidentiality. To further protect confidentiality, the study team assigned pseudonyms to all participants.

Certificates of Confidentiality

There are situations in which confidentiality can create tensions between researchers and legal or other authorities, especially if participants engage in criminal or dangerous activity (e.g., substance abuse). To avoid the possibility of forced, involuntary disclosure of sensitive research information (e.g., through a court order or subpoena), researchers in the United States can apply for a **Certificate of Confidentiality** from the National Institutes of Health (Lutz et al., 2000; Wolf et al., 2012). Any research that involves the collection of personally identifiable, sensitive information is potentially eligible for a Certificate, even if the study is not federally funded. Information is considered sensitive if its release might damage participants' financial standing, employability, or reputation or might lead to discrimination; information about a person's mental health, as well as genetic information, is also considered sensitive. A Certificate allows researchers to refuse to disclose identifying information on study participants in any civil, criminal, administrative, or legislative proceeding at the federal, state, or local level.

A Certificate of Confidentiality helps researchers to achieve their research objectives without threat of involuntary disclosure and can be helpful in recruiting participants. Researchers who obtain a Certificate should alert prospective participants about this valuable protection in the consent form and should note any planned exceptions to those protections. For example, a researcher might decide to voluntarily comply with state child abuse reporting laws even though the Certificate would prevent authorities from punishing researchers who chose not to comply.

Example of Obtaining a Certificate of Confidentiality: Mallory and Hesson-McInnis (2013) pilot tested an HIV prevention intervention with incarcerated and other high-risk women. The women were asked about various sensitive topics, and so the researchers obtained a Certificate of Confidentiality.

Debriefings, Communications, and Referrals

Researchers can show their respect—and proactively minimize emotional risks—by carefully attending to the nature of their interactions with participants. For example, researchers should always be gracious and polite, should phrase questions tactfully, and should be considerate with regard to cultural and linguistic diversity.

Researchers can also use more formal strategies to communicate respect and concern for participants' well-being. For example, it is sometimes useful to offer **debriefing** sessions after data collection is completed to permit participants to ask questions or air complaints. Debriefing is especially important when the data collection has been stressful or when ethical guidelines had to be "bent" (e.g., if any deception was used in explaining the study).

Example of Debriefing: Payne (2013) evaluated the effectiveness of a diabetes support group for indigenous women in Australia. Information was obtained before and after implementing the support group. At the end of the study,

"a final group debriefing was implemented for ethical closure" (p. 41).

It is also thoughtful to communicate with participants after the study is completed to let them know that their participation was appreciated. Researchers sometimes demonstrate their interest in study participants by offering to share study findings with them once the data have been analyzed (e.g., by mailing them a summary or advising them of an appropriate website).

Finally, in some situations, researchers may need to assist study participants by making referrals to appropriate health, social, or psychological services.

Example of Referrals: Simwaka and colleagues (2014) studied the perceptions of women living in villages in Malawi regarding the caring behaviors of nurse-midwives during perinatal loss. To minimize psychological distress, participants were told that a qualified community nurse and her students would be available in the community from time to time to provide professional support as they grieved their loss.

Treatment of Vulnerable Groups

Adherence to ethical standards is often straightforward, but additional procedures may be required to protect the rights of special **vulnerable groups**. Vulnerable populations may be incapable of giving fully informed consent (e.g., cognitively impaired people) or may be at risk of unintended side effects because of their circumstances (e.g., pregnant women). Researchers interested in studying high-risk groups should understand guidelines governing informed consent, risk/benefit assessments, and acceptable research procedures for such groups. Research with vulnerable groups should be undertaken only when the risk/benefit ratio is low or when there is no alternative (e.g., studies of childhood development require child participants).

Among the groups that nurse researchers should consider vulnerable are the following:

- *Children*. Legally and ethically, children do not have competence to give informed consent, so the informed consent of their parents or legal guardians must be obtained. It is appropriate, however—especially if the child is at least 7 years old—to obtain the child's assent as well. **Assent** refers to the child's agreement to participate. If the child is mature enough to understand basic informed consent information (e.g., a 12-year-old), it is advisable to obtain written consent from the child as well, as evidence of respect for the child's right to self-determination. Kanner and colleagues (2004) and Lambert and Glacken (2011) provide some guidance on children's assent and consent to participate in research. The U.S. government has issued special regulations (Code of Federal Regulations, 2009, Subpart D) for additional protections of children as study participants.

- *Mentally or emotionally disabled people*. Individuals whose disability makes it impossible for them to weigh the risks and benefits of participation (e.g., people affected by cognitive impairment or coma) also cannot legally or ethically provide informed consent. In such cases, researchers should obtain the written consent of a legal guardian. To the extent possible, informed consent or assent from participants themselves should be sought as a supplement to a guardian's consent. NIH guidelines note that studies involving people whose autonomy is compromised by disability should focus in a direct way on their condition.

- *Severely ill or physically disabled people.* For patients who are very ill or undergoing certain treatments, it might be prudent to assess their ability to make reasoned decisions about study participation. For certain disabilities, special procedures for obtaining consent may be required. For example, with deaf participants, the entire consent process may need to be in writing. For people who have a physical impairment preventing them from writing or for participants who cannot read and write, alternative procedures for documenting informed consent (e.g., videorecording consent proceedings) should be used.

- *The terminally ill.* Terminally ill people who participate in studies seldom expect to benefit personally from the research, and so the risk/benefit ratio needs to be carefully assessed. Researchers must take steps to ensure that the health care and comfort of terminally ill participants are not compromised.

- *Institutionalized people.* Particular care is required in recruiting institutionalized people because they depend on health care personnel and may feel pressured into participating or may believe that their treatment would be jeopardized by failure to cooperate. Inmates of prisons and other correctional facilities, who have lost their autonomy in many spheres of activity, may similarly feel constrained in their ability to withhold consent. The U.S. government has issued specific regulations for the protection of prisoners as study participants (see Code of Federal Regulations, 2009, Subpart C). Researchers studying institutionalized groups need to emphasize the voluntary nature of participation.

- *Pregnant women.* The U.S. government has issued additional requirements governing research with pregnant women and fetuses (Code of Federal Regulations, 2009, Subpart B). These requirements reflect a desire to safeguard both the pregnant woman, who may be at heightened physical and psychological risk, and the fetus, who cannot give informed consent. The regulations stipulate that a pregnant woman cannot be involved in a study unless its purpose is to meet the health needs of the pregnant woman, and risks to her and the fetus are minimized or there is only a minimal risk to the fetus.

Example of Research with a Vulnerable Group: Nyamathi and colleagues (2012) studied the impact of a nursing intervention on decreasing substance use among homeless youth. The participants were recruited from a drop-in agency in California. A community advisory board contributed to the design of the intervention. Research staff met with homeless youth who were interested in the study to assist them in reading and understanding informed consent. Participants completed two consent forms—one prior to screening for eligibility and the second prior to actual participation in one of two programs.

It should go without saying that researchers need to proceed with great caution in conducting research with people who might fall into two or more vulnerable categories (e.g., incarcerated youth).

External Reviews and the Protection of Human Rights

Researchers, who often have a strong commitment to their research, may not be objective in their risk/benefit assessments or in their procedures to protect participants' rights. Because of the possibility of a biased self-evaluation, the ethical dimensions of a study should normally be subjected to external review.

Most institutions where research is conducted have formal committees for reviewing proposed research plans. These committees are sometimes called *human subjects committees*, *ethical advisory boards*, or *research ethics committees*. In the United States, the committee usually is called an **Institutional Review Board (IRB)**, whereas in Canada, it is called a **Research Ethics Board (REB)**.

TIP: You should find out early what an institution's requirements are regarding ethics, in terms of its forms, procedures, and review schedules. It is wise to allow a generous amount of time for negotiating with IRBs, which may require procedural modifications and re-review.

Qualitative researchers in various countries have expressed concerns that standard ethical review procedures are not sensitive to special issues and circumstances faced in qualitative research. There is concern that regulations were " . . . created for quantitative work, and can actually impede or interrupt work that is not hypothesis-driven 'hard science'" (van den Hoonaard, 2002, p. i). Qualitative researchers may need to take care to explain their methods, rationales, and approaches to review board members unfamiliar with qualitative research.

Institutional Review Boards

In the United States, federally sponsored studies are subject to strict guidelines for evaluating the treatment of human participants. (Guidance on human subject's issues in grant applications is provided in Chapter 31.) Before undertaking such a study, researchers must submit research plans to the IRB and must also go through a formal training on ethical conduct and a certification process that can be completed online.

The duty of the IRB is to ensure that the proposed plans meet federal requirements for ethical research. An IRB can approve the proposed plans, require modifications, or disapprove the plans. The main requirements governing IRB decisions may be summarized as follows (Code of Federal Regulations, 2009, §46.111):

- Risks to participants are minimized.
- Risks to participants are reasonable in relation to anticipated benefits, if any, and the importance of the knowledge that may reasonably be expected to result.
- Selection of participants is equitable.
- Informed consent will be sought, as required, and appropriately documented.
- Adequate provision is made for monitoring the research to ensure participants' safety.
- Appropriate provisions are made to protect participants' privacy and confidentiality of the data.
- When vulnerable groups are involved, appropriate additional safeguards are included to protect their rights and welfare.

Example of IRB Approval: Deitrick and co-researchers (2015) compared the effectiveness of two different doses of promethazine for the treatment of postoperative nausea and vomiting in an American teaching hospital. Approval to conduct the study was obtained from the university's Institutional Review Board.

Many studies require a full IRB review at a meeting with a majority of IRB members present. An IRB must have five or more members, at least one of whom is not a researcher (e.g., a member of the clergy or a lawyer may be appropriate). One IRB member must be a person who is not affiliated with the institution and is not a family member of an affiliated person. To protect against potential biases, the IRB cannot comprise entirely men, women, or members from a single profession.

For certain research involving no more than minimal risk, the IRB can use expedited review procedures, which do not require a meeting. In an **expedited review**, a single IRB member (usually the IRB chairperson) carries out the review. An example of research that qualifies for an expedited IRB review is minimal-risk research " . . . employing survey, interview, oral history, focus group, program evaluation, human factors evaluation, or quality assurance methodologies" (Code of Federal Regulations, 2009, §46.110).

Federal regulations also allow certain types of research in which there are no apparent risk to participants to be exempt from IRB review. The website of the Office for Human Research Protections, in its policy guidance section, includes decision charts designed to clarify whether a study is exempt.

→ TIP: Researchers seeking a Certificate of Confidentiality must first obtain IRB approval because such approval is a prerequisite for the Certificate. Applications for the Certificate should be submitted at least 3 months before participants are expected to enroll in the study.

Data and Safety Monitoring Boards

In addition to IRBs, researchers in the United States may have to communicate information about ethical aspects of their studies to other groups. For example, some institutions have established separate **Privacy Boards** to review researchers' compliance with provisions in HIPAA, including review of authorization forms and requests for waivers.

For researchers evaluating interventions in clinical trials, NIH also requires review by a **data and safety monitoring board** (DSMB). The purpose of a DSMB is to oversee the safety of participants, to promote data integrity, and to review accumulated outcome data on a regular basis to determine whether study protocols should be altered, or the study stopped altogether. Members of a DSMB are selected based on their clinical, statistical, and methodologic expertise. The degree of monitoring by the DSMB should be proportionate to the degree of risk involved. Slimmer and Andersen (2004) offer suggestions on developing a DSM plan. Artinian and colleagues (2004) provided good descriptions of their data and safety monitoring plan for a study of a nurse-managed telemonitoring intervention and discussed how IRBs and DSMBs differ.

Building Ethics into the Design of the Study

Researchers need to give thought to ethical requirements while planning a study and should ask themselves whether intended safeguards for protecting humans are sufficient. They must continue their vigilance throughout the course of the study as well because unforeseen ethical dilemmas may arise. Of course, first steps in doing ethical research include ensuring that the research question is clinically significant and designing the study to yield sound evidence—it can be construed as unethical to do weakly designed research because it would be a poor use of people's time.

The remaining chapters of the book offer advice on how to design studies that yield high-quality evidence for practice. Methodologic decisions about rigor, however, must be made within the context of ethical requirements. Box 7.2 presents some examples of the

---

BOX 7.2 Examples of Questions for Building Ethics into a Study Design

RESEARCH DESIGN
- Will participants get allocated fairly to different treatment groups?
- Will steps to reduce bias or enhance integrity add to the risks participants will incur?
- Will the setting for the study protect against participant discomfort?

INTERVENTION
- Is the intervention designed to maximize good and minimize harm?
- Under what conditions might a treatment be withdrawn or altered?

SAMPLE
- Is the population defined so as to unwittingly and unnecessarily exclude important segments of people (e.g., women or minorities)?
- Will potential participants be recruited into the study equitably?

DATA COLLECTION
- Will data be collected in such a way as to minimize respondent burden?
- Will procedures for ensuring confidentiality of data be adequate?
- Will data collection staff be appropriately trained to be sensitive and courteous?

REPORTING
- Will participants' identities be adequately protected?

kinds of questions that might be posed in thinking about ethical aspects of study design.

→ **TIP:** After study procedures have been developed, researchers should undertake a self-evaluation of those procedures to determine if they meet ethical requirements. Box 7.3 later in this chapter provides some guidelines that can be used for such a self-evaluation.

OTHER ETHICAL ISSUES

In discussing ethical issues relating to the conduct of nursing research, we have given primary consideration to the protection of human participants. Two other ethical issues also deserve mention: the treatment of animals in research and research misconduct.

Ethical Issues in Using Animals in Research

Some nurse researchers work with animals rather than human beings as their subjects, typically focusing on biophysiologic phenomena. Despite some opposition to such research by animal rights activists, researchers in health fields likely will continue to use animals to explore physiologic mechanisms and interventions that could pose risks to humans.

Ethical considerations are clearly different for animals and humans; for example, the concept of *informed consent* is not relevant for animal subjects. Guidelines have been developed governing treatment of animals in research. In the United States, the Public Health Service has issued a policy statement on the humane care and use of laboratory animals. The guidelines articulate nine principles for the proper treatment of animals used in biomedical and behavioral research. These principles cover such issues as alternatives to using animals, pain and distress in animal subjects, researcher qualifications, use of appropriate anesthesia, and euthanizing animals under certain conditions. In Canada, researchers who use animals in their studies must adhere to the policies and guidelines of the Canadian Council on Animal Care (CCAC) as articulated in their *Guide to the Care and Use of Experimental Animals.*

Holtzclaw and Hanneman (2002) noted several important considerations in the use of animals in nursing research. First, there must be a compelling reason to use an animal model—not simply convenience or novelty. Second, study procedures should be humane, well planned, and well funded. Animal studies are not necessarily less costly than those with human participants, and they require serious consideration to justify their use.

Example of Research with Animals: Moes and Holden (2014) studied changes in spontaneous activity and skeletal muscle mass with Sprague-Dawley rats that had received chronic constriction injury surgery. The University of Michigan's Committee on the Use and Care of Animals approved all procedures, and the study adhered to guidelines of the Association for Assessment and Accreditation of Laboratory Animal Care.

Research Misconduct

Ethics in research involves not only the protection of human and animal subjects but also protection of the public trust. The issue of **research misconduct** (or *scientific misconduct*) has received greater attention in recent years as incidents of researcher fraud and misrepresentation have come to light. Currently, the U.S. agency responsible for overseeing efforts to improve research integrity and for handling allegations of research misconduct is the Office of Research Integrity (ORI) within DHHS. Researchers seeking funding from NIH must demonstrate that they have received training on research integrity and the responsible conduct of research.

Research misconduct is defined by U.S. Public Health Service regulation (42 CFR Part 93.103) as "fabrication, falsification, or plagiarism in proposing, performing, or reviewing research, or in reporting research results." To be construed as misconduct, there must be a significant departure from accepted practices in the research community, and the misconduct must have been committed intentionally and knowingly. *Fabrication* involves making up data or study results. *Falsification* involves manipulating research materials, equipment, or processes; it also involves changing or omitting data or distorting results such that the results are not accurately represented in reports. *Plagiarism* involves the appropriation of someone's ideas, results, or words without giving due credit, including information obtained through the confidential review of research proposals or manuscripts.

Example of Research Misconduct: In 2008, the U.S. Office of Research Integrity ruled that a nurse engaged in scientific misconduct in a study supported by the National Cancer Institute. The nurse falsified and fabricated data that were reported to the National Surgical Adjuvant Breast and Bowel Project (NIH Notice Number NOT-OD-08-096).

Although the official definition focuses on only three types of misconduct, there is widespread agreement that research misconduct covers many other issues including improprieties of authorship, poor data management, conflicts of interest, inappropriate financial arrangements, failure to comply with governmental regulations, and unauthorized use of confidential information.

Research integrity is an important concern in nursing. Jeffers and Whittemore (2005), for example, engaged in work to identify and describe research environments that promote integrity. In a study that focused on ethical issues faced by editors of nursing journals, Freda and Kearney (2005) found that 64% of 88 editors reported some type of ethical dilemma, such as duplicate publication, plagiarism, or conflicts of interest. Habermann and colleagues (2010) studied 1,645 research coordinators' experiences with research misconduct in their clinical environments. More than 250 coordinators, most of them nurses, said they had firsthand knowledge of scientific misconduct that included protocol violations, consent violations, fabrication, falsification, and financial conflicts of interest.

CRITIQUING THE ETHICS OF RESEARCH STUDIES

Guidelines for critiquing ethical aspects of a study are presented in Box 7.3. Members of an ethics committee should be provided with sufficient information to answer all these questions. Research journal articles, however, do not always include

BOX 7.3 Guidelines for Critiquing the Ethical Aspects of a Study

1. Was the study approved and monitored by an Institutional Review Board, Research Ethics Board, or other similar ethics review committee?
2. Were participants subjected to any physical harm, discomfort, or psychological distress? Did the researchers take appropriate steps to remove, prevent, or minimize harm?
3. Did the benefits to participants outweigh any potential risks or actual discomfort they experienced? Did the benefits to society outweigh the costs to participants?
4. Was any type of coercion or undue influence used to recruit participants? Did they have the right to refuse to participate or to withdraw without penalty?
5. Were participants deceived in any way? Were they fully aware of participating in a study and did they understand the purpose and nature of the research?
6. Were appropriate informed consent procedures used? If not, were there valid and justifiable reasons?
7. Were adequate steps taken to safeguard participants' privacy? How was confidentiality maintained? Were Privacy Rule procedures followed (if applicable)? Was a Certificate of Confidentiality obtained? If not, *should* one have been obtained?
8. Were vulnerable groups involved in the research? If yes, were special precautions used because of their vulnerable status?
9. Were groups omitted from the inquiry without a justifiable rationale, such as women (or men), minorities, or older people?

detailed information about ethics because of space constraints. Thus, it is not always possible to critique researchers' adherence to ethical guidelines, but we offer a few suggestions for considering a study's ethical aspects.

Many research reports acknowledge that study procedures were reviewed by an IRB or ethics committee, and some journals require such statements. When a report specifically mentions a formal review, it is usually safe to assume that a group of concerned people did a conscientious review of the study's ethical issues.

You can also come to some conclusions based on a description of the study methods. There may be sufficient information to judge, for example, whether participants were subjected to harm or discomfort. Reports do not always specifically state whether informed consent was secured, but you should be alert to situations in which the data could not have been gathered as described if participation were purely voluntary (e.g., if data were gathered unobtrusively).

In thinking about ethical issues, you should also consider who the study participants were. For example, if a study involved vulnerable groups, there should be more information about protective procedures. You might also need to attend to who the study participants were *not*. For example, there has been considerable concern about the omission of certain groups (e.g., minorities) from clinical research.

It is often difficult to determine whether the participants' privacy was safeguarded unless the researcher mentions pledges of confidentiality or anonymity. A situation requiring special scrutiny arises when data are collected from two people simultaneously (e.g., a husband/wife or parent/child who are jointly interviewed). As noted by Forbat and Henderson (2003), ethical issues arise when two people in an intimate relationship are interviewed about a common issue, even when they are interviewed privately. They described the potential for being "stuck in the middle" when trying to get two viewpoints and facing the dilemma of how to ask one person probing questions after having been given confidential information about the issue by the other.

RESEARCH EXAMPLES

Two research examples that highlight ethical issues are presented in the following sections.

Research Example from a Quantitative Study

Study: Effects of a healthy eating intervention on Latina migrant farmworker mothers (Kilanowski & Lin, 2013)

Study Purpose: The purpose of the study was to pilot test an intervention, the Dietary Intake and Nutrition Education (DINE) program, to promote healthy eating among migrant Latina farmworking mothers and their children in the United States. The hypothesis was that the mothers in the intervention would have improved nutrition knowledge and their children would have a decreased body mass index (BMI) percentiles and improved eating patterns.

Research Methods: The educational intervention, which involved three 1-hour classes, was made available to an intervention group of 34 mothers; 25 mothers working at different farms and not receiving the intervention were used as a comparison group. The data for the study, collected before and after the intervention, included mothers' self-reports on food security, self-efficacy, food patterns, and food knowledge. Height and weight measurements were obtained for children aged 2 to 12 years, behind a privacy screen.

Ethics-Related Procedures: The study was approved by Capital University's IRB by expedited review. The study also underwent a cultural assessment that evaluated the study methods and their congruence with cultural norms. Participating families were recruited through the cooperation of gatekeepers at farms in two Midwestern states. Mothers who were interested in participating approached researchers who answered their questions. Parents were asked to complete informed consent forms. Children who were 8 or older were also asked for verbal assent. Consent and assent procedures were implemented by bilingual research team members prior to the intervention. All forms and instruments were sensitive to low literacy levels and were available in English and Spanish. To enhance privacy, most instruments were administered using audio-enhanced personal digital assistants (PDAs), with questions read to the participants as they listened on personal headphones. All data collection and the intervention classes were conducted at agricultural work camps after working hours. In appreciation of the mothers' time, a national chain superstore gift card was given to them at both data collection sessions as well as at intervention sessions they attended. They were also allowed to keep the headphones used in data collection.

Key Findings: Positive results were observed with regard to the mothers' nutritional knowledge, and children in the intervention group had decreased BMI percentiles.

Research Example from a Qualitative Study

Study: Grief interrupted: The experience of loss among incarcerated women (Harner et al., 2011)

Study Purpose: The purpose of the study was to explore the experiences of grief among incarcerated women following the loss of a loved one.

Study Methods: The researchers used phenomenologic methods in this study. They recruited 15 incarcerated women who had experienced the loss of a loved one during their confinement. In-depth interviews about the women's experience of loss lasted 1 to 2 hours.

Ethics-Related Procedures: The researchers recruited women by posting flyers in the prison's dayroom. The flyers were written at the 4.5 grade level. Because the first author was a nurse practitioner at the prison, the researchers used several strategies to "diffuse any perceived coercion" (p. 457), such as not posting flyers near the health services unit and not offering any monetary or work-release incentives to participate. Written informed consent was obtained, but because of high rates of illiteracy, the informed consent document was read aloud to all potential participants. During the consent process and during the interviews, the women were given opportunities to ask questions. They were informed that participation would have no effect on sentence length, sentence structure, parole, or access to health services. They were also told they could end the interview at any time without fear of reprisals. Furthermore, they were told that the researcher was a mandated reporter and would report any indication of suicidal or homicidal ideation. Participants were not required to give their names

to the research team. During the interview, efforts were made to create a welcoming and nonthreatening environment. The research team received approval for their study from a university IRB and from the Department of Corrections Research Division.

Key Findings: The researchers revealed four themes, which they referred to as existential lifeworlds: Temporality: frozen in time; Spatiality: no place, no space to grieve; Corporeality: buried emotions; and Relationality: never alone, yet feeling so lonely.

SUMMARY POINTS

- Researchers face **ethical dilemmas** in designing studies that are both ethical and rigorous. **Codes of ethics** have been developed to guide researchers.

- Three major ethical principles from the *Belmont Report* are incorporated into most guidelines: beneficence, respect for human dignity, and justice.

- **Beneficence** involves the performance of some good and the protection of participants from physical and psychological harm and exploitation.

- **Respect for human dignity** involves participants' **right to self-determination**, which means they are free to control their own actions, including voluntary participation.

- **Full disclosure** means that researchers have fully divulged participants' rights and the risks and benefits of the study. When full disclosure could bias the results, researchers sometimes use **covert data collection** (the collection of information without the participants' knowledge or consent) or **deception** (providing false information).

- **Justice** includes the **right to fair treatment** and the **right to privacy**. In the United States, privacy has become a major issue because of the Privacy Rule regulations that resulted from the Health Insurance Portability and Accountability Act (HIPAA).

- Various procedures have been developed to safeguard study participants rights. For example, researchers can conduct a **risk/benefit assessment** in which the potential benefits of the study to participants and society are weighed against the costs.

- **Informed consent** procedures, which provide prospective participants with information needed to make a reasoned decision about participation, normally involve signing a **consent form** to document voluntary and informed participation.

- In qualitative studies, consent may need to be continually renegotiated with participants as the study evolves, through **process consent** procedures.

- Privacy can be maintained through **anonymity** (wherein not even researchers know participants' identities) or through formal **confidentiality procedures** that safeguard the information participants provide.

- U.S. researchers can seek a **Certificate of Confidentiality** that protects them against the forced disclosure of confidential information (e.g., by a court order).

- Researchers sometimes offer **debriefing** sessions after data collection to provide participants with more information or an opportunity to air complaints.

- **Vulnerable groups** require additional protection. These people may be vulnerable because they are unable to make a truly informed decision about study participation (e.g., children), because of diminished autonomy (e.g., prisoners), or because circumstances heighten the risk of physical or psychological harm (e.g., pregnant women).

- External review of the ethical aspects of a study by an ethics committee, Research Ethics Board (REB), or **Institutional Review Board (IRB)** is often required by either the agency funding the research or the organization from which participants are recruited.

- In studies in which risks to participants are minimal, an **expedited review** (review by a single member of the IRB) may be substituted for a full board review; in cases in which there are no anticipated risks, the research may be exempted from review.

- Researchers need to give careful thought to ethical requirements throughout the study's planning and implementation and to ask themselves continually whether safeguards for protecting humans are sufficient.

- Ethical conduct in research involves not only protection of the rights of human and animal subjects but also efforts to maintain high standards of integrity and avoid such forms of **research misconduct** as *plagiarism*, *fabrication* of results, or *falsification* of data.

STUDY ACTIVITIES

Chapter 7 of the *Resource Manual for Nursing Research: Generating and Assessing Evidence for Nursing Practice, 10th edition*, offers study suggestions for reinforcing concepts presented in this chapter. In addition, the following questions can be addressed in classroom or online discussions:

1. For one of the two studies described in the research example section (Kilanowski & Lin, 2013, or Harner et al., 2011), draft a consent form that includes required information, as described in the section on informed consent.

2. Answer the relevant questions in Box 7.3 regarding the Kilanowski and Lin (2013) study. Also consider the following questions: (a) Could the data for this study have been collected anonymously? Why or why not? (b) Might a Certificate of Confidentiality have been helpful in this study?

3. Answer the relevant questions in Box 7.3 regarding the Harner et al. (2011) study. Also consider the following questions: (a) The researchers did not offer any stipend—was this ethically appropriate? (b) Might the researchers have benefitted from obtaining a Certificate of Confidentiality for this research?

STUDIES CITED IN CHAPTER 7

American Nurses Association (2015). *Code of ethics for nurses with interpretive statements* (2nd ed.). Silver Spring, MD: ANA.

Artinian, N., Froelicher, E., & Wal, J. (2004). Data and safety monitoring during randomized controlled trials of nursing interventions. *Nursing Research, 53*, 414–418.

Beck, C. T., LoGiudice, J., & Gable, R. K. (2015). A mixed methods study of secondary traumatic stress in certified nurse-midwives: Shaken belief in the birth process. *Journal of Midwifery and Women's Health*, *60*, 16–23.

Carlsson, E., Paterson, B., Scott-Findley, S., Ehnfors, M., & Ehrenberg, A. (2007). Methodological issues in interviews involving people with communication impairments after acquired brain damage. *Qualitative Health Research*, *17*, 1361–1371.

Dale, C., Angus, J., Seto Nielsen, L., Kramer-Kile, M., Pritlove, C., Lapum, J., . . . Clark, A. (2015). "I'm no superman": Understanding diabetic men, masculinity, and cardiac rehabilitation. *Qualitative Health Research*. Advance online publication. doi:10.1177/1049732314566323

Darcy, L., Björk, M., Enskär, K., & Knuttson, S. (2014). The process of striving for an ordinary, everyday life, in young children with cancer, at six months and one year post diagnosis. *European Journal of Oncology Nursing*, *18*, 605–612.

Deitrick, C., Mick, D., Lauffer, V., Prostka, E., Nowak, D., & Ingersoll, G. (2015). A comparison of two differing doses of promethazine for the treatment of postoperative nausea and vomiting. *Journal of Perianesthesia Nursing*, *30*, 5–13.

*Edwards, P., Roberts, I., Clarke, M., Diguiseppi, C., Wentz, R., Kwan, I., . . . Pratap, S. (2009). Methods to increase response to postal and electronic questionnaires. *Cochrane Database of Systematic Reviews*, (8), MR000008.

Eide, P., & Kahn, D. (2008). Ethical issues in the qualitative researcher-participant relationship. *Nursing Ethics*, *15*, 199–207.

Ellett, M., Lane, L., & Keffer, J. (2004). Ethical and legal issues of conducting nursing research via the Internet. *Journal of Professional Nursing*, *20*, 68–74.

Flesch, R. (1948). New readability yardstick. *Journal of Applied Psychology*, *32*, 221–223.

Forbat, L., & Henderson, J. (2003). "Stuck in the middle with you": The ethics and process of qualitative research with two people in an intimate relationship. *Qualitative Health Research*, *13*, 1453–1462.

Freda, M. C., & Kearney, M. (2005). Ethical issues faced by nursing editors. *Western Journal of Nursing Research*, *27*, 487–499.

Gennaro, S. (2014). Conducting important and ethical research. *Journal of Nursing Scholarship*, *46*, 2.

*Habermann, B., Broome, M., Pryor, E., & Ziner, K. W. (2010). Research coordinators' experiences with scientific misconduct and research integrity. *Nursing Research*, *59*, 51–57.

Harner, H., Hentz, P., & Evangelista, M. (2011). Grief interrupted: The experience of loss among incarcerated women. *Qualitative Health Research*, *21*, 454–464.

Holmes, S. (2009). Methodological and ethical considerations in designing an Internet study of quality of life. *International Journal of Nursing Studies*, *46*, 392–405.

Holtzclaw, B. J., & Hanneman, S. (2002). Use of non-human biobehavioral models in critical care nursing research. *Critical Care Nursing Quarterly*, *24*, 30–40.

*Horgas, A., Yoon, S., Nichols, A., & Marsiske, M. (2008). The relationship between pain and functional disability in black and white older adults. *Research in Nursing & Health*, *31*, 341–354.

Jeffers, B. R., & Whittemore, R. (2005). Research environments that promote integrity. *Nursing Research*, *54*, 63–70.

Johnson, K. E., & McRee, A. (2015). Health-risk behaviors among high-school athletes and preventive services provided during sports physicals. *Journal of Pediatric Health Care*, *29*, 17–27.

Kanner, S., Langerman, S., & Grey, M. (2004). Ethical considerations for a child's participation in research. *Journal for Specialists in Pediatric Nursing*, *9*, 15–23.

*Kilanowski, J., & Lin, L. (2013). Effects of a healthy eating intervention on Latina migrant farmworker mothers. *Family and Community Health*, *36*, 350–362.

Lambert, V., & Glacken, M. (2011). Engaging with children in research: Theoretical and practical implications of negotiating informed consent/assent. *Nursing Ethics*, *18*, 781–801.

Lutz, K. F., Shelton, K., Robrecht, L., Hatton, D., & Beckett, A. (2000). Use of certificates of confidentiality in nursing research. *Journal of Nursing Scholarship*, *32*, 185–188.

Mallory, C., & Hesson-McInnis, M. (2013). Pilot test results of an HIV prevention intervention for high-risk women. *Western Journal of Nursing Research*, *35*, 313–329.

Moes, J., & Holden, J. (2014). Characterizing activity and muscle atrophy changes in rats with neuropathic pain. *Biological Research for Nursing*, *16*, 16–22.

Munhall, P. L. (2012). *Nursing research: A qualitative perspective* (5th ed.). Sudbury, MA: Jones & Bartlett.

*Nishimura, A., Carey, J., Erwin, P., Tilburt, J., Murad, M., & McCormick, J. (2013). Improving understanding in the research informed consent process: A systematic review of 54 interventions tested in randomized control trials. *BMC Medical Ethics*, *14*, 28.

*Nyamathi, A., Branson, C., Kennedy, B., Salem, B., Khalilifard, F., Marfisee, M., . . . Leake, B. (2012). Impact of nursing intervention on decreasing substances among homeless youth. *The American Journal on Addictions*, *21*, 558–565.

Olsen, D. P. (2003). HIPAA privacy regulations and nursing research. *Nursing Research*, *52*, 344–348.

Payne, C. (2013). A diabetes support group for Nywaigi women to enhance their capacity for maintaining physical and mental wellbeing. *Contemporary Nurse*, *46*, 41–45.

Polit, D. F., & Beck, C. T. (2009). International gender bias in nursing research, 2005–2006: A quantitative content analysis. *International Journal of Nursing Studies*, *46*, 1102–1110.

Polit, D. F., & Beck, C. T. (2013). Is there still gender bias in nursing research? An update. *Research in Nursing & Health*, *36*, 75–83.

Rothstein, W., & Phuong, L. (2007). Ethical attitudes of nurse, physician, and unaffiliated members of institutional review boards. *Journal of Nursing Scholarship*, *39*, 75–81.

Silva, M. C. (1995). *Ethical guidelines in the conduct, dissemination, and implementation of nursing research*. Washington, DC: American Nurses Association.

Simpson, C. (2010). Decision-making capacity and informed consent to participate in research by cognitively impaired individuals. *Applied Nursing Research*, *23*, 221–226.

*Simwaka, A., de Kok, B., & Chilemba, W. (2014). Women's perceptions of nurse-midwives' caring behaviours during perinatal loss in Lilongwe, Malawi. *Malawi Medical Journal, 26*, 8–11.

Slimmer, L., & Andersen, B. (2004). Designing a data and safety monitoring plan. *Western Journal of Nursing Research, 26*, 797–803.

van den Hoonaard, W. C. (2002).*Walking the tightrope: Ethical issues for qualitative researchers.* Toronto, Canada: University of Toronto Press.

*Wolf, L. E., Dame, L., Patel, M., Williams, B., Austin, J., & Beskow, L. (2012). Certificates of confidentiality: Legal counsels' experience with and perspectives on legal demands for research data. *Journal of Empirical Research on Human Research Ethics, 7*, 1–9.

Yates, B., Dodendorf, D., Lane, J., LaFramboise, L., Pozehl, B., Duncan, K., & Knodel, K. (2009). Testing an alternative informed consent process. *Nursing Research, 58*, 135–139.

A link to this open-access journal article is provided in the Toolkit for this chapter in the accompanying Resource Manual. ✲

8 | Planning a Nursing Study

Advance planning is required for all research and is especially important for quantitative studies because the study design usually is finalized before the study proceeds. This chapter provides advice for planning qualitative and quantitative studies.

TOOLS AND CONCEPTS FOR PLANNING RIGOROUS RESEARCH

This section discusses key methodologic concepts and tools in meeting the challenges of doing rigorous research.

Inference

Inference is an integral part of doing and evaluating research. An **inference** is a conclusion drawn from the study evidence, taking into account the methods used to generate that evidence. Inference is the attempt to come to conclusions based on limited information, using logical reasoning processes.

Inference is necessary because researchers use proxies that "stand in" for the things that are fundamentally of interest. A sample of participants is a proxy for an entire population. A study site is a proxy for all relevant sites in which the phenomena of interest could unfold. A control group that does not receive an intervention is a proxy for what would happen to the *same* people if they simultaneously received *and* did not receive the intervention.

Researchers face the challenge of using methods that yield good and persuasive evidence in support of inferences that they wish to make.

Reliability, Validity, and Trustworthiness

Researchers want their inferences to correspond with the *truth*. Research cannot contribute evidence to guide clinical practice if the findings are inaccurate, biased, or fail to represent the experiences of the target group. Consumers of research need to assess the quality of a study's evidence by evaluating the conceptual and methodologic decisions the researchers made, and those who do research must strive to make decisions that result in evidence of the highest possible quality.

Quantitative researchers use several criteria to assess the rigor of a study, sometimes referred to as its **scientific merit**. Two especially important criteria are reliability and validity. **Reliability** refers to the accuracy and consistency of information obtained in a study. The term is most often associated with the methods used to measure variables. For example, if a thermometer measured Alan's temperature as 98.1°F 1 minute and as 102.5°F the next minute, the reliability of the thermometer would be highly suspect. The concept of reliability is also important in interpreting statistical results. *Statistical reliability* refers to the probability that the results would hold with a wider group than the people who participated in the study—that is, the results support an inference about what is true in a population.

Validity is a more complex concept that broadly concerns the *soundness* of the study's evidence—that is, whether the findings are unbiased and well grounded. Like reliability, validity is an important criterion for evaluating methods to measure variables. In this context, the validity question is whether the methods are really measuring the concepts that they purport to measure. Is a self-reported measure of depression *really* measuring depression? Or is it measuring something else, such as loneliness or stress? Researchers strive for solid conceptual definitions of research variables and valid methods to operationalize them.

Validity is also relevant with regard to inferences about the effect of the independent variable on the dependent variable. Did a nursing intervention *really* bring about improvements in patients' outcomes—or were other factors responsible for patients' progress? Researchers make numerous methodologic decisions that influence this type of study validity.

Qualitative researchers use different criteria (and different terminology) in evaluating a study's quality. Qualitative researchers pursue methods of enhancing the **trustworthiness** of the study's data (Lincoln & Guba, 1985). Trustworthiness encompasses several dimensions—credibility, transferability, confirmability, dependability, and authenticity—which are described in detail in Chapter 25.

Credibility, an especially important aspect of trustworthiness, is achieved to the extent that the research methods inspire confidence that the results and interpretations are truthful. Credibility in a qualitative study can be enhanced through various approaches, but one strategy merits early discussion because it has implications for the design of all studies, including quantitative ones. **Triangulation** is the use of multiple sources or referents to draw conclusions about what constitutes the truth. In a quantitative study, this might mean having multiple measures of an outcome variable to see if predicted effects are consistent. In a qualitative study, triangulation might involve trying to reveal the complexity of a phenomenon by using multiple means of data collection to converge on the truth (e.g., having in-depth discussions with study participants as well as watching their behavior in natural settings). Or, it might involve triangulating the interpretations of multiple researchers working together as a team. Nurse researchers are increasingly triangulating across paradigms—that is, integrating both qualitative and quantitative data in a single study to enhance the validity of the conclusions (Chapter 26).

Example of Triangulation: Hallrup (2014) studied the lived experiences of adults with intellectual disabilities living in institutional care in Sweden. During several years of fieldwork, Hallrup interviewed residents and observed them in their everyday lives to gain a deep understanding of their experiences.

Nurse researchers need to design their studies in such a way that the reliability, validity, and trustworthiness of their studies are maximized. This book offers advice on how to do this.

Bias

A **bias** is an influence that produces a distortion or error. Bias can threaten a study's validity and trustworthiness and is a major concern in designing a study. Biases can affect the quality of evidence in both qualitative and quantitative studies.

Bias can result from factors that need to be considered in planning a study. These include the following:

- *Participants' lack of candor.* Sometimes people distort their behavior or statements—consciously or subconsciously—so as to present themselves in the best light.
- *Researcher subjectivity.* Investigators may distort inferences in the direction of their expectations, or in line with their own experiences—or they may unintentionally communicate their expectations to participants and thereby induce biased behavior or responses to questions.
- *Sample imbalances.* The sample itself may be biased; for example, if a researcher studying abortion attitudes included only members of right-to-life (or pro-choice) groups in the sample, the results would be distorted.
- *Faulty methods of data collection.* An inadequate method of capturing key concepts can

lead to biases; for example, a flawed measure of patient satisfaction with nursing care may exaggerate or underestimate patients' concerns.

- *Inadequate study design.* A researcher may structure the study in such a way that an unbiased answer to the research question cannot be achieved.
- *Flawed implementation.* Even a well-designed study can sustain biases if the design (or an intervention) is not carefully implemented. Monitoring for bias throughout the study is important.

Example of Respondent Bias: Collins and colleagues (2005) studied interview transcripts from three phenomenologic studies and searched for instances in which participants may have distorted their responses in a manner that would make them "look good," or that would flatter the interviewers. They identified only six potential instances of what they called "problematic interviewee behavior." Nevertheless, they concluded that "it is probably not a good idea for nurses to interview patients to whom they have personally delivered (or will deliver) care" (p. 197).

A researcher's job is to reduce or eliminate bias to the extent possible, to establish mechanisms to detect or measure it when it exists, and to take known biases into account in interpreting study findings. The job of consumers is to scrutinize methodologic decisions to reach conclusions about whether biases undermined the study evidence.

Unfortunately, bias can seldom be avoided totally because the potential for its occurrence is pervasive. Some bias is haphazard and affects only small data segments. As an example of such **random bias** (or *random error*), a handful of participants might provide inaccurate information because of fatigue. When error is random, distortions are as likely to bias results in one direction as the other. **Systematic bias**, on the other hand, is consistent and distorts results in a single direction. For example, if a scale consistently measured people's weights as being 2 pounds heavier than their true weight, there would be systematic bias in the data on weight.

Researchers adopt a variety of strategies to eliminate or minimize bias and strengthen study rigor. Triangulation is one such approach, the idea being that multiple sources of information or points of view can help counterbalance biases and offer avenues to identify them. Methods that quantitative researchers use to combat bias often involve research control.

Research Control

A central feature of quantitative studies is that they usually involve efforts to control aspects of the research. **Research control** most typically involves holding constant other influences on the dependent variable so that the true relationship between the independent and dependent variables can be understood. In other words, research control attempts to eliminate contaminating factors that might obscure the relationship between the variables of central interest.

Contaminating factors—called **confounding** (or **extraneous**) **variables**—can best be illustrated with an example. Suppose we were studying whether urinary incontinence (UI) leads to depression. Prior evidence suggests a link, but the question is whether UI itself (the independent variable) contributes to higher levels of depression or whether there are other factors that can account for the relationship between UI and depression. We need to design a study so as to control other determinants of the outcome—determinants that are also related to the independent variable, UI.

One confounding variable in this situation is age. Levels of depression tend to be higher in older people, and people with UI tend to be older than those without this problem. In other words, perhaps age is the *real* cause of higher depression in people with UI. If age is not controlled, then any observed relationship between UI and depression could be caused by UI or by age.

Three possible explanations might be portrayed schematically as follows:

1. UI→depression
2. Age→UI→depression
3.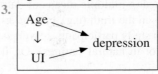

The arrows here symbolize a causal mechanism or an influence. In Model 1, UI directly affects depression, independently of any other factors. In Model 2, UI is a **mediating variable**—the effect of age on depression is *mediated* by UI. According to this representation, age affects depression *through* the effect that age has on UI. In Model 3, both age and UI have separate effects on depression, and age also increases the risk of UI. Some research is specifically designed to test paths of mediation and multiple causation, but in the present example, age is extraneous to the research question. We want to design a study so that the first explanation can be tested. Age must be controlled if our goal is to explore the validity of Model 1, which posits that, no matter what a person's age, having UI makes a person more vulnerable to depression.

How can we impose such control? There are a number of ways, as we discuss in Chapter 10, but the general principle is that the confounding variables must be *held constant*. The confounding variable must somehow be handled so that, in the context of the study, it is not related to the independent variable or the outcome. As an example, let us say we wanted to compare the average scores on a depression scale for those with and without UI. We would want to design a study in such a way that the ages of those in the UI and non-UI groups are comparable, even though, in general, the groups are not comparable in terms of age.

By exercising control over age in this example, we would be taking a step toward explaining the relationship between variables. The world is complex, and many variables are interrelated in complicated ways. When studying a particular problem in a quantitative study, it is difficult to examine this complexity directly; researchers usually must analyze a couple of relationships at a time and put pieces together like a jigsaw puzzle. Modest quantitative studies can contribute evidence, but the value of the evidence is often related to how well researchers control confounding influences. In the present example, we identified one variable (age) that could affect depression, but dozens of others might be relevant (e.g., social support, self-efficacy). Researchers need to isolate the independent and dependent variables in which they are interested and then identify confounding variables that need to be controlled.

It is unnecessary to control all variables that affect the dependent variable. Confounding variables need to be controlled only if they simultaneously are related to both the dependent and independent variables. Information in the Supplement to this chapter on thePoint® explains this in greater detail.

Research control is a critical tool for managing bias and enhancing validity in quantitative studies. There are situations, however, in which too much control can introduce bias. For example, if researchers tightly control the ways in which key study variables are manifested, it is possible that the true nature of those variables will be obscured. In studying phenomena that are poorly understood or whose dimensions have not been clarified, an approach that allows flexibility and exploration is more appropriate. Research rooted in the constructivist paradigm does not impose controls. With their emphasis on holism and individual human experience, some qualitative researchers believe that imposing controls removes some of the meaning of reality.

Randomness

For quantitative researchers, a powerful tool for eliminating bias involves **randomness**—having certain features of the study established by chance rather than by design or researcher preference. When people are selected at random to participate in the study, for example, each person in the initial pool has an equal probability of being selected. This in turn means that there are no systematic biases in the makeup of the sample. Men and women have an equal chance of being selected, for example. Similarly, if participants are allocated randomly to groups that will be compared (e.g., an intervention and "usual care" group), then there can be no systematic biases in the composition of the groups. Randomness is a compelling method of controlling confounding variables and reducing bias.

Example of Randomness: Adderley and Stubbs (2014) compared the standard treatment for venous leg ulcers (four-layer bandaging) to two-layer compression stockings. A total of 454 patients were randomly assigned to either bandages or stockings, and the researchers compared the groups 12 months later in terms of both clinical outcomes (ulcer recurrence rates) and treatment costs.

Qualitative researchers almost never consider randomness a desirable tool. Qualitative researchers tend to use information obtained early in the study in a purposeful (nonrandom) fashion to guide their inquiry and to pursue information-rich sources that can help them expand or refine their conceptualizations. Researchers' judgments are viewed as indispensable vehicles for uncovering the complexities of phenomena of interest.

Reflexivity

Qualitative researchers do not use research control or randomness, but they are as interested as quantitative researchers in discovering the truth about human experience. Qualitative researchers often rely on reflexivity to guard against personal bias in making judgments. **Reflexivity** is the process of reflecting critically on the self and of analyzing and making note of personal values that could affect data collection and interpretation.

Schwandt (2007) has described reflexivity as having two aspects. The first concerns an acknowledgment that the researcher is part of the setting, context, or social phenomenon under study. The second involves the process of self-reflection about one's own biases, preferences, stakes in, and fears about the research and theoretical inclinations. Qualitative researchers are encouraged to explore these issues, to be reflexive about every decision made during the inquiry, and to note their reflexive thoughts in personal journals and memos.

Reflexivity can be a useful tool in quantitative as well as qualitative research. Self-awareness and introspection can enhance the quality of any study.

Example of Reflexivity: Farrell and Comiskey (2014) studied the experiences of HIV-infected individuals who are co-infected with the hepatitis C virus. During the collection of their data, the researchers made efforts to recognize their own biases and assumptions by maintaining a reflexive journal.

Generalizability and Transferability

Nurses increasingly rely on evidence from research in their clinical practice. Evidence-based practice is based on the assumption that study findings are not unique to the people, places, or circumstances of the original research (Polit & Beck, 2010).

Generalizability is a criterion used in quantitative studies to assess the extent to which findings can be applied to other groups and settings. How do researchers enhance the generalizability of a study? First and foremost, they must design studies strong in reliability and validity. There is no point in wondering whether results are generalizable if they are not accurate or valid. In selecting participants, researchers must also give thought to the types of people to whom the results might be generalized—and then select participants in such a way that the sample reflects the population of interest. If a study is intended to have implications for male and female patients, then men and women should be included as participants. Chapters 10 and 12 describe issues to consider to enhance generalizability.

Qualitative researchers do not specifically aim for generalizability, but they do want to generate knowledge that could be useful in other situations. Lincoln and Guba (1985), in their influential book on naturalistic inquiry, discussed the concept of **transferability**, the extent to which qualitative findings can be transferred to other settings, as an aspect of a study's trustworthiness. An important mechanism for promoting transferability is the amount of rich descriptive information qualitative researchers provide about the contexts of their studies. The issue of transferability in qualitative research is discussed in Chapter 22.

> ⊘ **TIP:** When planning a study, it is wise to keep a sharp focus on your study's potential for evidence-based nursing practice. Make an effort to think about generalizability and transferability throughout the study.

OVERVIEW OF RESEARCH DESIGN FEATURES

A study's research design spells out the basic strategies that researchers adopt to develop evidence that is accurate and interpretable. The research design incorporates some of the most important methodologic decisions that researchers make, particularly in quantitative studies. It is important to understand design options when planning a research project.

Table 8.1 describes seven design features that typically need to be considered in planning a quantitative study, and several are also pertinent in qualitative studies. These features include the following:

- Whether or not there will be an *intervention*
- How confounding variables will be *controlled*
- Whether *blinding* will be used to avoid biases

- What the relative timing of collecting data on dependent and independent variables will be
- What types of *comparisons* will be made to enhance interpretability
- What the *location* of the study will be
- What *time frames* will be adopted

This section discusses the last three features because they are relevant in planning both qualitative and quantitative studies. Chapters 9 and 10 elaborate on the first four.

TABLE 8.1 • Key Research Design Features in Quantitative Studies

FEATURE	KEY QUESTIONS	DESIGN OPTIONS
Intervention	Will there be an intervention? What will the intervention entail? What specific design will be used?	Experimental (randomized controlled trial), quasi-experimental (controlled trial), nonexperimental (observational) design
Control over confounding variables	How will confounding variables be controlled? Which confounding variables will be controlled?	Matching, homogeneity, blocking, crossover, randomization, statistical control
Blinding (masking)	From whom will critical information be withheld to avoid bias?	Open versus closed study; single-blind, double-blind (with blinded groups specified)
Relative timing	When will information on independent and dependent variables be collected—looking backward or forward?	Retrospective, prospective design
Comparisons	What type of comparisons will be made to illuminate key processes or relationships? What is the nature of the comparison?	Within-subject design, between-subject design, mixed design, external comparisons
Location	Where will the study take place?	Single site versus multisite; in the field versus controlled setting
Time frames	How often will data be collected? When, relative to other events, will data be collected?	Cross-sectional, longitudinal design; repeated measures design

Note. Several terms in this table are explained in subsequent chapters.

⊜ **TIP:** Design decisions affect the believability of your findings. In some cases, the decisions will influence whether you receive funding (if you seek financial support) or whether you are able to publish your findings (if you submit to a journal). Therefore, a great deal of care and thought should go into these decisions during the planning phase.

Comparisons

In most quantitative (and some qualitative) studies, researchers incorporate comparisons into their design to provide a context for interpreting results. Most quantitative research questions are phrased in terms of a comparison, either an explicit or an implicit one. For example, if our research question asks, what is the effect of massage on anxiety in hospitalized patients, the implied comparison is massage versus no massage—that is, the independent variable.

Researchers can structure their studies to examine various types of comparison, the most common of which are as follows:

1. *Comparison between two or more groups.* For example, if we were studying the emotional consequences of having a mastectomy, we might compare the emotional status of women who had a mastectomy with that of women with breast cancer who did not have a mastectomy. Or, we might compare those receiving a special intervention with those receiving "usual care." In a qualitative study, we might compare mothers and fathers with respect to their experience of having a child diagnosed with schizophrenia.

2. *Comparison of one group's status at two or more points in time.* For example, we might want to compare patients' levels of stress before and after introducing a new procedure to reduce preoperative stress. Or, we might want to compare coping processes among caregivers of patients with AIDS early and later in the caregiving experience.

3. *Comparison of one group's status under different circumstances.* For example, we might com-

pare people's heart rates during two different types of exercise.

4. *Comparison based on relative rankings.* If, for example, we hypothesized a relationship between the pain level and degree of hopefulness in patients with cancer, we would be asking whether those with high levels of pain felt less hopeful than those with low levels of pain. This research question involves a comparison of those with different rankings—higher versus lower—on both variables.

5. *Comparison with external data.* Researchers may directly compare their results with results from other studies or with **norms** (standards from a large and representative sample), sometimes using statistical procedures. This type of comparison often supplements rather than replaces other comparisons. In quantitative studies, this approach is useful primarily when the dependent variable is measured with a widely accepted method (e.g., blood pressure readings, or scores on a standard measure of depression).

Example of Using Comparative Data from External Sources: Okajima and colleagues (2013) studied the health-related quality of life of Japanese patients with primary lymphedema. They used a measure of health and well-being for which national comparison data were available (the Short-Form 36), which enabled them to compare their sample's outcomes to national norms for women of similar age in Japan.

Research designs for quantitative studies can be categorized based on the type of comparisons that are made. Studies that compare different people (as in examples 1 and 4) are **between-subjects designs**. Sometimes, however, it is preferable to make comparisons for the *same* participants at different times or under difference circumstances, as in examples 2 and 3. Such designs are **within-subjects designs**. When two or more groups of people are followed over time, the design is sometimes called a **mixed design** because comparisons can be both within groups over time, or between groups.

Comparisons are often a central focus of a quantitative study, but even when they are not, they provide a context for interpreting the findings. In example 1 regarding the emotional status of women who had a mastectomy, it would be difficult to know whether the women's emotional state was worrisome without comparing it to that of others—or without comparing it to their state at an earlier time (e.g., prior to diagnosis). In designing a study, quantitative researchers choose comparisons that will best illuminate the central issue under investigation.

Qualitative researchers sometimes plan to make comparisons when they undertake an in-depth study, but comparisons are rarely their primary focus. Nevertheless, patterns emerging in the data often suggest that certain comparisons have rich descriptive value.

> **TIP:** Try not to make design decisions single-handedly. Seek the advice of faculty, colleagues, or consultants. Once you have made design decisions, it may be useful to write out a rationale for your choices and share it with others to see if they can find flaws in your reasoning or if they can suggest improvements. A worksheet for documenting design decisions and rationales is available as a Word document in the Toolkit section of the accompanying *Resource Manual.*

Research Location

An important planning task is to identify sites for the study. In some situations, the study site is a "given," as might be the case for a clinical study conducted in a hospital or institution with which researchers are affiliated, but in other studies, the identification of an appropriate site involves considerable effort.

Planning for this aspect of the study involves two types of activities—selecting the site or sites, and gaining access to them. While some of the issues we discuss here are of particular relevance to qualitative researchers working in the field, many quantitative studies also need to attend to these matters in planning a project, especially in intervention studies.

Site Selection

The primary consideration in site selection is whether the site has people with the behaviors, experiences, or characteristics of interest. The site must also have a sufficient *number* of these kinds of people and adequate *diversity* or mix of people to achieve research goals. In addition, the site must be one in which access to participants will be granted. Both methodologic goals (e.g., ability to exert needed controls) and ethical requirements (e.g., ability to ensure privacy and confidentiality) need to be achieved in the chosen site. The site also should be one in which the researcher will be allowed to maintain an appropriate role vis-à-vis study participants and clinical staff for the duration of the study.

> **TIP:** Before searching for a suitable site, it might be helpful to jot down the site characteristics that you would ideally like to have, so that you can more clearly assess the degree to which the reality matches the ideal. Once you have compiled a list, it might be profitable to brainstorm with colleagues, advisors, or other professionals about your needs to see if they can help you to identify potential sites.

Researchers sometimes must decide *how many* sites to include. Having multiple sites is advantageous for enhancing the generalizability of the study findings, but multisite studies are complex and pose management and logistic challenges. Multiple sites are a good strategy when several co-investigators from different institutions are working together on a project.

Site visits to potential sites and clinical fieldwork are useful to assess the "fit" between what the researcher needs and what the site has to offer. In essence, site visits involve "prior ethnography" (Erlandson et al., 1993) in which the researcher makes observations and converses with key gatekeepers or stakeholders in the site to better understand its characteristics and constraints. Buckwalter and colleagues (2009) have noted particular issues of concern when working in sites that are "unstable" research environments, such as critical care units or long-term care facilities.

Gaining Entrée

Researchers must gain entrée into the sites deemed suitable for the study. If the site is an entire community, a multitiered effort of gaining acceptance from gatekeepers may be needed. For example, it may be necessary to enlist the cooperation first of community leaders and subsequently of administrators and staff in specific institutions (e.g., domestic violence organizations) or leaders of specific groups (e.g., support groups).

Because establishing *trust* is a central issue, gaining entrée requires strong interpersonal skills as well as familiarity with the site's customs and language. Researchers' ability to gain the gatekeepers' trust can best occur if researchers are candid about research requirements and express genuine interest in and concern for the people in the site. Gatekeepers are most likely to be cooperative if they believe that there will be direct benefits to them or their constituents.

Information to help gatekeepers make a decision about granting access usually should be put in writing, even if the negotiation takes place in person. An information sheet should cover the following points: (1) the purpose and significance of the research, (2) why the site was chosen, (3) what the research would entail (e.g., study time frames, how much disruption there might be, what resources are required), (4) how ethical guidelines would be maintained, including how results would be reported, and (5) what the gatekeeper or others at the site have to gain from cooperating in the study. Figure 8.1 ⊗ presents an example of a letter of inquiry for gaining entrée into a facility.

Gaining entrée may be an ongoing process of establishing relationships and rapport with gatekeepers and others at the site, including prospective informants. The process might involve *progressive entry*, in which certain privileges are negotiated at first and then are subsequently expanded (Erlandson et al., 1993). Morse and Field (1995) advised ongoing communication with gatekeepers between the time that access is granted and the startup of the study, which may be a lengthy period if funding

decisions or study preparations (e.g., instrument development) are time-consuming. It is not only courteous to keep people informed but it may also prove critical to the success of the project because circumstances (and leadership) at the site can change.

Bernard (2006) offered five guidelines for entering the field: (1) If you have a choice, select a field site that gives you the easiest access to data; (2) bring along multiple copies of written documentation about yourself and your study; (3) if you have personal contacts, use them to help you enter the field site; (4) be prepared to address questions about yourself and your study; and (5) take time to become familiar with the physical and social layout of your field site.

Time Frames

Research designs designate when, and how often, data will be collected. In many studies, data are collected at one point in time. For example, patients might be asked on a single occasion to describe their health-promoting behaviors. Some designs, however, call for multiple contacts with participants, often to assess changes over time. Thus, in planning a study, researchers must decide on the number of data collection points needed to address the research question properly. The research design also designates *when*, relative to other events, data will be collected. For example, the design might call for measurement of cholesterol levels 4 weeks and 8 weeks after an exercise intervention.

Designs can be categorized in terms of study time frames. The major distinction, for both qualitative and quantitative researchers, is between cross-sectional and longitudinal designs.

Cross-Sectional Designs

Cross-sectional designs involve the collection of data once the phenomena under study are captured at a single time point. Cross-sectional studies are appropriate for describing the status of phenomena or for describing relationships among phenomena at a fixed point in time. For example, we might be interested in determining whether psychological symptoms in women going through menopause correlate contemporaneously with physiologic symptoms.

Ms. Wendy Smith, R.N.
Family Birth Place
General Hospital
Hartford, CT

Dear Ms. Smith:

   I am the Principal Investigator of a study whose primary goal is to improve the detection of postpartum depression in Hispanic mothers. The study will involve testing a standard Spanish version of the Postpartum Depression Screening Scale (PDSS). Postpartum depression is a cross-cultural mental illness that can have devastating effects for 10%–15% of new mothers and their families. It has been estimated that up to 50% of all cases go undetected. Non–English-speaking women in this country may be even more disadvantaged and isolated in their environments and may thus be at even higher risk for depression than English-speaking women, and thus effective screening with a valid instrument may be especially important.

   Your hospital would be a desirable site for this research because of the high percentage of Hispanic women who deliver at your Family Birth Place. The research would require a sample of 75 Hispanic mothers 18 years of age or older who have given birth within the past 3 months. Each mother would complete the PDSS-Spanish Version and would participate in a diagnostic interview for *DSM-IV* depressive disorders, conducted by a female Hispanic psychologist. If a woman is diagnosed with postpartum depression, she would be referred for psychiatric follow-up. Each mother would be given a gift certificate for $25.00 for participating in the study.

   If feasible, I would like to approach the 75 Hispanic women to invite them to participate in the study soon after delivery, while they are on the postpartum unit. The mothers would be recruited by a Hispanic research assistant who is an RN. Prospective participants will be asked to sign an informed consent form, which will be available in both English and Spanish (whichever language version participants prefer). Confidentiality will be strictly maintained. No name or identifying information will be written on any of the data collection forms. All data will be kept in a locked file cabinet in my office at the University of Connecticut.

   Results of the study will be presented at research conferences and in a nursing research journal. The study findings will provide you with a more complete picture of your own Hispanic population and the percentage suffering from postpartum depression. A Spanish version of the PDSS will be made available for your use for screening Hispanic mothers at your hospital.

   If it is possible, I would like to schedule an appointment with you so that we can discuss the possibility of my conducting this research on your unit.

Sincerely,
Cheryl Tatano Beck, DNSc, CNM, FAAN
Professor

FIGURE 8.1   Sample letter of inquiry for gaining entrée into a research site (fictitious).

Example of a Cross-Sectional Qualitative Study: Axelsson and co-researchers (2015) studied the meanings of being a close relative of a severely ill family member receiving hemodialysis approaching end of life. Interviews at a single point in time were conducted with 14 close relatives of deceased patients, who were asked to reflect retrospectively on their experiences.

   Cross-sectional designs are sometimes used for time-related purposes, but the results may be equivocal. For example, we might test the hypothesis, using cross-sectional data, that a determinant of excessive alcohol consumption is low impulse control, as measured by a psychological test. When both alcohol consumption and impulse control are measured concurrently, however, it is difficult to know which variable influenced the other, if either. Cross-sectional data can best be used to infer time sequence under two circumstances: (1) when a cogent theoretical rationale guides the analysis or (2) when there is evidence or logical reasoning indicating that one variable preceded the other. For example, in a study of the effects of low birth weight on morbidity in school-aged children, it is clear that birth weight came first.

   Cross-sectional studies can be designed to permit inferences about processes evolving over time, but such designs are usually less persuasive than longitudinal ones. Suppose, for example, we were studying changes in children's health promotion activities between ages 10 and 13. One way to study this would be to interview children at age 10 and then 3 years later at age 13—a longitudinal design. On the other hand, we could use a cross-sectional design by interviewing *different* children ages 10 and 13 and then comparing their responses. If 13-year-olds engaged in more health-promoting activities than 10-year-olds, it might be inferred that children improve in making healthy choices as they age. To make this kind of inference, we would have to assume that the older children would have responded like the younger ones had they been questioned 3 years earlier, or, conversely, that 10-year-olds would report more health-promoting activities if they were questioned again 3 years later. Such a design, which involves a comparison of multiple age cohorts, is sometimes called a **cohort comparison design**.

Cross-sectional studies are economical, but inferring changes over time with such designs is problematic. In our example, 10- and 13-year-old children may have different attitudes toward health promotion, independent of maturation. Rapid social and technologic changes may make it risky to assume that differences in the behaviors or traits of different age groups are the result of time passing rather than of cohort or generational differences. In cross-sectional studies designed to explore change, there are often alternative explanations for the findings—and that is precisely what good research design tries to avoid.

> **Example of a Cross-Sectional Study with Inference of Change Over Time:** Logan and Barksdale (2013) studied the relationship between age and arterial stiffness in a sample of Korean American adults. The carotid-femoral pulse wave velocity (PWV) was measured for participants in four age groups: 21-30, 31-40, 41-50, and 51-60. Average PWVs was found to increase in successively older groups.

Longitudinal Designs

A study in which researchers collect data at more than one point in time *over an extended period* is

a **longitudinal design**. There are four situations in which a longitudinal design is appropriate:

1. *Studying time-related processes.* Some research questions specifically concern phenomena that evolve over time (e.g., healing, physical growth).
2. *Determining time sequences.* It is sometimes important to establish how phenomena are sequenced. For example, if it is hypothesized that infertility affects depression, then it would be important to ascertain that the depression did not precede the fertility problem.
3. *Assessing changes over time.* Some studies examine whether changes have occurred over time. For example, an experimental study might examine whether an intervention had both short-term and long-term benefits. A qualitative study might explore the evolution of grieving in the spouses of palliative care patients.
4. *Enhancing research control.* Quantitative researchers sometimes collect data at multiple points to enhance the interpretability of the results. For example, when two groups are being compared with regard to the effects of alternative interventions, the collection of pre-intervention data allows the researcher to learn about initial group comparability.

There are several types of longitudinal designs. Most involve collecting data from one group of study participants multiple times, but others involve different samples. **Trend studies**, for example, are investigations in which samples from a population are studied over time with respect to some phenomenon. Trend studies permit researchers to examine patterns and rates of change and to predict future developments. Many trend studies document trends in public health issues, such as smoking, obesity, child abuse, and so on.

> **Example of a Trend Study:** Gowing and colleagues (2015) studied trends in trauma injuries over a 10-year period in a large hospital in Northern Australia. They examined changes over time in terms of patient demographics and the nature of the traumatic injuries.

In a more typical longitudinal study, the *same* people provide data at two or more points in time. Longitudinal studies of general (nonclinical) populations are sometimes called **panel studies**. The term *panel* refers to the sample of people providing data. Because the same people are studied over time, researchers can examine different patterns of change (e.g., those whose health improved or deteriorated). Panel studies are intuitively appealing as an approach to studying change, but they are expensive.

Example of a Panel Study: The U.S. government sponsors numerous large-scale panel studies, and many nurse researchers have analyzed data from these studies. For example, Everett (2014) studied the relationship between *changes* in neighborhood characteristics during the panel members' transition from adolescence to young adulthood on the one hand and levels of depression on the other among sexual minorities.

Follow-up studies are undertaken to examine the subsequent development of individuals who have a specified condition or who have received a specific intervention. For example, patients who have received a particular nursing intervention or clinical treatment may be followed to ascertain long-term effects. Or, in a qualitative study, patients initially interviewed shortly after a diagnosis of prostate cancer may be followed to assess their experiences during or after treatment decisions have been made.

Example of a Qualitative Follow-Up Study: Dysvik and colleagues (2013) followed up a sample of 34 outpatients who had participated in an 8-week pain management program. The qualitative component of this mixed methods study involved asking participants twice about their experiences with the pain management program. The first time was right after they completed the program and the second time was 6 months later.

Some longitudinal studies are called **cohort studies**, in which a group of people (the cohort) is tracked over time to see if subsets with exposure to different factors differ in terms of subsequent outcomes or risks. For example, in a cohort of women, those with or without a history of childbearing

could be tracked to examine differences in rates of ovarian cancer. This type of study, often called a *prospective study*, is discussed in Chapter 9.

Longitudinal studies are appropriate for studying the trajectory of a phenomenon over time, but a major problem is **attrition**—the loss of participants after initial data collection. Attrition is problematic because those who drop out of the study often differ in important ways from those who continue to participate, resulting in potential biases and difficulty in generalizing to the original population.

In longitudinal studies, researchers make decisions about the number of data collection points and the intervals between them based on the nature of the study. When change or development is rapid, numerous time points at short intervals may be needed to document it. Researchers interested in outcomes that may occur years after the original data collection must use longer term follow-up. However, the longer the interval, the greater the risk of attrition and resulting biases.

Repeated Measures Designs

Studies with multiple points of data collection are sometimes described as having a **repeated measures design**, which usually signifies a study in which data are collected three or more times. Longitudinal studies, such as follow-up and cohort studies, sometimes use a repeated measures design.

Repeated measures designs, however, can also be used in studies that are essentially cross-sectional. For example, a study involving the collection of postoperative patient data on vital signs hourly over an 8-hour period would not be described as longitudinal because the study does not involve an extended time perspective. Yet, the design could be characterized as repeated measures. Researchers are especially likely to use the term *repeated measures design* when they use a repeated measures approach to statistical analysis (see Chapter 17).

Example of a Repeated Measures Study: Asgar Pour and Yavuz (2014) studied the effects of peripheral cold application (PCA) on body temperature, blood pressure, and oxygen saturation. Measurements of these outcomes were made before PCA, immediately after PCA, and 30 minutes later.

TIP: In making design decisions, you will often need to balance various considerations, such as time, cost, ethical issues, and study integrity. Try to get a firm understanding of your "upper limits" before finalizing your design. That is, what is the *most* money that can be spent on the project? What is the *maximal amount* of time available for conducting the study? What is the limit of acceptability with regard to attrition? These limits often eliminate some design options. With these constraints in mind, the central focus should be on designing a study that maximizes the rigor or trustworthiness of the study.

PLANNING DATA COLLECTION

In planning a study, researchers must select methods to gather their research data. This section provides an overview of various methods of data collection for qualitative and quantitative studies.

Overview of Data Collection and Data Sources

As in the case of research designs, there is an array of alternative data collection methods and approaches from which to choose. Most often, researchers collect new data, and one key planning decision concerns the basic types of data to gather. Three approaches have been used most frequently by nurse researchers: self-reports, observation, and biophysiologic measures. In some cases, researchers may be able to use data from existing sources, such as records.

Self-Reports (Patient-Reported Outcomes)

A good deal of information can be gathered by questioning people directly, a method known as **self-report**. In the medical literature, the self-report method is often referred to as **patient-reported outcomes** or **PROs**, but some self-reports are not about patients (e.g., self-reports about nurses' burnout) and some are not *outcomes* (self-reports about attitudes toward abortion). The majority of nursing studies involve data collected by self-report. The

unique ability of humans to communicate verbally makes direct questioning a particularly important part of nurse researchers' data collection repertoire.

Self-reports are strong in directness and versatility. If we want to know what people think, believe, or plan to do, the most efficient means of gathering information is to ask them about it. The strongest argument that can be made for the self-report method is that it can yield information that would be impossible to gather by any other means. Behaviors can be observed, but only if participants engage in them publicly. Furthermore, observers can observe only those behaviors occurring at the time of the study. Through self-reports, researchers can gather *retrospective data* about events occurring in the past or information about behaviors in which people plan to engage in the future. Information about feelings or values can sometimes be inferred through observation, but actions and feelings do not always correspond exactly. Self-report methods can capture psychological characteristics and outcomes through direct communication with participants.

Despite these advantages, verbal report methods have some weaknesses. The most serious issue concerns their validity and accuracy: Can we be sure that people feel or act the way they say they do? Investigators often have no alternative but to assume that participants have been frank. Yet we all have a tendency to want to present ourselves positively, and this may conflict with the truth. Researchers who gather self-report data should recognize these limitations and take them into consideration when interpreting the results.

Example of a Study Using Self-Reports: Chao and colleagues (2015) explored how cancer patients receiving radiotherapy adapt to the treatment process. The data came from in-depth interviews with eight newly diagnosed patients who received radiotherapy as their primary treatment.

Self-report methods normally depend on respondents' willingness to share personal information, but **projective techniques** are sometimes used to obtain data about people's way of thinking indirectly. Projective techniques present participants with a stimulus of low structure, permitting them to "read in" and then describe their own interpretations. The Rorschach test is one example of a projective technique. Other projective methods encourage self-expression through the construction of some product (e.g., drawings). The assumption is that people express their needs, motives, and emotions by working with or manipulating materials. Projective methods are used infrequently by nurse researchers, the major exception being studies using expressive methods to explore sensitive topics with children.

Example of a Study Using Projective Methods: Tunney and Boore (2013) tested the effectiveness of a storybook (*The Tale of Woody's Tonsils*) on reducing anxiety in children undergoing tonsillectomy. Some children received the storybook intervention and others did not. Anxiety was assessed using a method called Child Drawing: Hospital, a projective technique based on the children's drawings.

Observation

For certain research problems, an alternative to self-reports is **observation** of people's behaviors or characteristics. Observation can be done directly through the human senses or with the aid of technical apparatus, such as video equipment, x-rays, and so on. Observational methods can be used to gather information about a wide range of phenomena, including the following: (1) characteristics and conditions of individuals (e.g., patients' sleep–wake state), (2) verbal communication (e.g., nurse–patient dialogue), (3) nonverbal communication (e.g., facial expressions), (4) activities and behavior (e.g., geriatric patients' self-grooming), (5) skill attainment (e.g., diabetic patients' skill in testing their urine), and (6) environmental conditions (e.g., architectural barriers in nursing homes).

Observation in health care environments is an important data-gathering strategy. Nurses are in an advantageous position to observe, relatively unobtrusively, the behaviors of patients, their families, and hospital staff. Moreover, nurses may, by training, be especially sensitive observers.

Observational methods may yield better data than self-reports when people are unaware of their own behavior (e.g., manifesting preoperative symp-

toms of anxiety), when people are embarrassed to report activities (e.g., displays of aggression), when behaviors are emotionally laden (e.g., grieving), or when people are not capable of describing their actions (e.g., young children). Furthermore, with an observational approach, humans—the observers—are used as measuring instruments and provide a uniquely sensitive and intelligent tool.

Shortcomings of observation include behavior distortions when participants are aware of being observed—a problem called **reactivity**. Reactivity can be eliminated if observations are made without people's knowledge, through some type of concealment—but this poses ethical concerns because of the inability to obtain truly informed consent. Another problem is **observer biases**. A number of factors (e.g., prejudices, emotions) can interfere with objective observations. Observational biases probably cannot be eliminated completely, but they can be minimized through careful training.

Example of a Study Using Observation: Brown and colleagues (2014) studied the effect of maternal behaviors on infant behaviors during a feeding. The dyads were video recorded and certain types of behavior were coded (e.g., maternal soothing, stimulation).

Biophysiologic Measures

Many clinical studies rely on the use of **biophysiologic measures**. Physiologic and physical variables typically are measured using specialized technical instruments and equipment. Because such equipment is available in health care settings, the costs of these measures to nurse researchers may be small or nonexistent.

A major strength of biophysiologic measures is their objectivity. Nurse A and nurse B, reading from the same spirometer output, are likely to record the same forced expiratory volume (FEV) measurements. Furthermore, two different spirometers are likely to produce the same FEV readouts. Another advantage of physiologic measurements is the relative precision they normally offer. By *relative*, we are implicitly comparing physiologic instruments with measures of psychological phenomena, such as self-report measures of anxiety or pain. Biophysiologic measures usually yield data of exceptionally high quality.

Example of a Study Using Biophysiologic Measures: Herrington and Chiodo (2014) evaluated the efficacy of gentle human touch on reducing pain responses to heel stick in infants in the NICU. The researchers analyzed the effect of gentle touch on heart rate, respiratory rate, and oxygen saturation.

Records

Most researchers create original data for their studies, but sometimes they take advantage of information available in **records**. Hospital records, patient charts, physicians' order sheets, care plan statements, and the like all constitute rich data sources to which nurse researchers may have access. Research data obtained from records and other documents are advantageous because they are economical: The collection of original data can be time-consuming and costly. Also, records avoid problems stemming from people's awareness of and reaction to study participation. Furthermore, investigators do not have to rely on participants' cooperation.

On the other hand, when researchers are not responsible for collecting data, they may be unaware of the records' limitations and biases. Two major types of bias in records are **selective deposit** and **selective survival**. If the available records are not the entire set of all possible such records, researchers must question how representative existing records are. Many record keepers *intend* to maintain an entire universe of records but may not succeed. Lapses may be the result of systematic biases, and careful researchers should attempt to learn what those biases may be. Gregory and Radovinsky (2012) have suggested some strategies for enhancing the reliability of data extracted from medical records, and Talbert and Sole (2013) offer advice about using large electronic health care databases and disease registries.

Other difficulties also may be relevant. Sometimes records have to be verified for their authenticity or accuracy, which may be difficult if the records are old. Researchers using records must be prepared to deal with systems they do not understand.

In using records to study trends, researchers should be alert to possible changes in record-keeping procedures. Another problem is the increasing difficulty of gaining access to institutional records. As mentioned in Chapter 7, federal legislation in the United States (HIPAA) has created some obstacles to accessing records for research purposes.

Thus, although records may be plentiful, inexpensive, and accessible, they should not be used without paying attention to potential problems. Moreover, it is often difficult to find existing data that are ideally suited to answering a research question.

Example of a Study Using Records: Staveski and colleagues (2014) studied whether the administration of as-needed sedative or analgesic medications on a pediatric cardiovascular intensive care unit varied by time of day. Their data source was medication administration records over a 4-month period.

Dimensions of Data Collection Approaches

Data collection methods vary along three key dimensions: structure, researcher obtrusiveness, and objectivity. In planning a study, researchers make decisions about where on these dimensions the data collection methods should fall.

Structure

In structured data collection, information is gathered from participants in a comparable, prespecified way. For example, most self-administered questionnaires are structured: They include a fixed set of questions to be answered in a specified sequence, usually with predesignated response options (e.g., agree or disagree). Structured methods give participants limited opportunities to qualify their answers or to explain the meaning of their responses. By contrast, qualitative studies rely mainly on unstructured methods of data collection.

There are advantages and disadvantages to both approaches. Structured methods often take considerable effort to develop and refine, but they yield data that are relatively easy to analyze because the data can be readily quantified. Structured methods are seldom appropriate for an in-depth examination of a phenomenon, however. Consider the following two methods of asking people about their levels of stress:

> *Structured*: During the past week, would you say you felt stressed:
>
> 1. rarely or none of the time,
> 2. some or a little of the time,
> 3. occasionally or a moderate amount of the time, or
> 4. most or all of the time?

> *Unstructured*: How stressed or anxious have you been this past week? Tell me about the kinds of tensions and stresses you have been experiencing.

Structured questions would allow researchers to compute what percentage of respondents felt stressed most of the time but would provide no information about the cause or circumstances of the stress. The unstructured question allows for deeper and more thoughtful responses but may pose difficulties for people who are not good at expressing themselves. Moreover, the unstructured question yields data that are much more difficult to analyze.

When data are collected in a structured fashion, researchers must develop (or borrow) a data collection **instrument**, which is the formal written document used to collect and record information, such as a questionnaire. When unstructured methods are used, there is typically no formal instrument, although there may be a list of the types of information needed.

Researcher Obtrusiveness

Data collection methods differ in the degree to which people are aware of the data gathering process. If people know they are under scrutiny, their behavior and responses may not be "normal," and distortions can undermine the value of the research. When data are collected unobtrusively, however, ethical problems may emerge, as discussed in Chapter 7.

Study participants are most likely to distort their behavior and their responses to questions under certain circumstances. Researcher obtrusiveness is likely to be most problematic when (1) a program

is being evaluated and participants have a vested interest in the evaluation outcome, (2) participants engage in socially unacceptable or unusual behavior, (3) participants have not complied with medical and nursing instructions, and (4) participants are the type of people who have a strong need to "look good." When researcher obtrusiveness is unavoidable under these circumstances, researchers should make an effort to put participants at ease, to stress the importance of candor and naturalistic behavior, and to adopt a nonjudgmental demeanor.

Objectivity

Objectivity refers to the degree to which two independent researchers can arrive at similar "scores" or make similar observations regarding concepts of interest. The goal of objectivity is to avoid biases. Some data collection approaches require more subjective judgment than others, and some research problems require a higher degree of objectivity than others.

Researchers with a positivist orientation usually strive for a reasonable amount of objectivity. In research based on the constructivist paradigm, however, the subjective judgment of investigators is considered an asset because subjectivity is viewed as essential for understanding human experiences.

Developing a Data Collection Plan

In planning a study, researchers make decisions about the type and amount of data to collect. The task involves weighing several factors, including costs, but a key goal is to identify the kinds of data that will yield accurate, valid, meaningful, and trustworthy information for addressing the research question.

Most researchers face the issue of balancing the need for extensive information against the risk of overburdening participants (and overtaxing the budget). In many studies, more data are collected than are needed or analyzed. Although it is better to have adequate data than to have unwanted omissions, minimizing *participant burden* should be an important goal. Careful advance planning to ensure good data coverage without placing undue demands on participants is essential. Specific guidance on developing a data collection plan is offered later in this book for quantitative studies (Chapter 13) and qualitative studies (Chapter 23).

ORGANIZATION OF A RESEARCH PROJECT

Studies typically take many months to complete and longitudinal studies require years of work. During the planning phase, it is a good idea to make preliminary estimates of how long various tasks will require. Having deadlines helps to delimit tasks that might otherwise continue indefinitely, such as problem selection and literature reviews.

Chapter 3 presented a sequence of steps that quantitative researchers follow in a study. The steps represented an idealized conception: The research process rarely follows a neatly prescribed sequence of procedures, even in quantitative studies. Decisions made in one step, for example, may require alterations in a previous activity. Iteration and backtracking are the norm. For example, sample size decisions may require rethinking how many sites are needed. Selection of data collection methods might require changes to how the population is defined, and so on. Nevertheless, preliminary time estimates are valuable. In particular, it is important to have a sense of how much total time the study will require and when it will begin.

TIP: We could not suggest even approximations for the relative percentage of time that should be spent on each task. Some projects need many months to recruit participants, whereas other studies can rely on an existing group, for example. Clearly, not all steps are equally time-consuming.

Researchers sometimes develop visual timelines to help them organize a study. These devices are especially useful if funding is sought because the schedule helps researchers to understand when and for how long staff support is needed (e.g., for transcribing interviews). This can best be illustrated with an example, in this case of a hypothetical quantitative study.

Suppose a researcher was studying the following problem: Is a woman's decision to have an annual mammogram related to her perceived susceptibility to breast cancer? Using the organization of steps outlined in Chapter 3, here are some of the tasks that might be undertaken:*

1. The researcher is concerned that many older women do not get mammograms regularly. Her specific *research question* is whether mammogram practices are different for women with different perceptions about their susceptibility to breast cancer.

2. The researcher *reviews the research literature* on breast cancer, mammography use, and factors affecting mammography decisions.

3. The researcher does *clinical fieldwork* by discussing the problem with nurses and other health care professionals in various clinical settings (health clinics, private obstetrics, and gynecology practices) and by informally discussing the problem with women in a support group for breast cancer patients.

4. The researcher seeks theories and models for her problem. She finds that the Health Belief Model is relevant, and this helps her to develop a *theoretical framework* and a conceptual definition of susceptibility to breast cancer.

5. Based on the framework, the following *hypothesis is developed*: Women who perceive themselves as not susceptible to breast cancer are less likely than other women to get an annual mammogram.

6. The researcher adopts a nonexperimental, cross-sectional, between-subjects *research design*. Her comparison strategy will be to compare women with different rankings on susceptibility to breast cancer. She designs the study to control the confounding variables of age, marital status, and health insurance status. Her research site will be Los Angeles.

7. There is no *intervention* in this study (the design is nonexperimental) and so this step is unnecessary.

---

*This is only a partial list of tasks and is designed to illustrate the flow of activities; the flow in this example is more orderly than would ordinarily be true.

8. The researcher designates that the *population* of interest is women between the ages of 50 and 65 years living in Los Angeles who have not been previously diagnosed as having any form of cancer.

9. The researcher will recruit 250 women living in Los Angeles as her *research sample*; they are identified at random using a telephone procedure known as random-digit dialing and so she does not need to gain entrée into any institution or organization.

10. *Research variables will be measured* by self-report; that is, the independent variable (perceived susceptibility), dependent variable (mammogram history), and confounding variables will be measured by asking participants a series of questions. The researcher will use existing instruments rather than developing new ones.

11. The IRB at the researcher's institution is asked to review the plans to ensure that the study *adheres to ethical standards*.

12. *Plans for the study are finalized*: The methods are reviewed and refined by colleagues with clinical and methodologic expertise and by the IRB; the data collection instruments are pretested, and interviewers who will collect the data are trained.

13. *Data are collected* by means of telephone interviews with women in the research sample.

14. *Data are prepared for analysis* by coding them and entering them onto a computer file.

15. *Data are analyzed* using statistical software.

16. The results indicate that the hypothesis is supported; however, the researcher's *interpretation* must take into consideration that many women who were asked to participate declined to do so.

17. The researcher presents an early report on her findings and interpretations at a conference of Sigma Theta Tau International. She subsequently publishes the report in the *Western Journal of Nursing Research*.

18. The researcher seeks out clinicians to discuss how the study findings can be *utilized in practice*.

The researcher plans to conduct this study over a 2-year period, and Figure 8.2 presents a hypothetical schedule. Many steps overlap or are undertaken concurrently; some steps are projected to involve little time, whereas others require months of work. (The Toolkit section of the accompanying *Resource Manual* includes the timeline in Figure 8.2 as a Word document for you to adapt for your study). ✪

In developing a time schedule, several considerations should be kept in mind, including methodologic expertise and the availability of funding or other assistance. In the present example, if the researcher needed financial support to help pay for the cost of hiring interviewers, the timeline would need to be expanded to accommodate the period required to prepare a proposal and await the funding decision. It is also important to consider the practical aspects of performing the study, which were not noted in the preceding section. Securing permissions, hiring staff, and holding meetings are all time-consuming, but necessary, activities.

In large-scale studies—especially studies in which there is an intervention—it is wise to incorporate a **pilot study** into the planning process. A pilot study is a trial run designed to test planned methods and procedures. Results and experiences from pilot studies help to inform many of decisions for larger and more rigorous projects. We discuss the important role of pilot studies as part of the planning process in Chapter 28.

Individuals differ in the kinds of tasks that appeal to them. Some people enjoy the preliminary phase, which has a strong intellectual component, whereas others are more eager to collect the data, a task that is more interpersonal. Researchers should, however, allocate a reasonable amount of time to do justice to each activity.

➲ **TIP:** Getting organized for a study has many dimensions beyond having a timeline. One especially important issue concerns having the right team and mix of skills for a research project, and developing plans for hiring and monitoring research staff (Kang et al., 2005; Nelson & Morrison-Beedy, 2008). We discuss research teams in connection with proposal development (Chapter 31).

Calendar Months:	1	2	3	4	5	6	7	8	9	10	11	12	13	14	15	16	17	18	19	20	21	22	23	24
Conceptual Phase																								
1. Problem identification	→																							
2. Literature review	→	→																						
3. Clinical fieldwork	→	→																						
4. Theoretical framework	→	→																						
5. Hypothesis formulation		→																						
Design/Planning Phase																								
6. Research design			→	→	→																			
7. Intervention protocols (NA)																								
8. Population specification				→	→																			
9. Sampling plan					→	→																		
10. Data collection plan				→	→	→																		
11. Ethics procedures						→	→																	
12. Finalization of plans					→	→	→																	
Empirical Phase																								
13. Collection of data										→	→	→	→	→										
14. Data preparation											→	→	→	→										
Analytic Phase																								
15. Data analysis														→	→	→								
16. Interpretation of results															→	→	→							
Dissemination Phase																								
17. Presentations/reports																			→	→	→	→	→	→
18. Utilization of findings																						→	→	→
Calendar Months:	1	2	3	4	5	6	7	8	9	10	11	12	13	14	15	16	17	18	19	20	21	22	23	24

FIGURE 8.2 Project timeline (in months) for a hypothetical study of women's mammography decisions.

CRITIQUING PLANNING ASPECTS OF A STUDY

Researchers typically do not describe the planning process or problems that arose during the study in journal articles. Thus, there is typically little that readers can do to critique the researcher's planning efforts. What *can* be critiqued, of course, are the outcomes of the planning—that is, the actual methodologic decisions themselves. Guidelines for critiquing those decisions are provided in subsequent chapters of this book.

There are, however, a few things that readers can be alert to relating to the planning of a study. First, evidence of careful conceptualization provides a clue that the project was well planned. If a conceptual map is presented (or implied) in the report, it means that the researcher had a "road map" that facilitated planning.

Second, readers can consider whether the researcher's plans reflect adequate attention to concerns about EBP. For example, was the comparison group strategy designed to reflect a realistic practice concern? Was the setting one that maximizes potential for the generalizability of the findings? Did the time frames for data collection correspond to clinically important milestones? Was the intervention sensitive to the constraints of a typical practice environment?

Finally, a report might provide clues about whether the researcher devoted sufficient time and resources in preparing for the study. For example, if the report indicates that the study grew out of earlier research on a similar topic, or that the researcher had previously used the same instruments, or had completed other studies in the same setting, this suggests that the researcher was not plunging into unfamiliar waters. Unrealistic planning can sometimes be inferred from a discussion of sample recruitment. If the report indicates that the researcher was unable to recruit the originally hoped-for number of participants, or if recruitment took months longer than anticipated, this suggests that the researcher may not have done adequate homework during the planning phase.

RESEARCH EXAMPLE

In this section, we describe the outcomes of a pilot study for a larger intervention study. Although this is not a very recent study, the "lessons learned" remain relevant.

Study: Tales from the field: What the nursing research textbooks will not tell you (Smith et al., 2008)

Purpose: The purpose of the article was to describe some of the setbacks and lessons learned in a pilot for an intervention study designed to test a multiphase management strategy for persons with dementia.

Pilot Study Methods: The researchers undertook a 1-year pilot study in the first phase of a multiyear project. The purpose of the pilot was to assess and refine data collection methods and procedures, review recruitment strategies and criteria used to select participants, evaluate the acceptability of the screening and outcome measures, and gather information for improving the intervention. The plan was to recruit and assess 20 people with probable or possible Alzheimer's disease living in assisted living facilities (ALF).

Pilot Study Findings: The researchers were faced with numerous challenges and setbacks in their study. Passive methods of recruiting family members who were needed for signing consent (placing posters and informational handouts in ALFs) yielded no participants, so other strategies had to be developed. Eventually, 17 participants were enrolled, but not a single one met the stringent criteria for inclusion in the study that the researchers had originally developed. Data collection took longer than anticipated. Staff at the ALF were not always cooperative. Problems with obtaining IRB approval resulted in months of delay.

Conclusions: The researchers found that "the information learned was quite valuable and was used to shape changes in subsequent research" (p. 235). They noted the value of undertaking pilot work and of doing a

systematic analysis about midway through the pilot. Other recommendations included doing good up-front assessments of study sites, allowing plenty of time for revisions for the IRB, and having a "Plan B" when things go awry.

SUMMARY POINTS

- Researchers face numerous challenges in planning a study. The major methodologic challenge is designing a study that is reliable and valid (quantitative studies) or trustworthy (qualitative studies).
- **Reliability** refers to the accuracy and consistency of information obtained in a study. **Validity** is a more complex concept that broadly concerns the *soundness* of the study's evidence—that is, whether the findings are cogent, convincing, and well grounded.
- **Trustworthiness** in qualitative research encompasses several different dimensions, including dependability, confirmability, authenticity, transferability, and credibility.
- **Credibility** is achieved to the extent that the research methods engender confidence in the truth of the data and in the researchers' interpretations. **Triangulation**, the use of multiple sources or referents to draw conclusions about what constitutes the truth, is one approach to establishing credibility.
- A **bias** is an influence that distorts study results. **Systematic bias** results when a bias operates in a consistent direction.
- In quantitative studies, **research control** is used to *hold constant* outside influences on the dependent variable so that its relationship to the independent variable can be better understood. Researchers use various strategies to control **confounding** (or **extraneous**) **variables**, which are extraneous to the study aims and can obscure understanding.
- In quantitative studies, a powerful tool to eliminate bias is **randomness**—having certain features of the study established by chance rather than by personal preference.
- **Reflexivity**, the process of reflecting critically on the self and of scrutinizing personal values

that could affect interpretation, is an important tool in qualitative research.

- **Generalizability** in a quantitative study concerns the extent to which findings can be applied to other groups and settings. **Transferability** is the extent to which qualitative findings can be transferred to other settings.
- In planning a study, researchers make many design decisions, including whether to have an intervention, how to control confounding variables, what type of comparisons will be made, where the study will take place, and what the time frames of the study will be.
- Quantitative researchers often incorporate comparisons into their designs to enhance interpretability. In **between-subjects designs**, different groups of people are compared. **Within-subjects designs** involve comparisons of the same people at different times or under different circumstances, and **mixed designs** involve comparisons of both.
- Site selection for a study often requires **site visits** to evaluate suitability and feasibility. Gaining entrée into a site involves developing and maintaining trust with gatekeepers.
- **Cross-sectional designs** involve collecting data at one point in time, whereas **longitudinal designs** involve data collection two or more times over an extended period.
- **Trend studies** have multiple points of data collection with different samples from the same population. **Panel studies** gather data from the same people, usually from a general population, more than once. In a **follow-up study**, data are gathered two or more times from a more well-defined group (e.g., those with a particular health problem). In a **cohort study**, a cohort of people is tracked over time to see if subsets with different exposures to risk factors differ in terms of subsequent outcomes.
- A **repeated measures design** typically involves collecting data three or more times, either in a longitudinal fashion or in rapid succession over a shorter time frame.
- Longitudinal studies are typically expensive and time-consuming, and risk **attrition** (loss of participants over time), but are essential for illuminating time-related phenomena.

- Researchers also develop a **data collection plan**. In nursing, the most widely used methods are self-report, observation, biophysiologic measures, and existing records.
- **Self-report** data (sometimes called **patient-reported outcomes** or **PROs**) are obtained by directly questioning people. Self-reports are versatile and powerful, but a drawback is the potential for respondents' deliberate or inadvertent misrepresentations.
- A wide variety of human activity and traits is amenable to direct **observation**. Observation is subject to **observer biases** and distorted participant behavior (**reactivity**).
- **Biophysiologic measures** tend to yield high-quality data that are objective and valid.
- Existing **records** and documents are an economical source of research data, but two potential biases in records are **selective deposit** and **selective survival**.
- Data collection methods vary in terms of structure, researcher obtrusiveness, and objectivity, and researchers must decide on these dimensions in their plan.
- Planning efforts should include the development of a timeline that provides estimates of when important tasks will be completed.

STUDY ACTIVITIES

Chapter 8 of the *Resource Manual for Nursing Research: Generating and Assessing Evidence for Nursing Practice, 10th edition*, offers study suggestions for reinforcing concepts presented in this chapter. In addition, the following questions can be addressed in classroom or online discussions:

1. Suppose you wanted to study how children's attitudes toward smoking change over time. Design a cross-sectional study to research this question, specifying the samples that you would want to include. Now design a longitudinal study to research the same problem. Identify the strengths and weaknesses of each approach.
2. Find a qualitative study that involved triangulation of multiple types of data. How did triangulation enhance the credibility of the findings?

STUDIES CITED IN CHAPTER 8

Adderley, U., & Stubbs, N. (2014). Stockings or bandages for leg-ulcer compression? *Nursing Times, 110*(15), 19–20.

Asgar Pour, H., & Yavuz, M. (2014). Effects of peripheral cold application on core body temperature and haemodynamic parameters in febrile patients. *International Journal of Nursing Practice, 20,* 156–163.

Axelsson, L., Klang, B., Lundh Hagelin, C., Jacobson, S. H., & Gleissman, S. A. (2015). Meanings of being a close relative of a family member treated with haemodialysis approaching end of life. *Journal of Clinical Nursing, 24,* 447–456.

Bernard, H. R. (2006). *Research methods in anthropology: Qualitative and quantitative approaches.* Lanham, MD: AltaMira Press.

*Brown, L. F., Pridham, K., & Brown, R. (2014). Sequential observation of infant regulated and dysregulated behavior following soothing and stimulating maternal behavior during feeding. *Journal for Specialists in Pediatric Nursing, 19,* 139–148.

*Buckwalter, K., Grey, M., Bowers, B., McCarthy, A., Gross, D., Funk, M., & Beck, C. (2009). Intervention research in highly unstable environments. *Research in Nursing & Health, 32,* 110–121.

Chao, Y. H., Wang, S., Hsu, T., & Wang, K. (2015). The desire to survive: The adaptation process of adult cancer patients undergoing radiotherapy. *Japanese Journal of Nursing Science, 12,* 79–86.

Collins, M., Shattell, M., & Thomas, S. P. (2005). Problematic interviewee behaviors in qualitative research. *Western Journal of Nursing Research, 27,* 188–199.

Dysvik, E., Kvaloy, J. T., & Furnes, B. (2013). A mixed-method study exploring suffering and alleviation in participants attending a chronic pain management programme. *Journal of Clinical Nursing, 23,* 865–876.

Erlandson, D. A., Harris, E. L., Skipper, B., & Allen, S. (1993). *Doing naturalistic inquiry: A guide to methods.* Thousand Oaks, CA: Sage.

Everett, B. (2014). Changes in neighborhood characteristics and depression among sexual minority young adults. *Journal of the American Psychiatric Nurses Association, 20,* 42–52.

Farrell, G., & Comiskey, C. (2014). Dualities of living with HIV/HCV co-infection: Patients' perspectives from those who are ineligible for or nonresponsive to treatment. *Journal of the Association of Nurses in AIDS Care, 25,* 9–22.

Gowing, C., McDermott, K., Ward, L., & Martin, B. (2015). Ten years of trauma in the "top end" of the Northern Territory, Australia. *International Emergency Nursing, 23,* 17–21.

*Gregory, K. E., & Radovinsky, L. (2012). Research strategies that result in optimal data collection from the patient medical record. *Applied Nursing Research, 25,* 108–116.

Hallrup, L. (2014). The meaning of the lived experiences of adults with intellectual disabilities in a Swedish institutional care setting: A reflective lifeworld approach. *Journal of Clinical Nursing, 23,* 1583–1592.

Herrington, C. J., & Chiodo, L. (2014). Human touch effectively and safely reduces pain in the newborn intensive care unit. *Pain Management Nursing, 15,* 107–115.

Kang, D. H., Davis, L., Habermann, B., Rice, M., & Broome, M. (2005). Hiring the right people and management of research staff. *Western Journal of Nursing Research, 27,* 1059–1066.

Lincoln, Y. S., & Guba, E. G. (1985). *Naturalistic inquiry.* Newbury Park, CA: Sage.

*Logan, J. G., & Barksdale, D. (2013). Pulse wave velocity in Korean American men and women. *Journal of Cardiovascular Nursing, 28,* 90–96.

Morse, J. M., & Field, P. A. (1995). *Qualitative research methods for health professionals* (2nd ed.). Thousand Oaks, CA: Sage.

*Nelson, L. E., & Morrison-Beedy, D. (2008). Research team training: Moving beyond job descriptions. *Applied Nursing Research, 21,* 159–164.

Okajima, S., Hirota, A., Kimura, E., Inagaki, M., Tamai, N., Iizaka, S., . . . Sanada, H. (2013). Health-related quality of life and associated factors in patients with primary lymphedema. *Japanese Journal of Nursing Science, 10,* 202–211.

Polit, D. F., & Beck, C. T. (2010). Generalization in qualitative and quantitative research: Myths and strategies. *International Journal of Nursing Studies, 47,* 1451–1458.

Schwandt, T. (2007). *The Sage dictionary of qualitative inquiry* (3rd ed.). Thousand Oaks, CA: Sage.

*Smith, M., Buckwalter, K., Kang, H., Schultz, S., & Ellingrod, V. (2008). Tales from the field: What the nursing research textbooks will not tell you. *Applied Nursing Research, 21,* 232–236.

Staveski, S., Tesoro, T., Cisco, M., Roth, S., & Shin, A. (2014). Sedative and analgesic use on night and day shifts in a pediatric cardiovascular intensive care unit. *AACN Advanced Critical Care, 25,* 114–118.

Talbert, S., & Sole, M. L. (2013). Too much information: Research issues associated with large databases. *Clinical Nurse Specialist, 27,* 73–80.

Tunney, A. M., & Boore, J. (2013). The effectiveness of a storybook in lessening anxiety in children undergoing tonsillectomy and adenoidectomy in Northern Ireland. *Issues in Comprehensive Pediatric Nursing, 36,* 319–335.

***A link to this open-access journal article is provided in the Toolkit for this chapter in the accompanying Resource Manual.** ✪

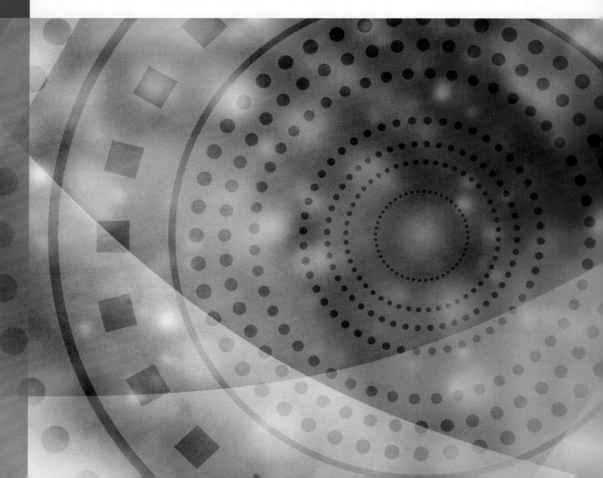

PART 3

DESIGNING AND CONDUCTING QUANTITATIVE STUDIES TO GENERATE EVIDENCE FOR NURSING

9 | Quantitative Research Design

GENERAL DESIGN ISSUES

Chapters 9 through 20 focus on methods of doing quantitative research. This chapter describes options for designing quantitative studies. We begin by discussing several broad issues.

Causality

As noted in Chapter 2, several broad categories of research questions are relevant to evidence-based nursing practice—questions about interventions (Therapy), Diagnosis and assessment, Prognosis, Etiology/harm, and Meaning or process (see Table 2.1). Questions about meaning or process call for qualitative approaches, which we describe in Chapters 21–25. Questions about diagnosis or assessment, as well as questions about the status quo of health-related situations, are typically descriptive. Many research questions, however, are about *causes* and *effects*:

- Does a telephone therapy intervention (I) for patients diagnosed with prostate cancer (P) *cause* improvements in their decision-making skills (O)? (Therapy question)
- Do birth weights less than 1,500 grams (I) *cause* developmental delays (O) in children (P)? (Prognosis question)
- Does a high-carbohydrate diet (I) *cause* dementia (O) in the elderly (P)? (Etiology/harm question)

Causality is a hotly debated philosophical issue, and yet we all understand the general concept of a **cause**. For example, we understand that lack of sleep *causes* fatigue and that high caloric intake *causes* weight gain.

Most phenomena have multiple causes. Weight gain, for example, can be the effect of high caloric consumption, but many other factors can cause weight gain. Causes of health-related phenomena usually are not *deterministic* but rather are *probabilistic*—that is, the causes increase the probability that an effect will occur. For example, there is ample evidence that smoking is a cause of lung cancer, but not everyone who smokes develops lung cancer, and not everyone with lung cancer has a history of smoking.

The Counterfactual Model

While it might be easy to grasp what researchers have in mind when they talk about a *cause*, what exactly is an **effect**? Shadish and colleagues (2002), who wrote an influential book on research design and causal inference, explained that a good way to grasp the meaning of an effect is by conceptualizing a counterfactual. In a research context, a **counterfactual** is what would have happened *to the same people* exposed to a causal factor if they *simultaneously* were *not* exposed to the causal factor. An effect represents the difference between what actually did happen with the exposure and what would have happened without it. A counterfactual clearly can never be realized, but it is a good model to keep in mind in designing a study to address cause-probing questions. As Shadish and colleagues (2002) noted, "A central task for all cause-probing research is to create reasonable approximations to this physically impossible counterfactual" (p. 5).

Criteria for Causality

Several writers have proposed criteria for establishing a *cause-and-effect relationship*. Three criteria are attributed to John Stuart Mill (Lazarsfeld, 1955).

1. *Temporal*: A cause must precede an effect in time. If we test the hypothesis that smoking causes lung cancer, we need to show that cancer occurred *after* smoking commenced.
2. *Relationship*: There must be an *empirical relationship* between the presumed cause and the presumed effect. In our example, we must show an association between smoking and cancer—that is, that a higher percentage of smokers than nonsmokers get lung cancer.
3. *No confounders*: The relationship cannot be explained as being *caused by a third variable*. Suppose that smokers tended also to live in urban environments. There would then be a possibility that the relationship between smoking and lung cancer reflects an underlying causal connection between the environment and lung cancer.

Additional criteria were proposed by Bradford-Hill (1971)—precisely as part of the discussion about the causal link between smoking and lung cancer. Two of Bradford-Hill's criteria foreshadow the importance of meta-analyses, techniques for which had not been fully developed when the criteria were proposed. The criterion of *coherence* involves having similar evidence from multiple sources, and the criterion of *consistency* involves having similar levels of statistical relationship in several studies. Another important criterion is *biologic plausibility*, that is, evidence from laboratory or basic physiologic studies that a causal pathway is credible.

Causality and Research Design

Researchers testing hypotheses about casual relationships must provide persuasive evidence about meeting these various criteria through their study designs. Some designs are better at revealing cause-and-effect relationships than others. In particular, experimental designs (randomized controlled trials or RCTs) are the best possible designs for illuminating causal relationships—but, it is not always possible to use such designs for various ethical or practical reasons. Much of this chapter focuses on designs for illuminating causal relationships.

Design Terminology

It is easy to get confused about terms used for research designs because there is inconsistency among writers. Also, design terms used by medical and epidemiologic researchers are often different from those used by social scientists. Early nurse researchers got their research training in social science fields such as psychology before doctoral training became available in nursing schools, and so social scientific design terms have prevailed in the nursing research literature.

Nurses interested in establishing an evidence-based practice must be able to understand studies from many disciplines. We use both medical and social science terms in this book. The first column of Table 9.1 shows several design terms used by social scientists and the second shows corresponding terms used by medical researchers.

EXPERIMENTAL DESIGN

A basic distinction in quantitative research design is between experimental and nonexperimental research. In an **experiment** (or **randomized controlled trial, RCT**), researchers are active agents, not passive observers. Early physical scientists learned that although pure observation is valuable, complexities in nature often made it difficult to understand relationships. This problem was addressed by isolating phenomena and controlling the conditions under which they occurred—procedures that were adopted by biologists in the 19th century. The 20th century witnessed the acceptance of experimental methods by researchers interested in human physiology and behavior.

Controlled experiments are considered the gold standard for yielding reliable evidence about causes and effects. Experimenters can be relatively confident in the authenticity of causal relationships because they are observed under controlled conditions and typically meet the criteria for establishing causality. Hypotheses are never *proved* by scientific methods, but RCTs offer the most convincing

TABLE 9.1 • Research Design Terminology in the Social Scientific and Medical Literature

SOCIAL SCIENTIFIC TERM	MEDICAL RESEARCH TERM
Experiment, true experiment, experimental study	Randomized controlled trial, randomized clinical trial, RCT
Quasi-experiment, quasi-experimental study	Controlled trial, controlled trial without randomization
Nonexperimental study, correlational study	Observational study
Retrospective study	Case-control study
Prospective nonexperimental study	Cohort study
Group or condition (e.g., experimental or control group/condition)	Group or arm (e.g., intervention or control arm)
Experimental group	Treatment or intervention group

evidence about whether one variable has a casual effect on another.

A true experimental or RCT design is characterized by the following properties:

- *Manipulation*: The researcher *does* something to at least some participants—that is, there is some type of intervention.
- *Control*: The researcher introduces controls over the research situation, including devising a counterfactual approximation—usually, a control group that does not receive the intervention.
- *Randomization*: The researcher assigns participants to a control or experimental condition on a random basis.

Design Features of True Experiments

Researchers have many options in designing an experiment. We begin by discussing several features of experimental designs.

Manipulation: The Experimental Intervention

Manipulation involves *doing* something to study participants. Experimenters manipulate the independent variable by administering a **treatment** (or **intervention** [I]) to some people and withholding it from others (C), or administering different treatments. Experimenters deliberately *vary* the

independent variable (the presumed cause) and observe the effect on the outcome (O)—often referred to as an **end point** in the medical literature.

For example, suppose we hypothesized that gentle massage is an effective pain relief strategy for nursing home residents (P). The independent variable, receipt of gentle massage, can be manipulated by giving some patients the massage intervention (I) and withholding it from others (C). We would then compare pain levels (the outcome [O] variable) in the two groups to see if receipt of the intervention resulted in group differences in average pain levels.

In designing RCTs, researchers make many decisions about what the experimental condition entails, and these decisions can affect the conclusions. To get a fair test, the intervention should be appropriate to the problem, consistent with a theoretical rationale, and of sufficient intensity and duration that effects might reasonably be expected. The full nature of the intervention must be delineated in formal *protocols* that spell out exactly what the treatment is. Among the questions researchers need to address are the following:

- What *is* the intervention, and how does it differ from usual methods of care?
- What specific procedures are to be used with those receiving the intervention?

- What is the dosage or intensity of the intervention?
- Over how long a period will the intervention be administered, how frequently will it be administered, and when will the treatment begin (e.g., 2 hours after surgery)?
- Who will administer the intervention? What are their credentials, and what type of special training will they receive?
- Under what conditions will the intervention be withdrawn or altered?

The goal in most RCTs is to have an identical intervention for all people in the treatment group. For example, in most drug studies, those in the experimental group are given the exact same ingredient, in the same dose, administered in exactly the same manner—all according to well-articulated protocols. There has, however, been some interest in **tailored interventions** or **patient-centered interventions** (PCIs) (Lauver et al., 2002). The purpose of PCIs is to enhance treatment efficacy by taking people's characteristics or needs into account. In tailored interventions, each person receives an intervention customized to certain characteristics, such as demographic traits (e.g., gender) or cognitive factors (e.g., reading level). Interventions based on the Transtheoretical (stages of change) Model (Chapter 6) usually are PCIs because the intervention is tailored to fit people's readiness to change their behavior. There is some evidence that tailored interventions can be very effective (e.g., K. Richards et al., 2007), but Beck and colleagues (2010) have noted the special challenges of conducting PCI research. More research in this area is needed because of the strong EBP-related interest in understanding not only *what* works but also what works for *whom*.

> **TIP:** Although PCIs are not universally standardized, they are typically administered according to well-defined procedures and guidelines, and the intervention agents are carefully trained in making decisions about who should get which type of treatment.

Manipulation: The Control Condition

Evidence about relationships requires making at least one comparison. If we were to supplement the diet of premature infants (P) with a special nutrient (I) for 2 weeks, their weight (O) at the end of 2 weeks would tell us nothing about treatment effectiveness. At a bare minimum, we would need to compare posttreatment weight with pretreatment weight to determine if, at least, their weight had increased. But let us assume that we find an average weight gain of 1 pound. Does this gain support the conclusion that the nutrition supplement (the independent variable) caused weight gain (the dependent variable)? No, it does not. Babies normally gain weight as they mature. Without a control group—a group that does *not* receive the supplement (C)—it is impossible to separate the effects of maturation from those of the treatment.

The term **control group** refers to a group of participants whose performance on an outcome is used to evaluate the performance of the treatment group on the same outcome. As noted in Table 9.1, researchers with training from a social science tradition use the term "group" or "condition" (e.g., the experimental group or the control condition) but medical researchers often use the term "arm," as in the "intervention arm" or the "control arm" of the study.

The control condition is a proxy for an ideal counterfactual. Researchers have choices about what to use as the counterfactual. Their decision is sometimes based on theoretical grounds but may be driven by practical or ethical concerns. In some research, control group members receive no treatment at all—they are merely observed with respect to performance on the outcome. This control condition is not usually feasible in nursing research. For example, if we wanted to evaluate the effectiveness of a nursing intervention for hospital patients, we would not devise an RCT in which patients in the control group received no nursing care at all. Possibilities for the counterfactual include the following:

1. An alternative intervention; for example, participants could receive two different types of distraction as alternative therapies for pain, such as music versus massage. (Sometimes the alternative is a previously tested effective treatment, in which case it is sometimes called a *positive control* design.)
2. Standard methods of care—that is, the usual procedures used to care for patients. This is the most typical control condition in nursing studies.

3. A **placebo** or pseudointervention presumed to have no therapeutic value; for example, in studies of the effectiveness of drugs, some patients get the experimental drug and others get an innocuous substance. Placebos are used to control for the nonpharmaceutical effects of drugs, such as the attention being paid to participants. (There can, however, be **placebo effects**—changes in the outcome attributable to the placebo condition—because of participants' expectations of benefits or harms.)

Example of a Placebo Control Group: In a study of the effectiveness of aromatherapy in relieving nausea and vomiting, Hodge and co-researchers (2014) randomly assigned patients with postoperative nausea to an aromatic inhaler or to a control group that received a placebo inhaler.

4. Different doses or intensities of treatment wherein all participants get some type of intervention, but the experimental group gets an intervention that is richer, more intense, or longer. This approach is attractive when there is a desire to analyze **dose-response effects**, that is, to test whether larger doses are associated with larger benefits, or whether a smaller (and less costly or burdensome) dose would suffice.

Example of Different Dose Groups: Lee and colleagues (2013) compared two treatments for the relief of lower back pain for women in labor. The women were randomly assigned to receive either a single intradermal sterile water injection or four injections.

5. **Wait-list control group**, with delayed treatment; the control group eventually receives the full experimental intervention, after all research outcomes are assessed.

Methodologically, the best test is between two conditions that are as different as possible, as when the experimental group gets a strong treatment and the control group gets no treatment. Ethically, the wait-list approach (number 5) is appealing but may be hard to do pragmatically. Testing two competing interventions (number 1) also has ethical appeal but

runs the risk of ambiguous results if both interventions are moderately effective.

Some researchers combine two or more comparison strategies. For example, they might test two alternative treatments (option 1) against a placebo (option 3). The use of multiple comparison groups is often attractive but adds to the cost and complexity of the study.

Example of a Three-Group Design: Silverman (2013) randomly assigned psychiatric inpatients to one of three conditions to assess effects on self-stigma and experienced stigma: music therapy (the main intervention), education (the alternative intervention), or a wait-list control condition.

Sometimes researchers include an **attention control** group when they want to rule out the possibility that intervention effects are caused by the special attention given to those receiving the intervention rather than by the actual treatment content. The idea is to separate the "active ingredients" of the treatment from the "inactive ingredients" of special attention.

Example of an Attention Control Group: Jenerette and co-researchers (2014) tested an intervention to decrease stigma in young adults with sickle cell disease. Participants were randomized to a care-seeking intervention that cultivated communication skills or to an attention control group that participated in life reviews.

The control group decision should be based on an underlying conceptualization of how the intervention might "cause" the intended effect and should also reflect consideration of what it is that needs to be controlled. For example, if attention control groups are being considered, there should be an underlying conceptualization of the construct of "attention" (Gross, 2005).

Whatever the control group strategy, researchers need to be careful in spelling it out. In research reports, researchers sometimes say that the control group got "usual methods of care" without explaining what that condition was and how different it was from the intervention being tested. In drawing on an evidence base for practice, nurses need to understand exactly what happened to study participants in different conditions. Barkauskas and colleagues (2005) and Shadish et al. (2002) offer useful advice about developing a control group strategy.

Randomization

Randomization (also called **random assignment** or **random allocation**) involves assigning participants to treatment conditions at random. *Random* means that participants have an equal chance of being assigned to any group. If people are placed in groups randomly, there is no systematic bias in the groups with respect to preintervention attributes that are potential confounders and could affect outcomes.

Randomization Principles. The overall purpose of random assignment is to approximate the ideal—but impossible—counterfactual of having the same people exposed to two or more conditions simultaneously. For example, suppose we wanted to study the effectiveness of a contraceptive counseling program for multiparous women who wish to postpone another pregnancy. Two groups of women are included—one will be counseled and the other will not. Women in the sample are likely to differ from one another in many ways, such as age, marital status, financial situation, and the like. Any of these characteristics could affect a woman's diligence in practicing contraception, independent of whether she receives counseling. We need to have the "counsel" and "no counsel" groups equal with respect to these confounding characteristics to assess the impact of counseling on subsequent pregnancies. Random assignment of people to one group or the other is designed to perform this equalization function.

Although randomization is the preferred method for equalizing groups, there is no *guarantee* that the groups will be equal. The risk of unequal groups is high when sample size is small. For example, with a sample of five men and five women, it is entirely possible that all five men would be assigned to the experimental and all five women to the control group. The likelihood of getting markedly unequal groups is reduced as the sample size increases.

You may wonder why we do not consciously control characteristics that are likely to affect

the outcome through *matching*. For example, if matching were used in the contraceptive counseling study, we could ensure that if there were a married, 38-year-old woman with five children in the experimental group, there would be a married, 38-year-old woman with five children in the control group. Matching is problematic, however. To match effectively, we must know the characteristics that are likely to affect the outcome, but this knowledge is often incomplete. Second, even if we knew the relevant traits, the complications of matching on more than two or three confounders simultaneously are prohibitive. With random assignment, *all* personal characteristics—age, income, health status, and so on—are likely to be equally distributed in all groups. Over the long run, randomized groups tend to be counterbalanced with respect to an infinite number of biologic, psychological, economic, and social traits.

Basic Randomization. The most straightforward randomization procedure, for a two-group design, is to simply allocate each person as they enroll into a study on a random basis—for example, by flipping a coin. If the coin comes up "heads," a participant would be assigned to one group; if it comes up "tails," he or she would be assigned to the other group. This type of randomization, with no restrictions, is sometimes called *complete randomization*. Each successive person has a 50-50 chance of being assigned to the intervention group. The problem with this approach is that large imbalances in group size can occur, especially when the sample size is small. For example, with a sample of 10 subjects, there is only a 25% probability that perfect balance (five per group) would result. In other words, three times out of four, the groups would be of unequal size, by chance alone. This method is not recommended when the sample size is less than 200 (Lachin et al., 1988).

Researchers often want treatment groups of equal size (or with predesignated proportions). *Simple randomization* involves starting with a known sample size and then prespecifying the proportion of subjects who will be randomly allocated to different treatment conditions. To illustrate how a simple randomization is performed, we turn to another example. Suppose we were testing two alternative interventions to reduce the anxiety of children who are about to undergo tonsillectomy. One intervention involves giving structured information about the surgical team's activities (procedural information); the other involves structured information about what the child will feel (sensation information). A third control group receives no special intervention. We have a sample of 15 children, and 5 will be randomly assigned to each group.

Before widespread availability of computers, researchers used a **table of random numbers** to randomize. A small portion of such a table is shown in Table 9.2. In a table of random numbers, any digit from 0 to 9 is equally likely to follow any other digit. Going in any direction from any point in the table produces a random sequence.

In our example, we would number the 15 children from 1 to 15, as shown in column 2 of Table 9.3, and then draw numbers between 01 and 15 from the random number table. To find a random starting point, you can close your eyes and let your finger fall at some point on the table. For this example, assume that our starting point is at number 52, bolded in Table 9.2. We can move in any direction from that point, selecting numbers that fall between

01 and 15. Let us move to the right, looking at two-digit combinations. The number to the right of 52 is 06. The person whose number is 06, Alex O., is assigned to group I. Moving along, the next number within our range is 11. (To find numbers in the desired range, we bypass numbers between 16 and 99.) Alaine J., whose number is 11, is also assigned to group I. The next three numbers are 01, 15, and 14. Thus, Kristina B., Christopher L., and Paul M. are assigned to group I. The next five numbers between 01 and 15 in the table are used to assign five children to group II, and the remaining five are put into group III. Note that numbers that have already been used often reappear in the table before the task is completed. For example, the number 15 appeared four times during this randomization. This is normal because the numbers are random.

We can look at the three groups to see if they are similar for one discernible trait, gender. We started out with eight girls and seven boys. Randomization did a fairly good job of allocating boys and girls similarly across the three groups: there are two, three, and three girls and three, two, and two boys in groups I through III, respectively. We must hope that other characteristics (e.g., age, initial anxiety)

TABLE 9.2 • Small Table of Random Digits

46	85	05	23	26	34	67	75	83	00	74	91	06	43	45
69	24	89	34	60	45	30	50	75	21	61	31	83	18	55
14	01	33	17	92	59	74	76	72	77	76	50	33	45	13
56	30	38	73	15	16	**52**	06	96	76	11	65	49	98	93
81	30	44	85	85	68	65	22	73	76	92	85	25	58	66
70	28	42	43	26	79	37	59	52	20	01	15	96	32	67
90	41	59	36	14	33	52	12	66	65	55	82	34	76	41
39	90	40	21	15	59	58	94	90	67	66	82	14	15	75
88	15	20	00	80	20	55	49	14	09	96	27	74	82	57
45	13	46	35	45	59	40	47	20	59	43	94	75	16	80
70	01	41	50	21	41	29	06	73	12	71	85	71	59	57
37	23	93	32	95	05	87	00	11	19	92	78	42	63	40
18	63	73	75	09	82	44	49	90	05	04	92	17	37	01
05	32	78	21	62	20	24	78	17	59	45	19	72	53	32
95	09	66	79	46	48	46	08	55	58	15	19	02	87	82
43	25	38	41	45	60	83	32	59	83	01	29	14	13	49
80	85	40	92	79	43	52	90	63	18	38	38	47	47	61
81	08	87	70	74	88	72	25	67	36	66	16	44	94	31
84	89	07	80	02	94	81	03	19	00	54	10	58	34	36

TABLE 9.3 • Example for Random Assignment Procedure

CHILD'S NAME	NUMBER	GROUP ASSIGNMENT
Kristina B.	01	I
Derek A.	02	III
Julia L.	03	III
Lauren J.	04	II
Grace S.	05	II
Alex O.	06	I
Norah J.	07	III
Cormac L.	08	III
Ronan B.	09	II
Rita T.	10	III
Alaine J.	11	I
Maren B.	12	II
Vadim B.	13	II
Paul M.	14	I
Christopher L.	15	I

are also well distributed in the randomized groups. The larger the sample, the stronger the likelihood that the groups will be balanced on factors that could affect the outcomes.

Researchers usually assign participants proportionately to groups being compared. For example, a sample of 300 participants in a two-group design would generally be allocated 150 to the experimental group and 150 to the control group. If there were three groups, there would be 100 per group. It is also possible (and sometimes desirable ethically) to have a different allocation. For example, if an especially promising treatment were developed, we could assign 200 to the treatment group and 100 to the control group. Such an allocation does, however, make it more difficult to detect treatment effects at statistically significant levels—or, to put it another way, the overall sample size must be larger to attain the same level of statistical reliability.

Computerized resources are available for free on the Internet to help with randomization. One such website is www.randomizer.org, which has a useful tutorial. Standard statistical software packages (e.g., SPSS or SAS) can also be used.

→ **TIP:** There is considerable confusion—even in research methods textbooks—about random assignment versus random sampling. Randomization (random assignment) is a *signature* of an experimental design. If there is no random allocation of participants to conditions, then the design is not a true experiment. Random *sampling*, by contrast, is a method of selecting people for a study (see Chapter 12). Random sampling is *not* a signature of an experimental design. In fact, most RCTs do *not* involve random sampling.

Randomization Procedures. The success of randomization depends on two factors. First, the allocation process should be truly random. Second, there must be strict adherence to the randomization schedule. The latter can be achieved if the allocation is unpredictable (for both participants and those enrolling them) and tamperproof. Random assignment should involve allocation concealment that prevents those who enroll participants from knowing upcoming assignments. **Allocation concealment** is intended to prevent biases that could stem from knowledge of allocations before assignments actually occur. As an example, if the person doing the enrollment knew that the next person enrolled would be assigned to a promising intervention, he or she might defer enrollment until a very needy patient enrolled.

Several methods of allocation concealment have been devised, several of which involve developing a randomization schedule before the study begins. This is advantageous when people do not enter a study simultaneously but rather on a *rolling enrollment* basis. One widely used method is to have sequentially numbered, opaque sealed envelopes (SNOSE) containing assignment information. As each participant enters the study, he or she receives the next envelope in the sequence (for procedural suggestions, see Vickers [2006], or Doig & Simpson [2005]). Envelope systems, however, can be subject to tampering (Vickers, 2006). A good method is to have treatment allocation performed by a person unconnected with enrollment or treatment and communicated to researchers by telephone or e-mail. Herbison and colleagues (2011) found, however, that trials with a SNOSE system had a comparable risk of bias as trials with centralized randomization.

➲ TIP: Downs and colleagues (2010) offer recommendations for avoiding practical problems in implementing randomization, and Padhye and colleagues (2009) have described an easy-to-use spreadsheet method for randomization in small studies.

The timing of randomization is also important. Study eligibility—whether a person meets the criteria for inclusion—should be ascertained before randomization. If **baseline data** (preintervention data) are collected to measure key outcomes, this should occur before randomization to rule out any possibility that group assignment in itself might affect baseline measurements. Randomization should occur as closely as possible to the start of the intervention to increase the likelihood that all randomized people will actually receive the condition to which they have been assigned. Figure 9.1 illustrates the sequence of steps that occurs in most RCTs, including the timing for obtaining informed consent.

Randomization Variants. Simple or complete randomization is used in many nursing studies, but variants of randomization offer advantages in terms

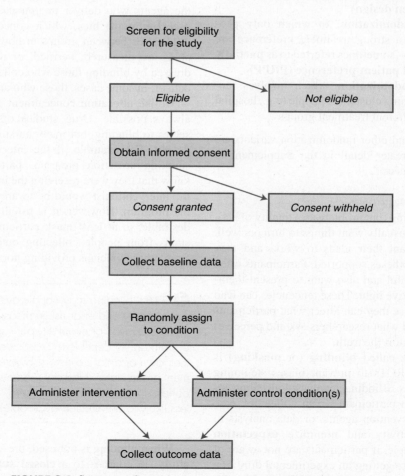

FIGURE 9.1 Sequence of steps in a conventional randomization design.

of ensuring group comparability or minimizing certain biases. These variants include the following:

- **Stratified randomization**, in which randomization occurs separately for distinct subgroups (e.g., males and females)
- **Permuted block randomization**, in which people are allocated to groups in small blocks to ensure a balanced distribution in each block
- **Urn randomization**, in which group balance is continuously monitored and the allocation probability is adjusted when an imbalance occurs (i.e., the probability of assignment becomes higher for the treatment condition with fewer participants)
- **Randomized consent**, in which randomization occurs prior to obtaining informed consent (also called a **Zelen design**)
- **Partial randomization**, in which only people without a strong treatment preference are randomized—sometimes referred to as **partially randomized patient preference (PRPP)**
- **Cluster randomization**, which involves randomly assigning clusters of people (e.g., hospital wards) to different treatment groups

These and other randomization variants are described in greater detail in the Supplement to Chapter 9 on thePoint®.

Blinding or Masking

A rather charming (but problematic) quality of people is that they usually want things to turn out well. Researchers want their ideas to work, and they want their hypotheses supported. Participants often want to be helpful and also want to present themselves in a positive light. These tendencies can lead to biases because they can affect what participants do and say (and what researchers ask and perceive) in ways that distort the truth.

A procedure called **blinding** (or **masking**) is often used in RCTs to prevent biases stemming from *awareness*. Blinding involves concealing information from participants, data collectors, care providers, intervention agents, or data analysts to enhance objectivity and minimize **expectation bias**. For example, if participants are not aware of whether they are getting an experimental drug or a placebo, then their outcomes cannot be influenced

by their expectations of its efficacy. Blinding typically involves disguising or withholding information about participants' status in the study (e.g., whether they are in the experimental or control group) but can also involve withholding information about study hypotheses, baseline performance on outcomes, or preliminary study results.

The absence of blinding can result in several types of bias. **Performance bias** refers to systematic differences in the care provided to members of different groups of participants, apart from any intervention. For example, those delivering an intervention might treat participants in groups differently (e.g., with greater attentiveness), apart from the intervention itself. Efforts to avoid performance bias usually involve blinding the participants and the agents who deliver treatments. **Detection** (or **ascertainment**) bias, which concerns systematic differences between groups in how outcome variables are measured, verified, or recorded, is addressed by blinding those who collect the outcome data or, in some cases, those who analyze the data.

Unlike allocation concealment, blinding is not always possible. Drug studies often lend themselves to blinding, but many nursing interventions do not. For example, if the intervention were a smoking cessation program, participants would know that they were receiving the intervention, and the interventionist would be aware of who was in the program. However, it is usually possible, and desirable, to at least mask participants' treatment status from people collecting outcome data and from other clinicians providing normal care.

> **TIP:** Blinding may not always be necessary if subjectivity and error risk in measuring the outcome are low. For example, participants' ratings of pain are susceptible to biases stemming from their own or data collectors' awareness of treatment group status. Hospital readmission and length of hospital stay, on the other hand, are variables less likely to be affected by people's awareness.

When blinding is not used, the study is an **open study**, in contrast to a **closed study** that results from masking. When blinding is used with only one group of people (e.g., study participants), it is sometimes described as a **single-blind study**. When it is possible to mask with two groups (e.g., those delivering an intervention and those receiving it), it is sometimes called **double-blind**. However, recent guidelines have recommended that researchers not use these terms without explicitly stating which groups were blinded because the term "double blind" has been used to refer to many different combinations of blinded groups (Moher et al., 2010).

The term *blinding*, although widely used, has fallen into some disfavor because of possible pejorative connotations, and some organizations (e.g., the American Psychological Association) have recommended using masking instead. Medical researchers, however, appear to prefer *blinding* unless the people in the study have vision impairments (Schulz et al., 2002). The vast majority of nurse researchers use the term *blinding* rather than *masking* (Polit et al., 2011).

Example of an Experiment with Blinding:
Kundu and colleagues (2014) studied the effect of Reiki therapy on postoperative pain in children undergoing dental procedures. Study participants were blinded—those in the control group received a sham Reiki treatment. Those who recorded the children's pain scores, the nurses caring for the children, and the children's parents, were also blinded to group assignments.

Specific Experimental Designs

Some popular experimental designs are summarized in Table 9.4. The second column (schematic diagram) depicts design notation from a classic monograph (Campbell & Stanley, 1963). In this notation, R means random assignment, O represents observations (i.e., data collected on the outcome), and X stands for exposure to the intervention. Each row designates a different group, and time is portrayed moving from left to right. Thus, in Row 2 (a basic pretest–posttest design), the top line represents the group that was randomly assigned (R) to an intervention (X) and from which data were collected prior to (O_1) and after (O_2) the intervention. The second row is the control group, which differs from the experimental group only by absence of the treatment (no X). (Some entries in

the "drawbacks" column of Table 9.4 are not discussed until Chapter 10.)

Basic Experimental Designs

Earlier in this chapter, we described a study that tested the effect of gentle massage on pain in nursing home residents. This example illustrates a simple design that is sometimes called a **posttest-only design** (or **after-only design**) because data on the dependent variable are collected only once—after randomization and completion of the intervention.

A second basic design involves the collection of baseline data, as shown in the flowchart, Figure 9.1. Suppose we hypothesized that convective airflow blankets are more effective than conductive waterflow blankets in cooling critically ill febrile patients. Our design involves assigning patients to the two blanket types (the independent variable) and measuring the outcome (body temperature) twice, before and after the intervention. This design allows us to examine whether one blanket type is more effective than the other in *reducing* fever—that is, with this design researchers can examine *change*. This design is a **pretest–posttest design** or a **before–after design**. Many pretest–posttest designs include data collection at multiple postintervention points (sometimes called *repeated measures designs*, as noted in Chapter 8). Designs that involve collecting data multiple times from two groups are mixed designs: Analyses can examine both differences *between* groups and changes *within* groups over time.

These basic designs can be "tweaked" in various ways—for example, the design could involve comparison of three or more groups or could have a wait-listed control group. These designs are included in Table 9.4.

Example of a Pretest–Posttest Experimental Design: Zhu and co-researchers (2014) tested the effects of a transtheoretical model-based exercise intervention on exercise behavior and self-efficacy in patients with coronary heart disease. The outcomes were measured at baseline and at a 3-month and 6-month follow-up.

Factorial Design

Most experimental designs involve manipulating only one independent variable and randomizing

TABLE 9.4 • Design Alternatives: Selected Experimental (Randomized) Designs

TYPE OF DESIGN	SCHEMATIC DIAGRAM	SITUATIONS THAT ARE BEST SUITED TO THIS DESIGN	DRAWBACKS OF THIS DESIGN
1. Basic posttest-only design	$R\ X\ O_1$ $R\ \ \ O_1$ **or** $R\ X_A\ O_1$ $R\ X_B\ O_1$	When the outcome is not relevant until after the intervention is complete (e.g., length of stay in hospital)	Does not permit an evaluation of whether the two groups were comparable at the outset on the outcome of interest
2. Basic pretest-posttest design (with optional repeated follow-ups)	$R\ O_1\ X\ O_2$ $R\ O_1\ \ \ O_2$ $R\ O_1\ X\ O_2\ O_3\ O_4$ $R\ O_1\ \ \ O_2\ O_3\ O_4$	a. When the focus of the intervention is on change (e.g., behaviors, attitudes) b. When the researcher wants to assess both group differences (experimental comparison), and change within groups (quasi-experimental)	Sometimes the pretest itself can affect the outcomes of interest
3. Multiple intervention design	$R\ O_1\ X_A\ O_2$ $R\ O_1\ X_B\ O_2$ $R\ O_1\ \ \ O_2$	Can be used to disentangle effects of different components of a complex intervention, or to test competing interventions	a. Requires larger sample than basic designs b. May be at risk to threats to statistical conclusion validity* if A and B are not very different (small effects)
4. Wait-list (delay of treatment) design	$R\ O_1\ X\ O_2\ O_3$ $R\ O_1\ \ \ O_2\ X\ O_3$	a. Attractive when there is patient preference for the innovative treatment b. Can strengthen inferences by virtue of replication aspect for the second group	a. Controls may drop out of study before they get deferred treatment b. Not suitable if key outcomes are measured long after treatment (e.g., mortality) or if there is an interest in assessing long-term effects (wait-list period is then too long)
5. Crossover design—participants serve as their own controls	$R\ O_1\ X_A\ O_2\ X_B\ O_3$ $R\ O_1\ X_B\ O_2\ X_A\ O_3$	a. Appropriate only if there is no expectation of carryover effects from one period to the next (effects should have rapid onset, short half-life) b. Useful when recruitment is difficult—smaller sample is needed; excellent for controlling confounding variables	a. Often cannot be assumed that there are no carryover effects b. If the first treatment received "fixes" a problem for participants, they may not remain in the study for the second one c. History threat* to internal validity a possibility
6. Factorial design	$R\ O_1\ X_{A1B1}\ O_2$ $R\ O_1\ X_{A1B2}\ O_2$ $R\ O_1\ X_{A2B1}\ O_2$ $R\ O_1\ X_{A2B2}\ O_2$	a. Efficient for testing two interventions simultaneously b. Can be useful in illuminating interaction effects, but most useful when strong synergistic/additive effects (or no interaction effects) are expected	Power needed to detect interactions could require larger sample size than when testing each intervention separately

KEY: R = Randomization
  X = Intervention (X_A = one treatment, X_B = alternative treatment, dose, etc.)
  O = Observation or measurement of the dependent variable/outcome
*Validity threats are discussed in Chapter 10.

Type of stimulation

		Auditory A1		Tactile A2	
Daily dose	15 Min. B1	A1	B1	A2	B1
	30 Min. B2	A1	B2	A2	B2
	45 Min. B3	A1	B3	A2	B3

FIGURE 9.2 Example of a 2 × 3 factorial design.

participants to different treatment groups—these are sometimes called *parallel-group designs*. It is possible, however, to manipulate two or more variables simultaneously. Suppose we wanted to compare two therapies for premature infants: tactile stimulation versus auditory stimulation. We also want to learn if the daily *amount* of stimulation (15, 30, or 45 minutes) affects infants' progress. The outcomes are measures of infant development (e.g., weight gain, cardiac responsiveness). Figure 9.2 illustrates the structure of this RCT.

This **factorial design** allows us to address three research questions:

1. Does auditory stimulation have a more beneficial effect on premature infants' development than tactile stimulation, or vice versa?
2. Is the duration of stimulation (independent of type) related to infant development?
3. Is auditory stimulation most effective when linked to a certain dose and tactile stimulation most effective when coupled with a different dose?

The third question shows the strength of factorial designs: They permit us to test not only **main effects** (effects from experimentally manipulated variables, as in questions 1 and 2) but also **interaction effects** (effects from combining treatments). Our results may indicate that 30 minutes of auditory stimulation is the most beneficial treatment. We could not have learned this by conducting two separate studies that manipulated one independent variable and held the second one constant.

In factorial experiments, people are randomly assigned to a specific combination of conditions. In our example (Figure 9.2), infants would be

assigned randomly to one of six **cells**—that is, six treatment conditions. The two independent variables in a factorial design are the **factors**. Type of stimulation is factor A, and amount of daily exposure is factor B. Level 1 of factor A is auditory, and level 2 of factor A is tactile. When describing the dimensions of the design, researchers refer to the number of **levels**. The design in Figure 9.2 is a 2 × 3 design: two levels in factor A times three levels in factor B. Factorial experiments with more than two factors are rare.

Example of a Factorial Design: Mosleh and colleagues (2014) used a factorial design in their study of communications to improve attendance in cardiac rehabilitation. In their 2 × 2 design, one factor was a standard invitation letter versus a letter with wording based on the Theory of Planned Behavior. The second factor was the inclusion or noninclusion of a leaflet with motivational messages.

Crossover Design

Thus far, we have described RCTs in which different people are randomly assigned to different conditions. For instance, in the previous example, infants exposed to auditory stimulation were not the same infants as those exposed to tactile stimulation. A **crossover design** involves exposing the same people to more than one condition. This type of within-subjects design has the advantage of ensuring the highest possible equivalence among participants exposed to different conditions—the groups being compared are equal with respect to age, weight, health, and so on because they are composed of the same people.

Because randomization is a signature characteristic of an experiment, participants in a crossover design must be randomly assigned to different *orderings* of treatments. For example, if a crossover design were used to compare the effects of auditory and tactile stimulation on infant development, some infants would be randomly assigned to receive auditory stimulation first, and others would be assigned to receive tactile stimulation first. When there are three or more conditions to which participants will be exposed, the procedure of **counterbalancing** can be used to rule out ordering effects.

For example, if there were three conditions (A, B, C), participants would be randomly assigned to one of six counterbalanced orderings:

A, B, C	A, C, B
B, C, A	B, A, C
C, A, B	C, B, A

Although crossover designs are extremely powerful, they are inappropriate for certain research questions because of the problem of **carryover effects**. When people are exposed to two different treatments or conditions, they may be influenced in the second condition by their experience in the first condition. As one example, drug studies rarely use a crossover design because drug B administered *after* drug A is not necessarily the same treatment as drug B administered *before* drug A. When carryover effects are a potential concern, researchers often have a **washout period** in between the treatments (i.e., a period of no treatment exposure).

Example of a Crossover Design: Lippoldt and colleagues (2014) used a randomized crossover design with a sample of healthy adults to test the effects of different bedrest elevations and different types of mattresses on peak interface pressures.

Strengths and Limitations of Experiments

In this section, we explore the reasons why experimental designs are held in high esteem and examine some limitations.

Experimental Strengths

An experimental design is the gold standard for testing interventions because it yields strong evidence about intervention effectiveness. Experiments offer greater corroboration than any other approach that, *if* the independent variable (e.g., diet, drug, teaching approach) is varied, *then* certain consequences in the outcomes (e.g., weight loss, recovery, learning) are likely to ensue. The great strength of RCTs, then, lies in the confidence with which causal relationships can be inferred. Through the controls imposed by manipulation, comparison, and randomization, alternative explanations can be discredited. It is because of these strengths that meta-analyses of RCTs, which integrate evidence

from multiple experimental studies, are at the pinnacle of evidence hierarchies for questions about treatment effects (see Figure 2.1).

Experimental Limitations

Despite the benefits of experiments, this type of design also has limitations. First, there are often constraints that make an experimental approach impractical or impossible. These constraints are discussed later in this chapter.

> **TIP:** Shadish and colleagues (2002) described 10 situations that are especially conducive to randomized experiments; these are summarized in a table in the Toolkit.

Experiments are sometimes criticized for their artificiality, which partly stems from the requirements for comparable treatment within randomized groups, with strict adherence to protocols. In ordinary life, by contrast, we interact with people in non-formulaic ways. Another criticism is the focus on only a handful of variables while holding all else constant—a requirement that has been criticized as artificially constraining human experience. Experiments that are undertaken without a guiding theoretical framework are sometimes criticized for suggesting causal connections without any explanation for *why* the intervention might affect outcomes.

A problem with RCTs conducted in clinical settings is that it is often clinical staff, rather than researchers, who administer an intervention, and therefore, it can sometimes be difficult to ascertain whether those in the intervention group actually received the treatment as specified and if those in the control group did not. Clinical studies are conducted in environments over which researchers may have little control—and control is a critical factor in RCTs. McGuire and colleagues (2000) have described some issues relating to the challenges of testing interventions in clinical settings.

Sometimes problems emerge when participants can "opt out" of the intervention. Suppose, for example, that we randomly assigned patients with HIV infection to a special support group intervention or to a control group. Intervention subjects who elect not to participate in the support groups, or who participate infrequently, actually are in a "condition" that looks more like the control condition than the experimental one. The treatment is diluted through nonparticipation, and it may become difficult to detect any treatment effects, no matter how effective it might otherwise have been. We discuss this at greater length in the next chapter.

Another potential problem is the **Hawthorne effect**, a placebo-type effect caused by people's expectations. The term is derived from a series of experiments conducted at the Hawthorne plant of the Western Electric Corporation in which various environmental conditions, such as light and working hours, were varied to test their effects on worker productivity. Regardless of what change was introduced, that is, whether the light was made better or worse, productivity increased. Knowledge of being included in the study (not just knowledge of being in a particular group) appears to have affected people's behavior, obscuring the effect of the treatments.

In sum, despite the superiority of RCTs for testing causal hypotheses, they are subject to a number of limitations, some of which may make them difficult to apply to real-world problems. Nevertheless, with the growing demand for evidence-based practice, true experimental designs are increasingly being used to test the effects of nursing interventions.

QUASI-EXPERIMENTS

Quasi-experiments, often called *controlled trials without randomization* in the medical literature, involve an intervention but they lack randomization, the signature of a true experiment. Some quasi-experiments even lack a control group. The signature of a quasi-experimental design, then, is an intervention in the absence of randomization.

Quasi-Experimental Designs

The most widely used quasi-experimental designs are summarized in Table 9.5, which depicts designs using the schematic notation we introduced earlier.

Nonequivalent Control Group Designs

The **nonequivalent control group pretest–posttest design** involves two groups of participants, for whom outcomes are measured before and after the intervention. For example, suppose we wished to study the effect of a new chair yoga intervention for older people. The intervention is being offered to everyone at a community senior center, and randomization is not possible. For comparative purposes, we collect outcome data in a different community senior center that is not instituting the intervention. Data on quality of life are collected from both groups at baseline and again 10 weeks after its implementation in one of the centers.

The first row of Table 9.5 depicts this study. The top line represents those receiving the intervention at the experimental site and the second row represents the elders at the comparison site. This diagram is identical to the experimental pretest–posttest design (second row of Table 9.4) *except* there is no "R"—participants have not been randomized to groups. The design in Table 9.5 is weaker because *it cannot be assumed that the experimental and comparison groups are initially equivalent.* Because there is no randomization, quasi-experimental comparisons are farther from an ideal counterfactual than experimental comparisons. The design is nevertheless strong because baseline data allow us to assess whether patients in the two centers had similar levels of quality of life at the outset. If the two groups are similar, on average, at baseline, we could be relatively confident inferring that any posttest difference in outcomes was the result of the yoga intervention. If quality of life scores are different initially, however, it will be difficult to interpret posttest differences. Note that in quasi-experiments, the term **comparison group** is often used in lieu of *control group* to refer to the group against which treatment group outcomes are evaluated.

Now suppose we had been unable to collect baseline data. This design, diagrammed in Row 2 of Table 9.5, has a major flaw. We no longer have information about initial equivalence of people in the two centers. If quality of life in the experimental senior center is higher than that in the comparison site

TABLE 9.5 • Design Alternatives: Selected Quasi-Experimental Designs

TYPE OF DESIGN	SCHEMATIC DIAGRAM	SITUATIONS THAT ARE BEST SUITED	DRAWBACKS
1. Nonequivalent control group, pretest–posttest design	$O_1 \ X \ O_2$ $O_1 \quad O_2$	Attractive when an entire unit must get the intervention and a similar unit not getting the intervention is available	a. Selection threat* remains a nearly intractable problem, but less so than when there is no pretest b. History threat* also a possibility
2. Nonequivalent control group, posttest-only design	$X \ O_1$ O_1	A reasonable choice only when there is some a priori knowledge about comparability of groups with regard to key outcomes	Extremely vulnerable to selection threat,* possibility of other threats as well, especially history threat*
3. One-group pretest–posttest design	$O_1 \ X \ O_2$	A reasonable choice only when intervention impact is expected to be dramatic and other potential causes have little credibility	Typically provides very weak support for causal inference—vulnerable to many internal validity threats (maturation, history, etc.)*
4. Time series design	$O_1 \ O_2 \ O_3 \ O_4 \ X \ O_5 \ O_6 \ O_7 \ O_8$	a. Good option when there are abundant data on key outcome in existing records b. Addresses maturation threat and change from secular trends and random fluctuation	a. Complex statistical analysis that is most appropriate with very large number of data points (100+) b. History threat* remains, and (sometimes) selection threat* if the population changes over time
5. Time series nonequivalent control group design	$O_1 \ O_2 \ O_3 \ O_4 \ X \ O_5 \ O_6 \ O_7 \ O_8$ $O_1 \ O_2 \ O_3 \ O_4 \quad O_5 \ O_6 \ O_7 \ O_8$	Attractive when an entire unit/institution adopts the intervention and a similar unit not adopting it is available, *and* if comparable data are readily available in records of both	a. Selection threat* remains, as two units or institutions are rarely identical b. Analyses may be very complex
6. Time series with withdrawn and reinstituted treatment	$O_1 \ O_2 \ X \ O_3 \ O_4 \ {-X} \ O_5 \ O_6 \ X \ O_7 \ O_8$	*Attractive if effects of an intervention are short-term	a. May be untenable to assume that there are no carryover effects b. May be difficult ethically to withdraw treatment if it is efficacious

KEY: X = Intervention
O = Observation or measurement of the dependent variable/outcome
*Validity threats are discussed in Chapter 10.

at posttest, can we conclude that the intervention *caused* improved quality of life? An alternative explanation for posttest differences is that the elders in the two centers differed at the outset. Campbell and Stanley (1963) called this *nonequivalent control group posttest-only design* preexperimental rather than quasi-experimental because of its fundamental weakness—although Shadish and colleagues (2002), in their more recent book on causal inference, simply called this a weaker quasi-experimental design.

> **Example of a Nonequivalent Control Group Pretest–Posttest Design:** Wang and co-researchers (2014) assessed the efficacy of narrowband ultraviolet B phototherapy in reducing renal pruritus in patients undergoing hemodialysis. Two groups were compared based on dates of receiving hemodialysis. One nonrandomized group received the intervention three times per week for 2 weeks, and the control group received usual care. Pruritus intensity was measured at baseline and on six subsequent occasions.

Sometimes researchers use *matching* in a pretest–posttest nonequivalent control group design to ensure that the groups are, in fact, equivalent on at least some key variables related to the outcomes. For example, if an intervention was designed to reduce patient anxiety, then it might be desirable to not only *measure* preintervention anxiety in the intervention and comparison group, but to take steps to ensure that the groups' anxiety levels were comparable by matching participants' initial anxiety. Because matching on more than one or two variables is unwieldy, a more sophisticated method of matching, called **propensity matching**, can be used by researchers with statistical sophistication. This method involves the creation of a single **propensity score** that captures the conditional probability of exposure to a treatment given various pre-intervention characteristics. Experimental and comparison group members can then be matched on this score (Qin et al., 2008). Both conventional and propensity matching are most easily implemented when there is a large pool of potential comparison group participants from which good matches to treatment group members can be selected.

In lieu of using a contemporaneous comparison group, researchers sometimes use a **historical comparison group**. That is, comparison data are gathered *before* implementing the intervention. Even when the people are from the same institutional setting, however, it is risky to assume that the two groups are comparable, or that the environments are comparable in all respects except for the new intervention. There remains the possibility that something other than the intervention could account for observed differences in outcomes.

> **Example of a Historical Comparison Group:** Cutler and Sluman (2014) assessed the effect of new oral hygiene protocols on the rates of ventilator-associated pneumonia (VAP) in a critical care unit. The incidence of VAP in 559 patients after the practice change was compared to that for 528 patients before the change.

Time Series Designs

In the designs just described, a control group was used but randomization was not, but some quasi-experimental studies have neither. Suppose that a hospital implemented rapid response teams (RRTs) in its acute care units. Administrators want to examine the effects on patient outcomes (e.g., unplanned admissions to the ICU, mortality rate) and nurse outcomes (e.g., stress). For the purposes of this example, assume no other hospital could serve as a good comparison. The only kind of comparison that can be made is a before–after contrast. If RRTs were implemented in January, one could compare the mortality rate (for example) during the 3 months before RRTs with the mortality rate during the subsequent 3-month period. The schematic representation of such a study is shown in Row 3 of Table 9.5.

This one-group pretest–posttest design seems straightforward, but it has weaknesses. What if either of the 3-month periods is atypical, apart from the innovation? What about the effects of any other policy changes inaugurated during the same period? What about the effects of external factors that influence mortality, such as a flu outbreak or seasonal migration? This design (also called preexperimental by Campbell and Stanley, 1963) cannot control these factors.

→ **TIP:** *One-group pretest–posttest designs* are sometimes adequate. For example, if a researcher tested a brief teaching intervention, with baseline knowledge measured immediately before the intervention and posttest knowledge measured immediately after it, it may be reasonable to infer that the intervention is a plausible explanation for knowledge gains.

In our RRT example, the design could be modified so that some alternative explanations for changes in mortality could be ruled out. One such design is the **time series design** (or *interrupted time series design*), diagrammed in Row 4 of Table 9.5. In a time series, data are collected over an extended period during which an intervention is introduced. In the diagram, O_1 through O_4 represent four separate instances of preintervention outcome measurement, X is the introduction of the intervention, and O_5 through O_8 represent four posttreatment observations. In our example, O_1 might be the number of deaths in January through March in the year before the new RRT system, O_2 the number of deaths in April through June, and so forth. After RRTs are introduced, data on mortality are collected for four consecutive 3-month periods, giving us observations O_5 through O_8.

Even though the time series design does not eliminate all interpretive challenges, the extended time period strengthens our ability to attribute change to the intervention. Figure 9.3 demonstrates why this is so. The two line graphs (*A* and *B*) in the figure show two possible outcome patterns for eight mortality observations. The vertical dotted line in the center represents the introduction of the RRT system. Patterns *A* and *B* both reflect a feature common to most time series studies—fluctuation from one data point to another. These fluctuations are normal. One would not expect that, if 480 patients died in a hospital in 1 year, the deaths would be spaced evenly with 40 per month. It is precisely because of these fluctuations that the one-group pretest–posttest design, with only one observation before and after the intervention, is so weak.

Let us compare the interpretations for the outcomes shown in Figure 9.3. In both patterns *A* and *B*, mortality decreased between O_4 and O_5, immediately after RRTs were implemented. In *B*, however, the number of deaths rose at O_6 and continued to rise at O_7. The decrease at O_5 looks similar to other apparently haphazard fluctuations in mortality.

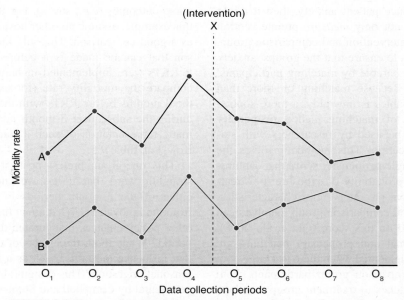

FIGURE 9.3 Two possible time series outcome patterns for quarterly mortality data.

In *A*, on the other hand, the number of deaths decreases at O_5 and remains relatively low for subsequent observations. There may well be other explanations for a change in the mortality rate, but the time series design permits us to rule out the possibility that the data reflect unstable measurements of deaths at only two points in time. If we had used a simple pretest–posttest design, it would have been analogous to obtaining the measurements at O_4 and O_5 of Figure 9.3 only. The outcomes in both *A* and *B* are the same at these two time points. The broader time perspective leads us to draw different conclusions about the effects of RRTs. Nevertheless, the absence of a comparison group means that the design does not yield an ideal counterfactual.

Time series designs are often especially important in *quality improvement studies*, because in such efforts randomization is rarely possible, and only one institution is involved in the inquiry.

Example of a Time Series Design: Burston and colleagues (2015) used a time series design to study the effect of a "transforming care" initiative on two patient outcomes—inpatient falls and hospital-acquired pressure ulcers. Patients who were discharged from surgical units of an acute care hospital over a 29-month period comprised the sample.

One drawback of a time series design is that a large number of data points—100 or more—are recommended for a traditional analysis (Shadish et al., 2002), and the analysis tends to be complex. Nurse researchers are, however, beginning to use a little-known but versatile and compelling approach called **statistical process control** to assess effects when they have collected data sequentially over a period of time before and after implementing an intervention or practice change (Polit & Chaboyer, 2012).

A particularly powerful quasi-experimental design results when the time series and nonequivalent control group designs are combined, as diagrammed in Row 5 of Table 9.5. In the example just described, a time series nonequivalent control group design would involve collecting data over an extended period from both the hospital introducing the RRTs and another similar hospital not implementing the system. Information from another comparable hospital would make any inferences

regarding the effects of RRTs more convincing because other external factors influencing the trends would presumably be similar in both cases.

Numerous variations on the simple time series design are possible. For example, additional evidence regarding the effects of a treatment can be achieved by instituting the treatment at several different points in time, strengthening the treatment over time, or instituting the treatment at one point in time and then withdrawing it at a later point, sometimes with reinstitution (diagrammed in the last row of Table 9.5).

A particular application of a time series approach is called **single-subject experiments** (sometimes called *N-of-1 studies*). Single-subject studies use time series designs to gather information about an intervention based on the responses of a single patient (or a small number of patients) under controlled conditions. In the literature on single-subject methods, the most basic design involves a baseline phase of data gathering (A) and an intervention phase (B), yielding what is referred to as an **AB design**. If the treatment is withdrawn, it would be an **ABA design**; and if a withdrawn treatment is reinstituted, it would be an **ABAB design**. Portney and Watkins (2009) and Duan and colleagues (2013) offer guidance about single-subject trials.

Example of a Single-Subject AB Design: Sheehy (2013) used an AB single-subject design to assess a nurse-coached exercise intervention with 10 patients with tetraplegic spinal cord injury. Participants completed three 3-hour sessions per week for more than 6 months. Data were collected multiple times on muscle strength, quality of life, and self-efficacy.

Other Quasi-Experimental Designs

Several other quasi-experimental designs offer alternatives to RCTs. Earlier in this chapter, we described partially randomized patient preference (PRPP). This strategy has advantages in terms of persuading people to participate in a study. Those without a strong preference are randomized, but those *with* a preference are given the condition they prefer and are followed up as part of the study. The two randomized groups are part of the true experiment, but the two groups who get their preference are part of a quasi-experiment. This type of design can yield valuable information about the kind of people who prefer one condition over another. The evidence of the effectiveness of the treatment is weak in the quasi-experimental segment because the people who elected a certain treatment likely differ from those who opted for the alternative— and these preintervention differences, rather than the alternative treatments, could account for any observed differences in outcomes. Yet, evidence from the quasi-experiment could usefully support or qualify evidence from the experimental portion of the study.

Example of a Partially Randomized Patient Preference Design: Coward (2002) used a PRPP design in a pilot study of a support group intervention for women with breast cancer. She found that the majority of women did *not* want to be randomized but rather had a strong preference for either being in or not being in the support group. Her article describes the challenges she faced.

Another quasi-experimental approach—sometimes embedded within a true experiment—is a **dose-response** design in which the outcomes of those receiving different doses of an intervention (not as a result of randomization) are compared. For example, in lengthy interventions, some people attend more sessions or get more intensive treatment than others. The rationale for a quasi-experimental dose-response analysis is that if a larger dose corresponds to better outcomes, the results provide supporting evidence that the treatment caused the outcome. The difficulty, however, is that people tend to get different treatment doses because of differences in motivation, physical function, or other characteristics that could be the true cause of outcome differences. Nevertheless, dose-response evidence may yield useful information, especially when a quasi-experimental dose-response analysis is conducted within an experiment.

Example of a Dose-Response Analysis: Barry and colleagues (2014) used a one-group design to examine the effects of community maternal and newborn family health meetings on the completeness of maternal and newborn care received in the early postnatal period in rural Ethiopia. A dose-response effect was observed between the number of meetings attended and greater completeness of care.

Quasi-Experimental and Comparison Conditions

Researchers using a quasi-experimental approach, like those adopting an experimental design, should strive to develop strong interventions and protocols documenting what the interventions entail. Researchers need to be especially careful in understanding and documenting the counterfactual in quasi-experiments. In the case of nonequivalent control group designs, this means understanding the conditions to which the comparison group is exposed (e.g., activities in the senior center without the yoga intervention in our example). In time series designs, the counterfactual is the conditions existing before implementing the intervention, and these should be understood. Blinding should be used, to the extent possible—indeed, this is often more feasible in a quasi-experiment than in an RCT.

Strengths and Limitations of Quasi-Experiments

A major strength of quasi-experiments is that they are practical. In clinical settings, it may be impossible to conduct true experimental tests of nursing interventions. Strong quasi-experimental designs introduce some research control when full experimental rigor is not possible.

Another advantage of quasi-experiments is that patients are not always willing to relinquish control over their treatment condition. Indeed, it appears that people are increasingly unwilling to volunteer to be randomized in clinical trials (Gross & Fogg, 2001; Vedelø & Lomborg, 2011). Quasi-experimental designs, because they do not involve random assignment, are likely to be acceptable to a broader group of people. This, in turn, has positive implications for the generalizability of the results—but the problem is that the results may be less conclusive.

Researchers using quasi-experimental designs should be cognizant of their weaknesses and should take steps to counteract the weaknesses or take them into account in interpreting results. When a quasi-experimental design is used, there usually are **rival hypotheses** competing with the intervention as explanations for the results. (This issue relates to *internal validity*, discussed further in Chapter 10.) Take as an example the case in which we administer a special diet to frail nursing home residents to assess its effects on weight gain. If we use no comparison group or a nonequivalent control group and then observe a weight gain, we must ask: Is it *plausible* that some other factor caused the gain? Is it *plausible* that pretreatment differences between the intervention and comparison groups resulted in differential gain? Is it *plausible* that the elders on average gained weight simply because the most frail patients died or were hospitalized? If the answer is "yes" to any of these questions, then inferences about the causal effect of the intervention are weakened. The plausibility of any particular rival explanation typically cannot be answered unequivocally. Because the conclusions from quasi-experiments ultimately depend in part on human judgment, rather than on more objective criteria, cause-and-effect inferences are less compelling.

NONEXPERIMENTAL/ OBSERVATIONAL RESEARCH

Many research questions—including ones seeking to establish causal relationships—cannot be addressed with an experimental or quasi-experimental design. For example, at the beginning of this chapter we posed this prognosis question: Do birth weights less than 1,500 grams *cause* developmental delays in children? Clearly, we cannot manipulate birth weight, the independent variable. Babies are born with weights that are neither random nor subject to research control. One way to answer this question is to compare two groups of infants—babies with birth weights above and below 1,500 grams at birth—in terms of their subsequent development. When researchers do not intervene by manipulating the independent variable, the study is **nonexperimental**, or, in the medical literature, **observational**.

Most nursing studies are nonexperimental, mainly because most human characteristics (e.g., birth weight, lactose intolerance) cannot be experimentally manipulated. Also, many variables that could *technically* be manipulated cannot be manipulated ethically. For example, if we were

studying the effect of prenatal care on infant mortality, it would be unethical to provide such care to one group of pregnant women while deliberately depriving a randomly assigned control group. We would need to locate a naturally occurring group of pregnant women who had not received prenatal care. Their birth outcomes could then be compared with those of women who had received appropriate care. The problem, however, is that the two groups of women are likely to differ in terms of many other characteristics, such as age, education, and income, any of which individually or in combination could affect infant mortality, independent of prenatal care. This is precisely why experimental designs are so strong in demonstrating cause-and-effect relationships. Many nonexperimental studies explore causal relationships when experimental work is not possible—although, some observational studies have primarily a descriptive intent.

Correlational Cause-Probing Research

When researchers study the effect of a potential *cause* that they cannot manipulate, they use **correlational designs** to examine relationships between variables. A **correlation** is a relationship or association between two variables, that is, a tendency for variation in one variable to be related to variation in another. For example, in human adults, height and weight are correlated because there is a tendency for taller people to weigh more than shorter people.

As mentioned earlier, one criterion for causality is that an empirical relationship (correlation) between variables must be demonstrated. It is risky, however, to infer causal relationships in correlational research. A famous research dictum is relevant: *Correlation does not prove causation.* The mere existence of a relationship between variables is not enough to warrant the conclusion that one variable caused the other, even if the relationship is strong. In experiments, researchers have direct control over the independent variable; the experimental treatment can be administered to some and withheld from others, and the two groups can be equalized with respect to everything except the independent variable through randomization. In correlational research, on the other hand, investigators do not control the independent variable, which often has already occurred. Groups being compared can differ in ways that affect outcomes of interest—that is, there are usually confounding variables. Although correlational studies are inherently weaker than experimental studies in elucidating causal relationships, different designs offer different degrees of supportive evidence.

Retrospective Designs

Studies with a **retrospective design** are ones in which a phenomenon existing in the present is linked to phenomena that occurred in the past. The signature of a retrospective study is that the researcher begins with the dependent variable (the effect) and then examines whether it is correlated with one or more previously occurring independent variables (potential causes).

Most early studies of the smoking–lung cancer link used a retrospective **case-control design**, in which researchers began with a group of people who had lung cancer (*cases*) and another group who did not (*controls*). The researchers then looked for differences between the two groups in antecedent circumstances or behaviors, such as smoking.

In designing a case-control study, researchers try to identify controls without the disease or condition who are as similar as possible to the cases with regard to key confounding variables (e.g., age, gender). Researchers sometimes use matching or other techniques to control for confounding variables. To the degree that researchers can demonstrate comparability between cases and controls with regard to confounding traits, inferences regarding the presumed cause of the disease are enhanced. The difficulty, however, is that the two groups are almost never totally comparable with respect to all potential factors influencing the outcome.

Example of a Case-Control Design: Hogan (2014) used a case-control design to assess demographic risk factors for infant sleep-related deaths. Infants who died within their first year were the cases, and infants who did not die were the controls.

Not all retrospective studies can be described as using a case-control design. Sometimes researchers use a retrospective approach to identify risk factors for different *amounts* of an outcome rather than

"caseness." For example, a retrospective design might be used to identify factors predictive of the length of time new mothers breastfed their infants. Such a design often is intended to understand factors that *cause* women to make different breastfeeding decisions.

Many retrospective studies are cross-sectional, with data on both the dependent and independent variables collected at a single point in time. In such studies, data for the independent variables often are based on recollection (retrospection)—or the researchers "assume" that the independent variables occurred before the outcome. One problem with retrospection is that recollection is usually less accurate than contemporaneous measurement.

Example of a Retrospective Design: Dang (2014) used cross-sectional data in a retrospective study designed to identify factors predictive of resilience in homeless youth. The independent variables included the youth's level of self-esteem and social connectedness with family, peers, and school.

Prospective Nonexperimental Designs

In correlational studies with a **prospective design** (called a **cohort design** in medical circles), researchers start with a presumed cause and then go forward in time to the presumed effect. For example, in prospective lung cancer studies, researchers start with a cohort of adults (P) that includes smokers (I) and nonsmokers (C) and then later compare the two groups in terms of lung cancer incidence (O). The strongest design for Prognosis questions, and for Etiology questions when randomization is impossible, is a cohort design (Table 9.6).

Prospective studies are more costly than retrospective studies, in part because prospective studies require at least two rounds of data collection. A substantial follow-up period may be needed before the outcome of interest occurs, as is the case in prospective studies of cigarette smoking and lung cancer. Also, prospective designs require large samples if the outcome of interest is rare. Another issue is that in a good prospective study, researchers take steps to confirm that all participants are free from the effect (e.g., the disease) at the time the independent variable is measured, and this may be difficult or expensive to do. For example, in prospective

TABLE 9.6 • Hierarchy of Designs for Different Cause-Probing Research Questions

TYPE OF QUESTION	HIERARCHY OF DESIGNS (MOST TO LEAST RIGOROUS)
Therapy	RCT/experimental > quasi-experimental > cohort > case-control > descriptive correlational
Prognosis	Cohort > case-control > descriptive correlational
Etiology/harm (prevention)	RCT/experimental* > quasi-experimental* > cohort > case-control > descriptive correlational

*Experimental or quasi-experimental designs are not always possible for Etiology questions.

smoking/lung cancer studies, lung cancer may be present initially but not yet diagnosed.

Despite these issues, prospective studies are considerably stronger than retrospective studies. In particular, any ambiguity about whether the presumed cause occurred before the effect is resolved in prospective research if the researcher has confirmed the initial absence of the effect. In addition, samples are more likely to be representative, and investigators may be in a position to impose controls to rule out competing explanations for the results.

TIP: The term "prospective" is not synonymous with "longitudinal." Although most nonexperimental prospective studies *are* longitudinal, prospective studies are not *necessarily* longitudinal. Prospective means that information about a possible cause is obtained prior to information about an effect. RCTs are inherently prospective because the researcher introduces the intervention and then determines its effect. An RCT that collected outcome data 1 hour after an intervention would be prospective but not longitudinal.

Some prospective studies are exploratory. Researchers sometimes measure a wide range of possible "causes" at one point in time and then examine an outcome of interest at a later point (e.g., length of stay in hospital). Such studies are usually stronger than retrospective studies if it can be determined that the outcome was not present initially because time sequences are clear. They are not, however, as powerful as prospective studies that involve specific *a priori* hypotheses and the comparison of cohorts known to differ on a presumed cause. Researchers doing exploratory retrospective or prospective studies are sometimes accused of going on "fishing expeditions" that can lead to erroneous conclusions because of spurious or idiosyncratic relationships in a particular sample of participants.

Example of a Prospective Nonexperimental Study: O'Donovan and colleagues (2014) obtained data from 866 pregnant women in their third trimester (e.g., about their anxiety, birthing expectations, any prior trauma) and used these data to predict who would develop posttraumatic stress disorder 4–6 weeks after childbirth.

Natural Experiments

Researchers are sometimes able to study the outcomes of a **natural experiment** in which a group exposed to a phenomenon with potential health consequences is compared with a nonexposed group. Natural experiments are nonexperimental because the researcher does not intervene, but they are called "natural *experiments*" if people are affected essentially at random. For example, the psychological well-being of people living in a community struck with a natural disaster (e.g., a volcanic eruption) could be compared with the well-being of people living in a similar but unaffected community to assess the toll exacted by the disaster (the independent variable).

Example of a Natural Experiment: Liehr and colleagues (2004) were in the midst of collecting data from healthy students over a 3-day period (September 10-12, 2001) when the events of September 11 unfolded. The researchers seized the opportunity to examine what people go through in the midst of stressful upheaval. Both pre- and post-tragedy data were available for the students' blood pressure, heart rate, and television viewing.

Path Analytic Studies

Researchers interested in testing theories of causation using nonexperimental data often use a technique called **path analysis** (or similar *causal modeling* techniques). Using sophisticated statistical procedures, researchers test a hypothesized causal chain among a set of independent variables, mediating variables, and a dependent variable. Path analytic procedures, described briefly in Chapter 18, allow researchers to test whether nonexperimental data conform sufficiently to the underlying model to justify causal inferences. Path analytic studies can be done within the context of both cross-sectional and longitudinal designs, the latter providing a stronger basis for causal inferences because of the ability to sort out time sequences.

Example of a Path Analytic Study: Chang and Im (2014) tested a causal model to explain older Korean adults' use of the Internet to seek health information. Their path analysis tested hypothesized causal pathways between prior experience with the Internet and their intentions to use it as resource on the one hand and actual information-seeking behavior on the other.

Descriptive Research

A second broad class of nonexperimental studies is **descriptive research**. The purpose of descriptive studies is to observe, describe, and document aspects of a situation as it naturally occurs and sometimes to serve as a starting point for hypothesis generation or theory development.

Descriptive Correlational Studies

Sometimes researchers simply describe relationships rather than infer causal pathways. Many research problems are cast in noncausal terms. We may ask, for example, whether men are less likely than women to seek assistance for depression, not whether a particular configuration of sex chromosomes *caused* differences in health behavior. Unlike other types of correlational research—such as the cigarette smoking and lung cancer investigations—the aim of **descriptive correlational research** is to describe relationships among variables rather than to support inferences of causality.

Example of a Descriptive Correlational Study: Kelly and colleagues (2015) conducted a descriptive correlational study to examine the relationship between the wellness and illness self-management skills of individuals in community corrections programs in the United States and such factors as gender, race, education, and mental health history.

Studies designed to address Diagnosis/assessment questions—that is, whether a tool or procedure yields accurate assessment or diagnostic information about a condition or outcome—typically involve descriptive correlational designs.

Univariate Descriptive Studies

The aim of some descriptive studies is to describe the frequency of occurrence of a behavior or condition rather than to study relationships. **Univariate descriptive studies** are not necessarily focused on a single variable. For example, a researcher might be interested in women's experiences during menopause. The study might describe the frequency of various symptoms, the average age at menopause, and the percentage of women using medications to alleviate symptoms. The study involves multiple variables, but the primary purpose is to describe the status of each and not to relate them to one another.

Two types of descriptive study come from the field of epidemiology. **Prevalence studies** are done to estimate the prevalence rate of some condition (e.g., a disease or a behavior, such as smoking) at a particular point in time. Prevalence studies rely on cross-sectional designs in which data are obtained from the population at risk of the condition. The researcher takes a "snapshot" of the population at risk to determine the extent to which the condition of interest is present. The formula for a **point prevalence rate** (PR) is:

$$\frac{\text{Number of cases with the condition}}{\text{Number in the population at risk}} \times K$$
$$\frac{\text{or disease at a given point in time}}{\text{of being a case}}$$

K is the number of people for whom we want to have the rate established (e.g., per 100 or per 1,000 population). When data are obtained from a sample (as would usually be the case), the denominator is the size of the sample, and the numerator is the number of cases with the condition, as identified in the study. If we sampled 500 adults living in a community, administered a measure of depression, and found that 80 people met the criteria for clinical depression, then the estimated prevalence rate of clinical depression would be 16 per 100 adults in that community.

Incidence studies estimate the frequency of developing *new* cases. Longitudinal designs are needed to estimate incidence because the researcher must first establish who is at risk of becoming a new case—that is, who is free of the condition at the outset. The formula for an **incidence rate (IR)** is:

$$\frac{\text{Number of new cases with the condition or disease over a given time period}}{\text{Number in the population at risk of being a case (free of condition at the outset)}} \times K$$

Continuing with our previous example, suppose in March 2016 we found that 80 in a sample of 500 people were clinically depressed (PR = 16 per 100). To determine the 1-year incidence rate, we would reassess the sample in March 2017. Suppose that, of the 420 previously deemed *not* to be clinically depressed in 2015, 21 were now found to meet the criteria for depression. In this case, the estimated 1-year incidence rate would be 5 per 100 [(21 ÷ 420) × 100 = 5].

Prevalence and incidence rates can be calculated for subgroups of the population (e.g., for men versus women). When this is done, it is possible to calculate another important descriptive index. **Relative risk** is an estimated risk of "caseness" in one group compared with another. Relative risk is computed by dividing the rate for one group by the rate for another. Suppose we found that the 1-year incidence rate for depression was 6 per 100 women and 4 per 100 men. Women's relative risk for developing depression over the 1-year period would be 1.5, that is, women would be estimated to be 1.5 times more likely to develop depression than men. Relative risk (discussed at greater length in Chapter 16) is an important index in assessing the contribution of risk factors to a disease or condition

(e.g., by comparing the relative risk for lung cancer for smokers versus nonsmokers).

Example of a Prevalence Study: Shahin and Lohrmann (2015) used data from nearly 10,000 hospitalized Austrian patients to estimate the prevalence of fecal incontinence and double (fecal and urinary) incontinence in patients with and without urinary catheters.

➜ **TIP:** The quality of studies that test hypothesized causal relationship is heavily dependent on design decisions—that is, how researchers design their studies to rule out competing explanations for the outcomes. Methods of enhancing the rigor of such studies are described in the next chapter. The quality of descriptive studies, by contrast, is more heavily dependent on having a good (representative) sample (Chapter 12).

Strengths and Limitations of Correlational Research

The quality of a study is not necessarily related to its approach; there are many excellent nonexperimental studies as well as flawed experiments. Nevertheless, nonexperimental correlational studies have several drawbacks.

Limitations of Correlational Research

Relative to experimental and quasi-experimental research, nonexperimental studies are weak in their ability to support causal inferences. In correlational studies, researchers work with preexisting groups that were not formed at random but rather through **self-selection** (also known as *selection bias*). A researcher doing a correlational study cannot assume that groups being compared are similar before the occurrence of the independent variable—the hypothesized cause. Preexisting differences may be a plausible alternative explanation for any group differences on the outcome variable.

The difficulty of interpreting correlational findings stems from the fact that, in the real world, behaviors, attitudes, and characteristics are interrelated (correlated) in complex ways. An example may help to clarify the problem. Suppose we conducted a cross-sectional study that examined the relationship between level of depression in cancer patients and their social support (i.e., assistance and emotional support from others). We hypothesize that social support (the independent variable) affects levels of depression (the outcome). Suppose we find that the patients with weak social support are significantly more depressed than patients with strong support. We could interpret this finding to mean that patients' emotional state is influenced by the adequacy of their social supports. This relationship is diagrammed in Figure 9.4A. Yet, there are alternative explanations. Perhaps a third variable influences *both* social support and depression, such as the patients' marital status. It may be that having a spouse is a powerful influence on how depressed cancer patients feel *and* on the quality of their social support. This set of relationships is diagrammed in Figure 9.4B. In this scenario, social support and depression are correlated simply because marital status affects both. A third possibility is reversed causality (Figure 9.4C). Depressed cancer patients may find it more difficult to elicit needed support from others than patients who are more cheerful or amiable. In this interpretation, the person's depression causes the amount of received social support and not the other way around. Thus, interpretations of most correlational results should be considered tentative, particularly if the research has no theoretical basis and if the design is cross-sectional.

Strengths of Correlational Research

Earlier, we discussed constraints that limit the application of experimental designs to many research problems. Correlational research will continue to play a crucial role in nursing research precisely because many interesting problems are not amenable to experimental intervention.

Despite our emphasis on causal inferences, it has already been noted that descriptive correlational research does not focus on understanding causal relationships. Furthermore, if the study is testing a causal hypothesis that has been deduced from an established theory, causal inferences may be possible, especially if strong designs (e.g., a prospective design) are used.

Correlational research is often efficient in that it may involve collecting a large amount of data about a problem. For example, it would be possible to collect extensive information about the health histories and eating habits of a large number of individuals. Researchers could then examine which health problems were associated with which diets, and could thus discover a large number of interrelationships in a relatively short amount of time. By contrast, an experimenter looks at only a few variables at a time. One experiment might manipulate foods high in cholesterol, whereas another might manipulate salt, for example.

Finally, correlational research is often strong in realism. Unlike many experimental studies, correlational research is seldom criticized for its artificiality.

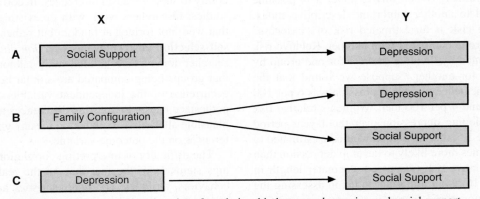

FIGURE 9.4 Alternative explanations for relationship between depression and social support in patients with cancer.

TIP: It can be useful to design a study with several relevant comparisons. In nonexperimental studies, multiple comparison groups can be effective in dealing with self-selection, especially if comparison groups are chosen to address competing biases. For example, in case-control studies of potential causes of lung cancer, cases would be people with lung cancer, one comparison group could be people with a different lung disease, and a second could be those with no lung disorder.

DESIGNS AND RESEARCH EVIDENCE

Evidence for nursing practice depends on descriptive, correlational, and experimental research. There is often a logical progression to knowledge expansion that begins with rich description, including description from qualitative research. Descriptive studies are valuable in documenting the prevalence, nature, and intensity of health-related conditions and behaviors and are critical in the development of effective interventions. Moreover, in-depth qualitative research may suggest causal links that could be the focus of controlled quantitative research. For example, Colón-Emeric and colleagues (2006) did case studies in two nursing homes. They looked at site differences in communication patterns among the medical and nursing staff in relation to differences in information flow. Their findings suggested that a "chain of command" type communication style may limit health care providers' ability to provide high-quality care. The study suggests possibilities for interventions—and indeed, Colón-Emeric and colleagues (2013) have conducted a pilot study of an intervention designed to improve nursing home staff's communication and problem solving. Thus, although qualitative studies are low on the standard evidence hierarchy for *confirming* causal connections (see Figure 2.1), they nevertheless serve an important function—an issue to which we will return in Chapter 27.

Correlational studies also play a role in developing an evidence base for causal inferences. Retrospective case-control studies may pave the way for more rigorous (but more expensive) prospective studies. As the evidence base builds, conceptual models may be developed and tested using path

analytic designs and other theory-testing strategies. These studies can provide hints about how to structure an intervention, who can most profit from it, and when it can best be instituted. Thus, nonexperimental studies can sometimes lead to innovative interventions that can be tested using experimental and quasi-experimental designs.

Many important research questions will never be answered using information from Level I (meta-analyses of RCTs) or Level II studies (RCTs) on the standard evidence hierarchy. An important example is the question of whether smoking causes lung cancer. Despite the inability to randomize people to smoking and nonsmoking groups, few people doubt that this causal connection exists. Thinking about the criteria for causality discussed early in this chapter, there is abundant evidence that smoking cigarettes is correlated with lung cancer and, through prospective studies, that smoking precedes lung cancer. The large number of studies conducted has allowed researchers to control for, and thus rule out, other possible "causes" of lung cancer. There has been a great deal of consistency and coherence in the findings. And, the criterion of biologic plausibility has been met through basic physiologic research.

Thus, it may be best to think of alternative evidence hierarchies for questions relating to causality. For Therapy questions, experimental designs are the "gold standard." On the next rung of the hierarchy for Therapy questions are strong quasi-experimental designs, such as nonequivalent control group pretest–posttest designs. Further down the hierarchy are weaker quasi-experimental designs and then correlational studies. This progression is depicted in Table 9.6, which summarizes a "hierarchy" of designs for answering different types of causal questions, and augments the evidence hierarchy presented in Figure 2.1 (see Chapter 2).

TIP: Studies have shown that evidence from RCTs, quasi-experimental, and observational studies often do not yield the same results. Often the relationship between "causes" and "effects" appears to be stronger in nonexperimental and quasi-experimental studies than in studies in which competing explanations are ruled out through randomization to different conditions.

For questions about Prognosis or about Etiology/harm, both of which concern causal relationships, strong prospective (cohort) studies are usually the best design (although sometimes, Etiology questions can involve randomization). Path analytic studies with longitudinal data and a strong theoretical basis can also be powerful. Retrospective case-control studies are relatively weak, by contrast. Systematic reviews of multiple prospective studies, together with support from theories or biophysiologic research, represent the strongest evidence for these types of question.

CRITIQUING GUIDELINES FOR STUDY DESIGN

The research design used in a quantitative study strongly influences the quality of its evidence and so should be carefully scrutinized. Researchers' design decisions have more of an impact on study quality than any other methodologic decision when the research question is about causal relationships.

Actual designs and some controlling techniques (randomization, blinding, allocation concealment)

BOX 9.1 Guidelines for Critiquing Research Designs in Quantitative Studies

1. What type of question (Therapy, Prognosis, etc.) was being addressed in this study? Does the research question concern a possible causal relationship between the independent and dependent variables?
2. What would be the strongest design for the research question? How does this compare to the design actually used?
3. Was there an intervention or treatment? Was the intervention adequately described? Was the control or comparison condition adequately described? Was an experimental or quasi-experimental design used?
4. If the study was an RCT, what specific design was used? Was this design appropriate, or could a stronger design have been used?
5. In RCTs, what type of randomization was used? Were randomization procedures adequately explained and justified? Was allocation concealment confirmed? Did the report provide evidence that randomization was successful—that is, resulted in groups that were comparable prior to the intervention?
6. If the design was quasi-experimental, what specific quasi-experimental design was used? Was there adequate justification for deciding not to randomize participants to treatment conditions? Did the report provide evidence that any groups being compared were equivalent prior to the intervention?
7. If the design was nonexperimental, was the study inherently nonexperimental? If not, is there adequate justification for not manipulating the independent variable? What specific nonexperimental design was used? If a retrospective design was used, is there good justification for not using a prospective design? What evidence did the report provide that any groups being compared were similar with regard to important confounding characteristics?
8. What types of comparisons were specified in the design (e.g., before–after? between groups?) Did these comparisons adequately illuminate the relationship between the independent and dependent variables? If there were no comparisons, or faulty comparisons, how did this affect the study's integrity and the interpretability of the results?
9. Was the study longitudinal? Was the timing of the collection of data appropriate? Was the number of data collection points reasonable?
10. Was blinding/masking used? If yes, who was blinded—and was this adequate? If not, was there an adequate rationale for failure to mask? Was the intervention a type that could raise expectations that in and of themselves could alter the outcomes?

were described in this chapter, and the next chapter explains in greater detail specific strategies for enhancing research control. The guidelines in Box 9.1 ✖ are the first of two sets of questions to help you in critiquing quantitative research designs.

RESEARCH EXAMPLES

In this section, we present descriptions of an experimental, quasi-experimental, and nonexperimental study.

Research Example of a Randomized Controlled Trial

Study: Clinical effectiveness of collaborative care for depression in UK primary care (CADET): Cluster randomised controlled trial (D. A. Richards et al., 2013)

Statement of Purpose: The purpose of the CADET trial was to assess the effectiveness of a collaborative care intervention for managing moderate to severe depression in primary care patients in the United Kingdom.

Treatment Groups: Collaborative care was delivered by a team of care managers, supervised by mental health specialists. Care managers were expected to have 6 to 12 face-to-face or telephone contacts with their patients over 14 weeks. The care involved antidepressant drug management, behavioral activation, symptom assessment, and communication with the patients' primary care physicians. Care workers, many of whom were nurses, received training specific to their roles. Participants in the control group received care from their physicians according to usual clinical practice.

Method: The study was a cluster randomized trial in which 51 primary care practices in three large metropolitan areas were randomized to either the collaborative care arm (24 practices) or the usual care arm (27 practices). The allocation sequence was concealed from those involved with recruiting the clinical practices. Patients in each practice were considered eligible to participate in the study if they were 18 or older, did not have severe mental health problems, and if their primary presenting problem was not drug or alcohol abuse. At baseline, 276 patients were enrolled in the intervention group and 305 were in the usual care group. The research team members who assessed patients for eligibility and who collected outcome data were blinded to the participants' treatment group status. The primary outcome was individual depression severity, measured at 4 months after baseline, and then again at 12 months. Secondary outcomes included quality of life, anxiety, and patient satisfaction. At the 12-month follow-up, data were obtained from 498 participants (86% retention).

Key Findings: In both groups, participants were predominantly female (72%), white (85%), middle-aged (average age = 45 years), had been prescribed antidepressants (83%), and had a secondary diagnosis of an anxiety disorder (98%). At both the 4-month and 12-month follow-ups, patients in the collaborative care group had significantly lower depression scores than those in the control group. There were no group differences in anxiety levels at either point. Participants in the intervention group were significantly more satisfied with their treatment than those in the control group.

Research Example of a Quasi-Experimental Study

Study: A study to promote breast feeding in the Helsinki Metropolitan area in Finland (Hannula et al., 2014)

Statement of Purpose: The purpose of the study was to test the effect of providing intensified support for breastfeeding during the perinatal period on the breastfeeding behavior of women in Finland.

Treatment Groups: The women in the intervention group were offered a free, noncommercial web-based service that provided intensified support for parenthood, child care, and breastfeeding from the 20th gestation week until the child was 1 year old. They were cared for by staff with specialized training who also provided individualized support. Women in the comparison group received usual care from midwifery and nursing professionals.

Method: The study was conducted in three public maternity hospitals in Helsinki. Two of the hospitals implemented the intensified support services, and the third hospital served as the control. Women who were 18–21 weeks gestation were recruited into the study if they were expecting a singleton birth. Altogether, 705 women participated in the study, 431 in the intervention group and 274 in the comparison group. Study participants completed questionnaires at baseline and at follow-up (at discharge or shortly afterward). The outcomes in the study were whether or not the mother breastfed exclusively in the hospital and scores on several scales measuring breastfeeding confidence, breastfeeding attitudes, and coping with breastfeeding.

Key Findings: The intervention and comparison group members were similar demographically in some respects (e.g., education, marital status), but several pre-intervention group differences were found. For example, patients in the intervention group were more likely to be primiparas and more likely to have participated in parenting education than women in the comparison group. To address this selection bias problem, these characteristics were controlled statistically, an approach discussed in the next chapter. Women in the intervention group were significantly more likely to breastfeed exclusively at the time of the follow-up (76%) than those in the comparison group (66%). The authors concluded that intensive support helped the mothers to breastfeed exclusively.

Research Example of a Correlational Study

Study: Factors associated with toileting disability in older adults without dementia living in residential care facilities (Talley et al., 2014)

Statement of Purpose: The purpose of the study was to estimate the prevalence of toileting disabilities in a population of older adults living in residential care facilities and to identify factors associated with such disabilities.

Method: Cross-sectional data from a previously conducted national survey of residents in residential care facilities in the United States were used in this study. The survey sample included 8,094 residents living in over 2,000 facilities. For this study, Talley and colleagues selected a subsample of 2,395 older adults (age 65+) without dementia. A resident was considered to have a toileting disability if he or she received any assistance using the bathroom. The data set for this retrospective study including numerous variables that were considered possible predictors of a toileting disability, such as demographic variables (age, gender, marital status), overall health status, pathologies (e.g., arthritis, heart disease), functional limitations (e.g., dressing), functional impairments (e.g., walking), and coexisting disability (activities of

daily living). Characteristics of the facility were also considered in the analysis (e.g., number of beds).

Key Findings: The prevalence of toileting disability in this population was 15%. The prevalence was higher among those resident reporting fair or poor health, those living in a for-profit facility, those having bowel and urinary incontinence, those with more physical impairments, and those with visual or hearing impairments.

SUMMARY POINTS

- Many quantitative nursing studies aim to elucidate *cause-and-effect relationships*. The challenge of research design is to facilitate inferences about causality.
- One criterion for causality is that the cause must precede the effect. Another is that a relationship between a presumed cause (independent variable) and an effect (dependent variable) cannot be explained as being caused by other (confounding) variables.
- In an idealized model, a **counterfactual** is what would have happened to the same people simultaneously exposed *and* not exposed to a causal factor. The *effect* is the difference between the two. The goal of research design is to find a good approximation to the idealized (but impossible) counterfactual.
- **Experiments** (or **randomized controlled trials, RCTs**) involve **manipulation** (the researcher manipulates the independent variable by introducing a **treatment** or **intervention**), control (including use of a **control group** that is not given the intervention and represents the comparative counterfactual), and **randomization** or **random assignment** (with people allocated to experimental and control groups at random so that they are equivalent at the outset).
- Subjects in the experimental group usually get the same intervention, as delineated in formal protocols, but some studies involve **patient-centered interventions (PCIs)** that are tailored to meet individual needs or characteristics.
- Researchers can expose the control group to various conditions, including no treatment, an alternative treatment, standard treatment

("usual care"), a **placebo** or pseudointervention, different doses of the treatment, or a *delayed treatment* (for a **wait-list** group).

- Random assignment is done by methods that give every participant an equal chance of being in any group, such as by flipping a coin or using a **table of random numbers**. Randomization is the most reliable method for equating groups on all characteristics that could affect study outcomes. Randomization should involve **allocation concealment** that prevents foreknowledge of upcoming assignments.
- Several variants to simple randomization exist, such as **permuted block randomization**, in which randomization is done for blocks of people—for example, six or eight at a time, in randomly selected block sizes.
- **Blinding** (or **masking**) is often used to avoid biases stemming from participants' or research agents' awareness of group status or study hypotheses. In **double-blind studies**, two groups (e.g., participants and investigators) are blinded.
- Many specific experimental designs exist. A **posttest-only (after-only) design** involves collecting data after an intervention only. In a **pretest–posttest (before–after) design**, data are collected both before and after the intervention, permitting an analysis of change.
- **Factorial designs**, in which two or more independent variables are manipulated simultaneously, allow researchers to test both **main effects** (effects from manipulated independent variables) and **interaction effects** (effects from combining treatments).
- In a **crossover design**, subjects are exposed to more than one condition, administered in a randomized order, and thus, they serve as their own controls.
- Experimental designs are the "gold standard" because they come closer than any other design in meeting criteria for inferring causal relationships.
- **Quasi-experimental designs** (*trials without randomization*) involve an intervention but lack randomization. Strong quasi-experimental designs include features to support causal inferences.
- The **nonequivalent control group pretest–posttest design** involves using a nonrandomized

comparison group and the collection of pretreatment data so that initial group equivalence can be assessed. Comparability of groups can sometimes be enhanced through *matching* on individual characteristics or by using **propensity matching**, which involves matching on a **propensity score** for each participant.
- In a **time series design**, information on the dependent variable is collected over a period of time before and after the intervention. Time series designs are often used in **single-subject (N-of-1) experiments**.
- Other quasi-experimental designs include quasi-experimental **dose-response analyses** and the quasi-experimental (nonrandomized) **arms** of a **partially randomized patient preference** (**PRPP**) randomization design (i.e., groups with strong preferences).
- In evaluating the results of quasi-experiments, it is important to ask whether it is plausible that factors other than the intervention caused or affected the outcomes (i.e., whether there are credible **rival hypotheses** for explaining the results).
- **Nonexperimental** (or **observational**) **research** includes **descriptive research**—studies that summarize the status of phenomena—and **correlational** studies that examine relationships among variables but involve no manipulation of independent variables (often because they *cannot* be manipulated).
- Designs for correlational studies include **retrospective (case-control) designs** (which look back in time for antecedent causes of "caseness" by comparing **cases** that have a disease or condition with controls who do not), **prospective (cohort) designs** (studies that begin with a presumed cause and look forward in time for its effect), **natural experiments** (in which a group is affected by a random event, such as a disaster), and **path analytic studies** (which test causal models developed on the basis of theory).
- **Descriptive correlational studies** describe how phenomena are interrelated without invoking a causal explanation. **Univariate descriptive studies** examine the frequency or average value of variables.

- Descriptive studies include **prevalence studies** that document the prevalence rate of a condition at one point in time and **incidence studies** that document the frequency of *new* cases, over a given time period. When the incidence rates for two groups are estimated, researchers can compute the **relative risk** of "caseness" for the two.
- The primary weakness of correlational studies for cause-probing questions is that they can harbor biases, such as **self-selection** into groups being compared.

STUDY ACTIVITIES

Chapter 9 of the *Resource Manual for Nursing Research: Generating and Assessing Evidence for Nursing Practice, 10th edition*, offers study suggestions for reinforcing concepts presented in this chapter. In addition, the following questions can be addressed in classroom or online discussions:

1. Assume that you have 10 people—Z, Y, X, W, V, U, T, S, R, and Q—who are going to participate in an RCT you are conducting. Using a table of random numbers, assign five individuals to group 1 and five to group 2.
2. Insofar as possible, use the questions in Box 9.1 to critique the three research examples described at the end of the chapter.
3. Discuss how you would design a prospective study to address the question posed in the Talley et al. (2014) retrospective study summarized at the end of the chapter.

STUDIES CITED IN CHAPTER 9

Barkauskas, V. H., Lusk, S. L., & Eakin, B. L. (2005). Selecting control interventions for clinical outcome studies. *Western Journal of Nursing Research*, 27, 346–363.

Barry, D., Frew, A., Mohammed, H., Desta, B., Tadesse, L., Aklilu, Y., . . . Sibley, L. (2014). The effect of community maternal and newborn health family meetings on type of birth attendant and completeness of maternal and newborn care received during birth and the early postnatal period in rural Ethiopia. *Journal of Midwifery & Women's Health*, 59, S44–S54.

*Beck, C., McSweeney, J., Richards, K., Robertson, P., Tsai, P., & Souder, E. (2010). Challenges in tailored intervention research. *Nursing Outlook*, 58, 104–110.

Bradford-Hill, A. (1971). *Principles of medical statistics* (9th ed.). New York: Oxford University Press.

Burston, S., Chaboyer, W., Gillespie, B., & Carroll, R. (2015). The effect of a transforming care initiative on patient outcomes in acute surgical units: A time series study. *Journal of Advanced Nursing*, 71, 417–429.

Campbell, D. T., & Stanley, J. C. (1963). *Experimental and quasi-experimental designs for research*. Chicago: Rand McNally.

Chang, S. J., & Im, E. O. (2014). A path analysis of Internet health information seeking behaviors among older adults. *Geriatric Nursing*, 35, 137–141.

*Colón-Emeric, C., Ammarell, N., Bailey, D., Corazzini, K., Lekan-Rutledge, D., Piven, M., . . . Anderson, R. A. (2006). Patterns of medical and nursing staff communication in nursing homes. *Qualitative Health Research*, 16, 173–188.

*Colón-Emeric, C., McConnell, E., Pinheiro, S., Corazzini, K., Porter, K., Earp, K., . . . Anderson, R. A. (2013). CONNECT for better fall prevention in nursing homes: Results from a pilot intervention study. *Journal of the American Geriatrics Society*, 61, 2150–2159.

Coward, D. (2002). Partial randomization design in a support group intervention study. *Western Journal of Nursing Research*, 24, 406–421.

Cutler, L. R., & Sluman, P. (2014). Reducing ventilator associated pneumonia in adult patients through high standards of oral care: A historical control study. *Intensive & Critical Care Nursing*, 30, 61–68.

Dang, M. T. (2014). Social connectedness and self-esteem: Predictors of resilience in mental health among maltreated homeless youth. *Issues in Mental Health Nursing*, 35, 212–219.

Doig, G., & Simpson, F. (2005). Randomization and allocation concealment: A practical guide for researchers. *Journal of Critical Care*, 20, 187–191.

Downs, M., Tucker, K., Christ-Schmidt, H., & Wittes, J. (2010). Some practical problems in implementing randomization. *Clinical Trials*, 7, 235–245.

Duan, N., Kravitz, R., & Schmid, C. (2013). Single-patient (n-of-1) trials: A pragmatic clinical decision methodology for patient-centered comparative effectiveness research. *Journal of Clinical Epidemiology*, 66, S21–S28.

Gross, D. (2005). On the merits of attention control groups. *Research in Nursing & Health*, 28, 93–94.

Gross, D., & Fogg, L. (2001). Clinical trials in the 21st century: The case for participant-centered research. *Research in Nursing & Health*, 24, 530–539.

Hannula, L. S., Kaunonen, M., & Puukka, P. (2014). A study to promote breast feeding in the Helsinki Metropolitan area in Finland. *Midwifery*, 30, 696–704.

Herbison, P., Hay-Smith, J., & Gillespie, W. (2011). Different methods of allocation to groups in randomized trials are associated with different levels of bias. A meta-epidemiological study. *Journal of Clinical Epidemiology*, 64, 1070–1075.

Hodge, N. S., McCarthy, M., & Pierce, R. (2014). A prospective randomized study of the effectiveness of aromatherapy for relief of postoperative nausea and vomiting. *Journal of Perianesthesia Nursing, 29,* 5–11.

Hogan, C. (2014). Socioeconomic factors affecting infant sleep-related deaths in St. Louis. *Public Health Nursing, 31,* 10–18.

Jenerette, C., Brewer, C., Edwards, L., Mishel, M., & Gil, K. (2014). An intervention to decrease stigma in young adults with sickle cell disease. *Western Journal of Nursing Research, 36,* 599–619.

Kelly, P. J., Ramaswamy, M., Chen, H., & Denny, D. (2015). Wellness and illness self-management skills in community corrections. *Issues in Mental Health Nursing, 36,* 89–95.

Kundu, A., Lin, Y., Oron, A., & Doorenbos, A. (2014). Reiki therapy for postoperative oral pain in pediatric patients: Pilot data from a double-blind, randomized clinical trial. *Complementary Therapies in Clinical Practice, 20,* 21–25.

Lachin, J. M., Matts, J., & Wei, L. (1988). Randomization in clinical trials: Conclusions and recommendations. *Controlled Clinical Trials, 9,* 365–374.

Lauver, D. R., Ward, S. E., Heidrich, S. M., Keller, M. L., Bowers, B. J., Brennan, P. F., . . . Wells, T. J. (2002). Patient-centered interventions. *Research in Nursing & Health, 25,* 246–255.

Lazarsfeld, P. (1955). Foreword. In H. Hyman (Ed.), *Survey design and analysis.* New York: The Free Press.

Lee, N., Webster, J., Beckmann, M., Gibbons, K., Smith, T., Stapleton, H., & Kildea, S. (2013). Comparison of a single vs. a four intradermal sterile water injection for relief of lower back pain for women in labour: A randomized controlled trial. *Midwifery, 29,* 585–591.

Liehr, P., Mehl, M., Summers, L., & Pennebaker, J. (2004). Connecting with others in the midst of stressful upheaval on September 11, 2001. *Applied Nursing Research, 17,* 2–9.

Lippoldt, J., Pernicka, E., & Staudinger, T. (2014). Interface pressure at different degrees of backrest elevation with various types of pressure-redistribution surfaces. *American Journal of Critical Care, 23,* 119–126.

McGuire, D., DeLoney, V., Yeager, K., Owen, D., Peterson, D., Lin, L., & Webster, J. (2000). Maintaining study validity in a changing clinical environment. *Nursing Research, 49,* 231–235.

*Moher, D., Hopewell, S., Schulz, K. F., Montori, V., Gøtzsche, P., Devereaux, P., . . . Altman D. G. (2010). CONSORT 2010 explanation and elaboration: Updated guidelines for reporting parallel group randomised trials. *British Medical Journal, 340,* c869.

Mosleh, S., Bond, C., Lee, A., Kiger, A., & Campbell, N. (2014). Effectiveness of theory-based invitations to improve attendance at cardiac rehabilitation: A randomized controlled trial. *European Journal of Cardiovascular Nursing, 13,* 201–210.

O'Donovan, A., Alcorn, K., Patrick, J., Creedy, D., Dawe, S., & Devilly, G. (2014). Predicting posttraumatic stress disorder after childbirth. *Midwifery, 30,* 935–941.

Padhye, N., Cron, S., Gusick, G., Hamlin, S., & Hanneman, S. (2009). Randomization for clinical research: An easy-to-use spreadsheet method. *Research in Nursing & Health, 32,* 561–566.

Polit, D. F., & Chaboyer, W. (2012). Statistical process control in nursing research. *Research in Nursing & Health, 35,* 82–93.

Polit, D., Gillespie, B., & Griffin, R. (2011). Deliberate ignorance: A systematic review of blinding in nursing clinical trials. *Nursing Research, 61,* 9–16.

Portney, L. G., & Watkins, M. (2009). *Foundations of clinical research: Applications to practice* (3rd ed.). Upper Saddle River, NJ: Prentice-Hall Health.

*Qin, R., Titler, M., Shever, L., & Kim, T. (2008). Estimating effects of nursing intervention via propensity score analysis. *Nursing Research, 57,* 444–452.

*Richards, D. A., Hill, J., Gask, L., Lovell, K., Chew-Graham, C., Bower, P., . . . Barkham, M. (2013). Clinical effectiveness of collaborative care for depression in UK primary care (CADET): Cluster randomised controlled trial. *British Medical Journal, 347,* f4913.

Richards, K., Enderlin, C., Beck, C., McSweeney, J., Jones, T., & Roberson, P. (2007). Tailored biobehavioral interventions: A literature review and synthesis. *Research and Theory for Nursing Practice, 21,* 271–285.

Schulz, K. F., Chalmers, I., & Altman, D. G. (2002). The landscape and lexicon of blinding in randomized trials. *Annals of Internal Medicine, 136,* 254–259.

Shadish, W. R., Cook, T. D., & Campbell, D. T. (2002). *Experimental and quasi-experimental designs for generalized causal inference.* Boston: Houghton Mifflin.

Shahin, E., & Lohrmann, C. (2015). Prevalence of fecal and double fecal and urinary incontinence in hospitalized patients. *Journal of Wound, Ostomy, & Continence Nursing, 42,* 89–93.

Sheehy, S. B. (2013). A nurse-coached exercise program to increase muscle strength, improve quality of life, and increase self-efficacy in people with tetraplegic spinal cord injuries. *Journal of Neuroscience Nursing, 45,* E3–E12.

Silverman, M. J. (2013). Effects of music therapy on self- and experienced stigma in patients on an acute care psychiatric unit: A randomized three-group effectiveness study. *Archives of Psychiatric Nursing, 27,* 223–230.

Talley, K., Wyman, J., Bronas, U., Olson-Kellogg, B., McCarthy, T., & Zhao, H. (2014). Factors associated with toileting disability in older adults without dementia living in residential care facilities. *Nursing Research, 63,* 94–104.

Vedelø, T. W., & Lomborg, K. (2011). Reported challenges in nurse-led randomised controlled trials: An integrative review of the literature. *Scandinavian Journal of the Caring Sciences, 25,* 194–200.

*Vickers, A. J. (2006). How to randomize. *Journal of the Society for Integrative Oncology, 4,* 194–198.

Wang, T. J., Lan, L. C., Lu, C., Lin, K., Tung, H., Wu, S., & Liang, S. (2014). Efficacy of narrowband ultraviolet phototherapy on renal pruritus. *Journal of Clinical Nursing, 23,* 1593–1602.

Zhu, L., Ho, S., Sit, J., & He, H. (2014). The effects of a transtheoretical model-based exercise stage-matched intervention on exercise behavior in patients with coronary heart disease: A randomized controlled trial. *Patient Education and Counseling, 95,* 384–392.

***A link to this open-access journal article is provided in the Toolkit for this chapter in the accompanying Resource Manual.** ⊗

10 | Rigor and Validity in Quantitative Research

VALIDITY AND INFERENCE

This chapter describes strategies for enhancing the rigor of quantitative studies, including ways to minimize biases and control confounding variables. Many of these strategies help to strengthen the inferences that can be made about cause-and-effect relationships.

Validity and Validity Threats

In designing a study, it is useful to anticipate the factors that could undermine the **validity** of inferences. Shadish and colleagues (2002) define validity in the context of research design as "the approximate truth of an inference" (p. 34). For example, inferences that an *effect* results from a hypothesized *cause* are valid to the extent that researchers can marshal strong supporting evidence. Validity is always a matter of degree, not an absolute.

Validity is a property of an inference, not of a research design, but design elements profoundly affect the inferences that can be made. **Threats to validity** are reasons that an inference could be wrong. When researchers introduce design features to minimize potential threats, the validity of the inference is strengthened, and thus, evidence is more persuasive.

Types of Validity

Shadish and colleagues (2002) proposed a taxonomy that identified four aspects of validity, and

catalogued dozens of validity threats. This chapter describes the taxonomy and summarizes major threats, but we urge researchers to consult this seminal work for further guidance.

The first type of validity, **statistical conclusion validity**, concerns the validity of inferences that there truly is an empirical relationship, or correlation, between the presumed cause and the effect. The researcher's job is to provide the strongest possible evidence that an observed relationship is *real*.

Internal validity concerns the validity of inferences that, given that an empirical relationship exists, it is the independent variable, rather than something else, that caused the outcome. Researchers must develop strategies to rule out the plausibility that some factor other than the independent variable accounts for the observed relationship.

Construct validity involves the validity of inferences "from the observed persons, settings, and cause and effect operations included in the study to the constructs that these instances might represent" (p. 38). One aspect of construct validity concerns the degree to which an intervention is a good representation of the underlying construct that was theorized as having the potential to cause beneficial outcomes. Another concerns whether the measures of the dependent variable are good operationalizations of the constructs for which they are intended.

External validity concerns whether inferences about observed relationships will hold over variations in persons, setting, time, or measures of the outcomes. External validity, then, is about the generalizability of causal inferences, and this is a critical concern for research that aims to yield evidence for evidence-based nursing practice.

These four types of validity and their associated threats are discussed in this chapter. Many validity threats concern inadequate control over confounding variables and so we briefly review methods of controlling confounders associated with participants' characteristics.

Controlling Confounding Participant Characteristics

This section describes six ways of controlling participant characteristics—characteristics that could compete with the independent variable as the cause of an outcome.

Randomization

As noted in Chapter 9, randomization is the most effective method of controlling individual characteristics. The function of randomization is to secure comparable groups—that is, to equalize groups with respect to confounding variables. A distinct advantage of random assignment, compared with other strategies, is that it can control *all* possible sources of confounding variation, *without any conscious decision about which variables need to be controlled.*

Crossover

Randomization within a crossover design is an especially powerful method of ensuring equivalence between groups being compared—participants serve as their own controls. Moreover, fewer participants usually are needed in such a design. Fifty people exposed to two treatments in random order yield 100 pieces of data (50 × 2); 50 people randomly assigned to two different groups yield only 50 pieces of data (25 × 2). Crossover designs are not appropriate for all studies, however, because of possible carryover effects: People exposed to two different conditions may be influenced in the second condition by their experience in the first.

Homogeneity

When randomization and crossover are not feasible, alternative methods of controlling confounding characteristics are needed. One method is to use only people who are homogeneous with respect to confounding variables—that is, confounding traits are not allowed to vary. Suppose we were testing the effectiveness of a physical fitness program on the cardiovascular functioning of elders. Our quasi-experimental design involves elders from two different nursing homes, with elders in one of them receiving the physical fitness intervention. If gender were an important confounding variable (and if the two nursing homes had different proportions of men and women), we could control gender by using only men (or only women) as participants.

The price of homogeneity is that research findings cannot be generalized to types of people who did not participate in the study. If the physical fitness intervention were found to have beneficial effects on the cardiovascular status of a sample of women 65 to 75 years of age, its usefulness for improving the cardiovascular status of men in their 80s would require a separate study. Indeed, one criticism of this approach is that researchers sometimes exclude people who are extremely ill, which means that the findings cannot be generalized to those who may be most in need of interventions.

Example of Control through Homogeneity: Bowles and co-researchers (2014) used a quasi-experimental design to examine the effect of a discharge planning decision support on time to readmission among older adult medical patients. Several variables were controlled through homogeneity, including age (all 55 or older), language (all spoke English), condition (none was on dialysis), and admission (none were in hospice or were admitted from an institution).

➲ TIP: The principle of homogeneity is often used to control (hold constant) external factors known to influence outcomes. For example, it may be important to collect outcome data at the same time of the day for all participants if time could affect the outcome (e.g., fatigue). As another example, it may be desirable to maintain **constancy of conditions** in terms of locale of data collection—for example, interviewing all respondents in their own homes rather than some in their places of work. In each setting, participants assume different roles (e.g., spouse and parent versus employee), and their responses to questions may be influenced to some degree by those roles.

Stratification/Blocking

Another approach to controlling confounders is to include them in the research design through stratification. To pursue our example of the physical fitness intervention with gender as the confounding variable, we could use a *randomized block design* in which men and women are assigned separately to treatment groups. This approach can enhance the likelihood of detecting differences between our experimental and control groups because the effect of the blocking variable (gender) on the outcome is eliminated. In addition, if the blocking variable is of interest substantively, researchers have the opportunity to study differences in groups created by the stratifying variable (e.g., men versus women).

Matching

Matching (also called **pair matching**) involves using information about people's characteristics to create comparable groups. If matching were used in our physical fitness example, and age and gender were the confounding variables, we would match a person in the intervention group with one in the comparison group with respect to age and gender. As noted in Chapter 9, matching is often problematic. To use matching, researchers must know the relevant confounders in advance. Also, it is difficult to match on more than two or three variables (unless propensity score matching is used), but typically many confounders can affect key outcomes. Thus, matching as the primary control technique should be used only when other, more powerful procedures are not feasible, as might be the case in some correlational studies (e.g., case-control designs).

Sometimes, as an alternative to pair matching, researchers use a *balanced design* with regard to key confounders. In such situations, researchers attempt only to ensure that the groups being compared have similar proportional representation on confounding variables rather than matching on a one-to-one basis. For example, if gender and age were the two variables of concern, we would strive to ensure that the same percentage of men and women were in the two groups and that the average age was comparable. Such an approach is less cumbersome than pair matching but has similar limitations. Nevertheless, both pair matching and balancing are preferable to failing to control participant characteristics at all.

Example of Control through Matching: Lee and colleagues (2014) studied whether the use of morphine treatment for patients with cancer is associated with increased risk of acute coronary syndrome (ACS). The researchers used a case-control design with subjects drawn from a very large database in Taiwan. All 499 patients who subsequently developed ACS were matched, in a 3:1 ratio, with patients who did not. Matching was done on the basis of age, sex, and year of cancer diagnosis.

Statistical Control

Another method of controlling confounding variables is through statistical analysis rather than research design. A detailed description of powerful **statistical control** mechanisms will be postponed until Chapter 18, but we will explain underlying principles with a simple illustration of a procedure called **analysis of covariance (ANCOVA)**.

In our physical fitness example, suppose we used a nonequivalent control group design with elders from two nursing homes, and resting heart rate was an outcome. We would expect individual differences in heart rate in the sample—that is, it would vary from one person to the next. The research question is, Can some of the individual differences in heart rate be attributed to program participation? We know that differences in heart rate are also related to other traits, such as age. In Figure 10.1, the large circles represent the total amount of individual variation for resting heart rate. A certain amount of variation can be explained by a person's age, depicted as the small circle on the left in Figure 10.1A. Another part of the variability may be explained by participation or nonparticipation in the program, represented as the small circle on the right. The two small circles (age and program participation) overlap, indicating a relationship between the two. In other words, people in the physical fitness group are, on average, either older

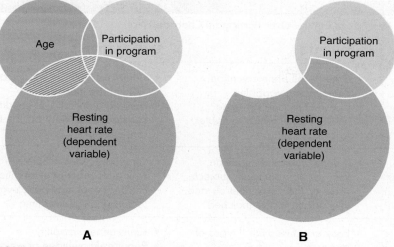

FIGURE 10.1 Schematic diagram illustrating the principle of analysis of covariance.

or younger than those in the comparison group, and so age should be controlled. Otherwise, we could not determine whether postintervention differences in resting heart rate are attributable to differences in age or program participation.

Analysis of covariance controls by statistically removing the effect of confounding variables on the outcome. In the illustration, the portion of heart rate variability attributable to age (the hatched area of the large circle in A) is removed through ANCOVA. Figure 10.1B shows that the final analysis assesses the effect of program participation on heart rate *after removing the effect of age.* By controlling heart rate variability resulting from age, we get a more accurate estimate of the effect of the program on heart rate. Note that even after removing variability due to age, there is still individual variation not associated with the program treatment—the bottom half of the large circle in B. This means that the study can probably be improved by controlling additional confounders, such as gender, smoking history, and so on. ANCOVA and other sophisticated procedures can control multiple confounding variables.

Example of Statistical Control: Chen and colleagues (2015) tested the effectiveness of a 6-month elastic band exercise program for older Taiwanese adults using wheelchairs in nursing homes.

In this cluster randomized trial, five nursing homes participated in the intervention, and five did not. The researchers compared physical fitness, lung capacity, and body flexibility of those in the intervention and control groups, statistically controlling for baseline values.

⊜ TIP: Confounding participant characteristics that need to be controlled vary from one study to another, but we can offer some guidance. The best variable is the outcome variable itself, measured before the independent variable occurs. In our physical fitness example, controlling preprogram measures of cardiovascular functioning through ANCOVA would be a good choice. Major demographic variables (e.g., age, race/ethnicity, education) and health indicators are usually good candidates to control. Confounding variables that need to be controlled—variables that correlate with the outcomes—should be identified through a literature review.

Evaluation of Control Methods

Table 10.1 summarizes benefits and drawbacks of the six control mechanisms. Randomization is the most effective method of managing confounding variables—that is, of approximating the ideal but unattainable counterfactual discussed in

TABLE 10.1 • Methods of Control Over Participant Characteristics

METHOD	BENEFITS	LIMITATIONS
Randomization	• Controls all preintervention confounding variables • Does not require advance knowledge of which variables to control	• Constraints (ethical, practical) on variables that can be manipulated. • Possible artificiality of conditions • Resistance by many people to being randomized
Crossover	• If done with randomization, very strong approach: subjects serve as their own controls and thus are perfectly "matched"	• Cannot be used if there are possible carry-over effect from one condition to the next • History threat may be relevant if external factors change over time
Homogeneity	• Easy to achieve in all types of research • Could enhance interpretability of relationships	• Limits generalizability • Requires knowledge of which variables to control • Range restriction could lower statistical conclusion validity
Stratification	• Enhances the ability to detect and interpret relationships • Offers opportunity to examine blocking variable as an independent variable	• Usually restricted to a few stratifying variables • Requires knowledge of which variables to control
Matching	• Enhances ability to detect and interpret relationships • May be easy if there is a large "pool" of potential available comparison subjects	• Usually restricted to a few matching variables (except with propensity matching) • Requires knowledge of which variables to match • May be difficult to find comparison group matches, especially if there are more than two matching variables
Statistical control	• Enhances ability to detect and interpret relationships • Relatively economical means of controlling several confounding variables	• Requires knowledge of which variables to control as well as measurement of those variables • Requires some statistical sophistication

Chapter 9—because it tends to cancel out individual differences on all possible confounders. Crossover designs are a useful supplement to randomization but are not always appropriate. The remaining alternatives have a common disadvantage: Researchers must know in advance the relevant confounding variables. To select homogeneous samples, stratify, match, or perform ANCOVA, researchers must know which variables need to be measured and controlled. Yet, when randomization is impossible, the use of any of these strategies is better than no control strategy at all.

STATISTICAL CONCLUSION VALIDITY

As noted in Chapter 9, one criterion for establishing causality is demonstrating that there is a relationship between the independent and dependent variable. Statistical methods are used to support inferences about whether relationships exist. Researchers can make design decisions that protect against reaching false statistical conclusions. Even for research that is not cause-probing, researchers need to attend to statistical conclusion validity: The issue is whether relationships that really exist can be reliably detected. Shadish and colleagues (2002) discussed nine threats to statistical conclusion validity. We focus here on three especially important threats.

Low Statistical Power

Statistical power refers to the ability to detect true relationships among variables. Adequate statistical power can be achieved in various ways, the most straightforward of which is to use a sufficiently large sample. When small samples are used, statistical power tends to be low, and the analyses may fail to show that the independent and dependent variables are related—*even when they are*. Power and sample size are discussed in Chapters 12 and 17.

Another aspect of a powerful design concerns how the independent variable is defined. Both statistically and substantively, results are clearer when differences between groups being compared are large. Researchers should aim to maximize group differences on the dependent variables by maximizing differences on the independent variable. Conn and colleagues (2001) offered good suggestions for enhancing the power and effectiveness of nursing interventions. Strengthening group differences is usually easier in experimental than in nonexperimental research. In experiments, investigators can devise treatment conditions that are as distinct as money, ethics, and practicality permit.

Another aspect of statistical power concerns maximizing **precision**, which is achieved through accurate measuring tools, controls over confounding variables, and powerful statistical methods. Precision can best be explained through an example. Suppose we were studying the effect of admission into a nursing home on depression by comparing elders who were or were not admitted. Depression varies from one elderly person to another for various reasons. We want to isolate—as precisely as possible—the portion of variation in depression attributable to nursing home admission. Mechanisms of research control that reduce variability from confounding factors can be built into the research design, thereby enhancing precision. The following ratio expresses what we wish to assess in this example:

$$\frac{\text{Variability in depression}}{\text{Variability in depression due to other factors}}$$
$$\text{(e.g., age, pain, medical condition)}$$

This ratio, greatly simplified here, captures the essence of many statistical tests. We want to make variability in the numerator (the upper half) as large as possible relative to variability in the denominator (the lower half), to evaluate precisely the relationship between nursing home admission and depression. The smaller the variability in depression due to confounding variables (e.g., age, pain), the easier it will be to detect differences in depression between elders who were or were not admitted to a nursing home. Designs that enable researchers to reduce variability caused by confounders can increase statistical conclusion validity. As a purely hypothetical illustration, we will attach some numeric values* to the ratio as follows:

$$\frac{\text{Variability due to nursing home admission}}{\text{Variability due to all confounding variables}} = \frac{10}{4}$$

If we can make the bottom number smaller, say by changing it from 4 to 2, we will have a more precise estimate of the effect of nursing home admission on depression, relative to other influences. Control mechanisms such as those described earlier help to reduce variability caused by extraneous variables and should be considered as design options in planning a study. We illustrate this by continuing our example, singling out age as a key

---

*You should not be concerned with how these numbers can be obtained. Analytic procedures are explained in Chapter 17.

confounding variable. Total variability in levels of depression can be conceptualized as having the following components:

$$\text{Total variability in depression} = \text{Variability due to nursing home admission} + \text{Variability due to age} + \text{Variability due to other confounding variables}$$

This equation can be taken to mean that part of the reason why elders differ in depression is that some were admitted to a nursing home and others were not; some were older and some were younger; and other factors, such as level of pain and medical condition also had an effect on depression.

One way to increase precision in this study would be to control age, thereby removing the variability in depression that results from age differences. We could do this, for example, by restricting age to elders younger than 80, thereby reducing the variability in depression due to age. As a result, the effect of nursing home admission on depression becomes greater, relative to the remaining variability. Thus, this design decision (homogeneity) enabled us to get a more precise estimate of the effect of nursing home admission on level of depression (although, of course, this limits generalizability). Research designs differ in the sensitivity with which effects under study can be detected statistically. Lipsey (1990) has prepared a good guide to enhancing the sensitivity of research designs.

Restriction of Range

Although the control of extraneous variation through homogeneity is easy to use and can help to clarify the relationship between key research variables, it can be risky. Not only does this approach limit generalizability, it can sometimes undermine statistical conclusion validity. When the use of homogeneity restricts the range of values on the outcome variable, relationships between the outcome and the independent variable will be *attenuated* and may therefore lead to the erroneous conclusion that the variables are unrelated.

In the example just used, we suggested limiting the sample of nursing home residents to elders younger than 80 to reduce variability in the denominator.

Our aim was to enhance the variability in depression scores attributable to nursing home admission, relative to depression variability due to other factors. But what if few elders under 80 were depressed? With limited variability, relationships cannot be detected—values in both the numerator and denominator are deflated. For example, if *everyone* had a depression score of 50, the scores would be unrelated to age, pain levels, nursing home admission, and so on. Thus, in designing a study, you should consider whether there will be sufficient variability to support the statistical analyses envisioned. The issue of *floor effects* and *ceiling effects*, which involve range restrictions at the lower and upper end of a measure, respectively, are discussed later in this book.

➲ TIP: In designing a study, try to anticipate nonsignificant findings and consider design adjustments that might affect the results. For example, suppose our study hypothesis is that environmental factors such as light and noise affect acute confusion in the hospitalized elderly. With a preliminary design in mind, imagine findings that *fail* to support the hypothesis. Then ask yourself what could be done to decrease the likelihood of getting such negative results, under the assumption that such results do not reflect the truth. Could power be increased by making differences in environmental conditions sharper? Could precision be increased by controlling additional confounding variables? Could bias be eliminated by better training of research staff?

Unreliable Implementation of a Treatment

The strength of an intervention (and statistical conclusion validity) can be undermined if an intervention is not as powerful in reality as it is "on paper." **Intervention fidelity** (or **treatment fidelity**) concerns the extent to which the implementation of an intervention is faithful to its plan. There is growing interest in intervention fidelity and considerable advice on how to achieve it (e.g., Dabbs et al., 2011; Eaton et al., 2011; Spillane et al., 2007).

Interventions can be weakened by various factors, which researchers can often influence.

One issue concerns whether the intervention is similar from one person to the next. Usually, researchers strive for constancy of conditions in implementing a treatment because lack of standardization adds extraneous variation. Even in tailored, patient-centered interventions, there are protocols, although different protocols are used with different people. Using the notions just described, when standard protocols are not followed, variability due to the intervention (i.e., in the numerator) can be suppressed, and variability due to other factors (i.e., in the denominator) can be inflated, possibly leading to the erroneous conclusion that the intervention was ineffective. This suggests the need for some standardization, the use of procedures manuals, thorough training of personnel, and vigilant monitoring (e.g., through observations of the delivery of the intervention) to ensure that the intervention is being implemented as planned—and that control group members have not gained access to the intervention.

Assessing whether the intervention was delivered as intended may need to be supplemented with efforts to ensure that the intervention was *received* as intended. This may involve a **manipulation check** to assess whether the treatment was in place, was understood, or was perceived in an intended manner. For example, if we were testing the effect of soothing versus jarring music on anxiety, we might want to determine whether participants themselves perceived the music as soothing and jarring. Another aspect of treatment fidelity for interventions designed to promote behavioral changes concerns the concept of *enactment* (Bellg et al., 2004). Enactment refers to participants' performance of the treatment-related skills, behaviors, and cognitive strategies in relevant real-life settings.

Example of Attention to Treatment Fidelity: Carpenter and co-researchers (2013) described their efforts to enhance treatment fidelity in a trial designed to improve the management of symptoms in menopausal women. Their treatment fidelity plan included monitoring to ensure that the treatments were properly delivered, using standardized packets of materials, maintaining logs when inadvertent unblinding occurred, careful training of staff, and following up with participants to ensure that they understood instructions.

Another issue is that participants often fail to receive the desired intervention due to lack of **treatment adherence**. It is not unusual for those in the experimental group to elect not to participate fully in the treatment—for example, they may stop going to treatment sessions. Researchers should take steps to encourage participation among those in the treatment group. This might mean making the intervention as enjoyable as possible, offering incentives, and reducing burden in terms of data collection (Polit & Gillespie, 2010). Nonparticipation in an intervention is rarely random, so researchers should document which people got what amount of treatment so that individual differences in "dose" can be examined in the analysis or interpretation of results.

TIP: Except for small-scale studies, every study should have a **procedures manual** that delineates the protocols and procedures for its implementation. The Toolkit section of the accompanying *Resource Manual* provides a model table of contents for such a procedures manual. The Toolkit also includes a model checklist to monitor delivery of an intervention through direct observation of intervention sessions.

INTERNAL VALIDITY

Internal validity refers to the extent to which it is possible to make an inference that the independent variable, rather than another factor, is truly causing variation in the outcome. We infer from an effect to a cause by eliminating (controlling) other potential causes. The control mechanisms reviewed earlier are strategies for improving internal validity. If researchers do not carefully manage confounding variation, the conclusion that the outcome was caused by the independent variable is open to challenge.

Threats to Internal Validity

True experiments possess a high degree of internal validity because manipulation and random assignment allows researchers to rule out most alternative explanations for the results. Researchers who use quasi-experimental or correlational designs must contend with competing explanations of what caused the outcomes. Major competing threats to internal validity are examined in this section.

Temporal Ambiguity

As noted in Chapter 9, a criterion for inferring a causal relationship is that the cause must precede the effect. In RCTs, researchers create the independent variable and then observe subsequent performance on an outcome, so establishing temporal sequencing is never a problem. In correlational studies, however, it may be unclear whether the independent variable preceded the dependent variable or vice versa—and this is especially true in cross-sectional studies.

Selection

Selection (self-selection) encompasses biases resulting from preexisting differences between groups. When individuals are not assigned to groups randomly, the groups being compared might not be equivalent. Differences on the outcomes could then reflect initial group differences rather than the effect of the independent variable. For example, if we found that women who were infertile were more likely to be depressed than women who were mothers, it would be impossible to conclude that the two groups differed in depression *because* of childbearing differences; women in the two groups might have been different in psychological well-being from the start. The problem of selection is reduced if researchers can collect data on participants' characteristics before the occurrence of the independent variable. In our example, the best design would be to collect data on women's depression before they attempted to become pregnant and then design the study to control early levels of depression. Selection bias is the most problematic and frequent threats to the internal validity of studies not using an experimental design.

History

The threat of **history** refers to the occurrence of external events that take place concurrently with the independent variable and that can affect the outcomes. For example, suppose we were studying the

effectiveness of an outreach program to encourage pregnant women in rural areas to improve health practices (e.g., smoking cessation, prenatal care). The program might be evaluated by comparing the average birth weight of infants born in the 12 months before the outreach program with the average birth weight of those born in the 12 months after the program was introduced, using a time series design. However, suppose that 1 month after the new program was launched, a well-publicized docudrama about the importance of prenatal care was aired on television. Infants' birth weight might now be affected by both the intervention and the messages in the docudrama, and it would be difficult to disentangle the two effects.

In a true experiment, history is not as likely to be a threat to a study's internal validity because we can often assume that external events are as likely to affect the intervention group as the control group. When this is the case, group differences on the dependent variables represent effects over and above those created by outside factors. There are, however, exceptions. For example, when a crossover design is used, an event external to the study may occur during the first half (or second half) of the experiment, and so treatments would be contaminated by the effect of that event. That is, some people would receive treatment A with the event and others would receive treatment A without it, and the same would be true for treatment B.

Selection biases sometimes interact with history to compound the threat to internal validity. For example, if the comparison group is different from the treatment group, then the characteristics of the members of the comparison group could lead them to have different intervening experiences, thereby introducing both history and selection biases into the design.

Maturation

In a research context, **maturation** refers to processes occurring within participants during the course of the study as a result of the passage of time rather than as a result of the independent variable. Examples of such processes include physical growth, emotional maturity, and fatigue. For instance, if we wanted to evaluate the effects of a sensorimotor program for developmentally delayed children, we would have to consider that progress occurs in these children even without special assistance. A one-group pretest–posttest design is highly susceptible to this threat.

Maturation is often a relevant consideration in health research. Maturation does not refer just to aging but rather to any change that occurs as a function of time. Thus, maturation in the form of wound healing, postoperative recovery, and other bodily changes could be a rival explanation for the independent variable's effect on outcomes.

Mortality/Attrition

Mortality is the threat that arises from attrition in groups being compared. If different kinds of people remain in the study in one group versus another, then these differences, rather than the independent variable, could account for observed differences on the dependent variables at the end of the study. The most severely ill patients might drop out of an experimental condition because it is too demanding, or they might drop out of the control group because they see no advantage to participation. In a prospective cohort study, there may be differential attrition between groups being compared because of death, illness, or geographic relocation. Attrition bias can also occur in single-group quasi-experiments if those dropping out of the study are a biased subset that make it look like a change in average values resulted from a treatment.

The risk of attrition is especially great when the length of time between points of data collection is long. A 12-month follow-up of participants, for example, tends to produce higher rates of attrition than a 1-month follow-up (Polit & Gillespie, 2009). In clinical studies, the problem of attrition may be especially acute because of patient death or disability.

If attrition is random (i.e., those dropping out of a study are comparable to those remaining in it), then there would not be bias. However, attrition is rarely random. In general, the higher the rate of attrition, the greater the likelihood of bias.

TIP: In longitudinal studies, attrition may occur because researchers cannot find participants rather than because they refused to stay in the study. One effective strategy to help **tracing** people is to obtain **contact information** from participants at each point of data collection. Contact information should include the names, addresses, and telephone numbers of two to three people with whom the participant is close (e.g., siblings, close friends)—people who could provide information if participants moved. A sample contact information form that can be adapted for your use is provided in the Toolkit of the accompanying *Resource Manual*.

Testing and Instrumentation

Testing refers to the effects of taking a pretest on people's performance on a posttest. It has been found, particularly in studies dealing with attitudes, that the mere act of collecting data from people changes them. Suppose a sample of nursing students completed a questionnaire about attitudes toward assisted suicide. We then teach them about various arguments for and against assisted suicide, outcomes of court cases, and the like. At the end of instruction, we give them the same attitude measure and observe whether their attitudes have changed. The problem is that the first questionnaire might sensitize students, resulting in attitude changes regardless of whether instruction follows. If a comparison group is not used, it may be impossible to segregate the effects of the instruction from the pretest effects. Sensitization, or testing, problems are more likely to occur when pretest data are from self-reports (e.g., through a questionnaire), especially if people are exposed to controversial or novel material in the pretest.

A related threat is **instrumentation**. This bias reflects changes in measuring instruments or methods of measurement between two points of data collection. For example, if we used one measure of stress at baseline and a revised measure at follow-up, any differences might reflect changes in the measuring tool rather than the effect of an independent variable. Instrumentation effects can occur even if the same measure is used. For example, if the measuring tool yields more accurate measures on a second administration (e.g., if data collectors are more experienced) or less accurate measures the second time (e.g., if participants become bored and answer haphazardly), then these differences could bias the results.

Internal Validity and Research Design

Quasi-experimental and correlational studies are especially susceptible to threats to internal validity. Table 10.2 lists specific designs that are *most* vulnerable to the threats just described—although it should not be assumed that threats are irrelevant in designs not listed. Each threat represents an alternative explanation that competes with the

TABLE 10.2 • Research Designs and Threats to Internal Validity

THREAT	DESIGNS MOST SUSCEPTIBLE
Temporal ambiguity	Case-control Other retrospective/ cross-sectional
Selection	Nonequivalent control group (especially, posttest-only) Case-control "Natural" experiments with two groups Time series, if the population changes over time
History	One-group pretest–posttest Time series Prospective cohort Crossover
Maturation	One-group pretest–posttest
Mortality/ Attrition	Prospective cohort Longitudinal studies (experimental and nonexperimental) One-group pretest–posttest
Testing	All pretest–posttest designs
Instrumentation	All pretest–posttest designs

independent variable as a cause of the outcome. The aim of a strong research design is to rule out competing explanations. (Tables 9.4 and 9.5 in Chapter 9 include information about internal validity threats for specific designs.)

An experimental design normally rules out most rival hypotheses, but even in RCTs, researchers must exercise caution. For example, if there is treatment infidelity or contamination between treatments, then history might be a rival explanation for any group differences (or lack of differences). Mortality can be a salient threat in true experiments. Because the experimenter does things differently with the experimental and control groups, people in the groups may drop out of the study differentially. This is particularly apt to happen if the experimental treatment is painful or inconvenient or if the control condition is boring or bothersome. When this happens, participants remaining in the study may differ from those who left, thereby nullifying the initial equivalence of the groups.

In short, researchers should consider how best to guard against and detect all possible threats to internal validity, no matter what design is used.

Internal Validity and Data Analysis

The best strategy for enhancing internal validity is to use a strong research design that includes control mechanisms and design features discussed in this chapter. Even when this is possible (and, certainly, when this is *not* possible), it is advisable to conduct analyses to assess the nature and extent of biases. When biases are detected, the information can be used to interpret substantive results. And, in some cases, biases can be statistically controlled.

Researchers need to be self-critics. They need to consider fully and objectively the types of biases that could have arisen—and then systematically search for evidence of their existence (while hoping, of course, that no evidence can be found). To the extent that biases can be ruled out or controlled, the quality of evidence the study yields will be strengthened.

Selection biases should always be examined. Typically, this involves comparing groups on pretest measures, when pretest data have been collected.

For example, if we were studying depression in women who delivered a baby by cesarean birth versus those who gave birth vaginally, selection bias could be assessed by comparing depression in these two groups during or before the pregnancy. If there are significant predelivery differences, then any postdelivery differences would have to be interpreted with initial differences in mind (or with differences controlled). In designs with no pretest measure of the outcome, researchers should assess selection biases by comparing groups with respect to key background variables, such as age, health status, and so on. Selection biases should be analyzed even in RCTs because there is no guarantee that randomization will yield perfectly equivalent groups.

Whenever the research design involves multiple points of data collection, researchers should analyze attrition biases. This is typically achieved through a comparison of those who did and did not complete the study with regard to baseline measures of the dependent variable or other characteristics measured at the first point of data collection.

Example of Assessing Selection Bias: Chao and colleagues (2014) used a cluster randomized design to study the effectiveness of an educational intervention in a sample of 500 Taiwanese patients with type 2 diabetes. Those who received the intervention were compared to those who did not on numerous background characteristics (e.g., age, gender, education) and clinical characteristics (e.g., HbA1C, blood pressure). A few group differences were found and were controlled in the multivariate analyses. Attrition in both groups at the 6-month follow-up was negligible.

When people withdraw from an intervention study, researchers are in a dilemma about whom to "count" as being "in" a condition. A procedure that is often used is a **per-protocol analysis**, which includes members in a treatment group only if they actually received the treatment. Such an analysis is problematic, however, because self-selection into a nontreatment condition could undo initial group comparability. This type of analysis will almost always be biased toward finding positive treatment effects. The "gold standard" approach is to use an **intention-to-treat analysis**, which

involves keeping participants who were randomized in the groups to which they were assigned (Polit & Gillespie, 2009, 2010). An intention-to-treat analysis may yield an underestimate of the effects of a treatment if many participants did not actually get the assigned treatment—but may be a better reflection of what would happen in the real world. Of course, one difficulty with an intention-to-treat analysis is that it is often difficult to obtain outcome data for people who have dropped out of a treatment, but there are strategies for estimating outcomes for those with missing data (Polit, 2010).

Example of Intention-to-Treat Analysis: Teresi and colleagues (2013) used a cluster randomized design to assess an intervention designed to sensitize nursing home staff to the issue of elder abuse. Key outcomes were staff knowledge and reporting at 6- and 12-months post-baseline. Analyses were conducted on an intent-to-treat basis.

In a crossover design, history is a potential threat both because an external event could differentially affect people in different treatment orderings and because the different orderings are in themselves a kind of differential history. *Substantive* analyses of the data involve comparing outcomes under treatment A versus treatment B. The analysis of bias, by contrast, involves comparing participants in the different orderings (e.g., A then B versus B then A). Significant differences between the two orderings are evidence of an **ordering bias**.

In summary, efforts to enhance the internal validity of a study should not end once the design strategy has been put in place. Researchers should seek additional opportunities to understand (and possibly to correct) the various threats to internal validity that can arise.

CONSTRUCT VALIDITY

Researchers conduct a study with specific exemplars of treatments, outcomes, settings, and people, which are stand-ins for broad constructs. Construct validity involves inferences from study particulars to the higher order constructs that they are intended to represent. Construct validity is important because constructs are the means for linking the operations used in a study to a relevant conceptualization and to mechanisms for translating the resulting evidence into practice. If studies contain construct errors, there is a risk that the evidence will be misleading.

Enhancing Construct Validity

The first step in fostering construct validity is a careful explication of the treatment, outcomes, setting, and population constructs of interest; the next step is to select instances that match those constructs as closely as possible. Construct validity is further cultivated when researchers assess the match between the exemplars and the constructs and the degree to which any "slippage" occurred.

Construct validity has most often been a concern to researchers in connection with the measurement of outcomes, an issue we discuss in Chapter 14. There is a growing interest, however, in the careful conceptualization and development of theory-based interventions in which the treatment itself has strong construct validity (see Chapter 27). It is just as important for the independent variable (whether it be an intervention or something not amenable to experimental manipulation) to be a strong instance of the construct of interest as it is for the measurement of the dependent variable to have strong correspondence to the outcome construct. In nonexperimental research, researchers do not create and manipulate the hypothesized cause, so ensuring construct validity of the independent variable is often more difficult.

Shadish and colleagues (2002) broadened the concept of construct validity to cover persons and settings as well as outcomes and treatments. For example, some nursing interventions specifically target groups that are characterized as "disadvantaged," but there is not always agreement on how this term is defined and operationalized. Researchers select specific people to represent the construct of a disadvantaged group about which inferences will be made, and so it is important that the specific people are good exemplars of the underlying construct. The construct "disadvantaged" must be carefully delineated before a sample is selected. Similarly, if a researcher is interested in such settings as "immigrant neighborhoods" or

"school-based clinics," these are constructs that require careful description—and the selection of exemplars that match those setting constructs. Qualitative description is often a powerful means of enhancing the construct validity of settings.

Threats to Construct Validity

Threats to construct validity are reasons that inferences from a particular study exemplar to an abstract construct could be erroneous. Such a threat could occur if the operationalization of the construct fails to incorporate all the relevant characteristics of the underlying construct, or it could occur if it includes extraneous content—both of which are instances of a mismatch. Shadish and colleagues (2002) identified 14 threats to construct validity (their Table 3.1) and several additional threats specific to case-control designs (their Table 4.3). Among the most noteworthy threats are the following:

1. *Reactivity to the study situation.* As discussed in Chapter 9, participants may behave in a particular manner because they are aware of their role in a study (the Hawthorne effect). When people's responses reflect, in part, their perceptions of participation in research, those perceptions become part of the treatment construct under study. There are several ways to reduce this problem, including blinding, using outcome measures not susceptible to reactivity (e.g., data from hospital records), and using preintervention strategies to satisfy participants' desire to look competent or please the researcher.

Example of a Possible Hawthorne Effect:
Eisenberg and colleagues (2013) evaluated the effect of ondansetron for the prevention of nausea and vomiting in patients receiving autologous stem cell transplantation infusion. Those receiving the treatment were compared to historic controls in terms of nausea scores and vomiting episodes. The researchers noted the possibility that the positive outcomes "may have been influenced by the Hawthorne Effect, whereby participants' responses are influenced by having study personnel focused on their nausea and vomiting" (p. 290).

2. *Researcher expectancies.* A similar threat stems from the researcher's influence on participant

responses through subtle (or not-so-subtle) communication about desired outcomes. When this happens, the researcher's expectations become part of the treatment construct that is being tested. Blinding can reduce this threat, but another strategy is to make observations during the study to detect verbal or behavioral signals of research staff expectations and correct them.

3. *Novelty effects.* When a treatment is new, participants and research agents alike might alter their behavior. People may be either enthusiastic or skeptical about new methods of doing things. Results may reflect reactions to the novelty rather than to the intrinsic nature of an intervention, and so the intervention construct is clouded by novelty content.

4. *Compensatory effects.* In intervention studies, *compensatory equalization* can occur if health care staff or family members try to compensate for the control group members' failure to receive a perceived beneficial treatment. The compensatory goods or services must then be part of the construct description of the study conditions. *Compensatory rivalry* is a related threat arising from the control group members' desire to demonstrate that they can do as well as those receiving a special treatment.

5. *Treatment diffusion or contamination.* Sometimes alternative treatment conditions get blurred, which can impede good construct descriptions of the independent variable. This may occur when participants in a control group condition receive services similar to those in the treatment condition. More often, blurring occurs when those in a treatment condition essentially put themselves into the control group by dropping out of the intervention. This threat can also occur in nonexperimental studies. For example, in case-control comparisons of smokers and nonsmokers, care must be taken during screening to ensure that participants are appropriately categorized (e.g., some people may consider themselves nonsmokers even though they smoke regularly but only on weekends).

Construct validity requires careful attention to what we *call* things (i.e., construct labels) so that appropriate construct inferences can be made. Enhancing construct validity in a study requires careful thought before a study is undertaken, in terms of a well-considered explication of constructs, and also requires poststudy scrutiny to assess the degree to which a match between operations and constructs was achieved.

EXTERNAL VALIDITY

External validity concerns the extent to which it can be inferred that relationships observed in a study hold true over variations in people, conditions, and settings. External validity has emerged as a major concern in an EBP world in which there is an interest in generalizing evidence from tightly controlled research settings to real-world clinical practice settings.

External validity questions may take several different forms. We may wish to ask whether relationships observed in a study sample can be generalized to a larger population—for example, whether results from a smoking cessation program found effective with pregnant teenagers in Boston can be generalized to pregnant teenagers throughout the United States. Many EBP questions, however, are about going from a study group to a *particular* client—for example, whether the pelvic muscle exercises found to be effective in alleviating urinary incontinence in one study are an effective strategy for Maryanna Stephens. Other external validity questions are about generalizing to types of people, settings, or treatments unlike those in the research (Polit & Beck, 2010). For example, can findings about a pain reduction treatment in a study of Australian women be generalized to men in Canada? Or, would a 6-week intervention to promote dietary changes in patients with diabetes be equally effective if the content were condensed into a 4-week program? Sometimes new studies are needed to answer questions about external validity, but external validity often can be enhanced by researchers' design decisions.

Enhancements to External Validity

One aspect of external validity concerns the *representativeness* of the participants used in the study.

For example, if the sample is selected to be representative of a population to which the researcher wishes to generalize the results, then the findings can more readily be applied to that population (Chapter 12). Similarly, if the settings in which the study occurs are representative of the clinical settings in which the findings might be applied, then inferences about relevance in those other settings can be strengthened.

An important concept for external validity is *replication*. Multisite studies are powerful because more confidence in the generalizability of the results can be attained if findings are replicated in several sites—particularly if the sites are different on dimensions considered important (e.g., size, nursing skill mix, and so on). Studies with a diverse sample of participants can test whether study results are replicated for subgroups of the sample—for example, whether benefits from an intervention apply to men *and* women or older *and* younger patients. Systematic reviews are a crucial aid to external validity precisely because they assess relationships in replication studies across different circumstances.

Another issue concerns attempts to use or create study situations as similar as possible to real-world circumstances. The real world is a "messy" place, lacking the standardization imposed in studies. Yet, external validity can be jeopardized if study conditions are too artificial. For example, if nurses require 5 days of training to implement a promising intervention, we might ask how realistic it would be for administrators to devote resources to such an intervention.

Threats to External Validity

In the previous chapter we discussed *interaction effects* that can occur in a factorial design when two treatments are simultaneously manipulated. The interaction question is whether the effects of treatment A hold (are comparable) for all levels of treatment B. Conceptually, questions regarding external validity are similar to this interaction question. Threats to external validity concern ways in which relationships between variables might interact with or be moderated by variations in people, settings, time, and conditions. Shadish and colleagues

(2002) described several threats to external validity, such as the following two:

1. *Interaction between relationship and people.* An effect observed with certain types of people might not be observed with other types of people. A common complaint about RCTs is that many people are excluded—not because they would not benefit from the treatment but because they cannot provide needed research data (e.g., cognitively impaired patients, non-English speakers). During the 1980s, the widely held perception that many clinical trials in the United States were conducted primarily with white males led to policy changes to ensure scrutiny of treatment and gender/ethnicity interactions.

2. *Interaction between causal effects and treatment variation.* An innovative treatment might be effective because it is paired with other elements, and sometimes those elements are intangible—for example, an enthusiastic project director. The same "treatment" could never be fully replicated, and thus, different results could be obtained in subsequent tests.

Shadish and colleagues (2002) noted that moderators of relationships are the norm, not the exception. With interventions, for example, it is normal for a treatment to "work better" for some people than for others. Thus, in thinking about external validity, the primary issue is whether there is constancy of a relationship (or constancy of causation) and not whether the *magnitude* of the effect is constant.

TRADE-OFFS AND PRIORITIES IN STUDY VALIDITY

Quantitative researchers strive to design studies that are strong with respect to all four types of study validity. Sometimes, efforts to increase one type of validity also benefit another type. In some instances, however, addressing one type of validity reduces the possibility of achieving others.

For example, suppose we went to great lengths to ensure intervention fidelity in an RCT. Our efforts might include strong training of staff, careful monitoring of intervention delivery, manipulation checks, and steps to maximize participants' adherence to treatment. Such efforts would have positive effects on statistical conclusion validity because the treatment was made as powerful as possible. Internal validity would be enhanced if attrition biases were minimized as a result of high adherence. Intervention fidelity would also improve the construct validity of the treatment because the content delivered and received would better match the underlying construct. But what about external validity? All of the actions undertaken to ensure that the intervention is strong, construct-valid, and administered according to plan are not consistent with the realities of clinical settings. People are not normally paid to adhere to treatments, nurses are not monitored and corrected to ensure that they are following a script, training in the use of new protocols is usually brief, and so on.

This example illustrates that researchers need to give careful thought to how design decisions may affect various aspects of study validity. Of particular concern is trade-offs between internal and external validity.

Internal Validity and External Validity

Tension between the goals of achieving internal validity and external validity is pervasive. Many control mechanisms that are designed to rule out competing explanations for hypothesized cause-and-effect relationships make it difficult to infer that the relationship holds true in uncontrolled real-life settings.

Internal validity was long considered the *sine qua non* of experimental research (Campbell & Stanley, 1963). The rationale was this: If there is insufficient evidence that an intervention really caused an effect, why worry about generalizing the results? This high priority given to internal validity, however, is somewhat at odds with the current emphasis on evidence-based practice. A reasonable question might be: If study results can't be generalized to real-world clinical settings, who *cares* if the study has strong internal validity? Clearly, both internal and external validity are important to building an evidence base for nursing practice.

There are several "solutions" to the conflict between internal and external validity. The first (and perhaps most prevalent) approach is to emphasize

one and sacrifice the other. Following a long tradition of field experimentation based on Campbell and Stanley's advice, it is often external validity that is sacrificed.

A second approach in some medical trials is to use a phased series of studies. In the earlier phase, there are tight controls, strict intervention protocols, and stringent criteria for including people in the RCT. Such studies are **efficacy studies**. Once the intervention has been deemed to be effective under tightly controlled conditions in which internal validity was the priority, it is tested with larger samples in multiple sites under less restrictive conditions, in **effectiveness studies** that emphasize external validity.

A third approach is to compromise. There has been recent interest in promoting designs that aim to achieve a balance between internal and external validity in a single intervention study. We discuss such *practical* (or *pragmatic*) *clinical trials* in Chapter 11.

The Supplement to this chapter on the**Point®** describes a framework that was developed to improve the generalizability of research evidence and has been used in some nursing projects: the **RE-AIM framework**.

TIP: The Toolkit section of the *Resource Manual* includes a table listing a number of strategies that can be used to enhance the external validity of a study. The table identifies the potential consequence of each strategy for other types of study validity.

Prioritization and Design Decisions

Unfortunately, it is impossible to avoid all possible threats to study validity. By understanding the various threats, however, you can reach conclusions about the trade-offs you are willing to make to achieve study goals. Some threats are more worrisome than others in terms of both likelihood of occurrence and consequences to the inferences you would like to make. And, some threats are more costly to avoid than others. Resources available for a study must be allocated so that there is a correspondence between expenditures and the importance of different types of validity. For example, with a fixed budget, you need to decide whether it is better to increase the size of the sample and hence power (statistical conclusion validity) or to use the money on efforts to reduce attrition (internal validity).

The point is that you should make conscious decisions about how to structure a study to address validity concerns. Every design decision has both a "payoff" and a cost in terms of study integrity. Being cognizant of the effects that design decisions have on the quality of research evidence is a responsibility that nurse researchers should attend to so that their evidence can have the largest possible impact on clinical practice.

➔ TIP: A useful strategy is to create a matrix that lists various design decisions in the first column (e.g., randomization, crossover design) and then use the next four columns to identify the potential impact of those options on the four

types of study validity. (In some cells, there may be no entry if there are no consequences of a design element for a given type of validity.) A sixth column could be added for estimates of the design element's financial implications, if any. The Toolkit section of the accompanying *Resource Manual* includes a model matrix as a Word document for you to use and adapt.

CRITIQUING GUIDELINES FOR STUDY VALIDITY

In critiquing a research report to evaluate its potential to contribute to nursing practice, it is crucial to make judgments about the extent to which threats to validity were minimized—or, at least, assessed and taken into consideration in interpreting the results. The guidelines in Box 10.1 focus on

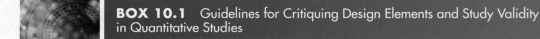

BOX 10.1 Guidelines for Critiquing Design Elements and Study Validity in Quantitative Studies

1. Was there adequate statistical power? Did the manner in which the independent variable was operationalized create strong contrasts that enhanced statistical power? Was precision enhanced by controlling confounding variables? If hypotheses were not supported (e.g., a hypothesized relationship was not found), is it possible that statistical conclusion validity was compromised?
2. In intervention studies, did the researchers attend to intervention fidelity? For example, were staff adequately trained? Was the implementation of the intervention monitored? Was attention paid to both the delivery and receipt of the intervention?
3. What evidence does the report provide that selection biases were eliminated or minimized? What steps were taken to control confounding participant characteristics that could affect the equivalence of groups being compared? Were these steps adequate?
4. To what extent did the study design rule out the plausibility of other threats to internal validity, such as history, attrition, maturation, and so on? What are your overall conclusions about the internal validity of the study?
5. Were there any major threats to the construct validity of the study? In intervention studies, was there a good match between the underlying conceptualization of the intervention and its operationalization? Was the intervention "pure" or was it confounded with extraneous content, such as researcher expectations? Was the setting or site a good exemplar of the type of setting envisioned in the conceptualization?
6. Was the context of the study sufficiently described to enhance its capacity for external validity? Were the settings or participants representative of the types to which results were designed to be generalized?
7. Overall, did the researcher appropriately balance validity concerns? Was attention paid to certain types of threats (e.g., internal validity) at the expense of others (e.g., external validity)?

validity-related issues to further help you to critique quantitative research designs. Together with the critiquing guidelines in the previous chapter, they are likely to be the core of a strong critical evaluation of the evidence that quantitative studies yield. From an EBP perspective, it is important to remember that drawing inferences about causal relationships relies not only on how high up on the evidence hierarchy a study is (Figure 2.1) but also, for any given level of the hierarchy, how successful the researcher was in managing study validity and balancing competing validity demands.

RESEARCH EXAMPLE

We conclude this chapter with an example of a study that demonstrated careful attention to many aspects of study validity.

Study: Investigation of standard care versus sham Reiki placebo versus actual Reiki therapy to enhance comfort and well-being in a chemotherapy infusion center (Catlin & Taylor-Ford, 2011)

Statement of Purpose: The purpose of the study was to evaluate the efficacy of Reiki therapy in enhancing comfort and well-being among patients undergoing outpatient chemotherapy. Reiki is a form of energy work that involves laying of hands over a fully clothed person to unblock energy centers.

Treatment Groups: Three groups of patients were compared: (1) an intervention group that received a Reiki intervention, (2) a placebo (attention control) group that received a sham Reiki treatment, and (3) a control group that got usual care only.

Method: The researchers used a design that addressed many validity concerns. In terms of internal validity, a sample of 189 participants from a single medical center was randomly assigned to one of the three groups. The researchers estimated how large a sample was needed to achieve adequate power for statistical conclusion validity, using a procedure called power analysis (Chapter 12). Patients in the intervention group received a 20-minute Reiki treatment during chemotherapy by an experienced Reiki therapist (an RN). For patients in the placebo group, the therapist pretended to perform a Reiki session. Patients in the control group received standard care.

Additional Study Validity Efforts: The intervention protocol was assessed by four certified Reiki instructors. The sham therapist, who was trained to move her hands in a specified manner, was selected to resemble the Reiki therapist, but she personally did not believe in the Reiki practice. In terms of intervention fidelity, actual sessions were not monitored, but sessions held before the study allowed other Reiki instructors to see that the actual therapist and the sham therapist approached patients in identical ways. All patients completed scales that measured their comfort and well-being, both prior to the treatment and again after the chemotherapy session. Infusion center nurses and patients themselves were blinded as to whether the sham or actual Reiki therapy was being administered. There was no attrition from the study, and so it was not necessary to perform an intention-to-treat analysis. A comparison of patients in the three study groups at baseline indicated that the three groups were comparable in terms of demographic characteristics (e.g., age, ethnicity) and treatment variables (e.g., round of chemotherapy), and so confounding variables did not need to be statistically controlled.

Key Findings: Improvements in both comfort and well-being were observed from baseline to posttest for patients in both the Reiki group and the placebo group, but not for those in the standard care group. The standard care group had significantly lower comfort and well-being scores at the end of the trial than those in the Reiki and placebo groups.

Conclusions: The researchers concluded that the presence of an RN providing one-on-one support during a chemotherapy session helped to improve comfort and well-being, with or without an attempted healing energy field.

SUMMARY POINTS

* Study validity concerns the extent to which appropriate inferences can be made. **Threats to validity** are reasons that an inference could be wrong. A key function of quantitative research design is to rule out validity threats.
* Control over confounding participant characteristics is key to managing many validity threats. The best control method is randomization to

treatment conditions, which effectively controls all confounding variables—especially in the context of a crossover design.

- When randomization is not possible, other control methods include **homogeneity** (the use of a homogeneous sample to eliminate variability on confounding characteristics); blocking or stratifying, as in the case of a *randomized block design*; **pair matching** participants on key variables to make groups more comparable (or **balancing** groups to achieve comparability); and **statistical control** to remove the effect of a confounding variable statistically (e.g., through **analysis of covariance**).

- Homogeneity, stratifying, matching, and statistical control share two disadvantages: Researchers must know in advance which variables to control, and can rarely control all of them.

- Four types of validity affect the rigor of a quantitative study: statistical conclusion validity, internal validity, construct validity, and external validity.

- **Statistical conclusion validity** concerns the validity of the inference that an empirical relationship between variables exists (most often, the presumed cause and the effect).

- Threats to statistical conclusion validity include low **statistical power** (the ability to detect true relationships among variables), low **precision** (the exactness of the relationships revealed after controlling confounding variables), and factors that undermine a strong operationalization of the independent variable (e.g., a treatment).

- **Intervention** (or **treatment**) **fidelity** concerns the extent to which the implementation of a treatment is faithful to its plan. Intervention fidelity is enhanced through standardized treatment protocols, careful training of intervention agents, monitoring of the delivery and receipt of the intervention, **manipulation checks**, and steps to promote **treatment adherence** and avoid **contamination of treatments**.

- **Internal validity** concerns inferences that outcomes were caused by the independent variable rather than by confounding factors. Threats to internal validity include temporal ambiguity (lack of clarity about whether the

presumed cause preceded the outcome), **selection** (preexisting group differences), **history** (the occurrence of external events that could affect outcomes), **maturation** (changes resulting from the passage of time), **mortality** (effects attributable to attrition), **testing** (effects of a pretest), and **instrumentation** (changes in the way data are gathered).

- Internal validity can be enhanced through judicious design decisions but can also be addressed analytically (e.g., through an analysis of selection or attrition biases). When people withdraw from a study, an **intention-to-treat analysis** (analyzing outcomes for all people in their original treatment conditions) is preferred to a **per-protocol analysis** (analyzing outcomes only for those who received the full treatment) for maintaining the integrity of randomization.

- **Construct validity** concerns inferences from the particular exemplars of a study (e.g., the specific treatments, outcomes, and settings) to the higher order constructs that they are intended to represent. The first step in fostering construct validity is a careful explication of those constructs.

- Threats to construct validity can occur if the operationalization of a construct fails to incorporate all relevant characteristics of the construct or if it includes extraneous content. Examples of such threats include *subject reactivity*, *researcher expectancies*, *novelty effects*, *compensatory effects*, and *treatment diffusion*.

- **External validity** concerns inferences about the extent to which study results can be generalized— that is, whether relationships observed in a study hold true over variations in people, settings, time, and treatments. External validity can be enhanced by selecting *representative* people and settings and through replication.

- Researchers need to prioritize and recognize trade-offs among the various types of validity, which sometimes compete with each other. Tensions between internal and external validity are especially prominent. One solution has been to begin with a study that emphasizes internal validity (**efficacy studies**) and then if a causal relationship can be inferred, to undertake **effectiveness studies** that emphasize external validity.

STUDY ACTIVITIES

Chapter 10 of the *Resource Manual for Nursing Research: Generating and Assessing Evidence for Nursing Practice*, 10th edition, offers exercises and study suggestions for reinforcing concepts presented in this chapter. In addition, the following study questions can be addressed:

1. How do you suppose the use of identical twins in a study could enhance control?
2. To the extent possible, apply the questions in Box 10.1 to the Reiki intervention study described at the end of the chapter (by Catlin & Taylor-Ford, 2011). Also, consider whether a crossover design would have been appropriate in this study.

STUDIES CITED IN CHAPTER 10

*Bellg, A., Borrelli, B., Resnick, B., Hecht, J., Minicucci, D., Ory, M., . . . Czajkowski, S. (2004). Enhancing treatment fidelity in health behavior change studies: Best practices and recommendations from the NIH Behavior Change Consortium. *Health Psychology, 23*, 443–451.

*Bowles, K., Hanlon, A., Holland, D., Potashnik, S., & Topaz, M. (2014). Impact of discharge planning decision support on time to readmission among older adult medical patients. *Professional Case Management, 19*, 29–38.

Campbell, D. T., & Stanley, J. C. (1963). *Experimental and quasi-experimental designs for research*. Chicago: Rand McNally.

*Carpenter, J. S., Burns, D., Wu, J., Yu, M., Ryker, K., Tallman, E., & Von Ah, D. (2013). Strategies used and data obtained during treatment fidelity monitoring. *Nursing Research, 62*, 59–65.

Catlin, A., & Taylor-Ford, R. (2011). Investigation of standard care versus sham Reiki placebo versus actual Reiki therapy to enhance comfort and well-being in a chemotherapy infusion center. *Oncology Nursing Forum, 38*, E212–E220.

Chao, Y., Usher, K., Buettner, P., & Holmes, C. (2014). Cluster randomized controlled trial: Educational self-care intervention with older Taiwanese patients with type 2 diabetes mellitus—Impact on blood glucose levels and diabetic complications. *Collegian, 21*, 43–51.

Chen, K., Li, C., Chang, Y., Huang, H., & Cheng, Y. (2015). An elastic band exercise program for older adults using wheelchairs in Taiwan nursing homes: A cluster randomized trial. *International Journal of Nursing Studies, 52*, 30–38.

Conn, V. S., Rantz, M. J., Wipke-Tevis, D. D., & Maas, M. L. (2001). Designing effective nursing interventions. *Research in Nursing & Health, 24*, 433–442.

*Dabbs, A. D., Song, M., Hawkins, R., Aubrecht, J., Kovach, K., Terhorst, L., . . . Callan, J. (2011). An intervention fidelity framework for technology-based behavioral interventions. *Nursing Research, 60*, 340–347.

*Eaton, L. H., Doorenbos, A., Schmitz, K., Carpenter, K., & McGregor, B. (2011). Establishing treatment fidelity in a web-based behavioral intervention study. *Nursing Research, 60*, 430–435.

Eisenberg, S., Wickline, M., Linenberger, M., Gooley, T., & Holmberg, L. (2013). Prevention of dimethylsulfoxide-related nausea and vomiting by prophylactic administration of ondansetron for patients receiving autologous cryopreserved peripheral blood stem cells. *Oncology Nursing Forum, 40*, 285–292.

Lee, C. W., Muo, C., Liang, J., Sung, F., & Kao, C. (2014). Modest increase in risk of acute coronary syndrome associated with morphine use in cancer patients: A population-based nested case-control study. *European Journal of Oncology Nursing, 18*, 295–298.

Lipsey, M. W. (1990). *Design sensitivity: Statistical power for experimental research*. Newbury Park, CA: Sage.

Polit, D. F. (2010). *Statistics and data analysis for nursing research* (2nd ed.). Upper Saddle River, NJ: Pearson.

Polit, D. F., & Beck, C. T. (2010). Generalization in qualitative and quantitative research: Myths and strategies. *International Journal of Nursing Studies, 47*, 1451–1458.

Polit, D. F., & Gillespie, B. (2009). The use of the intention-to-treat principle in nursing clinical trials. *Nursing Research, 58*, 391–399.

Polit, D. F., & Gillespie, B. (2010). Intention-to-treat in randomized controlled trials: Recommendations for a total trial strategy. *Research in Nursing and Health, 33*, 355–368.

Shadish, W. R., Cook, T. D., & Campbell, D. T. (2002). *Experimental and quasi-experimental designs for generalized causal inference*. Boston: Houghton Mifflin.

Spillane, V., Byrne, M., Byrne, M., Leathen, C., O'Malley, M., & Cupples, M. (2007). Monitoring treatment fidelity in a randomized controlled trial of a complex intervention. *Journal of Advanced Nursing, 60*, 343–352.

*Teresi, J., Ramirez, M., Ellis, J., Silver, S., Boratgis, G., Kong, J., . . . Lachs, M. (2013). A staff intervention targeting resident-to-resident elder mistreatment (R-REM) in long-term care increased staff knowledge, recognition and reporting: Results from a cluster randomized trial. *International Journal of Nursing Studies, 50*, 644–656.

A link to this open-access journal article is provided in the Toolkit for this chapter in the accompanying Resource Manual. ✳

11 | Specific Types of Quantitative Research

All quantitative studies can be categorized as experimental, quasi-experimental, or nonexperimental in design (Chapter 9). This chapter describes types of research that vary in study purpose rather in research design. The first two types (clinical trials and evaluations) involve interventions, but methods for each have evolved separately because of their disciplinary roots. Clinical trials are associated with medical research, and evaluation research is associated with the fields of education, social work, and public policy. There is overlap in approaches, but to acquaint you with relevant terms, we discuss each separately. Chapter 27 describes the emerging tradition of intervention research that is more clearly aligned with nursing.

CLINICAL TRIALS

Clinical trials are studies designed to assess clinical interventions. The terms associated with clinical trials are used by many nurse researchers.

Phases of a Clinical Trial

In medical and pharmaceutical research, clinical trials often adhere to a well-planned sequence of activities. Clinical trials undertaken to test a new drug or an innovative therapy often are designed in a series of four phases, as follows:

Phase I occurs after initial development of the drug or therapy and is designed primarily to establish safety and tolerance and to determine optimal dose. This phase typically involves small-scale studies using simple designs (e.g., before–after without a control group). The focus is on developing the best possible (and safest) treatment.

Phase II involves seeking preliminary evidence of treatment effectiveness. During this phase, researchers assess the feasibility of launching a rigorous test, seek evidence that the treatment holds promise, look for signs of possible side effects, and identify refinements to improve the intervention. This phase, essentially a pilot test of the treatment, may be designed either as a small-scale experiment or as a quasi-experiment. (Pilot tests for an intervention are described in more detail in Chapter 28.)

Example of an Early Phase Clinical Trial:
Northouse and co-researchers (2014) translated an existing nurse-delivered program for cancer survivors into a tailored, dyadic web-based format. They undertook a Phase II test of the new format with 38 dyads of patients and their family caregivers, using a before–after design.

Phase III is a full test of the treatment—an RCT with randomization to treatment groups under controlled conditions. The goal of this phase is to develop evidence about treatment *efficacy*— that is, whether the treatment is more efficacious than usual care (or an alternative counterfactual). Adverse effects are also monitored.

Phase III RCTs often involve a large and heterogeneous sample of participants, sometimes selected from multiple sites to ensure that findings are not unique to a single setting.

Example of a Multisite Phase III RCT: Robb and colleagues (2014) undertook a Phase III randomized controlled trial to test a therapeutic music video intervention for adolescents and young adults undergoing hematopoietic stem cell transplant. Patients in eight sites were randomized to either the intervention or to a "low dose" control group that received audiobooks.

Phase IV clinical trials are studies of the *effectiveness* of an intervention in a general population. The emphasis is on the external validity of an intervention that has shown promise of efficacy under controlled (but often artificial) conditions. Phase IV efforts may also examine the cost-effectiveness of new treatments. In pharmaceutical research, Phase IV trials typically focus on postapproval safety surveillance and on long-term consequences over a larger population and timescale than was possible in earlier phases.

Noninferiority and Equivalence Trials

The vast majority of RCTs are **superiority trials**, in which the researchers hypothesize that the intervention is "superior" to (more effective than) the control condition. Standard statistical analysis does not permit a straightforward testing of the null hypothesis, as we describe in Chapter 19. Yet, there are circumstances in which it is desirable to evaluate whether a new (and perhaps less costly or less painful) intervention results in similar outcomes to a standard intervention. In a **noninferiority trial**, the goal is to test whether a new intervention is no worse than a reference treatment (typically, the standard of care). Other trials are called **equivalence trials**, in which the goal is to test the hypotheses that the outcomes from two interventions are equal. In a noninferiority trial, it is necessary to specify in advance the smallest margin of inferiority on a primary outcome (e.g., 1%) that would be tolerated to accept the hypothesis of noninferiority.

In equivalence trials, a margin (or *tolerance*) must be established for the nonsuperiority of one treatment over the other, and the statistical test is two-sided—meaning that equivalence is accepted if the two are not different (in either direction) by no more than the specified tolerance. Both noninferiority and equivalence trials require statistical sophistication and very large samples to ensure statistical conclusion validity. Further information is provided by Christensen (2007) and Piaggio et al. (2012).

Example of a Noninferiority Trial: Albert and colleagues (2015) conducted a noninferiority trial to test whether disposable electrocardiographic (ECG) lead wires are no worse than (not inferior to) reusable ECG lead wires in terms of alarm event rates.

TIP: In a traditional Phase III trial, it may take months to recruit and randomize a sufficiently large sample, and years to arrive at results about efficacy (i.e., until all data have been collected and analyzed). In a **sequential clinical trial**, experimental data are continuously analyzed as they become available, and the trial can be stopped when the evidence is strong enough to support a conclusion about the intervention's efficacy. More information about sequential trials is provided by Bartroff et al. (2013) and Jennison and Turnbull (2000).

Practical Clinical Trials

A problem with traditional Phase III RCTs is that, in efforts to enhance internal validity and support causal inference, the designs are so tightly controlled that their relevance to real-life applications can be questioned. Concern about this situation has led to a call for **practical** (or **pragmatic**) **clinical trials**, which strive to maximize external validity with minimal negative effect on internal validity (Glasgow et al., 2005). Tunis and colleagues (2003), in an often-cited paper, defined practical clinical trials (PCTs) as "trials for which the hypotheses and study design are formulated based on information needed to make a decision" (p. 1626).

Practical clinical trials (sometimes contrasted with more traditional *explanatory trials* that are conducted under optimal conditions) address practical questions about the benefits and risks of an intervention—as well as its costs—as they would unfold in routine clinical practice. PCTs are thus sensitive to the issues under scrutiny in effectiveness (Phase IV) studies, but there is an increasing interest in developing strategies to bridge the gap between efficacy and effectiveness and to address issues of practicality earlier in the evaluation of promising interventions. As Godwin and colleagues (2003) have noted, achieving a creative tension between generalizability and internal validity is crucial.

Tunis and co-authors (2003) made these recommendations for PCTs: enrollment of diverse populations with fewer exclusions of high-risk patients, recruitment of participants from a variety of practice settings, follow-up over a longer period, inclusion of economic outcomes, and comparisons of clinically viable alternatives. Glasgow and colleagues (2005) have proposed several research designs for pragmatic trials, including cluster randomization and delayed treatment designs. Thorpe and colleagues (2009) have developed a tool with 10 criteria to help researchers determine how pragmatic their trial is.

Clearly, the efforts of those who pursue pragmatic trials are part of the larger movement to promote EBP and to facilitate the translation of research findings into real-world settings (see Chapter 2).

Example of a Practical Clinical Trial: Broderick and a multidisciplinary team of researchers (2014) undertook a multisite RCT in which the intervention involved nurse practitioners teaching pain coping skills to osteoarthritis patients. The study sites were doctors' offices, and the team used "methods favoring external validity, consistent with pragmatic effectiveness research" (p. 1743).

TIP: Godwin and colleagues (2003) prepared a table that contrasts features of an explanatory trial (i.e., a traditional Phase III RCT) and a pragmatic trial. The table can be accessed at www.biomedcentral.com/content/supplementary/1471-2288-3-28-S1.doc. This and other websites with material relevant to this chapter are included in the Toolkit of the accompanying *Resource Manual* so that you can "click" on them directly.

EVALUATION RESEARCH

Evaluation research focuses on developing information needed by decision makers about whether to adopt, modify, or abandon a program, practice, procedure, or policy. Evaluations often try to answer broader questions than whether an intervention is effective—for example, they often involve efforts to improve the program (as in Phase II of a clinical trial) or to learn how the program actually "works" in practice. When a program is multidimensional, involving several distinct features or elements, evaluations may address *black box questions*—that is, what is it about the program that is driving observed effects?

Evaluations are often the cornerstone of **policy research**. Nurses have become increasingly aware of the potential contribution their research can make to the formulation of national and local health policies and thus are undertaking evaluations that have implications for policies that affect the allocation of funds for health services (Fyffe, 2009).

Evaluation researchers often evaluate a program or practice that is embedded in an existing organizational context—and so they may confront problems that are organizational or interpersonal. Evaluation research can be threatening. Even when the focus of an evaluation is on a nontangible entity, such as a program, it is *people* who are implementing it. People tend to think that they, or their work, are being evaluated and may feel that their jobs or reputations are at stake. Thus, evaluation researchers need to have more than methodologic skills—they need to be adept in interpersonal relations with people.

Evaluations may involve several components to answer a variety of questions. Good resources for learning more about evaluation research include the books by Patton (2012) and Rossi and colleagues (2004).

Process/Implementation Analyses

A **process** or **implementation analysis** provides descriptive information about the process by which a program gets implemented and how it actually functions. A process analysis is typically designed to address such questions as the following: Does the program operate the way its designers intended? How does the program differ from traditional practices? What were the barriers to its implementation? What do staff and clients like most/least about the intervention?

A process analysis may be undertaken with the aim of improving a new or ongoing program (a *formative evaluation*). In other situations, the purpose of the process analysis is primarily to describe a program carefully so that it can be replicated by others—or so that people can better understand why the program was or was not effective in meeting its objectives. In either case, a process analysis involves an in-depth examination of the operation of a program, often involving the collection of both qualitative and quantitative data. Process evaluations often overlap with efforts to monitor intervention fidelity.

Example of an Implementation Analysis: F. Harris and colleagues (2013) undertook a process evaluation of the early implementation of a suicide prevention intervention. Process analyses, which involved questionnaires and interviews with multiple stakeholders as well as observations, were undertaken in four European countries.

Outcome Analyses

Evaluations often focus on whether a program or policy is meeting its objectives. Evaluations that assess the worth of a program are sometimes called *summative evaluations*, in contrast to formative evaluations. The intent of such evaluations is to help people decide whether the program should be continued or replicated.

Some evaluation researchers distinguish between an outcome analysis and an impact analysis. An **outcome analysis** (or *outcome evaluation*) does not use a rigorous experimental design. Such an analysis simply documents the extent to which the goals of the program are attained, that is, the extent to which positive outcomes occur. For example,

a program may be designed to encourage women in a poor rural community to obtain prenatal care. In an outcome analysis, the researchers might document the percentage of pregnant women who had obtained prenatal care, the average month in which prenatal care was begun, and so on, and perhaps compare this information to preintervention community data.

Example of an Outcome Analysis: Potter and colleagues (2013) reported on the development and evaluation of a program for compassion fatigue (a combination of secondary traumatic stress and burnout) for oncology nurses. The evaluation examined changes for program participants for several outcomes, such as burnout, compassion satisfaction, and secondary traumatic stress.

Impact Analysis

An **impact analysis** assesses a program's **net impacts**—impacts that can be attributed to the program, over and above effects of a counterfactual (e.g., standard care). Impact analyses use an experimental or strong quasi-experimental design because their aim is to permit causal inferences about program effects. In the example cited earlier, suppose that the program to encourage prenatal care involved having nurses make home visits to women in rural communities to explain the benefits of early care. If the visits could be made to pregnant women randomly assigned to the intervention, the labor and delivery outcomes of the group of women receiving the home visits could be compared to those not receiving them to assess the intervention's net impacts, that is, the percentage *increase* in receipt of prenatal care among the experimental group relative to the control group.

Example of an Impact Analysis: Deechakawan and co-researchers (2014) tested the impact of nurse-delivered self-management interventions for patients with irritable bowel syndrome on patients' anxiety, depression, and catecholamine levels, using a randomized design.

Cost Analysis

New programs or policies are often expensive to implement, but existing programs also may be costly.

In our current situation of spiraling health care costs, evaluations (as well as clinical trials) may include a **cost analysis** (or **economic analysis**) to determine whether the benefits of a program outweigh the monetary costs. Administrators and public policy officials make decisions about resource allocations for health services based not only on whether something "works" but also on whether it is economically viable. Cost analyses are typically done in connection with impact analyses and Phase III clinical trials, that is, when researchers establish strong evidence about program efficacy.

There are several different types of cost analyses (Chang & Henry, 1999), the two most common of which in nursing research are the following:

Cost–benefit analysis, in which monetary estimates are established for both costs and benefits. One difficulty with such an analysis is that it is sometimes difficult to quantify benefits of health services in monetary terms. There is also controversy about methods of assigning dollar amounts to the value of human life.

Cost-effectiveness analysis, which is used to compare health outcomes and resource costs of alternative interventions. Costs are measured in monetary terms, but outcome effectiveness is not. Such analyses estimate what it costs to produce impacts on outcomes that cannot easily be valued in dollars, such as quality of life. Without information on monetary benefits, though, such research may face challenges in persuading decision makers to make changes.

Example of a Cost-Effectiveness Analysis: Bensink and colleagues (2013) wrote an article describing methods of undertaking cost-effectiveness analysis for nursing research. They illustrated key features with an example from an RCT that tested the efficacy of a nurse-led pain and symptom management intervention in rural communities.

Cost–utility analyses, although uncommon when Chang and Henry did their analysis in 1999, are now appearing in the nursing literature. This approach is preferred when morbidity and mortality are outcomes of interest, or when quality of life is a major concern. An index called the **quality-adjusted life year (QALY)** is frequently an important outcome indicator in cost–utility analyses.

Example of a Cost–Utility Analysis: O'Neill and colleagues (2014) described their protocol for an RCT designed to test the efficacy of an exercise program for survivors of a critical illness following discharge from the ICU. The research will include a cost–utility analysis to assess cost-effectiveness of the program compared to standard care. The outcome of the analysis will be the cost per quality-adjusted life year.

Researchers doing cost analyses must document what it costs to operate both the new program and its alternative. In doing cost–benefit analyses, researchers must often think about an array of possible short-term costs (e.g., clients' days of work missed within 6 months after the program) and long-term costs (e.g., lost years of productive work life). Often the cost–benefit analyst examines economic gains and losses from several different accounting perspectives—for example, for the target group, the hospitals implementing the program, taxpayers, and society as a whole. Distinguishing these different perspectives is crucial if a particular program effect is a loss for one group (e.g., taxpayers) but a gain for another (e.g., the target group).

Nurse researchers are increasingly becoming involved in cost analyses. A useful resource for further guidance is the internationally acclaimed textbook by Drummond and colleagues (2005).

HEALTH SERVICES AND OUTCOMES RESEARCH

Health services research is the broad interdisciplinary field that studies how organizational structures and processes, health technologies, social factors, and personal behaviors affect access to health care, the cost and quality of health care, and, ultimately, people's health and well-being.

Outcomes research, a subset of health services research, comprises efforts to understand the end results of particular health care practices and to assess the effectiveness of health care services.

Outcomes research overlaps with evaluation research, but evaluation research typically focuses on a specific program or policy, whereas outcomes research is a more global assessment of nursing and health care services.

Outcomes research represents a response to the increasing demand from policy makers, insurers, and the public to justify care practices and systems in terms of improved patient outcomes and costs. The focus of outcomes research in the 1980s was predominantly on patient health status and costs associated with medical care, but there is a growing interest in studying broader patient outcomes in relation to nursing care—and a greater awareness that evidence-based nursing practice can play a role in quality improvement and health care safety, despite the many challenges (M. Harris et al., 2009).

Although many nursing studies examine patient outcomes, specific efforts to appraise and document the quality of nursing care—as distinct from the care provided by the overall health care system—are less common. A major obstacle is attribution—that is, linking patient outcomes to specific nursing actions or interventions, distinct from the actions of other members of the health care team. It is also difficult in some cases to attribute a causal link between outcomes and health care interventions because other factors (e.g., patient characteristics) affect outcomes in complex ways.

Outcomes research has used a variety of traditional designs and methodologic approaches (primarily quantitative ones) but is also developing a rich array of methods that are not within the traditional research framework. The complex and multidisciplinary nature of outcomes research suggests that this evolving area will offer opportunities for methodologic creativity in the years ahead.

Models of Health Care Quality

In appraising quality in nursing services, various factors need to be considered. Donabedian (1987), whose pioneering efforts created a framework for outcomes research, emphasized three factors: structure, process, and outcomes. The *structure* of care refers to broad organizational and administrative features. Structure can be appraised in terms of

such attributes as size, range of services, technology, organizational structure, and organizational climate. Nursing skill mix and nursing experience are two structural variables that have been found to correlate with patient outcomes. *Processes* involve aspects of clinical management, decision making, and clinical interventions. *Outcomes* refer to the specific clinical end results of patient care. Mitchell and co-authors (1998) noted that "the emphasis on evaluating quality of care has shifted from structures (having the right things) to processes (doing the right things) to outcomes (having the right things happen)" (p. 43).

Several modifications to Donabedian's framework for appraising health care quality have been proposed, the most noteworthy of which is the Quality Health Outcomes Model developed by the American Academy of Nursing (Mitchell et al., 1998). This model is less linear and more dynamic than Donabedian's original framework and takes client and system characteristics into account. This model does not link interventions and processes directly to outcomes. Rather, the effects of interventions are seen as mediated by client and system characteristics. This model, and others like it, are increasingly forming the conceptual framework for studies that evaluate quality of care (Mitchell & Lang, 2004).

Outcomes research usually focuses on various linkages within such models rather than on testing the overall model. Some studies have examined the effect of health care structures on various health care processes and outcomes, for example, and reliable methods to measure aspects of organizational structure and nurses' practice environments have been developed (Bonneterre et al., 2008; Warshawsky & Havens, 2011). Most outcomes research in nursing, however, has focused on the process-patient-outcomes nexus, often using large-scale data sets.

Example of Research on Structure: Pitkäaho and colleagues (2015) studied the relationship between nurse staffing (proportion of RNs and skill mix) on the one hand and patient outcomes (length of hospital stay) on the other in 35,306 patient episodes in acute care units of a Finnish hospital.

Nursing Processes and Interventions

To demonstrate nurses' effects on health outcomes, nurses' clinical actions and behaviors must be carefully described and documented, both quantitatively and qualitatively. Examples of nursing process variables include nurses' problem solving, clinical decision making, clinical competence, nurses' autonomy and intensity, clinical leadership, and specific activities or interventions (e.g., communication, touch).

The work that nurses do is increasingly documented in terms of established classification systems and taxonomies that are amenable to computerized systems. Indeed, in the United States, the standard use of electronic health records to record all health care events has been mandated. A number of research-based classification systems of nursing interventions have been developed, refined, and tested. Among the most prominent are the Nursing Diagnoses Taxonomy of the North American Nursing Diagnosis Association or NANDA (NANDA International, 2011) and the Nursing Intervention Classification or NIC, developed at the University of Iowa (Bulechek et al., 2013). NIC consists of over 400 interventions for all nursing specialties, and each is associated with a definition and a detailed set of activities that a nurse undertakes to implement the intervention.

Patient Risk Adjustment

Patient outcomes vary not only because of the care they receive but also because of differences in patient conditions and comorbidities. Adverse outcomes can occur no matter what nursing intervention is used. Thus, in evaluating the effects of nursing interventions on outcomes, there needs to be some way of controlling or taking into account patients' risks for poor outcomes, or the mix of risks in a caseload.

Risk adjustments have been used in a number of nursing outcomes studies. These studies typically involve the use of global measures of patient risks or patient acuity, such as the Acute Physiology and Chronic Health Evaluation (APACHE I, II, III, or IV) system for critical care environments. Wheeler (2009) has discussed the pros and cons of the different versions of the system.

Example of Outcomes Research with Risk Adjustment: Hickey and colleagues (2013) explored the amount of clinical experience of pediatric critical care nurses in relation to pediatric cardiac surgery mortality. The Risk Adjustment for Congenital Heart Surgery method was used to adjust for baseline differences in patient risk.

Nursing-Sensitive Outcomes

Measuring outcomes and linking them to nursing actions is critical in developing an evidence-based practice and in launching improvement efforts. Outcomes of relevance to nursing can be defined in terms of physical or physiologic function (e.g., heart rate, blood pressure, complications), psychological function (e.g., comfort, life quality, satisfaction), or social function (e.g., parenting competence). Outcomes of interest to nurses may be either temporary (e.g., postoperative body temperature) or more long-term and permanent (e.g., return to regular employment). Furthermore, outcomes may be defined in terms of the end results to individual patients receiving care, or to broader units such as a community or our entire society, including cost factors.

Just as there have been efforts to develop classifications of nursing interventions, work has progressed on developing nursing-sensitive outcome classification systems. **Nursing-sensitive outcomes** are patient outcomes that improve if there is greater quantity or quality of nurses' care. Examples include pressure ulcers, falls, and intravenous infiltrations. The American Nurses Association has developed a database of nursing-sensitive indicators, the National Database of Nursing Quality Indicators or NDNQI (Montalvo, 2007). Also, the Nursing Outcomes Classification (NOC) has been developed by nurses at the University of Iowa College of Nursing to complement the Nursing Intervention Classification (Moorhead et al., 2013).

Example of Outcomes Research: Staggs and Dunton (2014) examined the relationship between levels of nurse staffing on five types of nursing units on the one hand and patient fall rates on the other.

SURVEY RESEARCH

A **survey** is designed to obtain information about the prevalence, distribution, and interrelations of phenomena within a population. Political opinion polls are examples of surveys. When a survey involves a sample, as is usually the case, it may be called a **sample survey** (as opposed to a **census**, which covers an entire population). Surveys rely on participants' **self-reports**—that is, participants respond to a series of questions posed by investigators. Surveys, which yield quantitative data primarily, may be cross-sectional or longitudinal (e.g., panel studies).

An advantage of survey research is its flexibility and broad scope. It can be applied to many populations, it can focus on a wide range of topics, and its information can be used for many purposes. Information obtained in most surveys, however, tends to be relatively superficial: Surveys rarely probe deeply into human complexities. Survey research is better suited to extensive rather than intensive analysis.

The content of a survey is limited only by the extent to which people are able and willing to respond to questions on the topic. Any information that can reliably be obtained by direct questioning can be gathered in a survey, although surveys include mostly questions that require brief responses (e.g., yes or no, always/sometimes/never). Surveys often focus on what people do: what they eat, how they care for their health, and so forth. In some instances, the emphasis is on what people plan to do—for example, the health screenings they plan to have done.

Survey data can be collected in a number of ways. The most respected method is through **personal interviews** (or *face-to-face interviews*), in which interviewers meet in person with respondents. Personal interviews tend to be costly because they involve a lot of personnel time. Nevertheless, personal interviews are regarded as the best method of collecting survey data because of the quality of information they yield and because refusal rates tend to be low.

Example of a Survey with Personal Interviews: Li and colleagues (2013) conducted face-to-face interviews with 550 older Chinese adults to explore their expectations regarding aging, leisure time exercise, and functional health status.

Telephone interviews are less costly than in-person interviews, but respondents may be uncooperative (or difficult to reach) on the telephone. Telephoning can be an acceptable method of collecting data if the interview is short, specific, and not too personal, or if researchers have had prior personal contact with respondents. For example, some researchers conduct in-person interviews in clinical settings at baseline and then conduct follow-up interviews on the telephone. Telephone interviews may be difficult for certain groups of respondents, including the elderly (who may have hearing problems).

Questionnaires, unlike interviews, are self-administered. Respondents read the questions and give their answers in writing. Because respondents differ in their reading levels and in their ability to communicate in writing, questionnaires are *not* merely a printed form of an interview schedule. Care must be taken in a questionnaire to word questions clearly and simply. Questionnaires are economical but are not appropriate for surveying certain populations (e.g., the elderly, children). In survey research, questionnaires can be distributed through the mail (sometimes called a *postal survey*) but are increasingly being distributed over the Internet. Further guidance on mailed and web-based surveys is provided in Chapter 13.

Example of a Mailed Survey: Lillie and co-researchers (2014) mailed questionnaires to a sample of about 700 partners of women who had undergone cancer treatment in Detroit or Los Angeles. The survey included questions about treatment decision making, decision outcomes, and decision regret from the partners' perspectives.

Survey researchers are using new technologies to assist in data collection. Most major telephone surveys now use **computer-assisted telephone interviewing (CATI)**, and growing numbers of in-person surveys use **computer-assisted personal interviewing (CAPI)** with laptop computers. Both procedures involve developing computer programs that present interviewers with the questions to be asked on the monitor; interviewers then enter coded responses directly onto a computer file. CATI and CAPI surveys, although costly, greatly facilitate data collection and improve data quality because there is less opportunity for interviewer error.

Example of Computer-Assisted Telephone Interviewing: Harden and colleagues (2013) conducted a survey, using CATI, to document the long-term effects of prostate cancer treatment on spouses' quality of life.

Audio-CASI (computer-assisted self-interview) technology is a state-of-the-art approach for giving respondents more privacy than is possible in an interview (e.g., to collect information about drug use) and is especially useful for populations with literacy problems (Jones, 2003). With audio-CASI, respondents sit at a computer and listen to questions over headphones. Respondents enter their responses (usually simple codes like 1 or 2) directly onto the keyboard, without the interviewer having to see the responses. This approach is also being extended to surveys with tablets and smartphones.

There are many excellent resources for learning more about survey research, including the classic books by Fowler (2014) and Dillman et al. (2015).

OTHER TYPES OF RESEARCH

The majority of quantitative studies that nurse researchers have conducted are the types described thus far in this chapter or in Chapter 9. However, nurse researchers have pursued a few other specific types of research. In this section, we provide a brief description of some of them. The Supplement for this chapter on thePoint® provides more details about each type. 🅢

• **Secondary analysis**. Secondary analyses involve the use of existing data from a previous or ongoing study to test new hypotheses or answer questions that were not initially envisioned. Most often, secondary analyses are based on quantitative data from a large data set (e.g., from national surveys), but secondary analyses of data from qualitative studies have also been undertaken as well. Several useful websites for locating publicly available data sets are provided in the Toolkit of the accompanying *Resource Manual*. ✴

• **Needs assessments**. Researchers conduct needs assessments to estimate the needs of a group, community, or organization. The aim of such studies is to assess the need for special services or to see if standard services are meeting the needs of intended beneficiaries.
• **Delphi surveys**. Delphi surveys were developed as a tool for short-term forecasting. The technique involves a panel of experts who are asked to complete several rounds of questionnaires focusing on their judgments about a topic of interest. Multiple iterations are used to achieve consensus.
• **Replication studies**. Researchers sometimes undertake a replication study, which is an explicit attempt to see if findings obtained in one study can be duplicated in another setting. A strong evidence-based practice requires replications.
• **Methodologic studies**. Nurse researchers have undertaken many methodologic studies, which are aimed at gathering evidence about strategies of conducting high-quality, rigorous research.

One further type of research-like endeavor is **quality improvement (QI)** projects. The purpose of quality improvement is to improve practices and processes within a specific organization or patient group—not to generate new knowledge that can be generalized beyond the specific context of the study. Yet, there are many similarities between quality improvement and health care research, and distinctions become more complex when efforts to undertake EBP projects are thrown into the mix. The supplement to this chapter discusses the distinctions and similarities between QI, EBP efforts, and research. 🅢

CRITIQUING STUDIES DESCRIBED IN THIS CHAPTER

It is difficult to provide guidance on critiquing the types of studies described in this chapter because they are so varied and because many of the fundamental methodologic issues that require a critique concern the overall design. Guidelines for critiquing design-related issues were presented in the previous two chapters.

BOX 11.1 Some Guidelines for Critiquing Studies Described in Chapter 11

1. Does the study purpose match the study design? Was the best possible design used to address the study purpose?
2. If the study was a clinical trial, was adequate attention paid to developing an appropriate intervention? Was the intervention adequately pilot tested?
3. If the study was a clinical trial or evaluation, was there an effort to understand how the intervention was implemented (i.e., a process-type analysis)? Were the financial costs and benefits assessed? If not, should they have been?
4. If the study was an evaluation (or a practical clinical trial), to what extent do the study results serve the practical information needs of key decision makers or intended users?
5. If the study was a survey, was the most appropriate method used to collect the data (i.e., in-person interviews, telephone interviews, mail or Internet questionnaires)?
6. If the study was a secondary analysis, to what extent was the chosen data set appropriate for addressing the research questions? What were the limitations of the data set, and were these limitations acknowledged and taken into account in interpreting the results?

Box 11.1 offers a few specific questions for critiquing the types of studies included in this chapter. Separate guidelines for critiquing economic evaluations, which are more technically complex, are offered in the Toolkit section of the accompanying *Resource Manual*.

RESEARCH EXAMPLE

This section describes a set of related studies that stemmed from a clinical trial. The research example at the end of the next chapter is a good example of an outcomes research project that has generated many secondary analyses.

Background: Dr. Claire Rickard has undertaken a series of studies in Australia relating to the replacement of peripheral intravenous catheters. The main study, which was based on results from smaller clinical trials (Rickard et al., 2010; Van Donk et al., 2009), was a large, multisite randomized controlled trial that included a cost-effectiveness analysis. The study also required some methodologic work. Data from the parent study has been used in secondary analyses.

Phase III Randomized Equivalence Trial: Rickard and colleagues (2012) hypothesized that patients who had intravenous catheters replaced when clinically indicated would have equivalent rates of phlebitis and complications (e.g., bloodstream infections) but a reduced number of catheter insertions, compared to patients whose catheters were removed according to the standard guideline of every 3 days. Adults with expected catheter use of more than 4 days were recruited into the trial. A sample of 3,283 adults from three hospitals were randomized to clinically indicated catheter replacement or to third daily routine replacement. The equivalence margin was set to 3%. Consistent with the hypothesis of equivalence, phlebitis was found to occur in 7% of the patients in both groups. No serious adverse events relating to the two insertion protocols were observed.

Cost-Effectiveness Study: A cost-effectiveness study was also undertaken in connection with the RCT (Tuffaha et al., 2014). The team collected data on resource use and associated costs. Patients in the "clinically indicated" group used significantly fewer catheters. The mean dwell time for catheters in situ on Day 3 was 99 hours when replaced as clinically indicated, compared to 70 hours when routinely replaced. The cost analysis concluded that the incremental net monetary benefit of clinically indicated replacement was approximately $8 per patient.

Methodologic Substudy: As described in a review paper (Ray-Barruel et al., 2014), Rickard and her team developed and tested a new method to measure the incidence of phlebitis in the RCT reliably.

Secondary Analysis: Wallis and a team of colleagues that included Rickard (2014) used the data from the trial in a secondary analysis. Data from all 3,283 patients was used to explore risk factors for peripheral intravenous catheter (PIVC) failure. The researchers found that some of the factors that predicted phlebitis were modifiable (e.g., large diameter PIVC, ward insertion versus insertion by operating room staff), but others were not (e.g., women were at higher risk).

SUMMARY POINTS

- **Clinical trials** designed to assess the effectiveness of clinical interventions can unfold in a series of phases. Features of the intervention are finalized in *Phase I. Phase II* involves seeking opportunities for refinements and preliminary evidence of efficacy. *Phase III* is a full experimental test of treatment *efficacy*. In *Phase IV*, researchers focus primarily on generalized *effectiveness* and evidence about costs and benefits.

- Most trials are **superiority trials**, in which it is hypothesized that an intervention will result in better outcomes than the counterfactual. In a **noninferiority trial**, the goal is to test whether a new intervention is no worse than a reference treatment. Other trials are called **equivalence trials**, in which the goal is to test the hypotheses that the outcomes from two treatments are equal.

- **Practical** (or **pragmatic**) **clinical trials** are designed to provide information to clinical decision makers. They involve designs that aim to reduce the gap between efficacy and effectiveness studies—that is, between internal and external validity.

- **Evaluation research** assesses the effectiveness of a program, policy, or procedure. **Process** or **implementation analyses** describe the process by which a program gets implemented and how it functions in practice. **Outcome analyses** describe the status of some condition after the introduction of a program. **Impact analyses** test whether a program caused **net impacts** relative to the counterfactual. **Cost** (**economic**) **analyses**

assess whether the monetary costs of a program are outweighed by benefits and include **cost–benefit analyses**, **cost-effectiveness analyses**, and **cost–utility analyses**.

- **Outcomes research** (a subset of **health services research**) examines the quality and effectiveness of health care and nursing services. A model of health care quality encompasses several broad concepts, including *structure* (factors such as nursing skill mix and organizational climate), *process* (e.g., nursing decisions and actions), client risk factors (e.g., illness severity, comorbidities), and *outcomes*. In nursing, researchers often focus on **nursing-sensitive outcomes**—patient outcomes that improve if there is greater quantity or quality of nurse care.

- **Survey research** involves studies of people's characteristics, behaviors, and intentions by asking them to answer questions. One survey method is through **personal interviews**, in which interviewers meet respondents face-to-face and question them. **Telephone interviews** are less costly but are inadvisable if the interview is long or if the questions are sensitive. **Questionnaires** are self-administered (i.e., questions are read by respondents, who then give written responses) and in survey research are usually distributed by mail or over the Internet.

- Other specific types of research include **secondary analysis** (in which researchers analyze previously collected data), **needs assessments** (designed to document the needs of a group or community), **Delphi surveys** (which involve several rounds of questioning with an expert panel to achieve consensus), **replication studies** (which duplicate a prior study to test if results can be repeated), and **methodologic studies** (in which the focus is to develop and test methodologic tools or strategies).

- Research is considered distinct from **quality improvement (QI)** projects, despite many similarities. The purpose of QI is to improve practices and processes within a specific context, not to generate new knowledge that can be generalized beyond the study context.

STUDY ACTIVITIES

Chapter 11 of the *Resource Manual for Nursing Research: Generating and Assessing Evidence for Nursing Practice, 10th edition*, offers exercises and study suggestions for reinforcing concepts presented in this chapter. In addition, the following study questions can be addressed:

1. Suppose you were interested in doing a survey of nurses' attitudes toward caring for AIDS patients. Would you use a personal interview, telephone interview, or a mailed/e-mailed questionnaire to collect your data? Defend your decision.

2. In the research example of the RCT by Rickard and colleagues (2010) described at the end of the chapter, what were the independent and dependent variables? What might the researchers have done to enhance intervention fidelity? Comment on the possibility of blinding in such a study. What were the independent and dependent variables in the secondary analysis by Wallis et al. (2014)?

STUDIES CITED IN CHAPTER 11

Albert, N. M., Murray, T., Bena, J., Slifcak, E., Roach, J., Spence, J., & Burkle, A. (2015). Differences in alarm events between disposable and reusable electrocardiography lead wires. *American Journal of Critical Care, 24*, 67–74.

Bartroff, J., Lai, T. L., & Shih, M. (2013). *Sequential experimentation in clinical trials.* New York: Springer.

*Bensink, M. E., Eaton, L., Morrison, M., Cook, W., Curtis, R., Gordon, D., . . . Doorenbos, A. (2013). Cost effectiveness analysis for nursing research. *Nursing Research, 62*, 279–285.

Bonneterre, V., Liaudy, S., Chatellier, G., Lang, T., & de Gaudemaris, R. (2008). Reliability, validity, and health issues arising from questionnaires used to measure psychosocial and organizational work factors (POWFs) among hospital nurses: A critical review. *Journal of Nursing Measurement, 16*, 207–230.

Broderick, J., Keefe, F., Bruckenthal, P., Junghaenel, D., Schneider, S., Schwartz, J., . . . Gould, E. (2014). Nurse practitioners can effectively deliver pain coping skills training to osteoarthritis patients with chronic pain: A randomized, controlled trial. *Pain, 155*, 1743–1754.

Bulechek, G., Butcher, H., & Dochterman, J. M., & Wagner, C. (2013). *Nursing interventions classification (NIC)* (6th ed.). St. Louis, MO: Mosby.

Chang, W., & Henry, B. M. (1999). Methodologic principles of cost analyses in the nursing, medical, and health services literature, 1990-1996. *Nursing Research, 48*, 94–104.

Christensen, E. (2007). Methodology of superiority vs. equivalence trials and non-inferiority trials. *Journal of Hepatology, 46*, 947–954.

Deechakawan, W., Heitkemper, M. M., Cain, K., Burr, R., & Jarrett, M. (2014). Anxiety, depression, and catecholamine levels after self-management intervention in irritable bowel syndrome. *Gastroenterology Nursing, 37*, 24–32.

Dillman, D. A., Smyth, J., & Christian, L. (2015). *Internet, phone, mail, and mixed-mode surveys: The tailored design method* (4th ed.). New York: Wiley.

Donabedian, A. (1987). Some basic issues in evaluating the quality of health care. In L. T. Rinke (Ed.), *Outcome measures in home care* (Vol. 1, pp. 3–28). New York: National League for Nursing.

Drummond, M., Sculpher, M. J., Torrance, G. W., O'Brien, B., & Stoddart, G. L. (2005). *Methods for the economic evaluation of health care programmes* (3rd ed.). Oxford, United Kingdom: Oxford University Press.

Fowler, F. J., Jr. (2014). *Survey research methods* (5th ed.). Thousand Oaks, CA: Sage.

Fyffe, T. (2009). Nursing shaping and influencing health and social care policy. *Journal of Nursing Management, 17*, 698–706.

Glasgow, R. E., Magid, D., Beck, A., Ritzwoller, D., & Estabrooks, P. (2005). Practical clinical trials for translating research to practice: Design and measurement recommendations. *Medical Care, 43*, 551–557.

*Godwin, M., Ruhland, L., Casson, I., MacDonald, S., Delva, D., Birtwhistle, R., . . . Seguin, R. (2003). Pragmatic controlled clinical trials in primary care: The struggle between external and internal validity. *BMC Medical Research Methodology, 3*, 28.

*Harden, J., Sanda, M., Wei, J., Yarandi, H., Hembroff, L., Hardy, J., & Northouse, L. (2013). Survivorship after prostate cancer treatment: Spouses' quality of life at 36 months. *Oncology Nursing Forum, 40*, 567–573.

*Harris, F., Maxwell, M., O'Connor, R., Coyne, J., Arensman, E., Szekely, A., & Hegerl, U. (2013). Developing social capital in implementing a complex intervention: A process evaluation of the early implementation of a suicide prevention intervention in four European countries. *BMC Public Health, 13*, 158.

Harris, M., Vanderboom, C., & Hughes, R. (2009). Nursing-sensitive safety and quality outcomes: The taming of a wicked problem. *Applied Nursing Research, 22*, 146–151.

Hickey, P. A., Gauvreau, K., Curley, M., & Connor, J. (2013). The effect of critical care nursing and organizational characteristics on pediatric cardiac surgery mortality in the United States. *Journal of Nursing Administration, 43*, 637–644.

Jennison, C., & Turnbull, B. (2000). *Group sequential methods with applications to clinical trials.* Boca Raton, FL: Chapman & Hall.

Jones, R. (2003). Survey data collection using Audio Computer Assisted Self-Interview. *Western Journal of Nursing Research, 25,* 349–358.

Li, X., Lv, Q., Li, C., Zhang, H., Li, C., & Jin, J. (2013). The relationship between expectation regarding aging and functional health status among older adults in China. *Journal of Nursing Scholarship, 45,* 328–335.

Lillie, S. E., Janz, N., Friese, C., Graff, J., Schwartz, K., Hamilton, A., . . . Hawley, S. (2014). Racial and ethnic variation in partner perspectives about the breast cancer treatment decision-making experience. *Oncology Nursing Forum, 41,* 13–20.

Mitchell, P., Ferketich, S., & Jennings, B. (1998). Quality health outcomes model. *Image: The Journal of Nursing Scholarship, 30,* 43–46.

Mitchell, P., & Lang, N. (2004). Framing the problem of measuring and improving healthcare quality: Has the Quality Health Outcomes Model been useful? *Medical Care, 42,* II4–II11.

*Montalvo, I. (2007). The National Database of Nursing Quality Indicators® (NDNQI®). *The Online Journal of Issues in Nursing, 12*(3).

Moorhead, S., Johnson, M., Maas, M., & Swanson, E. (2013). *Nursing Outcomes Classification (NOC)* (5th ed.). St. Louis, MO: Mosby.

NANDA International. (2011). *NANDA International Nursing Diagnoses: Definitions and Classification 2012–2014* (9th ed.). Oxford, United Kingdom: Wiley-Blackwell.

Northouse, L., Schafenacker, A., Barr, K., Katapodi, M., Yoon, H., Brittain, K., . . . An, L. (2014). A tailored web-based psychoeducational intervention for cancer patients and their family caregivers. *Cancer Nursing, 37,* 321–330.

*O'Neill, B., McDowell, K., Bradley, J., Blackwood, B., Mullan, B., Lavery, G., . . . McAuley, D. (2014). Effectiveness of a programme of exercise on physical function in survivors of critical illness following discharge from the ICU: Study protocol for a randomised controlled trial (REVIVE). *Trials, 15,* 146.

Patton, M. Q. (2012). *Essentials of utilization focused evaluation.* Thousand Oaks, CA: Sage.

Piaggio, G., Elbourne, D., Pocock, S., Evans, S., & Altman, D. (2012). Reporting of noninferiority and equivalence randomized trials: Extension of the CONSORT 2010 statement. *Journal of the American Medical Association, 308,* 2594–2604.

Pitkäaho, T., Partanen, P., Miettinen, M., & Vehviläinen-Julkunen, K. (2015). Non-linear relationships between nurse staffing and patients' length of stay in acute care units: Bayesian dependence modelling. *Journal of Advanced Nursing, 71,* 458–473.

Potter, P., Deshields, T., & Rodriguez, S. (2013). Developing a systemic program for compassion fatigue. *Nursing Administration Quarterly, 37,* 326–332.

Ray-Barruel, G., Polit, D., Murfield, J., & Rickard, C. M. (2014). Infusion phlebitis assessment measures: A systematic review. *Journal of Evaluation in Clinical Practice, 20,* 191–202.

*Rickard, C. M., McCann, D., Munnings, J., & McGrail, M. (2010). Routine resite of peripheral intravenous devices every 3 days did not reduce complications compared with clinically indicated resite. *BMC Medicine, 8,* 53.

Rickard, C. M., Webster, J., Wallis, M., Marsh, N., McGrail, M., French, V., . . . Whitby, M. (2012). Routine versus clinically indicated replacement of peripheral intravenous catheters: A randomised controlled equivalence trial. *The Lancet, 380,* 1066–1074.

Robb, S., Burns, D., Stegenga, K., Haut, P., Monahan, P., Meza, J., . . . Haase, J. (2014). Randomized clinical trial of therapeutic music video intervention for resilience outcomes in adolescents undergoing hematopoietic stem cell transplant: A report from the Children's Oncology Group. *Cancer, 120,* 909–917.

Rossi, P., Lipsey, M., & Freeman, H. (2004). *Evaluation: A systematic approach* (7th ed.). Thousand Oaks, CA: Sage.

*Staggs, V. S., & Dunton, N. (2014). Associations between rates of unassisted inpatient falls and levels of registered and non-registered nurse staffing. *International Journal for Quality in Health Care, 26,* 87–92.

*Thorpe, K., Zwarenstein, M., Oxman, A., Treweek, S., Furberg, C., Altman, D., . . . Chalkidou, K. (2009). A pragmatic-explanatory continuum indicator summary (PRECIS): A tool to help trial designers. *Journal of Clinical Epidemiology, 62,* 464–475.

Tuffaha, H. W., Rickard, C. M., Webster, J., Marsh, N., Gordon, L., Wallis, M., & Scuffham, P. (2014). Cost-effectiveness of clinically indicated versus routine replacement of peripheral intravenous catheters. *Applied Health Economics and Health Policy, 12,* 51–58.

Tunis, S. R., Stryer, D., & Clancy, C. (2003). Practical clinical trials: Increasing the value of clinical research for decision making in clinical and health policy. *Journal of the American Medical Association, 290,* 1624–1632.

Van Donk, P., Rickard, C. M., McGrail, M., & Doolan, G. (2009). Routine replacement versus clinical monitoring of peripheral intravenous catheters in a regional hospital in the home program: A randomized controlled trial. *Infection Control and Hospital Epidemiology, 30,* 915–917.

Wallis, M., McGrail, M., Webster, J., Marsh, N., Gowardman, J., Playford, E., & Rickard, C. M. (2014). Risk factors for peripheral intravenous catheter failure: A multivariate analysis of data from a randomized controlled trial. *Infection Control and Hospital Epidemiology, 35,* 63–68.

Warshawsky, N. E., & Havens, D. (2011). Global use of the Nursing Work Index. *Nursing Research, 60,* 17–31.

Wheeler, M. M. (2009). APACHE: An evaluation. *Critical Care Nursing Quarterly, 32,* 46–48.

***A link to this open-access journal article is provided in the Toolkit for this chapter in the accompanying* Resource Manual. ⊗**

12 | Sampling in Quantitative Research

Researchers almost always obtain data from samples. In testing the efficacy of a new falls prevention program for hospital patients, researchers reach conclusions without testing it with *every* patient worldwide, or even every patient in a given hospital. But researchers must be careful not to draw conclusions based on a flawed sample.

Quantitative researchers seek to select samples that will allow them to achieve statistical conclusion validity and to generalize their results beyond the sample used. They develop a **sampling plan** that specifies in advance how participants are to be selected and how many to include. Qualitative researchers, by contrast, make sampling decisions during the course of data collection and typically do not have a formal sampling plan. This chapter discusses sampling for quantitative studies.

BASIC SAMPLING CONCEPTS

We begin by reviewing some terms associated with sampling—terms that are used primarily (but not exclusively) in quantitative research.

Populations

A **population** (the "P" of PICO questions) is the entire aggregation of cases in which a researcher is interested. For instance, if we were studying American nurses with doctoral degrees, the population could be defined as all U.S. citizens who are registered nurses (RNs) and who have a PhD, DNSc, DNP, or other doctoral-level degree. Other possible populations might be all patients who had cardiac surgery in Princess Alexandria Hospital in 2015, all women with irritable bowel syndrome in Sweden, or all children in Canada with cystic fibrosis. Populations are not restricted to humans. A population might consist of all hospital records in a particular hospital or all blood samples at a particular laboratory. Whatever the basic unit, the population comprises the aggregate of elements in which the researcher is interested.

It is sometimes useful to distinguish between target and accessible populations. The **accessible population** is the aggregate of cases that conform to designated criteria *and* that are accessible for a study. The **target population** is the aggregate of cases about which the researcher would like to generalize. A target population might consist of all diabetic people in New York, but the accessible population might consist of all patients with diabetes who attend a particular clinic. Researchers usually sample from an accessible population and hope to generalize to a target population.

> **TIP:** Many quantitative researchers fail to identify their target population or to discuss the generalizability of the results. The population of interest needs to be carefully considered in planning and reporting a study.

249

Eligibility Criteria

Researchers must specify criteria that define who is in the population. Consider the population American nursing students. Does this population include students in all types of nursing programs? How about RNs returning to school for a bachelor's degree? Or students who took a leave of absence for a semester? Do foreign students enrolled in American nursing programs qualify? Insofar as possible, the researcher must consider the exact criteria by which it could be decided whether an individual would or would not be classified as a member of the population. The criteria that specify population characteristics are the **eligibility criteria** or **inclusion criteria**. Sometimes, a population is also defined in terms of characteristics that people must *not* possess (i.e., **exclusion criteria**). For example, the population may be defined to exclude people who cannot speak English.

In thinking about ways to define the population and delineate eligibility criteria, it is important to consider whether the resulting sample is likely to be a good exemplar of the population construct in which you are interested. A study's construct validity is enhanced when there is a good match between the eligibility criteria and the population construct.

Of course, eligibility criteria for a study often reflect considerations other than substantive concerns. Eligibility criteria may reflect one or more of the following:

- *Costs*. Some criteria reflect cost constraints. For example, when non-English-speaking people are excluded, this does not usually mean that researchers are uninterested in non-English speakers but rather that they cannot afford to hire translators or multilingual data collectors.
- *Practical constraints*. Sometimes, there are other practical constraints, such as difficulty including people from rural areas, people who are hearing impaired, and so on.
- *People's ability to participate in a study*. The health condition of some people may preclude their participation. For example, people with cognitive impairments, who are in a coma, or who are in an unstable medical condition may need to be excluded.

- *Design considerations*. As noted in Chapter 10, it is sometimes advantageous to define a homogeneous population as a means of controlling confounding variables.

The criteria used to define a population for a study have implications for the interpretation and generalizability of the findings.

Example of Inclusion and Exclusion Criteria: Schallom and colleagues (2015) studied the relationship between gastric reflux and pulmonary aspiration in hospitalized patients receiving gastric tube feedings. To be eligible, patients had to have a confirmed gastric location of a feeding tube, be mechanically ventilated, and be aged 18 years or older. Patients were excluded if they were pregnant, had a documented history of GERD, had any airborne infectious disease, or had oral trauma.

Samples and Sampling

Sampling is the process of selecting cases to represent an entire population, to permit inferences about the population. A **sample** is a subset of population **elements**, which are the most basic units about which data are collected. In nursing research, elements most often are humans.

Samples and sampling plans vary in quality. *Two key considerations in assessing a sample in a quantitative study are its representativeness and size*. A **representative sample** is one whose key characteristics closely approximate those of the population. If the population in a study of patients who fall is 50% male and 50% female, then a representative sample would have a similar gender distribution. If the sample is not representative of the population, the study's external validity and construct validity are at risk.

Certain sampling methods are less likely to result in biased samples than others, but a representative sample can never be guaranteed. Researchers operate under conditions in which error is possible. Quantitative researchers strive to minimize errors and, when possible, to estimate their magnitude.

Sampling designs are classified as either probability sampling or nonprobability sampling. **Probability sampling** involves random selection of elements. In probability sampling, researchers can specify the probability that an element of the population will be included in the sample. Greater confidence can be placed in the representativeness of probability samples. In **nonprobability samples**, elements are selected by nonrandom methods. There is no way to estimate the probability that each element has of being included in a nonprobability sample, and every element usually does *not* have a chance for inclusion.

Strata

Sometimes, it is useful to think of populations as consisting of subpopulations, or **strata**. A stratum is a mutually exclusive segment of a population, defined by one or more characteristics. For instance, suppose our population was all RNs in the United Kingdom. This population could be divided into two strata based on gender. Or, we could specify three strata of nurses younger than 30 years of age, nurses aged 30 to 45 years, and nurses 46 years or older. Strata are often used in sample selection to enhance the sample's representativeness.

Staged Sampling

Samples are sometimes selected in multiple phases, in what is called **multistage sampling**. In the first stage, large units (such as hospitals or nursing homes) are selected. Then, in the next stage, individuals are sampled. In staged sampling, it is possible to combine probability and nonprobability sampling. For example, the first stage can involve the deliberate (nonrandom) selection of study sites. Then, people within the selected sites can be selected through random procedures.

Sampling Bias

Researchers work with samples rather than with populations because it is cost-effective to do so. Researchers seldom have the resources to study all members of a population. It may be possible to obtain reasonably accurate information from a sample, but data from samples *can* be erroneous. Finding 100 people willing to participate in a study may be easy, but it is usually hard to select 100 people who are an unbiased subset of the population.

Sampling bias refers to the systematic over- or underrepresentation of a population segment on a characteristic relevant to the research question.

As an example of consciously biased selection, suppose we were investigating patients' responsiveness to nurses' touch and decide to recruit the first 50 patients meeting eligibility criteria. We decide, however, to omit Mr. Z from the sample because he has been hostile to nursing staff. Mrs. X, who has just lost a spouse, is also bypassed. These decisions to exclude certain people do not reflect bona fide eligibility criteria. This can lead to bias because responsiveness to nurses' touch (the outcome variable) may be affected by patients' feelings about nurses or their emotional state.

Sampling bias often occurs unconsciously, however. If we were studying nursing students and systematically interviewed every 10th student who entered the nursing school library, the sample would be biased in favor of library-goers, even if we are conscientious about including every 10th student regardless of age, gender, or other traits.

> **⟶ TIP:** Internet surveys are attractive because they can be distributed to geographically dispersed people. However, there is an inherent bias in such surveys, unless the population is defined as people who have easy access to, and comfort with, a computer and the Internet.

Sampling bias is partly a function of population homogeneity. If population elements were all identical on key attributes, then any sample would be as good as any other. Indeed, if the population were completely homogeneous—exhibited no variability at all—then a *single* element would be sufficient. For many physiologic attributes, it may be safe to assume reasonably high homogeneity. For example, the blood in a person's veins is relatively homogeneous and so a single blood sample is adequate. For most human attributes, however, homogeneity is the exception rather than the rule. Age, health status, stress, motivation—all these attributes reflect human heterogeneity. When variation occurs in the population, then similar variation should be reflected, to the extent possible, in a sample.

➔ **TIP:** One easy way to increase a study's generalizability is to select participants from multiple sites (e.g., from different hospitals, nursing homes, communities). Ideally, the different sites would be sufficiently divergent that good representation of the population would be obtained.

Example of a Convenience Sample: Krueger and colleagues (2015) studied fetal response (fetal heart rate and movement) to live and recorded maternal speech following a history of fetal exposure to a passage spoken by the mother. The study participants were a convenience sample of 21 pregnant women.

NONPROBABILITY SAMPLING

Nonprobability sampling is less likely than probability sampling to produce representative samples. Despite this fact, most studies in nursing and other health disciplines rely on nonprobability samples.

Convenience Sampling

Convenience sampling entails using the most conveniently available people as participants. For example, a nurse who conducts a study of teenage risk-taking at a local high school is relying on a convenience sample. The problem with convenience sampling is that those who are available might be atypical of the population with regard to critical variables.

Sometimes, researchers seeking people with certain characteristics place an advertisement in a newspaper, put up signs in clinics, or post messages on online social media. These "convenient" approaches are subject to bias because people select themselves as volunteers in response to posted notices and likely differ from those who do not volunteer.

Snowball sampling (also called *network sampling* or *chain sampling*) is a variant of convenience sampling. With this approach, early sample members (called **seeds**) are asked to refer other people who meet the eligibility criteria. This approach is often used when the population involves people who might otherwise be difficult to identify (e.g., people who are afraid of hospitals).

Convenience sampling is the weakest form of sampling. In heterogeneous populations, there is no other sampling approach in which the risk of sampling bias is greater. Yet, convenience sampling is the most commonly used method in many disciplines.

➔ **TIP:** Rigorous methods of sampling *hidden populations*, such as the homeless or injection drug users, are emerging. Because standard probability sampling is inappropriate for such hidden populations, a method called **respondent-driven sampling (RDS)**, a variant of snowball sampling, has been developed. RDS, unlike traditional snowballing, allows the assessment of relative inclusion probabilities based on mathematical models (Magnani et al., 2005). McCreesh and colleagues (2012) have undertaken a recent evaluation of RDS.

Quota Sampling

A **quota sample** is one in which the researcher identifies population strata and determines how many participants are needed from each stratum. By using information about population characteristics, researchers can ensure that diverse segments are represented in the sample, in the proportion in which they occur in the population.

Suppose we were interested in studying nursing students' attitude toward working with AIDS patients. The accessible population is a school of nursing with 500 undergraduate students; a sample of 100 students is desired. The easiest procedure would be to distribute questionnaires in classrooms through convenience sampling. Suppose, however, that we suspect that male and female students have different attitudes. A convenience sample might result in too many men or women. Table 12.1 presents fictitious data showing the gender distribution for the population and for a convenience sample (second and third columns). In this example, the convenience sample overrepresents women and underrepresents men. We can, however, establish "quotas" so that the sample includes the appropriate number of participants from both strata.

TABLE 12.1 • Numbers and Percentages of Students in Strata of a Population, Convenience Sample, and Quota Sample

STRATA	POPULATION	CONVENIENCE SAMPLE	QUOTA SAMPLE
Male	100 (20%)	5 (5%)	20 (20%)
Female	400 (80%)	95 (95%)	80 (80%)
Total	500 (100%)	100 (100%)	100 (100%)

The far-right column of Table 12.1 shows the number of men and women required for a quota sample for this example.

You may better appreciate the dangers of a biased sample with a concrete example. Suppose a key study question was, "Would you be willing to work on a unit that cared exclusively for AIDS patients?" The number and percentage of students in the population who would respond "yes" are shown in the first column of Table 12.2. We would not know these values—they are shown to illustrate a point. Within the population, men are more likely than women to say they would work on a unit with AIDS patients, yet men were underrepresented in the convenience sample. As a result, population and sample values on the outcome are discrepant: Nearly twice as many students in the population are favorable toward working with AIDS patients (20%) than we would conclude based on results from the convenience sample (11%). The quota sample does a better job of reflecting the views of the population (19%). In actual research situations, the distortions from a convenience sample may be

smaller than in this example but could be larger as well.

Quota sampling does not require sophisticated skills or a lot of effort. Many researchers who use a convenience sample could profitably use quota sampling. Stratification should be based on variables that would reflect important differences in the dependent variable. Variables such as gender, ethnicity, education, and medical diagnosis may be good stratifying variables.

Procedurally, quota sampling is like convenience sampling. The people in any subgroup are a convenience sample from that population stratum. For example, the initial sample of 100 students in Table 12.1 constituted a convenience sample from the population of 500. In the quota sample, the 20 men are a convenience sample of the 100 men in the population. Quota sampling can share similar weaknesses as convenience sampling. For instance, if a researcher is required by a quota sampling plan to interview 10 men between the ages of 65 and 80 years, a trip to a nursing home might be the most convenient method of obtaining participants.

TABLE 12.2 • Students Willing to Work on an AIDS Unit, in the Population, Convenience Sample, and Quota Sample

	POPULATION	CONVENIENCE SAMPLE	QUOTA SAMPLE
Willing males (number)	28	2	6
Willing females (number)	72	9	13
Total number of willing students	100	11	19
Total number of all students	500	100	100
Percentage willing	20%	11%	19%

Yet this approach would fail to represent the many older men living independently in the community. Despite its limitations, quota sampling is a major improvement over convenience sampling.

> **Example of a Quota Sample:** Lam and colleagues (2012) studied the relationship between pedometer-determined physical activity and body composition in a quota sample of 913 working Chinese adults. The stratifying variable was occupational category (e.g., manager, professional, clerk).

Consecutive Sampling

Consecutive sampling involves recruiting *all* of the people from an accessible population who meet the eligibility criteria over a specific time interval, or for a specified sample size. For example, in a study of ventilator-associated pneumonia in ICU patients, if the accessible population were patients in an ICU of a specific hospital, a consecutive sample might consist of all eligible patients admitted to that ICU over a 6-month period. Or, it might be the first 250 eligible patients admitted to the ICU, if 250 were the targeted sample size.

Consecutive sampling is a far better approach than sampling by convenience, especially if the sampling period is sufficiently long to deal with potential biases that reflect seasonal or other time-related fluctuations. When all members of an accessible population are invited to participate in a study over a fixed time period, the risk of bias is greatly reduced. Consecutive sampling is often the best possible choice when there is "rolling enrollment" into a contained accessible population.

> **Example of a Consecutive Sample:** Balzer and colleagues (2014) studied whether characteristics of patients affected nurses' judgments about pressure ulcer risks. A consecutive sample of 106 patients who met the eligibility criteria at a university hospital in Germany comprised the study sample.

Purposive Sampling

Purposive sampling uses researchers' knowledge about the population to make selections. Researchers might decide purposely to select people who are judged to be particularly knowledgeable about the issues under study, for example, as in the case of a Delphi survey. A drawback is that this approach seldom results in a typical or representative sample. Purposive sampling is sometimes used to good advantage in two-staged sampling. That is, sites can first be sampled purposively, and then people can be sampled in some other fashion.

> **Example of Purposive Sampling:** Hewitt and Cappiello (2015) conducted a Delphi survey of nurse experts to identify the essential competencies in American nursing education for prevention and care related to unintended pregnancy. Purposive sampling was used to recruit 100 panelists representing all 50 U.S. states.

Evaluation of Nonprobability Sampling

Except for some consecutive samples, nonprobability samples are rarely representative of the population. When every element in the population does not have a chance of being included in the sample, it is likely that some segment of it will be systematically underrepresented. When there is sampling bias, the results could be misleading, and efforts to generalize to a broader population could be misguided.

Nonprobability samples will continue to predominate, however, because of their practicality. Probability sampling requires skill and resources, so there may be no option but to use a nonprobability approach. Strict convenience sampling without explicit efforts to enhance representativeness, however, should be avoided. Indeed, it has been argued that quantitative researchers would likely do better at achieving representative samples for generalizing to a population if they had an approach that was more purposeful (Polit & Beck, 2010).

Quota sampling is a semipurposive sampling strategy that is far superior to convenience sampling because it seeks to ensure sufficient representation within key strata of the population. Another purposive strategy for enhancing generalizability is deliberate multisite sampling. For instance, a convenience sample could be obtained from two communities known to differ socioeconomically so that the sample would reflect the experiences of both lower and middle-class participants. In other words, if the population is known to be heterogeneous, you should take steps to capture important variation in the sample.

Even in one-site studies in which convenience sampling is used, researchers can make an effort to explicitly add cases to correspond more closely to population traits. For example, if half the population is known to be male, then the researcher can check to see if approximately half the sample is male and use outreach to recruit more males if necessary.

Quantitative researchers using nonprobability samples must be cautious about the inferences they make. When there are efforts to deliberately enhance representativeness and to interpret results conservatively—and when the study is replicated with new samples—then nonprobability samples may work reasonably well.

PROBABILITY SAMPLING

Probability sampling involves the random selection of elements from a population. **Random sampling** involves a selection process in which each element in the population has an equal, independent chance of being selected. Probability sampling is a complex, technical topic, and books such as those by Thompson (2012) offer further guidance for advanced students.

> **TIP:** Random sampling should not be (but often is) confused with random assignment, which was described in connection with experimental designs (Chapter 9). Random assignment is the process of allocating people to different treatment conditions at random. Random *assignment* is unrelated to how people in an RCT were selected in the first place.

Simple Random Sampling

Simple random sampling is the most basic probability sampling design. In simple random sampling, researchers establish a **sampling frame**, the technical name for the list of elements from which the sample will be chosen. If nursing students at the University of Connecticut were the accessible population, then a roster of those students would be the sampling frame. If the sampling unit were 300-bed or larger hospitals in Taiwan, then a list of all such hospitals would be the sampling frame.

Sometimes, a population is defined in terms of an existing sampling frame. For example, if we wanted to use a voter registration list as a sampling frame, we would have to define the community population as residents who had registered to vote.

Once a sampling frame has been developed, elements are numbered consecutively. A table of random numbers or computer-generated list of random numbers would then be used to draw a sample of the desired size. An example of a sampling frame for a population of 50 people is shown in Table 12.3, and we wish to randomly sample 20 people. We could find a starting place in a random numbers

TABLE 12.3 • Sampling Frame for Simple Random Sampling Example

(1.) N. Alexander	(26.) C. Ball
2. D. Brady	27. L. Chodos
3. D. Carroll	28. K. DiSanto
4. M. Dakes	29. B. Eddy
(5.) H. Edelman	(30.) J. Fishon
(6.) L. Forester	(31.) R. Griffin
7. J. Galt	32. B. Hebert
8. L. Hall	(33.) C. Joyce
9. R. Ivry	(34.) S. Kane
10. A. Janosy	35. C. Lace
11. J. Kettlewell	36. M. Montanari
12. L. Lack	37. B. Nicolet
(13.) B. Mastrianni	(38.) T. Opitz
(14.) K. Nolte	39. J. Portnoy
15. N. O'Hara	40. G. Queto
16. T. Piekarz	41. A. Ryan
(17.) J. Quint	42. S. Singleton
(18.) M. Riggi	(43.) L. Tower
19. M. Solomons	44. V. Vaccaro
20. S. Thompson	(45.) B. Wilmot
(21.) C. VanWagner	(46.) D. Abraham
22. R. Walsh	47. V. Brusser
(23.) J. Yepsen	48. O. Crampton
(24.) M. Zimmerman	49. R. Davis
25. A. Arnold	(50.) C. Eldred

table by blindly placing our finger at some point on the page to find a two-digit combination between 1 and 50. For this example, suppose that we began with the first number in the random number table of Table 9.2 (p. 189), which is 46. The person corresponding to that number, D. Abraham, is the first person selected to participate in the study. Number 05, H. Edelman, is the second selection, and number 23, J. Yepsen, is the third. This process would continue until 20 participants are chosen. The selected elements are circled in Table 12.3.

A sample selected randomly in this fashion is unbiased. Although there is no guarantee that a random sample will be representative, random selection ensures that differences in the attributes of the sample and the population are purely a function of chance. The probability of selecting an unrepresentative sample decreases as the size of the sample increases.

Simple random sampling tends to be laborious. Developing a sampling frame, numbering all elements, and selecting elements are time-consuming chores, particularly if the population is large. In actual practice, simple random sampling is used infrequently because it is relatively inefficient. Furthermore, it is not always possible to get a listing of every element in the population, so other methods may be required.

Example of a Simple Random Sample: Scott and colleagues (2014) mailed questionnaires to a random sample of 3,500 critical care nurses drawn from a membership list of about 14,000 full-time staff nurses. The researchers examined the relationship between nurses' regrets about decisions they had made on the one hand and their levels of fatigue on the other.

Stratified Random Sampling

In **stratified random sampling**, the population is first divided into two or more strata, with the goal of enhancing representativeness. Researchers using stratified random sampling subdivide the population into homogeneous subsets (e.g., based on gender or illness severity), from which elements are selected at random.

In stratified sampling, a person's status in a stratum must be known before random selection, which can be problematic. Patient listings or organizational directories may contain information for meaningful stratification (e.g., about a person's gender), but many lists do not. Quota sampling does not have the same problem because researchers can ask people questions that determine their eligibility for a particular stratum.

The most common procedure for drawing a stratified sample is to group together elements belonging to a stratum and to select the desired number of elements randomly. To illustrate, suppose that the list in Table 12.3 consisted of 25 men (numbers 1 through 25) and 25 women (numbers 26 through 50). Using gender as the stratifying variable, we could guarantee a sample of 10 men and 10 women by randomly sampling 10 numbers from the first half of the list and 10 from the second half. As it turns out, simple random sampling did result in 10 people being chosen from each half-list, but this was purely by chance. It would not have been unusual to draw, say, 8 names from one half and 12 from the other. Stratified sampling can guarantee the appropriate representation of different population segments.

Stratification usually divides the population into unequal subpopulations. For example, if the person's race were used to stratify the population of U.S. citizens, the subpopulation of white people would be larger than that of nonwhite people. In **proportionate stratified sampling**, participants are selected in proportion to the size of the population stratum. If the population was students in a nursing school that had 10% African American, 10% Hispanic, 10% Asian, and 70% white students, then a proportionate stratified sample of 100 students, with race/ethnicity as the stratifier, would draw 10, 10, 10, and 70 students from the respective strata.

Proportionate sampling may result in insufficient numbers for making comparisons among strata. In our example, it would be risky to draw conclusions about Hispanic nursing students based on only 10 cases. For this reason, researchers may use **disproportionate sampling** when comparisons are sought between strata of greatly unequal size. In the example, the sampling proportions might be altered to select 20 African American, 20 Hispanic, 20 Asian, and 40 white students. This design would ensure a more adequate representation of the three racial/ethnic minorities. When disproportionate sampling is used, however, it is necessary to make an adjustment to arrive at the best estimate of *overall* population values. This adjustment, called **weighting**, is a simple mathematic computation described in textbooks on sampling.

Stratified random sampling enables researchers to sharpen a sample's representativeness. Stratified sampling, however, may be impossible if information on the critical variables is unavailable. Furthermore, a stratified sample requires even more labor and effort than simple random sampling because the sample must be drawn from multiple enumerated listings.

Example of Stratified Random Sampling: LoBiondo-Wood and colleagues (2014) conducted a survey of members of the Oncology Nursing Society regarding their views on priorities for oncology nursing research. All members with a doctoral degree were invited to participate. The survey was also sent to a stratified random sample of all other members, with educational credential as the stratifying variable.

Multistage Cluster Sampling

For many populations, it is impossible to obtain a listing of all elements. For example, the population of full-time nursing students in Canada would be difficult to list and enumerate for the purpose of drawing random sample. Large-scale surveys almost never use simple or stratified random sampling; they usually rely on multistage sampling, beginning with clusters.

Cluster sampling involves selecting broad groups (clusters) rather than selecting individuals—typically the first stage of a multistage approach. For a sample of nursing students, we might first draw a random sample of nursing schools and then draw a sample of students from the selected schools. The usual procedure for selecting samples from a general population in the United States is to sample successively such administrative units as census tracts, then households, and then household members. The resulting design can be described in terms of the number of stages (e.g., three-stage sampling). Clusters can be selected by simple or stratified methods. For instance, in selecting nursing schools, one could stratify on geographic region.

For a specified number of cases, multistage sampling tends to be less accurate than simple or stratified random sampling. Yet, multistage sampling is more practical than other types of probability sampling, particularly when the population is large and widely dispersed.

Example of Multistage Sampling: De Gouveia Santos and colleagues (2014) analyzed data regarding self-reported fecal incontinence from a sample of over 2,000 adults in a Brazilian city. Participants in this study were from randomly selected households, sampled from 390 census tracts, which had been randomly selected, with stratification on region of the city.

Systematic Sampling

Systematic sampling involves selecting every *k*th case from a list, such as every 10th person on a patient list or every 25th person on a student roster. When this sampling method is applied to a sampling frame, an essentially random sample can be drawn, using the following procedure.

The desired sample size is established at some number (n). The size of the population must be known or estimated (N). By dividing N by n, a sampling interval (k) is established. The **sampling interval** is the standard distance between sampled elements. For instance, if we wanted a sample of 200 from a population of 40,000, then our sampling interval would be as follows:

$$k = \frac{40,000}{200} = 200$$

In other words, every 200th element on the list would be sampled. The first element should be selected randomly. Suppose that we randomly selected number 73 from a random number table. People corresponding to numbers 73, 273, 473, and so on would be sampled.

Systematic sampling yields essentially the same results as simple random sampling but involves less work. Problems can arise if a list is arranged in such a way that a certain type of element is listed at intervals coinciding with the sampling interval. For instance, if every 10th nurse listed in a nursing staff roster was a head nurse and the sampling interval was 10, then head nurses would either always or never be included in the sample. Problems of this type are rare, fortunately. Systematic sampling can also be applied to lists that have been stratified.

➔ **TIP:** Systematic sampling is sometimes used to sample every *k*th person entering a store or leaving a hospital. In such situations, unless the population is narrowly defined as all those people entering or leaving, the sampling is essentially a sample of convenience.

Example of a Systematic Sample: Ridout and colleagues (2014) studied the incidence of failure to communicate vital information as patients progressed through the perioperative process. From a population of 1,858 patient records in a health care system meeting eligibility criteria, the researchers selected every sixth case, for a sample of 294 cases.

Evaluation of Probability Sampling

Probability sampling is the best method of obtaining representative samples. If all the elements in a population have an equal probability of being selected, then the resulting sample is likely to do a good job of representing the population. Another advantage is that probability sampling allows researchers to estimate the magnitude of sampling error. **Sampling error** refers to differences between sample values (e.g., the average age of the sample) and population values (the average age of the population).

The drawback of probability sampling is its impracticality. It is beyond the scope of most studies to draw a probability sample, unless the population is narrowly defined—and if it *is* narrowly defined, probability sampling might be "overkill." Probability sampling is the preferred and most respected method of obtaining sample elements but is often unfeasible.

➔ **TIP:** The quality of the sampling plan is of particular importance in survey research because the purpose of surveys is to obtain information about the prevalence or average values for a population. All national surveys, such as the National Health Interview Survey in the United States, use probability samples. Probability samples are rarely used in intervention studies.

SAMPLE SIZE IN QUANTITATIVE STUDIES

Quantitative researchers need to pay attention to the sample size needed to achieve statistical conclusion validity. A procedure called **power analysis** (Cohen, 1988) can be used to estimate sample size needs, but some statistical knowledge is needed before this procedure can be explained. In this section, we offer guidelines to beginning researchers; advanced students can read about power analysis in Chapter 17 or in a sampling or statistics textbook (e.g., Polit, 2010).

Sample Size Basics

There are no simple formulas that can tell you how large a sample you will need in a given study, but as a general recommendation, you should use as large a sample as possible. The larger the sample, the more representative of the population it is likely to be. Every time researchers calculate a percentage or an average based on sample data, they are estimating a population value. The larger the sample, the smaller the sampling error.

Let us illustrate this with an example of monthly aspirin consumption in a nursing home (Table 12.4). The population consists of 15 residents whose aspirin consumption averages 16.0 aspirins per month, as shown in the top row of the table. We drew 8 simple random samples—two each with sample sizes of 2, 3, 5, and 10. Each sample average represents an estimate of the population average (here, 16.0). With a sample size of two, our estimate might have been wrong by as many as eight aspirins (sample 1B, average of 24.0), which is 50% greater than the population value. As the sample size increases, the averages get closer to the true population value, *and* the differences in the estimates between samples A and B get smaller as well. As sample size increases, the probability of getting a markedly deviant sample diminishes. Large samples provide an opportunity to counterbalance atypical values. In the absence of a power analysis, the safest procedure is to obtain data from as large a sample as is feasible.

Large samples are no assurance of accuracy, however. When nonprobability sampling is used, even large samples can harbor bias. A famous

TABLE 12.4 • Comparison of Population and Sample Values and Averages: Nursing Home Aspirin Consumption Example

NUMBER OF PEOPLE IN GROUP	GROUP	INDIVIDUAL DATA VALUES (NUMBER OF ASPIRINS CONSUMED, PRIOR MONTH)	AVERAGE
15	Population	2, 4, 6, 8, 10, 12, 14, 16, 18, 20, 22, 24, 26, 28, 30	16.0
2	Sample 1A	6, 14	10.0
2	Sample 1B	20, 28	24.0
3	Sample 2A	16, 18, 8	14.0
3	Sample 2B	20, 14, 26	20.0
5	Sample 3A	26, 14, 18, 2, 28	17.6
5	Sample 3B	30, 2, 26, 10, 4	14.4
10	Sample 4A	22, 16, 24, 20, 2, 8, 14, 28, 20, 4	15.8
10	Sample 4B	12, 18, 8, 10, 16, 6, 28, 14, 30, 22	16.4

example is the 1936 American presidential poll conducted by the magazine *Literary Digest*, which predicted that Alfred Landon would defeat Franklin D. Roosevelt by a landslide. About 2.5 million people participated in this poll. Biases resulted from the fact that this large sample was drawn from telephone directories and automobile registrations during a depression year when only the affluent (who preferred Landon) had a car or telephone. Thus, a large sample cannot correct for a faulty sampling design. Nevertheless, a large nonprobability sample is preferable to a small one.

Because practical constraints such as time and resources often limit sample size, many nursing studies are based on relatively small samples. Most nursing studies use samples of convenience, and many are based on samples that are too small to provide an adequate test of research hypotheses. Quantitative studies typically are based on samples of fewer than 200 participants, and many have fewer than 100 people (e.g., Polit & Gillespie, 2009). Power analysis is not routinely used by nurse researchers, and research reports often offer no justification for sample size. When samples are too small, quantitative researchers run the risk of gathering data that will not support their hypotheses,

even when their hypotheses are correct, thereby undermining statistical conclusion validity.

Factors Affecting Sample Size Requirements in Quantitative Research

Sample size requirements are affected by various factors, some of which we discuss in this section.

Effect Size

Power analysis builds on the concept of an **effect size**, which expresses the strength of relationships among research variables. If there is reason to expect that the independent and dependent variables will be strongly related, then a relatively small sample may be adequate to reveal the relationship statistically. For example, if we were testing a powerful new drug, it might be possible to demonstrate its effectiveness with a small sample. Typically, however, nursing interventions have small to moderate effects. When there is no *a priori* reason for believing that relationships will be strong, then small samples are risky.

Homogeneity of the Population

If the population is relatively homogeneous, a small sample may be adequate. The greater the variability, the greater is the risk that a small sample will not adequately capture the full range of variation. For most nursing studies, it is probably best to assume a fair degree of heterogeneity, unless there is evidence from prior research to the contrary.

Cooperation and Attrition

In most studies, not everyone invited to participate in a study agrees to do so. Therefore, in developing a sampling plan, it is good to begin with a realistic, evidence-based estimate of the percentage of people likely to cooperate. Thus, if your targeted sample size is 200 but you expect a 50% refusal rate, you would have to recruit about 400 eligible people.

In studies with multiple points of data collection, the number of participants usually declines over time. Attrition is most likely to occur if the time lag between data collection points is great, if the population is mobile, or if the population is at risk of death or disability. If the researcher has an ongoing relationship with participants, then attrition might be low—but it is rarely 0%. Therefore, in estimating sample size needs, researchers should factor in anticipated loss of participants over time.

Attrition problems are not restricted to longitudinal studies. People who initially agree to cooperate in a study may be subsequently unable or unwilling to participate for various reasons, such as death, deteriorating health, early discharge, discontinued need for an intervention, or simply a change of heart. Researchers should expect participant loss and recruit accordingly.

TIP: Polit and Gillespie (2009) found, in a sample of over 100 nursing RCTs, that the average participant loss was 12.5% for studies with follow-up data collection between 31 and 90 days after baseline and was 18% when the final data collection was more than 6 months after baseline.

Subgroup Analyses

Researchers sometimes wish to test hypotheses not only for an entire population but also for subgroups. For example, suppose we were interested

in assessing whether a structured exercise program is effective in improving infants' motor skills. We might also want to test whether the intervention is more effective for certain infants (e.g., low birth weight versus normal birth weight infants). When a sample is divided to test for **subgroup effects**, the sample must be large enough to support analyses with subsets of the sample.

IMPLEMENTING A QUANTITATIVE SAMPLING PLAN

This section provides some practical guidance about implementing a sampling plan.

Steps in Sampling in Quantitative Studies

The steps to be undertaken in drawing a sample vary somewhat from one sampling design to the next, but a general outline of procedures can be described.

1. *Identify the population.* You should begin with a clear idea about the target population to which you would like to generalize your results. Unless you have extensive resources, you are unlikely to have access to the full target population, so you will also need to identify the population that is accessible to you. Researchers sometimes *begin* by identifying an accessible population and then decide how best to characterize the target population.
2. *Specify the eligibility criteria.* The criteria for eligibility in the sample should then be spelled out. The criteria should be as specific as possible with regard to characteristics that might exclude potential participants (e.g., extremes of poor health, inability to read English). The criteria might lead you to redefine the target population.
3. *Specify the sampling plan.* Next, you must decide the method of drawing the sample and how large it will be. If you can perform a power analysis to estimate the needed number of participants, we highly recommend that you do so. Similarly, if probability sampling is a viable option, that option should be exercised. If you are not in a position to do either, we recommend using as large a sample as possible and

taking steps to build representativeness into the design (e.g., by using quota or consecutive sampling).

4. *Recruit the sample.* The next step is to recruit prospective participants (after any needed institutional permissions have been obtained) and ask for their cooperation. Issues relating to participant recruitment are discussed next.

Sample Recruitment

Recruiting people to participate in a study involves two major tasks: identifying eligible candidates and persuading them to participate. Researchers must consider the best sources for recruiting potential participants. Researchers must ask such questions as, Where do large numbers of people matching my population construct live or obtain care? Will I have direct access, or will I need to work through gatekeepers? Will there be sufficiently large numbers in one location, or will multiple sites be necessary? During the recruitment phase, it may be necessary to create a **screening instrument**, which is a brief form that allows researchers to determine whether a prospective participant meets the study's eligibility criteria.

The next task involves gaining the cooperation of people who have been deemed eligible. There is considerable evidence that the percentage of people willing to cooperate in clinical trials and surveys is declining, and so it is critical to have an effective recruitment strategy.

A lot of recent methodologic research in health fields has focused on strategies for effective recruitment. Researchers have found that rates of cooperation can often be enhanced by means of the following: face-to-face recruitment, multiple contacts and requests, monetary and nonmonetary incentives, brief data collection, inclusion of questions perceived as having high relevance to participants, assurances of anonymity, and endorsement of the study by a respected person or institution.

The supplement to Chapter 12 on the**Point** offers more detailed guidance on recruitment (and retention) strategies, with special emphasis on clinical trials and surveys. Also, the Toolkit of the accompanying *Resource Manual* for this chapter offers examples of recruitment materials.

➔ **TIP:** Participant recruitment often proceeds at a slower pace than researchers anticipate. Once you have determined your sample size needs, it is useful to develop contingency plans for recruiting more people, should the initial plan prove overly optimistic. For example, a contingency plan might involve relaxing the eligibility criteria, identifying another institution through which participants could be recruited, offering incentives to make participation more attractive, or lengthening the recruitment period. When such plans are developed at the outset, it reduces the likelihood that you will have to settle for a less-than-desirable sample size.

Generalizing from Samples

Ideally, the sample is representative of the accessible population, and the accessible population is representative of the target population. By using an appropriate sampling plan, researchers can be reasonably confident that the first part of this ideal has been realized. The second part of the ideal entails greater risk. Are diabetic patients in Boston representative of diabetic patients in the United States? Researchers must exercise judgment in assessing the degree of similarity.

The best advice is to be realistic and conservative and to ask challenging questions: Is it reasonable to assume that the accessible population is representative of the target population? In what ways might they differ? How would such differences affect the conclusions? If differences are great, it would be prudent to specify a more restricted target population to which the findings could be meaningfully generalized.

Interpretations about the generalizability of findings can be enhanced by comparing sample characteristics with population characteristics, when this is possible. Published information about the characteristics of many populations may be available to help in evaluating sampling bias. For example, if you were studying low-income children in Chicago, you could obtain information on the Internet about salient characteristics (e.g., race/ethnicity, age distribution) of low-income American children from the U.S. Census Bureau. Population characteristics could then be compared with sample characteristics and differences taken into account in interpreting the findings. Sousa and colleagues (2004) provide suggestions for drawing conclusions about whether a convenience sample is representative of the population.

> **Example of Comparing Sample and Population Characteristics:** Griffin and colleagues (2008) conducted a survey of over 300 pediatric nurses, whose names had been randomly sampled from a list of 9,000 nurses. Demographic characteristics of the sample (e.g., gender, race/ethnicity, education) were compared to characteristics of a nationally representative sample of nurses.

CRITIQUING SAMPLING PLANS

In coming to conclusions about the quality of evidence that a study yields, you should carefully scrutinize the sampling plan. If the sample is seriously biased or too small, the findings may be misleading or just plain wrong.

You should consider two issues in your critique of a study's sampling plan. The first is whether the researcher adequately described the sampling strategy. Ideally, research reports should include a description of the following:

- The type of sampling approach used (e.g., convenience, simple random)
- The study population and eligibility criteria for sample selection
- The number of participants and a rationale for the sample size, including whether a power analysis was performed
- A description of the main characteristics of sample members (e.g., age, gender, medical condition, etc.) and, ideally, of the population
- The number and characteristics of potential participants who declined to participate in the study

If the description of the sample is inadequate, you may not be able to come to conclusions about whether the researcher made good sampling decisions. And, if the description is incomplete, it will be difficult to know whether the evidence can be applied in your clinical practice.

Sampling plans should be scrutinized with respect to their effects on the construct, internal, external, and statistical conclusion validity of the study. If a sample is small, statistical conclusion validity will likely be undermined. If the eligibility criteria are restrictive, this could benefit internal validity—but possibly to the detriment of construct and external validity.

We have stressed that a key criterion for assessing the adequacy of a sampling plan in quantitative research is whether the sample is representative of the population. You will never know for sure, but if the sampling strategy is weak or if the sample size is small, there is reason to suspect some bias. When researchers adopt a sampling plan in which the risk for bias is high, they should take steps to estimate the direction and degree of this bias so that readers can draw some informed conclusions.

Even with a rigorous sampling plan, the sample may be biased if not all people invited to participate in a study agree to do so—which is almost always the case. If certain segments of the population refuse to participate, then a biased sample can result, even when probability sampling is used. Research reports should provide information about **response rates** (i.e., the number of people participating in a study relative to the number of people sampled) and about possible **nonresponse bias**—differences between participants and those who declined to participate (also sometimes referred to as *response bias*). In longitudinal studies, attrition bias should be reported.

Quantitative researchers make decisions about the specification of the population as well as the selection of the sample. If the target population is defined broadly, researchers may have missed opportunities to control confounding variables, and the gap between the accessible and the target population may be too great. One of your jobs as reviewer is to come to conclusions about the reasonableness of generalizing the findings from the researcher's sample to the accessible population and from the accessible population to a target population. If the sampling plan is seriously flawed, it may be risky to generalize the findings at all without replicating the study with another sample.

BOX 12.1 Guidelines for Critiquing Quantitative Sampling Designs

1. Is the study population identified and described? Are eligibility criteria specified? Are the sample selection procedures clearly delineated?
2. Do the sample and population specifications (eligibility criteria) support an inference of construct validity with regard to the population construct?
3. What type of sampling plan was used? Was the sampling plan one that could be expected to yield a representative sample? Would an alternative sampling plan have yielded a better sample?
4. If sampling was stratified, was a useful stratification variable selected? If a consecutive sample was used, was the time period long enough to address seasonal or temporal variation? In a multisite study, were sites selected in a manner that enhanced representativeness?
5. How were people recruited into the sample? Does the method suggest potential biases? Were efforts made to enhance rates of recruitment?
6. Is it likely that some factor other than the sampling plan (e.g., a low response rate, recruitment problems) affected the representativeness of the sample?
7. Are possible sample biases or other sampling deficiencies identified by the researchers?
8. Are key characteristics of the sample described (e.g., mean age, percentage of female)?
9. Is the sample size sufficiently large to support statistical conclusion validity? Was the sample size justified on the basis of a power analysis or other rationale?
10. Does the sample support inferences of external validity? To whom can the study results reasonably be generalized?

Box 12.1 presents some guiding questions for critiquing the sampling plan of a quantitative research report.

RESEARCH EXAMPLE

In this section, we describe in some detail the sampling plan of a quantitative nursing study.

Studies: Several studies using a data set created by Dr. Barbara A. Mark

Purpose: Barbara A. Mark, with funding from NINR, launched a large multisite study called the Outcomes Research in Nursing Administration Project-II (ORNA-II). The overall purpose was to investigate relationships of hospital context and structure on the one hand and patient, nurse, and organization outcomes on the other. Data from this project have been used in numerous studies, three of which are cited here.

Design: The project was designed as a prospective correlational study.

Plan: Sampling was multistaged. In the first stage, 146 acute care hospitals were randomly selected from

a list of hospitals accredited by The Joint Commission on Accreditation of Health Organizations. To be included, hospitals had to have at least 99 licensed beds. Hospitals were excluded if they were federal, for-profit, or psychiatric facilities. Then, from each selected hospital, two medical, surgical, or medical-surgical units were selected to participate in the study. Units were excluded if they were critical care, pediatric, obstetric, or psychiatric units. Among hospitals with only two eligible units, both participated. Among hospitals with more than two eligible units, an on-site study coordinator selected two to participate. Ultimately, 281 nursing units in 143 hospitals participated in the study. Data from each hospital were gathered in three rounds of data collection over a 6-month period. On each participating unit, all RNs with more than 3 months of experience on that unit were asked to respond to three sets of questionnaires. The response rates were 75% of nurses at Time 1 (4,911 nurses), 58% at Time 2 (3,689 nurses), and 53% at Time 3 (3,272 nurses). Patients were also invited to participate at Time 3. Ten patients on each unit were randomly selected to complete a questionnaire. Patients were included if they were 18 years of age or older, had been hospitalized for at least 48 hours, were able to speak and read English, and were not scheduled for immediate discharge. A total of 2,720 patients participated, and the response rate was 91%.

Key Findings:

- In an analysis focusing on errors, it was found that nurses in Magnet hospitals were more likely to communicate about errors and participate in error-related problem solving than those in non-Magnet hospitals (Hughes et al., 2012).
- In an analysis of nurses' job satisfaction, a positive relationship was found between racial/ethnic workplace diversity among nurses and nurses' job satisfaction (Gates & Mark, 2012).
- In an analysis of medication errors, nursing units with a strong learning climate were found to have fewer errors (Chang & Mark, 2011).

SUMMARY POINTS

- **Sampling** is the process of selecting a portion of the **population**, which is an entire aggregate of cases, for a study. An **element** is the most basic population unit about which information is collected—usually humans in nursing research.
- **Eligibility criteria** are used to establish population characteristics and to determine who can participate in a study—either who can be included (**inclusion criteria**) or who should be excluded (**exclusion criteria**).
- Researchers usually sample from an **accessible population** but should identify the **target population** to which they want to generalize their results.
- A sample in a quantitative study is assessed in terms of **representativeness**—the extent to which the sample is similar to the population and avoids bias. **Sampling bias** refers to the systematic over- or underrepresentation of some segment of the population.
- Methods of **nonprobability sampling** (wherein elements are selected by nonrandom methods) include convenience, quota, consecutive, and purposive sampling. Nonprobability sampling designs are practical but usually have strong potential for bias.

- **Convenience sampling** uses the most readily available or convenient group of people for the sample. **Snowball sampling** is a type of convenience sampling in which referrals for potential participants are made by those already in the sample.
- **Quota sampling** divides the population into homogeneous **strata** (subpopulations) to ensure representation of subgroups; within each stratum, people are sampled by convenience.
- **Consecutive sampling** involves taking *all* of the people from an accessible population who meet the eligibility criteria over a specific time interval, or for a specified sample size.
- In **purposive sampling**, elements are hand-picked to be included in the sample based on the researcher's knowledge about the population.
- **Probability sampling** designs, which involve the random selection of elements from the population, yield more representative samples than nonprobability designs and permit estimates of the magnitude of **sampling error**.
- **Simple random sampling** involves the random selection of elements from a **sampling frame** that enumerates all the population elements; **stratified random sampling** divides the population into homogeneous strata from which elements are selected at random.
- **Cluster sampling** involves sampling of large units. In **multistage random sampling**, there is a successive, multistaged selection of random samples from larger units (clusters) to smaller units (individuals) by either simple random or stratified random methods.
- **Systematic sampling** is the selection of every *k*th case from a list. By dividing the population size by the desired sample size, the researcher establishes the **sampling interval**, which is the standard distance between the selected elements.
- In quantitative studies, researchers should use a **power analysis** to estimate **sample size** needs. Large samples are preferable to small ones because larger samples enhance statistical conclusion validity and tend to be more representative, but even large samples do not *guarantee* representativeness.

STUDY ACTIVITIES

Chapter 12 of the *Resource Manual for Nursing Research: Generating and Assessing Evidence for Nursing Practice, 10th edition,* offers exercises and study suggestions for reinforcing concepts presented in this chapter. In addition, the following study questions can be addressed:

1. Answer relevant questions from Box 12.1 with regard to sampling plan for the ORNA studies, described at the end of the chapter. Also consider the following additional questions: (a) How many stages would you say were involved in the sampling plan? (b) What are some of the likely sources of sampling bias in the final sample of 3,272 nurses?

2. Use the table of random numbers in Table 9.2 to select 10 names from the list of people in Table 12.3. How many names did you draw from the first 25 names and from the second 25 names?

STUDIES CITED IN CHAPTER 12

Balzer, K., Kremer, L., Junghans, A., Halfens, R., Dassen, T., & Kottner, J. (2014). What patient characteristics guide nurses' clinical judgement on pressure ulcer risk? A mixed methods study. *International Journal of Nursing Studies, 51,* 703–716.

*Chang, Y., & Mark, B. A. (2011). Effects of learning climate and registered nurse staffing on medication errors. *Nursing Research, 60,* 32–39.

Cohen, J. (1988). *Statistical power analysis for the behavioral sciences* (2nd ed.). Hillsdale, NJ: Lawrence Erlbaum Associates.

de Gouveia Santos, V. L., de Cássia Domansky, R., Hanate, C., Matos, D., Benvenuto, C., & Jorge, J. (2014). Self-reported fecal incontinence in a community-dwelling, urban population in southern Brazil. *Journal of Wound, Ostomy, & Continence Nursing, 41,* 77–83.

*Gates, M. G., & Mark, B. A. (2012). Demographic diversity, value congruence, and workplace outcomes in acute care. *Research in Nursing & Health, 35,* 265–276.

Griffin, R., Polit, D., & Byrne, M. (2008). Nurse characteristics and inferences about children's pain. *Pediatric Nursing, 34,* 297–305.

Hewitt, C., & Cappiello, J. (2015). Essential competencies in nursing education for prevention and care related to unintended pregnancy. *Journal of Obstetric, Gynecologic & Neonatal Nursing, 44,* 69–76.

Hughes, L., Chang, Y., & Mark, B. (2012). Quality and strength of patient safety climate on medical-surgical units. *Journal of Nursing Administration, 42,* S27–S36.

Krueger, C., Cave, E., & Garvan, C. (2015). Fetal response to live and recorded maternal speech. *Biological Research for Nursing, 17,* 112–120.

Lam, S., Lee, L., Wong, S., & Wong, A. (2012). Pedometer-determined physical activity and body composition in Chinese working adults. *Journal of Nursing Scholarship, 44,* 205–214.

LoBiondo-Wood, G., Brown, C., Knobf, M., Lyon, D., Mallory, G., Mitchell, S., . . . Fellman, B. (2014). Priorities for oncology nursing research: The 2013 national survey. *Oncology Nursing Forum, 41,* 67–76.

Magnani, R., Sabin, K., Saidel, T., & Heckathorn, D. (2005). Review of sampling hard-to-reach and hidden populations for HIV surveillance. *AIDS, 19,* S67–S72.

*McCreesh, N., Frost, S., Seeley, J., Katongole, J., Tarsh, M., Ndunguse, R., . . . White, R. G. (2012). Evaluation of respondent-driven sampling. *Epidemiology, 23,* 138–147.

Polit, D. F. (2010). *Statistics and data analysis for nursing research* (2nd ed.). Upper Saddle River, NJ: Pearson.

Polit, D. F., & Beck, C. T. (2010). Generalization in qualitative and quantitative research: Myths and strategies. *International Journal of Nursing Studies, 47,* 1451–1458.

Polit, D. F., & Gillespie, B. (2009). The use of the intention-to-treat principle in nursing clinical trials. *Nursing Research, 58,* 391–399.

Ridout, J., Aucoin, J., Browning, A., Piedra, K., & Weeks, S. (2014). Does perioperative documentation transfer reliably? *Computers, Informatics, Nursing, 32,* 37–42.

Schallom, M., Orr, J., Metheny, N., Kirby, J., & Pierce, J. (2015). Gastric reflux: Association with aspiration and oral secretion pH as marker of reflux. *Dimensions of Critical Care Nursing, 34,* 84–90.

Scott, L. D., Arslanian-Engoren, C., & Engoren, M. (2014). Association of sleep and fatigue with decision regret among critical care nurses. *American Journal of Critical Care, 23,* 13–23.

Sousa, V., Zauszniewski, J., & Musil, C. (2004). How to determine whether a convenience sample represents the population. *Applied Nursing Research, 17,* 130–133.

Thompson, S. K. (2012). *Sampling* (3rd ed.). New York: Wiley.

***A link to this open-access journal article is provided in the Toolkit for this chapter in the accompanying* Resource Manual.**

13 | Data Collection in Quantitative Research

Both the study participants and those collecting the data are constrained during the collection of structured quantitative data. The goal is to achieve consistency in what is asked and how answers are reported, in an effort to reduce biases and facilitate analysis. Major methods of collecting structured data are discussed in this chapter. We begin by discussing broad planning issues.

DEVELOPING A DATA COLLECTION PLAN

Data collection plans for quantitative studies ideally yield accurate, valid, and meaningful data. This is a challenging goal, typically requiring considerable time and effort to achieve. Steps in developing a data collection plan are described in this section. (A flowchart illustrating the sequence of steps is available in the Toolkit of the accompanying *Resource Manual*.)

Identifying Data Needs

Researchers usually begin by identifying the types of data needed for their study. In quantitative studies, researchers may need data for the following purposes:

1. *Testing hypotheses, addressing research questions.* Researchers must include one or more measures of all key variables. Multiple measures of some variables may be needed if a variable is complex or if there is an interest in corroboration.

2. *Describing the sample.* Information should be gathered about major demographic and health characteristics. We advise gathering data about participants' age, gender, race or ethnicity, and education (or income). This information is critical in interpreting results and understanding the population to whom findings can be generalized. If the sample includes participants with a health problem, data on the nature of that problem also should be gathered (e.g., severity, treatments, time since diagnosis).

> **TIP:** Asking demographic questions in the right way is more difficult than you might think. Because the need to collect information about sample characteristics is nearly universal, we have included a demographic form and guidelines in the Toolkit of the accompanying *Resource Manual*. The demographic questionnaire can be adapted as needed.

3. *Controlling confounding variables.* Several approaches to controlling confounding variables require measuring those variables. For example, for analysis of covariance, variables that are statistically controlled must be measured.

4. *Analyzing potential biases.* Data that can help to identify potential biases should be collected. For example, researchers should gather information that would help them understand selection or attrition biases.

5. *Understanding subgroup effects.* It is often desirable to answer research questions for key subgroups of participants. For example, we may wish to know if a special intervention for pregnant women is equally effective for primiparas and multiparas. In such a situation, we would need to collect data about the participants' childbearing history.

6. *Interpreting results.* Researchers should try to anticipate alternative results and then consider what types of data would help in interpreting them. For example, if we hypothesized that the presence of school-based clinics in high schools would lower the incidence of sexually transmitted diseases among students but found that the incidence remained constant after the clinic opened, what type of information would help us interpret this result (e.g., information about the students' frequency of intercourse, number of partners, and so on)?

7. *Assessing treatment fidelity.* In intervention studies, it is useful to monitor treatment fidelity and to assess whether the intended treatment was actually received.

8. *Assessing costs.* In intervention studies, information about costs and financial benefits of alternative treatments is often useful.

9. *Obtaining administrative information.* It is usually necessary to gather administrative data—for example, dates of data collection and contact information in longitudinal studies.

The list of possible data needs may seem daunting, but many categories overlap. For example, participant characteristics for sample description are often useful for bias analysis, for controlling confounders, or for creating subgroups. If resource constraints make it impossible to collect the full range of variables, then researchers must prioritize data needs.

➔ TIP: In prioritizing data needs, it may be useful to develop a matrix so that data collection decisions can be made in a systematic way. Such a matrix can help to identify "holes" and redundancies. A partial example of such a matrix is included in the Toolkit of the *Resource Manual* for you to use and adapt.

Selecting Types of Measures

After data needs have been identified, the next step is to select a data collection method (e.g., self-report, records) for each variable. It is not unusual to combine self-reports, observations, physiologic, or records data in a single study.

Data collection decisions must also be guided by ethical considerations (e.g., whether covert data collection is warranted), cost constraints, availability of assistants to help with data collection, and other issues discussed in the next section. Data collection is often the costliest and most time-consuming portion of a study. Because of this, researchers often have to make a few compromises about the type or amount of data collected.

Selecting and Developing Instruments

Once preliminary data collection decisions have been made, researchers should determine if there are instruments available for measuring study variables, as will often be the case. Potential data collection **instruments** should then be assessed. The primary consideration is conceptual relevance: Does the instrument correspond to your conceptual definition of the variable? Another important criterion is whether the instrument will yield high-quality data. Approaches to evaluating data quality of quantitative measures are discussed in Chapter 14. Additional factors that may affect decisions in selecting an instrument are as follows:

1. *Resources.* Resource constraints sometimes prevent the use of the highest quality measures. There may be some direct costs associated with the measure (e.g., some scales must be purchased), but the biggest expense is for compensating the people collecting the data if you cannot do it single-handedly. In such a situation, the instrument's length may determine whether it is a viable option. Also, it is often advantageous to pay a participant stipend to encourage participation. Data collection costs should be carefully considered, especially if the use of expensive methods means that you will be forced to cut costs elsewhere (e.g., using a smaller sample).

2. *Availability and familiarity.* You may need to consider how readily available various instruments are. Data collection strategies with which

you have had experience are often preferable to new ones because administration is usually smoother and more efficient in such cases.

3. *Population appropriateness*. Instruments must be chosen with the characteristics of the target population in mind. Characteristics of special importance include participants' age and literacy levels. If there is concern about participants' reading skills, the *readability* of a prospective instrument should be assessed. If participants include members of minority groups, you should strive to find instruments that are culturally appropriate. If non-English-speaking participants are included in the sample, then the selection of an instrument may be based on the availability of a translated version.

4. *Norms and comparisons*. It may be desirable to select an instrument that has relevant norms. **Norms** indicate the "normal" values on the measure for a specified population and thus offer a good comparison. Also, it may be advantageous to select an instrument because it was used in other similar studies to facilitate interpretation of study findings.

5. *Administration issues*. Some instruments have special requirements. For example, obtaining information about the developmental status of children may require the skills of a professional psychologist. Some instruments require stringent conditions with regard to the time of administration, privacy of the setting, and so on. In such a case, requirements for obtaining valid measures must match attributes of the research setting.

6. *Reputation*. Instruments designed to measure the same construct often differ in the reputation they enjoy among specialists in a field, even if they are comparable with regard to documented quality. Thus, it may be useful to seek the advice of knowledgeable people, preferably ones with personal, direct experience using the instruments.

If existing instruments are not suitable for some variables, you may be faced with either adapting an instrument or developing a new one. Creating a new instrument should be a last resort, especially for novice researchers, because it is challenging to develop accurate and valid measuring tools (see Chapter 15).

If you are fortunate to locate a suitable instrument, your next step likely will be to obtain the authors' permission to use it. In general, copyrighted materials require permission. Instruments that have been developed under a government grant are often in the public domain and may not require permission. When in doubt, it is best to obtain permission. By contacting the instrument's author for permission, you can also request more information about the instrument and its quality. (A sample letter requesting permission to use an instrument is in the Toolkit. 💿)

→ **TIP:** In finalizing decisions about instruments, it may be necessary to consider the trade-offs between data quality and data quantity (i.e., the number of instruments or questions). If compromises have to be made, it is usually preferable to forego quantity—especially because long instruments tend to depress participant cooperation.

Pretesting the Data Collection Package

Researchers who develop a new instrument usually subject it to rigorous **pretesting** so that it can be evaluated and refined. Even when the data collection plan involves existing instruments, however, it is wise to conduct a pretest with a small sample of people (usually 10 to 20) who are similar to actual participants.

One purpose of a pretest is to see how much time it takes to administer the entire instrument package. Typically, researchers use multiple instruments and it may be difficult to estimate how long it will take to administer the complete set. Time estimates are often required for informed consent purposes, for developing a budget, and for assessing participant burden.

Pretests can serve many other purposes, including the following:

- Identifying parts of the instrument package that are hard for participants to read or understand
- Identifying questions that participants find objectionable or offensive
- Assessing whether the sequencing of questions or instruments is sensible
- Evaluating training needs for data collectors
- Evaluating whether the measures yield data with sufficient variability

With regard to the last purpose, researchers need to ensure that there is sufficient variation on key variables with the instruments they select. In a study of the link between depression and a miscarriage, for example, depression would be compared for women who had or had not experienced a miscarriage. If the entire pretest sample looks very depressed (or not at all depressed), however, it may be advisable to pretest a different measure of depression.

Example of Pretesting: Nyamathi and colleagues (2012) studied the factors associated with depressive symptoms in a sample of 156 homeless young adults. The study involved collecting an extensive array of data via self-reports. All of the instruments had been previously tested, modified, and validated for homeless populations, including pretests to evaluate clarity and sensitivity to the population.

Developing Data Collection Forms and Procedures

After the instrument package is finalized, researchers face several administrative tasks, such as the development of various forms (e.g., screening forms to assess eligibility, informed consent forms, records of attempted contacts with participants). It is prudent to design forms that are attractively formatted, legible, and inviting to use, especially if they are to be used by participants themselves. Care should also be taken to design forms to ensure confidentiality. For example, identifying information (e.g., names, addresses) is often recorded on a page that can be detached and kept separate from other data.

→ TIP: Whenever possible, try to avoid reinventing the wheel. It is inefficient and unnecessary to start from scratch—not only in developing instruments but also in creating forms, training materials, and so on. Ask seasoned researchers if they have materials you could borrow or adapt.

In most quantitative studies, researchers develop **data collection protocols** that spell out procedures

to be used in data collection. These protocols describe such things as the following:

- Conditions for collecting the data (e.g., Can others be present during data collection? Where must data collection occur?)
- Specific procedures for collecting the data, including requirements for sequencing instruments and recording information
- Information for participants who ask routine questions about the study (i.e., answers to FAQs). Examples include the following: How will the information from this study be used? How did you get my name? How long will this take? Who will have access to this information? Can I see the study results? Whom can I contact if I have a complaint? Will I be paid or reimbursed for expenses?
- Procedures to follow in the event that a participant becomes distraught or disoriented or for any other reason cannot complete the data collection

Researchers also need to decide how to actually gather, record, and manage their data. Technologic advances continue to offer new options—some of which we discuss later in the chapter. Some suggestions about new technology for data collection are offered by Courtney and Craven (2005), Guadagno et al. (2004), and Hardwick et al. (2007).

→ TIP: Document all major actions and decisions as you develop and implement your data collection plan. You may need the information later when you write your research report, request funding for a follow-up study, or help other researchers with a similar study.

STRUCTURED SELF-REPORT INSTRUMENTS

The most widely used data collection method by nurse researchers is structured self-report, which involves a formal instrument. The instrument is an **interview schedule** when questions are asked orally in face-to-face or telephone interviews. It is called a **questionnaire** or an SAQ (self-administered questionnaire) when respondents complete the instrument themselves, either in a paper-and-pencil format or on a computer. This section discusses the development and administration of structured self-report instruments.

Types of Structured Questions

Structured instruments consist of a set of questions (often called **items**) in which the wording of both the questions and, in most cases, **response options** are predetermined. Participants are asked to respond to the same questions, in the same order, and with a fixed set of response options. Researchers developing structured instruments must devote careful effort to the content, form, and wording of questions.

Open and Closed Questions

Structured instruments vary in degree of structure through different combinations of open-ended and closed-ended questions. **Open-ended questions** allow people to respond in their own words, in narrative fashion. The question "What was your biggest challenge after your surgery?" is an example of an open-ended question. In questionnaires, respondents are asked to give a written reply to open-ended items, and so adequate space must be provided to permit a full response. Interviewers are expected to quote oral responses verbatim or as closely as possible.

Closed-ended (or *fixed-alternative*) **questions** offer response options, from which respondents choose the one that most closely matches the appropriate answer. The alternatives may range from a simple *yes* or *no* ("Have you smoked a cigarette within the past 24 hours?") to complex expressions of opinion or behavior.

Both open- and closed-ended questions have certain strengths and weaknesses. Good closed-ended items are often difficult to construct but easy to administer and, especially, to analyze. With closed-ended questions, researchers need only tabulate the number of responses to each alternative to gain descriptive information. The analysis of open-ended items is more difficult and time-consuming. The usual procedure is to develop categories and code open-ended responses into the categories. That is, researchers essentially transform open-ended

responses to fixed categories in a post hoc fashion so that tabulations can be made.

Closed-ended items are more efficient than open-ended questions, that is, respondents can answer more closed- than open-ended questions in a given amount of time. In questionnaires, participants may be less willing to compose written responses than to check off a response alternative. Closed-ended items are also preferred if respondents are unable to express themselves well verbally. Furthermore, some questions are less intrusive in closed form than in open form. Take the following example:

1. What was your family's total annual income last year?
2. In what range was your family's total annual income last year?
   - ❏ 1. Under $50,000,
   - ❏ 2. $50,000 to $99,999, or
   - ❏ 3. $100,000 or more

The second question gives respondents greater privacy than the open-ended question and is less likely to go unanswered.

A drawback of closed-ended questions is the risk of failing to include key responses. Such omissions can lead to inadequate understanding of the issues or to outright bias if respondents choose an alternative that misrepresents their position. Another objection to closed-ended items is that they tend to be superficial. Open-ended questions allow for a richer and fuller perspective on a topic, if respondents are verbally expressive and cooperative. Some of this richness may be lost when researchers tabulate answers they have categorized, but direct excerpts from open-ended responses can be valuable in imparting the flavor of the replies. Finally, some people object to being forced to choose from response options that do not reflect their opinions well. Open-ended questions give freedom to respondents and, therefore, offer the possibility of spontaneity and elaboration.

Decisions about the mix of open- and closed-ended questions are based on such considerations as the sensitivity of the questions, respondents' verbal ability, and the amount of time available. Combinations of both types can be used to offset the strengths and weaknesses of each. Questionnaires typically use closed-ended questions primarily, to minimize respondents' writing burden. Interview schedules, on the other hand, tend to be more variable in their mixture of these two question types.

Specific Types of Closed-Ended Questions

The analytic advantages of closed-ended questions are often compelling. Various types of closed-ended questions, illustrated in Table 13.1, are described here.

- **Dichotomous questions** require respondents to make a choice between two response alternatives, such as yes/no or male/female. Dichotomous questions are especially useful for gathering factual information.

- **Multiple-choice questions** offer three or more response alternatives. Graded alternatives are preferable to dichotomous items for attitude questions because researchers get more information (intensity as well as direction of opinion).

- **Rank-order questions** ask respondents to rank concepts along a continuum, such as most to least important. Respondents are asked to assign a 1 to the concept that is most important,

TABLE 13.1 • Examples of Closed-Ended Questions

QUESTION TYPE	EXAMPLE
1. Dichotomous question	Have you ever been pregnant? 1. Yes 2. No
2. Multiple-choice question	How important is it to you to avoid a pregnancy at this time? 1. Extremely important 2. Very important 3. Somewhat important 4. Not important
3. Rank-order question	People value different things in life. Below is a list of things that many people value. Please indicate their order of importance to you by placing a "1" beside the most important, "2" beside the second-most important, and so on. ____ Career achievement/work ____ Family relationships ____ Friendships, social interactions ____ Health ____ Money ____ Religion
4. Forced-choice question	Which statement most closely represents your point of view? 1. What happens to me is my own doing. 2. Sometimes I feel I don't have enough control over my life.
5. Rating question	On a scale from 0 to 10, where 0 means "extremely dissatisfied" and 10 means "extremely satisfied," how satisfied were you with the nursing care you received during your hospitalization? 0 1 2 3 4 5 6 7 8 9 10 Extremely Extremely dissatisfied satisfied

a 2 to the concept that is second in importance, and so on. Rank-order questions can be useful, but some respondents misunderstand them so good instructions are needed. Rank-order questions should involve 10 or fewer rankings.

• **Forced-choice questions** require respondents to choose between two statements that represent polar positions.

• **Rating scale questions** ask respondents to evaluate something on an ordered dimension. Rating questions are typically on a **bipolar scale**, with end points specifying opposite extremes on a continuum. The end points and sometimes intermediary points along the scale are verbally labeled. The number of gradations or points along the scale can vary but often is an odd number, such as 5, 7, 9, or 11, to allow for a neutral midpoint. (In the example in Table 13.1, the rating question has 11 points, numbered 0 to 10.)

• **Checklists** include several questions with the same response options. A checklist is a two-dimensional matrix in which a series of questions is listed on one dimension (usually vertically) and response options are listed on the other. Checklists are relatively efficient and easy to understand, but because they are difficult to read orally, they are used more frequently in SAQs than in interviews. Figure 13.1 presents an example of a checklist.

• **Visual analog scales** (VASs) are used to measure subjective experiences, such as pain, fatigue, and dyspnea. The VAS is a straight line, the end anchors of which are labeled as the extreme limits of the sensation or feeling being measured. People are asked to mark a point on the line corresponding to the amount of sensation experienced. Traditionally, the VAS line is 100 mm in length, which facilitates the derivation of a score from 0 to 100 through simple measurement of the distance from one end of the scale to the person's mark on the line. An example of a VAS is shown in Figure 13.2.

Researchers sometimes collect information about activities and dates using an **event history calendar** (Martyn & Belli, 2002). Such calendars are matrixes that plot time on one dimension (usually horizontally) and events or activities on the other. The person recording the data (either the participant or an interviewer) draws lines to indicate the stop and start dates of the specified events or behaviors. Event history calendars are especially useful in collecting information about the occurrence and sequencing of events retrospectively. Data quality about past occurrences is enhanced because the calendar helps participants relate the timing of some events to the timing of others. An example of an event history calendar is included in the Toolkit section of the accompanying *Resource Manual*.

An alternative to collecting event history data retrospectively is to ask participants to maintain information in an ongoing structured **diary** over a specified time period. This approach is often used to collect quantitative information about sleeping, eating, or exercise behavior.

The next question is about things that may have happened to you personally. Please indicate how recently, if ever, these things happened to you:

	Yes, within past 12 months	Yes, 2–3 years ago	Yes, more than 3 years ago	No, never
a. Has someone ever yelled at you all the time or put you down on purpose?	1	2	3	4
b. Has someone ever tried to control your every move?	1	2	3	4
c. Has someone ever threatened you with physical harm?	1	2	3	4
d. Has someone ever hit, slapped, kicked, or physically harmed you?	1	2	3	4

FIGURE 13.1 Example of a checklist (matrix question).

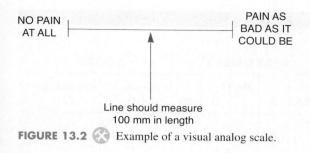

FIGURE 13.2 ⚙ Example of a visual analog scale.

Example of a Structured Diary: Oliva and colleagues (2014) studied nausea, vomiting, and well-being following chemotherapy in women with breast cancer. A structured 10-day diary of symptoms and experiences was used to collect the data.

Composite Scales and Other Structured Self-Reports

Several special types of structured self-reports are used by nurse researchers. The most important are *composite multi-item scales*. A **scale** provides a numeric score to place respondents on a continuum with respect to an attribute, such as a scale for measuring people's weight. Scales are used to discriminate quantitatively among people with different attitudes, symptoms, conditions, and needs. In the medical literature, when there is reference to a *patient-reported outcome* (PRO), it is usually about a self-report scale.

Likert-Type Summated Rating Scales

A widely used scaling technique is the **Likert scale**, named after the psychologist Rensis Likert. A traditional Likert scale consists of several declarative items that express a viewpoint on a topic. Respondents are asked to indicate the degree to which they agree or disagree with the opinion expressed by the statement.

Table 13.2 illustrates a 6-item Likert-type scale for measuring attitudes toward condom use. Likert-type scales often include more than six items; the example in Table 13.2 is shown to illustrate key features. After respondents complete a Likert scale, their responses are scored. Typically, agreement with positively worded statements and disagreement with negatively worded ones are assigned higher scores. (See Chapter 15, however, for a discussion of

problems in including both positive and negative items on a scale.) The first statement in Table 13.2 is positively worded; agreement indicates a favorable attitude toward condom use. Thus, a higher score would be assigned to those agreeing with this statement than to those disagreeing with it. With five response options, a score of 5 would be given to those strongly agreeing, 4 to those agreeing, and so forth. The responses of two hypothetical respondents are shown by a check or an X, and their scores are shown in far right columns. Person 1, who agreed with the first statement, has a score of 4, whereas person 2, who strongly disagreed, has a score of 1. The second statement is negatively worded, and so scoring is reversed—a 1 is assigned to those who strongly agree, and so on. This reversal is needed so that a high score consistently reflects positive attitudes toward condom use. A person's total score is computed by adding together individual item scores. Such scales are often called **summated rating scales** because of this feature. The total scores of both respondents are shown at the bottom of Table 13.2. The scores reflect a much more positive attitude toward condoms for person 1 than person 2.

The summation feature of such scales makes it possible to make fine discriminations among people with different points of view. A single question allows people to be put into only five categories. A 6-item scale, such as the one in Table 13.2, permits finer gradation—from a minimum possible score of 6 (6×1) to a maximum possible score of 30 (6×5).

Summated rating scales can be used to measure a wide array of attributes. In such cases, the bipolar scale usually is not on an agree/disagree continuum but might be always/never, likely/unlikely, and so on. Constructing a good summated rating scale requires considerable skill and work. Chapter 15 describes the steps involved in developing and testing such scales.

Example of a Likert Scale: Ranse and colleagues (2015) studied factors influencing the provision of end-of-life care in critical care settings and created a 58-question Likert-type scale. Examples of statements include the following: "Patients at the end-of-life require little nursing care" and "I feel a sense of personal failure when a patient dies." Responses were on a 5-point scale: strongly disagree, disagree, neutral, agree, strongly agree.

TABLE 13.2 • Example of a Likert Scale

| DIRECTION OF SCORING* | ITEM | RESPONSES† | | | | | SCORE | |
		SA	A	?	D	SD	Person 1 (✔)	Person 2 (✕)
+	1. Using a condom shows you care about your partner.		✔			✕	4	1
−	2. My partner would be angry if I talked about using condoms.			✕		✔	5	3
−	3. I wouldn't enjoy sex as much if my partner and I used condoms.			✕	✔		4	2
+	4. Condoms are a good protection against AIDS and other sexually transmitted diseases.			✔	✕		3	2
+	5. My partner would respect me if I insisted on using condoms.	✔				✕	5	1
−	6. I would be too embarrassed to ask my partner about using a condom.			✕		✔	5	2
	Total score						26	11

*Researchers would not indicate the direction of scoring on a Likert scale administered to study participants. The scoring direction is indicated in this table for illustrative purposes only.
†SA, strongly agree; A, agree; ?, uncertain; D, disagree; SD, strongly disagree.

> **TIP:** Most nurse researchers use existing scales rather than developing their own. Some websites for finding scales are included in the Toolkit. Another place to look for existing instruments is in the Health and Psychosocial Instruments (HaPI) database. Increasingly, there are also systematic reviews of instruments for specific constructs in the health care literature.

Cognitive and Neuropsychological Tests

Nurse researchers sometimes assess study participants' cognitive skills by asking questions. There are several different types of **cognitive tests**. For example, *intelligence tests* evaluate a person's global ability to solve problems and *aptitude tests* measure a person's potential for achievement. Nurse researchers are most likely to use ability tests in studies of high-risk groups, such as low birth weight children.

Some cognitive tests are specially designed to assess neuropsychological functioning among people with potential cognitive impairments, such as the Mini-Mental Status Examination (MMSE). These tests capture varying types of competence, such as the ability to concentrate and the ability to remember. Nurses have used such tests extensively in studies of elderly patients. A good source for learning more about ability tests is the book by the Buros Institute (Carlson et al., 2014).

Example of a Study Assessing Neuropsychological Function: Tappen and Hain (2014) tested the effect of in-home cognitive training on the functional performance of individuals with mild cognitive impairment. They used several cognitive tests, including the MMSE and the Fuld Object Memory Evaluation.

Other Types of Structured Self-Reports

Nurse researchers have used a few other types of structured self-report instruments but with lower frequency. A brief description of these data collection methods is offered here, and further information is presented in the Supplement to this chapter on thePoint®. 🔵

- **Semantic differential (SD) scales** are another technique for measuring attitudes. With the SD, respondents are asked to rate concepts (e.g., dieting, exercise) on a series of *bipolar adjectives*, such as good/bad, effective/ineffective, important/unimportant.
- **Q sorts** present participants with a set of cards on which statements are written. Participants are asked to sort the cards along a specified dimension, such as most helpful/least helpful, never true/always true.
- **Vignettes** are brief descriptions of events or situations (fictitious or actual) to which respondents are asked to react and provide information about how they would handle the situation described.
- **Ecologic momentary assessments (EMA)** involves repeated assessments of people's current behaviors, feelings, and experiences in real time, within their natural environment, using contemporary technologies such as text messaging.

Questionnaires versus Interviews

In developing their data collection plans, researchers need to decide whether to collect self-report data through interviews or questionnaires. Each method has advantages and disadvantages.

Advantages of Questionnaires

Self-administered questionnaires, which can be distributed in person, by mail, on a tablet, or over the Internet, offer some advantages. The strengths of questionnaires include the following:

- *Cost.* Questionnaires, relative to interviews, are much less costly. Distributing questionnaires to groups (e.g., nursing home residents) is inexpensive and expedient. And, with a fixed amount of funds or time, a larger and more geographically diverse sample can be obtained with mailed or Internet questionnaires than with interviews.
- *Anonymity.* Unlike interviews, questionnaires offer the possibility of complete anonymity. A guarantee of anonymity can be crucial in obtaining candid responses if questions are sensitive. Anonymous questionnaires often result in a higher proportion of responses revealing socially undesirable viewpoints or behaviors than interviews.
- *Interviewer bias.* The absence of an interviewer ensures that there will be no interviewer bias. Interviewers ideally are neutral agents through whom questions and answers are passed. Studies have shown, however, that this ideal is difficult to achieve. Respondents and interviewers interact as humans, and this interaction can affect responses.

Internet data collection is especially economical and can yield a data set directly amenable to analysis, without requiring someone to enter data onto a file (the same is also true for computer-assisted personal and telephone interviews, i.e., CAPI and CATI). Internet surveys also provide opportunities for providing participants with customized feedback and for prompts that can minimize missing responses.

Advantages of Interviews

It is true that interviews are costly, prevent anonymity, and bear the risk of interviewer bias. Nevertheless, interviews are considered superior to questionnaires for most research purposes because of the following advantages:

- *Response rates.* Response rates tend to be high in face-to-face interviews. People are less likely to refuse to talk to an interviewer who solicits their cooperation than to ignore a mailed questionnaire or an e-mail. A well-designed interview study normally achieves response rates in the vicinity of 80% to 90%, whereas mailed and Internet questionnaires typically achieve response rates of less than 50%. Because nonresponse is not random, low response rates can introduce bias. However, if questionnaires are personally distributed in a particular setting—for example, to patients in a cardiac rehabilitation program—reasonably good response rates often can be achieved. (S) (The Supplement to Chapter 12 on thePoint® reviews evidence on strategies to enhance response rates in mail and Internet surveys.)

- *Audience.* Many people cannot fill out a questionnaire. Examples include young children and blind, elderly, illiterate, or uneducated individuals. Interviews, on the other hand, are feasible with most people. For Internet questionnaires, an important drawback is that not everyone has access to computers or uses them regularly—but this problem is declining.
- *Clarity.* Interviews offer some protection against ambiguous or confusing questions. Interviewers can provide needed clarifications. With questionnaires, misinterpreted questions can go undetected.
- *Depth of questioning.* Information obtained from questionnaires tends to be more superficial than from interviews, largely because questionnaires usually contain mostly closed-ended items. Open-ended questions are avoided in questionnaires because most people dislike having to compose a reply. Furthermore, interviewers can enhance the quality of self-report data through *probing*, a topic we discuss later in this chapter.
- *Missing information.* Respondents are less likely to give "don't know" responses or to leave a question unanswered in an interview than on a questionnaire.
- *Order of questions.* In an interview, researchers have control over question ordering. Questionnaire respondents can skip around from one section to another—although this can be prevented in Internet questionnaires. A different ordering of questions from the one intended could bias responses.
- *Supplementary data.* Face-to-face interviews can yield additional data through observation. Inter-

viewers can observe and assess respondents' level of understanding, degree of cooperativeness, living conditions, and so forth. Such information can be useful in interpreting responses.

Some advantages of face-to-face interviews also apply to telephone interviews. Long or detailed interviews or ones with sensitive questions are not well suited to telephone administration, but for relatively brief instruments, telephone interviews are economical and tend to yield a higher response rate than mailed or Internet questionnaires.

Designing Structured Self-Report Instruments

Assembling a high-quality structured self-report instrument is challenging. To design useful instruments, researchers must carefully analyze the research requirements and attend to minute details. We have discussed major steps for developing structured self-report instruments earlier in this chapter, but a few additional considerations should be mentioned.

Related constructs should be clustered into *modules* or areas of questioning. For example, an interview schedule may consist of a module on demographic information, another on health symptoms, and a third on health-promoting activities. Thought needs to be given to sequencing modules, and questions within modules, to arrive at an order that is psychologically meaningful and encourages candor. The schedule should begin with questions that are interesting and not too sensitive. Whenever both general and specific questions about a topic are included, general questions should be placed first to avoid "coaching."

Instruments should be prefaced by introductory comments about the nature and purpose of the study. In interviews, introductory information is communicated by the interviewer, who typically follows a script. In questionnaires, the introduction takes the form of an accompanying **cover letter**. The introduction should be carefully constructed because it is an early point of contact with potential respondents. An example of a cover letter for a mailed questionnaire is presented in Figure 13.3. (This cover letter is included in the Toolkit for you to adapt. ✪)

Dear Mr. O'Hara,

We are conducting a study to understand how men who are nearing retirement age (55 to 65 years old) manage their health. This study, sponsored by the National Institutes of Health, will enable health care providers to better meet the needs of men in your age group. Would you please assist us by completing the enclosed questionnaire? Your opinions and experiences are needed to give an accurate picture of men's health.

Your name was selected at random from a list of residents in your area. The questionnaire is completely anonymous—so, we hope you will feel comfortable giving your honest opinions. If you have any comments or concerns about any questions, feel free to contact me by e-mail (dfp1@grifuni.edu) or by phone (518-587-3994).

A postage-paid return envelope is enclosed for your convenience. Please take a few minutes to complete and return the questionnaire to us. It should only take about 15 minutes of your time. In appreciation for your help, I am enclosing $2. Please return your questionnaire by May 12.

Your participation in the study is completely voluntary. By returning your study booklet, you will be granting your consent to participate in the study. Thank you in advance for your assistance.

Sincerely,
Denise F. Polit, Ph.D.
Professor*

*This cover letter could be readily adapted for an email message inviting people to participate in a web-based survey.

FIGURE 13.3 Example of a cover letter for a mailed questionnaire.

When a first draft of the instrument is in reasonably good order, it should be reviewed by experts in questionnaire construction, by substantive content area specialists, and by someone capable of detecting spelling mistakes or grammatical errors. When these various people have provided feedback, the instrument can be pretested.

In the remainder of this section, we offer some specific suggestions for designing high-quality self-report instruments. Additional guidance is offered in the books by Fowler (2014) and Bradburn and colleagues (2004).

Tips for Wording Questions

We all are accustomed to asking questions, but the proper phrasing of questions for a study is not easy. In wording questions, researchers should keep four important considerations in mind.

1. *Clarity.* Questions should be worded clearly and unambiguously. This is usually easier said than

done. Respondents do not always have the same mind-set as the researchers.
2. *Ability of respondents to give information.* Researchers need to consider whether respondents can be expected to understand the question or are qualified to provide meaningful information.
3. *Bias.* Questions should be worded in a manner that will minimize the risk of response biases.
4. *Sensitivity.* Researchers should strive to be courteous, considerate, and sensitive to respondents' circumstances, especially when asking questions of a private nature.

Here are some specific suggestions with regard to these four considerations (additional guidance on wording items for composite scales is provided in Chapter 15):

• Clarify in your own mind the information you are seeking. The question, "When do you usually eat your evening meal?" might elicit such responses as "around 6 pm," or "when my son gets home from soccer practice," or "when I feel like cooking." The question itself contains no words that are difficult, but the question is unclear because the researcher's intent is not apparent.

- Avoid jargon or technical terms (e.g., edema) if lay terms (e.g., swelling) are equally appropriate. Use words that are simple enough for the *least* educated sample members.
- Do not assume that respondents will be aware of, or informed about, issues in which you are interested—and avoid giving the impression that they *ought* to be informed. Questions on complex issues sometimes can be worded in such a way that respondents will be comfortable admitting ignorance (e.g., "Many people have not had a chance to learn much about factors that increase the risk of diabetes. Do you happen to know of any contributing factors?"). Another approach is to preface a question by a short explanation about terminology or issues.
- Avoid leading questions that suggest a particular answer. A question such as, "Do you agree that nurse-midwives play an indispensable role in the health team?" is not neutral.
- State a range of alternatives within the question itself when possible. For instance, the question, "Do you prefer to get up early in the morning on weekends?" is more suggestive of the "right" answer than "Do you prefer to get up early in the morning or to sleep late on weekends?"
- For questions that deal with controversial topics or socially unacceptable behavior (e.g., excessive drinking), closed-ended questions may be preferred. It is easier to check off having engaged in socially disapproved actions than to verbalize those actions in response to open-ended questions. When controversial behaviors are presented as options, respondents are more likely to conclude that their behavior is not unique, and admissions of such behavior become less difficult.
- Impersonal wording of questions is sometimes useful in encouraging honesty. For example, compare these two statements with which respondents might be asked to agree or disagree: (1) "I am dissatisfied with the nursing care I received during my hospitalization," (2) "The quality of nursing care in this hospital is unsatisfactory." A respondent might feel more comfortable admitting dissatisfaction with nursing care in the less personally worded second question.

Tips for Preparing Response Options

If closed-ended questions are used, researchers also need to develop response alternatives. Below are some suggestions for preparing them.

- Response options should cover all significant alternatives. If respondents are forced to choose from options provided by researchers, they should feel comfortable with the available options. As a precaution, researchers often have as a response option a phrase such as "Other—please specify."
- Alternatives should be mutually exclusive. The following categories for a question on a person's age are *not* mutually exclusive: 30 years or younger, 30-50 years, or 50 years or older. People who are exactly 30 or 50 would qualify for two categories.
- Response options should be ordered rationally. Options often can be placed in order of decreasing or increasing favorability, agreement, or intensity (e.g., strongly agree, agree). When options have no "natural" order, alphabetic ordering can avoid leading respondents to a particular response (e.g., see the rank order question in Table 13.1).
- Response options should be brief. One sentence or phrase for each option is usually sufficient to express a concept. Response alternatives should be about equal in length.

Tips for Formatting an Instrument

The appearance and layout of an instrument may seem a matter of minor administrative importance. Yet, a poorly designed format can have substantive consequences if respondents (or interviewers) become confused, miss questions, or answer questions they should have omitted. The format is especially important in questionnaires because respondents cannot ask for help. The following suggestions may be helpful in laying out an instrument:

- Do not compress questions into too small a space. An extra page of questions is better than a form that appears dense and confusing and that provides inadequate space for responses to open-ended questions.

- Set off the response options from the question or stem. Response alternatives are often aligned vertically (Table 13.1). In questionnaires, respondents can be asked either to circle their answer or to check the appropriate box.
- Give care to formatting **filter questions**, which route respondents through different sets of questions depending on the responses. In interview schedules, **skip patterns** instruct interviewers to skip to a specific question for a given response (e.g., SKIP TO Q10). In SAQs, skip instructions can be confusing. It is often better to put questions appropriate to a subset of respondents apart from the main series of questions, as illustrated in Box 13.1, part B. An important advantage of CAPI, CATI, audio-CASI, and Internet surveys is that skip patterns are built into the computer program, leaving no room for human error.
- Avoid forcing all respondents to go through inapplicable questions in an SAQ. That is, suppose question 2 in Box 13.1 part B had been worded as follows: "If you are a member of the American Nurses Association, for how long have you been a member?" Nonmembers may not be sure how to handle this question and may be annoyed at having to read through irrelevant material.

Administering Structured Self-Report Instruments

Administering interview schedules and questionnaires involves different considerations and requires different skills.

Collecting Interview Data

The quality of interview data relies on interviewer proficiency. Interviewers for large survey organizations receive general training in addition to specific training for each study. Although we cannot in this introductory book cover all the principles of good interviewing, we can identify some major issues. Additional guidance can be found in Fowler (2014).

A primary task of interviewers is to put respondents at ease so that they will feel comfortable in

BOX 13.1 Examples of Formats for a Filter Question

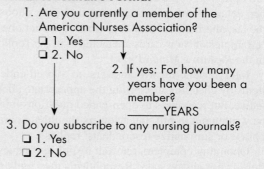

A. Interview Format

1. Are you currently a member of the American Nurses Association?
   - ❑ 1. Yes
   - ❑ 2. No (SKIP TO Q3)
2. For how many years have you been a member?
   _____YEARS
3. Do you subscribe to any nursing journals?
   - ❑ 1. Yes
   - ❑ 2. No

B. Questionnaire Format

1. Are you currently a member of the American Nurses Association?
   - ❑ 1. Yes
   - ❑ 2. No
        2. If yes: For how many years have you been a member?
        _____YEARS
3. Do you subscribe to any nursing journals?
   - ❑ 1. Yes
   - ❑ 2. No

expressing their views honestly. Respondents' reactions to interviewers can affect their level of cooperation. Interviewers should always be punctual (if an appointment has been made), courteous, and friendly. Interviewers should strive to appear unbiased and to create an atmosphere that encourages candor. All opinions of respondents should be accepted as natural; interviewers should not express surprise, disapproval, or even approval.

Example of Well-Trained Interviewers: Nyamathi and colleagues (2015) gathered data relating to the risk for incarceration among homeless young adults. The baseline questionnaire was "administered by the research staff well trained in confidential data collection, which included respecting each individual as a person, not judging the participant on reported behaviors, and in administering the questionnaire in a private location" (p. 803).

With a structured interview schedule, interviewers should follow question wording precisely. Interviewers should not offer spontaneous explanations of what questions mean. Repetition of a question is usually adequate to dispel misunderstandings, especially if the instrument has been pretested. Interviewers should not read questions mechanically. A natural, conversational tone is essential in building rapport, and this tone is impossible to achieve if interviewers are not thoroughly familiar with the questions.

When closed-ended questions have lengthy or complex response alternatives, or when a series of questions has the same response options, interviewers should hand respondents a **show card** that lists the options. People cannot be expected to remember detailed unfamiliar material and may choose the last alternative if they cannot recall earlier ones. (Examples of show cards are included in the Toolkit in the *Resource Manual* 🞮.)

Interviewers record answers to closed-ended items by checking or circling the appropriate alternative, but responses to open-ended questions must be written out in full. Interviewers should not paraphrase or summarize respondents' replies.

Obtaining complete, relevant responses to questions is not always easy. Respondents may reply to seemingly straightforward questions with partial answers. Some may say, "I don't know" to avoid giving their opinions on sensitive topics or to stall while they think over the question. In such cases, the interviewers' job is to **probe**. The purpose of a probe is to elicit more useful information than respondents volunteered initially. A probe can take many forms; sometimes it involves repeating the question, and sometimes it is a long pause intended to communicate to respondents that they should continue. Frequently, it is necessary to encourage a more complete response to open-ended questions by a nondirective supplementary question, such as, "How is that?" Interviewers must be careful to use only *neutral* probes that do not influence the content of a response. Box 13.2 gives some examples of neutral, nondirective probes used by professional interviewers to get more complete responses to questions. The ability to probe well is perhaps the greatest test of an interviewer's skill. To know

BOX 13.2 Examples of Neutral, Nondirective Probes

- Is there anything else?
- Go on.
- Are there any other reasons?
- How do you mean?
- Could you please tell me more about that?
- Would you tell me what you have in mind?
- There are no right or wrong answers; I'd just like to get your thinking.
- Could you please explain that?
- Could you please give me an example?

when to probe and how to select the best probes, interviewers must understand the purpose of each question. (The Toolkit for Chapter 14 🞮 has material relating to interviewer training that might be useful.)

Guidelines for telephone interviews are essentially the same as those for face-to-face interviews, but additional effort usually is required to build rapport over the telephone. In both cases, interviewers should strive to make the interview a pleasant and satisfying experience in which respondents are made to understand that the information they are providing is valued.

Example of a Telephone Survey: Hosek and co-researchers (2014) conducted a telephone survey of low-income pregnant women concerning their perceptions of care after being discharged from the hospital with a diagnosis of false or latent labor.

Collecting Questionnaire Data through In-Person Distribution

Questionnaires can be distributed by personal distribution, through the mail, and over the Internet. The most convenient procedure is to distribute questionnaires to a group of people who complete the instrument at the same time. This approach has the obvious advantages of maximizing the number of completed questionnaires and allowing respondents to ask questions. Group administrations may be possible in educational settings and in some clinical situations.

Researchers can also hand out questionnaires to individual respondents. Personal contact has a positive effect on response rates, and researchers can answer questions. Individual distribution of questionnaires in clinical settings is often inexpensive and efficient and can yield a relatively high rate of response.

> **Example of Personal Distribution of Questionnaires:** Yeo and Logan (2014) studied exercise and daily activities of 816 low-income pregnant women. Questionnaires were distributed at 13 county health departments by clinic nurses.

Collecting Questionnaire Data through the Mail

For surveys of a broad population, questionnaires can be mailed. A *mail* (or *postal*) *survey* approach is cost-effective for reaching geographically dispersed respondents, but it tends to yield low response rates. With low response rates, the risk is that people who did not complete a questionnaire would have answered questions differently from those who did return it. With response rates greater than 65%, the risk of bias may be small, but lower response rates are the norm. Response rates can be affected by the manner in which the questionnaires are designed and mailed. The standard procedure for distributing mailed questionnaires is to include a stamped, addressed return envelope.

> **TIP:** People are more likely to complete a mailed questionnaire if they are encouraged to do so by someone whose name they recognize. If possible, obtain an endorsement of a well-known person, or write the cover letter on the stationery of a respected organization, such as a university.

Follow-up reminders are effective in improving response rates for mailed (and Internet) questionnaires. This procedure involves additional mailings urging nonrespondents to complete and return their forms. Follow-up reminders should be sent about 5 to 10 days after the initial mailing. Sometimes, reminders simply involve a postcard of encouragement to nonrespondents, but it is preferable to send another copy of the questionnaire because many nonrespondents will have misplaced or discarded the original. With anonymous questionnaires, researchers may be unable to distinguish respondents and nonrespondents for the purpose of sending follow-up letters. In such a situation, the best procedure is to send out a follow-up reminder to everyone, thanking those who have already answered and asking others to cooperate. Dillman and colleagues (2014) offer excellent advice regarding mailed (and Internet and telephone) surveys.

> **Example of Mailed Questionnaires:** Von Vogelsang and co-researchers (2014) studied the transitional experiences of patients after an intra-cranial aneurysm rupture. Data were collected by a mail survey at 6 months, 1 year, and 2 years after the rupture. Telephone calls were made to those who had not returned a questionnaire within 2 weeks.

Collecting Questionnaire Data via the Internet

The Internet is a very economical means of distributing questionnaires. Internet surveys appear to be a promising approach for accessing groups of people interested in specific topics. There are a growing number of resources for doing such surveys.

Surveys can be administered through the Internet in several ways. One method is to design a questionnaire in a word processing program, as would be the case for mailed questionnaires. The file with the questionnaire is then attached to an e-mail message and distributed. Respondents can complete the questionnaire and return it as an e-mail attachment or print it and return it by mail or fax. This method may be problematic if respondents have trouble opening attachments or if they use a different word processing program. Surveys sent via e-mail also run the risk of not getting delivered to the intended party, either because e-mail addresses have changed or because the e-mail messages are blocked by Internet security filters. Blocks are especially common for messages with attachments.

Increasingly, researchers are collecting data through **web-based surveys**. This approach requires researchers to have a website on which the survey is placed or to use a service such as SurveyMonkey (http://www.surveymonkey.com/) or Qualtrics (http://www.qualtrics.com/). Respondents typically access the website by clicking on a hypertext link. For example, respondents may be invited to participate in the survey through an e-mail message that includes the link to the survey, or they may be invited to participate when they enter a website related in content to the survey (e.g., the website of a cancer support organization).

Web-based forms are designed for online response, and some can be programmed to include interactive features. By having dynamic features, respondents can receive as well as give information—a feature that can increase motivation to participate. For example, respondents can be given information about their own responses (e.g., how they scored on a scale) or aggregated information about previous participants. A major advantage of web-based surveys is that the data are directly amenable to analysis.

Example of a Web-Based Survey: Augustin and colleagues (2014) used SurveyMonkey to gather information about the breastfeeding experiences of mothers 6 months after delivery. The survey link was sent to 806 mothers, and the response rate was 50%.

→ TIP: When sending out an e-mail invitation, avoid using the word "survey" or "questionnaire" in the subject line—these might discourage people from opening the e-mail. There is some evidence that the best time to send out e-mail invitations is Monday afternoons.

Internet surveys have proliferated. They are inexpensive and can reach a broad audience. However, samples are almost never representative, and response rates tend to be low—often even lower than mailed questionnaires. Several references are available to help researchers who wish to launch an Internet survey. For example, the books by Dillman et al. (2014), Tourangeau et al. (2013), and Fitzpatrick and Montgomery (2004) provide useful information.

Evaluation of Structured Self-Reports

Structured self-reports are a powerful data collection method. They are versatile and yield information that can be readily analyzed statistically. Structured questions can be carefully worded and rigorously pretested. In an unstructured interview, by contrast, respondents may answer different questions, and there is no way to know whether question wording affected responses. On the other hand, the questions tend to be much more superficial than questions in unstructured interviews because structured questions usually are closed-ended.

Structured self-reports are susceptible to the risk of various **response biases**—many of which are also possible in unstructured self-reports. Respondents may give biased answers in reaction to the interviewers' behavior or appearance, for example. Perhaps the most pervasive problem is people's tendency to present a favorable image of themselves. **Social desirability response bias** refers to the tendency of some individuals to misrepresent themselves by giving answers that are congruent with prevailing social values. This problem is often difficult to combat. Subtle, indirect, and delicately worded questioning sometimes can help to minimize this response bias. Creating a nonjudgmental atmosphere and providing anonymity also encourage frankness. In an interview situation, interviewer training is essential.

Some response biases, called **response sets**, are most commonly observed in composite scales. **Extreme responses** are a bias reflecting consistent selection of extreme alternatives (e.g., "strongly agree"). These extreme responses distort the findings because they do not necessarily signify the most intense feelings about the phenomenon under study but rather capture a trait of the respondent.

Some people have been found to agree with statements regardless of content. Such people are called **yea-sayers**, and the bias is known as the **acquiescence response set**. A less common problem is the opposite tendency for other individuals, called **nay-sayers**, to disagree with statements independently of question content.

Researchers who construct scales should attempt to eliminate or minimize response set biases. If an instrument or scale is being developed for general use by others, evidence should be gathered to demonstrate that the scale is sufficiently free from response biases to measure the critical variable. Users should consider such evidence in selecting existing scales.

STRUCTURED OBSERVATION

Structured observation is used to record behaviors, actions, and events. Structured observation involves using formal instruments and protocols that specify what to observe, how long to observe it, and how to record information. The challenge of structured observation lies in formulating a system for accurately recording observations.

Methods of Recording Structured Observations

Researchers recording structured observations typically use either a checklist or a rating scale. Both types of record-keeping instruments are designed to produce numeric information.

Category Systems and Checklists

Structured observation often involves constructing a category system to classify observed phenomena. A **category system** represents an attempt to designate in a systematic fashion the qualitative behaviors and events transpiring in the observational setting.

Some category systems are constructed so that *all* observed behaviors within a specified domain (e.g., utterances) can be classified into one and only one category. In such an exhaustive system, the categories are mutually exclusive.

Example of Exhaustive Categories: Liaw and colleagues (2012) studied caregiving and positioning effects on preterm infants' sleep–wake states. The infants' respirations, eye movements, muscle tone, and motor activity in 1-minute segments were used to classify their sleep–wake state into one of six mutually exclusive categories (e.g., quiet sleep, quiet and active sleep, quiet awake).

When observers use an exhaustive system— that is, when all behaviors of a certain type, such

as verbal interaction, are observed and recorded— researchers must be careful to define categories so that observers know when one behavior ends and a new one begins. Another essential feature is that referent behaviors should be mutually exclusive, as in the previous example. The underlying assumption in using such a category system is that behaviors, events, or attributes that are allocated to a particular category are equivalent to every other behavior, event, or attribute in that same category.

A contrasting technique is to develop a system in which only particular types of behavior (which may or may not be manifested) are categorized. For example, if we were studying autistic children's aggressive behavior, we might develop such categories as "strikes another child," or "kicks/hits walls or floor." In such a category system, many behaviors—all the ones that are nonaggressive—would not be classified. Nonexhaustive systems are often adequate, but one risk is that resulting data might be difficult to interpret. Problems may arise if a large number of behaviors are not categorized or if long segments of the observation sessions do not involve the target behaviors. In such situations, investigators need to record the amount of time in which the target behaviors occurred, relative to the total time under observation.

Example of Nonexhaustive Categories: Nilsen and colleagues (2014) conducted a study of nursing care quality that involved observations of communication between nurses and mechanically ventilated patients in an intensive care unit. Among many different types of observations made, observers recorded instances of positive and negative nurse behaviors, according to carefully defined criteria. Nurse behaviors that were neutral were not categorized.

A critical requirement for a good category system is the careful definition of behaviors or characteristics to be observed. Each category must be explained in detail so that observers have relatively clear-cut criteria for identifying the occurrence of a specified phenomenon. Even with detailed definitions of categories, observers often are faced with making numerous on-the-spot inferences. Virtually all category systems require observer inference, to greater or lesser degree.

Example of Moderately Low Observer Inference: Tsai and colleagues (2011) examined factors that could predict osteoarthritic pain in elders, including nonverbal cues measured through observation. One predictor was motor patterns, which were videotaped in 10-minute sessions in which elders engaged in a set of activities. Observers coded for the presence of five behaviors (e.g., active rubbing of the knee or hip, joint flexion, rigidity) in 30-second intervals.

In this observational system, assuming that observers were properly trained, relatively little inference would be required to code motor patterns. Other category systems, however, require more inference, as for example in the coding of nurse and patient behaviors as negative or positive in the previously mentioned Nilsen et al. (2014) study. The decision concerning degree of observer inference depends on a number of factors, including the research purpose and the observers' skills. Beginning researchers are advised to construct or use category systems that require low to moderate inference.

Category systems are used to construct a **checklist**, which is the instrument observers use to record observed phenomena. The checklist is usually formatted with the list of behaviors or events from the category system on the left and space for tallying the frequency or duration of occurrence of behaviors on the right. With nonexhaustive category systems, categories of behaviors that may or may not be manifested by participants are listed on the checklist. The observer's tasks are to watch for instances of these behaviors and to record their occurrence.

With exhaustive checklists, the observers' task is to place all behaviors in only one category for each element. By **element**, we refer either to a unit of behavior, such as a sentence in a conversation, or to a time interval. To illustrate, suppose we were studying the problem-solving behavior of a group of public health staff discussing an intervention for the homeless. Our category system involves eight categories: (1) seeks information, (2) gives information, (3) describes problem, (4) offers suggestion, (5) opposes suggestion, (6) supports suggestion, (7) summarizes, and (8) miscellaneous. Observers would be required to classify every group member's contribution—using, for example, each sentence as the element—in terms of one of these eight categories.

Another approach with exhaustive systems is to categorize relevant behaviors at regular time intervals. For example, in a category system for infants' motor activities, the researcher might use 10-second time intervals as the element; observers would categorize infant movements within 10-second periods.

Rating Scales

An alternative to a checklist for recording structured observations is a **rating scale** that requires observers to rate a phenomenon along a descriptive continuum that is typically bipolar. The ratings are quantified for subsequent analysis.

Observers may be required to rate behaviors or events at specified intervals throughout the observational period (e.g., every 5 minutes). Alternatively, observers may rate entire events or transactions after observations are completed. Postobservation ratings require observers to integrate a number of activities and to judge which point on a scale most closely fits their interpretation of the situation. For example, suppose we were observing children's behavior during a scratch test for allergies. After each session, observers might be asked to rate the children's overall anxiety during the procedure on a *graphic rating scale* such as the following:

Rate how calm or nervous the child appeared to be during the procedure:

1	2	3	4	5	6	7
Extremely calm			Neither calm nor nervous			Extremely nervous

⟶ **TIP:** Observational rating scales are sometimes incorporated into structured interviews. For example, in a study of the health problems of 4,000 low-income mothers, interviewers were asked to rate the safety of children's home environment with regard to potential health hazards on a 5-point scale, from completely safe to extremely unsafe (Polit et al., 2001).

Rating scales can also be used as an extension of checklists, in which observers not only record the occurrence of a behavior but also rate some qualitative aspect of it, such as its intensity. When rating scales are coupled with a category scheme, considerable information about a phenomenon can be obtained, but it places a big burden on observers, particularly if there is extensive activity.

Example of Observational Ratings:
The NEECHAM Confusion Scale, an observational measure to detect the presence and severity of acute confusion, relies on ratings of behavior. For example, one rating concerns alertness/responsiveness, and the ratings are from 0 (responsiveness depressed) to 4 (full attentiveness). The NEECHAM has been used for both clinical and research purposes. For example, Ono and colleagues (2011) used NEECHAM scores as a measure of postoperative delirium in their study that tested the usefulness of bright light therapy after esophagectomy.

TIP: It is useful to spend a period of time with participants before the actual observation and recording of data. Having a warm-up period helps to relax people (especially if audio or video equipment is being used) and can be helpful to observers (e.g., if participants have a linguistic style to which observers must adjust, such as a strong regional accent).

Constructing versus Borrowing Structured Observational Instruments

Compared to the abundance of books that provide guidance in developing self-report instruments, there are relatively few resources for researchers who want to design their own observational instruments. Yoder and Symons (2010) provide one resource for observational measurements of behavior.

As with self-report instruments, however, we encourage researchers to search for available observational instruments, rather than creating one themselves. The use of an existing instrument saves considerable work and time and also facilitates cross-study comparisons. The best source for existing instruments is recent research literature on the study topic. For example, if you were conducting an observational study of infant pain, a good place to begin would be recent research on this topic to obtain information on how infant pain was operationalized.

Sampling for Structured Observations

Researchers must decide when and for how long structured observational instruments will be used. Observations are usually done for a specific amount of time, and the amount of time is standardized across participants.

Sometimes *sampling* is needed so as to obtain representative examples of behaviors without having to observe for prolonged periods. Observational sampling concerns the selection of behaviors or activities to be observed, not the selection of participants.

With **time sampling**, researchers select time periods during which observations will occur. The time frames may be selected systematically (e.g., 60 seconds at 5-minute intervals) or at random. For example, suppose we were studying mothers' interactions with their children in a clinic. During a 30-minute observation period, we sample moments to observe rather than observing continuously. Let us say that observations are made in 2-minute segments. If we used systematic sampling, we would observe for 2 minutes and then cease observing for a prespecified period, say 3 minutes. With this scheme, a total of six 2-minute observations would be made for each dyad. A second approach is to sample randomly 2-minute periods from the total of 15 such periods in a half hour; a third is to use all 15 periods. Decisions about the length and number of periods for creating a good sample must be consistent with research aims. In establishing time units, a key consideration is determining a psychologically meaningful time frame. Pretesting with different sampling plans is usually necessary.

Example of Time Sampling: Dellefield and colleagues (2012) studied how nurses spent clinical time in a nursing home. Observations of work activities were made for 30-second intervals every 5 minutes.

Event sampling uses integral behavior sets or events for observation. Event sampling requires that the investigator either have knowledge about the occurrence of events or be in a position to wait for (or arrange) their occurrence. Examples of integral events suitable for event sampling include shift changes of hospital nurses or cast removals of pediatric patients. This approach is preferable to time sampling when events of interest are infrequent and are at risk of being missed. Still, when behaviors and events of interest are frequent, time sampling can enhance the representativeness of observed behaviors.

Example of Event Sampling: Jackson and colleagues (2014) studied cues associated with violence toward nurses in an acute care setting. During periods of 4 to 6 hours in public areas, observers used a behavior observation instrument whenever a patient displayed one or more of 18 violence cues.

Technical Aids in Observations

A wide array of technical devices is available for recording behaviors and events, making analysis or categorization at a later time possible. When the target behavior is auditory, recordings can be used to obtain a permanent record. Technologic advances have vastly improved the quality, sensitivity, and unobtrusiveness of recording equipment. Auditory recordings can also be analyzed by speech software analysis to obtain objective quantitative measures of certain features (e.g., volume, pitch).

Video recording can be used when permanent visual records are desired. Video recordings can capture complex behaviors that might elude on-the-spot observers. Video recordings make it possible to check the accuracy of coders and so are useful as a training aid. Finally, cameras are often less obtrusive than a human observer. Video records have a few drawbacks, some of which are technical, such as lighting requirements, lens limitations, and so on. Sometimes the camera angle can present a lopsided view of an event. Also, some participants may be self-conscious in front of a video camera. Still, for many applications, visual records offer unparalleled opportunities to expand the scope of observational studies. Haidet and colleagues (2009) offer valuable advice on improving data quality of video-recorded observations.

There is a growing technology for assisting with the encoding and recording of observations. For example, there is equipment that permits observers to enter observational data directly into a computer as the observation occurs, and in some cases, the equipment can record physiologic data concurrently.

Example of Using Equipment: Pecanac and colleagues (2015) described the use of handheld technology to capture continuous observations of behavior, which they referred to as "timed event sequential data." The technology, which could be used to capture both patients' and nurses' behaviors, can address such questions as "When does this behavior occur? How long does the behavior last?" (p. 67). They illustrated with a study designed to answer the question: "What are the frequency, duration, and sequence of nursing care related to mobilizing older patients in acute care settings?" (p. 68).

Structured Observations by Nonresearch Observers

The observations discussed thus far are made and recorded by research team members. Sometimes, however, researchers ask people not connected with the research to provide structured data, based on their observations of others. This method has much in common (in terms of format and scoring) with self-report instruments; the primary difference is that the person answering questions is asked to describe the attributes and behaviors of *another* person. For example, a mother might be asked to describe the behavior problems of her preschool child.

Obtaining observational data from nonresearchers is economical compared with using trained observers. For example, observers might have to watch children for hours or days to describe the nature and intensity of behavior problems, whereas parents or teachers could do this readily. Some behaviors might never lend themselves to outsider observation because they occur in private situations, or are infrequent (e.g., sleepwalking).

On the other hand, such methods may have the same problems as self-reports (e.g., response-set bias) in addition to observer bias. Observer bias may in some cases be extreme, such as may happen when parents provide information about their children. Nonresearch observers are typically not trained, and interobserver agreement usually cannot be assessed. Thus, this approach has some problems but will continue to be used because, in many cases, there are no alternatives.

Example of Observations by Nonresearch Personnel: Oswalt and colleagues (2013) analyzed data from a randomized controlled trial aimed at reducing anxiety of children born preterm. Mothers complete the Child Behavior Checklist for children aged 1-3. A key outcome was the children's anxiety scores derived from this measure.

Evaluation of Structured Observation

Structured observation is an important data collection method, particularly for recording aspects of people's behaviors when they are not capable of reliable self-report. Observational methods are particularly valuable for gathering data about infants and children, older people who are confused or agitated, or people whose communication skills are impaired.

Observations, like self-reports, are vulnerable to biases. One source of bias comes from those being observed. Participants may distort their behaviors in the direction of "looking good." They may also behave atypically because of their awareness of being observed (*reactivity*) or their shyness in front of strangers or a camera.

Biases can also reflect human perceptual errors. Observation and interpretation are demanding tasks. To make and record observation in a completely objective fashion is challenging and perhaps impossible. The risk of bias is especially great when a high degree of observer inference is required.

Several types of observational bias are particularly common. One bias is the **enhancement of contrast effect**, in which observers distort observations in the direction of dividing content into clear-cut entities. The converse effect—a bias toward **central tendency**—occurs when extreme events are distorted toward a middle ground. With **assimilatory biases**, observers distort observations in the direction of identity with previous inputs. This bias would have the effect of miscategorizing information in the direction of regularity and orderliness. Assimilation to the observer's expectations and attitudes also occurs.

With regard to rating scales, the **halo effect** is the tendency of observers to be influenced by one characteristic in judging other, unrelated characteristics. For example, if we had a positive general impression of a person, we might rate that person as intelligent, loyal, and dependable simply because these traits are positively valued. Ratings may reflect observers' personality. The **error of leniency** is the tendency for observers to rate everything positively, and the **error of severity** is the contrasting tendency to rate too harshly.

The careful construction and pretesting of checklists and rating scales, and the thorough training and preparation of observers, play an important role in minimizing biases. To become a good instrument for collecting observational data, observers must be trained to make consistent, accurate observations. Even when the lead researcher is the primary observer, self-training and dry runs are essential. The setting during the trial period should resemble as closely as possible the settings that will be the focus of actual observations.

Training should include practice sessions in which the comparability of observers' classifications and rates is assessed. That is, two or more independent observers should watch a trial situation, and observational coding should then be compared. *Interrater reliability* of structured observations is described in the next chapter.

> **TIP:** People being observed are less likely to behave typically if they think they are being critically appraised. Even positive cues (such as nodding approval) should be avoided because approval may induce repetition of a behavior that might not otherwise have occurred.

BIOPHYSIOLOGIC MEASURES

Settings in which nurses work are typically filled with a wide variety of technical instruments for measuring physiologic functions. Nurse researchers have used biophysiologic measures for a wide variety of purposes. Examples include studies of basic biophysiologic processes, explorations of the ways in which nursing actions and interventions affect physiologic outcomes, studies to evaluate the accuracy of biophysiologic information gathered by nurses, and studies of the correlates of physiologic functioning in patients with health problems.

It is beyond the scope of this book to describe the many kinds of biophysiologic measures available to nurse researchers. Our goals are to present an overview of biophysiologic measures, to illustrate their use in research, and to note considerations in decisions to use them.

Types of Biophysiologic Measures

Physiologic measurements are either in vivo or in vitro. **In vivo measurements** are performed directly in or on living organisms. Examples include measures of oxygen saturation, blood pressure, and body temperature. An **in vitro measurement**, by contrast, is performed outside the organism's body, as in the case of measuring serum potassium concentration in the blood.

In vivo instruments have been developed to measure all bodily functions, and technologic improvements continue to advance our ability to measure biophysiologic phenomena more accurately, conveniently, and rapidly than ever before. The uses to which such instruments have been put by nurse researchers are richly diverse.

Example of a Study with In Vivo Measures: Uzelli and Yapucu Güneş, (2015) tested the effectiveness of a 5% oral solution on several outcomes in infants undergoing intramuscular injection. In addition to assessing the impact on pain, the researchers measured the effect of the solution on oxygen saturation and heart rate.

With in vitro measures, data are gathered by extracting physiologic material from people and submitting it for laboratory analysis. Usually, each laboratory establishes a range of normal values for each measurement (a *reference range*), and this information helps in interpreting the results. Several classes of laboratory analysis have been used by nurse researchers, including chemical measurements (e.g., measures of potassium levels), microbiologic measures (e.g., bacterial counts), and cytologic *or* histologic measures (e.g., tissue biopsies). Laboratory analyses of blood and urine

samples are the most frequently used in vitro measures in nursing investigations.

Example of a Study with In Vitro Measures: Koniak-Griffin and co-researchers (2015) studied the effects of a community health worker–led lifestyle behavior intervention for Latina women, using a randomized design. The researchers used a number of outcome variables in this trial, including lipid and blood glucose measurements.

Selecting a Biophysiologic Measure

The most basic issue in selecting a physiologic measure is whether it will yield good information about key research variables. In some cases, researchers need to consider whether the variable should be measured by observation or self-report instead of (or in addition to) using biophysiologic equipment. For example, stress could be measured by asking people questions (e.g., using the State-Trait Anxiety Inventory); by observing their behavior during exposure to stressful stimuli; or by measuring heart rate, blood pressure, or levels of adrenocorticotropic hormone in urine samples.

Several other considerations should be kept in mind in selecting a biophysiologic measure. Some key questions include the following:

- Is the equipment or laboratory analysis you need readily available to you?
- Can you operate the required equipment and interpret its results or do you need training? Are resources available to help you with operation and interpretation?
- Will you have difficulty obtaining permission from an Institutional Review Board or other institutional authority?
- Is a single measurement of the outcome sufficient or are multiple measurements needed for a reliable estimate? If the latter, what burden does this place on participants?
- Are your measures likely to be influenced by reactivity (i.e., participants' awareness of their status)?
- Are you thoroughly familiar with rules and safety precautions, such as grounding procedures, especially when using electrical equipment?

Evaluation of Biophysiologic Measures

Biophysiologic measures offer the following advantages to nurse researchers:

• Biophysiologic measures are accurate and precise compared with psychological measures (e.g., self-report measures of anxiety).
• Biophysiologic measures are objective. Two nurses reading from the same sphygmomanometer are likely to obtain the same blood pressure measurements, and two different sphygmomanometers are likely to produce the same readouts. Patients cannot easily distort measurements of biophysiologic functioning.
• Biophysiologic instruments provide valid measures of targeted variables: Thermometers can be depended on to measure temperature and not blood volume, and so forth. For self-report and observational measures, it is often more difficult to be certain that the instrument is really measuring the target concept.

Biophysiologic measures also have a few disadvantages:

• The cost of collecting some types of biophysiologic data may be low or nonexistent, but when laboratory tests are involved, they may be more expensive than other methods (e.g., assessing smoking status by means of cotinine assays versus self-report).
• The measuring tool may affect the variables it is attempting to measure. The presence of a sensing device, such as a transducer, located in a blood vessel partially blocks that vessel and, hence, alters the pressure–flow characteristics being measured.
• Energy must often be applied to the organism when taking the biophysiologic measurements; extreme caution must continually be exercised to avoid the risk of damaging cells by high-energy concentrations.

The difficulty in choosing biophysiologic measures for nursing studies lies not in their shortage, nor in their questionable utility, nor in their inferiority to other methods. Indeed, they are plentiful, often highly reliable and valid, and extremely useful in clinical nursing studies. Care must be exercised, however, in selecting instruments or laboratory analyses with regard to practical, ethical, medical, and technical considerations.

PERFORMANCE TESTS

Patients' abilities and skills are sometimes measured with **performance tests**. For example, the 6-Minute Walk Test (6MWT) is a widely used measure of physical functioning for patients with various cardiovascular, respiratory, or neurologic diseases, or those in need of surgical or rehabilitative intervention. The measure is the distance walked in a 6-minute period, typically involving the use of a treadmill. Many other physical performance tests have been devised to measure such attributes as balance, mobility, endurance, and flexibility.

> **Example of Performance Testing:** Wang and colleagues (2014) tested the effects of a Health-Belief Model nursing intervention on Chinese patients with COPD. One of their outcomes was patients' performance on the 6-Minute Walk Test.

IMPLEMENTING A DATA COLLECTION PLAN

Data quality in a quantitative study is affected by both the data collection plan and how the plan is implemented.

Selecting Research Personnel

An important decision concerns who will actually collect the research data. In small studies, the lead researcher usually collects the data personally, but in large studies, this is seldom feasible. When data are collected by others, it is important to select appropriate people. In general, they should be neutral agents—their characteristics or behavior should not affect the substance of the data. Here are some considerations to keep in mind when selecting research personnel:

• *Experience.* Research staff ideally have had prior experience collecting data (e.g., prior interviewing experience). If this is not feasible, look for people who can readily acquire the necessary skills (e.g., interviewers should have good verbal and social skills).
• *Congruence with sample characteristics.* If possible, data collectors should match participants with respect to racial or cultural background

and gender. The greater the sensitivity of the questions, the greater the desirability of congruence.

- *Unremarkable appearance*. Extremes of appearance should be avoided. For example, data collectors should not dress very casually (e.g., in tee shirts) nor formally (e.g., in designer clothes). Data collectors should not wear anything that conveys their political, social, or religious views.
- *Personality*. Data collectors should be pleasant (but not effusive), sociable (but not overly talkative), and nonjudgmental (but not unfeeling about participants' lives). The goal is to have nonthreatening data collectors who can put participants at ease.

In some situations, researchers cannot select research personnel. For example, the data collectors may be staff nurses employed at a hospital. Training of the data collection staff is particularly important in such situations. Even if researchers collect their own data, they should self-monitor their demeanor and prepare for their role with care.

Training Data Collectors

Depending on prior experience, training will need to cover both general procedures (e.g., how to probe in an interview) and ones specific to the study (e.g., how to ask a particular question or how to categorize a behavior). Training can often be done in a single day, but complex projects require more time. The lead researcher is usually the best person to conduct the training and to develop training materials.

Data collection protocols usually are a good foundation for a **training manual**. The manual normally includes background materials (e.g., the study aims), general instructions, specific instructions, and copies of all data forms.

→ **TIP:** A table of contents for a training manual for a self-report study is included in the Toolkit of the accompanying *Resource Manual*. Models for some of the sections in this table of contents (a section on avoiding interviewer bias and another on how to probe) are also in the Toolkit. If you are collecting the data yourself, you may not need a training manual, but you should learn techniques of professional interviewing.

Training often includes demonstrations of high-quality fictitious data collection sessions, performed either live or on videotape. Also, training usually involves having trainees do trial runs of data collection (e.g., *mock interviews*) in front of the trainers to demonstrate their understanding of the instructions. Thompson and colleagues (2005) provide some additional tips relating to the training of research personnel.

Example of Data Collector Training: In a two-wave panel study of the health of 4,000 low-income families, Polit and colleagues (2001) trained about 100 interviewers in four research sites. Each training session lasted 3 days, including a half day of training on the use of CAPI. At the end of the training, several trainees were not hired as interviewers because they did not show good interviewing skills in the mock interviews.

CRITIQUING STRUCTURED METHODS OF DATA COLLECTION

Most decisions that researchers make about data collection methods and procedures can affect data quality and hence overall study quality. These decisions should be critiqued in evaluating the study's evidence to the extent possible. The critiquing guidelines in Box 13.3 focus on global decisions about the design and implementation of a data collection plan ✪. Unfortunately, data collection procedures are often not described in detail in research reports, owing to space constraints in journals. A full critique of data collection plans is rarely feasible.

A second set of critiquing guidelines is presented in Box 13.4. These questions focus on the specific methods of collecting research data in quantitative studies. ✪ Further guidance on drawing conclusions about data quality in quantitative studies is provided in the next chapter.

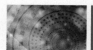

BOX 13.3 Guidelines for Critiquing Data Collection Plans in Quantitative Studies

1. Was the collection of structured data (versus unstructured data) consistent with study aims?
2. Were the right methods used to collect the data (self-report, observation, etc.)? Was triangulation of methods used appropriately? Should supplementary data collection methods have been used?
3. Was the right amount of data collected? Were data collected to address the varied needs of the study? Was *too much* data collected, resulting in participant burden—and, if so, how might this have affected data quality?
4. Did the researcher select good instruments, in terms of congruence with underlying constructs, data quality, reputation, efficiency, and so on? Were new instruments developed without a justifiable rationale?
5. Were data collection instruments adequately pretested?
6. Did the report provide sufficient information about data collection procedures?
7. Who collected the data? Were data collectors judiciously chosen with traits that were likely to enhance data quality?
8. Was the training of data collectors described? Was the training adequate? Were steps taken to improve data collectors' ability to produce high-quality data or to monitor their performance?
9. Where and under what circumstances were data gathered? Was the setting for data collection appropriate?
10. Were other people present during data collection? Could the presence of others have resulted in any biases?
11. Were data collectors blinded to study hypotheses or to participants' group status?

BOX 13.4 Guidelines for Critiquing Structured Data Collection Methods

1. If self-report data were collected, did the researcher make good decisions about the specific method used to solicit self-report information (e.g., mix of open- and closed-ended questions, use of composite scales, and so on)?
2. Was the instrument package adequately described in terms of conceptual appropriateness, reading level of the questions, length of time to complete it, and so on?
3. Was the mode of obtaining the self-report data appropriate (e.g., in-person interviews, mailed questionnaires, Internet questionnaires)?
4. Were self-report data gathered in a manner that promoted high-quality and unbiased responses (e.g., in terms of privacy, efforts to put respondents at ease, etc.)?
5. If observational methods were used, did the report adequately describe the specific constructs that were observed? What was the unit of observation?
6. Was a category system or rating system used to organize and record observations? Was the category system exhaustive? How much inference was required of the observers? Were decisions about exhaustiveness and degree of observer inference appropriate?
7. What methods were used to sample observational units? Was the sampling approach a good one, and did it likely yield a representative sample of behavior?
8. To what degree were observer biases controlled or minimized?
9. Were biophysiologic measures used in the study and was this appropriate? Did the researcher appear to have the skills necessary for proper interpretation of biophysiologic measures?
10. Were performance measures used in the study and was this appropriate?

RESEARCH EXAMPLE

In the study described next, a variety of data collection approaches was used to measure study variables.

Study: Predicting children's response to distraction from pain (Dr. Ann McCarthy and Dr. Charmaine Kleiber, principal investigators, NINR grant 1-R01-NR005269)

Statement of Purpose: Drs. McCarthy and Kleiber developed and tested an intervention to train parents as coaches to distract their children during insertion of an intravenous (IV) catheter. The overall study purpose was to test the effectiveness of the intervention in reducing children's pain and distress, to identify factors that predicted which children benefitted from the distraction, and to identify characteristics of parents who were successful in distracting their children.

Design: In this multisite clinical trial, 542 parents were randomly assigned to an intervention group or a usual-care control group. Their children, aged 4 to 10, were scheduled to undergo an IV insertion for a diagnostic medical procedure. Parents in the intervention group received 15 minutes of training regarding effective methods of distraction before the child's IV insertion.

Data Collection Plan: The researchers collected a wide range of data both prior to and following the intervention and IV procedure, using self-report, observational, and biophysiologic measures. The data collection plan included the use of formal instruments to describe sample characteristics, to assess key child outcomes, to measure parent and child factors they hypothesized would predict the intervention's effectiveness, to capture characteristics of the IV procedure, and to evaluate treatment fidelity. The researchers undertook a thorough literature review to identify factors influencing children's responses to a painful procedure and developed a model that guided their data collection efforts. Before proceeding with the full-scale study, the instruments were pretested (Kleiber & McCarthy, 2006). The pretest was used to assess whether the instruments were understandable, to evaluate the quality of data they would yield, and to explore interrelationships among study variables. Because of the extensiveness of their data collection plan, we describe only a few specific measures here.

Self-Report Instruments: Both parents and children provided self-report data. For example, the Oucher Scale was used as a self-report measure of children's pain. Children also reported their level of anxiety on a visual analog scale. Another child self-report instrument (Child Behavioral Style Scale) measured their coping style, using a vignette-type approach with four stressful scenarios. Parents completed self-administered questionnaires that incorporated scales to measure parenting style (Parenting Dimensions Inventory) and anxiety (State-Trait Anxiety Inventory). They also completed instruments that described their children's temperament (Dimensions of Temperament Survey).

Observational Instruments: A research assistant videotaped the parent and the child during their time in the treatment room. Videotapes were entered into a computerized video editing program and divided into 10-second intervals for analysis. The authors coded the parents' behavior in terms of the quality and frequency of distraction coaching, using an observational instrument that the researchers carefully developed, the Distraction Coaching Index (Kleiber et al., 2007). The videotapes were also used to code the children's behavioral distress, using the Observation Scale of Behavioral Distress.

Biophysiologic Measures: Children's stress was measured using salivary cortisol levels. Children chewed a piece of sugarless gum as a salivary stimulant. After discarding the gum, the children spat saliva into a collection tube. Each child provided four salivary cortisol samples: before IV insertion, 20 minutes after IV insertion, and two home samples to assess baseline cortisol levels. Care was taken to ensure the integrity of the samples and to control conditions under which they were obtained (McCarthy et al., 2009).

Key Findings: Reports on the results of the intervention study indicated that parents in the intervention group had significantly higher scores than those in the control group for distraction coaching frequency and quality (Kleiber et al., 2007), and children with the highest level of distraction coaching had the lowest levels of distress (McCarthy et al., 2010b). In another paper, the researchers identified several factors (the child's age, parental expectation of distress) that predicted children's pain and distress (McCarthy et al.,

2010a). In another analysis, McCarthy and colleagues (2011) compared behavioral distress and baseline salivary cortisol levels for children with and without attention-deficit/hyperactivity disorder (ADHD). They found significantly lower cortisol levels on the clinic day in the ADHD group of children. In another use of the data set, Hanrahan et al. (2012) developed a predictive model to predict children's risk of distress. In another analysis, McCarthy et al. (2014) explored the effects of three different doses of the distraction intervention for children at high and medium risks for distress.

SUMMARY POINTS

- Quantitative researchers develop a **data collection plan** before they begin to collect their data. For structured data, researchers use formal data collection **instruments** that place constraints on those collecting data and those providing them.
- An early step in developing a data collection plan is the identification and prioritization of data needs. Then, measures of the variables must be located. The selection of existing instruments should be based on conceptual suitability, data quality, cost, population appropriateness, and reputation.
- Even when existing instruments are used, the instrument package should be **pretested** to assess its length, clarity, and overall adequacy.
- Structured self-report instruments (**interview schedules** or **questionnaires**) can include open- and closed-ended questions. **Open-ended questions** permit respondents to reply in narrative fashion, whereas **closed-ended** (or *fixed-alternative*) **questions** offer **response options** from which respondents must choose.
- Types of closed-ended questions include (1) **dichotomous questions**, which require a choice between two options (e.g., yes/no); (2) **multiple-choice questions**, which offer a range of alternatives; (3) **rank-order questions**, in which respondents are asked to rank concepts on a continuum; (4) **forced-choice questions**,

which require respondents to choose between two competing options; (5) **rating questions**, which ask respondents to make graded ratings along a bipolar dimension; (6) **checklists** that include several questions with the same response format; and (7) **visual analog scales** (VASs), which are continually used to measure subjective experiences such as pain. **Event history calendars** and *diaries* are used to capture data about the occurrence of events.

- Composite psychosocial **scales** are multi-item self-report tools for measuring the degree to which individuals possess or are characterized by target attributes. Traditional **Likert scales** (**summated rating scales**) comprise a series of statements (**items**) about a phenomenon. Respondents rate their reaction to the item along a bipolar continuum (e.g., strongly agree/disagree). A total score is computed by summing item scores, each of which is scored for the intensity and direction of favorability expressed.
- Other self-report methods include **semantic differentials** (SDs), which consist of a set of bipolar rating scales on which respondents indicate reactions toward a phenomenon; **Q sorts**, in which people sort a set of card statements into piles according to specified criteria; **vignettes**, which descriptions of an event or situation to which respondents are asked to react; and **ecologic momentary assessments**, which involve repeated assessments of people's current behaviors or experiences in real time.
- Questionnaires are less costly and time-consuming than interviews and offer the possibility of anonymity. Interviews have higher response rates, are suitable for a wider variety of people, and yield richer data than questionnaires.
- Data quality in interviews depends on interviewers' interpersonal skills. Interviewers must put respondents at ease and build rapport, and need to **probe** skillfully for additional information when respondents give incomplete responses.
- Group administration is the most economical way to distribute questionnaires. Another approach is to mail them. Questionnaires can be distributed via the Internet, most often as a **web-based survey** that is accessed through a

hypertext link. Both types of questionnaires, especially those distributed over the Internet, tend to have low **response rates**, which can result in bias. Techniques such as **follow-up reminders** and good **cover letters** increase response rates to questionnaires.

• Structured self-reports are vulnerable to the risk of biases. **Response set biases** reflect the tendency of some people to respond to questions in characteristic ways, independently of content. Common response sets include **social desirability**, **extreme response**, and **acquiescence (yea-saying)**.

• Methods of **structured observation** impose constraints on observers to enhance the accuracy and objectivity of observations and to obtain an adequate representation of phenomena of interest.

• **Checklists** are used in observations to recording the occurrence or frequency of designated behaviors, events, or characteristics. Checklists are based on **category systems** for encoding observed phenomena into discrete categories. When using **rating scales**, observers rate phenomena along a dimension that is typically bipolar (e.g., passive/aggressive).

• **Time sampling** involves the specification of the duration and frequency of observational periods and intersession intervals. **Event sampling** selects integral behaviors or events of a special type for observation.

• Observational methods are an excellent way to operationalize some constructs but are subject to various biases. The greater the degree of observer inference, the more likely that distortions will occur.

• **Biophysiologic measures** comprise **in vivo measurements** (those performed within or on living organisms, such as blood pressure measurement) and **in vitro measurements** (those performed outside the organism's body, such as blood tests).

• Biophysiologic measures are objective, accurate, and precise, but care must be taken in using such measures with regard to practical, technical, and ethical considerations.

• When researchers cannot collect the data without assistance, they should carefully select data collection staff and formally train them.

STUDY ACTIVITIES

Chapter 13 of the *Resource Manual for Nursing Research*: *Generating and Assessing Evidence for Nursing Practice*, *10th edition*, offers exercises and study suggestions for reinforcing concepts presented in this chapter. In addition, the following study questions can be addressed:

1. Suppose you were planning to conduct a statewide study of the work plans and intentions of nonemployed registered nurses in your state. Would you ask mostly open-ended or closed-ended questions? Would you adopt an interview or questionnaire approach? If a questionnaire, how would you distribute it?

2. Suppose that the study of nonemployed nurses were done by a mailed questionnaire. Draft a cover letter to accompany it.

3. A nurse researcher is planning to study temper tantrums displayed by hospitalized children. Would you recommend using a time sampling approach? Why or why not?

STUDIES CITED IN CHAPTER 13

Augustin, A., Donovan, K., Lozano, E., Massucci, D., & Wohlgemuth, F. (2014). Still nursing at 6 months: A survey of breastfeeding mothers. *MCN: The American Journal of Maternal/Child Nursing, 39*, 50–55.

Bradburn, N., Sudman, S., & Wansink, B. (2004). *Asking questions: The definitive guide for questionnaire design—For market research, political polls, and social and health questionnaires.* San Francisco, CA: Jossey-Bass.

Carlson, J., Geisinger, K., & Jonson, J. (Eds.). (2014). *The nineteenth mental measurements yearbook.* Lincoln, NE: The Buros Institute.

Courtney, K., & Craven, C. (2005). Factors to weigh when considering electronic data collection. *Canadian Journal of Nursing Research, 37*(3), 150–159.

Dellefield, M. E., Harrington, C., & Kelly, A. (2012). Observing how RNs use clinical time in a nursing home: A pilot study. *Geriatric Nursing, 33*, 256–263.

Dillman, D., Smyth, J., & Christian, L. M. (2014). *Internet, phone, mail, and mixed-mode surveys: The tailored design method* (4th ed.). New York: Wiley.

Fitzpatrick, J. J., & Montgomery, K. S. (2004). *Internet for nursing research: A guide to strategies, skills, and resources.* New York: Springer.

Fowler, F. J. (2014). *Survey research methods* (5th ed.). Thousand Oaks, CA: Sage.

Guadagno, L., VandeWeerd, C., Stevens, D., Abraham, I., Paveza, G., & Fulmer, T. (2004). Using PDAs in data collection. *Applied Nursing Research, 17,* 283–291.

*Haidet, K. K., Tate, J., Divirgilio-Thomas, D., Kolanowski, A., & Happ, M. (2009). Methods to improve reliability of video-recorded behavioral data. *Research in Nursing & Health, 32,* 465–474.

*Hanrahan, K., McCarthy, A. M., Kleiber, C., Ataman, K., Street, W., Zimmerman, M., & Ersig, A. (2012). Building a computer program to support children, parents, and distraction during healthcare interventions. *Computers, Informatics, Nursing, 30,* 554–561.

Hardwick, M. E., Pulido, P., & Adelson, W. (2007). The use of handheld technology in nursing research and practice. *Orthopedic Nursing, 26,* 251–255.

Hosek, C., Faucher, M., Lankford, J., & Alexander, J. (2014). Perceptions of care in women sent home in latent labor. *MCN: American Journal of Maternal/Child Nursing, 39,* 115–121.

Jackson, D., Wilkes, L., & Luck, L. (2014). Cues that predict violence in the hospital setting: Findings from an observational study. *Collegian, 21,* 65–70.

Kleiber, C., & McCarthy, A. M. (2006). Evaluating instruments for a study on children's responses to a painful procedure when parents are distraction coaches. *Journal of Pediatric Nursing, 21,* 99–107.

Kleiber, C., McCarthy, A. M., Hanrahan, K., Myers, L., & Weathers, N. (2007). Development of the Distraction Coaching Index. *Children's Health Care, 36,* 219–235.

Koniak-Griffin, D., Brecht, M., Takayanagi, S., Villegas, J., Melendrez, M., & Balcazar, H. (2015). A community health worker-led lifestyle behavior intervention for Latina (Hispanic) women: Feasibility and outcomes of a randomized controlled trial. *International Journal of Nursing Studies, 52,* 75–87.

Liaw, J., Yang, L., Lo, C., Yuh, Y., Fan, H., Chang, Y., & Chao, S. (2012). Caregiving and positioning effects on preterm infant states over 24 hours in a neonatal unit in Taiwan. *Research in Nursing & Health, 35,* 132–145.

Martyn, K., & Belli, R. (2002). Retrospective data collection using event history calendars. *Nursing Research, 51,* 270–274.

*McCarthy, A. M., Hanrahan, K., Kleiber, C., Zimmerman, M. B., Lutgendorf, S., & Tsalikian, E. (2009). Normative salivary cortisol values and responsivity in children. *Applied Nursing Research, 22,* 54–62.

*McCarthy, A. M., Hanrahan, K., Scott, L., Zemblidge, N., Kleiber, C., & Zimmerman, M. (2011). Salivary cortisol responsivity to an intravenous catheter insertion in children with attention-deficit/hyperactivity disorder. *Journal of Pediatric Psychology, 36,* 902–910.

*McCarthy, A. M., Kleiber, C., Hanrahan, K., Zimmerman, M., Westhus, N., & Allen, S. (2010a). Factors explaining children's responses to intravenous needle insertions. *Nursing Research, 59,* 407–416.

McCarthy, A. M., Kleiber, C., Hanrahan, K., Zimmerman, M., Westhus, N., & Allen, S. (2010b). Impact of parent-provided distraction on child responses to an IV insertion. *Children's Health Care, 39,* 125–141.

McCarthy, A. M., Kleiber, C., Hanrahan, K., Zimmerman, M., Ersig, A., Westhus, N., & Allen, S. (2014). Matching doses of distraction with child risk for distress during a medical procedure: A randomized clinical trial. *Nursing Research, 63,* 397–407.

Nilsen, M., Sereika, S., Hoffman, L., Barnato, A., Donovan, H., & Happ, M. (2014). Nurse and patient interaction behaviors' effects on nursing care quality for mechanically ventilated older adults in the ICU. *Research in Gerontological Nursing, 5,* 113–125.

*Nyamathi, A., Marfisee, M., Slagle, A., Greengold, B., Liu, Y., & Leake, B. (2012). Correlates of depressive symptoms among homeless young adults. *Western Journal of Nursing Research, 34,* 97–117.

Nyamathi, A., Reback, C., Salem, B., Zhang, S., Shoptaw, S., Branson, C., & Leake, B. (2015). Correlates of self-reported incarceration among homeless gay and bisexual stimulant-using young adults. *Western Journal of Nursing Research, 37,* 799–811.

Oliva, D., Sandgren, A., Nilsson, M., & Lewin, F. (2014). Variations in self-reported nausea, vomiting, and well-being during the first 10 days postchemotherapy in women with breast cancer. *Clinical Journal of Oncology Nursing, 18,* E32–E36.

Ono, H., Taguchi, T., Kido, Y., Fujino, Y., & Doki, Y. (2011). The usefulness of bright light therapy for patients after oesophagectomy. *Intensive and Critical Care Nursing, 27,* 158–166.

*Oswalt, K., McClain, D., & Melnyk, B. (2013). Reducing anxiety among children born preterm and their young mothers. *MCN: The American Journal of Maternal/Child Nursing, 38,* 144–149.

Pecanac, K., Doherty-King, B., Yoon, J., Brown, R., & Schiefelbein, T. (2015). Using timed event sequential data in nursing research. *Nursing Research, 64,* 67–71.

Polit, D. F., London, A. S., & Martinez, J. M. (2001). *The health of poor urban women: Findings from the Project on Devolution and Urban Change.* New York: MDRC.

Ranse, K., Yates, P., & Coyer, F. (2015). Factors influencing the provision of end-of-life care in critical care settings: Development and testing of a survey instrument. *Journal of Advanced Nursing, 71,* 697–709.

Tappen, R., & Hain, D. (2014). The effect of in-home cognitive training on functional performance with mild cognitive impairment and early-stage Alzheimer's disease. *Research in Gerontological Nursing, 7,* 14–24.

*Thompson, A., Pickler, R., & Reyna, B. (2005). Clinical coordination of research. *Applied Nursing Research, 18,* 102–105.

Tourangeau, R., Conrad, F., & Couper, M. (2013). *The science of web surveys.* New York: Oxford University Press.

Tsai, P., Kuo, Y., Beck, C., Richards, K., Means, K., Pate, B., & Keefe, F. (2011). Non-verbal cues to osteoarthritis knee and/or hip pain in elders. *Research in Nursing & Health, 34,* 218–227.

Uzelli, D., & Yapucu Güneş, Ü. (2015). Oral glucose solution to alleviate pain induced by intramuscular injections in preterm infants. *Journal of Specialists in Pediatric Nursing, 20,* 29–35.

Von Vogelsang, A., Wenström, Y., Svensson, M., & Forsberg, C. (2014). Transitional experiences in patients following intracranial aneurysm rupture. *Journal of Clinical Nursing, 23,* 1263–1273.

Wang, Y., Zang, X., Bai, J., Liu, S., Zhao, Y., & Zhang, Q. (2014). Effect of a Health Belief Model-based nursing intervention on Chinese patients with moderate to severe chronic obstructive pulmonary disease: A randomised controlled trial. *Journal of Clinical Nursing, 23,* 1342–1353.

Yeo, S., & Logan, J. (2014). Preventing obesity: Exercise and daily activities of low-income pregnant women. *Journal of Perinatal & Neonatal Nursing, 28,* 17–25.

Yoder, P., & Symons, F. (2010). *Observational measurement of behavior.* New York: Springer.

***A link to this open-access journal article is provided in the Toolkit for this chapter in the accompanying Resource Manual.** ⊗

14 | Measurement and Data Quality

In quantitative studies, an ideal data collection procedure is one that measures a construct accurately, soundly, and with precision. Biophysiologic methods have a higher chance of success in attaining these goals than self-report or observational methods, but no method is flawless. In this chapter, we discuss criteria for evaluating the quality of data obtained by measuring constructs with structured instruments. We note that the field of measurement in health fields is evolving; a fuller discussion of the new directions and controversies, and a more detailed presentation of statistical issues in measurement, is provided in Polit and Yang (2015). We begin by discussing principles of measurement.

MEASUREMENT

Quantitative studies obtain data through the measurement of constructs. Clinicians also require that phenomena of interest be measured. **Measurement** involves assigning numbers to represent the amount of an attribute present in a person or object. Attributes are not constant: They vary from day to day or from one person to another. Variability is presumed to be capable of a numeric expression signifying *how much* of an attribute is present. The purpose of assigning numbers is to differentiate between people with varying degrees of the attribute.

Rules and Measurement

Measurement involves assigning numbers according to rules. *Rules* are necessary to promote consistency

and interpretability. The rules for measuring temperature, weight, and other physical attributes are familiar to us. Rules for measuring constructs such as nausea or quality of life, however, have to be invented. Whether the data are collected by observation, self-report, or some other method, researchers must specify criteria for assigning numeric values to the characteristic of interest. When researchers or clinicians invent a set of rules to gauge a construct, they create a **measure** of the construct. Measures yield **scores**—numeric values that communicate *how much* of an attribute is present or whether it is present at all.

The rules for measuring constructs must be evaluated to see if they are *good* rules. It is not enough to have rules—the rules must yield quantitative information that truly and accurately corresponds to different amounts of the targeted trait. New measurement rules reflect hypotheses about how attributes vary. The adequacy of the hypotheses—that is, the worth of the measurements—needs to be assessed empirically.

Researchers (and clinicians) work with fallible measures. Instruments that measure psychosocial phenomena by means of self-reports or observation are more error-prone than physical measures, but few measurements are error-free.

Advantages of Measurement

What exactly does measurement accomplish? Consider how handicapped health care professionals

297

would be in the absence of measurement. For example, what if there were no measures of body temperature or blood pressure? A major strength of measurement is that it removes subjectivity and guesswork. Because measurement is based on explicit rules, resulting information tends to be objective—that is, it can be independently verified. Two people measuring a person's weight using the same scale would likely get identical results. Most measures incorporate mechanisms for minimizing subjectivity.

Measurement also makes it possible to obtain reasonably precise information. Instead of describing Alex as "rather tall," we can depict him as being 6 feet 3 inches tall. With precise measures, researchers can differentiate among people with different degrees of an attribute.

Finally, measurement is a language of communication. Numbers are less vague than words. If a researcher reported that the average oral temperature of a sample of patients was "high," different readers might interpret the sample's physiologic state differently. However, if the researcher reported an average temperature of 99.8°F, there would be no ambiguity.

Theories of Measurement

Psychometrics is the branch of psychology concerned with the theory and methods of psychological measurement. Health measurement has been strongly influenced by psychometrics, although differences in aims and conceptualizations have begun to emerge. When new measures are developed and tested, researchers often say that they are undertaking a *psychometric assessment*.

Within psychometrics (and health measurement), two theories of measurement have been influential. **Classical test theory (CTT)** is a psychometric theory of measurement that has been dominant until fairly recently. CTT has been used as a basis for developing multi-item measures of health constructs and is also appropriate for conceptualizing all types of measurements (e.g., biophysiologic measures). An alternative measurement theory (**item response theory** or **IRT**) gaining in popularity is discussed in Chapter 15. Unlike CTT, IRT is an appropriate framework only for multi-item scales and tests.

Errors of Measurement

Procedures for obtaining measurements, as well as the objects being measured, are susceptible to influences that can alter the resulting data. Some influences can be controlled or minimized, and attempts should be made to do so, but such efforts are rarely completely successful.

Instruments that are not perfectly accurate yield measurements containing some error. Within classical test theory, an **observed** (or **obtained**) **score** can be conceptualized as having two parts—an error component and a true component. This can be written as follows:

$$\text{Obtained score} = \text{True score} \pm \text{Error}$$

or

$$X_O = X_T \pm X_E$$

The first term in the equation is an observed score—for example, a score on an anxiety scale. X_T is the value that would be obtained with an infallible measure. The **true score** is hypothetical—it can never be known because measures are *not* infallible. The final term is the **error of measurement**. The difference between true and obtained scores results from factors that distort the measurement.

Decomposing obtained scores in this manner highlights an important point. When researchers measure an attribute, they are also measuring attributes that are not of interest. The true score component is what they wish to isolate; the error component is a composite of other factors that are also being measured, contrary to their wishes. We illustrate with an exaggerated example. Suppose a researcher measured the weight of 10 people on a spring scale. As participants step on the scale, the researcher places a hand on their shoulders and applies pressure. The resulting measures (the X_Os) will be biased upward because scores reflect both actual weight (X_T) and pressure (X_E). Errors of measurement are problematic because their value is unknown and also because they often are variable. In this example, the amount of pressure applied likely would vary from one person to the next. In other words, the proportion of true score component in an obtained score varies from one person to the next.

Many factors contribute to errors of measurement. Some errors are random, while others are systematic, reflecting *bias*. Common sources of measurement error include the following:

1. *Transient personal factors*. A person's score can be influenced by such personal states as fatigue or mood. In some cases, such factors directly affect the measurement, as when anxiety affects pulse rate measurement. In other cases, personal factors alter scores by influencing people's motivation to cooperate, act naturally, or do their best.
2. *Situational contaminants*. Scores can be affected by the conditions under which they are produced. A participant's awareness of an observer's presence (reactivity) is one source of bias. Environmental factors, such as temperature, lighting, and time of day, are potential sources of measurement error.
3. *Response-set biases*. Relatively enduring characteristics of people can interfere with accurate measurements. Response sets such as social desirability or acquiescence are potential biases in self-report measures (Chapter 13).
4. *Administration variations*. Alterations in the methods of collecting data from one person to the next can result in score variations unrelated to variations in the target attribute. For example, if some physiologic measures are taken before a feeding and others are taken after a feeding, then measurement errors can potentially occur.
5. *Instrument clarity*. If the directions on an instrument are poorly understood, then scores may be affected. For example, questions in a self-report instrument may be interpreted differently by different respondents, leading to a distorted measure of the variable.
6. *Item sampling*. Errors can be introduced as a result of the sampling of items used in the measure. For example, a nursing student's score on a 100-item test of critical care nursing knowledge will be influenced by *which* 100 questions are included. A person might get 94 questions correct on one test but 92 right on another similar test.

> **TIP:** The Toolkit section of Chapter 14 of the *Resource Manual* includes a list of suggestions for enhancing data quality and minimizing measurement error in quantitative studies.

Major Types of Measures

Measurements for nursing research and practice can vary in a number of ways. For example, measurements can vary in terms of information source (i.e., self-reports, observation, etc.), complexity (e.g., a simple visual analog scale or a multidimensional scale with dozens of items), and type of scores they yield (e.g., continuous scores, categorical scores). Some measures are designed to be *generic*—that is, broadly applicable across different clinical or nonclinical populations; other measures are *specific*—that is, designed for use with specific groups of people. For example, there are self-efficacy scales that are generic, but there are many disease-specific self-efficacy scales (e.g., for diabetes or asthma).

Static and Adaptive Measures

Multi-item measures also differ with regard to whether they are static or adaptive. A **static measure** is administered in a comparable manner for everyone being measured. For a static composite scale, people complete an entire set of items and then are scored based on responses to all items. Most health-related measures are static. As an example, a widely used generic measure of depression is called the Center for Epidemiologic Studies Depression Scale, the CES-D (Radloff, 1977). Total scores on the CES-D rely on responses to the same 20 questions for everyone. Much of this book uses static scales to illustrate key measurement concepts.

An **adaptive measure**, by contrast, involves using responses to early questions to guide the selection of subsequent questions. Dynamic adaptive measures are becoming popular as a way to obtain precise information about an attribute with minimum respondent burden. Adaptive testing has its origin in measurement advances from item response theory. *Item banks* with hundreds of items have been created for broad health topics, such as physical function, pain, or sleep disturbance. The most important example of item banking is **PROMIS**® (Patient Reported Outcomes Measurement Information System), developed with support from the U.S. National Institutes of Health (Cella et al., 2007). An approach called **computerized adaptive testing (CAT)** uses these item banks to create measurements that are tailored to individuals. With such tailoring, the set of items used to measure a construct can be different for each patient. Despite item differences, cross-patient comparisons can be made because the testing places people along a dimension of interest.

Reflective Scales and Formative Indexes

An important distinction is whether a multi-item measure is formative or reflective, which concerns the nature of the relationship between a construct and the measure of the construct. Constructs are not directly observable—they must be inferred by the effects they have on observables, such as responses to items on a patient-reported outcome (PRO) or behaviors witnessed and recorded on an observational scale. Most health scales are **reflective scales**: The items are viewed as *reflections* of the construct. For example, on the CES-D, it is presumed that a person's underlying level of depression *causes* him or her to respond in a certain way to the items about sleep disturbance, sadness, and so on. The items on a reflective scale share a common cause—in this case, level of depression. Items on reflective scales are expected to be interrelated because they all reflect (are caused by) the construct.

Not all multi-item instruments, however, are reflective. A multi-item measure can be conceptualized as having items that "cause" or define the attribute (rather than being the effect of the attribute). Such measures are called **formative measures**. Several writers advocate using the term *scale* for multi-item reflective measures, and the term **index** for multi-item formative measures (DeVellis, 2012; Streiner, 2003). A formative index involves constructs that are *formed* by its components, rather than causing them.

A good illustration of a formative index is the Holmes-Rahe Social Readjustment Scale, which is a measure of stress. Psychiatrists Holmes and Rahe studied whether stressful life events might cause illness and devised an index that asked patients to indicate which of 43 life events they had experienced in the previous year (Holmes & Rahe, 1967). Examples of life event items include death of a spouse, pregnancy, and change in residence. The life events are assigned different weights or "life change units" (e.g., 100 for death of a spouse, 20 for a change in residence), and the units are then added together. The sum of life change units defines the construct of stressful life events. The items are not the "effect" of the construct—for example, having high stress does not "cause" the death of a spouse or a residential move.

Because the items on an index are not *caused* by an underlying construct, they are not necessarily intercorrelated. In fact, items with modest correlations that capture different aspects of an attribute are often desired in a formative index. Many screening tools are formative and are composed of components that independently predict an outcome.

The development of reflective scales and formative indexes is necessarily different. For example, because the items on a formative index define the attribute, the specific items matter very much. If the item "I had crying spells" on the CES-D scale was removed, for example, the other 19 items could carry most of the burden of measuring depression. But if the item "Death of a spouse" was removed from the Holmes-Rahe index, the score would misrepresent the stress levels of people who had lost a spouse. Another consequence of having noncorrelated items on a formative index is that some of the standard assessment methods associated with CTT are not appropriate, as we explain later in this chapter.

⊃ TIP: Formative indexes are seldom created using standard psychometric approaches. Formative indexes are sometimes developed within the field of **clinimetrics**, which is devoted to the development of measures of clinical phenomena. Polit and Yang (2015) have written a chapter on clinimetrics in their measurement book.

MEASUREMENT PROPERTIES: AN OVERVIEW

In making decisions about how to measure their constructs, careful researchers select instruments that are known to be psychometrically sound—that is, ones that have good **measurement properties**. Psychometricians have traditionally focused on two measurement properties when assessing the quality of a measure: reliability and validity. Measurement experts in health disciplines, however, have taken a broader view of the measurement properties of an instrument.

A Measurement Taxonomy

The field of health measurement was in some turmoil for many years with regard to measurement terminology and definitions. Recently, a working group in the Netherlands used a Delphi-type approach with a panel of health measurement experts to identify key measurement properties and to develop a taxonomy and definitions of those properties. The result was

the creation of **COSMIN**, the **Co**nsensus-based **S**tandards for the selection of health **M**easurement **In**struments (Mokkink et al., 2010a, 2010b; Terwee et al., 2012). (Information about COSMIN can be accessed at http://www.cosmin.nl.) Polit and Yang (2015), building on the groundbreaking COSMIN work, made small modifications to the taxonomy to more clearly incorporate a time perspective. A graphic depiction of the Polit-Yang measurement taxonomy is shown in Figure 14.1.

In this taxonomy, there are four measurement property domains. Two are cross-sectional—that is, they concern the quality of measurements at one point in time. These cross-sectional domains are *reliability* and *validity*, the properties used for decades by psychometricians. Two other domains in the taxonomy concern longitudinal measurement—that is,

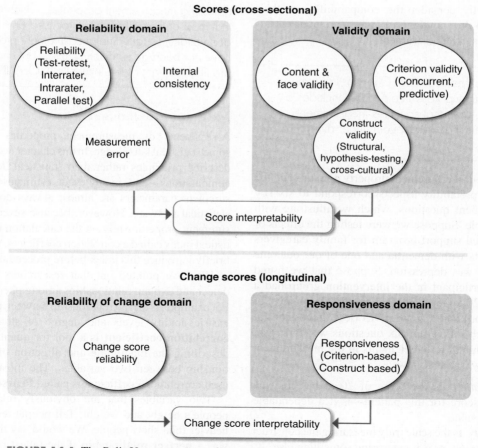

FIGURE 14.1 The Polit-Yang taxonomy of measurement properties.

the quality of measurements capturing changes over time. These two domains are called the *reliability of change scores* and *responsiveness*. New measures that are likely to be used to measure a construct at a single point *and* to assess how the construct changed over time ideally would be evaluated for all four measurement properties. The taxonomy also incorporates another concept—interpretability—that has relevance for both point-in-time scores and change scores.

Each measurement property can be evaluated by estimating **measurement parameters** that quantify the degree to which the scores on the measure have desirable properties. These estimates are the means by which conclusions can be drawn about an instrument's quality. Estimates of measurement properties are relevant for particular applications and particular populations, and so researchers need to carefully consider the comparability of their sample to the sample used in measurement assessments of a given instrument.

⊘ **TIP:** The Toolkit for Chapter 14 in the accompanying *Resource Manual* includes a summary table that specifies measurement parameters that are relevant under different scenarios.

The four measurement property domains and the two interpretability aspects correspond to six key measurement questions, which we illustrate with an example. Suppose we were testing the effects of a nurse-led support program for family caregivers of patients with dementia and one of our outcome variables was depression. Suppose that we found that a participant in the intervention group had a score of 20 on the CES-D at baseline (high level of depression) and a score of 15 (less depression) at a 6-month follow-up. Six questions we could ask, corresponding to the elements in the measurement taxonomy, are as follows:

1. *Reliability*: Is the score of 20 at baseline the right score for this patient—is it a dependable score value?
2. *Validity*: Is the scale truly measuring the construct depression, or is it measuring something else?

3. *Interpretation of a score*: What does a score of 20 *mean*? Is it high or low?
4. *Reliability of change*: Is the change from 20 to 15 a *real* change, or does it merely reflect random fluctuations in measurement?
5. *Responsiveness*: Does the change from 20 to 15 correspond to a commensurate improvement in degree of depression?
6. *Interpretation of a change score*: What does a 5-point improvement *mean*? Is the improvement large enough to be considered clinically significant?

This chapter describes the four domains in the measurement taxonomy. Issues relating to interpretation are discussed in Chapters 15 and 20.

⊘ **TIP:** Nurse researchers have mainly followed standard psychometric approaches to assessing measurement properties, which means that most of their efforts have focused on reliability and validity. Longitudinal measurement properties have not been given much scrutiny, but changes are likely in light of the influential COSMIN work.

Measurement and Statistics

Assessments of measurement properties require some statistical knowledge. In this chapter, we mainly describe principles rather than statistical details or computations—and, in any event, estimates of measurement parameters are almost always done with statistical software. However, because several measurement properties rely on the calculation of a statistical index called a correlation coefficient, we must briefly introduce this index before proceeding.

We have pointed out that researchers seek to detect and explain relationships among phenomena. For example, is there a relationship between patients' gastric acidity levels and degree of stress? The **correlation coefficient** is a tool for quantitatively describing the magnitude and direction of a relationship between two variables. The most widely used correlation coefficient is called **Pearson's r**.

Two variables that are obviously related are people's height and weight. Tall people tend to be heavier than short people. We would say that there was a **perfect relationship** if the tallest person in a population were the heaviest, the second tallest person were the second heaviest, and so forth. Correlation coefficients summarize how perfect a relationship is. The possible values for a correlation coefficient range from -1.00 through .00 to $+1.00$. If height and weight were perfectly correlated, the correlation coefficient expressing this relationship would be $+1.00$. Because the relationship exists but is not perfect, the correlation coefficient is in the vicinity of $+.50$ or $+.60$ (which would typically be written as .50 and .60). The relationship between height and weight is a **positive relationship** because *increases* in height tend to be associated with *increases* in weight.

When two variables are totally unrelated, the correlation coefficient equals zero. One might expect that women's height is unrelated to their intelligence. Tall women are as likely to perform well on IQ tests as short women. The correlation coefficient summarizing such a relationship would presumably be in the vicinity of .00.

Correlation coefficients running from .00 to -1.00 express **inverse** or **negative relationships**. When two variables are inversely related, increases in one variable are associated with *decreases* in the second variable. Suppose that there is an inverse relationship between people's age and the amount of sleep they get. This means that, on average, the older the person, the fewer the hours of sleep. If the relationship were perfect (e.g., if the oldest person in a population slept the fewest hours, and so on), the correlation coefficient would be -1.00. In actuality, the relationship between age and sleep is probably modest—in the vicinity of $-.15$ or $-.20$. A correlation coefficient of this magnitude describes a weak relationship: Older people *tend* to sleep fewer hours and younger people *tend* to sleep more, but nevertheless, some younger people sleep few hours, and some older people sleep a lot.

Correlation coefficients are important statistical tools in evaluating the quality of measuring instruments.

RELIABILITY

The reliability of a quantitative measure is a major criterion for assessing its quality. **Reliability**, broadly speaking, is the extent to which scores are free from measurement error. However, from an operational perspective, an extended definition is more useful. Adapting slightly from COSMIN, we offer this definition:

• Reliability is the extent to which scores for people *who have not changed* are the same for repeated measurements, under several situations, including repetition on different occasions, by different persons, or on different versions of a measure, or in the form of different items on a multi-item instrument (internal consistency).

In other words, reliability concerns consistency— the *absence* of variation—in measuring a stable attribute for an individual. In all types of assessments, reliability involves a *replication* to evaluate the extent to which scores for a stable trait are the same. Assessments to evaluate the degree of consistency require a heterogeneous sample of people from a population because the role of a reliable measure is to allow people to be distinguished from one another.

In our taxonomy shown in Figure 14.1, as well as in the COSMIN taxonomy, the cross-sectional reliability domain encompasses three components: reliability, internal consistency, and measurement error. We briefly discuss each component and describe the measurement parameters corresponding to each component.

Reliability

The first component within the broad reliability domain is simply called reliability. It covers four different approaches to reliability assessment, including the following:

• **Test–retest reliability**: administration of the same measure to the same people on two occasions (repetition over occasions)
• **Interrater reliability**: measurements by two or more observers or raters using the same instrument (repetition over persons)
• **Intrarater reliability**: measurements by the same observer or rater on two or more occasions (repetition over occasions)
• **Parallel test reliability**: measurements of the same attribute using alternate versions of the same instrument, with the same people (repetition over versions)

Assessments of reliability involve the calculation of a statistic broadly called a **reliability coefficient**, sometimes symbolized as *R*. These coefficients, calculated from sample data, are estimates of how reliable the scores are. Different types of coefficients are used in different situations, but they typically range from a low of 0.00 (signifying no reliability) to a high of 1.00 and are thus similar to correlation coefficients that are not negative in value. The higher the coefficient, the more reliable are the scores. Perfect reliability—a coefficient of 1.00—is virtually impossible to obtain, but it is the goal for reliability assessments.

Test–Retest Reliability

In **test–retest reliability**, replication takes the form of administering a measure to the same people on two occasions. If a measure yields a good estimate of the true scores of an attribute, ideally, it will do so comparably on separate administrations. The assumption is that for traits that have not changed, any differences in people's scores on the two testings are the result of measurement error. When score differences across waves are small, reliability is high. This type of reliability is sometimes called *stability* or *reproducibility*—the extent to which scores can be reproduced on repeated administrations.

To illustrate, suppose we were interested in the test–retest reliability of a 16-item self-esteem scale. Self-esteem is a fairly stable attribute that does not fluctuate much from day to day, so we would expect a reliable measure of it to yield consistent scores on two occasions. To check the instrument's reliability, we administer the scale 2 weeks apart. Fictitious data for this example are shown in Table 14.1 for a small sample of 10 people; in a real assessment, the sample would be much larger. It can be seen that, in general, differences in scores on the two testings are not large. The person who scored highest at Time 1 (Participant 3) also scored highest at Time 2, for example.

When a measure yields continuous scores, as in this example, the preferred reliability parameter for test–retest reliability is the **intraclass correlation coefficient** or **ICC**. It is beyond the scope of this book to explain how the ICC is computed, but in

TABLE 14.1 • Fictitious Data for 2-Week Test–Retest Reliability of Self-Esteem Scale

PARTICIPANT NUMBER	TIME 1	TIME 2	
1	55	57	
2	49	46	
3	78	74	
4	37	35	
5	44	46	
6	50	56	
7	58	55	
8	62	66	
9	48	50	
10	67	63	ICC = .95

Note. ICC = intraclass coefficient.

our example, the value of the ICC is .95.* ICCs be completed in major statistical software packages, such as IBM SPSS Statistics (SPSS), previously known as the Statistical Package for the Social Sciences.

> **TIP:** Many nurse researchers compute a Pearson's correlation coefficient (*r*) as the reliability estimate in retest situations. However, measurement experts consider Pearson's correlation inappropriate for estimating reliability (e.g., De Vet et al., 2011), even though the values of the ICC and *r* are usually close. In our example of self-esteem scores, the value of the Pearson's *r* coefficient was also .95.

Test–retest reliability can be assessed with virtually all measures, including biophysiologic measures, observational measures, performance tests,

---

*ICCs can be computed using several different formulas, and the values of the coefficient can vary from one formula to the next. As explained more fully in Polit and Yang (2015), a main distinction is between what is called ICC for agreement versus ICC for consistency. In our example in Table 14.1, the reliability estimate is .951 for $ICC_{Consistency}$ and .956 for $ICC_{Agreement}$. Researchers reporting the value of ICC should state which ICC was calculated.

1-item measures (e.g., visual analog scales, single demographic questions), formative indexes, and reflective scales. Nevertheless, retest reliability assessment can be problematic. One issue is that many traits *do* change over time, independently of the measure's stability. Attitudes, knowledge, skills, and so on can be modified by experiences between testings—and true change would make a measure look less reliable than it actually is. For this reason, a major issue in retest reliability assessment is finding the right interval between testings.

Another issue is that people's responses on a second administration can be influenced by their memory of initial responses, regardless of the actual values the second time. Such memory interference (called a *carryover effect*) could result in spuriously high reliability coefficients. Another difficulty is that people may actually change *as a result of* the first administration. Finally, people may not be as careful using the same instrument a second time. If they find the process boring on the second occasion, then responses could be haphazard, resulting in a spuriously low estimate of reliability. Other complications relating to retest reliability assessments, and strategies to deal with them, have been described by Polit (2014).

The myriad problems of retest reliability assessment led some measurement experts to discourage using the test–retest approach, including noted psychometricians Nunnally and Bernstein (1994): "We recommend that the retest method generally not be used to estimate reliability" (p. 255). Health care researchers, however, have disagreed with this viewpoint and have put strong emphasis on retest reliability—perhaps because of its role in coming to conclusions about true changes in scores. Because nurse researchers have often pursued standard psychometric methods, those who have developed scales have not always estimated test–retest reliability, but this likely will change in the years ahead.

Example of Test–Retest Reliability: Chow and Wong (2014) tested the reliability of the Chinese version of the Short-Form Chronic Disease Self-Efficacy Scale. In a 2-week retest, the value of the ICC was .98.

> **TIP:** Many reflective scales and formative indexes contain two or more **subscales**, each of which measures distinct but related concepts (e.g., a measure of fatigue might include subscales for mental and physical fatigue). The reliability of each subscale should be assessed. If subscale scores are summed for a total score, the scale's overall reliability is also estimated.

Interrater and Intrarater Reliability

When measurements involve the use of an observer who makes scoring judgments, a key source of measurement error can stem from the person making the measurements. This is a familiar situation for observational instruments (e.g., scales to measure agitation in nursing home residents) and is also true for some biophysiologic measurements (e.g., skinfold measurement) and performance tests (balance tests). In such situations, it is important to evaluate how reliably the measurements reflect attributes of the person being rated rather than attributes of the raters. Developers of new observational measures need to know how capable their instruments are of yielding reliable scores with trained observers. And, users of such measures—including clinicians and clinical trialists—often want to know whether they or their staff can reliably apply the measure and how much training is needed to achieve adequate reliability. In these reliability assessment situations, replication is necessary.

The most typical approach is to undertake an **interrater** (or *interobserver*) **reliability** assessment, which involves having two or more observers independently applying the instrument with the same people. Reliability assessment involves comparing the observers' scores to see if the scores are comparable.

A less frequently used approach—but one that is appropriate in many clinical situations—is an **intrarater reliability** assessment in which the *same* rater makes the measurements on two or more occasions, blinded to the ratings assigned previously. Intrarater reliability is an index of self-consistency. It is analogous to retest reliability, except that the focus in retest situations is the consistency of the person *being measured*, and intrarater reliability concerns the consistency of the person *making the measurements*. Like retest reliability, intrarater reliability assessments require a carefully selected interval between testings.

Estimates of inter- or intrarater reliability can be obtained by computing an ICC if the measurements yield continuous scores. In other situations, however, observers are asked to *classify* their observations into categories. When ratings are categorical, one procedure is to calculate the **proportion of agreement**, using the following equation:

$$\frac{\text{Number of agreements}}{\text{Number of agreements + disagreements}}$$

This formula unfortunately tends to overestimate agreements because it fails to account for agreement by chance. If a behavior being observed were coded for absence versus presence, the observers would agree 50% of the time by chance alone. A widely used statistic in this situation is Cohen's **kappa**, which adjusts for chance agreement. Values of kappa usually range from .00 to 1.00. Different standards have been proposed for acceptable levels of kappa, but there is some agreement that a value of .60 is minimally acceptable and that values of .75 or higher are very good.

Example of Interrater Reliability: Nilsen and colleagues (2014) tested interrater reliability on the Communication Interaction Behavior Instrument (CIBI), an observational measure for rating the quality of communication (positive/negative) between nurses and mechanically ventilated ICU patients. Proportion of agreement on individual items ranged from .73 to 1.00 for nurse behaviors and .68 to 1.00 for patient behaviors. Kappa coefficients ranged from .13 to 1.00, suggesting further refinement of some items was needed.

Parallel Test Reliability

Multi-item *parallel tests* (or *alternative-form tests*) are not common in health care measurement, but there are a few examples. For instance, the latest version of the Mini-Mental State Examination (MMSE-2), a measure of cognitive impairment, has alternate forms (Folstein et al., 2010). Parallel tests can be created by randomly sampling two sets of items from a carefully developed item pool. If the two tests are, indeed, parallel, then they are replicates whose true scores are identical. Having measures that are parallel is useful when researchers expect to make measurements in a fairly short period of time and want to avoid carryover biases.

Similar to test–retest reliability, **parallel test reliability** involves administration of the parallel tests to the same people on two separate occasions, and then estimating a reliability parameter, which would be the intraclass correlation coefficient. Unlike retest reliability, however, parallel test reliability is appropriate only for reflective multi-item scales. With formative indexes, the specific items are important and cannot be construed as a random sample of interrelated items.

Interpretation of Reliability Coefficients

Reliability coefficients are important indicators of an instrument's quality. Unreliable measures reduce statistical power and hence affect statistical conclusion validity. If data fail to support a hypothesis, one possibility is that the instruments were unreliable—not necessarily that the expected relationships do not exist.

For group-level comparisons, reliability coefficients in the vicinity of .70 may be adequate (especially for subscales), but coefficients of .80 or greater are desirable. By group-level comparisons, we mean that researchers compare scores of groups, such as males versus females or experimental versus control participants. The reliability coefficients for measures used for making decisions about individuals ideally should be .90 or better. For instance, if a score was used to make decisions about a patient's eligibility for a special intervention, then the test's reliability would be of critical importance.

Reliability coefficients have a special interpretation that relates to the decomposition of observed scores into error and true score components. Suppose we administered a scale that measures hopefulness to 50 patients with cancer. The scores would vary from one person to another—that is, some people would be more hopeful than others. Some variability in scores is true variability, reflecting real individual differences in hopefulness; some variability, however, is measurement error. Thus,

$$V_O = V_T + V_E$$

where V_O = observed total variability in scores
V_T = true variability
V_E = variability owing to error

A reliability coefficient is directly associated with this equation. *Reliability is the proportion of true variability to the total obtained variability*, or

$$R = \frac{V_T}{V_O}$$

If, for example, the reliability coefficient were .85, then 85% of the variability in obtained scores would represent true individual differences, and 15% of the variability would reflect extraneous fluctuations. Looked at in this way, it should be clear why instruments with reliability lower than .70 are risky to use.

Factors Affecting Reliability

Several factors under the control of researchers can affect the value of reliability coefficients. With observational scales, for example, reliability can be improved by greater precision in defining categories, or greater clarity in explaining the underlying construct. An excellent means of enhancing reliability for observational measures is thorough observer training.

A measure's reliability is related to the heterogeneity of the sample with which it is tested. The more homogeneous the sample (i.e., the more similar their scores), the lower the reliability coefficient will be. This is because instruments are designed to measure differences among those being measured. If the sample is homogeneous, then it is more difficult for the instrument to discriminate reliably among those who possess varying degrees of the attribute. For example, suppose that the self-esteem scores shown in Table 14.1 were changed for two individuals. If Participant 3 (the high scorer) had scores of 58 and 54 (rather than 78 and 74) and if Participant 4 (the low scorer) had scores of 57

and 55 (rather than 37 and 35), the ICC would be .85 rather than .95 because now the range of scores is smaller (44 to 67 versus 37 to 78).

An important thing to keep in mind in computing or interpreting reliability coefficients within the CTT framework—or in selecting an instrument for use in a study—is that *reliability is not a fixed property of an instrument*. For a given measure, reliability will vary from one population to another or from one situation to another. It is better to think of reliability as a property of a particular set of scores than as a property of a measure itself. Users of an instrument need to consider how similar their population is to the population used to estimate reliability parameters. If the populations are similar, then the reliability estimate calculated by the scale developer is probably a reasonably good index of the instrument's accuracy in the new research. But if the population is very different, new estimates of reliability should be computed.

Internal Consistency

Another component within the reliability domain of the measurement taxonomy (see Figure 14.1) is **internal consistency**. Our reliability definition supports including internal consistency within the reliability domain: Reliability is the extent to which scores for patients who have not changed are the same for repeated measurements. For internal consistency, replication involves people's responses to multiple items during a single administration. Whereas reliability estimates described in the previous section assess a measure's degree of consistency across time, raters, and versions of a measure, internal consistency captures consistency across items.

Single items are often inadequate for measuring a construct—indeed, the low reliability of single items is the reason for constructing multi-item scales. In responding to an item, people are influenced not only by the underlying construct but also by idiosyncratic reactions to the words. By sampling multiple items with various wordings, item irrelevancies are expected to cancel each other out. An instrument is said to be internally consistent to the extent that its items measure the same trait.

The most widely used statistic for evaluating internal consistency is **coefficient alpha** (or **Cronbach's alpha**). Coefficient alpha estimates the extent to which different subparts of an instrument (i.e., items) are reliably measuring the critical attribute, and greater internal consistency is obtained with a set of items that are highly intercorrelated. Coefficient alpha can be interpreted like other reliability coefficients: The normal range of values is between .00 and +1.00, and higher values reflect better internal consistency. Coefficients of .80 or higher are considered especially desirable. It is beyond the scope of this text to explain computations of coefficient alpha, but information is available in measurement textbooks (e.g., Nunnally & Bernstein, 1994; Polit & Yang, 2015). Most standard statistical software such as SPSS can be used to calculate alpha.

An important feature of internal consistency is that the value of coefficient alpha is partly a function of the scale's length. To improve internal consistency, more items tapping the same construct should be added.

Internal consistency has been the most widely reported aspect of reliability assessment among nurse researchers. Its popularity reflects the fact that it is economical (it requires only one administration) and is a means of assessing an important source of measurement error in psychosocial instruments, the sampling of items.

Internal consistency is a relevant measurement property only for multi-item reflective scales, however. It is *not* relevant for formative indexes, which are composed of items that are not necessarily intercorrelated. For formative indexes, only retest reliability should be estimated. For most multi-item reflective scales (whether they are self-report scales or observational scales), both internal consistency and retest reliability should be assessed by the scale developer. Users of an existing scale should also re-evaluate coefficient alpha whenever research data are collected.

> **Example of Internal Consistency Reliability:**
> Choe (2014) developed and assessed a scale to measure hope in people with schizophrenia. The 9-item scale had high internal consistency, with coefficient alpha = .92.

> **⊃ TIP:** Reliability estimates vary according to the procedures used to obtain them. A scale's test–retest reliability coefficient (ICC) should not be expected to be the same or even similar in value to an internal consistency estimate (alpha).

Measurement Error

Measurement error is another component within the reliability domain of our taxonomy. The concepts of measurement error and reliability are inextricably connected: Unless a reliability coefficient is 1.0 (which is virtually never the case), measurement error is present. Yet, measurement error statistics yield information that reliability coefficients do not provide. For example, measurement error statistics can be used to estimate the precision of a continuous score—that is, the range within which the true score probably lies.

The Standard Error of Measurement

The most widely used index of measurement error is the **standard error of measurement (SEM)**. The SEM can be thought of as quantifying "typical error" on a measure. It is an index that can be computed in connection with estimates of either reliability (e.g., test–retest reliability) or internal consistency.

Reliability coefficients, which typically range from 0.0 to 1.0, are not in the units of measurement associated with the actual measure. A reliability coefficient is a *relative* index that varies from sample to sample and across populations. SEMs, by contrast, are in the measurement units of the instrument. The SEM for a body weight would be in pounds (or grams), and the SEM for a scale such as the CES-D would be in the units of points on the CES-D scale. SEMs are more stable than reliability coefficients and not as affected by sample homogeneity.

The SEM can be estimated from one of several formulas. A popular and easy formula involves taking the square root of 1 minus the reliability coefficient $(1 - R)$ and multiplying that value by an index summarizing how variable the sample scores are.[†] (R could be either the ICC estimate from a

---

[†]Specifically, this formula for the SEM is: $SEM = SD\sqrt{(1 - R)}$.

test–retest analysis or alpha from an internal consistency analysis.) Unfortunately, the SEM is not computed in many major software packages, which might explain why it is not more routinely reported in instrument development papers.

For the self-esteem scores shown in Table 14.1, the SEM is 2.65 at Time 1 (and 2.49 at Time 2). Knowing the value of the SEM allows us to state the probability that a person's true score lies within a certain range. For example, Participant 1 had a score of 55 at Time 1. Knowing that the SEM is 2.65, we could state that there is a 95% probability that his or her true score at Time 1 was between about 50 and 60 (i.e., roughly twice the SEM on either side of the obtained score).

Limits of Agreement

An alternative index of measurement error is called the **limits of agreement (LOA)**, derived from work done by Bland and Altman (1986). *Bland-Altman plots* are widely used by medical researchers to examine aspects of both reliability and validity of measures but are seldom used by psychometricians or nurse researchers. A Bland-Altman plot is a useful device for visually interpreting and differentiating random measurement error and systematic error (bias) in retest or interrater assessments when scores are continuous. Limits of agreement as an index of measurement error cannot be computed when only internal consistency has been estimated.

Like the SEM, the LOA provides information about the precision of scores. Limits of agreement are easy to compute but are not routinely calculated in standard statistical software packages such as SPSS.[‡] For the self-esteem scores in Table 14.1, the limit of agreement is about ± 7.0 around a difference score (i.e., the value differentiating Time 1 and Time 2 scores). This means that any difference in a person's score that is greater than 7 is beyond what we would expect for measurements of a stable trait. None of the score differences in Table 14.1 is greater than 7. A Bland-Altman plot showing the

LOA for the data in Table 14.1 is presented in the Toolkit of the accompanying *Resource Manual*. ⊗

> **Example of Measurement Error Information:** Vellone and colleagues (2014) evaluated a 9-item version of the European Heart Failure Self-Care Behavior Scale. The average score on the scale was 58.3, and the value of the SEM was 4.3.

> ➲ **TIP:** Measurement error is routinely estimated for multi-item measures developed with item response theory (IRT) methods. Indeed, estimating measurement error typically replaces efforts to estimate internal consistency or reliability. One problem with measurement error in standard CTT measures is that the estimate is the same for everyone in a sample, whereas measurement error can be estimated for each individual using IRT models. In computerized adaptive tests, a "stopping rule" is established at a desired level of precision (i.e., for a maximum allowable amount of measurement error), and the stopping rule dictates how many items each respondent completes.

VALIDITY

A second domain in the taxonomy of measurement properties is validity. **Validity** in a measurement context is defined as the degree to which an instrument is measuring the construct it purports to measure. When researchers develop a scale to measure *resilience*, they need to be sure that the resulting scores validly reflect this construct and not something else, such as self-efficacy, hope, or perseverance. Assessing the validity of abstract constructs requires a careful conceptualization of the construct—as well as a conceptualization of what the construct is *not*.

Like reliability, validity has different aspects and assessment approaches. As shown in Figure 14.1, the three major components within the validity domain are content and face validity, criterion validity, and construct validity. Unlike reliability, however, an instrument's validity is difficult to gauge. There are no equations that can easily be applied to the

---

[‡]Limits of agreement can be computed using output from a paired *t*-test analysis. For 95% confidence, the LOA is 1.96 times the standard deviation of difference between the test and the retest.

scores of a resilience scale to estimate how good a job the scale is doing in measuring the critical variable. Validation is an evidence-building enterprise, in which the goal is to assemble sufficient evidence from which validity can be inferred. The greater the amount of evidence supporting validity, the more sound the inference.

⮕ **TIP:** Reliability and validity are not totally independent properties of an instrument. A measuring device that is unreliable cannot be valid. An instrument cannot validly measure an attribute if it is inconsistent.

Content and Face Validity

Face validity refers to whether the instrument *looks* like it is measuring the target construct. Although face validity is not considered strong evidence of validity, it is helpful for a measure to have face validity if other types of validity have also been demonstrated. Face validity is typically not considered a critical measurement property, but it can be important if patients' resistance to being measured reflects the view that the scale is not relevant to their problems or situations. One reason for developing disease-specific measures, in fact, is that general measures sometimes lack face validity.

Example of Face Validity: Gaugler and co-researchers (2013) developed and tested the CARES Observation Tool for assessing person-centered dementia care. Face validity was assessed through consultation with several sets of experts in dementia care.

Content validity may be defined as the extent to which an instrument's content adequately captures the construct—that is, whether an instrument has an appropriate sample of items for the construct being measured. Although content validity has not always been paid great attention, a guiding document for patient-reported outcomes issued by the U.S. Food and Drug Administration (2009) placed strong emphasis on content validity. It is increasingly

recognized that evaluating and enhancing a measure's content validity is a critical early step in enhancing the construct validity of an instrument (e.g., Strauss & Smith, 2009). If the content of an instrument is a good reflection of a construct, then the instrument has a greater likelihood of achieving its measurement objectives.

Three issues are pertinent in a content validation, which typically involves consultations with experts: relevance, comprehensiveness, and balance.

- *Relevance.* An assessment for relevance involves feedback on the relevance of individual items and the overall set of items. For each item, one needs to know: Is this item relevant to the construct, or to a specific dimension of the construct? Another consideration is whether the items have relevance for the target population.
- *Comprehensiveness.* The flip side of asking experts about the relevance of items is to ask them if there are notable omissions. To be content valid, a measure should comprehensively encompass the full complexity of the construct.
- *Balance.* An instrument that is content valid represents the domains of the construct in a balanced manner. In a multi-item scale, a sufficient number of items is needed for each dimension to ensure high internal consistency of the subscales.

Researchers designing a new instrument should begin with a thorough conceptualization of the construct so the instrument can capture the full content domain. Such a conceptualization might be based on rich first-hand knowledge, an exhaustive literature review, consultation with experts, and in-depth conversations with members of the target population. Specific advice about the application of qualitative methods to content validity efforts was offered by Brod and colleagues (2009).

Example of Using Qualitative Data to Enhance Content Validity: Miller and colleagues (2015) developed the Life Changes in Epilepsy Scale to measure perceived changes in social functioning, somatic health, and subjective well-being since epilepsy onset. The scale items were based in part on in-depth qualitative research with patients with adult-onset epilepsy.

An instrument's content validity is necessarily based on judgment. There are no objective methods of ensuring adequate content coverage on an instrument. Researchers often rely on a panel of experts to evaluate the content validity of new instruments. There are various approaches to assessing content validity using an expert panel, but nurse researchers have been in the forefront in developing an approach that involves the calculation of a **content validity index (CVI)**. The experts are asked to evaluate individual items on a draft of the new measure as well as the overall instrument.

At the item level, a common procedure is to have experts rate items on a 4-point scale of relevance. There are several variations of labeling the 4 points, but the scale used most often is as follows: 1 = *not relevant*, 2 = *somewhat relevant*, 3 = *quite relevant*, 4 = *highly relevant*. Then, for each item, the **item CVI (I-CVI)** is computed as the number of experts giving a rating of 3 or 4, divided by the number of experts—that is, the proportion in agreement about relevance. For example, an item rated as "quite" or "highly" relevant by 4 out of 5 experts would have an I-CVI of .80, which is considered an acceptable value. Items with an I-CVI below .78 should be carefully scrutinized and either revised or discarded (Polit et al., 2007).

There are two approaches to calculating **scale CVIs (S-CVIs)**, and unfortunately instrument development papers seldom indicate which approach was used (Polit & Beck, 2006). The preferred approach is to compute the S-CVI by averaging I-CVIs. We suggest a value of .90 for the S-CVI/Averaging as the standard for establishing excellent content validity (Polit et al., 2007). Content validation should be done with at least three experts, but a larger group is preferable. Further guidance is offered in Chapter 15.

Example of Using a Content Validity Index: Hawkins and colleagues (2014) developed a scale to measure patient satisfaction with anesthesia care. A panel of 13 nurse anesthetists served as experts and evaluated the content validity of the items and the scale. I-CVI values ranged from .83 to 1.0, and the S-CVI (averaging) was .98.

Criterion Validity

Criterion validity is the extent to which the scores on an instrument are a good reflection of a "gold standard"—that is, a criterion considered an ideal measure of the construct. Not all measures can be validated using a criterion approach because there is not always a "gold standard" to use as the criterion.

One might reasonably ask: If there is an established criterion, why do we need the focal measure at all—why not simply use the gold standard? Reasons for creating a new measure fall primarily into five categories.

- *Expense*. A new measure that is a good reflection of a criterion may be desired because the gold standard is too expensive to administer routinely. For example, a self-report measure of physical function is less costly than a battery of physical performance tests.
- *Efficiency*. A related reason is the desire to create a measure that is more efficient than the gold standard. For instance, if a 2-minute walk test yields comparable information to the 6-minute walk test, then the 2-minute walk test sometimes might be preferred.
- *Risk and discomfort*. Sometimes the criterion involves a measurement that puts people at risk or is invasive, and a substitute is desired to lower risks or pain.
- *Criterion unavailable*. A measure may be needed because criterion measures are difficult or impossible to obtain routinely in clinical settings. For example, for a measure of children's aggressiveness, the criterion might be conduct problems in school or police records, which are often inaccessible.
- *Prediction*. One other reason for developing an instrument that can be validated against a criterion is that the criterion cannot be measured until a future point in time. In such situations, the measure is designed to predict the occurrence of the criterion.

A requirement for criterion validation is the availability of a reliable and valid criterion with which measures on the focal instrument can be compared. When a criterion is unavailable, however, other validation approaches must be used to persuade potential users that scores on the measure validly reflect the attribute of interest. For example, it might be difficult to identify a valid and reliable external criterion for such attributes as patients' satisfaction with care, quality of life, or fearfulness. When this is the case, researchers rely on construct validity methods.

Criterion validation always involves testing a hypothesis, although it is usually implicit. The hypothesis is that the focal measure yields score information that is as good as that obtained from the criterion. This in turn means that scores on the two are hypothesized to be correlated or consistent with each other. When such a hypothesis is upheld through formal testing, users gain some assurance that the measure will support appropriate inferences regarding the attribute in question when used with the target population in a similar context.

Two types of criterion validity exist. **Concurrent validity** is the type of criterion validity that is assessed when the measurements of the criterion and the new instrument occur at the same time. In such a situation, the implicit hypothesis is that the new measure is an adequate substitute for a contemporaneous criterion. In **predictive validity**, the focal measure is tested against a criterion that is measured in the future. Screening scales are often tested against some future criterion—namely, the occurrence of the phenomenon for which a screening tool is sought.

A broad array of statistical procedures can be used to test whether the criterion validity hypothesis is supported by data from a relevant sample. The choice of statistics depends on whether the focal measure and the criterion are measured as a continuous score value or as categorical ones. Three situations are especially common.

Criterion Validity with a Continuous Measure and a Continuous Criterion

The first situation is when both the focal measure being tested and the criterion are continuous scores. For example, suppose we were assessing the criterion validity of a 2-minute walk test as a measure of functional performance, and we used the well-established 6-minute walk test as the criterion. In this situation, we would obtain measures of both tests from a sample of patients and compute a Pearson's r (the correlation coefficient) between the two sets of scores. The higher the value of r, the better the evidence of criterion validity.

Example of Concurrent Validity Using Correlations: Hammash and colleagues (2013) tested a short (9-item) measure of depressive symptoms for patients with heart failure. In a sample of 322 patients, scores on the focal measure (the PHQ-9) were correlated with scores on a widely used but longer measure of depression, the Beck Depression Inventory. The correlation coefficient was .80.

Criterion Validity with a Dichotomous Measure and a Dichotomous Criterion

When both the focal measure and the criterion are dichotomous, several statistical methods can be used but, most often, methods of assessing **diagnostic accuracy** are applied. **Sensitivity** is the ability of a measure to identify a "case" correctly, that is, to screen in or diagnose a condition correctly. A measure's sensitivity is its rate of yielding "true positives." **Specificity** is the measure's ability to identify noncases correctly, that is, to screen *out* those without the condition. Specificity is an instrument's rate of yielding "true negatives." Sensitivity and specificity are important criterion validity parameters and highly useful to potential users of the measure. Of course, to evaluate an instrument's sensitivity and specificity, researchers need a reliable and valid criterion of "caseness" against which scores on the instrument can be assessed.

To illustrate, suppose we wanted to evaluate the validity of adolescents' self-reports about their smoking, and we asked 100 teenagers whether they had smoked a cigarette in the previous 24 hours. The "gold standard" for nicotine consumption is cotinine levels in a body fluid, so we also performed a urinary cotinine assay. Some fictitious data are shown in Table 14.2. Sensitivity is calculated as the proportion of teenagers who said they smoked *and* who had high concentrations of cotinine (e.g., ≥ 200 ng/mL), divided by all real smokers according to the urine test. Put another way, it

TABLE 14.2 • Example Illustrating Sensitivity, Specificity, and Likelihood Ratios

SELF-REPORTED SMOKING	URINARY COTININE LEVEL (CRITERION)		
	Positive	Negative	Total
Yes	Cell A: true positives 30	Cell B: false positives 5	35 (A + B)
No	Cell C: false negatives 10	Cell D: true negatives 55	65 (C + D)
Total	40 (A + C)	60 (B + D)	100 (A + B + C + D)

Sensitivity: A ÷ (A + C) = .75
Specificity: D ÷ (B + D) = .92
Positive predictive value (PPV): A ÷ (A + B) = .86
Negative predictive value (NPV): D ÷ (C + D) = .85
Likelihood ratio-positive (LR+): Sensitivity ÷ (1 − Specificity) = 9.04
Likelihood ratio-negative (LR−): (1 − Sensitivity) ÷ Specificity = 0.27

is the true positives divided by all positives. In this case, there was some apparent underreporting of smoking, and so the sensitivity of the self-report was .75. Specificity is the proportion of teenagers who accurately reported they did not smoke, or the true negatives divided by all negatives. In our example, specificity is .92. There was less over-reporting of smoking ("faking bad") than underre-porting ("faking good"). We would conclude that the sensitivity of the self-reports was moderate, but the specificity was good.

Often, other related indicators are calculated with such data. **Predictive values** are posterior probabilities—the probability of an outcome after the results are known. A **positive predictive value** (or PPV) is the proportion of people with a positive result who have the target outcome. In our example, the PPV is the proportion of teens who said they smoke who actually *do* smoke, according to the cotinine test results. Thirty out of 35 of those who reported smoking had high concentrations of cotinine, and so PPV = .86. A **negative predictive value** (NPV) is the proportion of people who have a negative "score" on the focal measure who

also have a negative result on the gold standard. As shown in Table 14.2, 55 out of the 65 teenagers who reported not smoking actually were nonsmok-ers, and so NPV in our example is .85.

Example of Sensitivity, Specificity, and Predictive Values: Tilahun and colleagues (2015) tested the predictive value of nasal screening for methicillin-resistant *Staphylococcus aureus* for lower respiratory tract infections. Sensitivity and specificity of nasal colonization with methicillin-resistant *Staphylococcus aureus* were 80% and 87%, respectively. Positive predictive value was 29%, and negative predictive value was 99%.

In the medical community, reporting **likelihood ratios** has come into favor because it summarizes the relationship between specificity and sensitivity in a single number. The likelihood ratio-positive (LR+) is the ratio of true positives to false posi-tives. The formula for LR+ is sensitivity, divided by 1 minus specificity. For the data in Table 14.2, LR+ is 9.04: We are nine times as likely to find that a self-report of smoking really *is* for a true smoker than it is for a nonsmoker. The likelihood ratio-negative (LR−) is the ratio of false-negative results to true-negative results. For the data in Table 14.2, the LR− is .27, indicating that we are substantially less likely to find that a self-report of nonsmoking is false than we are to find that it reflects a true nonsmoker.

These criterion validity indicators are often used when a *cutpoint* on a continuous focal measure is used to classify patients into two categories, which we discuss next.

Criterion Validity with a Continuous Measure and a Dichotomous Criterion

When the measure being assessed is continuous and the criterion is dichotomous, sometimes a simple statistical test (a *t*-test, described in Chapter 17) is used to compare average score values for two groups (e.g., *cases* versus *noncases*). However, criterion validation in this situation often uses an approach that involves plotting each score on the index measure against its specificity and sensitivity for correct classification based on the dichotomous criterion.

The indicators we calculated for the data in Table 14.2 are contingent upon the critical value that we established for cotinine concentration.

Sensitivity and specificity would be different if we used 100 ng/mL as indicative of smoking status, rather than 200 ng/mL. There is almost invariably a trade-off between the sensitivity and specificity of a measure. When sensitivity is increased to include more true positives, the proportion of true negatives declines. Therefore, a common task in developing new measures for which there is a continuous "gold standard" is to find an appropriate cutoff point (or *cutpoint*), that is, a score to distinguish cases and noncases.

Researchers usually use a **receiver operating characteristic curve** (**ROC curve**) to identify the best cutoff point. In an ROC curve, the sensitivity of an instrument (i.e., the rate of correctly identifying a case vis-à-vis an established criterion) is plotted against the false-positive rate (i.e., the rate of incorrectly classifying someone as a case, which is the inverse of its specificity) over a range of different scores on the focal measure. The score (cutoff point) that yields the best balance between sensitivity and specificity can then be determined. The optimum cutoff is at or near the shoulder of the ROC curve.

Figure 14.2 presents an ROC curve from a study in which a goal was to establish cutoff points

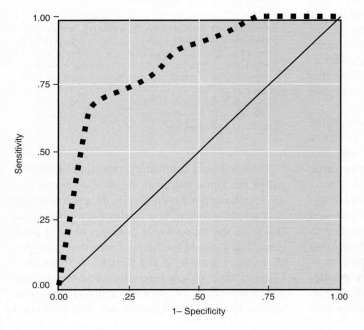

FIGURE 14.2 Receiver operating characteristic (ROC) curve for Braden Q Scale. (From Curley, M. A. Q., Razmus, I. S., Roberts, K. E., & Wypij, D. [2003]. Predicting pressure ulcer risk in pediatric patients: The Braden Q Scale. *Nursing Research, 52,* 22–33).

for scores on the Braden Q scale for predicting pressure ulcer risk in children (Curley et al., 2003). In this figure, sensitivity and 1 minus specificity are plotted for each possible score of the Braden Q scale. The upper left corner represents sensitivity at its highest possible value (1.0) and false positives at its lowest possible value (.00). Measures that do an excellent job of discriminating vis-à-vis the criterion have points that crowd close to the upper left corner, which indicates that as sensitivity increases, there is relatively little loss in specificity.

In ROC analyses, the **area under the curve (AUC)** can be used as a validity parameter. AUC values close to 1.00 are desirable and are found when the curve hugs close to the upper left corner. When the curve is close to the diagonal, the AUC value is .50, indicating that the measure cannot differentiate between those who are positive and negative on the criterion. Values of .70 are usually considered evidence of adequate validity. The AUC for the data portrayed in Figure 14.2 is .83. The cutoff score for the Braden Q in this example was established at 16. At this cutoff value, sensitivity was .88 and specificity was .58. The researchers used these preliminary analyses to improve the Braden Q scale and achieved even better results.

→ TIP: In Chapter 1, we discussed categories of EBP-related questions, such as therapy, prognosis, and so on. One category concerns the accuracy of diagnostic or screening tests. The methods discussed in this section on criterion validity are especially important for providing Level II evidence for this type of EBP question. Standards for reporting studies about diagnostic accuracy have been proposed, called GRADE, as described by Schünemann and colleagues (2008).

Construct Validity

For many abstract, unobservable human attributes (constructs), no gold-standard criterion exists, and so other validation avenues must be pursued.

The third component within the validity domain of our measurement taxonomy (see Figure 14.1) is construct validity. The construct validity question is basically this: What attribute is *really* being measured? Borrowing from the writings of esteemed methodologists Cook and Campbell (e.g., Shadish et al., 2002), we define **construct validity** as the degree to which evidence about a measure's scores in relation to other scores supports the inference that the construct has been appropriately represented. Construct validity is especially relevant for abstract constructs that are measured either by self-report or through observational methods but may also be relevant for performance tests.

Evidence for construct validity comes from tests of hypotheses about the nature of the construct and the scores on the focal measure. The researcher must speculate: If this instrument is, in fact, really measuring construct X, then how would we expect the scores to perform? In a construct validation, the instrument developer must have a firm conceptualization not only of the construct itself (as is true in a content validity effort) but also of how the construct is related to other constructs. In other words, there needs to be an overarching conceptual model of processes and traits of relevance to the construct.

Construct validity is complex and encompasses multiple aspects: hypothesis-testing construct validity, structural validity, and cross-cultural validity.

→ TIP: If an instrument developer has taken careful steps to ensure the content validity of the instrument, construct validity will also be strengthened.

Hypothesis-Testing Construct Validity

Hypothesis-testing validity concerns the extent to which it is possible to corroborate hypotheses regarding how scores on a measure function in relation to scores on measures of other constructs (or the same construct). All hypothesis-testing construct validations follow a similar path: Hypotheses are developed about a relationship between scores on the focal measure and scores on other constructs, data are collected to test the hypotheses with a sample from a specified population, and then validity conclusions are reached based on the hypothesis tests. A successful construct validation effort requires in-depth understanding of the construct, and it also requires insight and creativity. Researchers must challenge themselves to develop diverse and complementary ways of testing whether their measure is, indeed, measuring the construct of interest.

Different types of evidence can be brought to bear on construct validity, leading to approaches that have been given different names. Unfortunately, there are inconsistencies in the measurement literature with regard to what some of those names are. Because the terms associated with different validation approaches are often confusing, Table 14.3 presents a quick summary chart, which includes previously discussed validity terms as well.

TABLE 14.3 • Types of Measurement-Related Validity

TYPE OF VALIDITY	EXPLANATION
Content validity	Concerns the adequacy of content for multi-component measures
Face validity	Concerns whether a measure "looks" as though it is measuring the relevant construct
Criterion Validity	
Concurrent validity	Tests whether a measure is consistent with a criterion (a gold standard), measured at the same time
Predictive validity	Tests whether a measure is consistent with a criterion (a gold standard), measured at a future point in time
Construct Validity: Hypothesis Testing	
Convergent validity	In the absence of a gold standard, tests the correlation between the focal measure and a measure of a construct with which conceptual convergence is expected
Known-groups (discriminative) validity	Tests the degree to which a measure can discriminate between groups known to differ with regard to the focal construct
Divergent (discriminant) validity	Tests that the focal measure is not a measure of a construct other than the one intended
Construct Validity: Other	
Structural validity	Tests whether a measure captures the hypothesized dimensionality of a construct
Cross-cultural validity	Concerns the extent to which a translated or adapted measure is equivalent to the original

Convergent Validity. **Convergent validity** is the degree to which scores on the focal measure are correlated with scores on measures of constructs with which there is a hypothesized relationship—that is, the degree to which there is conceptual convergence. Sometimes the other measure is a different measure of the same construct (but not a measure that could be construed as a "gold standard"). For example, if we were developing a new, specific measure of fatigue in patients with cancer, we might predict that scores on our new scale would correlate fairly strongly and positively with patients' scores on a general measure of fatigue, such as the Piper Fatigue Scale.

From a broader perspective, convergent validity concerns the extent to which the focal measure correlates with variables in a manner consistent with an underlying theory or conceptual model. For example, we might hypothesize that inadequate social support is a factor contributing to postpartum depression. We could test the construct validity of a postpartum depression (PPD) scale by examining the correlation between scores on this scale with those on a measure of social support. In essence, researchers reason as follows:

- According to theory or prior evidence, construct X is positively related to construct Y.
- Instrument A is a measure of construct X; instrument B is a valid measure of construct Y.
- Scores on A and B are correlated positively, as predicted.
- Therefore, it is inferred that A is a valid measure of X.

This logical analysis does not constitute proof of construct validity but yields important evidence. Construct validation is essentially an ongoing evidence-building enterprise. With convergent validity, the validity parameter is typically the correlation coefficient between two measures—most often Pearson's r.

Example of Convergent Validity: Bekhet and Zauszniewski (2013) assessed the psychometric adequacy of an existing scale (the Depressive Cognition Scale) in a new population, caregivers of people with autism spectrum disorder. In their construct validation efforts, they hypothesized that

scores on the scale would correlate positively with a measure of caregiver burden and negatively with a measure of resourcefulness. Their hypotheses were supported ($r = .59$ and $-.57$, respectively).

Known-Groups Validity. **Known-groups validity**, which has also been called *discriminative validity*, relies on hypotheses concerning a measure's ability to discriminate between two or more groups known (or expected) to differ with regard to the construct of interest. For example, we might hypothesize that women who had planned their pregnancy would have more favorable scores on a PPD scale than women whose pregnancy was unwanted. If the scores on the PPD measure do not differ for the two groups, one might question the scale's validity, given the existing evidence that women whose pregnancies are planned and wanted are less susceptible than other women to postpartum depression. We would not necessarily expect large differences; some women in both groups would likely suffer from PPD. We would, however, hypothesize differences in *average* group scores. The known-groups approach is one of the most widely used methods of testing construct validity.

A key difference between convergent validity and known-groups validity concerns how the validation variable is measured. Continuous scores on a comparator construct can be used to create "known" groups by dividing the sample into subgroups for known-groups validity, or the continuous scores can be used to test a correlation for convergent validity. It is probably best to divide sample members into subgroups for a known-groups validation when there is a well-established cutpoint for "caseness."

Example of the Known-Groups Technique: Peters and colleagues (2014) evaluated the validity of an existing scale, the Trust in Provider Scale, for a new population, namely, pregnant African American women. Consistent with hypotheses, women who had experienced racism in health care had significantly lower scores on the trust scale than women who had not.

Divergent Validity. **Divergent validity** (which is often called *discriminant validity*) concerns evidence that a measure is *not* a measure of a different construct, distinct from the focal construct. We use the term *divergent* because it is a good contrast with *con*vergent validity and also because of possible confusion between the terms discriminant and discriminative (known-groups) validity.

In a divergent validation, researchers typically measure both the focal attribute and a similar—but distinct—attribute as a means of ensuring that the two are not really measures of the same construct but with different labels. Thus, in a divergent validation, the hypothesis is that the two measures are only weakly correlated.

Hypotheses for construct validations sometimes are stated in relative rather than absolute terms, especially when there are both convergent and divergent hypotheses. For example, an absolute hypothesis for a new PPD scale might predict that scores would correlate only modestly with scores on a measure of anxiety about maternal role performance to distinguish the PPD construct from maternal anxiety. For a relative hypothesis, we might predict that scores on a PPD scale would correlate more strongly with scores on a general measure of depression (convergent validity) than with scores on the maternal anxiety scale (divergent validity).

The primary approach to divergent validation is to compute correlation coefficients. Researchers should stipulate in advance how "weak" a correlation would need to be as evidence of divergent validity, either in absolute or relative terms.

> **Example of Convergent and Discriminant Validity:** Curley and colleagues (2013) undertook a validity assessment of the Family-Centered Care Scale (FCCS), a measure of parents' experience of nursing care. They hypothesized that scores on the FCCS would be more highly correlated with scores on certain subscales of the Pediatric Inpatient Experience Survey (those that measured nursing care and parent involvement) than with scores for other subscales measuring non-nursing aspects of care (e.g., the hospital environment). The correlation analysis was consistent with these hypotheses.

TIP: An approach known as the **multitrait–multimethod matrix method** (**MTMM**) is a significant construct validation tool (Campbell & Fiske, 1959). This procedure involves tests of both convergent and divergent validity. Few nurse researchers have used an MTMM in its full form, but several have applied parts of the approach. The MTMM is explained more fully in Polit and Yang (2015).

Construct Validity Evidence. Most researchers identify multiple hypotheses for their construct validity work and include several different types of validation approaches in a single study. As a result, drawing conclusions about a measure's construct validity is typically more complex than interpreting results for other measurement properties, such as reliability. For many measurement parameters, only a single number needs to be interpreted. For example, when an intraclass correlation coefficient (ICC) is computed with test–retest data, that value *is* the estimated reliability. However, there is seldom a single "validity coefficient" in construct validation because typically many hypotheses are tested. Indeed, the more supporting evidence there is, the greater the confidence one can have about the measure's validity. An instrument does not possess or lack validity; it is a question of degree. An instrument's validity is not proved, established, demonstrated, or verified but rather is supported to a greater or lesser extent by evidence. However, when there are multiple hypotheses, results may be "mixed"—some hypotheses are supported and others are not. This fact means that it is wise for researchers to establish a priori standards for how much confirmatory evidence is considered sufficient.

Structural Validity

Another aspect of construct validity is called structural validity. **Structural validity** refers to the extent to which the structure of a multi-item scale adequately reflects the hypothesized dimensionality of the construct being measured. Structural validity concerns which dimensions of a broader construct are captured by the instrument and whether the dimensions are consistent with theory. For example, we might conceptualize pain as having two dimensions: pain severity and pain interference. After developing a scale based on this conceptualization, we would want to test whether we were successful in capturing and distinguishing the two dimensions.

Content validity work ideally paves the way for a good conceptualization of a construct's multiple dimensions.

Assessments of structural validity rely on a statistical procedure called factor analysis. Although factor analysis, which we discuss in Chapter 15, is computationally complex, it is conceptually fairly simple. **Factor analysis** is a method for identifying clusters of related items—that is, dimensions underlying a broad construct. Each dimension, or **factor**, represents a relatively unitary attribute. The procedure is used to identify and group together different items measuring an underlying attribute. In effect, factor analysis constitutes another means of testing hypotheses about the interrelationships among variables and for formulating evidence of convergence and divergence at the item level.

As we discuss in the next chapter, there are two broad classes of factor analysis—exploratory and confirmatory. *Exploratory factor analysis* is an important tool in the development and refinement of multi-item scales. *Confirmatory factor analysis*, however, is the preferred method for testing structural validity hypotheses about the dimensionality of a scale.

It is important to note that information about a measure's structural validity does not constitute sufficient evidence of a measure's construct validity. Factor analysis can confirm a hypothesis that a complex construct has, for example, three underlying dimensions, but such an analysis does not in and of itself address the central construct validity question: Does this instrument really measure the construct it purports to measure?

Example of Structural Validation: S. W. Chen and colleagues (2015) developed and tested the Energy Retention Behavior Scale for Children (the ERB-C Scale). Responses to the scale's 14 items by a sample of 371 children were factor analyzed to assess structural validity. Confirmatory factor analyses confirmed a 2-factor structure.

TIP: Structural validity is an aspect of construct validity that is only relevant for multi-item reflective scales and not formative indexes. Factor analysis requires items with strong intercorrelations.

Cross-Cultural Validity

In our measurement taxonomy, a third type of construct validity is called cross-cultural validity, which is relevant for measures that have been translated or adapted for use with a different cultural group than that for the original instrument. We define **cross-cultural validity** as the degree to which the components (e.g., items) of a translated or culturally adapted measure perform adequately and equivalently, individually and collectively, relative to their performance on the original instrument.

Developing a high-quality and cross-culturally valid instrument requires even more time and effort than starting from scratch with a new instrument. Yet, without such efforts, it would be impossible to understand health outcomes globally. If, for example, we want to learn whether health-related quality of life differs across countries, comparisons cannot be made with disparate instruments. Several coordinated multinational efforts have been undertaken to adapt widely used English-language health scales, such as the Mini-Mental State Examination and a quality-of-life scale called the SF-36. Also, many item banks of health outcomes have been translated for use in computerized adaptive testing as part of the PROMIS® initiative.

Even within a single country, increased multiculturalism often necessitates the adaptation of well-validated instruments. For example, understanding health disparities in countries such as the United States requires the use of measures with cross-cultural validity for different ethnic and language groups.

The methods used in cross-cultural validation are complex and multi-faceted, and many of them require high levels of statistical sophistication. An overview of some of these methods, together with some guidance on undertaking a translation or adaptation of an instrument, is presented in the Supplement to this chapter on thePoint®. Fuller explanations are offered in Polit and Yang (2015).

RELIABILITY OF CHANGE SCORES

Two domains in our measurement taxonomy relate to measurements over time. Both of these domains concern change scores, so we briefly discuss the issue of measuring change.

Measuring Change

How does one measure whether a change in a construct has occurred? For some attributes, there is only one option: measuring it on two occasions and comparing the values—in other words, subtracting one value from the other to calculate a **change score** that represents the amount of change between two scores. If we want to learn, for example, whether a patient's blood pressure has decreased, we need to know what it was initially and what it is now, and calculate the difference. For patient-reported outcomes, there are two alternatives: asking patients directly whether a change has occurred and asking them to report retrospectively what their status was previously and then comparing it to their current status. Unfortunately, all three methods have potential problems. We focus on problems with change scores.

In clinical trials, statisticians have argued against using change scores as the dependent variables in the analysis of treatment effects. When patients are randomized to groups, it is recommended that scores at the posttest be used as the outcome variables, rather than change scores. A major emphasis in randomized trials is on *difference scores* (the difference between the randomized groups at posttest), rather than on *change scores*.

Yet, it is of inherent substantive interest to understand how much patients in all arms of a trial have changed. Moreover, some nonexperimental studies seek to describe outcomes over the course of an illness, which requires a direct examination of how scores have evolved. And, at the level of an individual patient, assessments of improvement, deterioration, or stability over time as measured by change scores may be the focus of clinical assessment and decision making.

Change scores can be affected by several factors that can threaten their accuracy and validity. A major concern with change scores concerns the fact that measurement error is inevitably present in all measurements. Change scores—the difference between an imperfectly reliable score at Time 1 and another imperfectly reliable score at Time 2—potentially can magnify a small change or mask a large one. The greater the degree of unreliability, the greater the risk that a change score will be misleading.

The reliability of change domain focuses on this issue: How do we know when a change score is a reliable one and not merely a random fluctuation? Except for measures created within an item response theory framework, reliable change has most often been assessed by computing one of two indexes: the smallest detectable change or the reliable change index.

The Smallest Detectable Change

The usual approach to assessing the reliability of group-level change is to test the statistical significance of a group's change in scores from one point in time to another—for example, using tests described in Chapter 17. From a measurement perspective, however, statistical significance may not be an informative way to understand change—and significance tells us nothing about whether a change was reliable for an individual.

Reliable change for continuous data often is estimated using an index called the **smallest detectable change (SDC)** or the *minimal detectable change (MDC)*.** An SDC can be defined as a change in scores that is beyond measurement error—a change of sufficient magnitude that the probability of it being the result of random error is low.

Operationally, the SDC is a change score that falls outside the limits of agreement (LOA) on a Bland-Altman plot. As noted earlier, the limits of agreement can be estimated using test–retest data from a stable population. The limits of agreement are an estimate of the probable range of score differences between a test and a retest for a stable population over a specified interval. If a change score falls outside the LOA, there can be greater confidence that the change is "real." High measurement error makes it more difficult to detect true change than when measurement error is small—further underscoring the importance of using measures with high reliability.

**The term "minimal detectable change" is often found in the medical literature. We use "smallest detectable change" to be consistent with COSMIN. The SDC has also been called the "smallest detectable *difference*" or "minimal detectable *difference*" but, like the COSMIN group, we prefer "smallest detectable *change*" to emphasize the focus on *change* scores.

Earlier we noted that the limits of agreement for the self-esteem scores in Table 14.1 were about 7.0 (actually, 7.1). Suppose that we evaluated an intervention designed to improve the self-esteem and mental health of adolescents. The scores in Table 14.1 are from a test–retest administration of the scale, but suppose that the Time 2 scores were baseline values for the intervention. Three months after the intervention, we would readminister the self-esteem scale (Time 3). Based on the LOA, any improvement in self-esteem scores of 7 points or greater in a participant's score would be considered indicative of real (reliable) improvement in self-esteem.

Example of the Smallest Detectable Change: Dawson and colleagues (2010) assessed a measure of back pain, the Oswestry Disability Index, with a sample of nursing students. The test–retest reliability was good (ICC = .88), but the researchers concluded that the high value for the smallest detectable change suggested that the "tool had limited ability to detect longitudinal change in disability in this population" (p. 604).

The Reliable Change Index

The SDC is similar to another index that is widely used in the field of psychotherapy. The **reliable change index (RCI)** was proposed by Jacobson and colleagues (Jacobson et al., 1984; Jacobson & Truax, 1991) as an element of a two-part process for assessing the clinical significance of patients' improvement during a psychotherapeutic intervention. Jacobson argued that, to be clinically meaningful, a change score on psychotherapy outcomes must pass the test of being "real"—that is, a change beyond measurement error.

Although we do not elaborate computation details, we note that the RCI is calculated by using a formula that includes the amount of measurement error for the scale, as estimated by the standard error of measurement.[††] The cutoff values for reliable change are similar (but not identical) for the RCI and the SDC. In our example of the self-esteem

scores in Figure 14.1, the SDC is 7.10 and the RCI is. 7.33. (The RCI is discussed in greater detail in the Supplement to Chapter 20 Ⓢ.)

Example of Using the Reliable Change Index: Moyle and colleagues (2013) conducted a pilot crossover trial to test the effects of a companion robot intervention on emotions in people with moderate to severe dementia. For each outcome measure (e.g., the Quality of Life in Alzheimer's Disease Scale), the researchers computed the RCI and then examined whether reliable change had occurred for study participants.

RESPONSIVENESS

The final domain in our measurement taxonomy also concerns measurements over time. We define the measurement property of **responsiveness** as the ability of a measure to detect change over time in a construct that has changed, commensurate with the amount of change that has occurred. Just as the measurement property of reliability can be extended to apply to change scores, responsiveness represents the extension of validity over time. Validity concerns whether a measure is truly capturing the intended construct, and responsiveness concerns whether a change score is truly capturing a real change in the construct.

The term *responsiveness* appears to have been introduced by Gordon Guyatt and colleagues (Guyatt et al., 1989; Kirshner & Guyatt, 1985). In the years following Guyatt's use of the term, responsiveness gained popularity as a measurement property, especially among quality-of-life researchers. Yet, there has been a marked lack of consensus about what it is or how to know when it has been achieved. Terwee and colleagues (2003) did a systematic review of the quality-of-life literature more than a decade ago and found 25 definitions of responsiveness and 31 ways to assess it. The COSMIN group can be credited with having brought together health measurement experts who reached agreement in defining responsiveness as the validity of change scores.

Validity and responsiveness share many features in common, the main difference being the time frame. The methods used to assess responsiveness overlap with methods used to assess validity.

[††]For 95% confidence, the formula for the RCI is 1.96 times $\sqrt{2} \times \text{SEM}^2$.

Validity and responsiveness are similar in another way: They both are challenging to assess. Assessments require researchers to be creative in developing useful hypotheses. Furthermore, both responsiveness and validity rely on ongoing evidence building. The more evidence that can be brought to bear on a measure's responsiveness, the greater the confidence one has in the measure's capacity to capture true change in a construct. This evidence-building feature of both cross-sectional and longitudinal validity (responsiveness) means that there is no single number to quantify its value.

Psychometricians have not traditionally considered responsiveness as a measurement property. The term is found nowhere in the writings of prominent psychometricians, nor in psychometric guides to scale construction. Streiner and Norman (2008), psychometricians who have worked in health measurement, have rejected responsiveness as a distinctive property, preferring to call it longitudinal construct validity. We agree with the COSMIN group, however, in believing that responsiveness merits independent consideration. Change is critically important to health care professionals who often hope to achieve improvements with clients. Little attention was paid to the issue of longitudinal construct validity before the concept of responsiveness was proposed. We think it is useful to use a separate label to identify a property of importance to health care practitioners because it can remind scale developers to incorporate the assessment of change score validity into their development plans.

Two broad approaches have been used in assessing responsiveness, and these are similar to approaches used in validity testing: a criterion approach and a construct approach.

The Criterion Approach to Responsiveness

Like criterion validation, the criterion approach to responsiveness requires a gold standard—a well-established and reliable criterion that indicates that a change in the target construct has occurred. This approach to responsiveness assessment has also been called an **anchor-based approach**, with the criterion serving as the anchor.

A criterion-based assessment of responsiveness sometimes involves an examination of the relationship between changes on the target measure and changes on the criterion, which corresponds directly to a longitudinal assessment of criterion validity. For example, earlier in the chapter, we used a study by Hammash and colleagues (2013) to illustrate criterion validity. These researchers correlated scores on a new short measure of depressive symptoms (the PHQ-9) with scores on a "gold standard" measure of depression, the Beck Depression Inventory (BDI). To assess the responsiveness of the PHQ-9, they could compute the correlation between *changes* in the PHQ-9 and *changes* in the BDI in a sample of people for whom change over time was expected. The implicit hypothesis in such a responsiveness assessment is that change scores on the focal measure are consistent with or correlated with change scores on the criterion. When formal testing supports such a hypothesis, then evidence of the focal measure's responsiveness (longitudinal validity) is obtained.

Another strategy for testing criterion-based responsiveness involves the use of a single-item **global rating scale** or **GRS** (also known as a **health transition rating**) as the criterion (De Vet et al., 2011). A GRS involves asking patients to rate directly the degree to which their status on the focal construct has changed over a time interval in which change is presumed to have occurred. Figure 14.3 provides an example of a 7-point GRS, which asks patients to rate changes in their ability

Please rate the changes you have experienced in the past three months with regard to *your ability to perform regular activities of daily living,* such as standing up from a sitting position or taking a bath or shower:

1. Very much better
2. Much better
3. A little better
4. No change
5. A little worse
6. Much worse
7. Very much worse

Shaded response options show one possible cut point on the criterion: Responses 1–3 (any improvement) versus 4–7 (no improvement)

FIGURE 14.3 Example of a global rating scale for a criterion-related assessment of responsiveness for an ADL scale.

to perform activities of daily living. Such a GRS would be relevant for assessing the responsiveness of a physical function or ADL scale—for example, for measuring improvements in patients' physical function several months after a health-promotion intervention known to be effective.

Let us suppose we were assessing the responsiveness of a physical function scale, such as the Barthel Index (BI). We might administer the BI just prior to an intervention and then 3 months later. At the 3-month point, patients would also be asked to complete the GRS shown in Figure 14.3. Several statistical approaches could then be used to test the BI's responsiveness. For example, the average BI change scores could be statistically compared for patients who said they had any improvement on the GRS (response options 1, 2, or 3) and patients who did not report improvements (response options 4-7). Alternatively, change scores on the BI could be plotted on an ROC curve against the sensitivity and specificity for predicting the GRS criterion: improved versus did not improve. The analysis is not focused on establishing a cutpoint on the BI but rather on evaluating the ability of the change scores to distinguish those who have and have not improved. Therefore, the area under the curve (AUC) would provide the estimate of responsiveness.

⮞ **TIP:** This GRS approach can lend supporting evidence of responsiveness, but it is not an ideal approach. Although a GRS has face validity, it is problematic as a gold standard. Indeed, if a GRS *were* a gold standard, there would be little apparent reason for developing the focal scale because nothing could be more efficient than a single change question. Multi-item scales are useful precisely because they are more reliable than one question. Thus, we would argue that if the GRS approach is used to assess responsiveness, it should be supplemented with other strategies.

The Construct Approach to Responsiveness

The construct approach to evaluating a measure's responsiveness is analogous to a hypothesis-testing

construct validation. Researchers develop and test hypotheses about changes on the focal measure in relation to other phenomena. Sometimes, the hypotheses concern an expected change on the construct resulting from a treatment of well-established efficacy (e.g., changes in quality of life after hip replacement). Alternatively, the hypotheses concern the nature and magnitude of relationship between changes on the focal measure on the one hand and changes on measures of constructs that are theoretically linked to the construct of interest on the other.

When hypotheses are developed about how changes in a focal measure are related to other measures, a full array of strategies and analytic methods can be used, analogous to those described in regard to hypothesis-testing construct validity. For example, some hypotheses are designed to support what might be called *convergent responsiveness*—the degree to which change scores on the focal measure are correlated with change scores on a measure of a construct with which a relationship is hypothesized. Similarly, it would be possible to hypothesize that changes on the focal construct, as captured in change scores on the focal measure, are *not* associated (or only weakly associated) with changes on another, unrelated measure (*divergent responsiveness*). Another option is *known-groups responsiveness*, the longitudinal extension of known-groups validity. In this approach, researchers test the hypothesis that changes on the focal measure are different for two or more groups known (or hypothesized) to have different amounts of change.

Although conceptually construct-focused responsiveness assessment is an extension of construct validation, procedurally there has been greater complexity in evaluating responsiveness—in part because of disputes about its definition. Many researchers have computed what they called a "responsiveness index" that purports to summarize the degree of responsiveness a measurement possesses. Many of so-called responsiveness indexes involve the calculation of an effect size index (see Chapter 17).[‡‡] These are often called **distribution-based methods** because they are based on change

[‡‡]One index used in connection with responsiveness is the effect size (ES) index described in Chapter 17. Another is called the *standardized response mean* (SRM).

score distributions. Given the definition of responsiveness as longitudinal validity, such indexes may serve as *evidence* of responsiveness, but they do encapsulate a fixed amount of longitudinal validity that a measure possesses.

Example of Responsiveness Assessment:
Y. Chen and co-researchers (2010) developed and tested a Short-Form Pulmonary Functional Status Scale (PFSS-11). The researchers tested the hypothesis that patients undergoing pulmonary rehabilitation would have improved scores at follow-up on the PFSS-11, and the hypothesis was supported.

→ TIP: When you select an instrument to use in a research project, you should seek evidence of the scale's psychometric soundness by examining the instrument developers' report. The report ideally would provide evidence regarding all the measurement properties discussed in this chapter—but information about reliability of change scores and responsiveness may be absent unless the scale was developed in a health discipline other than nursing. You should also consider evidence about the quality of the measure from others who have used it. Each time the scale "performs" as hypothesized, this constitutes supplementary evidence for its validity and possibly its responsiveness.

CRITIQUING DATA QUALITY IN QUANTITATIVE STUDIES

If data are seriously flawed, a study cannot contribute useful evidence. Therefore, in drawing conclusions about a study's evidence, you should consider whether researchers have taken appropriate steps to ensure high-quality measurements of key constructs. Research consumers need to ask: Can I trust the data in this study? Are the measurements of key constructs reliable and valid, and are change scores reliable and responsive?

Information about data quality should be provided in every quantitative research report because it is not possible to come to conclusions about the

quality of study evidence without such information. Reliability estimates are usually reported because they are easy to communicate. Ideally—especially for composite scales—the report should provide reliability or internal consistency coefficients based on data from the study itself, not just from previous research. Interrater or interobserver reliability is especially crucial for coming to conclusions about data quality in observational studies. The values of the reliability coefficients should be sufficiently high to support confidence in the findings. It is especially important to scrutinize reliability information in studies with nonsignificant findings because the unreliability of measures can undermine statistical conclusion validity.

Validity is more difficult to document in a report than reliability. At a minimum, researchers should defend their choice of existing measures based on validity information from the developers, and they should cite the relevant publication. If a study used a screening or diagnostic measure, information should also be provided about its sensitivity and specificity.

Box 14.1 ✪ provides some guidelines for critiquing aspects of data quality of quantitative measures. The guidelines are available in the Toolkit of the accompanying *Resource Manual* for your use and adaptation.

→ TIP: Methodologic studies that focus on the development and testing of new measures need careful scrutiny as well. Some guidelines for critiquing scale development papers are presented in Chapter 15.

●●●●●●●●●●●●●●●●●●●●●●●●●●

RESEARCH EXAMPLE

In this section, we describe a study that used both self-report and observational measures. We focus on the researchers' excellent documentation of data quality in their study. The report was published as an open-access article, and a link to it is provided in the Toolkit.

Study: Communication and outcomes of visits between older patients and nurse practitioners (Gilbert & Hayes, 2009)

BOX 14.1 Guidelines for Critiquing Measurement and Data Quality in Quantitative Studies

1. Was there congruence between the research variables as conceptualized (i.e., as discussed in the introduction of the report) and as operationalized (i.e., as described in the method section)?
2. If operational definitions (or scoring procedures) were specified, did they clearly indicate the rules of measurement? Do the rules seem sensible? Were data collected in such a way that measurement errors were minimized (e.g., ample training of data collectors)?
3. Did the report describe the measurement properties of the instruments used to measure key study constructs? Was a rationale offered for why the instruments were selected (e.g., better measurement properties than alternative measures of the same construct)?
4. Did the report offer evidence of the reliability of the measures used in the study? Did the evidence come from the research sample itself, or was it based on other studies? If the latter, is it reasonable to conclude that data quality would be similar for the research sample as for the reliability sample (e.g., are sample characteristics similar)?
5. If reliability was reported, which estimation method was used? Was this method appropriate? Should an alternative or additional method of reliability appraisal have been used? Was the appropriate reliability coefficient computed (e.g., an ICC for test–retest reliability)? Is the reliability sufficiently high? Was measurement error reported?
6. Did the report offer evidence of the validity of the measures? Assuming validity evidence came from other studies, is it reasonable to believe that data quality would be similar for the research sample as for the validity sample (e.g., are the sample characteristics similar)?
7. If validity information was reported, which validity approach was used? Was this method appropriate? Does the validity of the instrument appear to be adequate?
8. If the study involved computing change scores, was information provided about the reliability of change scores? Was evidence about the responsiveness of change scores provided?
9. If there was information about the measurement properties of key instruments used in the study, what conclusion can you reach about the quality of the data in the study?
10. Were the research hypotheses supported? If not, might data quality have played a role in the failure to confirm the hypotheses?

Statement of Purpose: The purpose of this nonexperimental study was to examine relationships between patient–clinician communication and background characteristics of the patients and the nurse practitioners (NPs) on the one hand and both proximal outcomes (e.g., patient satisfaction) and longer term patient outcomes (e.g., changes in patients' physical and mental health) on the other.

Design: Visits between 31 NPs and 155 patients were video recorded, and various aspects of patient and NP behaviors were coded. Proximal outcomes were measured by self-report after the visits. Four weeks later, changes in patients' health outcomes were assessed using self-report measures.

Instruments and Data Quality: Communications during the visits were measured using the Roter Interaction

Analysis System (RIAS) for verbal interaction and a checklist for nonverbal behaviors. The Roter system involves coding for both the content of the communication and relationship aspects, using a system of 69 categories for all utterances (only 43 were used in this study). The researchers noted that evidence of the predictive validity of the RIAS in previous research was strong. In the present study, trained members of the research team achieved an average interrater reliability of .95 (apparently using Pearson's r) for the 43 coded behavior categories. For the nonverbal behavior checklist, various actions (e.g., gazes, nods, smiles) were coded in 1-second segments over a 30-second sample of activities. Two coders independently coded all segments and any discrepancies in coding were resolved by a third party. Several variables were measured by patients' self-report, including both 1-item measures (e.g., satisfaction with the visit) and multi-item reflective scales (e.g., physical and mental health). For example, patient satisfaction with the NP visit was measured using one item, previously used in a large national survey, which asked for ratings of perceived quality of care on a 10-point scale from 1 (*worst care possible*) to 10 (*best care possible*). The authors concluded that a correlation of .72 between the ratings and the average of several other satisfaction items provided some evidence for the adequacy of the single item. Physical and mental health were measured with a 12-item scale called the SF-12 Health Survey, a widely used instrument for which there is strong evidence of reliability and validity. The test developer had reported Cronbach's alpha values of .89 for physical health and .82 for mental health among people 65 years and older. In the present study, the researchers computed the internal consistency to be .87 and .72 for physical and mental health, respectively. No information was provided in the report regarding the measures' responsiveness or the reliability of change scores, despite the fact that changes in physical and mental health on the SF-12 were key outcomes. The researchers also directly measured patients' perceptions of change in the status of presenting problems, using 7-point health ratings (from *gotten a lot worse* to *improved a lot*). The quality of those ratings appears not to have been assessed. As noted earlier, nurse researchers are only beginning to consider longitudinal measurement issues.

Key Findings: Among the many findings reported in this study, the researchers found that better patient outcomes were associated with a higher amount of communication content involving seeking and giving biomedical and psychosocial information and with a relationships component of more positive talk and greater trust and receptivity.

SUMMARY POINTS

- Measurement is a key feature of quantitative research. **Measurement** involves assigning numbers to objects to represent the amount of an attribute that is present, using a specified set of rules. When researchers invent a set of rules

to capture a construct, they create a **measure** of the construct.

- **Psychometrics** is the branch of psychology concerned with the theory and methods of psychological measurement, and many aspects of psychometrics have influenced health measurement. **Classical test theory (CTT)** is one major psychometric theory of measurement and **item response theory (IRT)** is another.

- Within CTT, **obtained scores** from a measure are conceptualized as having a **true score** component (the value that would be obtained for a hypothetical perfect measure of the attribute) and an error component, or **error of measurement**, that represents measurement inaccuracies.

- Quantitative measuring instruments are rarely infallible. Sources of measurement error include situational contaminants, response-set biases, and transient personal factors, such as fatigue.

- Measures can vary in many different ways, including whether they are *generic* (broadly applicable) or *specific* to certain types of people, such as disease-specific measures. Measures can be **static** (the same instrument and scoring for everyone) or **adaptive**, with different questions from an *item bank* being administered to different people, usually using **computerized adaptive testing**.

- For multi-item measures, another distinction is important. In **reflective scales**, the items are viewed as being *caused by* the construct—responses are reflections of the underlying attribute. In a **formative index**, the items are viewed as defining the construct.

- The **COSMIN** initiative was undertaken by a panel of health measurement experts to classify and define key **measurement properties**. The taxonomy presented in this book slightly modified the COSMIN taxonomy to include two cross-sectional measurement properties (reliability and validity) and two longitudinal measurement properties (reliability of change scores and responsiveness).

- Each measurement property can be assessed by computing a statistic that estimates a **measurement parameter**. Several parameter estimates involve computing a **correlation coefficient** that indicates the magnitude and direction of a relationship between two variables. Correlation coefficients can range from −1.00 (a **perfect negative relationship**) through zero to +1.00 (a **perfect positive relationship**).

- **Reliability** is the extent to which scores for people *who have not changed* are the same for repeated measurements, under several situations, including repetition on different occasions (test–retest and intrarater reliability), by different persons (interrater reliability), on different versions of a measure (parallel test reliability), or in the form of different items on a multi-item instrument (internal consistency).
- Assessments of **test–retest reliability** involve administering a measure on two occasions to assess the stability of scores over a short time interval. When scores are continuous, the preferred index of test–retest reliability is the **intraclass correlation coefficient (ICC)**. Reliability coefficients like the ICC usually range from .00 to 1.00, with higher values reflecting greater reliability.
- **Interrater reliability** involves assessing the congruence of ratings or classifications of two or more independent observers. When observers make classifications, interrater agreement is usually assessed using the **kappa** statistic, which is an index of chance-adjusted **proportion in agreement**.
- **Internal consistency**, a component in the reliability domain, concerns the extent to which all the instrument's items are measuring the same attribute; it is usually assessed by **Cronbach's alpha**. Internal consistency is not relevant for formative indexes.
- A third component in the reliability domain is measurement error, for which there are two indexes that indicate the precision of a score. The **standard error of measurement (SEM)**, which quantifies "typical error" on a measure, is in the units of measurement of the measure itself. Another index is called the **limits of agreement (LOA)** on a *Bland-Altman plot*. The LOA can be used to identify how much a difference is scores in a retest study is reasonable if the attribute has in fact not changed.

- **Validity**, a second domain in the measurement taxonomy, is the degree to which an instrument measures what it purports to measure. Validity has multiple components.
- **Face validity** refers to whether the instrument appears, on the face of it, to be measuring the appropriate construct.
- **Content validity** is the extent to which an instrument's content (its items) adequately and comprehensively captures the construct being measured. Expert ratings on the relevance of items can be used to compute **content validity index (CVI)** information. **Item CVIs (I-CVIs)** represent the proportion of experts rating each item as relevant. A **scale CVI (S-CVI)** using the averaging calculation method is the average of all I-CVI values.
- **Criterion-related validity** (which includes both **predictive validity** and **concurrent validity**) is the extent to which scores on an instrument are an adequate reflection of a "gold standard" criterion. When both the focal measure and the criterion are continuous measures, correlation coefficients are used as estimates of criterion validity.
- Criterion-related validity is often assessed with indexes associated with evaluations of diagnostic accuracy, namely, sensitivity and specificity. **Sensitivity** is the instrument's ability to identify a case correctly (i.e., its rate of yielding true positives). **Specificity** is the instrument's ability to identify noncases correctly (i.e., its rate of yielding true negatives).
- Sensitivity is sometimes plotted against specificity in a **receiver operating characteristic curve (ROC curve)** to determine the optimum **cutoff point** for caseness. An ROC yields an index called the **area under the curve (AUC)** that can be used as an index of criterion validity.
- **Construct validity**, a third component in the validity domain, concerns what abstract construct an instrument is actually measuring. One aspect is **hypothesis-testing construct validity**: The extent to which hypotheses about what the instrument is measuring can be supported. The key approaches include **convergent validity**, the degree to which there is conceptual convergence between scores on the focal measure and another measure; **known-groups**

validity, the extent to which hypotheses about groups expected to differ on a measure are supported; and **divergent validity**, the extent to which hypotheses about what an instrument does *not* measure are supported.

- Another aspect of construct validity is **structural validity**, which concerns the extent to which evidence supports hypotheses about the dimensionality of a complex construct.
- **Cross-cultural validity**, another aspect of construct validity, concerns the degree to which the items on a translated or culturally adapted scale perform adequately and equivalently in relation to their performance on the original instrument.
- Change is often measured by computing a **change score** that is the difference in value between two measurements. A major issue with change scores is that they tend to amplify measurement error; and hence, a third domain in the taxonomy concerns the **reliability of a change score**.
- Two indexes can be used to summarize whether a change in a person's score over time is reliable or merely reflects random fluctuations. One is the **smallest detectable change (SDC)**, which is a value that is outside the limits of agreement. The **reliable change index (RCI)** is a similar index that is based on a formula using the standard error of measurement.
- The final domain in the measurement taxonomy is **responsiveness**, which refers to the ability of a measure to detect change over time in a construct that has changed. Responsiveness, the longitudinal analog of validity, can be assessed by testing hypotheses about how changes in the focal measure are consistent with changes in other measures.
- Assessments of responsiveness, such as validity, can involve a criterion approach or a construct approach. Some researchers used **health transition ratings** (also called **global rating scales**) as the criterion for change.

STUDY ACTIVITIES

Chapter 14 of the *Resource Manual for Nursing Research: Generating and Assessing Evidence for*

Nursing Practice, 10th edition, offers exercises and study suggestions for reinforcing concepts presented in this chapter. In addition, the following study questions can be addressed:

1. Explain in your own words the meaning of the following correlation coefficients:
   a. The relationship between intelligence and grade-point average was found to be .72.
   b. The correlation coefficient between age and gregariousness was −.20.
   c. It was revealed that patients' compliance with nursing instructions was related to their length of stay in the hospital ($r = -.50$).
2. Use the critiquing guidelines in Box 14.1 to evaluate data quality in the study by Gilbert and Hayes (2009), referring to the original study if possible.

STUDIES CITED IN CHAPTER 14

Bekhet, A. K., & Zauszniewski, J. (2013). Psychometric assessment of the Depressive Cognition Scale among caregivers of persons with autism spectrum disorder. *Archives of Psychiatric Nursing, 27*, 96–100.

Bland, J. M., & Altman, D. G. (1986). Statistical methods for assessing agreement between two methods of clinical measurement. *Lancet, 327*, 307–310.

Brod, M., Tesler, L., & Christensen, T. (2009). Qualitative research and content validity: Developing best practices based on science and experience. *Quality of Life Research, 18*, 1263–1278.

*Campbell, D. T., & Fiske, D. W. (1959). Convergent and discriminant validation by the multitrait-multimethod matrix. *Psychological Bulletin, 56*, 81–105.

Cella, D., Gershon, R., Lai, J., & Choi, S. (2007). The future of outcome measurement: Item banking, tailored short forms, and computerized adaptive assessment. *Quality of Life Research, 16*(Supp. 1), 133–141.

Chen, S. W., Cheng, C., Wang, R., Jian, S., & Chen, M. (2015). Development and psychometric testing of an energy retention behavior scale for children. *Journal of Nursing Research, 23*, 47–55.

Chen, Y., Narsavage, G. L., Culp, S., & Weaver, T. (2010). The development and psychometric analysis of the Short-Form Pulmonary Functional Status Scale (PFSS-11). *Research in Nursing & Health, 33*, 477–485.

Choe, K. (2014). Development and preliminary testing of the Schizophrenia Hope Scale, a brief scale to measure hope in people with schizophrenia. *International Journal of Nursing Studies, 51*, 927–933.

Chow, S. K., & Wong, F. K. (2014). The reliability and validity of the Chinese version of the Short-Form Chronic Disease Self-Efficacy Scales for older adults. *Journal of Clinical Nursing, 23*, 1095–1104.

Curley, M. A., Hunsberger, M., & Harris, S. (2013). Psychometric evaluation of the Family-Centered Care Scale for pediatric acute care nursing. *Nursing Research, 62*, 160–168.

Curley, M. A., Razmus, I. S., Roberts, K. E., & Wypij, D. (2003). Predicting pressure ulcer risk in pediatric patients: The Braden Q Scale. *Nursing Research, 52*, 22–33.

Dawson, A. P., Steele, E., Hodges, P., & Stewart, S. (2010). Utility of the Oswestry Disability Index for studies of back pain related disability in nurses: Evaluation of psychometric and measurement properties. *International Journal of Nursing Studies, 47*, 604–607.

DeVellis, R. F. (2012). *Scale development: Theory and applications* (3rd ed.). Thousand Oaks, CA: Sage.

De Vet, H. C. W., Terwee, C., Mokkink, L. B., & Knol, D. L. (2011). *Measurement in medicine: A practical guide*. Cambridge, United Kingdom: Cambridge University Press.

Folstein, M., Folstein, S., White, T., & Messer, M. (2010). *Mini-Mental State Examination: User's manual* (2nd ed.). Lutz, FL: Psychological Assessment Resources.

*Gaugler, J. E., Hobday, J., & Savik, K. (2013). The CARES observational tool: A valid and reliable instrument to assess person-centered dementia care. *Geriatric Nursing, 34*, 194–198.

*Gilbert, D. A., & Hayes, E. (2009). Communication and outcomes of visits between older patients and nurse practitioners. *Nursing Research, 58*, 283–293.

Guyatt, G. H., Deyo, R., Charlson, M., Levine, M., & Mitchell, A. (1989). Responsiveness and validity in health status measurement: A clarification. *Journal of Clinical Epidemiology, 42*, 403–408.

Hammash, M., Hall, L., Lennie, T., Heo, S., Chung, M., Lee, K., & Moser, D. (2013). Psychometrics of the PHQ-9 as a measure of depressive symptoms in patients with heart failure. *European Journal of Cardiovascular Nursing, 12*, 446–453.

Hawkins, R. J., Swanson, B., Kremer, M., & Fogg, L. (2014). Content validity testing of questions for a patient satisfaction with general anesthesia care questionnaire. *Journal of Perianesthesia Nursing, 29*, 28–35.

Holmes, T. H., & Rahe, R. (1967). The Social Readjustment Rating Scale. *Journal of Psychosomatic Research, 11*, 213–218.

Jacobson, N. S., Follette, W. C., & Revenstorf, D. (1984). Psychotherapy outcome research: Methods for reporting variability and evaluating clinical significance. *Behavior Therapy, 15*, 336–352.

Jacobson, N. S., & Truax, P. (1991). Clinical significance: A statistical approach to defining meaningful change in psychotherapy research. *Journal of Consulting and Clinical Psychology, 59*, 12–19.

Kirshner, B., & Guyatt, G. (1985). A methodological framework for assessing health indices. *Journal of Chronic Diseases, 38*, 27–36.

Miller, W., Bakas, T., Weaver, M., Buelow, J., & Sabau, D. (2015). The Life Changes in Epilepsy Scale: Development and establishment of content and face validity. *Clinical Nurse Specialist, 29*, 95–99.

*Mokkink, L. B., Terwee, C., Patrick, D., Alonso, J., Stratford, P., Knol, D. L., . . . De Vet, H. C. W. (2010a). The COSMIN checklist for assessing the methodological quality of studies on measurement properties of health status instruments: An international Delphi study. *Quality of Life Research, 19*, 539–549.

Mokkink, L. B., Terwee, C., Patrick, D., Alonso, J., Stratford, P., Knol, D. L., . . . De Vet, H. C. W. (2010b). The COSMIN study reached international consensus on taxonomy, terminology, and definitions of measurement properties for health-related patient-reported outcomes. *Journal of Clinical Epidemiology, 63*, 737–745.

Moyle, W., Cooke, M., Beattie, E., Jones, C., Klein, B., Cook, G., & Gray, C. (2013). Exploring the effect of companion robots on emotional expression in older adults with dementia: A pilot randomized controlled trial. *Journal of Gerontological Nursing, 39*, 46–53.

Nilsen, M., Happ, M., Donovan, H., Barnato, A., Hoffman, L., & Sereika, S. (2014). Adaptation of a communication interaction behavior instrument for use in mechanically ventilated, nonvocal older adults. *Nursing Research, 63*, 3–13.

Nunnally, J., & Bernstein, I. H. (1994). *Psychometric theory* (3rd ed.). New York: McGraw-Hill.

Peters, R. M., Benkert, R., Templin, T., & Cassidy-Bushrow, A. (2014). Measuring African American women's trust in provider during pregnancy. *Research in Nursing & Health, 37*, 144–154.

Polit, D. F. (2014). Getting serious about test-retest reliability: A critique of retest research and some recommendations. *Quality of Life Research, 23*, 1713–1720.

Polit, D. F. (2015). Assessing measurement in health: Beyond reliability and validity. *International Journal of Nursing Studies*. Advance online publication. doi:10.1007/s11136-014-0632-9

Polit, D. F., & Beck, C. T. (2006). The content validity index: Are you sure you know what is being reported? Critique and recommendations. *Research in Nursing & Health, 29*, 489–497.

Polit, D. F., Beck, C. T., & Owen, S. V. (2007). Is the CVI an acceptable indicator of content validity? Appraisal and recommendations. *Research in Nursing & Health, 30*, 459–467.

Polit, D. F., & Yang, F. M. (2015). *Measurement and the measurement of change: A primer for health professionals*. Philadelphia: Lippincott Williams & Wilkins.

Radloff, L. S. (1977). The CES-D scale: A self-rating depression scale for research in the general population. *Applied Psychological Measurement, 1*, 385–401.

*Schünemann, H., Oxman, A., Brozek, J., Glasziou, P., Jaeschke, P., Vist, G., . . . Guyatt, G. (2008). Grading quality of evidence and strength of recommendations for diagnostic tests and strategies. *British Medical Journal, 336*, 1106–1110.

Shadish, W. R., Cook, T. D., & Campbell, D. T. (2002). *Experimental and quasi-experimental designs for generalized causal inference*. Boston: Houghton Mifflin.

*Strauss, M. E., & Smith, G. T. (2009). Construct validity: Advances in theory and methodology. *Annual Review of Clinical Psychology, 5*, 1–25.

Streiner, D. L. (2003). Being inconsistent about consistency: When coefficient alpha does and doesn't matter. *Journal of Personality Assessment, 80*, 217–222.

Streiner, D. L., & Norman, G. R. (2008). *Health measurement scales: A practical guide to their development and use* (4th ed.). Oxford, United Kingdom: Oxford University Press.

Terwee, C. B., Dekker, F., Wiersinga, W., Prummel, M., & Bossuyt, P. (2003). On assessing responsiveness of health-related quality of life instruments: Guidelines for instrument evaluation. *Quality of Life Research, 12*, 349–362.

*Terwee, C. B., Mokkink, L. B., Knol, D. L., Ostelo, R., Bouter, L. M., & De Vet, H. C. W. (2012). Rating the methodological quality in systematic reviews of studies on measurement properties: A scoring system for the COSMIN checklist. *Quality of Life Research, 21*, 651–657.

Tilahun, B., Faust, A., McCorstin, P., & Ortegon, A. (2015). Nasal colonization and lower respiratory tract infections with methicillin-resistant *Staphylococcus aureus. American Journal of Critical Care, 24*, 8–12.

*U.S. Food and Drug Administration. (2009). *Guidance for industry patient-reported outcome measures: Use in medical product development to support labeling claims.* Washington, DC: U.S. Department of Health and Human Services.

Vellone, E., Jaarsma, T., Stromberg, A., Fida, R., Arestiedt, K., Rocco, G., . . . Alvaro, R. (2014). The European Heart Failure Self-Care Behaviour Scale: New insights into factorial structure, reliability, precision and scoring procedure. *Patient Education and Counseling, 94*, 97–102.

***A link to this open-access journal article is provided in the Toolkit for this chapter in the accompanying Resource Manual.** ✪

15 | Developing and Testing Self-Report Scales

Researchers sometimes are unable to identify an appropriate instrument to operationalize a construct. This may occur when the construct is new, but often it is due to limitations of existing instruments. Because this situation occurs fairly often, this chapter provides an overview of the steps involved in developing high-quality self-report scales.

The scope of this chapter is fairly narrow, but it covers instruments that nurse researchers often use. Specifically, we focus on *multi-item* reflective scales and primarily scales rooted in classical test theory.

> **TIP:** The development of high-quality scales is a lengthy, labor-intensive process that requires some statistical sophistication. We urge you to think carefully about embarking on a scale development endeavor and to consider involving a psychometric consultant if you proceed.

BEGINNING STEPS: CONCEPTUALIZATION AND ITEM GENERATION

Conceptualizing the Construct

The importance of a sound, thorough conceptualization of the construct to be measured cannot be overemphasized. You will not be able to quantify an attribute adequately unless you thoroughly understand the **latent trait** (the underlying construct) you wish to capture. For reflective scales, the unobservable latent trait is the *cause* of people's responses and hence their scores on the measure. You cannot develop items to produce the right score, and you cannot expect good content and construct validity, if you are unclear about the construct and its nuances. Thus, the first step in scale development is to become an *expert* on the construct.

Complex constructs have a number of different facets or dimensions, and it is important to identify and understand each one. This is partly a content validity consideration: For the scale to be content valid, there must be items representing all facets of the construct. All scales—or subscales of a broader scale—need to be *unidimensional* (measuring a single construct or facet of a construct) and internally consistent. Thus, an adequate number of items (operational definitions) of each dimension need to be developed. For instruments that are being developed for use by others, it is useful to establish an expert panel to review domain specifications, in an early effort to ensure the content validity of the scale.

During the early conceptualization, you also need to think about related constructs that should be differentiated from the target construct. If you are measuring, say, self-esteem, you have to be sure you can differentiate it from similar but distinct constructs, such as self-confidence. In thinking about the dimensions of the target construct, you should be sure that they are truly aspects of the construct and not a different construct altogether.

You should also have an explicit conceptualization of the population for whom the scale is intended. For example, a general anxiety scale may not be suitable for measuring childbearing anxiety in pregnant women. There are arguments for developing patient-specific scales, particularly with respect to item relevance and face validity. On the other hand, a highly focused scale reduces the scale's generalizability and the ability to make comparisons across populations. The point is that you should have a clear view of how and with whom the scale will be used.

Understanding the population for whom the scale is intended is critical for developing good items. Without a good grasp of the population, it will be difficult to consider such issues as reading levels and cultural appropriateness in wording the items.

Deciding on the Type of Scale

Before items can be generated, you need to decide on the type of scale you wish to create because item characteristics vary by scale type. Our focus is restricted to the multi-item reflective scales, which are also the focus of several other books on scale development that can be consulted for greater elaboration (DeVellis, 2012; McCoach et al., 2013; Polit & Yang, 2015; Streiner & Norman, 2008). Two broad categories of scales fall into this category: traditional summated rating (Likert-type) scales and latent trait scales.

Traditional summated rating scales (Chapter 13) are based in classical test theory (CTT). In CTT, items are presumed to be roughly comparable indicators of the underlying construct. The items gain strength in approximating a hypothetical true score through their aggregation. Traditional scales rely on items that are deliberately redundant, in the hope that multiple indicators of the construct will converge on the true score and balance out error.

Item response theory (IRT) is an alternative to CTT that is growing in popularity for scale development. IRT methods are complex and require statistical sophistication and access to special software. We note a few characteristics of IRT;

further information is provided in the Supplement to this chapter on thePoint®.

In CTT, traits are modeled at the level of the observed scale score, whereas in IRT, the models are at the level of the observed item response. The goal of IRT is to allow researchers to gain understanding of the characteristics of items independent of the people who complete them. *Latent trait scales* using IRT models can use items like the ones used in CTT, such as items in a Likert-type format—in fact, a person completing a scale would likely not know whether it had been developed within the CTT or IRT framework. But a person *developing* a scale must decide which measurement theory is being used. Items on a CTT scale are designed to be similar to each other to tap the underlying construct in a comparable manner, but items on a latent-trait IRT scale tap different levels of the attribute being measured.

As an example, suppose we were developing a scale to measure risk-taking behavior in adolescents. In a CTT scale, the items might include statements about risk taking of similar intensity, to which respondents would respond with graded responses corresponding to frequency or intensity of endorsement. The aggregate of responses would array respondents along a continuum indicating varying propensity to take risks. In an IRT scale, the items themselves would be chosen to reflect different levels of risk taking (e.g., not eating vegetables, smoking cigarettes, having unprotected sex, texting while driving). Each item could be described as having a different *difficulty*. It is "easier" to agree with or admit to lower risk items than higher risk items. Measurements based on an IRT model result in information about the *location* of both items and people on a trait continuum. If a pool of unidimensional items can readily be ordered into a hierarchy of difficulty, then a good IRT model fit is plausible. Item difficulty is one of several parameters that can be analyzed in IRT scale development.

Generating an Item Pool: Getting Started

An early step in scale construction is to develop a pool of possible items for the scale. Items—which collectively constitute the operational definition of the construct—need to be carefully crafted to reflect the latent variable they are designed to measure.

This is often easier to do as a team effort because different people articulate a similar idea in diverse ways. Regardless of whether you are doing this alone or with a team, you may be asking: Where do scale items come from? Here are some possible sources for generating an **item pool**:

1. *Existing instruments.* Sometimes it is possible to adapt an existing instrument rather than starting from scratch. Adaptations may require adding and deleting items or may involve rewording them— for example, to make them more culturally appropriate, or to simplify wording for a population with low reading skills. Permission from the author of the original scale should be sought because published scales are copyright protected.
2. *The literature.* Ideas for item content often come from a thorough understanding of prior research.
3. *Concept analysis.* A related source of ideas is a concept analysis. Walker and Avant (2011) offer concept analysis strategies that could be used to develop items for a scale.
4. *In-depth qualitative research.* In-depth inquiry relating to the key construct is a particularly rich source for scale items. A qualitative study can help you to understand the dimensions of a phenomenon and can also give you actual words for items. If you are unable to undertake an in-depth study yourself, be sure to pay particular attention to the verbatim quotes in published qualitative reports about your construct.
5. *Clinical observations.* Patients in clinical settings may be an excellent source of items. Ideas for items may come from direct observation of patients' behaviors in relevant situations or from listening to their comments and conversations.

Example of Sources of Items: Choe (2014) developed a scale to measure hope in people with schizophrenia. Forty items were initially developed, based on concept clarification research, a qualitative study, and an extensive literature review.

DeVellis (2012) urged scale developers to get started writing scale items without a lot of editing and critical review in the early stages. Perhaps a good way to begin if you are struggling is to develop a simple statement with the key construct mentioned in it. For example, if the construct is test anxiety, you might start with, "I get anxious when I take a test." This could be followed by similar statement worded differently (e.g., "Taking tests makes me nervous.").

Making Decisions about Item Features

In preparing to write items, you need to make decisions about such issues as the number of items to develop, the number and form of the response options, whether to include positively and negatively worded items, and how to deal with time.

Number of Items

In the CTT framework, a **domain sampling model** is assumed, which involves the random sampling of a homogeneous set of items from a hypothetical universe of items on the construct. Of course, sampling from a *universe* of all possible items does not happen in reality. The idea is to generate a fairly exhaustive set of item possibilities, given the construct's theoretical demands. For a traditional scale, redundancy (except for trivial word substitutions) is a good thing. The goal is to measure the construct with a set of items that capture its essence in slightly different ways so that irrelevant idiosyncrasies of individual items will cancel each other out.

There is no magic formula for how many items should be developed, but our advice is to generate a very large pool of items. As you proceed, many items will be discarded. Longer scales tend to be more reliable, so starting with a large number of items promotes the likelihood that you will eventually have an internally consistent scale. DeVellis (2012) recommends starting with 3 to 4 times as many items as you will have in your final scale (e.g., 30 to 40 items for a 10-item scale), but the minimum should be 50% more (e.g., 15 items for a 10-item scale).

Response Options

Scale items involve both a *stem* (often a declarative statement) and *response options*. Traditional Likert scales involve response options on a continuum of agreement, but other continua are possible, such as frequency (never/always), importance (very important/unimportant), quality (excellent/very poor), and likelihood (highly likely/impossible).

How many response options should there be? There is no simple answer, but keep in mind the goal is to array people on a continuum, and so variability is essential. Variability can be enhanced by including a lot of items, by offering numerous response options, or both. However, there is not much merit in creating the illusion of precision when it does not exist. With a 1–15 range of response options, for example, the difference between a 12 and a 13 might not be meaningful. Also, it has been found that too many options can be confusing to some people.

Most scales have five to seven options, with verbal descriptors attached to each option and, often, numbers placed under the descriptors to further help respondents find an appropriate place on the continuum. An odd number of response options gives respondents an opportunity to be neutral or ambivalent (i.e., to choose a midpoint). Some scale developers prefer an even number (e.g., four or six) to force even slight tendencies and to avoid equivocation. However, some respondents may actually *be* neutral or ambivalent, so a midpoint option allows them to express it. The midpoint can be labeled with such phrases as "neither agree nor disagree," "undecided," "agree and disagree equally," or simply "?".

➲ **TIP:** Here are some frequently used words for response options, with midpoint terms not listed:

- Strongly disagree, disagree, agree, strongly agree
- Never, almost never (or rarely), sometimes (or occasionally), often (or frequently), almost always (or always)
- Very important, important, somewhat important, of little importance, unimportant
- Definitely not, probably not, possibly, probably, very probably, definitely
- With no trouble, with a little trouble, with some trouble, with a lot of trouble, not able to do

Positive and Negative Stems

A generation ago, psychometricians advised scale developers to deliberately include both positively and negatively worded statements and to reverse score negative items. As an example, consider these two items for a scale of depression: "I frequently feel blue," and "I don't often feel sad." The objective was to include items that would minimize the possibility of an acquiescence response set—the tendency to agree with statements regardless of their content.

Many experts currently advise again including negative and positive items on a scale. Some respondents are confused by reversing polarities. Responding to item with negative stems appears to be an especially difficult cognitive task for younger respondents. Some research suggests that acquiescence can be minimized by putting the most positive response options (e.g., strongly agree) at the end of the list rather than at the beginning.

Item Intensity

In a traditional summated rating scale, the intensity of the statements (stems) should be similar and fairly strongly worded. If items are worded such that almost anyone would agree with them, the scale will not be able to discriminate between people with different amounts of the underlying trait. For example, an item such as "Good health is important" would generate almost universal agreement. On the other hand, statements should not be so extremely worded as to result in universal rejection. For a latent trait scale, scale developers seek a range of item intensities. Yet, even on an IRT-based scale, there is no point in including items with which almost everyone would either agree or disagree.

Item Time Frames

Some items make an explicit reference to a time frame (e.g., "In the past week I have had trouble falling asleep"), but others do not (e.g., "I have trouble falling asleep"). Sometimes instructions to a scale can designate a temporal frame of reference (e.g., "In answering the following questions, please indicate how you have felt in the past week"). And yet other scales ask respondents to respond in terms of a time frame: "In the past week, I have had trouble falling asleep: Every day, 5–6 days . . . Never."

A time frame should not emerge as a consequence of item development. You should decide in advance, based on your conceptual understanding of the construct and the needs for which the scale is being constructed, how to deal with time.

Example of Handling Time in a Scale: The Postpartum Depression Screening Scale asks respondents to indicate their emotional state in the previous 2 weeks—for example, over the last 2 weeks I: ". . . had trouble sleeping even when my baby was asleep" and ". . . felt like a failure as a mother" (Beck & Gable, 2000, 2001). The 2-week period was chosen because it parallels the duration of symptoms required for a diagnosis of major depressive episode according to the DSM-V criteria.

Wording the Items

Items should be worded in such a manner that every respondent is answering the same question. In addition to the suggestions on question wording we provided in Chapter 13, some additional tips specific to scale items are as follows:

1. *Clarity.* Scale developers should strive for clear, unambiguous items. Words should be carefully chosen with the educational and reading level of the target population in mind. In most cases, this will mean developing a scale at the 6th- to 7th-grade reading level. Even beyond reading level, you should strive to select words that everyone understands and to have everyone reach the same conclusion about what the words mean.
2. *Jargon.* Jargon should be avoided. Be especially cautious about using terms that might be well-known in health care circles (e.g., lesion) but not familiar to the average person.
3. *Length.* Avoid long sentences or phrases. In particular, eliminate unnecessary words. For example, "It is fair to say that in the scheme of things I do not get enough sleep," could more simply be worded, "I usually do not get enough sleep."
4. *Double negatives.* It is preferable to word things affirmatively ("I am usually happy") than negatively ("I am not usually sad"), but double negatives should always be avoided ("I am not usually *un*happy").
5. *Double-barreled items.* Avoid putting two or more ideas in a single item. For example, "I am afraid of insects and snakes" is a bad item because a person who is afraid of insects but not snakes (or vice versa) would not know how to respond.

→ **TIP:** When scale developers anticipate a possible translation into another language, they should consider the following tips for crafting items: (1) avoid metaphors, idioms, and colloquialisms; (2) use specific words rather than ones open to interpretation, such as "daily" rather than "frequently"; (3) avoid pronouns—repeat nouns if necessary to avoid ambiguity; (4) write in the present tense and avoid the subjunctive mode, such as "should"; and (5) use words with a Latin root if translation into a Romance language such as Spanish is expected (Hilton & Skrutkowski, 2002).

PRELIMINARY EVALUATION OF ITEMS

Internal Review

Once a large item pool has been generated, it is time for critical appraisal. Care should be devoted to such issues as whether individual items capture the construct and are grammatical and well-worded. The initial review should also consider whether the items taken together adequately embrace the full nuances of the construct.

It is imperative to assess the scale's **readability**, unless the scale is intended for a highly educated population. There are different approaches for assessing the reading level of written documents, but many methods are either time-consuming or require several hundreds of words of text, and thus are not suited to evaluating scale items (Streiner & Norman, 2008).

Many word processing programs provide some information about readability. In Microsoft Word, for example, you could type your items on a list and then get readability statistics for the items as a whole or for individual items, as described in Chapter 7. For example, take the following two sets of items for tapping fatigue:

Set A	Set B
I am frequently exhausted.	I am often tired.
I invariably get insufficient sleep.	I don't get enough sleep.

The Word software tells us that the items in set A have a *Flesch-Kincaid grade level* of 12.0 and a *Flesch reading ease score* of 4.8. (Reading ease scores rate text on a 100-point scale, with higher values associated with greater ease, using a formula that considers average sentence length and average number of syllables.) Set B, by contrast, has a grade level of 1.8 and a reading ease score of 89.4. Streiner and Norman (2008) warn that word processing–based readability scores be interpreted cautiously, but it is clear from the foregoing analysis that the second set of items would be superior for a population that includes people with limited education. A general principle is to avoid long sentences and words with four or more syllables.

Example of Assessing Readability: Ruiz and colleagues (2015) examined the readability and psychometric properties of a scale (the Brief COPE) to measure coping in pregnant minority women. Using the Flesch-Kincaid reading level test, the researchers found that the scale was at the sixth-grade reading level.

Input from the Target Population

In the next step, the initial pool of items is pretested. In a conventional pretest of a new instrument, a small sample of people (20 to 40 or so) representing the target population is invited to complete the items. In analyzing pretest data, researchers look for items with high rates of nonresponse, items with limited variability, items with numerous midpoint responses (fence-sitting). Such items are candidates for deletion or revision, or items with a high proportion of responses at one extreme (*floor effects* or *ceiling effects*).

Developments in cognitive science over the past 25 years have paved the way for a different approach to pretesting, often used to supplement standard pretests. In **cognitive interviews**, people are asked to reflect upon their interpretation of the items and their answers so that the underlying process of response selection is better understood.

There are two basic approaches to cognitive interviewing. One is called the **think-aloud method**, wherein respondents are asked to explain step by step how they processed the question and arrived at an answer. A second approach is to conduct an interview in which the interviewer uses a series of targeted **probes** that encourage reflection about underlying cognitive processes. (The Toolkit offers suggestions for cognitive questioning 🗗.)

Example of Cognitive Questioning: Andersen and colleagues (2014) translated the COMFORT behavioral rating scale (an observational scale for rating distress with pediatric patients) into Norwegian. As part of the translation process, cognitive interviews were conducted with eight nurses, three physicians, and a nurse assistant. Both the think-aloud method and structured probes were used to identify problems with the scale and the translation.

➔ **TIP:** When questioning pretest respondents about the clarity or meaning of the items, avoid using the word "item," which is research jargon (e.g., do not say, "Are there *items* that confused you?").

As an alternative or supplement to pretests, *focus groups* can also be used at this stage in scale development. Two or three groups can be convened to discuss whether, from the respondents' perspective, the items are understandable, linguistically and culturally appropriate, inoffensive, and relevant to the construct.

External Review by Experts

External review of the revised items by a panel of experts should be undertaken to assess the scale's content validity. It is advisable to undertake two rounds of review, if feasible—the first to refine or weed out faulty items or to add new items to cover the domain adequately and the second to formally assess the content validity of the items and scale. We discuss some procedures in such a two-step strategy, although the two steps are sometimes combined.

Selecting and Recruiting the Experts

The panel of experts should include people with strong credentials with regard to the construct being measured. Experts also should be knowledgeable about the target population. In the first review, it is also desirable to include experts on scale construction.

In the initial phase of a two-part review, we advise having an expert panel of 8 to 12 members, with a good mix in terms of roles (e.g., clinicians, faculty, researchers) and disciplines. For example, for a scale designed to measure fear of dying in the elderly, the experts might include nurses, gerontologists, and psychiatrists. If the scale is intended for broad use, it might also be advantageous to recruit experts from various countries or areas of a country, because of possible regional variations in language. The second panel for formally assessing the content validity of a more refined set of items should consist of three to five experts in the content area.

Example of an Expert Panel: Gaugler and colleagues (2013) developed an observational tool (CARES) to measure whether person-centered care is delivered to patients with dementia. In the content validity assessment, a panel of nine nationally recognized experts was recruited. The panel reflected a range of disciplines: advance practice nursing, occupational therapy, social work, and psychology.

Experts are typically sent a packet of materials, including a strong cover letter, background information about the construct and target population, reviewer instructions, and a questionnaire soliciting their opinion. A critical component of the packet is a careful explanation of the conceptual underpinnings of the construct, including an explication of the various dimensions encompassed by the construct to be captured in subscales. The panel may also be given a brief overview of the literature as well as a bibliography.

→ **TIP:** The Toolkit section of the *Resource Manual* includes, as Word documents, a sample cover letter and other material relating to expert review that can be adapted.

Preliminary Expert Review: Content Validation of Items

The experts' job is to evaluate individual items and the overall scale (and any subscales), using guidelines established by the scale developer. The first panel of experts is usually invited to rate each item in terms of several characteristics, such as clarity of wording; relevance of the item to the construct; and appropriateness for the target population (e.g., developmental or cultural appropriateness). Experts can be asked to make judgments dichotomously (e.g., ambiguous/clear) or along a continuum. As noted in the previous chapter, relevance is most often rated as follows: 1 = *not relevant*, 2 = *somewhat relevant*, 3 = *quite relevant*, 4 = *highly relevant*. Figure 15.1 🔅 shows a possible format for a content validation assessment of relevance.

The questionnaire usually asks for detailed comments about items judged to be unclear, not relevant, or not appropriate, such as how wording might be improved, or why the item is deemed to be not relevant. Another question that could be included for each item in a first phase evaluation concerns an overall recommendation—for example, retain the item exactly as worded, make minor revisions to the item, make major revisions to the item, and drop the item entirely.

In addition to evaluating each item, the initial expert panel should be asked to consider whether the items taken as a whole adequately cover the construct domain. The items on a scale constitute the operational definition of the construct, so it is important to assess whether the operational definition taps each dimension adequately. Experts should be asked for specific guidance on items or subdomains that should be added. For scales constructed within an IRT framework, the experts can also be asked whether the items span a continuum of difficulty.

The formula for evaluating agreement among experts on individual items is the number agreeing, divided by the number of experts. When the aspect being rated is relevance, the standard method for computing an item-level content validity index (I-CVI) is the number giving a rating of 3 or 4 on the 4-point relevance scale, divided by the number of experts. For example, if five experts rated an item as 3 and one rated the item as 2, the I-CVI would be .83. Because of the risk of chance agreement, we recommend I-CVIs of .78 or higher (Polit et al., 2007). This means that there must be 100% agreement among raters when there are four or fewer experts. When there are five to eight experts, one rating of "not relevant" can be tolerated.

The scale items shown below have been developed to measure one dimension of the construct of safe sexual behaviors among adolescents, namely **assertiveness**. Please read each item and score it for its relevance in representing this concept.

Assertiveness is defined as the use of verbal and interpersonal skills to negotiate protection during sexual activities.

Item	**Relevance Rating**			
	Not Relevant	Somewhat Relevant	Quite Relevant	Highly Relevant
1. I ask my partner about his/her sexual history before having intercourse.	1	2	3	4
2. I don't have sex without asking the person if he/she has been tested for HIV/AIDS.	1	2	3	4
3. When I am having sex with someone for the first time, I insist that we use a condom.	1	2	3	4
4. I don't let my partner talk me into having sex without knowing something about how risky it would be.	1	2	3	4

Please comment on any of these items, including possible revisions or substitutions, or your thoughts about why an item is not relevant to the concept of assertiveness. Please suggest any additional items you feel would improve the measurement of assertiveness relating to adolescents' safe sexual behaviors.

FIGURE 15.1 Example of a content validation form.

Items with lower than desired I-CVIs need careful scrutiny. It may be necessary to recontact the experts to better understand genuine differences of opinion or to strive for greater consensus. If there are legitimate disagreements among the experts on individual items (or if there is agreement about lack of relevance), the items should be revised or dropped.

Content Validation of the Scale

In the second round of content validation, a smaller group of experts (three to five) can be used to evaluate the relevance of the revised set of items and to compute the scale content validity (S-CVI). Although it is possible to use a new group of experts, we recommend using a subset from the first panel because then information from the first round can be used to select the most qualified judges. With information from round 1, for example, you can perhaps identify experts who did not understand the task, who had a tendency to give high (or low) ratings, who were not as familiar with the construct as you thought, or who otherwise seemed biased. In other words, data from the first round can be

analyzed with a view toward evaluating the performance of the experts, not just the items. This analysis might also require discussion with some of the experts to fully understand the reason for incongruent or anomalous ratings.

In terms of selecting experts based on their ratings in the first round, here are some suggestions. First, experts who rated every item as "highly relevant" (or "not relevant") may not be sufficiently discriminating. Second, an expert who gave high ratings to items that were judged by most others to not be relevant might be problematic. Third, the proportion of items judged relevant should be computed for all judges. For example, if an expert rated 8 out of 10 items as relevant, the proportion for that judge would be .80. The pattern across experts can be examined for "outliers." If the average proportion across raters is, for example, .80, you might consider not inviting back for a second round of experts whose average proportion was either very low (e.g., .50) or very high (e.g., 1.0). Qualitative feedback from an expert in round 1 in the form of useful comments might indicate both content capability and a commitment to the project. Finally, items known not to be relevant can be included in the first round to identify judges who rate irrelevant items as relevant and thus may not really be experts after all.

After ratings of relevance are obtained for a revised set of items, the S-CVI can be computed. There is more than one way to compute an S-CVI, as noted in Chapter 14. We recommend the approach that averages across I-CVIs. On a 10-item scale, for example, if the I-CVIs for 5 items were .80 and the I-CVIs for the remaining 5 items were 1.00, then the S-CVI/Ave would be .90. An S-CVI/Ave of .90 or higher is desirable.

In summary, we recommend that for a scale to be judged as having excellent content validity, it would be composed of items that had I-CVIs of .78 or higher and an S-CVI (using the averaging approach) of .90 or higher. This requires strong items, outstanding experts, and clear instructions to the experts regarding the underlying constructs and the rating task.

→ TIP: When you describe content validation in a report, be specific about your criteria for accepting items (i.e., the cutoff value for your I-CVIs) and the scale (the S-CVI). The report should indicate the range of obtained I-CVI values and the method used to compute the S-CVI.

FIELD TESTING THE INSTRUMENT

At this point, you will have whittled down and refined your items based on your own and others' careful scrutiny. The next step in scale development is to undertake a quantitative assessment of the items, which requires that they be administered to a fairly large assessment sample. As with content validation, this may involve a two-part process, with preliminary assessment occurring in the first phase and subsequent efforts to evaluate the scale's psychometric adequacy in the second.

Testing a new instrument is a full study in and of itself, and care must be taken to design the study to yield useful evidence about the scale's worth. Important steps include the development of a sampling plan and data collection strategy.

Developing a Sampling Plan

The sample for testing the scale should be representative of the population for whom the scale has been devised and should be large enough to support complex analyses. If it is not possible to administer the items to a random sample (as is typical), it is advantageous to recruit a sample from multiple sites to enhance representativeness and to assess geographic variation in responding to items. Other strategies to enhance representativeness should be sought, as well—for example, making sure that the sample includes older and younger respondents, men and women, people with varying educational and ethnic backgrounds, and so on, if these characteristics are relevant. You should also consider taking steps to ensure that the sample includes the right subsets of people for a "known groups" analysis.

How large is a "large" sample? There is neither consensus among experts nor hard-and-fast rules. Some suggest that 300 is an adequate number to support a factor analysis (Nunnally & Bernstein, 1994), while others offer guidance in terms of a ratio of items to respondents. Recommendations range from 3-4 people per item to 40-50 per item, with 10 per item often being recommended. That means that if you have 20 items, your sample should be at least 200. Having a sufficiently large sample is essential to ensure stability in estimating inter-item relationships. Note that if you plan to conduct an assessment of test–retest reliability (and you probably should), it is common to involve a smaller subsample of participants (e.g., 50 to 100) in the retest effort.

Finally, you should make efforts to recruit a heterogeneous sample with regard to the target attribute. Reliability and internal consistency estimates can be dampened if the scores are not sufficiently diverse.

Developing a Data Collection Plan

Decisions have to be made concerning how to administer the instrument (e.g., by mailed or distributed questionnaires, over the Internet) and what to include in the instrument. In deciding on a mode of administration, you should choose an approach that best approximates how the scale typically would be administered after it is finalized.

The instrument should include the scale items and basic demographic information. If the intent is to estimate test–retest reliability, then contact information would need to be obtained for scheduling the second administration—and the same would be true if the reliability of change scores and responsiveness were being assessed.

Thought should also be given to including other measures on the instrument—which would be essential if you do not plan to undertake a separate study to evaluate the scale's validity. As discussed in Chapter 14, various validation approaches can be used to assess a new instrument, but they all require additional measures. For example, measures of other constructs hypothesized to be correlated with the target construct should be included. If the data confirm a relationship predicted by theory or prior research, this would lend evidence to the new scale's validity. Also, it may be useful to include measures to assess response biases, especially social desirability. Item correlations with a measure of social desirability could suggest potentially biased items. (More complex approaches to evaluating and addressing the effects of social desirability and "faking bad" biases are discussed in Streiner and Norman [2008], Chapter 6.)

TIP: In deciding on what other measures to administer, keep in mind that respondents' willingness to cooperate may decline as the instrument package gets longer.

Preparing for Data Collection

As in all data collection efforts, care should be taken to make the instrument attractive, professional-looking, and easy to understand. Colleagues, mentors, or family members should be asked to evaluate the appearance of the instrument before it is reproduced.

Instructions for completing the instrument should be clear, and a readability assessment of the instructions is useful. There should be no ambiguity about what is expected of respondents. Guidance in understanding the end points of response options should be provided if points along the continuum are not explicitly labeled. The instructions should encourage candor. Sometimes social desirability can be minimized by stating that there are no right or wrong answers. Pett and colleagues (2003) offer useful suggestions for laying out an instrument and for developing instructions to respondents.

One other consideration is how to sequence the items in the instrument. At issue is something that is called a *proximity effect*, the tendency to be influenced in responding to an item by the response given to the previous item. This effect would tend to artificially inflate estimates of internal consistency. One approach to deal with this is the random ordering of items. An alternative, for scales designed to measure several related dimensions, is to systematically alternate items that are expected to be scored into different subscales.

ANALYSIS OF SCALE DEVELOPMENT DATA

The analysis of data from multi-item scales is a topic about which entire books have been written. We provide only an overview here. We assume that readers of this section have basic familiarity with statistics. Those who need a refresher should consult Chapters 16 through 18.

Basic Item Analysis

The performance of each item on the preliminary scale needs to be evaluated empirically. Within classical test theory, what is desired is an item that has a high correlation with the true score of the underlying construct. We cannot assess this directly, but if each item is a measure of that construct, then the items should correlate with one another.

The degree of **inter-item correlation** can be assessed by inspecting the correlation matrix of all the items. If there are items with substantial negative intercorrelations, some should perhaps be *reverse-scored*. Unless intentional, however, negative correlations are likely to reflect problems and may signal the desirability of removing some items. For items on the same subscale, inter-item correlations between .30 and .70 are often recommended, with correlations lower than .30 suggesting little congruence with the underlying construct and ones higher than .70 suggesting over-redundancy.

However, the evaluation depends on the number of items in the scale. An average inter-item correlation of .57 is needed to achieve a coefficient alpha of .80 on a 3-item scale, but an average of only .29 is needed for a 10-item scale (DeVellis, 2012).

A next step is to compute preliminary total scale or subscale scores and then calculate correlations between items and total scores on the scales they are intended to represent. If item scores do not correlate well with scale scores, it is probably measuring something else and will lower the reliability of the scale. There are two types of **item–scale correlations**, one in which the total score includes the item under consideration (*uncorrected*) and another in which the item is removed in calculating the total scale score. The latter (*corrected*) approach is preferable because the inclusion of the item on the scale inflates the correlation coefficients. The standard advice is to eliminate items whose item–scale correlation is less than .30.

Basic descriptive information for each item should also be examined. Items should have good variability—without it, they will not correlate with the total scale and will not fare well in a reliability analysis. Means for the items that are close to the center of the range of possible scores are also desirable (e.g., a mean near 4 on a 7-point scale). Items with means near one extreme or the other tend not to discriminate well among respondents—and may perform poorly if a goal is to assess changes over time because there may be no room for further improvement or deterioration (i.e., if there are *floor* or *ceiling effects*).

Example of Item Analysis: Grassley and colleagues (2013) undertook an item analysis in their field testing of the Supportive Needs of Adolescents Breastfeeding Scale. They eliminated two items whose corrected item–total correlation was less than .35. The remaining 18 items had corrected item–total correlations ranging from .35 to .55.

Exploratory Factor Analysis

A set of items is not necessarily a scale—the items form a scale only if they measure a common underlying construct. **Factor analysis** disentangles complex interrelationships among items and identifies items that "go together" as unified concepts. This section deals with a type of factor analysis known as **exploratory factor analysis (EFA)**, which essentially assumes no *a priori* hypotheses about dimensionality of a set of items. Another type—confirmatory factor analysis—uses more complex modeling and estimation procedures, as described later.

Suppose we developed 50 items measuring women's attitudes toward menopause. We could form a scale by adding together scores from several individual items, but which items should be combined? Would it be reasonable to combine all 50 items? Probably not, because the 50 items are not all tapping the same thing—there are various *dimensions* to women's attitude toward menopause. One dimension may relate to aging, and another to loss of reproductive ability. Other items may involve sexuality, and others may concern avoidance of monthly menstruation. These multiple dimensions to women's attitudes toward menopause should be captured on separate subscales. Women's attitude on one dimension may be independent of their attitude on another. Dimensions of a construct are usually identified during initial conceptualization and content validation. Preconceptions about dimensions, however, do not always "pan out" when tested against actual responses. Factor analysis offers an objective method of clarifying the underlying dimensionality of a set of items. Underlying dimensions thus identified are called **factors**, which are weighted combinations of items in the analysis.

➲ **TIP:** Before undertaking an EFA, you should evaluate the *factorability* of your set of items. Procedures for a factorability assessment are described in Polit (2010) and Polit and Yang (2015).

Factor Extraction

EFA involves two phases. The first phase (**factor extraction**) condenses items into a smaller number of factors and is used to identify the number of underlying dimensions. The goal is to extract clusters of highly interrelated items from a correlation matrix. There are various methods of performing the first step, each of which uses different criteria for assigning weights to items. A widely used factor extraction method is **principal components analysis (PCA)** and another is **principal-axis factor analysis**. The pros and cons of alternative approaches to factor extraction have been nicely summarized by Pett and colleagues (2003). Our discussion focuses mostly on PCA, although the two methods often lead to the same conclusion about dimensionality.

Factor extraction yields an *unrotated factor matrix*, which contains coefficients or *weights* for all original items on each extracted factor. Each extracted factor is a weighted linear combination of all the original items. For example, with three items, a factor would be item 1 (times a weight) + item 2 (times a weight) + item 3 (times a weight). In the PCA method, weights for the first factor are computed such that the average squared weight is maximized, permitting a maximum amount of variance to be extracted by the first factor. The second factor, or linear weighted combination, is formed so that the highest possible amount of variance is extracted from what *remains* after the first factor has been taken into account. The factors thus represent independent sources of variation in the data matrix.

Factoring should continue until no further meaningful variance is left, and so a criterion must be applied to decide when to stop extraction and move on to the next phase. Several of the possible criteria can be described by illustrating information from a factor analysis. Table 15.1 presents fictitious values for eigenvalues, percentages of variance accounted for, and cumulative percentages of variance accounted for, for 10 factors. **Eigenvalues** are equal to the sum of the squared item weights for the factor. Many researchers establish as their cutoff point for factor extraction eigenvalues greater than 1.00. In our example, the first five factors meet this criterion. Another cutoff benchmark, called the *scree test*, is based on a principle of discontinuity: A sharp drop in the percentage of explained variance indicates a possible termination point. In Table 15.1, we might argue that there is considerable discontinuity between the third and fourth factors—that is, that three factors should be extracted. Another guideline concerns the amount of variance explained by the factors. Some advocate that the number of factors extracted should account for at least 60% of the total variance and that for any factor to be meaningful, it must account for at least 5% of the variance. In our table, the first three factors account for 68.1% of the total variance. Six factors contribute 5% or more to the total variance.

So, should we extract three, five, or six factors? One approach is to see whether there is any convergence among the criteria. In our example, two of them (the scree test and total variance test) suggest three factors. Another approach is to see whether any of the rules yields a number consistent with

TABLE 15.1 • Summary of Factor Extraction Results

FACTOR	EIGENVALUE	PERCENTAGE OF VARIANCE EXPLAINED	CUMULATIVE PERCENTAGE OF VARIANCE EXPLAINED
1	12.32	29.2	29.2
2	8.57	23.3	52.5
3	6.91	15.6	68.1
4	2.02	8.4	76.5
5	1.09	6.2	82.7
6	.98	5.8	88.5
7	.80	4.5	93.0
8	.62	3.1	96.1
9	.47	2.2	98.3
10	.25	1.7	100.0

our original conceptualization. In our example, if we had designed the items to represent three theoretically meaningful subscales, we might consider three factors to be the right number because the data provide sufficient support for that conclusion.

> **TIP:** Polit (2010) provides a "walk-through" demonstration of how decisions are made in undertaking an exploratory factor analysis.

Factor Rotation

The second phase of factor analysis—**factor rotation**—is performed on factors that have met extraction criteria, to make the factors more interpretable. The concept of rotation can be best explained graphically. Figure 15.2 shows two coordinate systems, marked by axes A1 and A2 and B1 and B2. The primary axes (A1 and A2) represent factors I and II, respectively, as defined *before* rotation. Points 1 through 6 represent six items in this two-dimensional space. The weights for each item

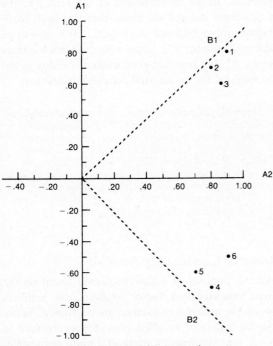

FIGURE 15.2 Illustration of factor rotation.

can be determined in reference to these axes. For instance, before rotation, item 1 has a weight of .80 on factor I and .85 on factor II and item 6 has a weight of −.45 on factor I and .90 on factor II. Unrotated axes account for a maximum amount of variance but may not provide a structure with conceptual meaning. Interpretability is enhanced by rotating the axes so that clusters of items are distinctly associated with a factor. In the figure, B1 and B2 represent rotated factors. After rotation, items 1, 2, and 3 have large weights on factor I and small weights on factor II, and the opposite is true for items 4, 5, and 6.

Researchers choose from two types of rotation. Figure 15.2 illustrates **orthogonal rotation**, in which factors are kept at right angles to one another. Orthogonal rotations maintain the independence of factors—that is, orthogonal factors are uncorrelated with one another. **Oblique rotations** permit rotated axes to depart from a 90-degree angle. In our figure, an oblique rotation would have put axis B1 between items 2 and 3 and axis B2 between items 5 and 6. This placement strengthens the clustering of items around an associated factor but results in correlated factors. Some writers argue that orthogonal rotation leads to greater theoretical clarity; others claim that it is unrealistic. Advocates of oblique rotation point out that if the concepts *are* correlated, then the analysis should reflect this fact. In developing a scale with multiple dimensions, we likely would expect the dimensions to be correlated, and so oblique rotation might well be more meaningful. This can be assessed empirically: If an oblique rotation is specified, the correlation between factors is computed. If the correlations are low (e.g., less than .15 or .20), an orthogonal rotation may be preferred because it yields a simpler model.

Researchers work with a **rotated factor matrix** in interpreting the factor analysis. As an example, Table 15.2 shows information from a factor analysis (principal components analysis) for the final 12 items on the Uncivil Behavior in Clinical Nursing Education (UBCNE) scale (Anthony et al., 2014). The entries under each factor are the weights, or **factor loadings**. For orthogonally rotated factors, factor loadings can range from −1.00 to +1.00 and can be interpreted like correlation coefficients—they express the correlation between

TABLE 15.2 • Factor Loadings: Uncivil Behavior in Clinical Nursing Education

HOW OFTEN HAVE YOU HAD A SITUATION WHERE A NURSE:	FACTOR 1	FACTOR 2
1. Embarrassed you . . .	**.83**[a]	.18
2. Rolled their eyes at you	**.73**	.30
3. Gave you an incomplete report	.02	**.70**
4. Used an inappropriate tone . . .	**.77**	.19
5. Avoided taking a report from you	.24	**.75**
6. Avoided giving you a report	.21	**.82**
7. Made snide remarks . . .	**.58**	.30
8. Raised their voice . . .	**.76**	.23
9. Did not involve you in a patient care decision . . .	.23	**.70**
10. Did not pass on patient information . . .	.18	**.78**
11. Told you that you were incompetent	**.82**	−.07
12. Refused to help you	**.77**	.18

[a]High loadings are bolded; these are the ones used to name and interpret the factors. Factor 1 was named *Hostile/Mean/Dismissive* and Factor 2 was named *Exclusionary Behavior.* Adapted from Table 6 and Appendix B of Anthony et al. (2014).

items and factors. In this example, item 1 is highly correlated with Factor 1, .83. By examining factor loadings, we can find which items "belong" to a factor. In this example, items 1, 2, 4, 7, 8, 11, and 12 had sizable loadings on Factor 1. Loadings with an absolute value of .40 or higher often are used as cutoff values, but somewhat smaller values may be acceptable if it makes theoretical sense to do so. The underlying dimensionality of the items can then be interpreted. By inspecting the content of these seven items, we can search for a common theme that makes the items go together. The developers of the UBCNE called this first factor *Hostile/Mean/Dismissive.* Items 3, 5, 6, 9, and 10 had high loadings on Factor 2, which they named *Exclusionary Behavior.* The naming of factors is a process of identifying underlying constructs—and this naming often would have occurred during the conceptualization phase.

The results of the factor analysis can be used not only to identify the dimensionality of the construct but also to make decisions about item retention and deletion. If items have low loadings on all factors, they likely are good candidates for deletion (or revision, if you can detect wording problems that may have caused different respondents to infer

different meanings). Items with fairly high loadings on multiple factors may also be candidates for deletion. In the development of the UBCNE, the researchers deleted six items that had high loadings on more than one factor (e.g., "Told you to go ask your instructor"). Items with marginal loadings (e.g., .35) but that had good content validity could be retained for the internal consistency analysis.

Example of an Exploratory Factor Analysis: Thomas and co-researchers (2013) developed a scale to measure parents' attitudes toward human papillomavirus vaccination (PHPVS). The 28-item scale was tested with 200 parents of children attending elementary and middle school in the United States. Exploratory factor analysis, using principal axis factor extraction and oblique rotation, yielded four theoretically meaningful factors.

Internal Consistency Analysis

After a final set of items is selected based on the item analysis and factor analysis, an analysis should be undertaken to calculate coefficient alpha. Alpha, it may be recalled, provides an estimate of a key measurement property of a multi-item scale, internal consistency.

Most general purpose statistical programs provide many item analysis diagnostics we described earlier. They also calculate the value of coefficient alpha for the scale—and for a hypothetical scale with each individual item removed. If the overall alpha is extremely high, it may be prudent to eliminate redundancy by deleting items that do not make a sizeable contribution to alpha. (Sometimes, removal of a faulty item actually *increases* alpha.) A modest reduction in reliability is sometimes worth the benefit of lowering respondent burden. Scale developers must consider the best trade-off between brevity and internal consistency.

One thing that should be kept in mind is that internal consistency estimates tend to capitalize on chance factors in a sample of respondents and so may well be lower in a new sample. Thus, you should aim for alphas that are a bit higher in the development sample than ones you would consider minimally acceptable so that if the alphas deteriorate they will still be adequate. This is especially true if the development sample is small.

→ TIP: If you have the good fortune to have a very large sample, you should consider dividing the sample in half, running the factor analysis and internal consistency analysis with one subsample, and then re-running them with the second as a cross-validation.

Test–Retest Reliability Analysis

Although test–retest reliability analysis has not been a standard feature of psychometric assessment in nursing research, we urge developers of new scales to gather information about both internal consistency and test–retest reliability. Indeed, the COSMIN group considers test–retest reliability a particularly important indicator of a scale's quality.

An issue of great importance in a retest study is the timing of the retest relative to the initial administration. Timing decisions must balance the risks for different potential sources of error. When the time interval is too brief, carryover effects (the memory of answers on the previous measurement and the desire to be consistent) can lead to

artificially high estimates of reliability. But other factors—including true change—could depress reliability coefficients. Some experts advise that the time interval between measurements should be in the vicinity of 1 to 2 weeks (e.g., Streiner & Norman, 2008). Polit (2014) has offered several suggestions for strategies to improve decision making about the retest interval, and for basing decisions on evidence or theory about an attribute's stability, rather than assumptions. She also provides guidance on how a test–retest analysis can be used to identify items that may benefit from revision.

SCALE REFINEMENT AND VALIDATION

In some scale development efforts, the bulk of work is over at this point. For example, if you developed a scale as part of a larger substantive project because you were unable to identify a good measure of a key construct, you may be ready to pursue your substantive analyses. If, however, you are developing a scale for others to use, a few more steps remain.

Revising the Scale

The analyses undertaken in the development study often suggest the need to revise or add items. For example, if subscale alpha coefficients are lower than .80 or so, consideration should be given to adding items for subsequent testing. In thinking about new items, a good strategy is to examine items that had high factor loadings because they may offer good clues for additional items.

Before deciding that your scale is finalized, it is a good idea to examine the content of the items in the scale. Sometimes alphas are inflated by items that have similar wording, so it is wise to make decisions about retaining or removing items based not only on their contribution to alpha but also on content validity considerations. It may be worthwhile to re-examine the I-CVIs of each item in making final decisions.

Scoring the Scale

Scoring a composite summated rating scale is easy: Item scores are typically just added together (with reverse scoring of items, if appropriate) to form subscale scores. Subscale scores are sometimes added together to form total scale scores—although this is not always justifiable. Some scale developers create a total score that is the *average* across items so that the total score is on the same scale as the items. In either case, the items are all weighted equally. Such scoring involves an implicit assumption that each item is equally important as a measure of the target construct. Sometimes, however, it may be attractive to have differential weighting of items to reflect differences in the items' contribution to the measure. Weighting usually has been found to have little effect on a scale's measurement properties (Streiner & Norman, 2008). Nevertheless, weighting may improve predictive validity—but at the cost of increased scoring complexity and thus possibly increased error. Moreover, weights are usually developed for a specific population and may be unsuitable when the instrument is used with a different population. Thus, unitary weighting of items is typical for most composite scales.

Conducting a Validation Study

Scales designed for use by others need to be subjected to validation efforts. Scale developers who are not able to undertake a separate validation study should strive to undertake many of the activities described in this section with data from the original development sample. Designing a validation study entails much of the same issues (and advice) as designing a development study, in terms of sample composition, sample size, and data collection strategies. The exception is that if efforts will be made to assess longitudinal measurement properties, a longitudinal design is needed. We focus here primarily on analyses undertaken in a validation study. Internal consistency should be recomputed in the validation sample.

Confirmatory Factor Analysis

Confirmatory factor analysis (CFA) is playing an increasingly important role in validation studies. CFA is preferable to EFA as an approach to construct (structural) validity because CFA is a hypothesis testing approach—testing the hypothesis that the items belong to specific factors, rather

than having the dimensionality of a set of items emerge empirically, as in EFA.

CFA is a subset of an advanced class of statistical techniques known as **structural equation modeling** (SEM). CFA differs from EFA in a number of respects, many of which are technical. One concerns the estimation procedure. As we explain in Chapter 18, many statistical procedures used by nurse researchers employ *least-squares estimation*. In SEM, the most frequently used estimation procedure is *maximum likelihood estimation*. (Maximum likelihood estimators are ones that estimate the parameters most likely to have generated the observed measurements.) Least-squares procedures have several stringent assumptions that are generally untenable—for example, the assumption that variables are measured without error. SEM approaches can accommodate measurement error and avoid other restrictions as well.

CFA involves testing a **measurement model**, which specifies the hypothesized relationships among underlying latent variables (constructs) and the *manifest variables*—that is, the items. The measurement model specifies the hypothesized factor structure. Loadings on the factors (the *latent variables*) provide a method for evaluating relationships between observed variables (the items) and unobserved variables (the factors or dimensions of a construct).

We illustrate with an example of a scale designed to measure two aspects of fatigue: physical fatigue and mental fatigue. In the example shown in Figure 15.3, both types of fatigue are captured by five items: items I1 to I5 for physical fatigue and items I6 to I10 for mental fatigue. According to the model, item responses are caused by respondents' level of physical and mental fatigue (the straight arrows indicate hypothesized causal paths) and are also affected by error (e_1 through e_{10}). It is also expected that the error terms are correlated, as indicated by the curved lines connecting the errors. Correlated measurement errors on items might arise from a person's desire to "look good" or to acquiesce—factors that would systematically affect all item scores. The two fatigue constructs also are predicted to be correlated.

The hypothesized measurement model would be tested against actual data. The analysis would

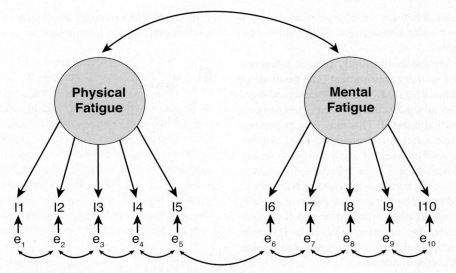

FIGURE 15.3 Example of a measurement model.

yield loadings of observed variables on the latent variables, the correlation between the two latent variables, and correlations among the error terms. The analysis would also indicate whether the overall model fit is good, based on several *goodness-of-fit statistics*.

CFA is a complex topic, and we have described only basic characteristics. Further reading on the topic is imperative for those wishing to pursue it (e.g., Brown, 2006; Kline, 2011).

Example of Confirmatory Factor Analysis: Pinto and colleagues (2012) assessed the psychometric properties of the Revised Attribution Questionnaire (r-AQ), a measure of mental illness stigma, in adolescents. The researchers' EFA had suggested a 1-factor structure, contrary to what had been found with adults. A CFA was used to test the hypothesis that the items formed a unitary scale, and the hypothesis was supported.

Other Validation Activities

A validation effort would not be complete without undertaking additional activities, such as ones described in Chapter 14. The assessment of criterion or construct validity primarily relies on correlational evidence. In criterion-related validity, scores on the new scale are correlated with an external criterion. In construct validity, scores on the scale can, for example, be correlated with measures of constructs hypothesized to be related to the target construct, or supplementary measures of the same construct (convergent validity), or measures of a closely related but distinguishable construct (divergent validity). Validation using a known-groups approach requires sampling people with membership in groups expected to be different, on average, on the scale. It is desirable to produce as much validity evidence as possible.

If a CFA is not possible (perhaps because of lack of training in CFA), it is still advisable to undertake a "confirmatory" factor analysis using an EFA with the validation sample. Comparisons between the original and new factor analyses can be made with respect to factor structure, loadings, variance explained, eigenvalues, and so on. In the new analysis, the number of factors to be extracted and rotated can be prespecified, since this is now the working hypothesis about the underlying dimensionality of the construct.

Longitudinal Measurement Properties

In both clinical work and research, measurements of health outcomes are often made on at least two occasions to assess whether a change has occurred. Scale developers who anticipate that their scales will be used to measure change should make efforts to assess the reliability of change scores on the measure and its responsiveness (longitudinal construct validity).

Such assessments inherently require a longitudinal design so that measurements can be made on two occasions. The study should be designed using a population in which change is expected to occur over a specified interval. This may be a population in which deterioration is anticipated (e.g., patients with a progressive disease) or a population receiving a treatment known to be effective. In terms of the time interval between measurements, enough time should have elapsed that one could reasonably expect change to have occurred on the focal construct for a sizeable subset of the sample. However, lengthy time periods may create several problems, including the risk of attrition.

Using our definition of responsiveness as longitudinal validity (Chapter 14), it follows that much of the advice we offered with regard to construct validation is relevant here. As with assessments of construct validity, multiple hypothesis tests are desirable for examining a measure's responsiveness—which typically means correlating change scores on the focal measure with change scores on other measures with which a relationship is expected. When a known-groups approach to responsiveness assessment is adopted, comparison groups whose change trajectories are expected to differ are needed. Further advice on testing responsiveness is offered in Polit and Yang (2015).

INTERPRETABILITY OF SCALE SCORES

In addition to the four measurement property domains identified in the taxonomy in Chapter 14 (Figure 14.1), another important aspect of measurement concern interpretability—that is, understanding what a score *means*. The COSMIN group defined **interpretability** as "the degree to which one can assign qualitative meaning—that is, clinical or commonly understood connotations—to an instrument's qualitative scores or change in scores" (Mokkink et al., 2010, p. 743).

A raw score on a scale is seldom directly interpretable. What does a score of 16 on the CES-D

scale mean, for example? We briefly discuss some ways to enhance the interpretability of scale scores.

→ TIP: If you expect the scale to be used by others, you should consider creating a manual for its use. Guidelines for preparing manuals are published in *Standards for Educational and Psychological Testing* (American Educational Research Association, American Psychological Association, & National Council on Measurement in Education, 2014). Scale developers should consider registering a copyright, even if they do not plan to publish the scale commercially.

Percentiles

Raw score values from a scale can be made more interpretable by converting them into percentiles. A **percentile** indicates the percentage of people who score below a particular score value. Percentiles provide information about how a person performs relative to others and are easily interpreted by most people. Percentiles can range from the 0th to the 99th percentile, and the 50th percentile corresponds to the median. Percentile values are most useful when they are determined on the basis of a large, representative sample.

Standard Scores

Standard scores transform raw scores into values that have been stripped of the original measurement metric. The transformation makes it possible to compare people on a measure along an easily interpretable scale, without needing to understand the raw score value. Standard scores also make it possible to compare a person's performance on multiple measures with different metrics (e.g., a 10-item fatigue scale and a 5-item pain scale).

Standard scores are expressed in terms of their relative distance from the mean, in standard deviation (*SD*) units. A standard score of 0.0 corresponds to a raw score exactly at the scale's mean—regardless of what that mean is. A standard score of 1.0 corresponds to a score 1 *SD* above the mean, and a standard score of −1.0 corresponds to a score 1 *SD* below the mean. Standard scores can be readily calculated from raw scores once the mean and *SD* have been computed, as we describe in Chapter 18.

It is often easier to work with score values that do not have negative values and decimal points. Standard scores can be transformed to have any desired mean and *SD*, and certain transformations are particularly common. In particular, standard scores with a mean of 50 and an *SD* of 10 are widely used and are often called **T scores**. With T scores, a score of, say, 60, is immediately interpretable, even without knowing much about the scale.

Norms

In some cases, it might be desirable to standardize a new scale and establish **norms**. This typically occurs if it is expected that the scale will be widely used by people who will rely on solid comparative information to help them evaluate scores. Norms are often established for key demographic characteristics, such as age and gender.

A good sampling plan is critical in a norming effort. The sample should be geographically dispersed and representative of the population for whom the scale is intended. A large standardization sample is required so that subgroup values are stable.

Norms are often expressed in terms of percentiles. For example, an adult male with a score of 72 on the scale might be at the 80th percentile, but a female with the same score might be at the 85th percentile. Guidelines for norming instruments have been developed by Nunnally and Bernstein (1994).

Cutoff Points

Interpretation of scores can often be facilitated when the instrument developer establishes *cutpoints* for classification purposes. Cutpoints are typically used as the basis for making decisions about needed treatments or further assessments. Sometimes cutpoints are defined in terms of percentiles. For example, for children's weights, those below the 5th percentile are often interpreted as underweight (or, in infants, "failure to thrive"), whereas those above the 95th percentile are considered overweight. In other cases, the cutpoints are designated with standard scores. For example, the World Health Organization defines

osteoporosis as a standard score on a bone mineral density test at or below −2.5—that is, 2½ *SDs* below the mean for women in their 30s. Cutpoints that are linked to the measure's distribution are considered *norm-referenced*.

Various methods—both empirical and subjective—have been developed for establishing cutoff points for raw scale scores. As described in Chapter 14, a frequently used method is the construction of receiver operating characteristic (ROC) curves to identify the cutpoint that maximizes and balances sensitivity and specificity. Scale developers who intend to develop ROC curves need to select highly reliable criteria for dividing people into groups (e.g., those with and those without the condition being screened), and the criteria must be independent of participants' responses on the scale.

➲ **TIP:** Norms and cutoff points can play an important role in evaluating the *clinical significance* of findings and so are extremely useful to users of a scale. Also, it may be important to develop guidelines for interpreting *change scores*. If you are developing a scale that will be used to capture change (e.g., as an outcome measure in an intervention study), then you should make an effort to establish the value of a *minimal important change* (MIC) for your scale, as well as the *smallest detectable change* (SDC), which we discuss in Chapter 14. Approaches to assessing clinical significance are described in Chapter 20.

CRITIQUING SCALE DEVELOPMENT STUDIES

Articles on scale development appear regularly in many nursing journals. If you are planning to use a scale in a substantive study, you should carefully review the methods used to construct the scale and test its measurement properties. And, of course, you should scrutinize whether the evidence regarding the scale's psychometric adequacy is sufficiently sound to merit its use. Remember that you run the risk of undermining the statistical conclusion validity of your study (i.e., of having insufficient power for testing your hypotheses) if you use a scale with

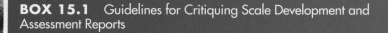

BOX 15.1 Guidelines for Critiquing Scale Development and Assessment Reports

1. Did the report offer a clear definition of the construct? Did it provide sufficient context for the study through a summary of the literature and discussion of relevant theory? Is the population for whom the scale intended adequately described?
2. Did the report indicate how items were generated? Do the procedures seem sound? Was information provided about the reading level of scale items?
3. Did the report describe content validation efforts, and was the description thorough? Is there evidence of good content validity?
4. Were appropriate efforts made to refine the scale (e.g., through pretests, item analysis)?
5. Was the development or validation sample of participants appropriate in terms of representativeness, size, and heterogeneity?
6. Was factor analysis used to examine or validate the scale's dimensionality? If yes, did the report offer evidence to support the factor structure and the naming of factors?
7. Were appropriate methods used to assess the scale's internal consistency and reliability? Were estimates of reliability and internal consistency sufficiently high?
8. Were appropriate methods used to assess the scale's criterion or construct validity? Is the evidence about the scale's validity persuasive? What other validation methods would have strengthened inferences about the scale's worthiness?
9. Were efforts made to assess the reliability of change scores and the responsiveness of the new measure?
10. Did the report provide information for scoring the scale and interpreting scale scores—for example, means and standard deviations, cutoff scores, norms?

weak reliability. And you can run the risk of poor construct validity in your study if your measures are not strong proxies for key constructs.

Box 15.1 provides broad guidelines for evaluating a research report on the development and validation of a scale. Additionally, many important evaluative questions with regard to reporting and study design for measurement studies have been incorporated into a series of checklists prepared by the COSMIN group (Terwee et al., 2012).

RESEARCH EXAMPLE

Studies: Postpartum Depression Screening Scale: Development and psychometric testing (Beck & Gable, 2000); Further validation of the Postpartum Depression Screening Scale (Beck & Gable, 2001); Postpartum Depression Screening Scale: Spanish version (Beck & Gable, 2003)

Background: Beck studied postpartum depression (PPD) in a series of qualitative studies, using both a phenomenologic approach and a grounded theory approach. Based on her in-depth understanding of PPD, she began in the late 1990s to develop a scale that could be used to screen for PPD, the Postpartum Depression Screening Scale (PDSS).

Statement of Purpose: Beck and an expert psychometrician undertook methodologic studies to develop, refine, and validate a scale to screen women for postpartum depression and to translate the scale into Spanish.

Scale Development: The PDSS is a summated rating scale designed to tap seven dimensions, such as sleeping/eating disturbances and mental confusion. A 56-item pilot form of the PDSS was initially developed with 8 items per dimension, using a 5-point response option scale. Beck's program of research on PPD and her knowledge of the literature were the basis for specifying the domain. Themes from Beck's qualitative research were used to develop seven dimensions and to craft the items to operationalize those dimensions. The reading level of the final PDSS was assessed to be at the third grade level and the Flesch reading ease score was 92.7.

Content Validity: Content validity was enhanced by using direct quotes from the qualitative studies as items on the scale (e.g., "I felt like I was losing my mind"). The pilot form was subjected to two content validation procedures with a panel of five content experts and a focus group of 15 expert nurses. Feedback from these procedures led to some item revisions.

Construct Validity: The PDSS was administered to a sample of 525 new mothers in six states (Beck & Gable, 2000). Preliminary item analyses resulted in the deletion of several items, based on item–total correlations. The PDSS was finalized as a 35-item scale with seven subscales, each with 5 items. This version of the PDSS was subjected to confirmatory factor analyses, which involved a validation of Beck's hypotheses about how individual items mapped onto underlying constructs, such as cognitive impairment. Item response theory analysis was also used and provided supporting evidence of the scale's construct validity. In a subsequent study, Beck and Gable (2001) administered the PDSS and two other depression scales to 150 new mothers and tested hypotheses about how scores on the PDSS would correlate with scores on other scales. The results indicated good convergent validity.

Internal Consistency: In both studies, Beck and Gable evaluated the internal consistency of the PDSS and its subscales. Subscale alphas were high, ranging from .83 to .94 in the first study and from .80 to .91 in the second study. Figure 15.4 shows a reliability analysis printout (from IBM SPSS Statistics, or SPSS, Version 17.0) for the five items on the Mental Confusion subscale from the first study. In Panel A, we see that the reliability for the 5-item subscale is high, .912. The first column of Panel B (Item Statistics) identifies subscale items by number: Item 11, Item 18, and so on. Item 11, for example, is the item "I felt like I was losing my mind." The item means and standard deviations for the 522 cases suggest a good amount of variability on each item. Panel C shows intercorrelations among the five items. The correlations are fairly high, ranging from .601 for item 25 with 53 to .814 for item 11 with 25. Panel D (Summary Item Statistics) presents descriptive item statistics. In Panel E, the fourth column ("Corrected Item–Total Correlation") presents correlation coefficients for the relationship between women's score on an item and their score on the subscale, after removing the item from the scale. Item 11 has a corrected item–total correlation of .799, which is very high; all five items have excellent correlations with the total subscale score. The final column shows what the internal consistency would be if an item were deleted. If Item 11 were removed from the subscale and only four items remained, the reliability coefficient would be .888—less than the reliability for all 5 items (.912). Deleting any of the items on the subscale would reduce its internal consistency but only by a rather small amount.

Criterion-Related Validity: In the second study, Beck and Gable correlated scores on the PDSS with an expert clinician's diagnosis of PPD for each woman. The coefficient was .70, which was higher than the correlations between the diagnosis and scores on other depression scales, indicating its superiority as a screening instrument. Additionally, ROC curves were constructed to examine the sensitivity and specificity of the PDSS at different cutoff points, using the expert diagnosis to establish PPD caseness. In this sample, 46 of the 150 mothers had a diagnosis of major or minor depression. To illustrate the trade-off the researchers made, the ROC curve (Figure 15.5) revealed that with a cutoff score of 95 on the PDSS, the sensitivity would be only .41, meaning that only 41% of the women actually diagnosed with PPD would be identified. A score of 95 has a specificity of 1.00, meaning that all cases *without* an actual PPD diagnosis would be accurately screened out. At the other extreme, a cutoff score of 45 would have 1.00 sensitivity but only .28 specificity (i.e., 72% false positive), an unacceptable rate of overdiagnosis. Beck and Gable recommended a cutoff score of 60, which would accurately screen in 91% of true PPD cases and would mistakenly screen in 28% who do not have PPD. Beck and Gable found that this cutoff point correctly classified 85% of their sample. In their ROC analysis, the area under the curve was excellent, .91.

Spanish Translation: Beck collaborated with translation experts to develop a Spanish version of the PDSS. Eight bilingual translators from four backgrounds (Mexican, Puerto Rican, Cuban, and South American) translated

A   **Reliability Statistics**

Cronbach's Alpha	Cronbach's Alpha Based on Standardized Items	N of Items
.912	.912	5

B   **Item Statistics**

	Mean	Std. Deviation	N
Item 11	2.36	1.424	522
Item 18	2.21	1.270	522
Item 25	2.21	1.374	522
Item 39	2.40	1.351	522
Item 53	2.28	1.349	522

C   **Inter-Item Correlation Matrix**

	Item 11	Item 18	Item 25	Item 39	Item 53
Item 11	1.000	.654	.814	.646	.649
Item 18	.654	1.000	.603	.659	.751
Item 25	.814	.603	1.000	.652	.601
Item 39	.646	.659	.652	1.000	.724
Item 53	.649	.751	.601	.724	1.000

D   **Summary Item Statistics**

	Mean	Minimum	Maximum	Range	Maximum / Minimum	Variance	N of Items
Item Means	2.292	2.205	2.399	.194	1.088	.008	5
Item Variances	1.835	1.612	2.029	.416	1.258	.023	5
Inter-Item Correlations	.675	.601	.814	.213	1.354	.006	5

E   **Item-Total Statistics**

	Scale Mean if Item Deleted	Scale Variance if Item Deleted	Corrected Item-Total Correlation	Squared Multiple Correlation	Cronbach's Alpha if Item Deleted
Item 11	9.09	21.371	.799	.715	.888
Item 18	9.24	23.006	.770	.623	.895
Item 25	9.25	22.097	.769	.691	.894
Item 39	9.06	22.290	.869	.610	.894
Item 53	9.18	22.176	.781	.666	.891

FIGURE 15.4 SPSS reliability analysis for the Mental Confusion subscale of the Postpartum Depression Screening Scale.

and back-translated the items. The translators met as a committee to review each other's wordings and to arrive at a consensus. The English and Spanish versions were then administered, in random order, to a bilingual sample. Scores on the two versions correlated highly (e.g., .98 on the "Sleeping/Eating Disturbances" subscale). Coefficient alpha was .95 for the total scale and ranged from .76 to .90 for subscales. Confirmatory factor analysis yielded information that was judged to indicate an adequate fit with the hypothesized measurement model, and screening performance was found to be good (Beck & Gable, 2005).

Other Translations: The PDSS has been translated into several other languages (e.g., Chinese, Portuguese, Turkish, Hungarian), and psychometric assessments in all cases suggest that the instrument has strong measurement properties. In the Turkish version of the PDSS, test–retest reliability, which was not reported in other papers, was high, $r = .86$ (Karaçam & Kitiş, 2008). In the Hungarian version, the parallel forms reliability for the English and Hungarian versions was .97 (Hegedus & Beck, 2012).

Responsiveness: Responsiveness of the PDSS was not assessed by the scale developers. There is, however, some

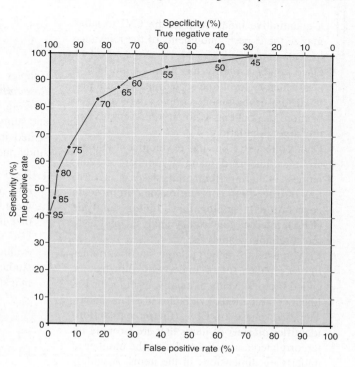

FIGURE 15.5 Receiver operating characteristic (ROC) curve for Postpartum Depression Screening Scale. (Used with permission from Beck, C. T., & Gable, R. K. [2001]. Further validation of the Postpartum Depression Screening Scale. *Nursing Research, 50,* 155–164.)

evidence that PPD as measured by the PDSS is sensitive to interventions, suggesting good responsiveness of the scale. For example, in a study of the effects of kangaroo mother care in Brazil, scores on the PDSS dropped dramatically during the time the infants were in the NICU, consistent with the researchers' hypotheses (de Alencar et al., 2009). Also, in a quasi-experimental analysis of the effects of a psychoeducation intervention for pregnant women with abuse-related posttraumatic stress, Rowe et al. (2014) reported a significant decrease in PDSS scores, consistent with the researchers' hypothesis.

SUMMARY POINTS

- Scale development begins with a sound conceptualization of the construct (the **latent trait**) to be measured, including its dimensionality.
- After deciding on the type of scale to construct, items must be generated; common sources for items include existing instruments, the research literature, concept analyses, qualitative studies, and clinical observations.
- In classical test theory, a **domain sampling model** is assumed; the basic notion is to sample a homogeneous set of items from a hypothetical universe of items.
- In generating items, a number of decisions must be made, including how many items to generate (typically a large number initially), what continuum to use for the response options, how many response options there should be, whether to include positive and negative item stems, how intensely worded the items should be, and what to do about references to time.
- Items should be inspected for clarity, length, inappropriate use of jargon, and good wording; the scale's **readability** should also be assessed.
- External review of the preliminary pool of items should also be undertaken, including review by members of the target population (e.g., via a small pretest that could include **cognitive questioning**).
- Content validity should be built into the scale through careful efforts to conceptualize the construct and through content validation by a panel of experts—including the calculation of

a quantitative index such as the CVI to summarize the experts' judgments of the relevance of scale items.

- Once content validity has been established at a satisfactory level, the scale must be administered to a development sample—typically 300 or more respondents who are representative of the target population.
- Data collected from the development sample are then analyzed using a number of techniques, including **item analysis** (e.g., a scrutiny of **inter-item correlations** and **item–scale correlations**); **exploratory factor analysis (EFA)**, internal consistency analysis, and test–retest reliability analysis.
- EFA is used to reduce a large set of variables into a smaller set of underlying dimensions, called **factors**. Mathematically, each factor is a linear combination of variables in a data matrix.
- The first phase of EFA (**factor extraction**) identifies clusters of items that are strongly intercorrelated and helps to define the number of underlying dimensions in the items. A widely used factor extraction method is **principal components analysis (PCA)**, another is **principal axis factor analysis**.
- The second phase of factor analysis involves **factor rotation**, which enhances the interpretability of the factors by aligning items more distinctly with a particular factor. Rotation can be either **orthogonal** (which maintains the independence of the factors) or **oblique** (which allows correlated factors). **Factor loadings** of the items on the rotated factor matrix are used to interpret and name the factors.
- After the scale is finalized based on the preliminary analyses, a second study is often undertaken to validate the scale, using a variety of validation techniques; one widely used approach to assess structural validity is **confirmatory factor analysis (CFA)**.
- CFA involves tests of a **measurement model**, which stipulates the hypothesized relationship between latent traits and *manifest variables* (items). CFA is a subset of sophisticated statistical techniques called **structural equation modeling**.

STUDY ACTIVITIES

Chapter 15 of the *Resource Manual for Nursing Research: Generating and Assessing Evidence for Nursing Practice, 10th edition*, offers exercises and study suggestions for reinforcing concepts presented in this chapter. In addition, the following study questions can be addressed:

1. Read a recent scale development paper and see how many of the steps discussed in this chapter were followed. Do omitted steps (if any) jeopardize the evidence about the scale's quality?
2. Use the critiquing guidelines in Box 15.1 to evaluate scale development procedures in the studies by Beck and Gable, referring to the original studies if possible.

STUDIES CITED IN CHAPTER 15

American Educational Research Association, American Psychological Association, & National Council on Measurement in Education. (2014). *Standards for educational and psychological testing* (5th ed.). Washington, DC: American Psychological Association.

Andersen, R. D., Jylli, L., & Ambuel, B. (2014). Cultural adaptation of patient and observational outcome measures: A methodological example using the COMFORT behavioral rating scale. *International Journal of Nursing Studies, 51*, 934–942.

Anthony, M., Yastik, J., MacDonald, D., & Marshall, K. (2014). Development and validation of a tool to measure incivility in clinical nursing education. *Journal of Professional Nursing, 30*, 48–55.

Beck, C. T., & Gable, R. K. (2000). Postpartum Depression Screening Scale: Development and psychometric testing. *Nursing Research, 49*, 272–282.

Beck, C. T., & Gable, R. K. (2001). Further validation of the Postpartum Depression Screening Scale. *Nursing Research, 50*, 155–164.

Beck, C. T., & Gable, R. K. (2003). Postpartum Depression Screening Scale: Spanish version. *Nursing Research, 52*, 296–306.

Beck, C. T., & Gable, R. K. (2005). Screening performance of the Postpartum Depression Screening Scale—Spanish version. *Journal of Transcultural Nursing, 16*, 331–338.

Brown, T. (2006). *Confirmatory factor analysis for applied research*. New York: Guilford Press.

Choe, K. (2014). Development and preliminary testing of the Schizophrenia Hope Scale, a brief scale to measure hope in people with schizophrenia. *International Journal of Nursing Studies*, *51*, 927–933.

de Alencar, A., Arraes, L., de Albuquerque, E., & Alves, J. (2009). Effect of kangaroo mother care on postpartum depression. *Journal of Tropical Pediatrics*, *55*, 36–38.

DeVellis, R. F. (2012). *Scale development: Theory and applications* (3rd ed.). Thousand Oaks, CA: Sage.

*Gaugler, J. E., Hobday, J., & Savik, K. (2013). The CARES® Observational Tool: A valid and reliable instrument to assess person-centered dementia care. *Geriatric Nursing*, *34*, 194–198.

Grassley, J. S., Spencer, B., & Bryson, D. (2013). The development and psychometric testing of the Supportive Needs of Adolescents Breastfeeding Scale. *Journal of Advanced Nursing*, *69*, 708–716.

Hegedus, K. S., & Beck, C. T. (2012). Development and psychometric testing of the Postpartum Depression Screening Scale: Hungarian version. *International Journal for Human Caring*, *16*, 54–58.

Hilton, A., & Skrutkowski, M. (2002). Translating instruments into other language: Development and testing processes. *Cancer Nursing*, *25*, 1–7.

Karaçam, Z., & Kitiş, Y. (2008). The Postpartum Depression Screening Scale: Its reliability and validity for the Turkish population. *Türk Psikiyatri Dergisi*, *19*, 187–196.

Kline, R. B. (2011). *Principles and practice of structural equation modeling* (3rd ed.). New York: Guilford Press.

McCoach, D. B., Gable, R. K., & Madura, J. P. (2013). *Instrument development in the affective domain* (3rd ed.). New York: Springer.

Mokkink, L. B., Terwee, C., Patrick, D., Alonso, J., Stratford, P., Knol, D. L., . . . de Vet, H. C. W. (2010). The COSMIN study reached international consensus on taxonomy, terminology, and definitions of measurement properties for health-related patient-reported outcomes. *Journal of Clinical Epidemiology*, *63*, 737–745.

Nunnally, J., & Bernstein, I. H. (1994). *Psychometric theory* (3rd ed.). New York: McGraw Hill.

Pett, M., Lackey, N., & Sullivan, J. (2003). *Making sense of factor analysis: The use of factor analysis for instrument development in health care research*. Thousand Oaks, CA: Sage.

*Pinto, M. D., Hickman, R., Logsdon, M., & Burant, C. (2012). Psychometric evaluation of the Revised Attribution Questionnaire (r-AQ) to measure mental illness stigma in adolescents. *Journal of Nursing Measurement*, *20*, 47–58.

Polit, D. F. (2010). *Statistics and data analysis for nursing research* (2nd ed.). Upper Saddle River, NJ: Pearson.

Polit, D. F. (2014). Getting serious about test-retest reliability: A critique of retest research and some recommendations. *Quality of Life Research*, *23*, 1713–1720.

Polit, D. F., Beck, C., & Owen, S. (2007). Is the CVI an acceptable indicator of content validity? Appraisal and recommendations. *Research in Nursing & Health*, *30*, 459–467.

Polit, D. F., & Yang, F. M. (2015). *Measurement and the measurement of change: A primer for health professionals*. Philadelphia: Lippincott Williams & Wilkins.

Rowe, H., Sperlich, M., Cameron, H., & Seng, J. (2014). A quasi-experimental outcomes analysis of a psychoeducation intervention for pregnant women with abuse-related posttraumatic stress. *Journal of Obstetric, Gynecologic & Neonatal Nursing*, *43*, 282–293.

Ruiz, R. J., Gennaro, S., O'Connor, C., Marti, C., Lulloff, A., Keshinover, T., . . . Melnyk, B. (2015). Measuring coping in pregnant minority women. *Western Journal of Nursing Research*, *37*, 257–275.

Streiner, D. L., & Norman, G. R. (2008). *Health measurement scales: A practical guide to their development and use* (4th ed.). Oxford, United Kingdom: Oxford University Press.

*Terwee, C. B., Mokkink, L. B., Knol, D. L., Ostelo, R., Bouter, L. M., & de Vet, H. C. W. (2012). Rating the methodological quality in systematic reviews of studies on measurement properties: A scoring system for the COSMIN checklist. *Quality of Life Research*, *21*, 651–657.

*Thomas, T. L., Strickland, O., DiClemente, R., Higgins, M., Williams, B., & Hickey, K. (2013). Parental Human Papillomavirus Vaccine Survey (PHPVS): Nurse-led instrument development and psychometric testing for use in research and primary care screening. *Journal of Nursing Measurement*, *21*, 96–109.

Walker, L. O., & Avant, K. C. (2011). *Strategies for theory construction in nursing* (5th ed.). Upper Saddle River, NJ: Prentice Hall.

A link to this open-access journal article is provided in the Toolkit for this chapter in the accompanying Resource Manual. ✇

16 | Descriptive Statistics

Statistical analysis enables researchers to organize, interpret, and communicate numeric information. Mathematic skill is not required to grasp statistics—only logical thinking ability is needed. In this book, we underplay computation. We focus on explaining which statistics to use in different situations and on how to understand what statistical results mean.

Statistics can be descriptive or inferential. **Descriptive statistics** are used to describe and synthesize data (e.g., a percentage). When a percentage or other descriptive statistic is calculated from population data, it is called a **parameter**. A descriptive index from a sample is a **statistic**. Research questions are about parameters, but researchers calculate statistics to estimate them and use **inferential statistics** to make inferences about the population. This chapter discusses descriptive statistics, and Chapter 17 focuses on inferential statistics. First we discuss levels of measurement because the analyses that can be performed depend on how variables are measured.

LEVELS OF MEASUREMENT

Scientists have developed a system for classifying measures. The four **levels of measurement** are nominal, ordinal, interval, and ratio.

Nominal Measurement

The lowest level of measurement is **nominal measurement**, which involves assigning numbers to classify characteristics into categories. In previous chapters, we referred to nominal measurement as *categorical*. Examples of variables amenable to nominal measurement include gender, blood type, and marital status.

Numbers assigned in nominal measurement have no quantitative meaning. If we code males as 1 and females as 2, the number 2 does not mean "more than" 1. The numbers are only symbols representing different values of gender. We easily could use 1 for females, 2 for males.

Nominal measurement provides no information about an attribute except equivalence and nonequivalence. If we were to "measure" the gender of Nate, Alan, Mary, and Anna by assigning them the codes 1, 1, 2, and 2, respectively, this means Nate and Alan are equivalent on the gender attribute but are not equivalent to Mary and Anna.

Nominal measures must have categories that are mutually exclusive and collectively exhaustive. For example, if we were measuring marital status, we might use these codes: 1 = married, 2 = separated or divorced, 3 = widowed. Each person must be classifiable into one and only one category. The requirement for collective exhaustiveness would not be met if there were people in a sample who had never been married.

Numbers in nominal measurement cannot be treated mathematically. It is not meaningful to calculate the average gender of a sample, but we can compute percentages. In a sample of 50 patients with 30 men and 20 women, we could say that 60% were male and 40% were female.

Ordinal Measurement

Ordinal measurement involves sorting people based on their relative ranking on an attribute. This measurement level goes beyond categorization: Attributes are *ordered* according to some criterion. Ordinal measurement captures not only equivalence but also relative rank.

Consider this ordinal scheme for measuring ability to perform activities of daily living: (1) completely dependent, (2) needs another person's assistance, (3) needs mechanical assistance, (4) completely independent. The numbers signify incremental ability to perform activities of daily living. People coded 4 are equivalent to each other with regard to functional ability *and*, relative to those in the other categories, have more of that attribute.

Ordinal measurement does not, however, tell us anything about how much greater one level is than another. We do not know if being completely independent is twice as good as needing mechanical assistance. Nor do we know if the difference between needing another person's assistance and needing mechanical assistance is the same as that between needing mechanical assistance and being completely independent. Ordinal measurement tells us only the relative ranking of the attribute's levels.

As with nominal measures, mathematic operations with ordinal-level data are restricted—for example, averages are usually meaningless. Frequency counts, percentages, and several other statistics to be discussed later are appropriate for ordinal-level data.

Interval Measurement

Interval measurement occurs when researchers can assume equivalent distance between rank ordering on an attribute. The Fahrenheit temperature scale is an example: A temperature of 60°F is 10°F warmer than 50°F. A 10°F difference similarly separates 40°F and 30°F, and the two differences in temperature are equivalent. Interval-level measures are more informative than ordinal ones, but interval measures do not communicate absolute magnitude. For example, we cannot say that 60°F is twice as hot as 30°F. The Fahrenheit scale uses an arbitrary zero point: Zero degrees does not signify an absence of heat. Most psychological and educational tests are assumed to yield interval-level data.

Interval scales expand analytic possibilities—in particular, interval-level data can be averaged meaningfully. It is reasonable, for example, to compute an average daily body temperature for hospital patients. Many statistical procedures require interval measurements.

Ratio Measurement

Ratio measurement is the highest measurement level. Ratio measures provide information about ordering on the critical attribute, the intervals between objects, *and* the absolute magnitude of the attribute because they have a rational, meaningful zero. Many physical measures provide ratio-level data. A person's weight, for example, is measured on a ratio scale. We can say that someone who weighs 200 pounds is twice as heavy as someone who weighs 100 pounds.

Because ratio measures have an absolute zero, all arithmetic operations are permissible. Statistical procedures suitable for interval-level data are also appropriate for ratio-level data. In previous chapters, we called variables that were measured on either the interval or ratio scale as *continuous*.

Example of Different Measurement Levels: Grønning and colleagues (2014) tested the effect of a nurse-led education program for patients with chronic inflammatory polyarthritis. Gender (male/female) and diagnosis (psoriatic, rheumatoid, or unspecified arthritis) were measured as nominal-level variables. Education (10 years, 11–12 years, 13+ years) was operationalized as an ordinal measurement in this particular study. Many outcomes (e.g., self-efficacy, coping, pain, hospital anxiety and depression) were measured on an interval-level scale. Several variables were measured on a ratio level (e.g., age, number of hospital admissions).

Comparison of the Levels

The four levels of measurement form a hierarchy, with ratio scales at the top and nominal measurement at the base. Moving from a higher to a lower level of measurement results in an information loss. For example, if we measured a woman's weight in pounds, this would be a ratio measure. If we categorized the weights into three groups (e.g., under 125, 125 to 175, and 176+), this would be an ordinal measure. With this scheme, we would not be able to differentiate a woman who weighed 125 pounds from one who weighed 175 pounds—we have much less information with the ordinal information. This example illustrates another point: With information at one level, it is possible to convert data to a lower level, but the converse is not true. If we were given only the ordinal measurements, we could not reconstruct actual weights.

It is not always easy to identify a variable's level of measurement. Nominal and ratio measures usually are discernible, but the distinction between ordinal and interval measures is more problematic. Some methodologists argue that most psychological measures that are treated as interval measures are really only ordinal measures. Although instruments such as Likert scales produce data that are, strictly speaking, ordinal, many analysts believe that treating them as interval measures results in too few errors to warrant using less powerful statistical procedures.

⮕ TIP: In operationalizing variables, it is best to use the highest measurement level possible because they are more powerful and precise. Sometimes, however, group membership is more informative than continuous scores, especially for clinicians who need "cut points" for making decisions. For example, for some purposes, it may be more relevant to designate infants as being of low versus normal birth weight (nominal level) than to use actual birth weight values (ratio level). But it is best to *measure* at the higher level and then convert to a lower level, if appropriate.

FREQUENCY DISTRIBUTIONS

When quantitative data are unanalyzed, it is not possible to discern even general trends. Consider the 60 numbers in Table 16.1, which are fictitious scores of 60 preoperative patients on a six-item measure of anxiety—scores that we will consider as interval level. Inspection of the numbers does not help us understand patients' anxiety.

A set of data can be described in terms of three characteristics: the shape of the distribution of values, central tendency, and variability. Central tendency and variability are dealt with in subsequent sections.

Constructing Frequency Distributions

Frequency distributions are used to organize numeric data. A **frequency distribution** is a systematic arrangement of values from lowest to highest, together with a count of the number of times each value was obtained. Our 60 anxiety scores are shown in a frequency distribution in Table 16.2. We can readily see the highest and lowest scores, the most common score, where the bulk of scores clustered, and how many patients were in the sample (total sample size is typically depicted as N). None of this was apparent before the data were organized.

Frequency distributions consist of two parts: observed score values (the Xs) and the frequency of cases at each value (the fs). Scores are listed in order in one column, and corresponding frequencies

TABLE 16.1 • Patients' Anxiety Scores

22	27	25	19	24	25	23	29	24	20
26	16	20	26	17	22	24	18	26	28
15	24	23	22	21	24	20	25	18	27
24	23	16	25	30	29	27	21	23	24
26	18	30	21	17	25	22	24	29	28
20	25	26	24	23	19	27	28	25	26

TABLE 16.2 • Frequency Distribution of Patients' Anxiety Scores

SCORE (X)	FREQUENCY (f)	PERCENTAGE (%)
15	1	1.7
16	2	3.3
17	2	3.3
18	3	5.0
19	2	3.3
20	4	6.7
21	3	5.0
22	4	6.7
23	5	8.3
24	9	15.0
25	7	11.7
26	6	10.0
27	4	6.7
28	3	5.0
29	3	5.0
30	2	3.3
	$N = 60 = \Sigma f$	$\Sigma\% = 100.0\%$

are listed in another. The sum of numbers in the frequency column must equal the sample size. In less verbal terms, $\Sigma f = N$, which means the sum of (signified by Greek sigma, Σ) the frequencies (f) equals the sample size (N).

It is useful to display percentages for each value, as shown in column 3 of Table 16.2. Just as the sum of all frequencies should equal N, the sum of all percentages should equal 100.

Frequency data can also be displayed graphically. Graphs for displaying interval- and ratio-level data include **histograms** and **frequency polygons**, which are constructed in a similar fashion. First, score values are arrayed on a horizontal dimension, with the lowest value on the left, ascending to the highest value on the right. Frequencies or percentages are displayed vertically. A histogram is constructed by drawing bars above the score classes to the height corresponding to the frequency for that score. Figure 16.1 shows a histogram for the anxiety score data. Frequency polygons are similar, but dots connected by straight lines are used to show frequencies. A dot corresponding to the frequency is placed above each score (Figure 16.2).

Shapes of Distributions

Frequency polygons can assume many shapes. A distribution is **symmetric** if, when folded over, the two halves are superimposed on one another. All the distributions in Figure 16.3 are symmetric. With real data sets, distributions are rarely perfectly symmetric, but minor discrepancies are ignored in characterizing a distribution's shape.

In **skewed** (asymmetric) distributions, the peak is off center and one tail is longer than the other.

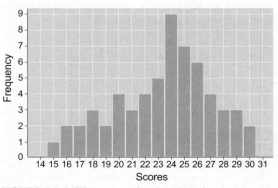

FIGURE 16.1 Histogram of patients' anxiety scores.

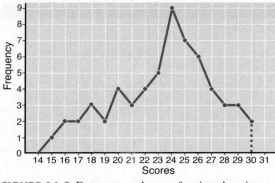

FIGURE 16.2 Frequency polygon of patients' anxiety scores.

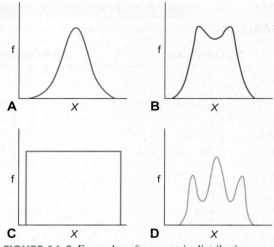

FIGURE 16.3 Examples of symmetric distributions.

When the longer tail points to the right, the distribution is **positively skewed** (Figure 16.4A). Personal income, for example, is positively skewed. Most people have low to moderate incomes, with relatively few people with high incomes in the tail. If the tail points to the left, the distribution is **negatively skewed** (Figure 16.4B). Age at death is an example of a negatively skewed attribute: Most people are at the upper end of the distribution, with relatively few dying at an early age. Patients' anxiety scores (see Figure 16.2) were negatively skewed, with high scores more common than low ones.

Modality is a second aspect of a distribution's shape. A **unimodal distribution** has only one peak (i.e., a value with high frequency), whereas a **multimodal distribution** has two or more peaks. A distribution with two peaks is **bimodal**. Figure 16.3A is unimodal, and multimodal distributions are illustrated in Figure 16.3B and D. Symmetry and modality are independent: Skewness is unrelated to how many peaks a distribution has.

Some distributions have special names. Of particular importance is the **normal distribution** (sometimes called a *Gaussian distribution* or *bell-shaped curve*). A normal distribution is symmetric, unimodal, and not too peaked, as shown in Figure 16.3A. Many human attributes (e.g., height, intelligence) approximate a normal distribution.

CENTRAL TENDENCY

Frequency distributions are a good way to organize data and clarify patterns, but often a pattern is of less interest than an overall summary. Researchers usually ask such questions as, "What is the average body temperature of infants during bathing?" or "What is the average weight loss of patients with cancer?" Such questions seek a single number that best represents a distribution of values. Because an index of typicalness is more likely to come from the center of a distribution

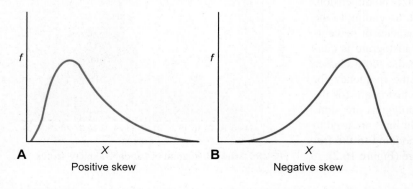

A Positive skew   **B** Negative skew

FIGURE 16.4 Examples of skewed distributions.

than from an extreme, such indexes are called measures of **central tendency**. Lay people use the term *average* to designate central tendency. Researchers avoid this term because there are three indexes of central tendency: the mode, the median, and the mean.

The Mode

The **mode** is the most frequently occurring score value in a distribution. In the following distribution, we can see that the mode is 53:

50 51 51 52 53 53 53 53 54 55 56

The score of 53 occurred four times, a higher frequency than for any other score. The mode of patients' anxiety scores (see Table 16.2) is 24. In multimodal distributions, there is more than one score value that has high frequencies. Modes are a quick way to determine a "popular" score but are rather unstable. By *unstable*, we mean that modes tend to fluctuate from sample to sample drawn from the same population.

The Median

The **median** is the point in a distribution above which and below which 50% of cases fall. As an example, consider the following set of values:

2 2 3 3 4 5 6 7 8 9

The value that divides the cases exactly in half is 4.5, the median for this set of numbers. The point that has 50% of the cases above and below it is halfway between 4 and 5. For the patient anxiety scores, the median is 24. An important characteristic of the median is that it does not take into account the quantitative values of scores—it is an index of average *position* in a distribution and is thus insensitive to extremes. In the above set of numbers, if the value of 9 were changed to 99, the median would remain 4.5. Because of this property, the median is often a preferred index of central tendency when a distribution is skewed. In research reports, the median may be abbreviated as **Md** or **Mdn**.

The Mean

The **mean**—often symbolized as M or $\bar{X}$—is the sum of all scores, divided by the number of scores. The mean is what people usually refer to as the

average. The mean of the patients' anxiety scores is 23.4 (1,405 ÷ 60). Let us compute the mean weight of eight people with the following weights: 85, 109, 120, 135, 158, 177, 181, and 195:

$$\bar{X} = \frac{85 + 109 + 120 + 135 + 158 + 177 + 181 + 195}{8} = 145$$

Unlike the median, the mean is affected by every score. If we were to exchange the 195-pound person in this example for one weighing 275 pounds, the mean would increase from 145 to 155. Such a substitution would leave the median unchanged.

The mean is the most widely used measure of central tendency. When researchers work with interval-level or ratio-level measurements, the mean, rather than the median or mode, is usually the statistic reported.

Comparison of the Mode, Median, and Mean

The mean is the most stable index of central tendency. If repeated samples were drawn from a population, means would fluctuate less than modes or medians. Sometimes, however, the primary interest is to understand what is typical, in which case a median might be preferred. If we wanted to know about the economic well-being of U.S. citizens, for example, we would get a distorted impression by considering mean income, which would be inflated by the wealth of a minority. The median would better reflect how a typical person fares financially.

When a distribution of scores is symmetric and unimodal, the three indexes of central tendency coincide. In skewed distributions, the values of the mode, median, and mean differ. The mean is always pulled in the direction of the long tail, as shown in Figure 16.5. A variable's level of measurement

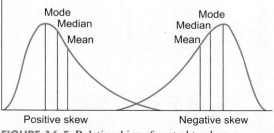

FIGURE 16.5 Relationships of central tendency indexes in skewed distributions.

plays a role in determining the appropriate index of central tendency to use. In general, the mode is most suitable for nominal measures, the mode or median is appropriate for ordinal measures, and the mean is appropriate for interval and ratio measures.

VARIABILITY

Two distributions with identical means could differ in **variability**—how spread out or dispersed the data are. Consider the two distributions in Figure 16.6, which represent fictitious scores for students from two schools on an IQ test. Both distributions have a mean of 100, but the score patterns differ. School A has a wide range of scores, from below 70 to above 130. In school B, by contrast, there are few low scores and few high scores. School A is more **heterogeneous** (i.e., more variable) than school B, and school B is more **homogeneous** than school A.

Researchers compute an index of variability to express the extent to which scores in a distribution differ from one another. Two common indexes are the range and standard deviation.

The Range

The **range** is simply the highest score minus the lowest score in a distribution. In the example of patients' anxiety scores, the range is 15 (30 − 15). In the examples shown in Figure 16.6, the range for school A is about 80 (140 − 60), and the range for school B is about 50 (125 − 75).

The chief virtue of the range is computational ease but, being based on only two scores, the range is unstable. From sample to sample from a population, the range tends to fluctuate widely. Another

limitation is that the range ignores variations in scores between the two extremes. In school B of Figure 16.6, suppose one student obtained a score of 60 and another obtained a score of 140. The range of both schools would then be 80, despite clear differences in heterogeneity. For these reasons, the range is used mainly as a gross descriptive index.

➲ TIP: Another index of variability is called the *interquartile range* (*IQR*), which is calculated on the basis of *quartiles*. The IQR indicates the range of scores within which the middle 50% of score values lie. IQRs are infrequently reported but play a role in detecting extreme values (*outliers*). For more detailed information, see Polit (2010).

The Standard Deviation

The most widely used measure of variability is the standard deviation. The **standard deviation** indicates the *average amount* of deviation of values from the mean and is calculated using every score. In research reports, the standard deviation is often abbreviated as *s* or *SD*.

A variability index needs to capture the degree to which scores deviate from one another. This concept of deviation is represented in the range by the minus sign, which produces an index of deviation, or difference, between two score points. The standard deviation is also based on score differences. In fact, the first step in calculating a standard deviation is to compute deviation scores for each case. A **deviation score** (symbolized as x) is the difference between an individual score and the mean, that is, $x = X - \bar{X}$. If a person weighed 150 pounds and the sample mean were 140, then the person's deviation score would be +10.

Because we want an *average* deviation, you might think that a good variability index could be computed by summing all deviation scores and then dividing by the number of cases. This gets us close to a good solution, but the problem is that the sum of a set of deviation scores is always zero. Table 16.3 presents deviation scores for

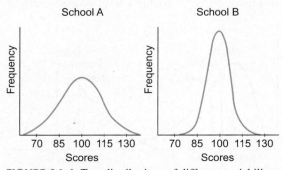

FIGURE 16.6 Two distributions of different variability.

TABLE 16.3 • Computation of a Standard Deviation

X	$x = X - \bar{X}$	$x^2 = (X - \bar{X})^2$
4	−3	9
5	−2	4
6	−1	1
7	0	0
7	0	0
7	0	0
8	1	1
9	2	4
10	3	9
$\Sigma X = 63$	$\Sigma x = 0$	$\Sigma x^2 = 28$
$\bar{X} = 7$		

$$SD = \sqrt{\frac{28}{8}} = \sqrt{3.50} = 1.87$$

nine numbers. As shown in the second column, the sum of the *x*s is zero. Deviations above the mean always balance exactly deviations below the mean.

The standard deviation overcomes this problem by squaring each deviation score before summing. After dividing by the number of cases (minus 1), the square root is taken to bring the index back to the original unit of measurement. The formula for the standard deviation is

$$SD = \sqrt{\frac{\Sigma x^2}{N - 1}}$$

➔ **TIP:** For calculating the SD of a *population*, the formula has N rather than N − 1 in the denominator. Differences in the results from the two formulas are negligible unless the sample size is small. (Statistical programs use N − 1 to compute SDs.)

A standard deviation has been worked out for the data in Table 16.3. First, a deviation score is calculated for each of the nine raw scores by subtracting the mean ($\bar{X} = 7$) from them. Each deviation

score is squared (column 3), converting all values to positive numbers. The squared deviation scores are summed ($\Sigma x^2 = 28$), divided by 8 (*N − 1*), and a square root taken to yield an *SD* of 1.87.

➔ **TIP:** The standard deviation often is shown in relation to the mean without a formal label. For example, patients' anxiety scores might be shown as M = 23.4 (3.7) or M = 23.4 ± 3.7, where 23.4 is the mean and 3.7 is the standard deviation.

A related index of variability is the **variance**, which is the value of the standard deviation before a square root has been taken. In other words, Variance = SD^2. In our example, the variance is 1.87^2, or 3.50. The variance is rarely reported because it is not in the same unit of measurement as the original data, but it is important in statistical tests we discuss in Chapter 17.

A standard deviation is more difficult to interpret than other statistics, like the mean or range. In our example, we calculated an *SD* of 1.87. One might well ask, 1.87 *what*? What does the number mean? First, the standard deviation is a variability index for a set of scores. If two distributions had a mean of 25.0, but one had an *SD* of 7.0 and the other had an *SD* of 3.0, we would know that the first sample was more heterogeneous.

Second, think of a standard deviation as an average of deviations from the mean. The mean tells us the single best value for summarizing a distribution; a standard deviation tells us how much, on average, scores deviate from that mean. A standard deviation can thus be interpreted as our degree of error when we use a mean to describe the entire sample.

The standard deviation can also be used to interpret individual scores in a distribution. Suppose we had weight data from a sample whose mean weight was 150 pounds with *SD* = 10. The *SD* provides a *standard* of variability. Weights greater than 1 *SD* away from the mean (i.e., greater than 160 or less than 140 pounds) are greater than the average in terms of variability in that distribution.

In normal and near-normal distributions, there are roughly 3 *SD*s above and 3 *SD*s below the

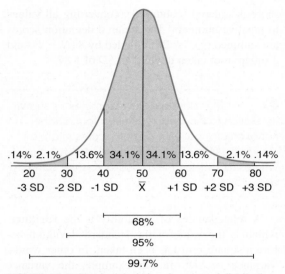

FIGURE 16.7 Standard deviations in a normal distribution.

usually used for this purpose. The Toolkit section of the accompanying *Resource Manual* includes some table templates for displaying descriptive information that can be "filled in" with descriptive results.

Example of Descriptive Statistics: Awoleke and co-researchers (2015) studied factors that predicted delays in seeking care for a ruptured tubal pregnancy in Nigeria. Sophisticated statistical analyses were performed, but the researchers also presented descriptive information about study participants' characteristics. For example, the mean age of the 92 women in the sample was 30.3 years (*SD* = 5.6), 76.9% were urban dwellers, 74.7% were married, and 27.5% had no prior births. The mean duration of amenorrhea before hospital presentation was 5.5 weeks (*SD* = 4.0).

mean. To illustrate, suppose we had normally distributed scores with a mean of 50 and an *SD* of 10 (Figure 16.7). In a normal distribution, a fixed percentage of cases falls within certain distances from the mean. Sixty-eight percent of cases fall within 1 *SD* of the mean (34% above and 34% below the mean). In our example, nearly 7 out of 10 scores fall between 40 and 60. Ninety-five percent of scores in a normal distribution fall within 2 *SD*s from the mean. Only a handful of cases—about 2% at each extreme—lie more than 2 *SD*s from the mean. In the figure, we can see that a person with a score of 70 had a higher score than about 98% of the sample.

In summary, the *SD* is a useful variability index for describing a distribution and interpreting individual scores. Like the mean, the standard deviation is a stable estimate of a parameter and is the preferred index of a distribution's variability.

> ➔ **TIP:** Descriptive statistics (e.g., percentages, means, standard deviations) are most often used to summarize sample characteristics, describe key research variables, and document methodologic features (e.g., response rates). They are seldom used to answer research questions—inferential statistics (Chapter 17) are

BIVARIATE DESCRIPTIVE STATISTICS

The mean, mode, and standard deviation are **univariate** (one-variable) **descriptive statistics** that describe one variable at a time. Most research is about relationships between variables, and **bivariate** (two-variable) **descriptive statistics** describe such relationships. Two commonly used methods of describing two-variable relationships are through crosstabs tables and correlation indexes.

Crosstabs Tables

A **crosstabs table** (or *contingency table*) is a two-dimensional frequency distribution in which the frequencies of two variables are crosstabulated. Suppose we had data on patients' gender and whether they were nonsmokers, light smokers (<1 pack of cigarettes a day), or heavy smokers (≥1 pack a day). The question is whether there is a tendency for men to smoke more heavily than women, or vice versa (i.e., whether there is a relationship between smoking and gender). Fictitious data on these two variables are shown in Table 16.4. Six **cells** are created by placing one variable (gender) on one dimension and the other variable (smoking status) on the other. Each sample member is allocated to a cell based on their status on the two variables. For example,

TABLE 16.4 • Contingency Table for Gender and Smoking Status Relationship

| | GENDER | | | | | |
| | WOMEN | | MEN | | TOTAL | |
SMOKING STATUS	*n*	%	*n*	%	*n*	%
Nonsmoker	10	45.4	6	27.3	16	36.4
Light smoker	8	36.4	8	36.4	16	36.4
Heavy smoker	4	18.2	8	36.4	12	27.3
TOTAL	22	100.0	22	100.0	44	100.0

a woman who does not smoke would be counted in the upper left of the six cells. After all participants are allocated to the appropriate cells, percentages are computed. The crosstab allows us to see that, in this sample, women were more likely than men to be nonsmokers (45.4% versus 27.3%) and less likely to be heavy smokers (18.2% versus 36.4%). Crosstabs tables are used with nominal data or ordinal data with few ranks. In the present example, gender is nominal, and smoking status, as defined, is ordinal.

Crosstabs tables are easily constructed, by hand or (more often) by commands to a computer. A key issue is which variable to put in the rows and which in the columns. Crosstabs tables are often set up such that the percentages in a column add to 100%, as in Table 16.4. However, cell percentages can be computed based on either row totals or column totals. In Table 16.4, the number 10 in the first cell (nonsmoking women) was divided by the *column* total (i.e., total number of women—22) to arrive at the percentage of women who were nonsmokers (45.4%). This cell *could* have shown 62.5%—the percentage of nonsmokers who were women (10 ÷ 16). Thus, care must be taken in reading crosstabs tables.

Example of Crosstabulations: Williamson and colleagues (2014) studied patient characteristics that were associated with incidents of aggression in a general ward of a metropolitan hospital.

They presented a table showing whether or not a patient had a "code grey" (aggressive) event in relation to such factors as their gender, marital status, and type of hospital admission. For example, 71.7% of the code grey patients (*n* = 78), compared to 55.7% of the non-code grey patients (*n* = 6,394) were male.

Correlation

Relationships between two variables are usually described through **correlation** procedures. Correlation coefficients, briefly described in Chapter 14, can be computed with two variables measured on the ordinal, interval, or ratio scale. The correlation question is: To what extent are two variables related to each other? For example, to what degree are anxiety scores and blood pressure readings related?

Correlations between two variables can be graphed on a **scatter plot** (*scatter diagram*) using a coordinate graph, with the two variables laid out at right angles. Values for one variable (*X*) are scaled on the horizontal axis, and values for the second variable (*Y*) are scaled vertically, as shown in Figure 16.8. This graph presents data for 10 people (a–j). For person a, the values for *X* and *Y* are 2 and 1, respectively. To graph person a's position, we go two units to the right along the *X* axis and one unit up on the *Y* axis. The letters on the plot are shown to help identify individuals, but normally only dots appear.

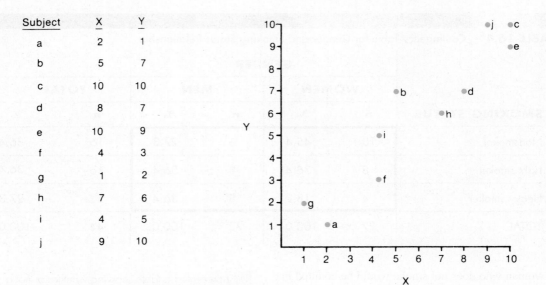

Subject	X	Y
a	2	1
b	5	7
c	10	10
d	8	7
e	10	9
f	4	3
g	1	2
h	7	6
i	4	5
j	9	10

FIGURE 16.8 Construction of a scatter plot.

In a scatter plot, the direction of the slope of points indicates the direction of the correlation. As noted in Chapter 14, a positive correlation occurs when high values on one variable are associated with high values on a second variable. If the slope of points begins at the lower left corner and extends to the upper right corner, the relationship is positive. In the current example, X and Y are positively related. People with high scores on variable X tended to have high scores on variable Y, and low scorers on X tended to score low on Y.

A negative relationship is one in which high values on one variable are related to low values on the other. Negative relationships on a scatter plot are depicted by points that slope from the upper left corner to the lower right corner, as in Figure 16.9A and D.

When relationships are *perfect*, it is possible to predict perfectly the value of one variable by knowing the value of the second. For instance, if all people who were 6 feet 2 inches tall weighed 180 pounds, and all people who were 6 feet 1 inch tall weighed 175 pounds, and so on, then weight and height would be perfectly, positively related. In such a situation, we would only need to know a person's height to know his or her weight, or vice versa. On a scatter plot, a perfect relationship is represented by a sloped straight line (Fig. 16.9C). When a relationship is not perfect, as is usually the case, one can interpret the *degree* of correlation by seeing how closely the points cluster around a straight line. The closer the points are around a diagonal slope, the stronger the correlation. When the points are scattered all over the graph, the relationship is low or nonexistent. Various degrees and directions of relationships are shown in Figure 16.9.

It is more efficient to express relationships by computing a correlation coefficient, an index with values ranging from −1.00 for a perfect negative correlation, through zero for no relationship, to +1.00 for a perfect positive correlation. The higher the absolute value of the coefficient (i.e., the value disregarding the sign), the stronger the relationship. A correlation of −.30, for instance, is stronger than a correlation of +.20.

The most widely used correlation statistic is the **product–moment correlation coefficient**, also called **Pearson's r**. This coefficient is computed with variables measured on an interval or ratio scale. **Spearman's rho** (ρ) is a correlation index for ordinal-level data. The calculation of these correlation statistics is laborious and seldom performed by hand. (Computational formulas are available in statistics textbooks, such as that by Polit, 2010.)

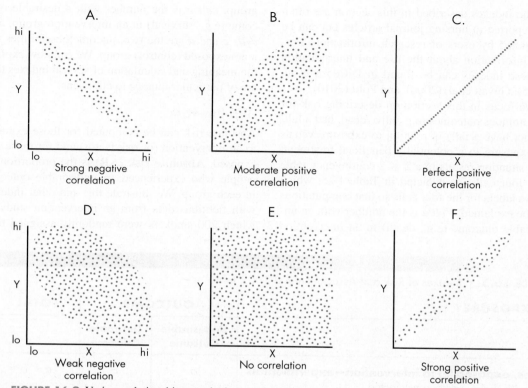

A.
Strong negative correlation

B.
Moderate positive correlation

C.
Perfect positive correlation

D.
Weak negative correlation

E.
No correlation

F.
Strong positive correlation

FIGURE 16.9 Various relationships graphed on scatter plots.

Few researchers compute statistics manually, even for relatively simple descriptive statistics such as means and percentages. The Supplement to this chapter illustrates printouts for a variety of descriptive statistics discussed in this chapter using widely used statistical software called *IBM SPSS Statistics* (SPSS).

It is difficult to offer guidelines on what to interpret as strong or weak relationships because it depends on the variables. If we measured patients' body temperatures orally and rectally, a correlation (*r*) of .70 between the two values would be low. For most psychosocial variables (e.g., stress and illness severity), an *r* of .70 is high; correlations between such variables are typically in the .30 to .40 range.

Correlation coefficients are often reported in tables displaying a two-dimensional **correlation matrix**, in which every variable is displayed in both a row and a column and coefficients are displayed

at the intersections. An example of a correlation matrix is presented at the end of this chapter.

TIP: Many statistics discussed in this chapter *can* be used for inferential as well as descriptive purposes, as we discuss in Chapter 17.

RISK INDEXES

Several descriptive statistical indexes can be used to facilitate clinical decision making. These indexes reflect the realization that risks and risk reduction must be interpreted within a context. If an intervention reduces the risk of an adverse event three times over, but the initial risk is miniscule, the intervention may have too high a cost/benefit ratio to be practical. Both absolute and relative differences in risks are important in clinical decision making.

The indexes described in this section are often not reported in nursing journal articles but can be calculated by users of research information. Further information about the use and interpretation of these indexes can be found in DiCenso et al. (2005), Guyatt et al. (2008), and Polit (2010).

We focus in this section on describing risk for dichotomous outcomes (e.g., alive/dead, had a fall/did not have a fall) in relation to exposure versus nonexposure to a potentially beneficial treatment. This situation results in a 2 × 2 contingency table with four cells, as depicted in Table 16.5, which shows labels for the four cells so that computations can be explained. *Cell a* is the number with an undesirable outcome (e.g., death) in an intervention

group, *cell b* is the number with a desirable outcome (e.g., survival) in an intervention group, and *cells c* and *d* are the two outcome possibilities for a nonexposed (control) group. We can now explain the meaning and calculation of several indexes that are of particular interest to clinicians.

Absolute Risk

Absolute risk can be computed for those exposed to an intervention (or risk factor) and for those not exposed. **Absolute risk (AR)** is the proportion of people who experienced an undesirable outcome in each group. We illustrate this and other indexes with fictitious data from an intervention study in which 200 smokers were randomly assigned to a

TABLE 16.5 • Indexes of Risk and Association in a 2 × 2 Table

EXPOSURE	OUTCOME		TOTAL
	Undesirable Outcome	**Desirable Outcome**	
Yes, exposed (E) to intervention—experimentals (or, NOT exposed to a risk factor)	a	b	a + b
No, not exposed (NE) to intervention—controls (or, exposed to a risk factor)	c	d	c + d
TOTAL	a + c	b + d	a + b + c + d

Absolute risk, exposed group (AR$_E$) = $a / (a + b)$

Absolute risk, nonexposed group (AR$_{NE}$) = $c / (c + d)$

Absolute risk reduction (ARR) = $AR_{NE} - AR_E$

Relative risk (RR) = $\dfrac{AR_E}{AR_{NE}}$

Relative risk reduction (RRR) = $\dfrac{ARR}{AR_{NE}}$

Odds, exposed group (Odds$_E$) = a / b

Odds, nonexposed group (Odds$_{NE}$) = c / d

Odds ratio (OR) = $\dfrac{Odds_E}{Odds_{NE}}$

Number needed to treat (NNT) = $\dfrac{1}{ARR}$

TABLE 16.6 • Hypothetical Data for Smoking Cessation Example Illustrating Risk Index Calculation

EXPOSURE TO SMOKING CESSATION INTERVENTION	OUTCOME		TOTAL
	Continued Smoking	**Stopped Smoking**	
Yes, exposed: E (Experimental group)	50 (a)	50 (b)	100
No, not exposed: NE (Control group)	80 (c)	20 (d)	100
TOTAL	130	70	200

Absolute risk, exposed group (AR_E)   =   50 / 100   =   .50
Absolute risk, nonexposed group (AR_{NE})   =   80 / 100   =   .80
Absolute risk reduction (ARR)   =   .80 − .50   =   .30
Relative risk (RR)   =   .50 / .80   =   .625
Relative risk reduction (RRR)   =   .30 / .80   =   .375
Odds ratio (OR) $= \dfrac{(50 / 50)}{(80 / 20)} =$ .25
Number needed to treat   =   1 / .30   =   3.33

smoking cessation intervention or to a control group (Table 16.6). Smoking status 3 months after the intervention is the outcome variable. In this example, the absolute risk of continued smoking was .50 in the intervention group and .80 in the control group. The risk of an undesirable outcome for a treatment group is sometimes called the *experimental event rate* (*EER*), and the risk of an adverse outcome for untreated people is sometimes called the *baseline risk rate*, or the *control event rate* (*CER*). In the absence of the intervention, 20% of those in the experimental group might have stopped smoking anyway, but the intervention boosted the rate to 50%.

⏺ **TIP:** The computations shown in Table 16.5 specifically reflect risk indexes that assume that the intervention exposure will be beneficial and that information for the *undesirable* outcome will be in cells a and c. If good outcomes rather than bad ones are put in cells a and c, formulas would have

to be modified. For example, AR_E would then be *b / (a + b)*, and so on. Similarly, if the research question involved the association between an adverse outcome and a hypothesized risk factor (e.g., the risk that smoking is associated with a cardiovascular accident), the group exposed to the risk factor (e.g., those who smoke) should be in the *bottom* row (cells c and d) and not the top row—or, again, the formulas would need to be adapted. As a general rule, to use the formulas shown in Table 16.6, the cell in the lower left corner (cell c) should be predicted to reflect the highest percentage of undesirable outcomes.

Absolute Risk Reduction

The **absolute risk reduction (ARR)**, sometimes called the *risk difference* or *RD*, represents a comparison of the two risks. It is computed by subtracting the absolute risk for the exposed group from the absolute risk for the untreated group. This index indicates the estimated proportion of people who would be spared the undesirable outcome through exposure to the intervention. In our example, the value of ARR is .30: Thirty percent of the control group participants would presumably have stopped smoking if they had received the intervention, over and above the 20% who stopped without it.

Relative Risk

Relative risk (RR), or the *risk ratio*, represents the estimated proportion of the original risk of an adverse outcome (in our example, continued smoking) that persists when people are exposed to the intervention. To compute an RR, the absolute risk for exposed people is divided by the absolute risk for nonexposed people. In our fictitious example, the RR is .625. This means that the risk of continued smoking after the smoking cessation intervention is estimated to be 62.5% of what it would have been in its absence.

Relative Risk Reduction

Relative risk reduction (RRR) is another useful index for evaluating the effectiveness of an intervention. RRR is the estimated proportion of untreated risk that is reduced through exposure to the intervention. This index is computed by dividing the ARR by the absolute risk for the control group. In our example, RRR = .375. This means that the smoking cessation intervention decreased the relative risk of continued smoking by 37.5%, compared to not having had the intervention.

Odds Ratio

The **odds ratio (OR)** is a widely reported index, even though it is less intuitively meaningful than RR as an index of risk. The **odds**, in this context, is the proportion of people *with* the adverse outcome relative to those *without* it. In our example, the odds of continued smoking for the experimental group is 50 (the number who continued smoking) divided by 50 (the number who stopped), or 1. The odds for the control group is 80 divided by 20, or 4. The odds ratio is the ratio of these two odds, or .25 in our example. The estimated odds of continuing to smoke are one

fourth as high among those in the intervention group as among those in the control group. Turned around, we could say that the estimated odds of continued smoking is 4 times higher among smokers who did not get the intervention as among those who did.

> **TIP:** Odds ratios can be computed when the independent variable is not dichotomous, using a statistical procedure described in Chapter 18. For example, we could estimate the odds ratio for obesity among adults in four different income groups, using one of the groups as a reference.

Number Needed to Treat

A final index of interest is the **number needed to treat (NNT)**, which represents an estimate of how many people would need to receive a treatment or intervention to prevent one undesirable outcome. NNT is computed by dividing 1 by the value of the absolute risk reduction. In our example, ARR = .30, and so NNT is 3.33. About three smokers would need to be exposed to the intervention to avoid one person's continued smoking. The NNT is inversely related to the RRR. An intervention that is twice as effective with regard to relative risk reduction will cut the number needed to treat in half. The NNT is especially valuable for decision makers because it can be integrated with monetary information to determine if an intervention is cost-effective.

> **Example of AR, RRR, and NNT:** Cutler and Sluman (2014) evaluated the impact of oral hygiene measures in an adult critical care unit on the incidence of ventilator-associated pneumonia (VAP). The incidence of VAP in 528 patients prior to the practice change was compared to the incidence in 559 patients after the change. The absolute risk in the control group was .09, compared to an AR of .04 among patients after the practice change. Relative risk reduction was .53, and the NNT was 21.

> **TIP:** Various tools on the Internet facilitate the calculation of risk indexes. Links to these and other useful websites are available in the Toolkit for you to "click" on directly.

BOX 16.1 Guidelines for Critiquing Descriptive Statistics

1. Did the report include descriptive statistics? Do these statistics sufficiently describe major characteristics of the sample?
2. Were descriptive statistics used appropriately—for example, were descriptive statistics used to describe sample characteristics, key variables, and methodologic features of the study, such as response rate or attrition rate? Were they used to answer research questions when inferential statistics would have been more appropriate?
3. Were the correct descriptive statistics used—for example, was a mean presented when percentages would have been more informative? Was the mean used without information about the median even though the distribution was severely skewed?
4. Was the descriptive information presented in a useful format—for example, were tables used effectively? Is information in the text and the tables redundant? Is information in the text and tables consistent with each other? Were the tables clear, with a good title, carefully labeled headings, and good table notes?
5. Were any risk indexes computed? If not, would they have been useful, to increase the clinical utility of the findings?

CRITIQUING DESCRIPTIVE STATISTICS

Descriptive statistics help to set the stage for understanding quantitative research evidence. Descriptive statistics are particularly useful for communicating information about the study sample. Readers of reports cannot draw inferences about the study's external validity without understanding who the participants were, especially with regard to key demographic characteristics and health-related attributes.

In addition to describing sample characteristics, descriptive statistics are useful in communicating information about the baseline values of key outcome variables in longitudinal or intervention studies, or correlations between a set of independent variables. Methodologic information about study quality also typically relies on descriptive statistics—for example, response rates and attrition rates are typically shown as percentages, and means are used to characterize such things as time elapsed between two interviews.

Descriptive statistics are sometimes used to directly address research questions in studies that are primarily descriptive. However, when only descriptive statistics are presented, readers should think about whether the inclusion of inferential statistics would have been appropriate. If a research question is about a *population*, and not just about the particular people who participated in the research, inferential statistics usually are needed.

In critiquing the researcher's use of descriptive statistics, readers can consider whether the information was adequate, whether the correct statistical indexes were used, and whether it was presented in a clear and efficient manner. Box 16.1 presents some guiding questions for critiquing the descriptive statistics in a research report.

RESEARCH EXAMPLE

Study: Predictors of medication adherence among HIV-positive women in North America (Tyer-Viola et al., 2014)

Statement of Purpose: The overall purpose of this study was to explore the relationships among contextual, environmental, and psychosocial factors on the one hand and antiretroviral (ARV) medication adherence on the other among women living with HIV.

Methods: The analysis for this paper was based on data from a subsample of participants from a large study of persons living with HIV who were recruited in 19 sites. The sample in this secondary analysis consisted of 338 North American women who were taking ARV medications at the time of the survey. Participants answered questions about their background characteristics and medication adherence and completed several psychosocial scales (e.g., depression, self-efficacy for adherence). Medication adherence was measured, for a 3-day and 30-day period, on a visual analog scale that asked participants to indicate on the 0 to 100 scale the percentage of time they were able to take their medications as prescribed.

Analysis and Findings: One table showed descriptive statistics for the main continuous study variables (e.g., adherence, depression scores). The table showed the means, *SD*s, the theoretical range for scaled variables, and coefficient alpha. A separate table showed frequency information for nominal-level characteristics (e.g., race) and ordinal-level variables (e.g., educational category). To conserve space, we collapsed some of the data from these two tables into Table 16.7. This table shows, for example, that about half of the participants (50.3%) were African American and that only a minority (23.1%) had education beyond a high school diploma; 58% of the women had been diagnosed with AIDS. In this sample, depression scores were high. The mean was 22.2 on a depression scale that categorizes people as "at risk" for depression with scores of 16 or higher. On average, women had high levels of medication adherence: 87% of the time for 3-day adherence and 83% for 30-day adherence.

TABLE 16.7 • Selected Demographic Characteristics and Clinical Variables for HIV-Positive Women in the Study Sample (*N* = 338)

SAMPLE CHARACTERISTIC	FREQUENCY (*n*)	PERCENT OR MEAN (*SD*)
Race		
African American	170	50.3%
Hispanic/Latina	55	16.3%
White/Anglo (not Hispanic)	72	21.3%
Other	38	11.2%
Education		
11th grade or less	126	37.2%
High school diploma or equivalency	134	39.6%
Postsecondary education	78	23.1%
AIDS diagnosis?		
Yes	196	58.0%
No	134	39.6%
Age		45.0 (9.1)
Depression scores (CES-D)		22.2 (11.9)
Adherence self-efficacy scores		92.5 (27.1)
Percentage of time adherent (3 days)		87.0 (22.0)
Percentage of time adherent (30 days)		83.0 (24.0)

CES-D, Center for Epidemiological Studies Depression Scale.
Adapted from Tables 1 and 2 of Tyer-Viola et al. (2014).

TABLE 16.8 • Correlation Matrix for Selected Study Variables: Medication Adherence in HIV-Positive Women

VARIABLE	1	2	3	4	5	6
1 Age	1.00					
2 Education	.14	1.00				
3 Depression score	−.10	−.09	1.00			
4 Self-efficacy for adherence scores	.05	.06	−.16	1.00		
5 3-day adherence	.13	.05	−.23	.42	1.00	
6 30-day adherence	.12	.04	−.25	.45	.70	1.00

Adapted from Table 2 of Tyer-Viola et al. (2014).

Findings relevant to the study purpose were presented in a correlation matrix. An adapted version of this matrix, with selected variables, is presented in Table 16.8.* This table lists, on the left, six variables: age, education, scores on the depression scale, scores on a scale of perceived self-efficacy for adherence, and the 3-day and 30-day adherence variables. The numbers in the top row correspond to the six variables: 1 is age, and so on. The correlation matrix shows, in the first column, the correlation coefficients (r) between age with all six variables. At the intersection of row 1 and column 1, we find the value 1.00, which simply indicates that age values are perfectly correlated with themselves. The next entry in the first column is the correlation between age and education. The value of .14 indicates a very modest positive relationship: Older women were somewhat more likely than younger ones to have more years of education. The next entry (−.10) indicates a modest negative relationship between age and depression: The older the patient, the *less* severe the depression, but only marginally so. In the bottom row, we see that 30-day adherence was highest for women who were less depressed ($r = -.25$) and for women who had a higher sense of self-efficacy for adherence ($r = .45$). Adherence was virtually unrelated to education ($r = .04$).

*Although we present only descriptive information in Table 16.8, Tyer-Viola et al. (2014) also presented inferential statistical information in their correlation matrix.

SUMMARY POINTS

- There are four **levels of measurement**: (1) **nominal measurement**—the classification of characteristics into mutually exclusive categories; (2) **ordinal measurement**—the ranking of objects based on their relative standing on an attribute; (3) **interval measurement**—indicating not only the ranking of objects but also the amount of distance between them; and (4) **ratio measurement**—distinguished from interval measurement by having a rational zero point.
- **Descriptive statistics** enable researchers to summarize and describe quantitative data.
- **Frequency distributions** impose order on raw data. Numeric values are ordered from lowest to highest, accompanied by a count of the number (or percentage) of times each value was obtained.
- **Histograms** and **frequency polygons** are two common methods of displaying frequency information graphically.
- Data for a variable can be completely described in terms of the shape of the distribution, central tendency, and variability.
- A distribution is **symmetric** if its two halves are mirror images of each other. A **skewed** distribution, by contrast, is asymmetric, with one tail longer than the other.
- In **positively skewed distributions**, the long tail points to the right (e.g., personal income);

in negatively skewed distributions, the long tail points to the left (e.g., age at death).

- The **modality** of a distribution refers to the number of peaks: A **unimodal distribution** has one peak, and a **multimodal distribution** has more than one peak.
- A **normal distribution** (*bell-shaped curve*) is symmetric, unimodal, and not too peaked.
- Measures of **central tendency** are indexes that represent the average or typical value of a set of scores. The **mode** is the value that occurs most frequently in a distribution. The **median** is the point above which and below which 50% of the cases fall. The **mean** is the arithmetic average of all scores. The mean is usually the preferred measure of central tendency because of its *stability* from sample to sample drawn from a population.
- Measures of **variability**—how spread out the data are—include the range and standard deviation. The **range** is the distance between the highest and lowest scores. The **standard deviation** (*SD*) indicates how much, on average, scores deviate from the mean.
- The *SD* is calculated by first computing **deviation scores**, which indicate the degree to which a person's score deviates from the mean. The **variance** is equal to the *SD* squared. In a normal distribution, 95% of scores fall within 2 *SD*s above and below the mean.
- **Bivariate descriptive statistics** describe relationships between two variables.
- A **crosstabs table** is a two-dimensional frequency distribution in which the frequencies of two nominal- or ordinal-level variables are crosstabulated.
- **Correlation coefficients** describe the direction and magnitude of a relationship between two variables. Researchers most often compute the **product–moment correlation coefficient** (Pearson's *r*), used with interval- or ratio-level variables. The **Spearman rho coefficient** is used with ordinal-level variables.
- Graphically, the relationship between two continuous variables can be displayed on a **scatter plot**.
- Several risk indexes describe outcomes in relation to exposures (to interventions or risk factors) for a two-group (e.g., experimental versus control) situation with dichotomous outcomes (e.g., alive/dead). These indexes provide useful information for making clinical decisions.
- **Absolute risk reduction (ARR)** expresses the estimated proportion of people who would be spared an adverse outcome through exposure to an intervention (or lack of exposure to a risk). **Relative risk (RR)** is the estimated proportion of the original risk of an adverse outcome that persists among people exposed to an intervention. **Relative risk reduction (RRR)** is the estimated proportion of untreated risk that is reduced through exposure to the intervention. The **odds ratio (OR)** is the ratio of the odds for the treated versus untreated group, with the **odds** reflecting the proportion of people with the adverse outcome relative to those without it. The **number needed to treat (NNT)** is an estimate of how many people would need to receive the intervention to prevent one adverse outcome.

STUDY ACTIVITIES

Chapter 16 of the *Resource Manual for Nursing Research*: *Generating and Assessing Evidence for Nursing Practice, 10th edition*, offers study suggestions for reinforcing concepts presented in this chapter. In addition, the following study questions can be addressed:

1. What are the mean, median, and mode for the following set of data?

   13 12 9 15 7 10 16 9 6 10

   Compute the range and standard deviation.

2. Suppose that 400 subjects (200 per group) were in the intervention study described in connection with Table 16.8 and that 60% of those in the experimental group and 90% of those in the control group continued smoking. Compute the various risk indexes for this scenario.

3. Apply relevant questions in Box 16.1 to the research example at the end of the chapter (Tyer-Viola et al., 2014), referring to the full journal article as necessary.

STUDIES CITED IN CHAPTER 16

*Awoleke, J., Adaniken, A., & Awoleke, A. (2015). Ruptured tubal pregnancy: Predictors of delays in seeking and obtaining care in a Nigerian population. *International Journal of Women's Health, 27*, 141–147.

Cutler, L. R., & Sluman, P. (2014). Reducing ventilator associated pneumonia in adult patients through high standards of oral care: A historical control study. *Intensive and Critical Care Nursing, 30*, 61–68.

DiCenso, A., Guyatt, G., & Ciliska, D. (2005). *Evidence-based nursing: A guide to clinical practice.* St. Louis, MO: Elsevier Mosby.

*Grønning, K., Rannestrad, T., Skomsvoll, J., Rygg, L., & Steinsbekk, A. (2014). Long-term effects of a nurse-led group and individual patient education programme for patients with chronic inflammatory polyarthritis. *Journal of Clinical Nursing, 23*, 1005–1017.

Guyatt, G., Rennie, D., Meade, M., & Cook, D. (2008). *Users' guides to the medical literature: Essentials of evidence-based clinical practice* (2nd ed.). New York: McGraw Hill.

Polit, D. F. (2010). *Statistics and data analysis for nursing research* (2nd ed.). Upper Saddle River, NJ: Pearson.

Tyer-Viola, L. A., Corless, I., Webel, A., Reid, P., Sullivan, K., & Nichols, P. (2014). Predictors of medication adherence among HIV-positive women in North America. *Journal of Obstetric, Gynecologic, and Neonatal Nursing, 43*, 168–178.

Williamson, R., Lauricella, K., Browning, A., Tierney, E., Chen, J., Joseph, S., . . . Hamilton, B. (2014). Patient factors associated with incidents of aggression in a general inpatient setting. *Journal of Clinical Nursing, 23*, 1144–1152.

A link to this open-access journal article is provided in the Toolkit for this chapter in the accompanying Resource Manual. 🟦

17 | Inferential Statistics

Inferential statistics, based on the **laws of probability**, provide a means for drawing conclusions about a population, given data from a sample. Inferential statistics would help us with such questions as, "What can I infer about 5-minute Apgar scores of premature babies (the population) after calculating a mean Apgar score of 7.5 in a sample of 300 premature babies?" Inferential statistics provide a framework for making objective judgments about the reliability of sample estimates. Different researchers applying inferential statistics to the same data are likely to draw the same conclusions.

SAMPLING DISTRIBUTIONS

To estimate population parameters, it is advisable to use representative samples, and probability samples are the best way to get representative samples (Chapter 12). Inferential statistics assume random sampling from populations, an assumption that is widely violated. The validity of statistical calculations does depend, however, on the extent to which results from the sample are similar to what you would have obtained had you randomly selected people from the population.

Even when random sampling *is* used, sample characteristics are seldom identical to population characteristics. Suppose we had a population of 50,000 nursing school applicants whose mean score on a standardized entrance exam was 500.0 with a standard deviation (*SD*) of 100.0. Suppose we had to estimate the population mean from the scores of a random sample of 25 students. Would we expect a mean of *exactly* 500.0 for the sample? Obtaining the exact population value is unlikely. Let us say the sample mean is 505.1. If a new random sample were drawn, we might obtain a mean of, say, 497.8. The tendency for statistics to fluctuate from one sample to another reflects **sampling error**. The challenge is to decide whether sample values are good estimates of population parameters.

Researchers compute statistics with only *one* sample, but to understand inferential statistics, we must perform a mental exercise. Consider drawing a sample of 25 students from the population of 50,000, calculating a mean, replacing the students, and drawing a new sample. Each mean is one datum. If we drew 10,000 such samples, we would have 10,000 means (data points) that could be used to construct a frequency polygon (Figure 17.1). This distribution is a **sampling distribution of the mean**. A sampling distribution is theoretical because in practice no one draws consecutive samples from a population and plots their means. Sampling distributions are the basis of inferential statistics.

Characteristics of Sampling Distributions

When an infinite number of samples is randomly drawn from a population, the sampling distribution of the mean has certain characteristics. (Our example of 10,000 samples is large enough to

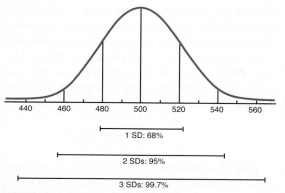

FIGURE 17.1 A sampling distribution.

approximate these characteristics.) Sampling distributions of means are normally distributed, and the mean of a sampling distribution with an infinite number of sample means always equals the population mean. In the example shown in Figure 17.1, the mean of the sampling distribution is 500.0, the same as the population mean.

Remember that when data are normally distributed, 68% of values fall between ±1 SD from the mean. Because a sampling distribution of means is normally distributed, we can say that the probability is 68 out of 100 that any randomly drawn sample mean lies between +1 SD and −1 SD of the population mean. Thus, if we knew the standard deviation of the sampling distribution, we could interpret the accuracy of a sample mean.

Standard Error of the Mean

The standard deviation of a sampling distribution of the mean is called the **standard error of the mean (SEM)**. The word *error* signifies that the various means in the sampling distribution have some error as estimates of the population mean. The smaller the SEM—that is, the less variable the sample means—the more accurate are the means as estimates of the population value.

No one actually constructs a sampling distribution, so how can its standard deviation be computed? Fortunately, there is a formula for estimating the SEM from a single sample, using two pieces of information: the sample's standard deviation and sample size. The equation for the SEM is: $SD/\sqrt{N}$. In our example, if we use this formula to calculate

the SEM for an SD of 100.0 with a sample of 25 students we obtain

$$SEM = \frac{100.0}{\sqrt{25}} = 20.0$$

The standard deviation of the sampling distribution in our example is 20.0, as shown in Figure 17.1. This SEM is an estimate of how much sampling error there is from one sample mean to another when samples of 25 are randomly drawn and the SD is 100.0.

Given that a sampling distribution of means follows a normal curve, we can estimate the probability of drawing a sample with a certain mean. With a sample size of 25 and a population mean of 500.0, the chances are about 95 out of 100 that any sample mean will fall between 460 and 540 (i.e., 2 SDs above and below the mean). Only 5 times out of 100 would the mean of a randomly selected sample exceed 540 or be less than 460. Only 5 times out of 100 would we get a sample whose mean deviated from the population mean by more than 40 points.

Because the SEM is partly a function of sample size, we need only increase sample size to increase the accuracy of our estimate. If we used a sample of 100 applicants, rather than 25, the SEM would be 10 (i.e., $100/\sqrt{100} = 10.0$). In this situation, the chances are about 95 out of 100 that a sample mean will be between 480 and 520. The chances of drawing a sample with a mean very different from the population mean is reduced as sample size increases because large numbers promote the likelihood that extreme values will cancel each other out.

ESTIMATION OF PARAMETERS

Statistical inference consists of two techniques: (1) estimation of parameters and (2) hypothesis testing. Parameter estimations have not traditionally been presented in nursing research reports, but that situation is changing. The emphasis on evidence-based practice (EBP) has heightened interest among practitioners in learning not only whether a hypothesis was supported (via hypothesis testing) but also the estimated value of a population parameter and the level of accuracy of the estimate (via parameter estimation). Many medical research journals *require* that estimation information be reported because it is more useful to clinicians (e.g., Brahman, 1991; Sackett et al., 2000). In this section, we present general concepts relating to parameter estimation and offer some examples based on one-variable descriptive statistics. We expand on this discussion throughout the chapter within the context of specific bivariate statistical tests.

Confidence Intervals

Parameter estimation is used to estimate a parameter—for example, a mean, a proportion, or a mean difference between two groups (e.g., experimental and control participants). Estimation can take two forms: point estimation or interval estimation. *Point estimation* involves calculating a single descriptive statistic to estimate the population parameter. To continue with the earlier example, if we calculated the mean entrance exam score for a sample of 25 applicants and found that it was 510.0, then this would be the point estimate of the population mean.

Point estimates convey no information about margin of error, however, and so we could not make inferences about the accuracy of the parameter estimate. *Interval estimation* is useful because it indicates a range of values within which the parameter has a specified probability of lying. With interval estimation, researchers construct a **confidence interval** (**CI**) around the estimate; the upper and lower limits are **confidence limits**. Constructing a confidence interval around a sample mean establishes a range of values for the population value as well as the probability of being right—the estimate is made with a certain degree of confidence. By convention, researchers usually use either a 95% or a 99% confidence interval.

➜ TIP: Confidence intervals address one of the key EBP questions for appraising evidence (see Box 2.2): How *precise* is the estimate of effects?

Confidence Intervals around a Mean

Calculating confidence limits around a mean involves using the *SEM*. In a normal distribution,

95% of the scores lie within about 2 *SD*s (more precisely, 1.96 *SD*s) from the mean. In our example, suppose the point estimate for mean entrance exam scores is 510.0, and the *SD* is 100.0. The *SEM* for a sample of 25 would be 20.0. We can build a 95% confidence interval with the following formula:

$$CI\ 95\% = (\bar{X} \pm 1.96 \times SEM)$$

That is, confidence is 95% that the population mean lies between the values equal to 1.96 times the *SEM*, above and below the sample mean. In the example at hand, we would obtain the following:

$$CI\ 95\% = [510.0 \pm (1.96 \times 20.0)]$$
$$CI\ 95\% = [510.0 \pm (39.2)]$$
$$CI\ 95\% = (470.8 \le \mu \le 549.2)$$

The final statement may be read as follows: the confidence is 95% that the population mean (symbolized by the Greek letter mu [μ] by convention) is between 470.8 and 549.2. This would be stated in a research report as 95% CI = 470.8 to 549.2, or 95% CI (470.8, 549.2).

Confidence intervals reflect the researchers' risk of being wrong. With a 95% CI, researchers accept the probability that they will be wrong 5 times out of 100. A 99% CI sets the risk at only 1% by allowing a wider range of possible values. The formula is as follows:

$$CI\ 99\% = (\bar{X} \pm 2.58 \times SEM)$$

The 2.58 reflects the fact that 99% of all cases in a normal distribution lie within ± 2.58 *SD* units from the mean. In the example, the 99% confidence interval would be:

$$CI\ 99\% = [510.0 \pm (2.58 \times 20.0)]$$
$$CI\ 99\% = [510.0 \pm (51.6)]$$
$$CI\ 99\% = (458.4 \le \mu \le 561.6)$$

In random samples with 25 subjects, 99 out of 100 confidence intervals so constructed would contain the population mean. The price of having a reduced risk of being wrong is reduced precision.

With a 95% interval, the range of the CI was about 80 points; with a 99% interval, the range is more than 100 points. The acceptable risk of error depends on the nature of the problem. In research with implications for the health of individual patients, a stringent 99% confidence interval might be used; for most studies, a 95% confidence interval is sufficient.

Confidence Intervals around Proportions and Risk Indexes

Calculating confidence intervals around a proportion or percentage is important in certain types of research, especially with regard to risk estimates. Consider, for example, this question: "What percentage of people exposed to a certain hazard will contract a disease?" This question calls for an estimated proportion (an absolute risk index, as described in Chapter 16) that is more useful if it is reported within a 95% confidence interval.

For proportions based on dichotomous variables, as implied in the above question (positive/negative for a disease), the applicable theoretical distribution is not a normal distribution but rather a **binomial distribution**. A binomial distribution is the probability distribution of the number of "successes" (e.g., heads) in a sequence of independent yes/no trials (e.g., a coin toss), each of which yields "success" with a specified probability.

Using binomial distributions to build confidence intervals around a proportion is computationally complex, and so we do not provide formulas here. Certain features of confidence intervals around proportions are, however, worth noting. First, the CI is rarely symmetric around a sample proportion. For example, if 3 out of 30 sample members were "positive" for an outcome, such as hospital readmission, the estimated population proportion would be .10 and the 95% CI for the proportion would be from .021 to .265. Second, the width of the CI depends on both the value of the proportion and the sample size. The larger the sample, the smaller the CI. Also, the closer the sample proportion is to .50, the wider the CI. For example, with a sample size of 30, the range for a 95% CI for a proportion of .50 is .374 (.313, .687), while that for a proportion of .10 is only .188 (.021, .265).

Finally, the CI for a proportion never extends below 0 or above 1.0, but a CI can be constructed around an *obtained* proportion of 0 or 1.0. For example, if 0 out of our 30 participants were readmitted to the hospital, the estimated proportion would be 0.0 and the 95% CI would be from 0.0 to .116.

It is possible—and advisable—to construct confidence intervals around all of the indexes of risk described in the previous chapter, such as the ARR, RRR, OR, and NNT. The computed value of these indexes from study data represents a single "best estimate," but confidence intervals convey important information about the precision of the estimate. Clearly, clinical inference is enhanced when information about a plausible range of values for risk indexes is presented. Formulas for constructing CIs around the major risk indexes are presented in an appendix of DiCenso et al. (2005), but an easier method for constructing 95% CIs around major risk indexes is to use an online calculator, such as the one by the Centre for Evidence-Based Medicine in Canada (http://ktclearinghouse.ca/cebm/practise/ca/calculators/statscalc). The calculator will compute various risk indexes and the 95% CIs, for different research scenarios, which can be selected from a dropdown menu.

> **Example of Confidence Intervals around Proportions:** Reed and colleagues (2014) studied the prevalence of foot and ankle musculoskeletal disorders (MSDs) experienced by nurses working in a pediatric hospital in Australia. Based on survey responses from 304 nurses, 43.8% of the nurses experienced foot/ankle MSDs in the previous 7 days (95% CI = 38.2%, 49.4%).

HYPOTHESIS TESTING

Statistical hypothesis testing provides objective criteria for deciding whether hypotheses are supported by data. Suppose we hypothesized that participation in a stress management program would reduce anxiety levels among patients with cancer. The sample is 25 patients in the control arm who do not participate in the program and 25 experimental patients who do. The mean posttreatment anxiety score for experimentals is 15.8 and that for controls is 17.9. Should we conclude that the hypothesis is correct? Group differences are in the predicted direction, but the results might reflect sampling fluctuations. With a new sample, group means might be nearly identical. Statistical hypothesis testing allows researchers to make objective decisions about whether study results likely reflect chance sample differences or true population differences.

The Null Hypothesis

Hypothesis testing is based on negative inference. In our example, patients participating in the intervention had lower mean anxiety scores than control group patients. There are two possible explanations: (1) the intervention was successful in reducing anxiety or (2) the differences resulted from chance factors, such as group differences in anxiety even before the treatment. The first explanation is our research hypothesis, and the second is the null hypothesis. The **null hypothesis**, it may be recalled, states that there is no relationship between variables. Statistical hypothesis testing is basically a process of rejection. It cannot be demonstrated directly that the research hypothesis is correct but, using theoretical sampling distributions, it can be shown that the null hypothesis has a high probability of being incorrect. Researchers seek to reject the null hypothesis through various **statistical tests**.

The null hypothesis in our example can be stated formally as follows:

$$H_0: \mu_E = \mu_C$$

The null hypothesis (H_0) is that the mean population anxiety score for experimental patients (μ_E) is the same as that for controls (μ_C). The **alternative**, or research, **hypothesis** (H_A) is that the means are *not* the same:

$$H_A: \mu_E \neq \mu_C$$

Null hypotheses are accepted or rejected based on sample data, but hypothesis testing is used to make inferences about the population.

Type I and Type II Errors

Researchers decide whether to accept or reject a null hypothesis by determining how *probable* it is that observed results are due to chance. Researchers cannot know with certainty whether a null hypothesis is or is not true based on data from a sample. They can only conclude that hypotheses are *probably* true or *probably* false, and there is always a risk of error.

Researchers can make two types of statistical error: rejecting a true null hypothesis or accepting a false null hypothesis. Figure 17.2 summarizes possible outcomes of researchers' decisions. Researchers make a **Type I error** by rejecting a null hypothesis that is, in fact, true. For instance, if we concluded that a drug was more effective than a placebo in reducing cholesterol, when in fact the observed differences in cholesterol levels resulted from sampling fluctuations, we would be making a Type I error—a false positive conclusion. Conversely, if we concluded that group differences in cholesterol resulted by chance, when in fact the drug *did* reduce cholesterol, we would be committing a **Type II error**—a false negative conclusion. In the context of drug testing, a good way to think about statistical error can be expressed as follows: A Type I error might allow an ineffective drug to come onto the market, but a Type II error might *prevent* an effective drug from coming onto the market.

		The actual situation is that the null hypothesis is:	
		True	False
The researcher calculates a test statistic and decides that the null hypothesis is:	True (Null accepted)	Correct decision	Type II error (False negative)
	False (Null rejected)	Type I error (False positive)	Correct decision

FIGURE 17.2 Outcomes of statistical decision making.

Level of Significance

Researchers never know when they have made an error in statistical decision making. The validity of a null hypothesis could be known only by collecting data from the population. Researchers control the *risk* of a Type I error by selecting a **level of significance**, which signifies the probability of incorrectly rejecting a true null hypothesis.

The two most frequently used significance levels (referred to as **alpha** or α) are .05 and .01. With a .05 significance level, we accept the risk that out of 100 samples drawn from a population, a true null hypothesis would be rejected 5 times. With a .01 significance level, the risk of a Type I error is *lower*: In only 1 sample out of 100 would we erroneously reject the null hypothesis. The minimum acceptable level for α usually is .05. A stricter level (e.g., .01 or .001) may be needed when the decision has important consequences.

Naturally, researchers want to reduce the risk of committing both types of error, but unfortunately, lowering the risk of a Type I error increases the risk of a Type II error. The stricter the criterion for rejecting a null hypothesis, the greater the probability of accepting a false null hypothesis. Researchers must deal with trade-offs in establishing criteria for statistical decision making, but the simplest way of reducing the risk of a Type II error is to increase sample size. Type II errors are discussed later in this chapter.

Critical Regions

By selecting a significance level, researchers establish a decision rule. That rule is to reject the null hypothesis if the test statistic falls at or beyond the limits that establish a **critical region** on an applicable theoretical distribution and to accept the null hypothesis otherwise. The critical region indicates whether the null hypothesis is *improbable*, given the results.

An example from our study of gender bias in nursing research (Polit & Beck, 2013) illustrates the statistical decision-making process. We examined whether males and females are equally represented as the study participants in nursing studies—that is, whether the average percentage of females across studies in four leading nursing research journals was 50.0. The null

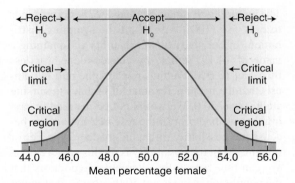

FIGURE 17.3 Critical regions in the sampling distribution for a two-tailed test: gender bias example.

hypothesis is H_0: $\mu = 50.0$, and the alternate hypothesis is H_A: $\mu \neq 50.0$. We found, using a consecutive sample of 300 studies published over a 2-year period, that the mean percentage of females was 74.1. Using statistical procedures, we tested the hypothesis that the mean of 74.1 was not merely a chance fluctuation from a population mean of 50.0.

In hypothesis testing, researchers assume the null hypothesis is true and then gather evidence to disprove it. Assuming a mean percentage of 50.0 for the population of nursing studies, a theoretical sampling distribution can be constructed. For simplicity, let us say that the standard error of the mean in this example is 2.0 (the actual *SEM* was less than 2.0), as shown in Figure 17.3.

Based on normal distribution characteristics,* we can determine *probable* and *improbable* values of sample means from the population of nursing studies. If, as is assumed in the null hypothesis, the population mean is 50.0, then 95% of all sample means would fall between 46.0 and 54.0, that is, within about 2 *SD*s above and below the mean of 50.0. The obtained sample mean of 74.1 lies in the critical region considered *improbable* if the null hypothesis were correct—in fact, any value greater than 54.0% female would be improbable if a true population mean of 50.0 is assumed and the criterion of improbability is an alpha of .05.

*Strictly speaking, the appropriate theoretical distribution in this example is the *t* distribution, but with a large *N*, the *t* and normal distribution are highly similar.

The *improbable* range beyond 2 *SD*s corresponds to only 5% (100% − 95%) of the sampling distribution. In our study, the probability of obtaining a value of 74.1% female by chance alone was less than 1 in 10,000. We thus rejected the null hypothesis that the mean percentage of females in nursing studies was 50.0. We would not be justified in saying that we had *proved* the research hypothesis because the possibility of having made a Type I error remains—but the possibility is, in this case, remote. We can thus *accept* the alternative hypothesis that the population mean is not 50.0—that is, that males and females are not equally represented as participants in nursing studies.

TIP: Levels of significance are analogous to the CI values described earlier—an alpha of .05 is analogous to the 95% CI, and an alpha of .01 is analogous to the 99% CI. In our example of gender bias, the 95% CI around the mean of 74.1 was 71.1 to 77.1.

Statistical Tests

Researchers do not compute critical regions on a sampling distribution. Rather, they compute **test statistics** with their data. For every test statistic, there is a related theoretical distribution. The value of the computed test statistic is compared to values of the critical limits for the applicable distribution.

When researchers calculate a test statistic that is beyond the critical limit, the results are said to be **statistically significant**. The word *significant* does not mean *important* or *clinically meaningful*. In statistics, *significant* means that obtained results are not likely to have been the result of chance at a specified level of probability. A **nonsignificant result** means that an observed result could reflect chance fluctuations.

TIP: When the null hypothesis is retained (i.e., when results are nonsignificant), this is sometimes referred to as a *negative result*. Negative results are often disappointing to researchers and may lead to rejection of a manuscript by journal editors. Research reports with negative

---

results are not rejected because editors are prejudiced against certain types of outcomes; they are rejected because negative results are usually inconclusive and difficult to interpret. A nonsignificant result indicates that the result *could* have occurred as a result of chance and provides no evidence that the research hypothesis is or is not correct.

One-Tailed and Two-Tailed Tests

In most hypothesis-testing situations, researchers use **two-tailed tests**. This means that both tails of the sampling distribution are used to determine improbable values. In Figure 17.3, for example, the critical region that contains 5% of the sampling distribution's area involves 2½% in one tail of the distribution and 2½% at the other. If the significance level were .01, the critical regions would involve ½% in each tail.

When researchers have a strong basis for a directional hypothesis, they sometimes use a **one-tailed test**. For example, if we did an RCT study involving a program to improve prenatal practices among rural women, we would expect birth outcomes for the two groups not to just be *different*; we would expect program participants to *benefit*. It might not make sense to use the tail of the distribution signifying *worse* outcomes in the intervention group.

In one-tailed tests, the critical region of improbable values is in only one tail of the distribution—the tail corresponding to the direction of the hypothesis, as illustrated in Figure 17.4. Using our earlier

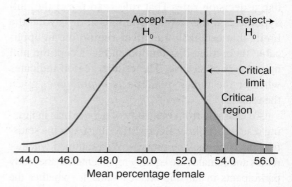

FIGURE 17.4 Critical region in the sampling distribution for a one-tailed test: gender bias example.

gender bias example, the research hypothesis being tested might be that the population mean is *greater than* 50.0—that is, that, on average, females are overrepresented in nursing studies. When a one-tailed test is used, the critical 5% area of "improbability" covers a bigger area of the specified tail, so one-tailed tests are less conservative. Thus, it is easier to reject the null hypothesis with a one-tailed test than with a two-tailed test. In our example, with an alpha of .05, a sample mean of 53.0 or greater would result in rejecting the null hypothesis for a one-tailed test rather than 54.0 for a two-tailed test.

One-tailed tests are controversial. Most researchers use a two-tailed test even if they have a directional hypothesis. In reading research reports, one can assume that two-tailed tests were used unless one-tailed tests are specifically mentioned. When there is a strong theoretical reason for a directional hypothesis and for assuming that findings in the opposite direction are virtually impossible, however, a one-tailed test might be warranted. In the remainder of this chapter, the examples are for two-tailed tests.

➲ TIP: You should choose a one-tailed test only if you state a directional hypothesis in advance of statistical testing. And, you must be prepared to attribute any observed group differences in the "wrong" direction to chance, even if the group differences are large.

Parametric and Nonparametric Tests
There are two broad classes of statistical tests, parametric and nonparametric. **Parametric tests** involve estimation of a parameter, require measurements on at least an interval scale, and involve several assumptions, such as the assumption that the variables are normally distributed in the population. **Nonparametric tests**, by contrast, do not estimate parameters. They involve less restrictive assumptions about the shape of the variables' distribution than do parametric tests. For this reason, nonparametric tests are sometimes called *distribution-free statistics*.

Parametric tests are more powerful than nonparametric tests and are usually preferred, but there

is some disagreement about the use of nonparametric tests. Purists insist that if the requirements of parametric tests are not met, they are inappropriate. Statistical studies have shown, however, that statistical decision making is not affected when the assumptions for parametric tests are violated if sample sizes are large. Nonparametric tests are most useful when data cannot in any manner be construed as interval-level, when the distribution is markedly non-normal, or when the sample size is very small.

➲ TIP: Some statisticians advise that when *N* is 50 or greater, it may not be necessary to use nonparametric statistics, unless the population has a markedly unusual distribution. Such advice invokes the **central limit theorem**, which, briefly, concerns the fact that when samples are large, the theoretical distribution of sample *means* tends to follow a normal distribution—*even if* the variable itself is not normally distributed in the population. With small *N*s, you cannot rely on the central limit theorem, so probability values could be wrong if a parametric test is used.

Between-Subjects Tests and Within-Subjects Tests
Another distinction in statistical tests concerns the nature of the comparisons. When comparisons involve different people (e.g., men versus women), the study uses a between-subjects design, and the statistical test is a **test for independent groups**. Other designs involve one group of people—for example, with a crossover design, participants are exposed to two or more treatments. In within-subjects designs, comparisons are not independent because the same people are used in all conditions, and the appropriate statistical tests are **tests for dependent groups**.

Overview of Hypothesis-Testing Procedures

This chapter describes several bivariate statistical tests. We have emphasized applications rather than computations but urge you to consult other references (e.g., Dancey et al., 2012; Gravetter &

Wallnau, 2013; Polit, 2010) for fuller explanations. In this research methods textbook, our goal is to provide an overview of the use and interpretation of some common statistical tests.

Each statistical test has a particular application, but the process of testing hypotheses is basically the same. The steps are as follows:

1. *Select an appropriate test statistic.* Figure 17.5 provides a quick reference guide for selecting many widely used bivariate statistical tests. (Multivariate tests are discussed in Chapter 18.) Researchers must consider such factors as which measurement levels were used, whether a parametric test is justified, whether a dependent groups test is needed, and whether the focus is correlations or group comparisons—and how many groups are being compared.
2. *Establish the level of significance.* Researchers establish the criterion for accepting or rejecting the null hypothesis. An α of .05 is usually acceptable.
3. *Select a one-tailed or two-tailed test.* In most cases, a two-tailed test should be used.
4. *Compute a test statistic.* Using collected data, researchers calculate a test statistic using appropriate computational formulas or instruct a computer to calculate the statistic.
5. *Determine the degrees of freedom* (symbolized as *df*). **Degrees of freedom** refers to the number of observations free to vary about a parameter. The concept is too complex for full elaboration here, but *df* is easy to compute.
6. *Compare the test statistic with a tabled value.* Theoretical distributions for test statistics enable researchers to determine whether obtained values of the test statistic (Step 4) are beyond the range of what is *probable* if the null hypothesis were true. Computed test statistic values are compared to values in a table. If the absolute value of the test statistic is larger than the tabled value, the results are statistically significant. If the computed value is smaller, the results are nonsignificant.

When analyses are done by a computer, as is usually the case, researchers follow only the first three steps and then give commands to the computer. The computer calculates the test statistic, degrees of freedom, and the *actual* probability that the null hypothesis is true. For example, the computer may show that the two-tailed probability (p) of an

Level of Measurement of Dependent Variable	Group Comparisons: Number of groups (the independent variable)				Correlational analyses (to examine relationship strength)
	2 Groups		3+ Groups		
	Independent Groups Tests	Dependent Groups Tests	Independent Groups Tests	Dependent Groups Tests	
Nominal (categorical)	χ^2 (or Fisher's exact test)	McNemar's test	χ^2	Cochran's Q	Phi coefficient (dichotomous) or Cramér's V (not restricted to dichotomous)
Ordinal (rank)	Mann-Whitney test	Wilcoxon signed ranks test	Kruskal-Wallis H test	Friedman's test	Spearman's rho (or Kendall's tau)
Interval or ratio (continuous)*	Independent group t-test	Paired t-test	ANOVA	RM-ANOVA	Pearson's r
	Multifactor ANOVA for 2+ independent variables				
	RM-ANOVA for 2+ groups x 2+ measurements over time				

*For distributions that are markedly non-normal or samples that are small, the nonparametric tests in the row above may be needed.

FIGURE 17.5 Quick guide to bivariate statistical tests.

intervention group being different from a control group by chance alone is .025. This means that only 25 times out of 1,000 would a group difference as large as the one obtained reflect chance differences rather than true intervention effects. The computed probability can then be compared with the desired significance level. If the significance criterion were .05, then the results would be significant, because .025 is more stringent than .05. By convention, any computed probability greater than .05 (e.g., .20) indicates nonsignificance (sometimes abbreviated *NS*)—that is, a result that could have occurred by chance in more than 5 out of 100 samples.

➔ **TIP:** The reference guide in Figure 17.5 does not include every test you may need, but it does include bivariate tests most often used by nurse researchers. Many resources are now available online to help with selecting an appropriate test, including interactive decision-tree tools. Links to useful websites are included in the Toolkit of the *Resource Manual* for you to click on directly.

In the sections that follow, several of the most common bivariate statistical tests and their applications are described. It is important to note that our introduction to inferential statistics is simplified and neglects important issues such as specific assumptions underlying various tests. We urge readers to have a good grasp of statistical principles before undertaking quantitative analyses.

TESTING DIFFERENCES BETWEEN TWO GROUP MEANS

A common research situation involves comparing two groups of participants on a continuous dependent variable. For instance, we might compare an experimental and control group of patients with regard to their mean blood pressure. Or, we might contrast men and women with regard to mean depression scores.

The parametric procedure for testing differences in group means is the *t*-test. A *t*-test can be used

when there are two independent groups (e.g., experimental versus control) and also when the sample is dependent (e.g., pretreatment and posttreatment scores for the same people).

➔ **TIP:** A **one-sample *t*-test** can be used to compare mean values of a single group to a hypothesized value. One-sample *t*-tests were used in Polit and Beck's (2013) study of gender bias in nursing studies, which tested obtained mean values to a hypothesized population value of 50.0.

t-Tests for Independent Groups

Suppose we wanted to test the effect of early discharge of maternity patients on perceived maternal competence. We administer a scale of perceived maternal competence at discharge to 20 primiparas who had a vaginal delivery: 10 who remained in the hospital 25 to 48 hours (regular-discharge group) and 10 who were discharged within 24 hours of delivery (early-discharge group). In Table 17.1, we see that mean scores for these two groups are 25.0

TABLE 17.1 • Fictitious Data for *t*-Test Example: Scores on a Perceived Maternal Competence Scale for Regular-Discharge and Early-Discharge Mothers

REGULAR-DISCHARGE MOTHERS	EARLY-DISCHARGE MOTHERS
30	23
27	17
25	22
20	18
24	20
32	26
17	16
18	13
28	21
29	14
Mean = 25.0	Mean = 19.0

$t = 2.86$: $df = 18$; $p = .011$

and 19.0, respectively. Are these differences *reliable* (i.e., Would they be found in the population of early-discharge and later-discharge mothers?), or do group differences reflect chance factors?

Note that the 20 scores in Table 17.1—10 per group—vary from one person to another. Some variability reflects individual differences in perceived maternal competence. Some variability might be due to measurement error (e.g., the scale's low reliability), some could result from participants' moods on a particular day, and so forth. The research question is: Can a portion of the variability reliably be attributed to the independent variable—time of discharge from the hospital? The *t*-test allows us to answer this question objectively. The hypotheses are

$$H_0: \mu_A = \mu_B \qquad H_A: \mu_A \neq \mu_B$$

To test these hypotheses, we would compute a *t*-statistic. The formula for the *t*-statistic uses group means, variability, and sample size to calculate a value for *t*. When the data from Table 17.1 are used in the formula, the value of *t* is 2.86. Next, degrees of freedom are calculated. In this situation, degrees of freedom equal the total sample size minus 2 ($df = 20 - 2 = 18$). A table of critical *t* values is shown in Table A.1, Appendix A. Degrees of freedom are listed in the left column, and different alpha values are shown in the top rows. The shaded column shows values for $\alpha = .05$ for a two-tailed test. We find in this column that for $df = 18$, the tabled value of *t* is 2.10. *This value establishes an upper limit to what is probable if the null hypothesis is true.* Thus, the calculated *t* of 2.86, which is larger than the tabled value of the statistic,[†] is improbable (i.e., statistically significant). We can now say that the primiparas discharged early had significantly lower perceptions of maternal competence than those who were not discharged early. The group difference in perceived maternal competence is sufficiently large that it is unlikely to reflect merely chance fluctuations. If a computer were used to analyze the data, the output would show the

exact probability, which is .011. This means that in only 11 out of 1,000 samples would we expect a group difference of 6.0 points by chance alone.

> **Example of Independent *t*-Tests:** White and colleagues (2014) studied the effect of a large-scale quality improvement program in Ireland (the Productive Ward: releasing time to care initiative) on the level of work engagement in hospital-based ward teams. The mean work engagement score was 4.33 among staff in the Productive group compared to 4.07 among those in the control group; an independent groups *t*-test revealed that this difference was statistically significant, $p = .01$.

When multiple tests are run with the same data—that is, when there are multiple dependent variables—the risk of a Type I error increases. One *t*-test with an $\alpha = .05$ has a 5% probability of a Type I error. Two *t*-tests with the same data set, however, have a probability of 9.75% of one spurious significant result, and with three tests, the risk goes up to 14.3%. Researchers sometimes apply a **Bonferroni correction** when they run multiple tests, to establish a more conservative alpha level. For example, if the desired α is .05, and there are three separate tests, the corrected alpha needed to reject the null hypothesis for *all* tests would be .017, not .05. The correction is computed by dividing the desired α by the number of tests—for example, $.05 / 3 = .017$. If we concluded that mean group differences were significant for three tests at or below $p = .017$, there would be only a 5% probability of wrongly rejecting the null across all three comparisons. The Bonferroni correction can, however, be problematic in that it tends to increase the risk of a Type II error—incorrectly concluding there is no statistical association when in fact there is one.

Confidence Intervals for Mean Differences

Confidence intervals can be constructed around the difference between two means, and the results provide information about both statistical significance (i.e., whether the null hypothesis should be rejected) and precision of the estimated difference. Because CI information is richer and more useful in clinical applications than *p* values, it is sometimes preferred—although nursing journals have not yet required it, as many medical journals have.

[†]The tabled *t* values should be compared to the absolute value of the calculated *t*. Thus, if the calculated *t* were −2.86, then the results would still be significant.

In the example in Table 17.1, the mean maternal competence scores were 25.0 in the regular discharge group and 19.0 in the early discharge group. Using a formula to compute the *standard error of the difference*, CIs can be constructed around the mean difference of 6.0. For a 95% CI, the confidence limits in our example are 1.6 and 10.4. This means that we can be 95% confident that the true difference in population means for early- and regular-discharge mothers lies somewhere between these limits.

In the *t*-test analysis, we obtained an estimate of mean group differences (6.0) and learned that the group differences were probably not spurious (*p* = .011). The CI information tells us the range within which the mean difference probably lies. We can see from the CI that the mean difference is significant at the .05 level *because the range does not include 0*. Given that there is a 95% probability that the mean difference is not lower than 1.6, this means that there is less than a 5% probability that there is no difference at all—thus, the null hypothesis can be rejected.

Because the CI does not give exact probabilities about the plausibility of the null hypothesis, it is often useful to present both parameter estimation and hypothesis testing information in reports. In the current example, the results could be reported as follows: "Mothers who were discharged early had significantly lower maternal competence scores (19.0) than mothers with a regular discharge (26.0) (*t* = 2.86, *df* = 18, *p* = .011). The mean difference of 6.0 had a 95% CI of 1.6 to 10.4." Such information is more conveniently displayed in tables when there are multiple dependent variables.

TIP: The Toolkit section of the accompanying *Resource Manual* has some table templates that may be useful for presenting findings from analyses described in this chapter.

Paired *t*-Tests

Researchers sometimes obtain two measurements from the same people or from paired sets of participants (e.g., siblings). When means for two sets of scores are not independent, researchers should use a **paired *t*-test**—a *t*-test for dependent groups.

Suppose we were studying the effect of a special diet on the cholesterol level of elderly men. A sample of 50 men is randomly selected, and their cholesterol levels are measured before and again after 2 months on the diet. The hypotheses being tested are

$$H_0: \mu_{x_1} = \mu_{x_2} \qquad H_A: \mu_{x_1} \neq \mu_{x_2}$$

where X_1 = pretreatment cholesterol levels
X_2 = posttreatment cholesterol levels

A *t*-statistic then would be computed from pretest and posttest data, using a different formula than for the independent group *t*-test. The obtained *t* would be compared with tabled *t* values. For this type of *t*-test, degrees of freedom equals the number of paired observations minus one (*df* = *N* − 1). Confidence intervals can be constructed around mean differences for paired as well as independent means.

Example of Paired *t*-Tests: Nicoteri and Miskovsky (2014) compared the body mass index (BMI) for 125 students in their freshman and senior years at a small U.S. college. A paired *t*-test indicated that there was no significant mean differences between admission BMI and the BMI 4 years later.

Nonparametric Two-Group Tests

In certain two-group situations, a nonparametric test may be needed—for example, if the dependent variable is on an ordinal scale or if the distribution is markedly non-normal. The **Mann-Whitney U test**, the nonparametric analog of an independent group's *t*-test, involves assigning ranks to the two groups of scores. The sum of the ranks for the two groups can be compared by calculating the *U* statistic. When ordinal-level data are paired (dependent), the Wilcoxon signed-rank test can be used. The **Wilcoxon signed-rank test** involves taking the difference between paired scores and ranking the absolute difference.

TESTING MEAN DIFFERENCES WITH THREE OR MORE GROUPS

Analysis of variance (ANOVA) is the parametric procedure for testing differences between means when there are three or more groups. The statistic computed in ANOVA is the **F-ratio**. ANOVA decomposes total variability in a dependent variable into two parts: (1) variability attributable to the independent variable and (2) all other variability, such as individual differences, measurement error, and so on. Variation *between* groups is contrasted to variation *within* groups to get an F-ratio. When differences between groups are large relative to variation within groups, the probability is high that the independent variable is related to, or has caused, group differences.

One-Way ANOVA

Suppose we were comparing the effectiveness of alternative interventions to help people stop smoking. One group of smokers receives intensive nurse counseling (group A), a second group is treated by a nicotine patch (group B), and a third control group receives no special treatment (group C). The dependent variable is 1-day cigarette consumption measured 1 month after the intervention. Thirty smokers who wish to quit smoking are randomly

assigned to one of the three conditions. **One-way ANOVA** tests the following hypotheses:

$$H_0: \mu_A = \mu_B = \mu_C \qquad H_A: \mu_A \neq \mu_B \neq \mu_C$$

The null hypothesis is that the population means for posttreatment cigarette smoking are the same for all three groups, and the alternative (research) hypothesis is inequality of means. Table 17.2 presents fictitious data for all participants. The mean numbers of posttreatment cigarettes consumed are 16.6, 19.2, and 34.0 for groups A, B, and C, respectively. These means are different, but are they significantly different—or do differences reflect random fluctuations?

In calculating an F-statistic, total variability in the data is broken down into two sources. The portion of the variance due to group status (i.e., exposure to different treatments) is reflected in the **sum of squares between groups**, or SS_B. The SS_B is the sum of squared deviations of individual group means from the overall **grand mean** for all participants. SS_B reflects variability in scores attributable to the independent variable, that is, group membership.

The second component is the **sum of squares within groups**, or SS_W. This index is the sum of the squared deviations of each individual score from its *own* group mean. SS_W indicates variability attributable to individual differences, measurement error, and so on.

TABLE 17.2 • Fictitious Data for a One-Way ANOVA: Number of Cigarettes Smoked in One Day, 1 Month Postintervention in Three Treatment Groups

GROUP A NURSE COUNSELING		GROUP B NICOTINE PATCH		GROUP C UNTREATED CONTROL	
28	19	0	27	33	35
0	24	31	0	54	0
17	0	26	3	19	43
20	21	30	24	40	39
35	2	24	27	41	36
$\bar{X}_A = 16.6$		$\bar{X}_B = 19.2$		$\bar{X}_C = 34.0$	

$F = 4.98$, $df = 2, 27$, $p = .01$

Recall from Chapter 16 that the formula for calculating a sample variance is $\Sigma x^2 \div N - 1$. The two sums of squares are like the numerator of this variance equation: Both SS_B and SS_W are sums of squared deviations from means. So, to compute variance within and variance between groups, we must divide the sums of squares by something similar to $N - 1$, namely, degrees of freedom for each sum of squares. For between groups, $df_B = G - 1$ (number of groups minus 1). For within groups, df_W is the number of participants less 1, for each group.

In an ANOVA context, the variance is conventionally referred to as the **mean square** (MS). The formulas for the mean square between groups and the mean square within groups are

$$MS_B = \frac{SS_B}{df_B} \qquad MS_W = \frac{SS_W}{df_W}$$

The F-ratio statistic is the ratio of these mean squares, or

$$F = \frac{MS_B}{MS_W}$$

The ANOVA summary table (Table 17.3) shows that the calculated F-statistic in our example is 4.98. For $df = 2$ and 27 and $\alpha = .05$, the tabled F-value is 3.35 (see Table A.2 in Appendix A for values from the theoretical F distribution). Because our obtained F-value of 4.98 exceeds 3.35, we reject the null hypothesis that the population means are equal. The *actual* probability, calculated by computer, is .014. Mean group differences in the number of posttreatment cigarettes smoked are beyond chance expectations. In only 14 samples out of 1,000 would differences this great be obtained by chance alone.

The data support the research hypothesis that different treatments were associated with different cigarette smoking, but we cannot tell from the test whether treatment A was significantly more effective than treatment B. Statistical analyses known as **multiple comparison procedures** (or **post hoc tests**) are needed. Their function is to isolate the differences between group means that are responsible for rejecting the overall ANOVA null hypothesis. Note that it is *not* appropriate to use a series of *t*-tests (group A versus B, A versus C, and B versus C) because this would increase the risk of a Type I error. Multiple comparison methods are described in most intermediate statistical textbooks, such as that by Polit (2010).

Example of a One-Way ANOVA: Park and colleagues (2014) conducted a randomized trial that compared text messages (TM) for medication reminders and education, TM for education only, or no TM among 90 patients with coronary heart disease. Using ANOVA, the researchers found that medication adherence for antiplatelets was significantly higher in the two TM groups for percentage of correct doses taken, $F(2, 41) = 3.29$, $p = .047$, and percentage of doses taken on schedule, $F(2, 41) = 3.53$, $p = .04$.

Two-Way ANOVA

One-way ANOVA is used to test the relationship between one categorical independent variable (e.g., different interventions) and a continuous dependent variable. Data from studies with multiple factors, as in a factorial design, are sometimes analyzed by *multifactor ANOVA*. In this section, we describe some principles underlying **two-way ANOVA**.

Suppose we wanted to test whether the two smoking cessation treatments (nurse counseling and a

TABLE 17.3 • ANOVA Summary Table for Posttreatment Smoking Example

SOURCE OF VARIANCE	SS	df	MEAN SQUARE	F	p
Between groups	1761.9	2	880.9	4.98	.014
Within groups	4772.0	27	176.7		
TOTAL	6533.9	29			

nicotine patch) were equally effective for men and women. We randomly assign women and men, separately, to the two treatment conditions. One month after the intervention, participants report the number of cigarettes they smoked the previous day. Fictitious data for this example are shown in Table 17.4.

With two independent variables, three hypotheses are tested. First, we are testing the effectiveness, for both men and women, of nurse counseling versus the nicotine patch. Second, we are testing whether postintervention smoking differs for men and women, regardless of treatment approach. These are tests for **main effects**. Third, we are testing for **interaction effects** (i.e., differential treatment effects on men and women). Interaction concerns whether the effect of one independent variable is consistent for all levels of a second independent variable.

The data in Table 17.4 reveal that participants in the Nurse Counseling group smoked less, on average, than those in Nicotine Patch group (19.0 versus 25.0); that women smoked less than men

after treatment (21.0 versus 23.0); and that men smoked less when exposed to nurse counseling, but women smoked less when exposed to the nicotine patch. By performing a two-way ANOVA on these data, we could learn whether the differences were statistically significant.

Multifactor ANOVA is not restricted to two-way analyses. In theory, any number of independent variables is possible but in practice studies with more than two factors are rare. Other statistical techniques typically are used with three or more independent variables, as we discuss in Chapter 18.

Repeated-Measures ANOVA

Repeated-measures ANOVA (RM-ANOVA) is used in several situations, one of which is when there are three or more measures of the same dependent variable for each participant. For instance, in some studies, physiologic measures such as blood pressure or heart rate might be collected before, during,

TABLE 17.4 • Fictitious Data for a Two-Way (2 × 2) ANOVA: Number of Cigarettes Smoked in One Day, 1 Month Postintervention for Gender × Treatment Groups

FACTOR B—GENDER	FACTOR A—TREATMENT			
	Nurse Counseling (1)		Nicotine Patch (2)	
Female (1)	24	25	27	23
	28	38	0	18
	2	21	45	20
	19	0	29	12
	27	36	22	4 — Female $\bar{X}_{B1} = 21.0$
	$\bar{X}_{A1B1} = 22.0$		$\bar{X}_{A2B1} = 20.0$	
Male (2)	10	16	36	27
	21	18	41	0
	17	3	28	49 — Male
	0	25	37	35
	33	17	5	42 — $\bar{X}_{B2} = 23.0$
	$\bar{X}_{A1B2} = 16.0$		$\bar{X}_{A2B2} = 30.0$	
Total	Treatment 1 $\bar{X}_{A1} = 19.0$		Treatment 2 $\bar{X}_{A2} = 25.0$	$\bar{X}_T = 22.0$

and after a medical procedure. In this situation, a one-way RM-ANOVA is an extension of a paired *t*-test. It can be used with a single group studied longitudinally, or in a crossover design with three or more different conditions. (In Chapter 18, we discuss RM-ANOVA for mixed designs.)

As an example, suppose we wanted to compare three interventions for preterm infants, with regard to effects on infants' feeding rates: (1) nonnutritive sucking, (2) nonnutritive sucking plus music, or (3) music alone. Using an experimental crossover design, the infants participating in the study are randomly assigned to different orderings of the three treatments. Bottle feeding rate, the dependent variable, is measured after each treatment. The null hypothesis for this study is that type of intervention is unrelated to feeding rate (i.e., $\mu_1 = \mu_2 = \mu_3$). The alternative hypothesis is that feeding rate and type of intervention are related (i.e., that the three population means are not all equal).

We would find in such a study that there was variability in feeding rates both across infants within each condition and across the three treatment conditions within infants. As was true with other ANOVA situations, total variability in the dependent variable is represented by the total sum of squares, which can be partitioned into contributing components. In RM-ANOVA, three sources of variation contribute to total variability:

$$SS_{total} = SS_{treatments} + SS_{subjects} + SS_{error}$$

Conceptually, *sum of squares–treatments* is analogous to sum of squares–between in regular ANOVA: It represents the effect of the independent variable. (When measurements are taken at multiple points without an intervention, it may be called *sum of squares–time*.) The *sum of squares–error* is similar to the sum of squares–within in regular ANOVA: Both represent variations associated with random fluctuations. The third component, *sum of squares–subjects*, has no counterpart in a simple ANOVA, because those being compared in regular ANOVA are not the same people. The $SS_{subjects}$ term captures individual differences, the effects of which are consistent across conditions. That is,

some infants tend to have high feeding rates and others tend to have low feeding rates, regardless of treatment. Because individual differences can be statistically isolated from the error term (random fluctuation), RM-ANOVA yields a more sensitive test of the relationship between the independent and dependent variables than between-subjects ANOVA. By statistical isolation, we mean that variability attributable to individual differences is removed from the denominator in computing the *F*-statistic.

Example of RM-ANOVA: Harrington and colleagues (2014) studied changes in body composition and metabolic profile in men who received androgen-deprivation therapy (ADT) compared to those not receiving ADT. Data were collected at baseline and at 3-month intervals for 1 year. The data were analyzed both for within group and between group changes over time using RM-ANOVA. One finding was that the ADT group experienced a significant but transient change in measures of insulin resistance at the 3-month point ($p < .02$).

Nonparametric "Analysis of Variance"

Nonparametric tests do not, strictly speaking, analyze variance, but there are nonparametric analogs to ANOVA when a parametric test is not appropriate. The **Kruskal-Wallis test** is a generalized version of the Mann-Whitney *U* test, based on assigning ranks to the scores of various groups. This test is used when the number of groups is greater than two- and a one-way test for independent samples is desired. When multiple measures are obtained from the same subjects, the **Friedman test** for "analysis of variance" by ranks can be used. Both tests are described in Polit (2010) and other statistics textbooks.

TESTING DIFFERENCES IN PROPORTIONS

Tests discussed thus far involve dependent variables measured on an interval or ratio scale, when group means are being compared. In this section, we examine tests of group differences when the dependent variable is on a nominal scale.

The Chi-Square Test

The **chi-square** (χ^2) **test** is used to test hypotheses about group differences in proportions, as when a crosstabs table has been created. Suppose we were studying the effect of nursing instruction on patients' compliance with a self-medication regimen. Nurses implement a new instructional strategy with 100 randomly assigned experimental patients, while 100 control group patients are cared for using usual instruction. The research hypothesis is that a higher proportion of people in the intervention group than in the control group will be compliant.

The chi-square statistic is computed by comparing observed frequencies (i.e., values observed in the data) and expected frequencies. **Observed frequencies** for our example are shown in Table 17.5. As this table shows, 60 experimental participants (60%), but only 40 controls (40%), reported self-medication compliance after the intervention. The chi-square test enables us to decide whether a difference in proportions of this magnitude is likely to reflect a real treatment effect or only chance fluctuations. **Expected frequencies** are the cell frequencies that would be found if there were *no* relationship between the two variables. In this example, if there were no relationship between the two groups, the expected frequency would be 50 people per cell because, overall, exactly half the participants (100 out of 200) complied.

The chi-square statistic is computed by summarizing differences between observed and expected frequencies for each cell. Formulas and computations are not shown here, but in our example, $\chi^2 = 8.00$. For chi-square tests, *df* equals the number of rows minus 1 times number of columns minus 1. In the current case, $df = 1 \times 1 = 1$. With 1 *df*, the tabled value (Table A.3 of Appendix A) from a theoretical chi-square distribution that must be exceeded to establish significance at the .05 level is 3.84. The obtained value of 8.00 is much larger than would be expected by chance (actual $p = .005$). We can conclude that a significantly larger proportion of experimental patients than control patients were compliant.

Example of Chi-Square Test: Hogan (2014) studied socioeconomic factors in relation to infant sleep-related deaths, using a case-control design. Chi-square analysis was used to test whether poverty status (poor/not poor) and race/ethnicity was related to a sleep-related death in the infants' first year of life. She found, for example, that a higher percentage of poor mothers (55.3%) experienced an infant death than nonpoor mothers (29.2%) ($\chi^2 = 5.11$, $p = .024$).

Confidence Intervals for Differences in Proportion

As with means, it is possible to construct confidence intervals around the difference between two proportions. To do this, we would need to calculate the *standard error of the difference of proportions*. In the example used to explain the chi-square statistic, the difference in proportions was .20 ($p < .01$),

TABLE 17.5 • Observed Frequencies for Chi-Square Example: Patient Compliance in Two Treatment Groups

PATIENT COMPLIANCE	GROUP		
	CONTROL	EXPERIMENTAL	TOTAL
Compliant	40	60	100
Noncompliant	60	40	100
TOTAL	100	100	200

$X^2 = 8.00$, $df = 1$, $p = .005$

and the *SE* of the difference is .069. The 95% CI in this example is .06 to .34. We can be 95% confident that the true population difference in compliance rates between those exposed to the intervention and those not exposed is between 6% and 34%. This interval does not include 0%, indicating that we can be 95% confident that group differences are "real."

Other Tests of Proportions

Sometimes a chi-square test is not appropriate. When the total sample size is small (total *N* of 30 or less) or when there are cells with small frequencies (five or fewer), **Fisher's exact test** should be used to test the significance of differences in proportions. When the proportions being compared are from two paired groups (e.g., when a pretest–posttest design is used to compare changes in proportions on a dichotomous variable), the appropriate test is **McNemar's test**.

TESTING CORRELATIONS

The statistical tests discussed thus far are used to test differences between *groups*—they involve situations in which the independent variable is a nominal-level variable. In this section, we consider statistical tests used when both the independent and the dependent variables are ordinal, interval, or ratio.

Pearson's *r*

Pearson's *r*, the correlation coefficient calculated when two variables are measured on at least the interval scale, is both descriptive and inferential. Descriptively, the correlation coefficient summarizes the magnitude and direction of a relationship between two variables. As an inferential statistic, *r* tests hypotheses about population correlations, which are symbolized as ρ, the Greek letter rho. The null hypothesis is that there is no relationship between two variables:

$$H_0: \rho = 0 \qquad H_A: \rho \neq 0$$

For instance, suppose we studied the relationship between patients' self-reported level of stress and the pH level of their saliva. In a sample of 50 people, we find that $r = -.29$, indicating a modest tendency for people with high stress scores to have low pH levels. But can we generalize this finding to the population? Does the coefficient of $-.29$ reflect a random fluctuation, observable only for the people in our sample, or is the relationship likely to be true in the population? We can compare our computed *r* to a tabled value from a theoretical distribution for *r*. Degrees of freedom for *r* equal the number of participants minus 2, or $(N - 2)$. With $df = 48$, the tabled value for *r* for a two-tailed test with $\alpha = .05$ (Table A.4 in Appendix A) is .2803. Because the absolute value of the calculated *r* is .29, the null hypothesis can be rejected. We accept the research hypothesis that the correlation between stress and saliva acidity in the population is not zero.

Pearson's *r* can be used in both within-group and between-group situations. The example about the relationship between stress scores and the pH levels is a between-group situation: The question is whether people with high stress scores tend to have significantly lower pH levels than *different* people with low stress scores. If stress scores were obtained both before and after surgery, however, the correlation between the two scores would be a within-group situation.

Example of Pearson's *r*: Kawano and Emori (2015) tested the hypothesis that mothers' postpartum psychological state is related to breast milk secretory immunoglobin A (SIgA). They found that breast milk SIgA was significantly negatively correlated with several measures of the mothers' psychological state, such as tension/anxiety ($r = -.33$, $p < .05$), anger/hostility ($r = -.39$, $p < .05$), and overall mental health ($r = -.63$, $p < .01$) in their sample of 81 Japanese mothers.

Other Tests of Bivariate Relationships

Pearson's *r* is a parametric statistic. When the assumptions for a parametric test are violated, or when the data are ordinal-level, then the appropriate coefficient of correlation is either **Spearman's rho** (r_S) or **Kendall's tau**. The values of these statistics range from -1.00 to $+1.00$, and their interpretation is similar to that of Pearson's r. Another correlation statistic that is used to correlate a dichotomous variable with a continuous one is called a **point-biserial correlation coefficient**. Interpretation of this statistic requires knowing how the dichotomous variable was coded (usually, it is 1 versus 0).

Indexes summarizing the magnitude of relationships can also be computed with nominal-level data. For example, the **phi coefficient** (Φ) is an index describing the relationship between two dichotomous variables. **Cramér's V** is an index of relationship applied to crosstabs tables larger than 2×2. Both statistics are based on the chi-square statistic and yield values that range between .00 and 1.00, with higher values indicating a stronger association between variables.

Inferential statistics are almost invariably calculated using statistical software. The Supplement to this chapter illustrates how *IBM SPSS Statistics* (SPSS) can be used to test hypotheses.

POWER ANALYSIS AND EFFECT SIZE

Many published nursing studies (and even more *un*published ones) have nonsignificant findings, and many of these could reflect Type II errors. As indicated earlier, researchers set the probability of committing a Type I error (a false positive) as the significance level, alpha (α). The probability of a Type II error (a false negative) is **beta** (β). The complement of beta ($1 - \beta$) is the *probability of detecting a true relationship or group difference* and is the **power** of a statistical test. Polit and Sherman (1990) found that many published nursing studies have insufficient power, placing them at risk for Type II errors—although a more recent study has found that, on average, power has improved in nursing studies, perhaps because greater attention has been paid to this topic (Gaskin & Happell, 2014). Nevertheless, even in the more recent analysis, many studies continued to be **underpowered**.

Power analysis is used to reduce the risk of Type II errors and strengthen statistical conclusion validity by estimating in advance how big a sample is needed. There are four components in a power analysis, three of which must be known or estimated:

1. *The significance criterion*, α. Other things being equal, the more stringent this criterion, the lower the power.
2. *The sample size, N*. As sample size increases, power increases.
3. *The effect size* (ES). ES is an estimate of how wrong the null hypothesis is, that is, how strong the relationship between the independent variable and the dependent variable is in the population.
4. *Power, or $1 - \beta$*. This is the probability of rejecting a false null hypothesis.

Researchers typically use power analysis at the outset of a study to estimate the sample size needed to avoid a Type II error. To estimate needed sample size (N), researchers must specify α, ES, and $1 - \beta$. Researchers usually establish the risk of a Type I error (α) as .05. The conventional standard for $1 - \beta$ is .80. With power equal to .80, there is a 20% risk of committing a Type II error. Although this risk may seem high, a stricter criterion requires sample sizes larger than many researchers could afford.

With α and $1 - \beta$ specified, the information needed to solve for N is ES, the estimated population effect size. The **effect size** is the magnitude of the relationship between the research variables. When relationships (effects) are strong, they can be detected at significant levels even with small samples. With modest relationships, large sample sizes are needed to avoid Type II errors.

In using power analysis to estimate sample size needs, the population effect size is not *known*; if it were known, there would be no need for the new study. Effect size must be estimated using available evidence and theory. In essence, the effect size estimate in a power analysis represents the researcher's *hypothesis* about how strong relationships are. Researchers sometimes use findings from a pilot study as a basis for the estimate—although we explain in Chapter 28 why this is risky. More often an effect size is calculated based on findings from earlier studies on a similar problem. When there are *no* relevant earlier findings and when theory offers only broad guidance, researchers use conventions based on expectations of a *small*, *medium*, or *large* effect. Most nursing studies have modest (small-to-medium) effects.

TIP: Researchers can usually find more than one study from which the effect size can be estimated. In such a case, the estimate should be based on the study with the most reliable results. Researchers can also estimate effect size by combining information from multiple high-quality studies through averaging or weighted averaging. If you are studying a problem that has been the focus of a meta-analysis, ES estimates will likely be readily available in the report.

Procedures for estimating effects and sample size needs vary from one statistical situation to another. We focus mainly on a two-group situation for which we can estimate mean values.

Sample Size Estimates for Testing Differences between Two Means

Suppose we were testing the hypothesis that cranberry juice reduces the urinary pH of diet-controlled patients. We plan to assign some patients randomly to a control condition (no cranberry juice) and others to an experimental condition in which they will be given 300 mL of cranberry juice for 5 days. How large a sample is needed for this study, given a desired α of .05 and power of .80?

To answer this, we must first estimate ES. In a two-group situation in which mean differences are of interest, ES is usually designated as **Cohen's *d***, the formula for which is

$$d = \frac{\mu_1 - \mu_2}{\sigma}$$

That is, the effect size (*d*) is the difference between the two population means, divided by the population standard deviation (σ). These population values are never known but must be estimated. For example, suppose we found an earlier nonexperimental study that compared the urinary pH of people who had or had not ingested cranberry juice

in the previous 24 hours. The earlier and planned studies are different in many respects, but the earlier study is a reasonable starting point. Suppose the results were as follows:

$$\overline{X}_1(\text{no cranberry juice}) = 5.70$$
$$\overline{X}_2(\text{cranberry juice}) = 5.50$$
$$SD = .50$$

Thus, the estimated value of *d* would be .40:

$$d = \frac{5.70 - 5.50}{.50} = .40$$

Table 17.6 presents approximate sample size requirements for various effect sizes and powers, for $\alpha = .05$ (for two-tailed tests), in a two-group mean-difference situation. We find in this table that the estimated *n* (number per group) to detect an effect size of .40 with power equal to .80 is 99 people. Assuming that the earlier study provided a good estimate of the population effect size, the total number of people needed in the new study would be about 200, with half assigned to the control group (no cranberry juice) and the other half assigned to the experimental group. With a sample size smaller than 200, there would be a greater than 20% chance of a false negative conclusion, that is, a Type II error. For example, a sample size of 128 (64 per group) would result in an estimated 40% chance of incorrect nonsignificant results.

If there is no prior research, researchers can, as a last resort, estimate whether the expected effect is small, medium, or large. By convention (Cohen, 1988), the value of *ES* in a two-group test of mean differences is estimated at .20 for small effects, .50 for medium effects, and .80 for large effects. With an α value of .05 and power of .80, the *n* (number of participants per group) for studies with expected small, medium, and large effects would be 394, 64, and 25, respectively. Most nursing studies cannot expect effect sizes in excess of .50; those in the range of .20 to .40 are most common. In Polit and Sherman's (1990) analysis of effect sizes for studies published in *Nursing Research* and *Research in Nursing & Health*, the average effect size for *t*-test situations was .35. Cohen (1988) noted that in new areas of research inquiry, effect sizes are likely to

TABLE 17.6 • Approximate Sample Sizes* per Group Needed to Achieve Selected Levels of Power as a Function of Estimated Effect Size for Test of Difference of Two Means, for $\alpha = .05$

POWER	ESTIMATED EFFECT SIZE (d)†										
	.10	.15	.20	.25	.30	.35	.40	.50	.60	.70	.80
.60	979	435	245	157	109	80	62	40	28	20	16
.70	1233	548	309	198	137	101	78	50	35	26	20
.80	1576	701	394	253	176	129	99	64	44	33	25
.90	2103	935	526	337	234	172	132	85	59	43	33
.95	2594	1154	649	416	289	213	163	105	73	53	41

*Sample size requirements for each group; total sample size would be twice the number shown.
†Estimated effect size (d) is the estimated population mean group difference divided by the estimated population standard deviation or $(\mu_1 - \mu_2)/\sigma$.

be small. A medium effect should be estimated only when the effect is so substantial that it can be detected by the naked eye (i.e., without formal research procedures).

> ⮊ **TIP:** Performing a power analysis based on estimates of an effect size is an *evidence-based* approach to designing a new study—that is, the new study uses evidence from earlier studies to estimate how many sample members will be needed to achieve an effect that seems plausible in light of what is already known. A useful supplementary approach is to ask, "How big an effect would be needed to be clinically relevant?" If effect size estimates are both evidence-based and clinically meaningful, the study will be stronger.

Sample Size Estimates for Other Bivariate Tests

Power analysis can be undertaken for the other statistical tests described in this chapter. It is relatively easy to do a power analysis online (we suggest several relevant websites in the Toolkit with the *Resource Manual* ⊛). Here we discuss only a few basic features for situations in which ANOVA, Pearson's *r*, or a chi-square situation would be the basis for doing the power analysis.

There are alternative approaches to doing a power analysis in an ANOVA context. The simplest approach is to estimate **eta-squared** (η^2), which is an ES index indicating the proportion of variance explained in ANOVA. Eta-squared equals the sum of squares between (SS_B) divided by the total sum of squares (SS_T) and can be used directly as the estimate of effect size if sum of square information is available. When eta-squared cannot be estimated, researchers can estimate whether effects are likely to be small, medium, or large. For ANOVA situations, the conventional estimates for small, medium, and large effects would be values of η^2 equal to .01, .06, and .14, respectively. Assuming $\alpha = .05$ and power = .80, this corresponds to sample size requirements of about 319, 53, or 22 subjects *per group* in a three-group study, and about 272, 44, and 19 *per group* in a four-group study.‡ (For the data in Table 17.2 and shown in an ANOVA summary table in Table 17.3, $\eta^2 = .27$, a large effect.)

For Pearson correlations, the estimated value of ES is ρ, the population correlation coefficient. Thus, the value of the correlation coefficient (*r*) from a relevant earlier study can be used directly as the estimated effect size. Table 17.7 shows sample

---

‡Power tables are not provided here for ANOVA and chi-square situations.

TABLE 17.7 • Approximate Sample Sizes Necessary to Achieve Selected Levels of Power as a Function of Estimated Population Correlation Coefficient, for $\alpha = .05$

POWER	ESTIMATED POPULATION CORRELATION COEFFICIENT (ρ)*										
	.10	.15	.20	.25	.30	.35	.40	.50	.60	.70	.80
.60	489	217	122	78	54	39	30	19	13	9	7
.70	614	272	152	97	67	49	37	23	16	11	8
.80	785	347	194	123	85	62	47	29	19	13	10
.90	1047	463	258	164	112	81	61	37	25	17	12
.95	1296	575	322	204	141	101	80	50	32	22	18

*Estimated effect size (r) is the estimated population correlation coefficient (ρ).

size requirements in situations in which Pearson's r is used for various effect sizes and powers when $\alpha = .05$. For example, if our estimated population correlation was .25, we would need a sample size of 123 for power = .80. With a sample this size, we can expect that we would wrongly reject a true null hypothesis 5 times out of 100 and wrongly retain a false null hypothesis 20 times out of 100. When prior estimates of effect size are unavailable, the conventional values of small, medium, and large effect sizes in a bivariate correlation situation are .10, .30, and .50, respectively (i.e., samples of 785, 85, and 29 for a power of .80 and a significance level of .05). In Polit and Sherman's (1990) study, the average correlation in nursing studies was found to be around .20.

Estimating sample size requirements for testing differences in proportions between groups is complex. The effect size for crosstabs tables is influenced not only by expected differences in proportions (e.g., 60% in one group versus 40% in another, a 20% point difference) but also by the absolute values of the proportions. Effect sizes are *larger* (and thus sample size needs are *smaller*) at the extremes than near the midpoint. A 20% point difference is easier to detect if the percentages are 10% and 30% than if they are near the middle, such as 60% and 40%. Because of this fact, it is difficult to offer information on values for small, medium, and large effects in this context. We can, however,

give *examples* of differences in proportions that conform to the conventions in a 2 × 2 situation:

Small: .05 versus .10, .20 versus .29, .40 versus .50, .60 versus .70, .80 versus .87
Medium: .05 versus .21, .20 versus .43, .40 versus .65, .60 versus .82, .80 versus .96
Large: .05 versus .34, .20 versus .58, .40 versus .78, .60 versus .92, .80 versus .96

As an example, if the expected proportion for a control group were .40, the researcher would need about 385, 70, and 24 per group if higher values were expected for the experimental group and the effect was expected to be small, medium, and large, respectively. As in other situations, researchers are encouraged to avoid using the conventions in favor of more precise estimates based on existing evidence. If the conventions cannot be avoided, conservative estimates should be used to minimize the risk of obtaining nonsignificant results.

Example of a Power Analysis: Wang and colleagues (2015) used a randomized design to test the effect of abdominal massage in reducing malignant ascites symptoms in end-stage cancer patients. Power calculations to estimate sample size were based on an assumed moderate effect size. With a power of .80 and $\alpha = .05$, the power analysis indicated a need for 40 patients in the experimental and control groups. Eighty patients with malignant ascites were recruited.

> **→ TIP:** Although power analysis is frequently used to estimate sample size needs when planning a study, an alternative is to use *precision estimation*, which uses a confidence interval framework to estimate an appropriate sample size (Corty & Corty, 2011; Hayat, 2013). Another approach is to include benchmarks for *clinical significance* (Chapter 20) when estimating sample size needs.

Effect Size Calculations in Completed Studies

Power analysis concepts are sometimes used *after* analyses are completed to calculate estimated population effects based on *actual N*s. In this situation, power, alpha, and *N* are known, and so the task is to solve for ES. Effect sizes provide readers and clinicians with estimates about the magnitude of effects—an important issue in EBP (see Table 2.1). Effect size information can be crucial because, with large samples, even tiny effects can be statistically significant. *P* values tell you whether results are likely to be *real*, but effect sizes can suggest whether they are important. Effect size estimates are needed in doing meta-analyses (see Chapter 29), and so when these values are presented directly in a report, they are helpful to meta-analysts.

> **Example of Calculated Effect Size:** Hooge and colleagues (2014) tested the effects of a parenting education program using a quasi-experimental pretest–posttest design. The mothers' change in scores on a test of parenting knowledge was statistically significant, $F(1, 158) = 184.09$, $p < .001$, and the effect size was large ($\eta^2 = .54$).

CRITIQUING INFERENTIAL STATISTICAL ANALYSES

It is difficult to critique researchers' data analysis decisions without good training in statistics. Nevertheless, there are certain things you can do to critically appraise statistical analyses even if your background in statistics is modest.

You can begin by asking whether the report presents the results of statistical tests for all study hypotheses and whether the researchers undertook analyses to address questions about the study's internal validity. For example, in an RCT or case-control study, was the comparability of the groups assessed (i.e., were analyses undertaken to test for selection biases)? Did groups differ with regard to attrition? As noted in Chapter 10, statistical analyses and design issues are sometimes intertwined, in the sense that both analytic and design decisions can affect statistical conclusion validity. When sample size is small, when an independent variable is weakly defined (or when participation in an intervention is low), and when a weak statistical procedure is used in lieu of a more powerful one, then the risk of drawing the wrong conclusion about the research hypotheses is heightened. Risks to statistical conclusion validity should be considered when research hypotheses are not supported.

Other issues important in a thorough critique are whether the researcher used the right statistical tests, whether the statistical information reported is adequate to meet readers' information needs, and whether the results were presented in a clear and thoughtful manner, with a judicious combination of information reported in the text and in well laid-out tables. ✖ Box 17.1 presents some guiding questions for critiquing the use of bivariate inferential statistics in a research report.

> **→ TIP:** You may find it helpful to consult the glossary of statistical symbols in the inside back cover if you find a symbol in a research report that you do not recognize. Not all symbols in this glossary are described in this book, and so it may be necessary to refer to a statistics textbook for further information.

RESEARCH EXAMPLE

Study: Neonatal neurobehavioral organization after exposure to maternal epidural analgesia in labor (Bell et al., 2010)

BOX 17.1 Guidelines for Critiquing Bivariate* Inferential Analyses

1. Did the report include any bivariate inferential statistics? Was a statistical test performed for each hypothesis or research question? If inferential statistics were not used, should they have been?
2. Were statistical tests used to strengthen inferences about the study's internal validity (e.g., to test for selection bias or attrition bias)? If not, should they have been?
3. Were the selected statistical tests appropriate, given the level of measurement of the variables and the nature of the hypotheses?
4. Were parametric tests used? Does it appear that the use of parametric tests was appropriate? If nonparametric tests were used, was a rationale provided, and does the rationale seem sound?
5. Was information provided about both hypothesis testing and estimation of parameters? Were effect sizes reported? Overall, did the statistical results provide sufficient information about the study's evidence?
6. In general, did the report provide a rationale for the use of the selected statistical tests? Did the report contain sufficient information for you to judge whether appropriate statistics were used?
7. Were the results of any statistical tests significant? What do the tests tell you about the plausibility of the research hypotheses? Were effects sizeable?
8. Were the results of any statistical tests nonsignificant? Is it plausible that these reflect Type II errors? What factors might have undermined the study's statistical conclusion validity?
9. Was an appropriate amount of statistical information reported? Are the findings clearly and logically organized?
10. Were tables or figures used judiciously to summarize large amounts of statistical information? Are the tables clearly presented, with good titles and carefully labeled column headings? Is the information in the text consistent with the information presented in the tables? Is the information totally redundant?

*Most of these questions are equally appropriate for critiquing the use of multivariate statistics, as described in Chapter 18.

Statement of Purpose: The purpose of this study was to explore relationships between exposure to epidural analgesia in labor and measures of neurobehavioral organization in infants at the initial feeding 1 hour after birth.

Methods: A sample of 52 mothers (18 who were unmedicated and 34 who opted for an epidural) and their term infants was recruited for the study. A nutritive sucking apparatus yielded data on the infants' total number of sucks over a 5-minute period and sucking pressure. Video recordings of the infants before and after the first feeding were coded for frequency of alertness over a 15-minute period by raters blinded to mothers' use of epidural analgesia.

Analysis and Findings: The researchers presented a table summarizing key demographic and clinical characteristics of the two groups. Group differences were tested using *t*-tests for continuous variables

(e.g., maternal age) and chi-square tests for categorical variables (e.g., infant gender). The two groups were found to be significantly different in many respects. For example, the unmedicated group was significantly older ($p = .03$), more likely to be multiparous ($p = .03$), and had a shorter mean duration of labor ($p = .03$). The groups were similar with regard to gestational age ($p = .87$), infant birth weight ($p = .83$), and Pitocin dosage ($p = .14$).

The mean number of sucks was 37.6 (95% CI = 28.8, 46.3) in the unmedicated group and 34.4 (95% CI = 26.0, 42.9) in the epidural group. The two groups were not significantly different with regard to mean number of sucks ($t = .51, p = .61$), nor in terms of mean sucking pressure ($t = -.16, p = .87$).

Two-way ANOVA was used to compare the mean number of sucks of three medication groups (unmedicated, high-dose, and low-dose epidural) and infant girls versus boys (a 3 × 2 analysis). A post hoc test indicated that girls in the unmedicated group had a significantly higher number of sucks than girls in the high-dose group. Chi-square tests were used to compare the three groups (unmedicated, low-dose, and high-dose), separately by infant gender, in terms of having a low versus high number of sucks. Unmedicated girls (but not boys) were significantly more likely to be classified in the high-number group, while girls in the high epidural dosage group were more likely to be in the low-number group ($\chi^2 = 10.80$, $p = .005$).

Because of highly skewed data, the researchers used the Mann-Whitney U test to examine differences between the no medication and epidural groups with regard to infants' frequency of alertness. No significant differences were found either before feeding ($p = .40$) or after feeding ($p = .79$).

SUMMARY POINTS

- **Inferential statistics**, which are based on **laws of probability**, allow researchers to make inferences about a population based on data from a sample; they offer a framework for deciding whether the **sampling error** that results from sampling fluctuations is too high to provide reliable population estimates.

- The **sampling distribution of the mean** is a theoretical distribution of the means of an infinite number of samples drawn from a population. The sampling distribution of means follows a normal curve, and so the probability that a given sample value will be obtained can be ascertained.

- The **standard error of the mean** (*SEM*)—the standard deviation of this theoretical distribution—indicates the degree of average error of a sample mean; the smaller the *SEM*, the more accurate are the sample estimates of the population mean.

- Statistical inference consists of two approaches: estimating parameters and testing hypotheses. **Parameter estimation** is used to estimate a population parameter from a sample statistic.

- **Point estimation** provides a descriptive value of the population estimate (e.g., a mean or

odds ratio). **Interval estimation** provides the upper and lower limits of a range of values—the **confidence interval (CI)**—between which the population value is expected to fall at a specified probability. A 95% CI indicates a 95% probability that the true population value lies between the upper and lower **confidence limits**.

- **Hypothesis testing** through statistical procedures enables researchers to make objective decisions about the validity of their hypotheses.

- The **null hypothesis** states that there is no relationship between research variables and that any observed relationship is due to chance. Rejection of the null hypothesis lends support to the research hypothesis.

- A **Type I error** occurs when a null hypothesis is incorrectly rejected (a false positive). A **Type II error** occurs when a null hypothesis is wrongly accepted (a false negative).

- Researchers control the risk of a Type I error by establishing a **level of significance** (or **alpha** [α] level), which is the probability that such an error will occur. The .05 level means that in only 5 out of 100 samples would the null hypothesis be rejected when it should have been accepted.

- In testing hypotheses, researchers compute a **test statistic** and then determine whether the statistic falls at or beyond the **critical region** on a relevant theoretical distribution. If the value of the test statistic indicates that the null hypothesis is "improbable," the result is **statistically significant** (i.e., obtained results are not likely to result from chance fluctuations at the specified level of significance).

- Most hypothesis testing involves **two-tailed tests**, in which both ends of the sampling distribution are used to define the region of improbable values; a **one-tailed test** may be appropriate if there is a strong rationale for an a priori directional hypothesis.

- **Parametric tests** involve the estimation of at least one parameter, the use of interval- or ratio-level data, and the assumption of normally distributed variables; **nonparametric tests** are used when the data are nominal or ordinal or when a normal distribution cannot be assumed—especially when samples are small.

- **Tests for independent groups** compare different groups of people (between-subjects design), and **tests for dependent groups** compare the same group of people over time or conditions (within-subjects designs).
- Two common statistical tests are the **t-test** and **analysis of variance** (**ANOVA**), both of which are used to test the significance of the difference between group means; ANOVA is used when there are three or more groups (**one-way ANOVA**) or when there is more than one independent variable (e.g., **two-way ANOVA**). **Repeated-measures ANOVA** (**RM-ANOVA**) is used when there are multiple means being compared over time.
- The **chi-square test** (χ^2) is used to test hypotheses about differences in proportions. For small samples or small cell sizes, **Fisher's exact test** should be used.
- Statistical tests to measure the magnitude of bivariate relationships and to test whether the relationship is significantly different from zero include **Pearson's r** for continuous data, Spearman's rho and **Kendall's tau** for ordinal-level data, and the **phi coefficient** and **Cramér's V** for nominal-level data. A **point-biserial correlation coefficient** can be computed when one variable is dichotomous and the other is continuous.
- Confidence intervals can be constructed around almost any computed statistic, including differences between means, differences between proportions, and correlation coefficients. CI information is valuable to clinical decision makers, who need to know more than whether differences are probably real.
- **Power analysis** is a method of estimating either the likelihood of committing a Type II error or sample size requirements. Power analysis involves four components: desired significance level (α), **power** ($1 - \beta$), sample size (N), and estimated **effect size** (ES). Effect size estimates convey important information about the magnitude of effects in a study and are a useful supplement to p values and CI values.

Cohen's d is a widely used effect size index summarizing mean-difference effects between two groups.

STUDY ACTIVITIES

Chapter 17 of the *Resource Manual for Nursing Research: Generating and Assessing Evidence for Nursing Practice, 10th edition*, offers exercises and study suggestions for reinforcing concepts presented in this chapter. In addition, the following study questions can be addressed:

1. Which inferential statistics would you choose for the following sets of variables? Explain your answers (refer to Figure 17.5).
   a. Variable 1 = weights of 100 patients; Variable 2 = patients' resting heart rate
   b. Variable 1 = patients' marital status; Variable 2 = patients' level of preoperative stress on a 10-item scale
   c. Variable 1 = whether an amputee has a leg removed above or below the knee; Variable 2 = whether or not the amputee shows signs of aggressive behavior during rehabilitation
2. Apply relevant questions in Box 17.1 to the research example at the end of the chapter (Bell et al., 2010), referring to the full journal article as necessary.

STUDIES CITED IN CHAPTER 17

Bell, A., White-Traut, R., & Medoff-Cooper, B. (2010). Neonatal neurobehavioral organization after exposure to maternal epidural analgesia in labor. *Journal of Obstetric, Gynecologic, & Neonatal Nursing, 39*, 178–190.

Brahman, L. (1991). Confidence intervals assess both clinical significance and statistical significance. *Annals of Internal Medicine, 114*, 515–517.

Cohen, J. (1988). *Statistical power analysis for the behavioral sciences* (2nd ed.). Hillsdale, NJ: Lawrence Erlbaum Associates.

Corty, E. W., & Corty, R. (2011). Setting sample size to ensure narrow confidence intervals for precise estimation of population values. *Nursing Research, 60*, 148–154.

Dancey, C., Reidy, J., & Rowe, R. (2012). *Statistics for the health sciences*. Thousand Oaks, CA: Sage.

DiCenso, A., Guyatt, G., & Ciliska, D. (2005). *Evidence-based nursing: A guide to clinical practice.* St. Louis, MO: Elsevier Mosby.

Gaskin, C., & Happell, B. (2014). Power, effects, confidence, and significance: An investigation of statistical practices in nursing research. *International Journal of Nursing Studies, 51,* 795–806.

Gravetter, F., & Wallnau, L. (2013). *Statistics for the behavioral sciences* (9th ed.). Belmont, CA: Wadsworth.

*Harrington, J., Schwenke, D., Epstein, D., & Bailey, D. (2014). Androgen-deprivation therapy and metabolic syndrome in men with prostate cancer. *Oncology Nursing Forum, 41,* 21–29.

Hayat, M. J. (2013). Understanding sample size determination in nursing research. *Western Journal of Nursing Research, 35,* 943–956.

Hogan, C. (2014). Socioeconomic factors affecting infant sleep-related deaths in St. Louis. *Public Health Nursing, 31,* 10–18.

Hooge, S. L., Benzies, K., & Mannion, C. (2014). Effects of a brief, prevention-focused parenting education program for new mothers. *Western Journal of Nursing Research, 36,* 957–974.

Kawano, A., & Emori, Y. (2015). The relationship between maternal postpartum psychological state and breast milk secretory immunoglobulin A level. *Journal of the American Psychiatric Nurses Association, 21,* 23–30.

Nicoteri, J., & Miskovsky, M. (2014). Revisiting the freshman "15": Assessing body mass index in the first college year and beyond. *Journal of the American Association of Nurse Practitioners, 26,* 220–224.

Park, L. G., Howie-Esquivel, J., Chung, M., & Dracup, K. (2014). A text messaging intervention to promote medication adherence for patients with coronary heart disease: A randomized controlled trial. *Patient Education and Counseling, 94,* 261–268.

Polit, D. F. (2010). *Statistics and data analysis for nursing research* (2nd ed.). Upper Saddle River, NJ: Pearson.

Polit, D. F., & Beck, C. T. (2013). Is there still gender bias in nursing research? An update. *Research in Nursing & Health, 36,* 75–83.

Polit, D. F., & Sherman, R. (1990). Statistical power in nursing research. *Nursing Research, 39,* 365–369.

*Reed, L., Battistutta, D., Young, J., & Newman, B. (2014). Prevalence and risk factors for foot and ankle musculoskeletal disorders experienced by nurses. *BMC Musculoskeletal Disorders, 15,* 196.

Sackett, D. L., Straus, S. E., Richardson, W. S., Rosenberg, W., & Haynes, R. B. (2000). *Evidence-based medicine: How to practice and teach EBM* (2nd ed.). Edinburgh, Scotland: Churchill Livingstone.

Wang, T., Wang, H., Yang, T., Jane, S., Huang., T., Wang, C., & Lin, Y. (2015). The effect of abdominal massage in reducing malignant ascites symptoms. *Research in Nursing & Health, 38,* 51–59.

*White, M., Wells, J., & Butterworth, T. (2014). The impact of a large-scale quality improvement programme on work engagement: Preliminary results from a national cross-sectional survey of the "Productive Ward." *International Journal of Nursing Studies, 51,* 1634–1643.

***A link to this open-access journal article is provided in the Toolkit for this chapter in the accompanying Resource Manual.** ⊗

18 | Multivariate Statistics

Phenomena of interest to nurse researchers usually are complex. Phenomena such as patients' spirituality or abrupt elevations of patients' temperature are multiply determined. Scientists, in efforts to explain or predict phenomena, have recognized that two-variable studies are often inadequate. The classic approach to data analysis and research design, which involved studying the effect of a single independent variable on a single dependent variable, is being replaced by sophisticated **multivariate* procedures**.

Multivariate statistics are computationally formidable. Our purpose is to provide a general understanding of how, when, and why multivariate statistics are used, without working out computations. Nevertheless, we must present more formulas than we did in the previous two chapters because, to read and create tables with results from multivariate procedures, you must understand underlying components. This chapter introduces a few frequently used multivariate techniques—although we readily acknowledge that many of the highly sophisticated analytic procedures that are coming increasingly into use—such as *generalized estimating equations (GEE)*—are not covered in this brief overview. Those needing more comprehensive coverage of multivariate statistics should consult books

such as those by Tabachnick and Fidell (2012) or Hair et al. (2010). Hardin and Hilbe (2013) offer detailed descriptions of generalized estimating equations.

Ⓢ Multivariate statistics are never computed manually. We present examples of output from several multivariate analyses using *IBM SPSS Statistics* (SPSS) in the Supplement to this chapter.

One widely used multivariate procedure is multiple regression analysis, which is used to analyze the effects of two or more independent variables on a continuous dependent variable. The terms **multiple correlation** and **multiple regression** will be used almost interchangeably, consistent with the strong bond between correlation and regression. To comprehend this bond, we first explain simple (i.e., bivariate) regression.

SIMPLE LINEAR REGRESSION

Regression analysis is used to predict outcomes. In simple regression, one independent variable (X) is used to predict a dependent variable (Y). For instance, we could use simple regression to predict stress levels from noise levels. The higher the correlation between two variables, the more accurate the prediction. If the correlation between diastolic and systolic blood pressure were perfect (i.e., if $r = 1.00$), we would need to measure only one to know the value of the other. Few variables

---

*We use the term multivariate in this chapter to refer to analyses with at least three variables.

are perfectly correlated, and so predictions made through regression analysis usually are imperfect.

The basic linear regression equation is

$$Y' = a + bX$$

where Y' = predicted value of variable Y
a = intercept constant
b = regression coefficient
X = actual value of variable X

Regression analysis solves for a and b, and so a prediction about Y can be made for any value of X. You may remember from high school algebra that the preceding equation is the algebraic equation for a straight line. **Linear regression** is used to determine a straight-line fit to the data that minimizes deviations from the line.

As an illustration, consider the data in Table 18.1 for five people on two strongly correlated variables, X and Y ($r = .90$). If we used the five pairs of X and Y values to solve for a and b in a regression equation, we would be able to predict Y values for a *new* group of people about whom we have information on variable X only.

We do not show the formulas for computing the values of a and b here, but suffice it to say they are straightforward calculations involving deviation scores from X and Y values. As shown at the bottom of Table 18.1, the solution to the regression equation is $Y' = 1.5 + .9X$. Now suppose that the X

values in column 1 are the only data we have, and we want to predict values for Y. For the first person, $X = 1$; we would predict that $Y = 1.5 + (.9)(1)$, or 2.4. Column 3 shows Y' values for each X. These numbers show that Y' does not equal Y, the actual values obtained (column 2). Most **errors of prediction** (e) are small, as shown in column 4. Errors of prediction occur because the correlation between X and Y is not perfect. Only when $r = 1.00$ or -1.00 does $Y' = Y$. The regression equation solves for a and b in a way that minimizes such errors. More precisely, the solution minimizes the sums of squares of prediction errors, and so standard regression analysis is said to use a **least-squares** criterion. Indeed, standard regression is sometimes called *ordinary least squares*, or *OLS*, regression. In column 5 of Table 18.1, the error terms—called **residuals**—have been squared and summed to yield a value of 7.60. Any values of a and b other than 1.5 and .9, respectively, would yield a larger sum of squared residuals.

Figure 18.1 shows the solution to this regression analysis graphically. Actual X and Y values are plotted with circles. The line running through these points represents the regression solution. The intercept (a) is the point at which the line crosses the Y axis, which is 1.5. The slope (b) is the angle of the line. With $b = .90$, the line slopes so that for every 4 units on the X axis, we must go up 3.6 units (.9 × 4) on the Y axis. The line thus embodies the

TABLE 18.1 • Example of Simple Linear Regression

(1) X	(2) Y	(3) Y'	(4) e	(5) e²
1	2	2.4	−.4	.16
3	6	4.2	1.8	3.24
5	4	6.0	−2.0	4.00
7	8	7.8	.2	.04
9	10	9.6	.4	.16
$\bar{X} = 5.0$	$\bar{Y} = 6.0$		0.0	$\Sigma e^2 = 7.60$

$r = .90$
$Y' = a + bX = 1.5 + .9X$

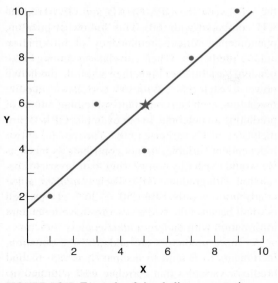

FIGURE 18.1 Example of simple linear regression.

regression equation. To predict a value for Y, we would go to the point on the X axis for an obtained X value, go up to vertically to the point on the regression line directly above the X score, and then read the predicted Y' value horizontally on the Y axis. For example, for an X value of 5, we would predict a Y' of 6, indicated by the star.

Correlation coefficients express how variation in one variable is associated with variation in another. The square of r (r^2) tells us the proportion of variance in Y that is accounted for by X. In our example, $r = .90$, so $r^2 = .81$. This means that 81% of the variability in Y values can be understood in terms of variability in X values. The remaining 19% is variability due to other factors. Thus, the stronger the correlation, the better the prediction; the stronger the correlation, the greater the percentage of variance explained.

MULTIPLE LINEAR REGRESSION

The correlation between two variables is rarely perfect, and so researchers often try to improve predictions of Y by including multiple independent variables—which are often called **predictor variables** in a multiple regression context.

Basic Concepts for Multiple Regression

Suppose we wanted to predict graduate nursing students' grade-point averages (GPAs). Not all applicants can be accepted, so we want to select those with the greatest likelihood of success. Suppose we had previously found that students with high scores on the verbal portion of an entrance exam (EE-V) tended to get better grades than those with lower EE-V scores. The correlation between EE-V and graduate GPAs is .50. With only 25% ($.50^2$) of the variance of graduate GPA accounted for, there will be many errors of prediction: Many admitted students will not perform as well as expected, and many rejected applicants would have made good students. It may be possible, by adding information, to make more accurate predictions through multiple regression. The basic multiple regression equation is

$$Y' = a + b_1X_1 + b_2X_2 + \ldots b_kX_k$$

where Y' = predicted value for variable Y
 a = intercept constant
 k = number of predictor (independent) variables
 b_1 to b_k = regression coefficients for the k variables
 X_1 to X_k = scores or values on the k independent variables

In our example of predicting graduate nursing students' GPAs, suppose we hypothesized that undergraduate GPA (GPA-U) and scores on the quantitative portion of the entrance exam (EE-Q) would improve the prediction of graduate GPA. Suppose the resulting equation were

$$Y' = .4 + .05(\text{GPA-U}) + .003(\text{EE-Q}) + .002(\text{EE-V})$$

For instance, suppose an applicant had an EE-V score of 600, an EE-Q score of 550, and a GPA-U of 3.2. The predicted graduate GPA would be

$$Y' = .4 + (.05)(3.2) + .003(550) + .002(600) = 3.41$$

We can assess the degree to which adding two independent variables improved our ability to predict graduate school performance through the multiple correlation coefficient. In bivariate correlation, the index is Pearson's r. With two or more independent variables, the index is the **multiple correlation coefficient**, or R. Unlike r, R does not have negative values. R varies from .00 to 1.00, showing the *strength* of relationship between several independent variables and a dependent variable but not *direction*. R, when squared (R^2), indicates the proportion of variance in Y accounted for by the combined, simultaneous influence of the independent variables.

R^2 provides a way to evaluate the accuracy of a prediction equation. Suppose that with the three predictors in the current example, the value of $R = .71$. This means that 50% ($.71^2$) of the variation in graduate GPA can be explained by the two EE scores and undergraduate grades. Adding two predictors doubled the variance accounted for by EE-V alone, from .25 to .50.

The multiple correlation coefficient is never less than the highest bivariate correlation between a predictor and the dependent variable. Table 18.2 presents a correlation matrix with the rs for all pairs of variables in this example. The predictor most strongly correlated with graduate grades is GPA-U, $r = .60$. The value of R could not be less than .60.

R is more readily increased when predictors have low correlations among themselves. In the current case, the correlations range from .40 (between EE-Q and GPA-U) and .70 (EE-Q and EE-V). All correlations are fairly substantial, which helps to explain why R is not much higher than the r between the GPA-GRAD and GPA-U alone (.71 compared with .60). This somewhat puzzling phenomenon reflects redundancy of information among predictors. When correlations among independent variables are high, they add little predictive power to each other. With low correlations among predictors, each can contribute something unique to predicting an outcome. In our example, GPA-U predicts 36% of Y's variance ($.60^2$). The remaining two independent variables do not contribute as much as we would expect by considering their bivariate correlation with graduate GPA. Their *combined* added contribution is only 14% ($.50 - .36 = .14$), which is small because the two test scores have redundant information with undergraduate grades.

As more predictors are added to the equation, increments to R tend to decline. It is rare to find predictor variables that correlate well with an outcome but negligibly with one another. Redundancy is difficult to avoid as more and more variables are added. The inclusion of independent variables beyond the first three or four typically does little to improve the proportion of variance accounted for or the accuracy of prediction.

TIP: When predictors are too highly correlated, the problem known as **multicollinearity** can occur, which can lead to unstable results. Most researchers therefore assess the risk of multicollinearity before finalizing their regression model. The Supplement shows how multicollinearity can be evaluated.

TABLE 18.2 • Correlation Matrix for Graduate Nursing Student Grade Example

	GPA-GRAD	GPA-U	EE-Q	EE-V
GPA-GRAD	1.00			
GPA-U	.60	1.00		
EE-Q	.55	.40	1.00	
EE-V	.50	.50	.70	1.00

GPA, grade point average; EE, entrance examination; GPA-GRAD, graduate GPA; GPA-U, undergraduate GPA; EE-Q, entrance examination quantitative score; EE-V, entrance examination verbal score.

Dependent variables in multiple regression analysis, as in ANOVA, should be measured on an interval or ratio scale. Independent variables, on the other hand, can either be interval- or ratio-level variables *or* categorical variables. Categorical variables usually are coded as dichotomous **dummy variables**, with the code of 1 designating the presence of an attribute and 0 designating its absence. For example, if males were coded 1 and females were coded 0, the code of 1 would represent "maleness." A text such as that by Polit (2010) can be consulted for information on how to use and interpret dichotomous dummy variables.

Tests of Significance

Multiple regression analysis is not used solely (or even primarily) to develop prediction equations. Researchers typically ask inferential questions about relationships in the analysis (e.g., Does *R* reflect chance fluctuations, or does it reflect true relationships in the population?) Several significance tests address different questions.

Tests of the Overall Equation and *R*

The basic null hypothesis in multiple regression is that the population multiple correlation coefficient equals zero. The test for the significance of *R* is based on principles analogous to those for ANOVA. With ANOVA, the *F*-ratio statistic is the ratio of the mean squares between divided by mean squares within. In multiple regression, the form is similar:

$$F = \frac{SS_{\text{due to regression}} / df_{\text{regression}}}{SS_{\text{of residuals}} / df_{\text{residuals}}}$$

$$= \frac{\text{Mean Square}_{\text{due to regression}}}{\text{Mean Square}_{\text{of residuals}}}$$

As in ANOVA, variance from independent variables is contrasted with variance attributable to other factors, or error. In our example of predicting graduate GPAs, suppose a multiple correlation coefficient of .71 ($R^2 = .50$) was calculated for a sample of 100 graduate students. The computed value of the *F*-statistic in this example is 32.05. The tabled value of *F* (with $df = 3$ and 96) for a significance

level of .01 is about 4.00; thus, the probability that $R = .71$ resulted from chance fluctuations is considerably less than .01.

> **Example of Multiple Regression:** Using multiple regression analysis, Morken and colleagues (2014) studied the relationship between symptoms of posttraumatic stress disorder (PTSD) in recipients of implantable cardioverter defibrillator and a range of clinical, demographic, and psychosocial predictors. They found that PTSD symptoms were predicted by such factors as shock anxiety, age, and nonconstructive support from health care staff. The R^2 for all predictors was .45, $p < .01$.

Tests for Adding Predictors

Another question researchers may want to answer is: Does *adding* X_k to the regression significantly improve the prediction of *Y* over that achieved with X_{k-1}? For example, does a third predictor increase our ability to predict *Y* after two predictors have been used? An *F*-statistic can be computed to answer this question.

In the current example, let us say that $X_1 = $ GPA-U; $X_2 = $ EE-Q; and $X_3 = $ EE-V. We can then symbolize various correlation coefficients as follows:

$R_{y.1}$ = the correlation of *Y* with GPA-U = .60
$R_{y.12}$ = the correlation of *Y* with GPA-U *and* EE-Q = .71
$R_{y.123}$ = the correlation of *Y* with all three predictors = .71

We can see that EE-V scores made no independent contribution to the multiple correlation coefficient. The value of $R_{y.12}$ is identical to the value of $R_{y.123}$. We cannot tell at a glance, however, whether adding X_2 to X_1 *significantly* increased the prediction of *Y*. What we want to know is whether X_2 would improve predictions in the population, or if its added predictive power in this sample resulted from chance. In the current example, the value of the *F*-statistic for testing whether adding EE-Q scores significantly improves our prediction of *Y* is 27.16. If we consulted a table for the theoretical distribution of *F* with $df = 1$ and 97 and a significance level of .01, we would find that the critical value is about 6.90. Therefore, adding EE-Q to the regression equation with GPA-U significantly improved the accuracy of predicting graduate GPA, beyond the .01 level.

Tests of the Regression Coefficients

When a regression coefficient (b) is divided by its standard error, the result is a value for the t statistic, which can be used to assess the significance of individual predictors. A significant t indicates that the regression coefficient (b) is significantly different from zero.

In simple regression, the value of b indicates the amount of change in predicted values of Y for a specified rate of change in X. In multiple regression, the coefficients represent the number of units the dependent variable is predicted to change for each unit change in an independent variable *when the effects of other predictors are held constant.* "Holding constant" other variables means that they are statistically controlled, a feature that can enhance a study's internal validity. If a regression coefficient is significant when confounding variables are included in the regression equation, it means that the predictor associated with the coefficient contributed significantly to the regression, even after confounding variables are taken into account.

Strategies for Handling Predictors in Multiple Regression

Three alternative strategies for entering predictor variables into regression equations are simultaneous, hierarchical, and stepwise regressions.

Simultaneous Multiple Regression

The most basic strategy, **simultaneous multiple regression**, enters all predictor variables into the regression equation at the same time. One regression equation is developed, and statistical tests indicate the significance of R and of individual regression coefficients. This strategy is most appropriate when there is no basis for considering any particular predictor as causally prior to another and when the predictors are of comparable importance to the research problem.

Hierarchical Multiple Regression

Many researchers use **hierarchical multiple regression**, which involves entering predictors into

the equation in a series of steps. Researchers control the order of entry, with the order typically based on theoretical considerations. For example, some predictors may be thought of as causally or temporally prior to others, in which case they could be entered in an early step. Another important reason for using hierarchical regression is to examine the effect of a key independent variable after first removing (controlling) the effect of confounding variables.

> **Example of Hierarchical Multiple Regression:** Majer and co-researchers (2014) studied predictors of HIV-risk sexual behaviors among ex-offenders completing inpatient substance dependence treatment. They used hierarchical regression to enter predictors in a series of three steps. Demographic variables (age, gender, race) were entered first, history of abuse was entered in the second step, and substance abuse and scores on the Psychiatric Severity Index were entered in the third block.

With hierarchical regression, researchers determine the number of steps and the number of predictors included in each step. When several variables are added as a block, as in the Majer et al. (2014) example, the analysis is a simultaneous regression for those variables at that stage. Thus, hierarchical regression can be considered a controlled sequence of simultaneous regressions.

Stepwise Multiple Regression

Stepwise multiple regression involves *empirically* selecting the combination of independent variables with the most predictive power. In stepwise multiple regression, predictors enter the regression equation in the order that produces the greatest increments to R^2. The first step selects the single best predictor of the dependent variable, that is, the independent variable with the highest bivariate correlation with Y. The second variable to enter the equation is the one that produces the largest increase to R^2 when used simultaneously with the variable selected in the first step. The procedure continues until no additional predictor significantly increases the value of R^2.

Figure 18.2 illustrates stepwise multiple regression. Suppose that the first variable (X_1), has a correlation of .60 with Y ($r^2 = .36$). Variable X_1

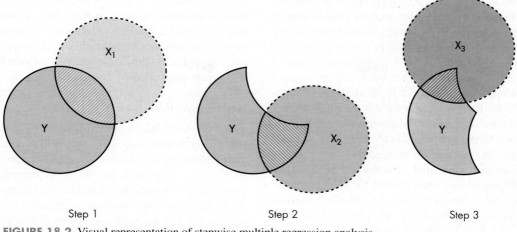

Step 1   Step 2   Step 3

FIGURE 18.2 Visual representation of stepwise multiple regression analysis.

accounts for the portion of the variability of Y represented by the hatched area in step 1 of the figure. This hatched area is, in effect, removed from further consideration, because this portion of Y's variability is explained. The variable chosen in step 2 is not always the X variable with the second largest correlation with Y. The selected predictor is the one that explains the largest portion of what *remains* of Y's variability after X_1 has been taken into account. Variable X_2, in turn, removes a second part of Y so that the independent variable selected in step 3 is the one that accounts for the most variability in Y after *both* X_1 and X_2 are removed.

Example of Stepwise Multiple Regression:
Ko and colleagues (2014) explored factors that predicted postpartum women's sleep quality in Taiwan. Variables that were stepped into the regression were physical symptoms, number of nighttime awakenings, co-sleeper disturbances, marital satisfaction, perceived stress, and poor sleep of the infant, respectively. Other variables (e.g., social support) did not enter the equation once these six variables were included. The final R^2 was .299.

➲ **TIP:** Stepwise regression is controversial because variables are entered into the regression equation based on statistical rather than theoretical criteria. If stepwise regression is used, cross-validation is recommended (e.g., by dividing

the sample in half and running two independent series of regressions).

Relative Contribution of Predictors

Scientists want not only to predict phenomena but also to explain them. Predictions can be made in the absence of understanding. For instance, in our graduate school example, we could predict performance moderately well without explaining *why* the factors contributed to students' success. For practical applications, it may be sufficient to make accurate predictions, but scientists typically want to understand phenomena.

In multiple regression, one approach to understanding a phenomenon is to explore the relative importance of independent variables. Unfortunately, determining the relative contributions of independent variables in predicting an outcome is a thorny issue. When predictor variables are correlated, as they usually are, there is no ideal way to disentangle the effects of variables in the equation.

It may appear that the solution is to compare the contributions of the Xs to R^2. In our graduate school example, GPA-U accounted for 36% of Y's variance; EE-Q explained an additional 14%. Should we conclude that undergraduate grades are more than twice as important as EE-Q scores in explaining graduate school grades? This conclusion would be inaccurate because the order of entry of variables in a regression equation affects their apparent contribution. If these two predictor variables were entered in reverse order (i.e., EE-Q first), R^2 would remain unchanged at .50; however, EE-Q's contribution would be .30 ($.55^2$), and GPA-U's contribution would be .20 ($.50 - .30$). This is because whatever variance the independent variables have in common is attributed to the first variable entered in the analysis.

Another approach to assessing the relative importance of the predictors is to compare regression coefficients. Earlier, we presented an equation for multiple regression that included a (the constant) and bs (regression coefficients) for each predictor. The b values cannot be directly compared because they are in the units of original scores, which differ from one X to another. X_1 might be in milliliters, X_2 in degrees Fahrenheit, and so forth. The use of **standard scores**[†] (or z **scores**) eliminates this problem by transforming all variables to scores with a mean of 0.0 and a standard deviation (SD) of 1.00. Transforming regular scores to z scores is easy—they are the difference between a score and the mean of that score divided by the standard deviation, or

$$z_x = \frac{X - \bar{X}}{SD_x}$$

In standard score form, the regression equation uses standard scores (zs) instead of raw scores (Xs), and the regression coefficients for each z are standardized regression coefficients, called **beta** [β] **weights**. With all the βs in the same measurement units, can their relative size shed light on the relative importance of predictors? Many researchers have interpreted beta weights in this fashion, but there are problems in doing so. These regression coefficients will be the same no matter what the order of entry of the variables. The difficulty, however, is that regression weights are unstable. Values of β tend to fluctuate from sample to sample. Moreover, when a variable is added to or subtracted from the equation, beta weights change. Because values of the regression coefficients fluctuate, it is difficult to attach theoretical importance to them.

One of the best solutions is to compare the **squared semipartial correlation coefficients (sr^2)**

of the predictors. It is beyond the scope of this book to explain this index in detail, but we note that the sr^2 is useful because it indicates a predictor's unique contribution to variability in the dependent variable—that is, the contribution after other predictors are controlled.

Regression Results

There are no standard table formats for presenting regression results, and different formats are relevant depending on whether standard, hierarchical, or stepwise regression has been performed. The most frequently reported elements are values of β, R^2, and p values. We illustrate a table of regression results using a study of predictors of Norwegian nurses' mental health problems, using data from a large longitudinal survey (Reknes et al., 2014). A key hypothesis in the study was that experiences of bullying in the workplace would be associated with worse mental health outcomes (anxiety, depression, and fatigue) at the time of a follow-up survey 1 year after the initial one. The researchers used a three-step hierarchical regression that allowed them to control for baseline mental health status (Step 1) and demographic and work-related factors (Step 2). Bullying was added in Step 3. Table 18.3 shows results for the final model in which all predictors were in the equation.

The first column of the table shows the order of entry of the six predictors (in blocks), which are listed in the second column. The next column shows values for bs, that is, the raw regression coefficients for each predictor. The next column shows the standard error (SE) of the regression coefficients, and the last column shows the standardized beta coefficients. In this table, t values are not shown, but some regression tables *do* present them. We can compute them, though, from information in the table; for example, the value of t for the first predictor (Time 1 anxiety symptoms) would be 32.5 (i.e., b / SE or .65 / .02). This is significant ($p < .01$), as shown by the asterisk in the last column: The probability (p) is less than 1 in 100 that the relationship between anxiety at Time 1 and Time 2 is spurious. Nurses with high anxiety initially tended to have high anxiety a year later. The results suggest that bullying experiences were significantly associated with higher symptoms of

---

[†]Standard scores were described in Chapter 15 of this book. For further information, see Polit (2010).

TABLE 18.3 • Multiple Regression Analysis Results: Predictors of Symptoms of Anxiety[a] in Norwegian Nurses (N = 1,552)

BLOCK[b]	PREDICTOR	b	SE b	BETA
1	Symptoms of anxiety at Time 1	.65	.02	.65**
2	Age	−.01	.01	−.02
2	Gender (female)	−.23	.23	−.02
2	Night work (number of night shifts prior year)	.00	.00	−.03
2	Job demands (scores on Job Demand Control Scale)	.04	.03	.03
3	Exposure to bullying behaviors (scores on Negative Acts Questionnaire)	.08	.03	.06**

For final regression: R^2 = .46, $p < .001$.

[a]Dependent variable = symptoms of anxiety measured at Time 2, 1 year after measurement of predictors.

[b]In this hierarchical regression, variables were entered in three blocks, as designated. Parameter estimates are shown for the Block 3 results only.

**p < .01.

Adapted from Table 2 of Reknes et al., 2014.

anxiety at Time 2, even after controlling for initial anxiety and other factors (gender, age, job demands, and working a night shift). These other factors were not independent predictors of anxiety at Time 2 at significant levels.

At the bottom of the table, we see that the value of R^2 for the final model was .46, which is significant at $p < .001$. Thus, 46% of the variance in nurses' anxiety symptoms are explained by the combined effect of the six predictors. The remaining 54% of variation is explained by factors not included in the regression model.

⊗ **TIP:** Some table templates for presenting multivariate results are included in the Toolkit of the accompanying *Resource Manual*.

Power Analysis for Multiple Regression

Small samples are especially problematic in multiple regression and other multivariate procedures. Inadequate sample size can lead to Type II errors and can also yield erratic and misleading regression coefficients.

One approach to estimating sample size needs concerns the ratio of predictor variables to total number of cases. Tabachnick and Fidell (2012) suggest this guideline: N should be greater than 50, plus 8 times the number of predictors. So, with five predictors, the sample size should be at least 90 (50 + [8 × 5]). Some experts recommend a ratio of 20 cases to 1 predictor for simultaneous and hierarchical regression and a ratio of 40 to 1 for stepwise. More cases are needed for stepwise regression because this procedure capitalizes on the idiosyncrasies of a specific data set.

Another way to estimate sample size needs is to perform a power analysis. The number of participants needed to reject the null hypothesis that R equals zero is estimated based on effect size, number of predictors, desired power, and the significance criterion. In multiple regression, the estimated effect size is a function of the value of R^2. Researchers must either predict the value of R^2 on the basis of earlier research, or use the convention that effect size will be small ($R^2 = .02$), moderate ($R^2 = .13$), or large ($R^2 = .30$).

Table 18.4 presents sample size estimates for 2 to 10 predictors and various values of R^2, for power = .80 and alpha = .05. As an example, suppose we were planning a study to predict functional ability in nursing home residents using five predictor variables. We estimate a moderate effect size

TABLE 18.4 • Power Analysis Table for Multiple Regression: Sample Size Estimates to Test the Null Hypothesis that R^2 = .00, for Power = .80, and α = .05 with 2–10 Predictor Variables

NO. OF PREDICTORS	ESTIMATED POPULATION R^2										
	.02	.04	.06	.08	.10	.13	.15	.20	.25	.30	.40
2	478	230	152	113	89	67	58	42	32	26	18
3	543	261	173	128	102	77	66	48	37	30	21
4	597	287	190	141	112	85	73	53	41	33	24
5	643	309	205	153	121	92	79	57	45	36	26
6	684	329	218	163	129	98	84	61	48	39	28
7	721	347	231	172	136	104	89	65	51	41	30
8	755	375	242	180	143	109	94	69	54	44	32
9	788	380	252	188	150	114	98	72	56	46	33
10	818	395	262	196	156	119	102	75	59	48	35

Shaded columns indicate conventions for small, medium, and large effect sizes.

(R^2 = .13) and want to achieve a power of .80 and α = .05. A sample of about 92 nursing home residents is needed to detect a population R^2 of .13 with five predictors, with a 5% chance of a Type I error and a 20% chance of a Type II error.

⊗ **TIP:** Several websites (many of which are in the Toolkit for you to click on) do instantaneous power calculations and sample size estimates for many multivariate procedures.

ANALYSIS OF COVARIANCE

Analysis of covariance (ANCOVA) has much in common with multiple regression, but it also has features of ANOVA. Like ANOVA, ANCOVA is used to compare the means of two or more groups, and the central question for both is the same: Are mean group differences likely to be *real* or spurious? Like multiple regression, however, ANCOVA allows researchers to control confounding variables statistically.

Uses of Analysis of Covariance

ANCOVA is especially useful in certain situations. For example, if a nonequivalent control group design is used to test an intervention, researchers must consider whether obtained results are influenced by preexisting group differences. When experimental control through randomization is lacking, ANCOVA offers post hoc statistical control. Even in true experiments, ANCOVA can result in more precise estimates of group differences because, even with randomization, there are typically slight differences between groups. ANCOVA adjusts for initial differences so that the results more precisely illuminate the effect of an intervention.

Strictly speaking, ANCOVA should not be used with existing groups because randomization is an underlying assumption of ANCOVA. This assumption is often violated, however. Random assignment should be done whenever possible, but when randomization is not feasible, ANCOVA can sometimes improve the internal validity of a study.

ANCOVA Procedures

Suppose we were testing the effectiveness of biofeedback therapy on patients' anxiety. A group in one hospital is exposed to the treatment, and a comparison group in another hospital is not. Patients' anxiety levels are measured both before and after the intervention, so pretest anxiety scores can be statistically controlled through ANCOVA. In such a situation, the dependent variable is the posttest anxiety scores, the independent variable is experimental/comparison group status, and the **covariate** is pretest anxiety scores. Covariates are usually continuous variables (e.g., anxiety scores) but can sometimes be dichotomous variables (male/female); the independent variable is a nominal-level variable.

ANCOVA tests the significance of differences between group means after adjusting scores on the dependent variable to remove the effect of covariates. In essence, the first step in ANCOVA is the same as the first step in hierarchical multiple regression. Variability in the dependent measure that can be explained by the covariate is removed from further consideration. ANOVA is performed on what remains of Y's variability to see whether, once the covariate is controlled, significant differences between group means exist.

Let us consider another example to explore further aspects of ANCOVA. Suppose we were testing the effectiveness of weight-loss diets, and we randomly assigned 30 people to one of three groups. ANCOVA, using pretreatment weight as the covariate, permits a more sensitive analysis of weight change than simple ANOVA. Some hypothetical data for such a study are shown in Table 18.5. Two aspects of the weight values in this table are discernible. First, despite random assignment to treatment groups, initial group means are different. Participants in diet B differ from those in diet C by

an average of 10 pounds (175 versus 185 pounds). This difference, reflecting chance fluctuations, is not significant ($F = .45$, $p = .64$). Second, posttreatment means are also different by a maximum of only 10 pounds (160 to 170). However, the mean number of pounds *lost* ranged from 10 pounds for diets A and B to 25 pounds for diet C.

When we perform an ordinary ANOVA testing group differences in posttreatment weights, we get an F of 0.55, indicating nonsignificant mean group differences ($p = .58$). Based on ANOVA, we would conclude that all three diets had equal effects on weight loss.

Now let us use ANCOVA to analyze the data. The first step breaks total variability in posttreatment weights into two components: (1) variability explained by the covariate (pretreatment weights) and (2) residual variability. The covariate accounts for a significant amount of variance, which is not surprising because there is a strong relationship between pretreatment and posttreatment weights: People who started out especially heavy tended to stay that way, relative to others in the sample. In the second step, residual variance is broken down to reflect between-group and within-group contributions. The resulting F of 17.54 ($df = 2, 26$) is significant beyond the .001 level. We can conclude that, after controlling for initial weight, there is a significant difference in weight attributable to exposure to different diets.

This fictitious example was contrived so that an ANOVA result of "no difference" would be altered by adding a covariate. Most actual results are much

TABLE 18.5 • Fictitious Data for ANCOVA Example: Comparison of Pre- and Posttreatment Weights for Three Diet Interventions

	DIET A	DIET B	DIET C	TOTAL
Pretreatment weight, mean (SD)	180.0 (23.5)	175.0 (22.5)	185.0 (24.6)	180.0 (23.1)
Posttreatment weight, mean (SD)	170.0 (21.7)	165.0 (22.0)	160.0 (20.3)	165.0 (20.0)

ANOVA $F(2, 27)$ for mean group differences in posttreatment weight = 0.55, $p = .58$

ANCOVA $F(1, 26)$ for covariate (pretreatment weight) = 309.88, $p < .001$
ANCOVA $F(2, 26)$ for mean group differences in posttreatment weight = 17.54, $p < .001$

less dramatic. Nonetheless, ANCOVA yields a more sensitive statistical test than ANOVA because the covariate reduces the error term (within-group variability), against which treatment effects are compared.

Theoretically, it is possible to use any number of covariates. It is seldom advisable, however, to use more than two or three. For one thing, a large number of covariates is often unnecessary because of the typically high degree of redundancy beyond the first few. Moreover, each covariate uses up a degree of freedom; fewer degrees of freedom means that a higher F is required for significance. For instance, with 2 and 26 *df*, an F of 5.53 is required for significance at the .01 level, but with 2 and 23 *df* (i.e., adding three covariates), an F of 5.66 is needed.

Selection of Covariates

Useful covariates are almost always available. Background characteristics, such as age and gender, are often good candidates, for example. However, it is important to select covariates that are correlated with the dependent variable. Background characteristics are especially important to control if they are predictors of the outcome and there are differences between the groups being compared. The literature is a good source of information about factors correlated with outcomes, and analyses to detect strong predictors in the research sample itself (e.g., through regression analyses) can also be undertaken.

A baseline measure of the outcome is an excellent covariate, invariably strongly correlated with the final outcome. However, RM-ANOVA is an alternative to ANCOVA when analyzing data from studies with pretest–posttest designs. Propensity scores, discussed briefly in Chapter 9, can be powerful covariates. Propensity scores capture group differences on a broad range of attributes because they represent an attempt to model group differences using available data. The use of propensity scores as covariates is described by Qin et al. (2008). In general, it is important to select covariates that have strong reliability. Measurement errors can lead to either overadjustments or underadjustments of the mean and can contribute to Type I or Type II errors.

Adjusted Means

In our example of the three diets, the significant ANCOVA F test indicates that at least one of the three groups had a posttreatment weight that is significantly different from the overall grand mean, after adjusting for pretreatment weights. It sometimes is useful to examine **adjusted means**, that is, group means on the dependent variable after adjusting for (i.e., removing the effect of) covariates. Adjusted means allow researchers to determine *net effects* (i.e., group differences on the dependent variable that are net of the effect of covariates). In our example of posttreatment weights for participants in three diet interventions, the adjusted means for Diets A, B, and C were 170.0, 169.4, and 155.6, respectively—values that more clearly indicate differences among those exposed to the different diets.

When ANCOVA results in a significant group F test, researchers can reject the null hypothesis that the adjusted group means are equal. As with ANOVA, further analysis is needed to assess which pairs of adjusted group means are significantly different from one another. In our example, post-hoc tests revealed that the mean for Diet C is significantly different from that for both Diets A and B, but Diets A and B are not significantly different from each other.

> **TIP:** For ANCOVA, an eta squared can be computed to summarize the magnitude of the *adjusted* effect of the independent variable on the dependent variable. Estimates of eta squared can be used in a power analysis to estimate sample size needs when planning a study. In general, when ANCOVA is used with carefully selected covariates, the analysis of group differences is more powerful than with ANOVA because error variance is reduced. In our example of the three diets, the value of adjusted eta squared is .57.

Example of ANCOVA: Budhrani and colleagues (2014) compared breast cancer survivors who were white (non-Hispanic) to those from racial/ethnic minorities in terms of sleep disturbances and physical and psychological symptoms. ANCOVA was used to compare outcomes for women in the two groups, after controlling for the effects of age.

OTHER LEAST-SQUARES MULTIVARIATE TECHNIQUES

Many of the multivariate statistics we have discussed thus far are related. For example, ANOVA and multiple regression are similar. Both techniques analyze total variability in a continuous dependent measure and contrast variability due to independent variables with that attributable to individual differences or error. By tradition, experimental data typically are analyzed by ANOVA, and correlational data are analyzed by regression. Yet, *any data for which ANOVA is appropriate can be analyzed by multiple regression*, although the reverse is not true.

A broad class of statistical techniques are subsumed under the **general linear model (GLM)**, which include techniques that fit data to straight-line (linear) solutions. The GLM is the foundation for such procedures as the *t*-test, ANOVA, and multiple regression. The GLM is an important model because of its generality and applicability to numerous research situations, but a thorough understanding of the GLM requires advanced statistical training. In this section, other GLM methods are briefly introduced. The intent is to acquaint you with research situations for which these methods are appropriate.

Repeated-Measures ANOVA for Mixed Designs

In Chapter 17, we discussed one-way repeated-measures ANOVA (RM-ANOVA), which is appropriate when one group of people is measured at multiple points. Many RCTs involve randomly assigning participants to different treatment groups and then collecting postintervention data several times. When there are only two data collection points (e.g., a pretest and a posttest), ANCOVA is often used to test the null hypothesis that groups means are equal, after removing the effect of pretest (baseline) scores. When data are collected three or

more times, a **repeated-measures ANOVA for mixed designs** is often used.

As an example, suppose we collected heart rate data at 2 hours (Time 1 or T1), 4 hours (T2), and 6 hours (T3) postsurgery for people in an experimental and control group. Structurally, the ANOVA for analyzing these data would look similar to a 2 × 3 multifactor ANOVA, but calculations would differ in this mixed design—mixed because it involves both a within-subject and a between-subject factor. An *F*-statistic would be computed to test for a *between-subjects effect* (i.e., differences between experimentals and controls). This statistic would indicate whether, across all time periods, mean heart rate differed in the two groups. Another *F*-statistic would be computed to test for a *within-subjects effect* or time factor (i.e., differences at T1, T2, and T3). This statistic would indicate whether, across both groups, mean heart rates differed over time. Finally, an **interaction effect** would be tested to assess whether group differences varied across time. In mixed design RM-ANOVA, the interaction effect usually is of primary importance. When people are randomized to treatment groups, we would expect their mean values at baseline to be equivalent—but if there are treatment effects, group means would differ at subsequent points of data collection, thus resulting in a time × treatment interaction.

Tests within the GLM have several basic assumptions, all of which are fully described in statistics textbooks. Assumptions such as normality of the distributions and the equality of variances apply to most GLM procedures, but ANOVA and most of its variants are fairly **robust** to violation of assumptions (i.e., violations tend not to affect the accuracy of statistical decision making). However, RM-ANOVA has some unique assumptions—the assumption of *sphericity* and the related assumption of *compound symmetry*, both of which are too complex to elaborate here. RM-ANOVA is not, unfortunately, robust to violations of these assumptions. Furthermore, there are different opinions about how to detect and address violations. Thus, RM-ANOVA tends to be more complex than many procedures discussed thus far. Polit (2010) and advanced statistical texts offer suggestions on using RM-ANOVA.

Multivariate Analysis of Variance

Multivariate analysis of variance (MANOVA) is
the extension of ANOVA to more than one dependent variable. MANOVA is used to test the significance of differences in group means for multiple
dependent variables considered simultaneously.
For instance, if we wanted to test the effect of
two methods of exercise on diastolic *and* systolic
blood pressure, MANOVA would be appropriate.
Researchers often analyze such data by performing
two separate ANOVAs. Strictly speaking, this practice is not appropriate. Separate ANOVAs imply
that the dependent variables were independent
when, in fact, they were obtained from the same
people and are correlated. MANOVA takes the intercorrelations of dependent variables into account.
ANOVA is, however, a more widely understood
procedure than MANOVA, and thus, its results may
be more easily communicated to a broad audience.

MANOVA can be readily extended in ways
analogous to ANOVA. For example, it is possible
to perform **multivariate analysis of covariance
(MANCOVA)**, which allows for the control of confounding variables (covariates) when there are two
or more dependent variables.

➲ **TIP:** If you elect to use simpler analyses
to enhance the utility of the evidence to clinical
audiences (e.g., three separate ANOVAs rather
than a MANOVA), you should run the analyses
both ways. Then, you could present bivariate
results (e.g., from ANOVAs) in the report,
but note whether the more complex analysis
(e.g., MANOVA) confirmed the conclusions.

comparison group of adolescents from the same
urban environment. Using MANOVA, the researchers
tested group differences in illness frequency and number of frequency of symptoms.

➲ **TIP:** In clinical trials, researchers often
undertake **subgroup analyses** to assess
whether the intervention had particularly strong
(or weak) effects for certain subgroups of people.
Much has been written about the abuse of
subgroup analyses in "fishing" for significant
effects, especially when overall group differences were not statistically significant. Subgroup
analyses should be limited to a few comparisons
that are specified in advance based on carefully
considered hypotheses. Such subgroup analyses
should involve an examination of the *interaction*
between the treatment variable and the subgroup
variable (Pocock et al., 2002).

LOGISTIC REGRESSION

Logistic regression is a widely used multivariate
technique. Like multiple regression, logistic regression analyzes the relationship between multiple independent variables and a dependent variable and
yields a predictive equation. Logistic regression,
however, relies on an estimation procedure that has
less restrictive assumptions than multivariate procedures within the GLM, which use least squares
estimation. Logistic regression is used to predict
categorical dependent variables.

➲ **TIP:** A least-squares procedure for predicting categorical outcomes is called *discriminant
analysis*. Although popular a decade ago,
discriminant analysis is infrequently used and has
been superseded by logistic regression.

Basic Concepts for Logistic Regression

Logistic regression uses **maximum likelihood
estimation (MLE)**. Maximum likelihood estimators are ones that estimate the parameters most

likely to have generated the observed data. Confirmatory factor analysis, discussed in Chapter 15, also uses MLE.

Logistic regression has few assumptions about the underlying distribution of variables. Logistic regression is also well suited to many clinical questions because it models the probability of an outcome. For example, we might be interested in modeling the probability of engaging in breast self-examination or the probability of a patient fall.

Logistic regression transforms the probability of an event occurring (e.g., that a woman will practice breast self-examination) into its odds. As discussed briefly in Chapter 16, **odds** reflect the ratio of two probabilities: the probability of an event occurring, to the probability that it will not occur. For example, if 40% of women practice breast self-examination, the odds would be .40 divided by .60, or .667.

Probabilities, which range between zero and one, are then transformed into continuous variables that range between zero and infinity. Because this range is still restricted, a further transformation is performed, namely, calculating the logarithm of the odds. The range of this new variable (the **logit**, short for *logi*stic probability un*it*) is from minus to plus infinity. Using the logit as the dependent variable, a maximum likelihood procedure estimates the coefficients of the independent variables, with the logit as a continuous dependent variable.

The solution yields an equation that predicts the logit from a weighted combination of independent variables, plus a constant, much like a multiple regression equation. The interpretation, however, is different because the equation does not predict *actual* values of the dependent variable. In logistic regression, a regression coefficient (*b*) can be interpreted as the change in the log odds associated with a one-unit change in the associated predictor variable.

The Odds Ratio

A logistic regression equation is hard to interpret because we do not think in terms of log odds. The equation can, however, be transformed back to yield information in terms of odds rather than log odds. The factor by which the odds change is the *odds ratio* (OR), the risk index we discussed in Chapter 16.

For example, suppose that we used logistic regression to predict the probability of performing breast self-examination. One of the independent variables might be whether or not the woman has had a family member (e.g., a sister) who had breast cancer. A logistic regression analysis might indicate that the *OR* was 12.1, with all other predictors in the equation held constant. (This is often called an *adjusted odds ratio*.) As noted previously, the odds ratio provides an estimate (around which confidence intervals can be built) of relative risk—the risk of an event occurring given one condition, versus the risk of it occurring given a different condition. In our example, we would estimate that the "risk" of performing breast self-examination is about 12 times greater if a woman has a family history of breast cancer than if she does not, with other factors in the model held constant (controlled).

→ **TIP:** Just as there is simple regression with least-squares estimation—that is, the prediction of a dependent variable based on a single independent variable—*bivariate logistic regression* is also possible. This is often done to produce estimates of *unadjusted* (or *crude*) odds ratios—that is, odds ratios without controlling other variables.

Variables in Logistic Regression

The dependent variable in logistic regression is a dichotomous variable. The dependent variable is typically coded 1 to represent an event or a characteristic (e.g., had a fall, is obese), and 0 to represent the absence of the event or characteristic (no fall, no obesity). Predictor variables can be continuous variables, categorical variables, or interaction terms. Although there are no strict limits to the number of predictors that can be included, it is best to achieve a parsimonious model with strong predictive power using a small set of good predictors.

When continuous variables are the predictors, the odds ratio is interpreted somewhat differently than with categorical variables. For example, suppose we were predicting whether a nursing home resident would or would not have a fall, and one predictor variable was age. Suppose we found, for example, that the *OR* associated with age was 1.15. This means that for every additional year of age, the odds of having a fall increased by 15%, with everything else in the model held constant.

Dummy-coded variables, also called *indicator variables*, are a common method of representing dichotomous predictors, such as smokes cigarettes (1) versus does not smoke cigarettes (0). For variables with more than two categories, a series of dummy variables is needed. For example, if marital status were a predictor variable in a logistic regression for predicting breast self-examination, a bivariate logistic analysis could provide estimates of the relative risk of different marital statuses (e.g., never married, married, formerly married) on breast self-examination. In such an analysis, one group would be the **reference group**, with an *OR* of 1.0, and the other two groups would have *OR*s in relation to the reference group. As a hypothetical example, if the *OR* for a never-married reference group was 1.0 and the *OR* for married was 1.23, this means that married women were 23% more likely to perform breast self-examination than never-married women.

As with multiple regression, predictors in multiple regression can be entered into the equation in different ways. The options include simultaneous, hierarchical, and stepwise entry.

TIP: When a categorical dependent variable is not dichotomous (e.g., three different types of chronic illness), *multinomial logistic regression* can be used (Kwak & Clayton-Matthews, 2002).

Significance Tests in Logistic Regression

Researchers usually want to assess the overall reliability of the model, that is, whether the set of predictors, taken as a whole, is significantly better than chance in predicting the probability of the outcome event. Unfortunately, assessing the goodness of fit of a logistic regression model can be confusing because there are several different tests, and different authors use different names for the tests. Another potential source of confusion is that some tests indicate goodness of fit by a significant result, and others indicate goodness of fit by a *non*significant

result. We briefly describe two approaches but recommend further reading in advanced textbooks such as Tabachnik and Fidell (2012) or Hosmer and Lemeshow (2013).

One statistic in logistic regression is called the **likelihood index**, which is the probability of the observed results, given parameters estimated in the analysis. If the overall model fits the data perfectly, the likelihood index is 1.0. Because the likelihood index is typically a small decimal, it is usually transformed by multiplying it by −2 times the log of the likelihood. The transformed index (**−2LL**) is a small number when the fit is good; in a perfect fit, the value is zero. The chi-square statistic is then used to test the null hypothesis that all of the *b* regression coefficients are zero, in what is sometimes called a **likelihood ratio test**. A **goodness-of-fit statistic**, which has a chi-squared distribution, is the analog of the overall *F* test in multiple regression. This statistic is based on the residuals for all cases in the analysis—which, in logistic regression is the difference between the observed probability of an event and the predicted probability. This statistic is thus a mechanism for evaluating the fit of the predictive model. The likelihood ratio test also can be used to evaluate the significance of *improvement* to −2LL with successive entry of predictors, when hierarchical or stepwise regression is performed.

An alternative approach to testing the overall model is the **Hosmer-Lemeshow test**, which compares the prediction model to a hypothetically "perfect" model. In brief, the perfect model is one that contains the exact set of predictors needed to duplicate the observed frequencies in the dependent variable. The full model can be tested against the perfect model by computing differences between observed frequencies and expected frequencies—that is, those expected in the perfect model. With this test, a *nonsignificant* chi-square is desired. A nonsignificant result indicates that the model being tested is not reliably different from the perfect model. In other words, nonsignificance supports the inference that the model adequately duplicates the observed frequencies of the outcome.

TIP: There is no consensus on which approach for an overall model test is better, but logistic regression software programs can perform both tests, and some researchers present both results.

It is also possible to test the significance of individual predictors in the model—just as the t statistic is used in multiple regression. A frequently used statistic for this purpose is the **Wald statistic**, which is distributed as a chi-square. Significance is also sometimes assessed by examining the confidence intervals around the odds ratios. If the 95% CI includes the value of 1.0, this indicates that the *OR* was not statistically significant at the .05 level.

Effect Size in Logistic Regression

Statisticians have worked on developing an effect size index for logistic regression that is analogous to R^2 in multiple regression. The main problem, however, is that R^2 in multiple regression can be interpreted as the percentage of variance in the dependent variable explained by the predictors, but this is more complex with a dichotomous outcome. Despite difficulties in achieving a good analog to least-squares-based R^2, several **pseudo R^2** measures have been proposed for logistic regression. These indexes should be reported as approximations to an R^2 from least-squares regression rather than as the percentage of variance explained. A statistic called the **Nagelkerke R^2** is the most frequently reported pseudo R^2 index.

Example of Logistic Regression: Hildingsson and co-researchers (2014) studied childbirth fear in a sample of 1,047 expectant fathers in Sweden. In their logistic regression model, they found that those with a high level of fear (compared to those with low or no fear) had less positive feelings about the impending birth ($OR = 3.4$), had been born in a country other than Sweden ($OR = 2.8$), had a preference for a cesarean birth ($OR = 2.1$), and were expecting a first baby ($OR = 1.8$).

SURVIVAL AND EVENT HISTORY ANALYSIS

Some dependent variables are time-related. **Survival analysis** is widely used by epidemiologists when the dependent variable is a time interval between an initial event (e.g., onset of a disease) and a terminal event (e.g., death). Survival analysis calculates a survival score, which compares survival time for one participant with that for others. When researchers are interested in group comparisons—for example, comparing the survival function of people in an experimental group versus a control group—a statistic can be computed to test the null hypothesis that the groups are sampled from the same survival distribution.

Survival analysis can be applied to many situations unrelated to mortality. For example, survival analysis could be used to analyze such time-related phenomena as length of time in labor, length of stay in hospital, or length of time breastfeeding. Survival analysis can be used when time-related data are **censored**, that is, the observation period does not cover all possible events. As an example, if the outcome were hospital readmission and data are collected 2 years after release, the data are censored because there will be readmissions beyond the 2-year period, and some will never be readmitted. Further information about survival analysis can be found in Hosmer and colleagues (2008).

Extensions of survival analysis have been developed that allow researchers to examine determinants of survival-type transitions in a multivariate (regression) framework. In these analyses, independent variables are used to model the risk (or hazard) of experiencing an event at a given point in time, given that one has not experienced the event before that time. The most common specification of the hazard is known as the **Cox proportional hazards model**. Further information may be found in O'Quigley (2008).

Example of Cox Regression: One of this book's authors (Polit) and co-researchers in Australia used Cox regression to test the effects of an intervention to reduce hospital admissions among residents of long-term care facilities presenting to an emergency department. Using Cox regression, they found that those in the intervention group had significantly shorter lengths of in-hospital stay than those in a usual care group, even after controlling for age, sex, and acuity (Crilly et al., 2011).

CAUSAL MODELING

Causal modeling involves testing a hypothesized causal explanation of a phenomenon, typically with data from nonexperimental (observational) studies. In a causal model, researchers posit causal linkages among three or more variables and then test whether hypothesized pathways from the causes to the effect are consistent with the data. Causal modeling is not a method for discovering causes; rather, it is a method applied to a prespecified model formulated on the basis of prior knowledge and theory.

Causal modeling is often referred to as **path analysis**. Until fairly recently, nurse researchers performed path analysis primarily using ordinary least-squares estimation. In fact, it is possible to conduct a path analysis with a series of multiple regression analyses. We begin our explanation of path analysis within an OLS framework.

In reports, path analytic results are usually displayed in a **path diagram**, and we use such a diagram (Figure 18.3) to illustrate key concepts. This model postulates that the dependent variable, patients' functional ability (V4), is influenced by patients' capacity for self-care (V3); this, in turn, is affected by nursing actions (V1) and the severity of their illness (V2). The model in Figure 18.3 is a **recursive model**, which means that the causal flow is unidirectional. It is hypothesized that V2 is a cause of V3 but not that V3 is a cause of V2.

Path analysis distinguishes exogenous and endogenous variables. Determinants of an **exogenous variable** lie outside the model. In Figure 18.3, nursing actions (V1) and illness severity (V2) are exogenous; no attempt is made in the model to elucidate what causes different nursing actions or different degrees of illness. An **endogenous variable**, by contrast, is one whose variation is hypothesized to be affected by other variables in the model. In our example, self-care capacity (V3) and functional ability (V4) are endogenous.

Causal linkages are shown on a path diagram by arrows drawn from presumed causes to presumed effects. In our illustration, severity of illness is hypothesized to affect functional ability both directly (path p_{42}) and indirectly through the *mediating variable* self-care capacity (paths p_{32} and p_{43}). Correlated exogenous variables are indicated by curved lines, as shown by the curved line between nursing actions and illness severity.

Ideally, the model would totally explain the outcome, but this almost never happens because there are other determinants, which are **residual variables**. The two boxes labeled e in Figure 18.3 denote a composite of all determinants of self-care capacity (e_3) and functional ability (e_4) that are not in the model. If we could identify and measure additional causes and incorporate them into the theory, the model could be strengthened.

Path analysis solves for **path coefficients**, which are the weights representing the effect of one variable on another. In Figure 18.3, causal paths indicate that one variable (e.g., V3) is caused by another (e.g., V2), yielding a path labeled p_{32}. In research

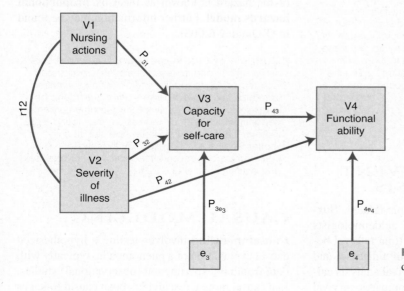

FIGURE 18.3 Example of a path diagram.

reports, path symbols would be replaced by actual path coefficients. Path coefficients are standardized partial regression slopes. For example, path p_{32} is equal to $\beta_{32.1}$—the beta weight between variables 2 and 3, holding variable 1 constant. Because path coefficients are in standard form, they indicate the proportion of a standard deviation difference in the caused variable that is directly attributable to a 1 *SD* difference in the specified causal variable. Thus, path coefficients provide an indication about the relative importance of various determinants.

Structural equations modeling (SEM) using maximum likelihood estimation is a more powerful approach to path analysis that avoids several problems in OLS estimation, notably difficulties in meeting assumptions. Unlike an OLS approach, SEM can accommodate measurement errors, correlated residuals, and **nonrecursive models** that allow for reciprocal causation. Another attractive feature of SEM is that it can be used to analyze causal models involving *latent variables*—a variable representing a construct that is not measured directly (Chapter 15). In SEM, latent variables are captured by two or more measured (manifest) variables that are indicators of a construct. A decade or so ago, the use of SEM by nurse researchers was hampered by the unavailability of user-friendly software, but that situation has changed.

When there are latent variables, SEM proceeds in two phases. In the first phase, which corresponds to a confirmatory factor analysis (CFA), a measurement model is tested (Chapter 15). When there is evidence of an adequate fit of the data to the hypothesized measurement model, the theoretical causal model is tested by structural equation modeling.

SEM yields information about the hypothesized causal parameters—that is, path coefficients that are presented as beta weights. The coefficients indicate the expected amount of change in the (latent) endogenous variable that is caused by a change in the (latent) causal variable. SEM programs yield information on the significance of individual paths. The overall fit of the model to the research data can be tested by means of several statistics, such as the **goodness-of-fit index** (**GFI**) and **adjusted goodness-of-fit index** (**AGFI**). For both indexes,

a value of .90 or greater indicates a good fit of the model to the data.

Path analysis using SEM has gained considerable popularity among nurse researchers but is a complex procedure. Readers interested in further information on SEM can consult Loehlin (2004) or Kline (2011).

Example of a Path Analysis: Chen and colleagues (2014) used path analysis (using SEM) to test a causal model predicting agitation in 405 nursing home residents in Taiwan. The complex model, which had a good fit, indicated that cognitive function and depression had direct effects on agitation; pain and functional ability affected agitation indirectly, through their effects on depression.

CRITIQUING MULTIVARIATE STATISTICS

As we advised in the previous chapter, it is difficult to critique researchers' statistical analysis without statistical skills. This caution is even more relevant when it comes to complex multivariate analyses.

As with bivariate statistics, one issue is whether the researcher selected the right tests. The selection of a multivariate procedure depends on several factors, including the nature of the research question and the measurement level of the variables. (It also depends on whether the data conformed to various assumptions underlying the tests—an issue we did not address in this brief chapter.) Table 18.6, which summarizes some of the major features of multivariate statistics discussed in this chapter, may be helpful in assessing the appropriateness of an analytic approach. It might also be noted that studies in which multivariate statistics were *not* used might well be critiqued in terms of whether or not they *should* have been used. As we illustrated, results from an ANOVA or *t*-test can sometimes be altered by controlling confounding variables. Conversely, some researchers apply multivariate statistics when their sample size is too small to justify their use.

No specific critiquing guidelines for multivariate statistics are presented in this chapter, but most of the questions presented in Box 17.1 are also relevant for researchers' use of the statistics discussed in this chapter.

TABLE 18.6 • Guide to Selected Multivariate Analyses

TEST NAME	PURPOSE	MEASUREMENT LEVEL[a] OF VARIABLES[b]			NUMBER OF VARIABLES[b]		
		IV	DV	CV	IVs	DVs	CV
Multiple regression/ correlation	To test the relationship between 2+ IVs and 1 DV; to predict a DV from 2+ IVs	Nominal, continuous	Continuous	—	2+	1	—
Analysis of covariance (ANCOVA)	To test the difference between the means of 2+ groups while controlling for 1+ covariate	Nominal	Continuous	Nominal, continuous	1+	1	1+
Mixed design RM-ANOVA	To test mean differences for 2+ groups for outcomes measured multiple times	Nominal	Continuous	Nominal, continuous	1+	1	1+
Multivariate analysis of variance (MANOVA)	To test the difference between the means of 2+ groups for 2+ DVs simultaneously	Nominal	Continuous	—	1+	2+	—
Multivariate analysis of covariance (MANCOVA)	To test the difference between the means of 2+ groups for 2+ DVs simultaneously, while controlling for 1+ covariate	Nominal	Continuous	Nominal, continuous	1+	2+	1+
Logistic regression	To test the relationship between 2+ IVs and 1 DV; to predict the probability of an event; to estimate relative risk	Nominal, continuous	Nominal	—	2+	1	—

[a]Measurement levels: Continuous = Interval- or Ratio-level.
[b]Variables: IV, independent variables; DV, dependent variable; CV, covariate.

●●●●●●●●●●●●●●●●●●●●●●●●
RESEARCH EXAMPLE

Study: Discharge clinical characteristics and 60-day readmission in patients hospitalized with heart failure (Anderson, 2014)

Statement of Purpose: The purpose of this study was to explore the clinical and diagnostic characteristics predictive of a re-hospitalization within 60 days of discharge from a hospital with a primary diagnosis of heart failure (HF).

Methods: The study sample included patients discharged from two U.S. hospitals over a 2-year period with a primary diagnosis of HF. A power analysis indicated that 134 individuals would provide 80% power to detect differences between patients who did and did not experience 60-day HF readmission. Data for the study were obtained from existing medical and health records, including information about demographic traits (age, gender) and clinical characteristics at discharge (e.g., dyspnea, vital signs). All patients readmitted within 60 days of an initial stay were included in the readmission group. In this case-control design, the comparison group was selected from those not readmitted within 60 days, matched to cases in terms of admission year and month and institution. The main analysis involved a hierarchical logistic regression.

Analysis and Findings: The researchers first tested bivariate relationships between readmission status and a wide range of possible predictors. They found statistically significant correlations between 60-day rehospitalization and, for example, congestion on chest radiograph, history of heart failure, crackles, need for assistance with activities of daily living (ADLs), and use of assistive devices for ambulation. Other characteristics (e.g., blood pressure, heart rate, discharge medications) were not significantly correlated with readmission status. A hierarchical logistic regression was performed, with order of entry based on theoretical and clinical considerations. Demographic variables (age and gender) were entered in the first step, followed by clinical variables (after removing some predictors that could cause multicollinearity). The final full model included age, gender, assistance with ADLs, crackles, and dyspnea at discharge. The researchers determined that the model correctly classified 77% of the sample as having or not having a 60-day readmission. The Hosmer-Lemeshow test suggested that the model fit the data adequately, and the value of the Nagelkerke R^2 for the model was .45. The two significant predictors in the model were needing assistance with ADLs ($OR = 10.26$, 95% CI $= 3.70$—28.44) and crackles ($OR = 5.41$, 95% CI $= 1.87$—15.61).

SUMMARY POINTS

- **Multivariate statistical procedures** are increasingly being used in nursing research to untangle complex relationships among three or more variables.

- Simple **linear regression** makes predictions about the values of one variable based on values of a second variable. **Multiple regression** is a method of predicting a continuous dependent variable on the basis of two or more independent (**predictor**) variables.

- **Multiple correlation coefficients** (R) can be squared (R^2) to estimate the proportion of variability in the dependent variable accounted for by the predictors. The F-statistic is used to test the overall regression model, as well as changes to R^2 as new predictors are introduced.

- The regression equation yields **regression coefficients** (**bs**) for each predictor that, when standardized, are called **beta weights** (βs).

- **Simultaneous multiple regression** enters all predictor variables into the regression equation at the same time. **Hierarchical multiple regression** enters predictors into the equation in a series of steps controlled by researchers. **Stepwise multiple regression** enters predictors in steps using a statistical criterion for order of entry.

- **Analysis of covariance** (**ANCOVA**), an extension of ANOVA, removes the effect of confounding variables (**covariates**) before testing whether mean group differences on the outcome variable are statistically significant.

- **Mixed design RM-ANOVA** is used to test mean differences between groups (between-subjects factor) over time (within-subjects factor). In mixed design RM-ANOVAs, the interaction term (time $\times$ group) usually is of primary interest.

- **Multivariate analysis of variance** (**MANOVA**) is the extension of ANOVA to situations in which there is more than one dependent variable.

- The **general linear model** (**GLM**) encompasses a broad class of frequently used statistical techniques that fit data to straight-line (linear) solutions, including t-tests, ANOVA, ANCOVA, and multiple regression.

- **Least-squares estimation** used within GLM minimizes the square of **errors of prediction** (the **residuals**). An alternative is **maximum likelihood estimation** (**MLE**), which estimates the parameters most likely to have generated observed data.

- **Logistic regression**, which is based on MLE, is used to predict the probability of an outcome. Logistic regression yields an **odds ratio** that is an index of relative risk for each predictor, that is, the risk of an outcome occurring given one condition, versus the risk of it occurring given a different condition, while controlling other predictors.
- The overall logistic regression model can be tested with a **likelihood ratio test** that uses a **goodness-of-fit chi-square** statistic. An alternative is the **Hosmer-Lemeshow** test that tests how close the model is to a perfect model. Individual predictors can be tested with the **Wald statistic**. Several **pseudo** R^2 indexes can be used to summarize overall effect size for logistic regression; the most widely reported is the **Nagelkerke R^2**.
- **Survival analysis** and other related event history methods such as **Cox regression** are used when the dependent variable of interest is a time interval (e.g., length of time in hospital).
- **Causal modeling** involves the development and testing of a hypothesized causal explanation of a phenomenon.
- **Path analysis**, a method for testing causal models, involves the preparation of a **path diagram** that stipulates hypothesized causal links among variables. Path analysis can be performed using least-squares estimation but currently is more likely to involve **structural equations modeling** (**SEM**), an MLE approach to causal modeling.

STUDY ACTIVITIES

Chapter 18 of the *Resource Manual for Nursing Research: Generating and Assessing Evidence for Nursing Practice, 10th edition*, offers exercises and study suggestions for reinforcing concepts presented in this chapter. In addition, the following study questions can be addressed:

1. A researcher has examined the relationship between preventive health care attitudes on the one hand and the person's educational level, age, and gender on the other. The multiple correlation coefficient is .62. Explain the meaning of this statistic. How much variation in attitudinal scores is explained by the three predictors? How much is *unexplained*? What other variables might improve the power of the prediction?

2. Using power analysis, determine the sample size needed to achieve power = .80 for α = .05, when (a) estimated R^2 = .15, and k = 5; and (b) estimated R^2 = .08, and k = 3.

STUDIES CITED IN CHAPTER 18

Anderson, K. M. (2014). Discharge clinical characteristics and 60-day readmission in patients hospitalized with heart failure. *Journal of Cardiovascular Nursing*, 29, 232–241.

*Budhrani, P., Lengacher, C., Kip, K., Tofthagen, C., & Jim, H. (2014). Minority breast cancer survivors: The association between race/ethnicity. Objective sleep disturbances, and physical and psychological symptoms. *Nursing Research and Practice*, 2014, 858403.

Chen, Y. H., Lin, L. C., Chen, K. B., & Liu, Y. C. (2014). Validation of a causal model of agitation among institutionalized residents with dementia in Taiwan. *Research in Nursing & Health*, 37, 11–20.

Crilly, J., Chaboyer, W., Wallis, M., Thalib, L., & Polit, D. (2011). An outcomes evaluation of an Australian Hospital in the Nursing Home admission avoidance programme. *Journal of Clinical Nursing*, 19, 1178–1187.

Hair, J. F., Tatham, R. L., Anderson, R., & Black, B. (2010). *Multivariate data analysis* (7th ed.). Upper Saddle River, NJ: Prentice-Hall.

Hardin, J. W., & Hilbe, J. M. (2013). *Generalized estimating equations* (2nd ed.). Boca Raton, FL: CRC Press.

Hildingsson, I., Johansson, M., Fenwick, J., Haines, H., & Rubertsson, C. (2014). Childbirth fear in expectant fathers: Findings from a regional Swedish cohort study. *Midwifery*, 30, 242–247.

Hosmer, D., & Lemeshow, S. (2013). *Applied logistic regression* (3rd ed.). New York: John Wiley & Sons.

Hosmer, D., Lemeshow, S., & May, S. (2008). *Applied survival analysis: Regression modeling of time to event data* (2nd ed.). New York: John Wiley & Sons.

Kline, R. (2011). *Principles and practice of structural equation modeling.* (3rd ed.). New York: Guilford Press.

Ko, S. H., Chen, C. H., Wang, H. H., & Su, Y. T. (2014). Postpartum women's sleep quality and its predictors in Taiwan. *Journal of Nursing Scholarship*, 46, 74–81.

Korhan, E. A., Khorshid, L., & Uyar, M. (2014). Reflexology: Its effects on physiological anxiety signs and sedation needs. *Holistic Nursing Practice*, 28, 6–23.

Kwak, C., & Clayton-Matthews, A. (2002). Multinomial logistic regression. *Nursing Research, 51,* 404–409.

Loehlin, J. C. (2004). *Latent variable models: An introduction to factor, path, and structural equation analysis* (4th ed.). Mahwah, NJ: Lawrence Erlbaum Associates.

Majer, J., Rodriguez, J., Bloomer, C., & Jason, L. (2014). Predictors of HIV-risk sexual behavior: Examining lifetime sexual and physical abuse histories in relation to substance use and psychiatric problem severity among ex-offenders. *Journal of the American Psychiatric Nurses Association, 20,* 138–146.

Morken, I., Bru, E., Norekvål, T., Larsen, A., Idsoe, T., & Karlsen, B. (2014). Perceived support from healthcare professionals, shock anxiety, and post-traumatic stress in implantable cardioverter defibrillator recipients. *Journal of Clinical Nursing, 23,* 450–460.

O'Quigley, J. (2008). *Proportional hazards regression.* New York: Springer.

Pocock, S. J., Assmann, S., Enos, L., & Kasten, L. (2002). Subgroup analysis, covariate adjustment and baseline comparisons in clinical trial reporting: Current practice and problems. *Statistics in Medicine, 21,* 2917–2930.

Polit, D. F. (2010). *Statistics and data analysis for nursing research* (2nd ed.). Upper Saddle River, NJ: Pearson.

*Qin, R., Titler, M., Shever, L., & Kim, T. (2008). Estimating effects of nursing intervention via propensity score analysis. *Nursing Research, 57,* 444–452.

Reknes, I., Pallesen, S., Magerøy, B., Moen, B., Bjorvatn, B., & Einarsen, S. (2014). Exposure to bullying behaviors as a predictor of mental health problems among Norwegian nurses: Results from the prospective SUSSH-survey. *International Journal of Nursing Studies, 51,* 479–487.

Schneiderman, J., Kools, S., Negriff, S., Smith, S., & Trickett, P. (2015). Differences in caregiver-reported health problems and health care use in maltreated adolescents and a comparison group from the same urban environment. *Research in Nursing & Health, 38,* 60–70.

Tabachnick, B. G., & Fidell, L. S. (2012). *Using multivariate statistics* (6th ed.). Upper Saddle River, NJ: Pearson Education.

***A link to this open-access journal article is provided in the Toolkit for this chapter in the accompanying Resource Manual.** ⊗

19 | Processes of Quantitative Data Analysis

In this chapter, we offer an overview of steps that are normally taken in preparing for the analysis of quantitative data. Most of the activities we describe in this chapter would be undertaken *before* performing the statistical analyses described in the last few chapters, but we have positioned this chapter here because some of the material requires some familiarity with statistics.

Figure 19.1 shows what the flow of tasks in a quantitative might look like, organized in phases. Progress in analyzing quantitative data is not always as linear as this figure suggests, but it provides a framework for discussing key steps in the analytic process.

PREANALYSIS PHASE

The first phase of a quantitative analysis involves various clerical and administrative tasks, such as logging in forms, reviewing data for completeness and legibility, retrieving pieces of missing information, and assigning identification (ID) numbers. Another task involves selecting statistical software for doing the data analyses. Two widely used statistical software packages are IBM SPSS Statistics and the Statistical Analysis System (SAS). Next, researchers must code the data and enter them onto computer files to create a **data set** (the total collection of data for all sample members) for analysis.

Coding Quantitative Data

Coding is the process of transforming data into symbols—usually numbers. Certain variables are inherently quantitative (e.g., age, body temperature) and do not require coding, unless the data are gathered in categories (e.g., younger than 50 years of age versus 50 or older). Even with "naturally" quantitative data, researchers need to inspect their data. All responses should be of the same form and precision. For example, for the variable *height* in the nonmetric system, researchers need to decide whether to record feet and inches as two separate "variables" or to convert the information entirely to inches. Whichever method is adopted, it must be used consistently for all participants. There must also be consistency in handling information reported by sample members with different degrees of precision (e.g., a decision about how to code a response such as 5 feet 2½ inches).

Most data from structured instruments can be precoded with codes designated before data are collected. For example, questions with fixed response alternatives can be preassigned a numeric code that is printed on the data collection form, such as under age 50 = 1 and 50 and older = 2. Codes are often arbitrary, as in the case of the variable gender. Whether a female subject is coded 1 or 2 has no analytic importance so long as females are consistently assigned one code and males another code.

Respondents sometimes can check off more than one response to a question, as in the following

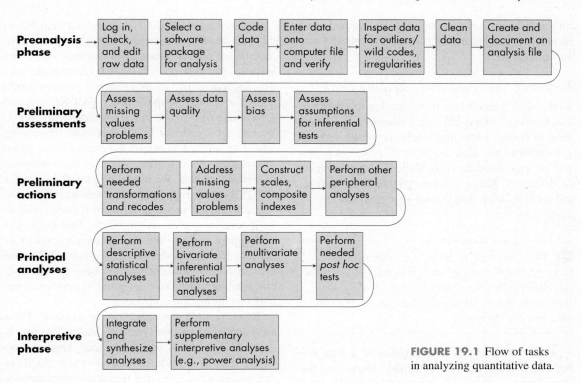

Preanalysis phase

Log in, check, and edit raw data → Select a software package for analysis → Code data → Enter data onto computer file and verify → Inspect data for outliers/ wild codes, irregularities → Clean data → Create and document an analysis file

Preliminary assessments

Assess missing values problems → Assess data quality → Assess bias → Assess assumptions for inferential tests

Preliminary actions

Perform needed transformations and recodes → Address missing values problems → Construct scales, composite indexes → Perform other peripheral analyses

Principal analyses

Perform descriptive statistical analyses → Perform bivariate inferential statistical analyses → Perform multivariate analyses → Perform needed *post hoc* tests

Interpretive phase

Integrate and synthesize analyses → Perform supplementary interpretive analyses (e.g., power analysis)

FIGURE 19.1 Flow of tasks in analyzing quantitative data.

question that might be used in a study about irritable bowel syndrome:

Which of the following symptoms have you experienced in the past week? (Check all that apply.)
- ❑ Abdominal pain
- ❑ Bloating
- ❑ Constipation
- ❑ Diarrhea
- ❑ Flatulence

With questions of this type, a 1-2-3-4-5 coding scheme cannot be used. Responses must be coded as though there were five separate questions: "Did you experience abdominal pain?" "Did you experience bloating?" and so on. Each check is treated as a "yes." The question yields five variables, with one code (e.g., 1) signifying "yes" and another code (e.g., 0) signifying "no."

If data from open-ended questions are going to be used in quantitative analysis, they must be coded. Sometimes researchers can develop codes ahead of time, but unstructured data often are collected because responses cannot be anticipated. In

such situations, researchers typically review a sizable portion of the data to understand content and then develop a coding scheme.

A code is needed for each variable for every sample member, even if there is no response. **Missing values** can be of various types. A person answering a question may be undecided, refuse to answer, or say, "Don't know." When skip patterns are used, there is missing information for those questions that are irrelevant to some respondents. A single missing values code may suffice, but it may be important to distinguish different types of missing data using different codes (e.g., distinguishing refusals and *don't knows*).

The choice of what code to use for missing data is often arbitrary, but missing values codes must be ones that have not been used for actual pieces of information. Some researchers use blanks, periods, or negative values for missing information. Some use 9 as the missing code because this value is out of the range of real codes for many variables.

Precise coding instructions should be documented in a coding manual. Coders, like observers and interviewers, must be properly trained, and intercoder (or intracoder) reliability checks are recommended.

Entering, Verifying, and Cleaning Data

Coded data typically are transferred onto a data file via keyboard entry, but other options (e.g., scanning of forms, importing electronic health records information) are also available. Various programs can be used for data entry, including spreadsheets or databases. Major software packages for statistical analysis have data editors that make data entry fairly easy.

TIP: Sometimes sample members enter their own data directly onto a computer file—for example, when they complete an online questionnaire. This is clearly advantageous in terms of efficiency and costs.

Figure 19.2 shows a screenshot of a data file for IBM SPSS Statistics (SPSS). These are the data from a fictitious intervention study used to illustrate analyses in the Supplements S to Chapters 16–18, and this screenshot appears in all three Supplements. This data file is very small: a 30 × 7 matrix, with 30 rows (one for each participant) and 7 columns for the variables—that is, one variable per column.

Each variable in a data set has to be named. Usually the variable name is abbreviated—for example, in Figure 19.2, we can see that the variable names are all short (GROUP, BWEIGHT, etc.). The software allows users to enter a more detailed description of each variable. For example, for the variable BWEIGHT, the extended label is "Infant birthweight in ounces." This full name would appear on all output rather than BWEIGHT. The Supplement to this chapter on thePoint' shows a screenshot with extended variable information. S

Each participant's unique ID should be entered along with actual data because this would allow you to go back to original sources if something needed to be verified. The ID number normally is entered as the first variable of the record, as in Figure 19.2.

The variables BWEIGHT, AGE, and PRIORS in this data set are ones that are "naturally" quantitative (number of ounces, years, prior pregnancies). Other variables had to be coded. GROUP, for example, uses a coding scheme of 1 for experimental group members and 2 for control group members. SMOKE is coded 1 for those who smoke and 0 for those who do not. We use a 1-2 code for GROUP because this coding would ensure that in output the experimental group information would be first, which is the convention in research reports. We used a dummy 0-1 code for SMOKE to make regression results easier to interpret.

Data entry is prone to error, so it is essential to verify entries and correct mistakes. One method is to compare visually the numbers on a printout of the data file with codes on the original source, and another is to double enter data. There are also special verifying programs designed to perform comparisons during direct data entry.

Even verified data need to be cleaned. **Data cleaning** involves two types of checks. The first is a check for outliers and wild codes. **Outliers** are values that lie outside the normal range. Outliers can be found by inspecting frequency distributions, paying special attention to the lowest and highest values. (Most researchers begin data analysis by constructing frequency distributions for all variables in their data set.) Some outliers are true, legitimate values (e.g., an income of $1 million in a distribution where the mean is $50,000), but sometimes they result from data entry errors.

Another problem is a **wild code**—that is, a code that is not possible. For example, the variable gender might have these three codes: 1 = female, 2 = male, and "blank" = missing. If someone was coded 3 for gender, there is an error. The computer could show the ID number of the faulty record, and the correct code could then be tracked down.

TIP: Such checks will never reveal all errors. If a male were incorrectly coded 1 for gender in the coding scheme just mentioned, the mistake might not be detected. Errors can have a big effect on the analysis and interpretation of data, so it is important to code, enter, verify, and clean data with care.

	ID	GROUP	AGE	PRIORS	SMOKE	BWEIGHT	REPEAT
1	1	1	17	1	1	107	1
2	2	1	14	0	0	101	0
3	3	1	21	3	0	119	0
4	4	1	20	2	0	128	1
5	5	1	15	1	1	89	0
6	6	1	19	0	1	99	0
7	7	1	19	1	0	111	0
8	8	1	18	1	1	117	1
9	9	1	17	0	0	102	1
10	10	1	20	0	0	120	0
11	11	1	13	0	1	76	0
12	12	1	18	0	1	116	0
13	13	1	16	0	0	100	1
14	14	1	18	0	0	115	0
15	15	1	21	2	1	113	0
16	16	2	19	0	0	111	1
17	17	2	21	1	0	108	0
18	18	2	19	2	1	95	0
19	19	2	17	0	1	99	0
20	20	2	19	0	0	103	1
21	21	2	15	0	1	94	0
22	22	2	17	1	0	101	1
23	23	2	21	2	0	114	0
24	24	2	20	1	0	97	0
25	25	2	18	0	1	99	1
26	26	2	18	0	1	113	0
27	27	2	19	1	0	89	0
28	28	2	20	0	0	98	0
29	29	2	17	0	0	102	0
30	30	2	19	1	1	105	0

Notes:

GROUP: Group status, 1 = Experimental group 2 = Control group
AGE: Mother's age in years
PRIORS: Number of prior pregnancies
SMOKE: Mother's smoking status, 1 = Smokes 0 = Does not smoke
BWEIGHT: Infant's birthweight, in ounces
REPEAT: Had repeat pregnancy within 18 months, 1 = Yes 0 = No

FIGURE 19.2 Fictitious data set for intervention study with low-income pregnant adolescents (screenshot of an SPSS data file).

A second data-cleaning procedure involves **consistency checks**, which focus on internal data consistency. In this task, researchers check for errors by testing compatibility of data within a case. For example, one question in a survey might ask current marital status, and another might ask number of marriages. If the data were internally consistent, respondents who answered "Single, never married" to the first question should have a zero (or a missing values code) for the second. Researchers should search for opportunities to check the consistency of entered data.

Osborne (2012) has devoted an entire book to a discussion of data cleaning. Another very useful resource is a brief open-access paper on this topic by Van den Broeck and colleagues (2005).

> **Example of Data Verification and Cleaning:** Minnick and colleagues (2013) described capacity issues for Doctor of Nursing Practice (DNP) programs based on a survey of nursing deans in U.S. nursing schools with DNP programs. Here is how they described preparing their data set for analysis: "After entry into an SPSS data file, all data were subjected to tests for outliers. We conducted >25 random checks of surveys returned by mail for data entry errors" (p. 95).

Creating and Documenting the Analysis Files

The decisions that researchers make about coding and variable naming should be fully documented. Memory should not be trusted; several weeks after coding, researchers may no longer remember if males were coded 1 and females were coded 2, or vice versa. Moreover, colleagues may wish to borrow the data for a secondary analysis. Documentation should always be sufficiently thorough that someone unfamiliar with the original study could use the data.

Documentation primarily involves preparing a codebook. A **codebook** is essentially a listing of each variable together with information about placement in the file, codes associated with the values of the variable, and other basic information. Codebooks can be generated by statistical or data entry programs.

PRELIMINARY ASSESSMENTS AND ACTIONS

Researchers typically undertake several preanalytic activities before they test their hypotheses. Several preparatory activities are discussed next.

Assessing and Handling Missing Values Problems

Researchers strive to have data values for all participants on all key variables—but usually find that their data sets have some missing values. Before they can deal with this problem, researchers must first understand their missing values. An appropriate solution depends on such factors as the extent of missing data, the role of the variable with missing data, and the pattern of missingness.

There are three missing values patterns. The first, and most desirable, is **missing completely at random** (MCAR), which occurs when cases with missing values are just a random subset of all cases. When data are MCAR, analyses remain unbiased—but missing values are seldom MCAR. Data are considered **missing at random** (MAR) if missingness is related to other variables in the data set (e.g., gender)—but *not* related to the value of the variable that has the missing values. For example, if missing values for depression occur more frequently for men than for women—but not for people who are most or least depressed—the pattern of missingness may be MAR. The third pattern is **missing not at random** (MNAR), a pattern in which the value of the variable that is missing *is* related to its missingness (e.g., those declining to report their income tend to be either rich or poor). Missing values that are MAR or MNAR can result in biased results, but solutions are most readily accomplished when missing data are MAR and not MNAR—although it is difficult to know for sure which of these two pattern applies.

A first step in analyzing missing data is to assess the extent of the problem by examining frequency distributions on a variable-by-variable basis. Another step is to examine the cumulative extent of missing values (e.g., what percentage of cases had no variables missing, one variable missing, and so on). Another task is to evaluate the randomness of missing values. A simple procedure is to divide the sample into two groups—those with and without missing data on a specified variable. The two groups can then be compared in terms of their characteristics to assess whether the two groups are comparable in terms of key demographic or clinical variables (e.g., Were men more likely than women to leave certain questions blank? Was the mean age of those with missing values different from that of people without missing values?).

Until recently, examining patterns of missingness was a tedious process, which may explain why some researchers simply ignore the problem of missing data (and therefore ignore the risk of bias that can be introduced). Now, however, programs in widely used statistical software have greatly simplified this important task. For example, the Missing Values Analysis (MVA) module within SPSS offers powerful means of detecting and addressing missing values.

Once researchers have assessed the extent and patterning of missing values, they must decide how to address the problem. There are three basic types of solutions: deletions, imputations, and mixed modeling within longitudinal data sets. We discuss the first two here; information about sophisticated modeling solutions are discussed in Shin (2009) and Son et al. (2012).

Missing Data and Deletions

Listwise deletion (also called *complete case analysis*) is simply the analysis of those cases for which there are no missing data. Listwise deletion is based on an implicit assumption of MCAR. Researchers who use this method typically have not made a formal assessment of the extent to which MCAR is probable but rather are simply disregarding the problem of missing data.

Perhaps the most widely used (but not the best) approach is to delete cases selectively, on a variable-by-variable basis by means of **pairwise deletion** (also called *available case analysis*). For example, in a test of an intervention to reduce patient anxiety, the dependent variables might be blood pressure and self-reported anxiety. If 10 people from the sample 100 failed to complete the anxiety scale, we might base the analyses of anxiety data on the

90 people who completed the scale, but use the full sample of 100 in the blood pressure analysis. If the number of cases fluctuates widely across outcomes, the results are difficult to interpret because the sample is essentially a "moving target."

➔ **TIP:** Computer programs like SPSS use either listwise or pairwise deletion as the **default** (i.e., the option that will be used in the analysis unless there are specific instructions to the contrary).

Researchers sometimes use pairwise deletion in analyses involving a correlation matrix. From one pair of variables in the matrix to another, the number of cases can vary substantially. Although such correlation matrixes may provide useful descriptive information, it is imprudent to use pairwise deletion for correlation-based multivariate analyses such as multiple regression or factor analysis because the correlations are calculated on nonidentical subsets of people.

Another deletion option is to delete a variable for all participants. This option may be suitable when a high percentage of cases have missing values on a variable that is not central to the analysis. Recommendations for how much missing data should drive this decision range from 15% to 40% of cases (Fox-Wasylyshyn & El-Masri, 2005).

Missing Data and Imputations

Preferred methods for addressing missing values involve **imputation**—that is, "filling in" missing data with values believed to be good estimates of what the values would have been, had they not been missing. An attractive feature of imputation is that it allows researchers to maintain full sample size, and thus, statistical power is not compromised. The risk is that the imputations will be poor estimates of real values, leading to biases of unknown magnitude and direction.

The simplest imputation procedure is **mean substitution** or *median substitution*, which involves using "typical" sample values to replace missing data that are continuous. For example, if a person's age were missing and if the average age of sample members were 45.2 years, we could substitute the value 45.2 in place of the missing values code. Mean substitution is, like listwise deletion, popular because of its simplicity. Yet, even though mean substitution increases sample size and leaves variable means unchanged, it is rarely the best approach. Regardless of what the underlying pattern of missingness is, mean imputation leads to underestimations of variance, and variance is what most statistical analyses are all about.

A refinement on mean substitution is to use the mean value for a relevant subgroup—called a **subgroup** (or *conditional*) **mean substitution**. The assumption is that a better estimate of the missing value can be obtained by making the substitution conditional on participants' characteristics. For example, rather than replacing a missing age value with 45.2, we could replace a man's missing value with men's mean age, and a woman's mean value with women's mean age. This is a better option than mean substitution because the substituted values are presumably closer to the real values and also because variance is not reduced as much. Nevertheless, conditional (subgroup) mean substitution is not a preferred approach, except when overall missingness is low.

➲ TIP: When data are missing for individual items on a multi-item scale, it may be appropriate to replace a missing value with the mean of other similar items from the person with the missing value, an approach that assumes that people are "internally consistent" across similar questions. Such **case mean substitution**, which uses person-specific information to inform the estimate, has the advantage of not throwing out data altogether (listwise deletion) and not assuming that a person is similar to all others in a sample or subgroup (mean substitution). Case mean substitution has been found to be an acceptable method of imputation at the item level, even compared to more sophisticated methods.

Researchers are increasingly using imputation methods that make more extensive use of data in the data set. One example is to use regression analysis to "predict" the correct value of missing data. Suppose we found that participants' age was correlated with gender, education, and health status. Based on data from those with complete data, age could be regressed on these three variables to predict age for people with missing age data, but whose values for the three other variables were not missing. Regression-based imputation is more accurate than previously discussed strategies, although variability remains underestimated using regression.

Even more sophisticated solutions have been developed. Maximum likelihood estimation is useful because it uses all data points in a data set to construct estimated replacement values. **Expectation (EM) maximization** involves using an iterative procedure with a maximum-likelihood-based algorithm to produce the best parameter estimates.

An approach called **multiple imputation (MI)** is currently considered the best method for addressing missing values problems. MI addresses a fundamental issue—the uncertainty of any given estimate—by imputing several (m) estimates of the missing data, and each estimate has an element of randomness introduced. Results from analyses across the m imputations are later pooled. MI has not often been used because of its complexity and the limited availability of appropriate software, but recent versions of the SPSS MVA module (version 17.0 and higher) do offer multiple imputation. Patrician (2002) has described multiple imputation is some detail.

Example of Handling Missing Values: Mejía and colleagues (2014) undertook a cost-effectiveness analysis of a nurse-facilitated intervention for patients with heart failure. Patients' resource use was measured using a wide array of information sources. Multiple imputation was used to impute missing values.

It might be noted that the issue of missingness has been given a lot of attention in the analysis of data from randomized controlled trials (RCTs) because attrition in trials is common. As noted in Chapter 10, the "gold standard" for analyzing data from RCTs is to use an **intention-to-treat (ITT) analysis**, which involves analyzing outcome data from all participants who were randomized, regardless of whether they dropped out of the study. A true ITT analysis is achieved only if there are no missing outcome data, or if missing values are accounted for in the analysis, such as through imputation. A resource for advice on how to achieve

ITT is offered in Polit and Gillespie (2010). Polit and Gillespie (2009) found, in their analysis of 124 nursing trials, that 75% of the RCTs had missing outcome data, and one out of four had 20% or more missing values. Listwise and pairwise deletion were the most common approaches; only about 10% of the studies used imputation or mixed effects modeling in their ITT analyses. The approach most often used to impute values for missing outcome variables in these RCTs was a procedure called **last observation carried forward (LOCF)**, which imputes the missing outcome using the previous measurement of that same outcome. For example, if data were collected 1 month and 3 months after the intervention, but data for the 3-month outcome were missing for some participants, the 1-month value would replace the missing value. LOCF is no longer considered the best approach.

Procedures for dealing with missing data are discussed at greater length in McKnight and colleagues (2007) and Polit (2010). Also, links to some open-access articles relating to the handling of missing values is available in the Toolkit ✷.

Assessing Data Quality

Assessing data quality is another early analytic task. For example, when a composite scale is used, researchers should assess its internal consistency (Chapter 14). The distribution of data values for key variables also should be examined to assess any anomalies, such as limited variability, extreme skewness, or the presence of ceiling or floor effects. A **ceiling effect** occurs when values for a variable are restricted at the upper end of a continuum, and a **floor effect** occurs when values are restricted at the lower end. For example, a vocabulary test for 10-year-olds likely would yield a clustering of high scores in a sample of 11-year-olds, creating a ceiling effect that would reduce correlations between test scores and other characteristics of the children. Conversely, there likely would be a clustering of low scores on the test with a sample of 9-year-olds, resulting in a floor effect with similar consequences. Floor and ceiling effects are of special concern when the goal is to measure change: If a measure has floor or ceiling effect, improvement (or deterioration) will not be adequately captured.

Earlier we discussed outliers in connection with efforts to clean a data set to ensure the accuracy of data entered into a file. Legitimate outliers—extreme scores that are true values—are a data quality issue. Outliers can distort study results and cause errors in statistical decision making, and so outliers should be scrutinized. By convention, a value is considered an **extreme outlier** if it is greater than 3 times the *interquartile range (IQR)* above the third quartile or below the first quartile. The IQR, as noted briefly in Chapter 16, is an index of variability. Methods for detecting and addressing outlier problems are discussed in Polit (2010).

Example of Data Quality Screening: Lee and co-researchers (2012) used an incident reporting system in a hospital to explore factors related to the prevention and management of pressure ulcers in 4,301 hospital cases in Taiwan. For each variable considered, a case was excluded as an outlier if the value was more than 3 standard deviations from the mean.

➲ **TIP:** For those using SPSS, the EXPLORE routine is invaluable in making assessments of data quality. We illustrate this in the Supplement to this chapter on the**Point**. Ⓢ

Assessing Bias

Researchers often undertake preliminary analyses to assess biases, including the following:

- *Nonresponse (volunteer) bias.* If possible, researchers should assess whether a biased subset of people participated in a study. If there is information about the characteristics of all people who were asked to participate (e.g., demographic information from hospital records), researchers should compare the characteristics of those who did and did not participate to assess the nature and direction of any biases and to inform conclusions about the study's generalizability.
- *Selection bias.* When nonrandomized comparison groups are used (e.g., in quasi-experimental studies), researchers should check for selection

biases by comparing the groups' baseline characteristics. Detected differences should, if possible, be controlled—for example, through analysis of covariance or regression—especially if a characteristic is a strong predictor of the dependent variable. Even when an experimental design has been used, researchers often check the success of randomization.

- *Attrition bias.* In studies with multiple points of data collection, it is important to check for attrition biases by comparing people who did and did not continue to participate in later waves of data collection, based on baseline characteristics.

In performing any of these analyses, significant group differences are often an indication of bias, and such bias must be taken into consideration in interpreting and discussing the results. The biases usually should be controlled in testing the principal hypotheses.

➲ **TIP:** It is not considered appropriate to test the significance of group differences on baseline variables in randomized controlled trials—even though this practice is adopted widely, and results are often reported in tables (Pocock et al., 2002). If randomization was done properly and the sample size is adequate, one would expect 5% of the group differences to be significant, when α = .05—and this does not signify a bias. Experts advise that it is preferable to control for significant predictors of the outcome, even if group differences are not significant, than to control for a baseline variable with significant group differences but weakly related to the outcome.

Example of Assessing Bias: Richmond and colleagues (2014) tested the hypothesis that postinjury depression for patients experiencing a minor injury was related to their quality of life in the year after the injury. They tested for attrition bias by comparing the characteristics of patients who did and did not provide follow-up data. Patients lost to follow-up were more likely to be men and had a lower mean number of years of education, for example.

Testing Assumptions for Statistical Tests

Most statistical tests are based on a number of assumptions—conditions that are presumed to be true and, when violated, can lead to erroneous conclusions. For example, parametric tests assume that variables are distributed normally. Frequency distributions, scatter plots, and other assessment procedures provide researchers with information about whether or not underlying assumptions for statistical tests have been upheld.

Graphic displays of frequency distributions can show whether the distribution of values is severely skewed, multimodal, too peaked, or too flat. There are statistical indexes of skewness or peakedness that test whether the shape of the distribution is significantly skewed or peaked or flat. Many software programs also include the *Kolmogorov-Smirnov test*, which tests that a distribution does not deviate significantly from a normal distribution.

Example of Testing Assumptions: Aghaie and colleagues (2014) tested the effect of nature-based sound therapy on the agitation and anxiety of coronary artery bypass graft patients. The Kolmogorov-Smirnov test was used to test for departures from normality of outcome variables. None deviated significantly from normality, and so repeated-measures ANOVA was used in the main analyses.

Performing Data Transformations

Raw data often need to be modified or transformed before hypotheses can be tested. Various **data transformations** can easily be handled through commands to the computer. For example, the scoring direction of some items on multi-item scales might need to be reversed before item scores can be summed. Some guidance on **item reversals** was presented in Chapter 15.

Sometimes researchers want to create a variable that is a cumulative **count** based on other variables in the data set. For example, suppose we asked people to indicate which types of illegal drug they had used in the past month, from a list of 10 options. Use of each drug would be answered independently in a yes (e.g., coded 1) or no (e.g., coded 0) fashion. We could create a new variable of number of different drugs used that represented a count of all the

"1" codes for the 10 drug items. Other transformations involve **recodes** of original values. Recoding is often used to create *dummy variables* for multivariate analyses.

Transformations also can be undertaken to render data appropriate for statistical tests. For example, if a distribution is non-normal, a transformation can sometimes help to make parametric procedures appropriate. A logarithmic transformation, for example, tends to normalize positively skewed distributions.

⟶ **TIP:** The Toolkit in the accompanying *Resource Manual* includes a table with data transformations that may help to correct skewed distributions. The table also identifies the SPSS functions that would be used for the transformations.

When you do transformations, it is important to check that they were done correctly by examining a sample of values for the original and transformed variables. This can be done by instructing the computer to list, for a sample of cases, the values of the newly created variables and the original variables used to create them.

Example of Transforming Variables: Tsai and co-researchers (2013) studied the relationship between daytime napping and sleep duration in a sample of pregnant women in Taiwan. Nap durations were not normally distributed, and so square root transformations were applied.

Performing Additional Peripheral Analyses

Depending on the study, additional peripheral analyses may be needed before proceeding to substantive analyses. It is impossible to catalog all such analyses, but we offer a few examples to alert readers to the kinds of issues that need to be given some thought.

Data Pooling

Researchers sometimes obtain data from more than one source, for example, when researchers recruit participants from multiple sites. The risk is that participants from different sites may not really be drawn from the same population, and so it is wise to evaluate whether **pooling** of data (combining data across sites) is warranted (Knapp & Brown, 2014). This involves comparing participants from the different sites in terms of key research variables, or comparing the extent to which correlations between key variables are similar across sites.

Example of Testing for Pooling: Metheny and colleagues (2012) studied methods used by critical care nurses to assess tolerance to gastric tube feedings. They pooled data from a mailed national survey with data from an online survey posted in a newsletter circulated to the American Association of Critical Care Nurses. They undertook analyses to assess whether pooling was justified.

Testing Cohort Effects

Nurse researchers sometimes accumulate a sample over an extended period of time to achieve adequate sample sizes. This can result in **cohort effects**, that is, differences in participant characteristics over time. This might occur because of changes in community characteristics or in health care services, for example. If the research involves an intervention, it may also be that the treatment itself changes—for example, if those administering the treatment get better at doing it. Thus, researchers with a long period of *sample intake* should consider testing for cohort effects because such effects can confound the results or even mask relationships. This activity usually involves examining correlations between entry dates and key variables.

Example of Testing for Cohort Effects: Polit and colleagues (2001), in their study of health problems among low-income mothers, analyzed survey data that were collected over a 12-month period from a sample of 4,000 women. They discovered that women interviewed later were significantly more disadvantaged than those interviewed early. In their analyses, timing of the interview was statistically controlled.

Testing Ordering (Carryover) Effects

When a crossover design is used (i.e., people are randomly assigned to different orderings of treatments), researchers should assess whether outcomes are different for people in the different treatment-order groups. That is, did getting A before B yield different outcomes than getting B before A? In essence, such tests offer evidence that it is legitimate to pool the data from alternative orderings.

> **Example of Testing for Ordering Effects:**
> Mackereth and colleagues (2009) compared the effects of reflexology versus progressive muscle relaxation training for people with multiple sclerosis, using a crossover design. Despite having a 4-week washout period, outcome measures such as salivary cortisol and blood pressure did not return to baseline levels, and an ordering effect was detected.

PRINCIPAL ANALYSES

At this point in the analysis process, researchers have a cleaned data set, with missing data problems resolved and transformations completed; they also have some understanding of data quality and biases. They can now proceed with more substantive data analyses.

Planning the Substantive Data Analysis

In many studies, researchers collect data on dozens of variables. They cannot analyze every variable in relation to all others, and so a plan to guide data analysis must be developed. One approach is to prepare a list of the analyses to be undertaken, specifying both the variables and the statistical test to be used. Another approach is to develop table shells. **Table shells** are layouts of how researchers envision presenting their findings, without numbers filled in. Once a table shell is prepared, researchers can do the analyses needed to complete the table. (The table templates in the Toolkit of the accompanying *Resource Manual*, for Chapters 16-18, can be used as a basis for table shells ⊗.) Researchers do not need to adhere rigidly to table shells, but they provide a good mechanism for organizing the analysis of large amounts of data.

Substantive Analyses

Substantive analyses typically begin with descriptive analyses. Researchers usually develop a profile of the sample and may look descriptively at correlations among variables. These initial analyses may suggest further analyses or further data

transformations that were not originally envisioned. They also give researchers an opportunity to become familiar with their data.

> ➔ **TIP:** When you explore your data, resist the temptation of going on a "fishing expedition," that is, hunting for *any* significant relationships. The facility with which computers can generate statistics makes it easy to run analyses indiscriminately. The risk is that you will serendipitously find significant correlations between variables as a function of chance. For example, in a correlation matrix with 10 variables—which results in 45 nonredundant correlations—there are likely to be two to three *spurious* significant correlations when alpha =.05 (i.e., .05 × 45 = 2.25).

Researchers then perform statistical analyses to test their hypotheses. Researchers whose data analysis plan calls for multivariate analyses (e.g., MANOVA) often begin with bivariate analyses (e.g., a series of ANOVAs). The primary statistical analyses are complete when all research questions are addressed and when table shells have the applicable numbers in them.

Supplementary Analyses

Sometimes supplementary analyses can facilitate interpretation of the results. For example, suppose our analyses revealed that an exercise intervention was successful in lowering blood pressure in hypertensive patients. In scrutinizing sample characteristics, however, we find that women were underrepresented, which might lead critics to suggest that the evidence for effectiveness in a mixed-gender population is weak. In this situation, we could examine experimental-control group differences for men and women separately. If the results are similar, it would strengthen inferences about the potential benefits of the intervention for both genders.

Another strategy is to undertake **sensitivity analyses**, which are analyses that test research hypotheses using different assumptions or different strategies. One example concerns testing alternative strategies to address missing values problems. Some strategies are appropriate under varying conditions, so sensitivity analyses to understand how different strategies affect substantive results are valuable. Another example of sensitivity analyses is running analyses with and without legitimate outliers to see if the results change. Thabane and colleagues (2013) offer a tutorial on sensitivity analyses.

Example of Sensitivity Analysis: Felisbino-Mendes and colleagues (2014) studied the relationship between maternal obesity and fetal deaths in Brazil. The evidence suggested that increases in maternal body mass index were associated with a higher risk of spontaneous abortion. A sensitivity analysis was conducted with women who had had only one pregnancy, and similar results were obtained.

RESEARCH EXAMPLE

We conclude this chapter with an example of a study that provided considerable detail about their data management and analyses.

Study: Randomized clinical trial of a school-based academic and counseling program for older school-age students (Kintner & Sikorskii, 2009)

Statement of Purpose: The purpose of this feasibility study was to gather preliminary evidence about the efficacy of an academic and counseling program for older elementary students with asthma, in terms of cognitive, behavioral, psychosocial, and quality of life outcomes.

Method: The researchers used a two-group cluster randomized design with a sample of fourth- to sixth-grade students aged 9 to 12 years. Three schools were randomly assigned to receive the Staying Healthy—Asthma Responsible and Prepared (SHARP) program, and two schools were assigned to a control group, in an effort to reduce contamination of treatments among students at a given school. A total of 66 students were included in the sample. Students in the SHARP program met weekly for 10 weeks during school hours to discuss asthma management. There was also a community component for family members, friends, and others. Data were collected at baseline and after the intervention for such outcomes

as knowledge of asthma, asthma health behaviors, acceptance of asthma, participation in life activities, and illness severity.

Analyses: The researchers collected and managed their data using laptop computers: "The system included quality-control methods to restrict field ranges and values, to provide internal consistency checks, to prevent entry of erroneous data, and to track missing data" (p. 326). Virtually no missing data were found in completed surveys. There were, however, four dropouts (all in the intervention group) before the Time 2 data collection, and data for one control group member could not be used. Reasons for all participant loss were reported. The researchers noted that "an intention-to-treat approach was adopted for analysis" (p. 326). The researchers looked at distributions for all variables to assess data quality and evaluate whether assumptions for statistical tests had been met. Internal consistency estimates were computed for all scales. The baseline characteristics of students in the two groups were compared to assess possible biases. Because the groups differed in terms of some baseline measures, baseline values were statistically controlled to estimate program effects. The researchers also compared the characteristics of those who completed the study and those who did not, and found no significant differences. Postintervention outcomes for the two groups were assessed using complex hierarchical models. The researchers computed adjusted mean scores, as well as effect size indexes, for all outcomes.

Results: Compared with students in the control group, students in the SHARP program had statistically significant improvements in asthma knowledge, use of risk reduction behaviors, and other outcomes, with sizeable effect sizes of d greater than .70. Moderate (but not statistically significant) effects (d between .30 and .50) were observed for two other outcomes.

SUMMARY POINTS

- Researchers who collect quantitative data typically progress through a series of steps in the analysis and interpretation of their data. Careful researchers lay out a data analysis plan in advance to guide that progress.

- Quantitative data typically must be **coded** into numerical values; codes need to be developed for legitimate data and for **missing values**. Decisions about coding and variable naming are documented in a **codebook**.
- **Data entry** is an error-prone process that requires verification and **data cleaning**. Cleaning involves checks for **outliers** (values that lie outside the normal range of values) and **wild codes** (codes that are not legitimate), as well as **consistency checks** (checks for internally consistent information).
- Decisions on handling missing values must be based on the amount of missing data and how missing data are patterned (i.e., the extent to which missingness is random). Addressing missing data is important for undertaking **intention-to-treat analyses**.
- The three missing values patterns are (1) **missing completely at random (MCAR)**, which occurs when cases with missing values are just a random subsample of all cases in the sample; (2) **missing at random (MAR)**, which occurs if missingness is related to other variables but *not* related to the value of the variable that has the missing values; and (3) **missing not at random (MNAR)**, a pattern in which the value of the variable that is missing is related to its missingness.
- Two basic missing values strategies involve **deletion** or **imputation**. Deletion strategies include deleting cases with missing values (i.e., **listwise deletion**), selective **pairwise deletion** of cases, or deleting variables with missing values. Imputation strategies include **mean substitution**, regression-based estimation of missing values, **expectation maximization (EM) imputation**, and **multiple imputation (MI)**, which is considered the best approach.
- Raw data often need to be transformed for analysis. Examples of **data transformations** include reversing the coding of items, recoding the values of a variable (e.g., for dummy variables), and transforming data to meet statistical assumptions (e.g., through logarithmic transformations to achieve normality).
- Researchers usually undertake additional steps to assess data quality, such as evaluating the internal consistency of scales, examining distributions for **extreme outliers** that are legitimate values, and analyzing the magnitude and direction of any biases, such as nonresponse bias, selection bias, and attrition bias.
- Another assessment may involve a scrutiny for possible **ceiling effects** (which occurs when values for a variable are restricted at the upper end of a continuum) or **floor effects** (which occurs when values are restricted at the lower end).
- Sometimes peripheral analyses involve tests to determine whether **pooling** of participants is warranted, and tests for **cohort effects** or **ordering effects**.
- Once the data are fully prepared for substantive analysis, researchers should develop a formal analysis plan, to reduce the temptation to go on a "fishing expedition." One approach is to develop **table shells**, that is, fully laid-out tables without numbers in them.
- Supplementary statistical analyses can sometimes facilitate interpretation (e.g., doing **sensitivity analyses** that test whether results hold true under different assumptions or different statistical procedures).

STUDY ACTIVITIES

Chapter 19 of the *Resource Manual for Nursing Research*: *Generating and Assessing Evidence for Nursing Practice*, *10th edition*, offers exercises and study suggestions for reinforcing concepts presented in this chapter. In addition, the following study questions can be addressed:

1. Read an article in a recent nursing research journal. Which analytic steps discussed in this chapter were described in the report? Why do you think the authors did not provide more information?
2. Read the following article and comment on the sensitivity analysis that was performed: Donnelly, J., Winder, J., Kernohan, W., & Stevenson, M. (2011). An RCT to determine the effect of a heel elevation device in pressure ulcer prevention post-hip fracture. *Journal of Wound Care*, *20*, 309–312.

STUDIES CITED IN CHAPTER 19

Aghaie, B., Rejeh, N., Heravi-Karimooi, M., Ebadi, A., Moradian, S., Vaismoradi, M., & Jasper, M. (2014). Effect of nature-based sound therapy on agitation and anxiety in coronary artery bypass graft patients during the weaning of mechanical ventilation: A randomised clinical trial. *International Journal of Nursing Studies*, *51*, 526–538.

*Felisbino-Mendes, M., Matozinhos, F., Miranda, J., Villamor, E., & Velasquez-Melendez, G. (2014). Maternal obesity and fetal deaths: Results from the Brazilian cross-sectional demographic health survey, 2006. *BMC Pregnancy & Childbirth*, *14*, 5.

Fox-Wasylyshyn, S., & El-Masri, M. (2005). Handling missing data in self-report measures. *Research in Nursing & Health*, *28*, 488–495.

*Kintner, E., & Sikorskii, A. (2009). Randomized clinical trial of a school-based academic and counseling program for older school-age students. *Nursing Research*, *58*, 321–331.

Knapp, T. R., & Brown, J. (2014). Ten statistics commandments that almost never should be broken. *Research in Nursing & Health*, *37*, 347–351.

Lee, T. T., Lin, K., Mills, M., & Kuo, Y. (2012). Factors related to the prevention and management of pressure ulcers. *Computers, Informatics, Nursing*, *30*, 489–495.

Mackereth, P., Booth, K., Hillier, V., & Caress, A. (2009). Reflexology and progressive muscle relaxation training for people with multiple sclerosis: A crossover trial. *Complementary Therapies in Clinical Practice*, *15*, 14–21.

McKnight, P., McKnight, K., Sidani, S., & Figueredo, A. (2007). *Missing data: A gentle introduction*. New York: Guilford Press.

Mejía, A., Richardson, G., Pattenden, J., Cockayne, S., & Lewin, R. (2014). Cost-effectiveness of a nurse facilitated, cognitive behavioural self-management programme compared with usual care using a CBT manual alone for patients with heart failure: Secondary analysis of data from the SEMAPHFOR trial. *International Journal of Nursing Studies*, *51*, 1214–1220.

Metheny, N. A., Mills, A., & Stewart, B. (2012). Monitoring intolerance to gastric tube feedings: A national survey. *American Journal of Critical Care*, *21*, e33–e40.

Minnick, A. F., Norman, L., & Donaghey, B. (2013). Defining and describing capacity issues in U.S. Doctor of Nursing Practice programs. *Nursing Outlook*, *61*, 93–101.

Osborne, J. W. (2012). *Best practices in data cleaning: A complete guide to everything you need to do before and after collecting your data*. Thousand Oaks, CA: Sage.

Patrician, P. A. (2002). Multiple imputation for missing data. *Research in Nursing & Health*, *25*, 76–84.

Pocock, S. J., Assmann, S., Enos, L., & Kasten, L. (2002). Subgroup analysis, covariate adjustment and baseline comparisons in clinical trial reporting: Current practice and problems. *Statistics in Medicine*, *21*, 2917–2930.

Polit, D. F. (2010). *Statistics and data analysis for nursing research* (2nd ed.). Upper Saddle River, NJ: Pearson.

Polit, D. F., & Gillespie, B. (2009). The use of the intention-to-treat principle in nursing clinical trials. *Nursing Research*, *58*, 391–399.

Polit, D. F., & Gillespie, B. (2010). Intention-to-treat in randomized controlled trials: Recommendations for a total trial strategy. *Research in Nursing & Health*, *33*, 355–368.

Polit, D. F., London, A. S., & Martinez, J. M. (2001). *The health of poor urban women*. New York: MDRC. Retrieved from http://www.mdrc.org

Richmond, T. S., Guo, W., Ackerson, T., Hollander, J., Gracias, V., Robinson, K., & Amsterdam, J. (2014). The effect of postinjury depression on quality of life following minor injury. *Journal of Nursing Scholarship*, *46*, 116–124.

Shin, J. H. (2009). Application of repeated-measures analysis of variance and hierarchical linear model in nursing research. *Nursing Research*, *58*, 211–217.

Son, H., Friedman, E., & Thomas, S. A. (2012). Application of pattern mixture models to address missing data in longitudinal data analysis using SPSS. *Nursing Research*, *61*, 195–203.

*Thabane, L., Mbuagbaw, L., Zhang, S., Samaan, Z., Marcucci, M., Ye, C., . . . Goldsmith, C. (2013). A tutorial on sensitivity analyses in clinical trials: The what, why, when, and how. *BMC Research Methodology*, *13*, 92.

Tsai, S. Y., Kuo, L., Lee, C., Lee, Y., & Landis, C. (2013). Reduced sleep duration and daytime naps in pregnant women in Taiwan. *Nursing Research*, *62*, 99–105.

*Van den Broeck, J., Cunningham, S., Eeckles, R., & Herbst, K. (2005). Data cleaning: Detecting, diagnosing, and editing data abnormalities. *PLoS Medicine*, *2*, 10.

A link to this open-access journal article is provided in the Toolkit for this chapter in the accompanying Resource Manual. ⊗

20 Clinical Significance and Interpretation of Quantitative Results

In this chapter, we discuss the issue of interpreting quantitative (statistical) results. We begin with some general interpretive guidelines. In the second part of this chapter, we pay particular attention to an important emerging topic in health research: clinical significance.

INTERPRETATION OF QUANTITATIVE RESULTS

The analysis of research data provides the **results** of the study. These results need to be evaluated and interpreted, giving thought to the aims of the study, its theoretical basis, the body of related research evidence, and limitations of the adopted research methods. Interpretation of statistical results forms the basis for the discussion section of quantitative research reports.

Issues in Interpretation

The interpretive task is complex, requiring strong methodologic and substantive skills. Although interpretation is difficult to teach, we offer some advice about ways of making sound inferences from study results.

The Interpretive Mind-Set

Evidence-based practice (EBP) encourages clinicians to make decisions based on a careful assessment of "best evidence." Thinking critically, and demanding evidence, are also part of a research interpreter's job. Just as clinicians must ask, "What *evidence* is there that this intervention or strategy will be beneficial?" so should interpreters ask, "What *evidence* is there that the results are real, true, and important?"

To be a good interpreter of research results, it is reasonable to adopt a skeptical attitude—much like in hypothesis testing, which begins with a null hypothesis that researchers want to reject. *The "null hypothesis" to be rejected in interpretation is that the results are wrong.* The "research hypothesis" in interpretation is that the evidence can be trusted and used in practice because the results reflect the truth. The greater the evidence that your design and methods were sound, the less plausible is the "null hypothesis" of faulty results.

⊃ **TIP:** You should ask such questions as, Is it *plausible* that my results were affected by selection biases? Is it *plausible* that if participants had been blinded to the treatment, the results would have been different? Is it *plausible* that if I had used a different instrument, or had gotten a larger sample, or had less attrition, my results would change? You hope that the answers to such questions are "no," but you should start with the working assumption that the answer is "yes" until you have satisfied yourself that this is not true.

Aspects of Interpretation

Interpreting the results of a study involves attending to different but overlapping considerations:

- The credibility and accuracy of the results
- The precision of the estimate of effects
- The magnitude of effects and importance of the results
- The meaning of the results, especially with regard to causality
- The generalizability of the results
- The implications of the results for practice, theory development, or further research

Credibility of Quantitative Results

One of the most important interpretive tasks is to assess whether the results are *correct*. This corresponds to the first EBP question we posed in Chapter 2 (Box 2.2): "What is the quality of the evidence—that is, how rigorous and reliable is it?" If the results are not credible, the remaining interpretive issues (meaning, magnitude, and so on) are not likely to be relevant.

Research findings are meant to reflect "truth in the real world." The findings are intended to be proxies for the true state of affairs in actual community or health care settings. Inference is the vehicle for linking results to the real world. Inferences about the real world are valid, however, to the extent that the researchers have made rigorous methodologic decisions. To come to a conclusion about whether the results closely approximate "truth in the real world," each aspect of the study—its research design, intervention design, sampling plan, measurement and data collection plan, and analytic approach—must be subjected to critical scrutiny.

There are various ways to assess credibility, including the use of the critiquing guidelines we have offered throughout this book. Here we share some additional perspectives.

Proxies and Credibility

Researchers begin with abstract constructs and then devise ways to operationalize them. Constructs are linked to realities in a series of approximations, each of which affects interpretation because at each step, there is a potential for misrepresentation. The better the proxies, the more credible results are likely to be. In this section, we illustrate successive proxies using sampling concepts to highlight the potential for inferential challenges.

When researchers formulate research questions or hypotheses, the population is typically broad and abstract. Population specifications are delineated later when eligibility criteria are defined. For example, suppose we wanted to test the effectiveness of an intervention to increase physical activity in low-income women. Figure 20.1 shows the series of steps between the abstract population construct (low-income women) and the *actual* women who participated in the study. Using data from the actual sample on the far right, the researcher would like to make inferences about the effectiveness of the intervention for a broader group, but each proxy along the way represents a potential problem for achieving the desired inference. In interpreting a study, readers must consider how *plausible* it is that the actual sample reflects the recruited sample, the accessible population, the target population, and then the population construct.

Table 20.1 presents a description of a hypothetical scenario in which the researchers moved from a population construct of low-income women to an actual sample of 161 women who participated in the study. The table shows some questions that a person trying to make inferences about the study results might ask—that is, inferential challenges.

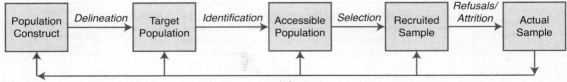

FIGURE 20.1 Inferences about populations: from the analysis sample to the population construct.

TABLE 20.1 • Successive Proxies in Sampling Example: From the Population Construct to the Analysis Sample

ELEMENT	DESCRIPTION	POSSIBLE INFERENTIAL CHALLENGES
Population construct	Low-income women	
Target population	All women who receive public assistance (cash welfare) in California	• Why only welfare recipients—why not the working poor? • Why California?
Accessible population	All women who receive public assistance in Los Angeles and who speak English or Spanish	• Why Los Angeles? • What about non-English/non-Spanish speakers?
Recruited sample	A consecutive sample of 300 female welfare recipients (English or Spanish speaking) who applied for benefits in January 2016 at two randomly selected welfare offices in Los Angeles	• Why only new applicants—what about women with long-term receipt? • Why only two offices? Are these representative? • Is January a typical month?
Actual sample	161 women from the recruited sample who fully participated in the study	• Who refused to participate (or was too ill, and so on) and why? • Who dropped out of the study, and why?

Answers to these questions would affect the interpretation of whether the intervention *really* is effective with low-income women—or only with motivated, cooperative welfare recipients from two neighborhoods of Los Angeles who recently got approved for public assistance.

As Figure 20.1 suggests, researchers in our example made a series of methodologic decisions that affect inferences, and these decisions must be carefully scrutinized in assessing study credibility. However, participant behavior and external circumstances also affect the results and need to be considered in the interpretation. In our example in Table 20.1, 300 women were recruited, but only 161 provided usable data for analysis. The final sample of 161 almost surely would differ in important ways from the 139 who were not in the study, and these differences affect inferences about the value of the study evidence.

We illustrated how successive proxies in a study, from the abstract to the concrete, can affect inferences with regard to sampling, but we could have chosen other aspects of a study. As another example, Figure 20.2 considers successive

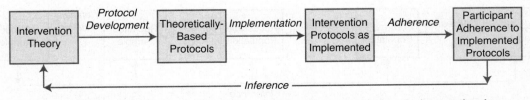

FIGURE 20.2 Inferences about interventions: from actual program operations to the intervention theory.

proxies for an intervention. As with our previous illustration, researchers move from an abstraction on the left (here, a theory about why an intervention might have beneficial outcomes), through the design of protocols that purport to operationalize the theory, to the actual implementation and use of the intervention on the right. Researchers want the right side to be a good proxy for the left side— and, in interpreting results, they must assess the plausibility that they were successful in the transformation.

Credibility and Validity

Studies inherently involve making inferences. We *infer* that scores on a depression scale are, in fact, capturing the depression construct. We *infer* that a sample can tell us something about a population. We use inferential statistics to make inferences about relationships observed in the data. Inference and validity are inextricably linked. Indeed, research methodology experts Shadish and colleagues (2002) defined validity as "the approximate truth of an inference" (p. 34). To be careful interpreters, researchers must seek evidence within their study that desired inferences are, in fact, valid.

In Chapter 10, we discussed four types of validity that play a key role in assessing the credibility of quantitative study results: statistical conclusion validity, internal validity, external validity, and construct validity. Let us use our sampling example (Figure 20.1 and Table 20.1) to demonstrate the relevance of methodologic decisions to all four types of validity—and hence to inferences about study results.

First, let us consider construct validity—a term that has relevance not only for the measurement of research constructs but also for many aspects of a study. In our example, the population construct was *low-income women*, which led to population eligibility criteria stipulating public assistance recipients in California. There are, however, other alternative operationalizations of the population construct (e.g., women living in families below the official poverty level). Construct validity, it may be recalled, involves inferences from the particulars of the study to higher order constructs. So it is fair to ask, "Do the specified eligibility criteria

adequately capture the population construct, low-income women?"

Statistical conclusion validity—the extent to which correct inferences can be made about whether relationships between key variables are "real"—is also affected by sampling decisions. Ideally, researchers would do a power analysis to estimate how large a sample is needed. In our example, let us say we estimated (based on previous research) a small-to-moderate effect size for the intervention, $d = .40$. For a power of .80, with risk of a Type I error set at .05, we would need a sample of about 200 participants. The actual sample of 161 yields a nearly 30% risk of a Type II error, that is, falsely concluding that the intervention was not successful.

External validity—the generalizability of the results—is also affected by sampling decisions. To whom would it be safe to generalize the results in this example—to the population construct of low-income women? to all welfare recipients in California? to all new welfare recipients in Los Angeles who speak English or Spanish? Inferences about the extent to which the study results correspond to "truth in the real world" must take sampling decisions and sampling problems (e.g., recruitment and retention difficulties) into account.

Finally, internal validity (the extent to which a causal connection between variables can be inferred) is also affected by sample composition. In particular (in this example), differential attrition would be a concern. Were those in the intervention group more likely (or less likely) than those in the control group to drop out of the study? If so, any observed differences in physical activity outcomes could be caused by individual differences in the two groups (e.g., differences in motivation) rather than by the intervention itself.

Methodologic decisions and the careful implementation of those decisions—whether they be about sampling, intervention design, measurement, research design, or analysis—inevitably affect study validity and the interpretation of the results.

Credibility and Bias

Part of a researcher's job in doing a study is to translate abstract constructs into plausible and meaningful proxies. Another job is to eliminate or reduce biases—or, as a last resort, to detect and understand them. In interpreting results, the risk for various biases should be assessed and factored into conclusions.

Biases are factors that create distortions and undermine researchers' efforts to capture and reveal "truth in the real world." Biases are pervasive. It is not so much a question of whether there *are* biases in a study, so much as what types of bias are present, and how extensive and systematic the biases are. We have discussed many types of bias—some reflect design inadequacies (e.g., selection bias), others reflect recruitment or sampling problems (nonresponse bias), others are related to measurement (social desirability bias). To our knowledge, there is no comprehensive listing of biases that might arise in a study, but Table 20.2 presents a list of some of the biases and errors mentioned in this book. This list is not all-inclusive but is meant to serve as a reminder of some of the problems to consider in interpreting study results.

> **TIP:** The Toolkit on the accompanying *Resource Manual* includes a longer list of biases with definitions and notes. It is important to recognize that different disciplines use different names for the same or similar biases. The actual names are not important—what is important is to understand how different forces can distort the results and affect inferences.

Credibility and Corroboration

Earlier we noted that research interpreters should seek evidence to disconfirm the interpretive "null hypothesis" that the research results were inaccurate. Some evidence to discredit the null hypothesis comes from the plausibility that proxies were good stand-ins for abstractions or idealized methods. Other evidence involves ruling out validity threats and biases. Yet another strategy is to seek corroboration for results.

Corroboration can come from both internal and external sources, and the concept of *replication* is

TABLE 20.2 • Selected List of Major Potential Biases or Errors in Quantitative Studies

RESEARCH DESIGN	SAMPLING	MEASUREMENT	ANALYSIS
Expectation bias	Sampling error	Social desirability bias	Type I error
Hawthorne effect	Volunteer bias	Acquiescence bias	Type II error
Performance bias	Nonresponse bias	Nay-sayers bias	
Detection bias		Extreme response set bias	
Contamination of treatments		Recall/memory bias	
Carryover (ordering) effects		Ceiling effects	
Noncompliance bias		Floor effects	
Selection bias		Reactivity	
Attrition bias		Observer biases	
History bias			

an important one in both cases. Interpretations are aided by considering prior research on the topic, for example. Interpreters can examine whether the study results replicate (are congruent with) those of other studies. Discrepancies in study results may lend support to the "null hypothesis" of erroneous results, while consistency across studies discredit it.

Researchers can pursue opportunities for replication themselves. For example, in multisite studies, if results are similar across sites, this suggests that something "real" is occurring with some regularity. Triangulation can be another form of replication and sometimes can help to corroborate results. For example, if results are similar across different measures of an outcome, then there can perhaps be greater confidence that the results are "real" and do not reflect some peculiarity of an instrument. If results are different, this could provide support for the null hypothesis of erroneous results—but it could also reflect a problem with one of the measures. When mixed results occur, interpreters must dig deeper to uncover the reason.

Finally, we are strong advocates of mixed methods studies, a special type of triangulation (Chapter 26). When findings from the analysis of qualitative data are consistent with the results of statistical analyses, internal corroboration can be especially powerful and persuasive.

Precision of the Results

The results of statistical hypothesis testing indicate whether an observed relationship or group difference is probably real and replicable. A p value in hypothesis testing indicates how unlikely it is that the null hypothesis is true—it is not an estimate of a numeric value of direct relevance to clinicians. A p value offers information that is important but incomplete.

Confidence intervals, by contrast, communicate information about how precise (or imprecise) the study results are. Dr. David Sackett, a founding father of the EBP movement, had this to say about confidence intervals: "P values on their own are . . . not informative . . . By contrast, CIs indicate the strength of evidence about quantities of direct interest, such as treatment benefit. They are thus of

particular relevance to practitioners of evidence-based medicine" (Sackett et al., 2000, p. 232). It is hoped nurse researchers will increasingly report CI information because of its value for interpreting study results and assessing their potential utility for nursing practice.

Magnitude of Effects and Importance

In quantitative studies, results that support the researcher's hypotheses are described as *significant*. A careful analysis of study results involves evaluating whether, in addition to being statistically significant, the effects are large and clinically important.

Attaining statistical significance does not necessarily mean that the results are meaningful to nurses and clients. Statistical significance indicates that the results are unlikely to be due to chance—not that they are necessarily important. With large samples, even modest relationships are statistically significant. For instance, with a sample of 500, a correlation coefficient of .10 is significant at the .05 level, but a relationship this weak may have little practical value. This issue concerns an important EBP question (Box 2.2): "What *is* the evidence—what is the magnitude of effects?" Estimating the magnitude and importance of effects is relevant to the issue of clinical significance, a topic we discuss later in this chapter.

Meaning of the Results

In quantitative studies, standard statistical results are in the form of p values, effect sizes, and confidence intervals, to which researchers must attach meaning once they have concluded that these results are credible. Many questions about the meaning of statistical results reflect a desire to interpret causal connections.

Interpreting what results mean usually is not challenging in descriptive studies. For example, suppose we found that, among patients undergoing electroconvulsive therapy (ECT), the percentage who experience an ECT-induced headache is 59.4% (95% CI = 56.3, 63.1). This result is directly meaningful and interpretable. But if we found that headache prevalence is significantly lower for patients in a cryotherapy intervention group than for patients given acetaminophen, we would need to interpret what the results mean. In particular, we need to interpret whether it is plausible that cryotherapy *caused* reductions in headaches. Even if the results are deemed to be "real," that is, statistically significant, interpretation involves coming to conclusions about internal validity when a causal inference is sought.

In this section, we discuss the interpretation of various research outcomes within a hypothesis-testing context, with an emphasis on causal interpretations. In thinking about causal interpretations, we encourage you to review the criteria for causal relationships (Chapter 9).

Interpreting Hypothesized Results

Interpreting statistical results is easiest when hypotheses are supported, i.e., when there are *positive results*. In this situation, interpretations have been partly achieved beforehand because researchers have brought together prior findings, a theoretical framework, and logical reasoning in developing hypotheses. This groundwork forms the context within which more specific interpretations are made.

Some caveats should be kept in mind, however. It is important to avoid the temptation of going beyond the data to explain what results mean. As an example, suppose we hypothesized that pregnant women's anxiety level about labor and delivery is correlated with the number of children they have borne. The data reveal a significant negative relationship between anxiety levels and parity ($r = -.30$). We interpret this to mean that increased experience with childbirth results in decreased anxiety. Is this conclusion supported by the data? The conclusion seems logical, but in fact, there is nothing in the data that leads to this interpretation. An important, indeed critical, research precept is *correlation does not prove causation*. The finding that two variables are related offers no evidence suggesting which of the two variables—if either—caused the other. In our example, perhaps causality runs in the opposite direction, that is, a woman's anxiety level influences how many children she bears. Or perhaps a third variable, such as the

woman's relationship with her husband, influences both anxiety and number of children. Inferring causality is especially difficult in studies that have not used an experimental design.

⊘ **TIP:** Froman and Owen (2014) have written a compelling paper about avoiding inappropriate causal language in research reports. For example, they point out that researchers often use misleading "loaded words" that suggest a causal link even when the study design does not support a causal inference—words like *impact*, *effect*, and *determinant*.

Alternative explanations for the findings should always be considered. Researchers sometimes can test rival hypotheses directly. If competing interpretations can be ruled out, so much the better, but every angle should be examined to see if one's own explanation has been given adequate competition. Threats to internal validity reflect competing explanations for what the results might mean and need thorough consideration.

Empirical evidence supporting research hypotheses never constitutes *proof* of their veracity. Hypothesis testing is probabilistic. There is always a possibility that observed relationships resulted from chance—that is, that a Type I error occurred. Researchers must be tentative about their results and about interpretations of them. Even when the results are in line with expectations, researchers should draw conclusions with restraint and should give due consideration to limitations identified in assessing the credibility of the results.

Example of Corroboration of a Hypothesis: Ngai and Ngu (2014) tested hypotheses (via a causal model) about the role that *family sense of coherence* plays in successful family adaptation during a transition to parenthood among Chinese childbearing couples. Consistent with the model, a measure of family sense of coherence was significantly related to family and marital functioning and depression. The researchers concluded that the study offered evidence that "family sense of coherence in parental transition plays a significant role in promoting family functioning and reducing depressive symptoms" (p. 82).

This study is an example of the challenges of interpreting findings in correlational studies, especially ones that are cross-sectional. The researchers' interpretation was that family sense of coherence was a factor that *promoted* marital functioning and *reduced* depressive symptoms—verbs that imply a causal interpretation. This is a conclusion supported by earlier research and consistent with a well-known theory (the Salutogenic Model). Yet nothing in the data rules out the possibility that a person's level of depression *reduced* the perception of family coherence, for example, or that a third factor caused both higher depression and lower sense of coherence. The researchers' interpretation is plausible and even likely to be correct, but their cross-sectional design makes it difficult to rule out other explanations. A major threat to the internal validity of the inference in this study is temporal ambiguity—that is, whether or not depression preceded perceptions of family sense of coherence.

TIP: A mistake that many researchers make is to qualitatively interpret the *p* values in statistical tests. A *p* value of .0001 is not "more significant" than a *p* value of .05. The outcome of a significance test is dichotomous: The result either is or is not significant. Similarly, a *p* value of .08 is not "marginally significant"; if one has established alpha = .05, the result is not significant (Hayat, 2010). Mechanisms other than *p* values are needed to interpret magnitude and importance, as we discuss in other sections of this chapter.

Interpreting Nonsignificant Results

Nonsignificant results pose interpretative problems because statistical tests are geared toward disconfirmation of the null hypothesis. Failure to reject a null hypothesis can occur for many reasons, and the real reason is usually difficult to discern. The null hypothesis *could* actually be true, for example. A nonsignificant result could accurately reflect the absence of a relationship among

research variables. On the other hand, the null hypothesis could be false, in which case a Type II error has been committed. Nonsignificant results are inconclusive.

Retention of a false null hypothesis can result from several methodologic problems, such as poor internal validity, an anomalous sample, a weak statistical procedure, or unreliable measures. In particular, failure to reject null hypotheses is often a consequence of insufficient power resulting from too small a sample size—and, often, a relatively small effect.

In any event, a retained null hypothesis should not be considered as proof of the *absence* of relationships among variables. *Nonsignificant results provide no evidence of the truth or the falsity of the hypothesis.* Interpreting nonsignificant results can, however, be aided by considering such factors as sample size and effect size estimates.

Example of Nonsignificant Results: Griffin and colleagues (2007) hypothesized that nurses' stereotypes about patients (based on gender, race, and attractiveness) would influence the nurses' pain treatment recommendations for children in pain. The hypotheses were not supported—that is, there was no evidence of stereotyping. The conclusion that stereotyping probably did not occur was bolstered by the fact that the sample was fairly large ($N = 334$), and nurses were blinded to the manipulation (children's characteristics). Extremely low effect sizes offered additional support for concluding that stereotyping was negligible.

Because statistical tests offer support for rejecting null hypotheses, they are not well-suited for testing *actual* research hypotheses about the absence of relationships or about group equivalence. Yet sometimes this is exactly what researchers want to do—and this is especially true in clinical situations in which the goal is to assess if one practice is as effective as another (an *equivalence trial*) or not less effective than another (a *noninferiority trial*). When the actual research hypothesis is null (i.e., a prediction of no group difference or no relationship), additional strategies must be used to provide supporting evidence. In particular, it is important to compute effect sizes and confidence intervals to show that the risk of a Type II error was small. There may also be clinical standards that can be used to corroborate that nonsignificant—but predicted—results are plausible. In noninferiority and equivalence trials, clinical parameters must be stipulated for undertaking a power analysis (Tunes da Silva et al., 2009).

Example of Support for a Hypothesized Nonsignificant Result: Lavender and colleagues (2013) conducted a noninferiority trial to test that a baby wash product formulated for newborn bathing is not inferior to bathing with water alone, in terms of transepidermal water loss, clinical observations of the skin, and other outcomes. In their sample of 307 healthy infants, none of the group differences was statistically significant.

Interpreting Unhypothesized Significant Results

Unhypothesized significant results can occur in two situations. The first involves exploring relationships that were not anticipated during the design of the study. For example, in examining correlations among variables in the data set, a researcher might notice that two variables that were not central to the research questions were nevertheless significantly correlated—and interesting. To interpret serendipitous findings, it is wise to consult the literature to see if similar relationships had been previously observed.

Example of a Serendipitous Significant Finding: Watt and colleagues (2012) examined the effect of a mother's delivery method (vaginal versus cesarean) on breastfeeding initiation in a sample of 2,560 Canadian women who delivered full-term infants. Method of delivery was unrelated to breastfeeding, but the researchers found that women whose delivery method was unexpected (i.e., an unplanned cesarean or an instrument-assisted vaginal delivery) had a significantly higher likelihood of initiating breastfeeding.

The second situation is more perplexing, and it does not happen often: obtaining results *opposite* to those hypothesized. For instance, a researcher might hypothesize that individualized teaching about AIDS risks is more effective than group instruction, but the results might indicate that group instruction was significantly better. Some researchers view such situations as awkward, but research should not be undertaken primarily to corroborate researchers' predictions but rather to arrive at truthful evidence.

When significant findings are opposite to what was hypothesized, it is less likely that the methods are flawed than that the underlying reasoning or theory is problematic. The interpretation of such findings should involve comparisons with other research, a consideration of alternative theories, and—if possible—in-depth interviews with a subsample of study participants.

Example of Significant Results Contrary to Hypotheses: Dotson and colleagues (2014) tested a model of nurse retention in a sample of 861 RNs. They predicted that higher levels of altruism would be associated with stronger intentions to stay in nursing, but the opposite was found to be true. They speculated that this might reflect the fact that some nurses "are no longer experiencing the fulfillment of their altruistic desires in the field of nursing" (p. 115).

Interpreting Mixed Results

Interpretation is often complicated by *mixed results*: Some hypotheses are supported by the data, but others are not. Or, a hypothesis may be accepted with one measure of the dependent variable but rejected with a different measure. When only some results run counter to a theoretical prediction, the research methods are the first aspect of the study deserving critical scrutiny. Differences in the validity and reliability of the various measures may account for such discrepancies, for example. Or, the sample size might be sufficiently large when effects are large but insufficient for more modest effects. On the other hand, mixed results may suggest that a theory needs to be qualified or that certain constructs within the theory need to be reconceptualized. Mixed results sometimes present opportunities for conceptual advances because efforts to make sense of disparate pieces of evidence may lead to a breakthrough.

In summary, interpreting the meaning of research results is a demanding task but offers the possibility of intellectual rewards. Interpreters must in essence play the role of scientific detectives, trying to make pieces of the puzzle fit together so that a coherent picture emerges.

Generalizability of the Results

Researchers are rarely interested in discovering relationships among variables for a specific group of people at a specific point in time. If a new nursing intervention is found to be successful, others may want to adopt it. Thus, an important interpretive question is whether the intervention will "work" or whether relationships will "hold" in other settings, with other people. Part of the interpretive process involves asking the question, "To what groups, environments, and conditions can the results of the study reasonably be applied?"

In interpreting the study with regard to the generalizability of the results, it is useful to consider our earlier discussion about proxies. For which higher order constructs, which populations, which settings, or which versions of an intervention were the study operations good "stand-ins"?

Implications of the Results

Once you have reached conclusions about the credibility, precision, importance, meaning, and generalizability of the results, you are ready to think about their implications. You might consider the implications with respect to future research (What should other researchers working in this area do—what is the right "next step"?) or theory development (What are the implications for nursing theory?). A key issue, though, is the implications of the evidence for nursing practice. How do the results contribute to a base of evidence to improve nursing? Specific suggestions for implementing the results of the study in a real nursing context are valuable in the EBP process.

⮕ TIP: In interpreting your data, remember that others will be reviewing your interpretation with a critical and perhaps even a skeptical eye. The job of consumers is to make decisions about the credibility and utility of the evidence, which is likely to be affected by how much support you offer for the validity and meaning of your results.

CLINICAL SIGNIFICANCE

It has long been recognized that statistical hypothesis testing provides limited information for interpretation purposes. In particular, attaining significance does not address the question of whether a finding is clinically meaningful or relevant. With a large enough sample, a trivial relationship or group difference can be statistically significant, and, conversely, some nonsignificant findings could potentially be clinically important. Broadly speaking, we define **clinical significance** as the practical importance of research results in terms of whether they have genuine, palpable effects on the daily lives of patients or on the health care decisions made on their behalf.

More than 20 years ago, LeFort (1993) wrote, in a prominent nursing journal, about the "recent interest" in clinical significance—but that interest has had a bigger impact on fields other than nursing. Relatively few nurse researchers comment on the clinical significance of their findings when discussing their results. When nurse researchers mention clinical significance, they often use the phrase loosely and ambiguously, or sometimes they establish a criterion for clinical significance without offering a rationale (Bruner et al., 2012).

In fields other than nursing, notably in medicine and psychotherapy, a lot of attention has been paid in the past few decades to two key challenges relating to clinical significance: developing a conceptual definition of what it means and developing ways to operationalize it. To be sure, there has been no consensus on either front, but there are a few conceptual and statistical solutions that are used with considerable regularity. Some of these solutions are relevant to nursing, and perhaps nurse researchers will work toward different or better solutions. In this section, we briefly describe recent advances in defining and operationalizing clinical significance in other health fields. Further information is available in Polit and Yang (2015).

In statistical hypothesis testing, a fair degree of consensus was reached decades ago—for better or worse—that a *p* value of .05 would be the standard for statistical significance. It is unlikely that a uniform standard will ever be adopted with regard to clinical significance, however, in part because it is a far more complex concept than statistical significance. For example, in some cases, *no change* over time could be clinically significant if it means that a group with a progressive disease has not experienced any deterioration. In other cases, clinical significance is associated with improvements. Another issue concerns whose *perspective* on clinical significance is considered. Sometimes clinicians' perspective is paramount because of implications for health management (e.g., regarding cholesterol levels or blood pressure values), whereas for other outcomes, the patient's view is what matters (e.g., about pain or quality of life). Two other issues concern whether clinical significance is about group-level findings or about individual patients, and whether clinical significance is attached to point-in-time outcomes or to change scores. Most of the work that has been done to date, and therefore most of our discussion here, is about the clinical significance of *change scores* for individual patients. We begin, however, with a brief discussion of group-level clinical significance.

Clinical Significance at the Group Level

Many studies concern group-level comparisons. For example, one-group pretest–posttest designs involve comparing a group at two (or more) points in time to examine whether or not a change in outcomes has occurred, on average. In randomized controlled trials (RCTs) and case-control studies, the central comparison is about average differences for different groups of people. It is these comparisons that are subjected to hypothesis-testing procedures, and statistical tests lead to conclusions about retention of the null hypothesis.

Group-level clinical significance (which is sometimes called *practical significance*) typically involves using statistical information other than *p* values to draw conclusions about the usefulness or importance of research findings. The most widely used statistics for this purpose are effect size (ES) indexes, confidence intervals (CIs), and number-needed-to-treat (NNT). Many medical journals insist that information about CIs and effect sizes be presented in results sections of papers. Yet, it has been found that only a minority of articles in top nursing research journal report on CIs or on effect sizes (Gaskin & Happell, 2014).

Effect size indexes summarize the magnitude of a change or a relationship and thus provide insights into how a group, *on average*, might benefit from a treatment (or be spared a harm). In most cases, a clinically significant finding at the group level means that the effect size is sufficiently large to be noticeable (i.e., measurable) and to have relevance for patients.

Confidence intervals are espoused by several writers as useful tools for understanding clinical significance (e.g., Fethney, 2010). CIs provide the most plausible range of values, at a given level of confidence, for the unknown population parameter (e.g., the mean value on an outcome after treatment). Fethney (2010) provided an example that illustrated how CIs were used in a study evaluating an intervention for premature infants. A weight gain value was established as clinically significant by a panel of experts, and then CIs around the obtained mean weight gain were calculated to see if the CI encompassed the designated value.

NNTs are sometimes promoted as useful indicators of clinical significance in clinical trials because the information is in a format that is relatively easy to understand. For example, if the NNT for an important outcome is found to be 2.0, only two patients have to receive a particular treatment in order for one patient to benefit. If the NNT is 10.0, however, 9 patients out of 10 receiving the treatment would get no benefit. Another advantage of NNTs is that they can fairly easily be linked to cost information so that feasibility can be assessed.

With any of the group-level indexes mentioned, researchers should designate in advance what would constitute clinical significance—just as they would establish an alpha value for statistical significance. For example, would an ES of

.20 (for the *d* index described in Chapter 17) be considered clinically significant? A *d* of .20 was described by Cohen (1988) as a "small" effect, but sometimes small improvements can have clinical relevance. Claims about attainment of clinical significance for groups should be based on reasonable criteria.

⬥ **TIP:** In Chapter 17, we discussed using a power analysis to estimate sample size needs during the planning stage of the study based on a goal of detecting statistical significance. However, a valuable approach is to estimate sample size needs that will support goals for both clinical and statistical significance.

Clinical Significance at the Individual Level

Clinicians usually are not interested in what happens in a *group* of people—they are concerned with individual patients. As noted in Chapter 2, a key goal in evidence-based practice (EBP) is to personalize "best evidence" into decisions for a specific patient's needs, within a particular clinical context. Efforts to come to conclusions about clinical significance at the individual level can thus be directly linked to EBP goals.

Dozens of approaches to defining and operationalizing clinical significance at the individual level have been developed, but they share one thing in common: They involve establishing a **benchmark** (or *threshold*) that designates the value on a measure (or the value of a change score) that would be considered meaningful or clinically important. With a benchmark for clinical significance, established based on an external standard, each person in a study can be classified as having or not having a score or change score that is clinically significant. Thus, efforts to operationalize clinical significance are linked to the interpretability of measures, which is one of the elements on our measurement property taxonomy described in Chapter 14 (Figure 14.1). Before looking at how the benchmarks have been established, we consider alternative definitions of clinical significance.

⬥ **TIP:** Some studies do not focus on change, but researchers may still be interested in linking the findings to a relevant threshold. For example, Al-Gamal and Yorke (2014) conducted a descriptive study of psychological distress in patients with COPD. The researchers used benchmarks that had been established as clinical cutpoints on well-validated scales to draw conclusions about the percentage of study participants with clinically significant levels of anxiety and depression.

Conceptual Definitions of Clinical Significance

Dozens of definitions of clinical significance can be found in the health literature, and most of these concern changes in measures of patient outcomes. The various definitions fall mainly into one of four categories.

One definitional category is linked to statistical issues discussed in Chapter 14, that is, whether a change score is statistically reliable. Some have reasoned that if a patient's improved score on an outcome is more than random error, the improvement has clinical significance.

Example of Defining Reliable Change as Clinical Significance: Dysvik and colleagues (2011) studied the effectiveness of a multidisciplinary pain program for patients with chronic pain. Their outcomes included pain level and health-related quality of life. The Reliable Change Index (RCI) was used with their primary outcome measures to distinguish patients who had or had not achieved reliable improvements.

Reliable change also figures into a definition of clinical significance that appeared in the psychotherapy literature in the early 1990s. Jacobson and Truax (1991) proposed that a clinically significant change for patients undergoing a psychotherapeutic intervention would involve a reliable improvement *and* a return to "normal" functioning. They proposed several ways of making a decision about whether individual patients in a study had changed sufficiently to meet this criterion of normalcy. Their approach, sometimes referred to as the *J-T approach*, has been used for outcomes other than those used in psychotherapy research, such as in studies using measures of physical function as key outcomes (e.g., Mann et al., 2012). The J-T approach is described more fully in the Supplement to this chapter on thePoint®. Ⓢ

Example of Using the J-T Approach: Bevan and colleagues (2013) used the J-T approach in a pilot study of an intervention for postpartum depression. Each patient was assessed with regard to the reliability of their change scores on measures of depression and anxiety, as well as whether the final score could be classified as being in the normal range, as established by cutpoints on the measures established in earlier research.

➔ **TIP:** In some health care applications, "normalcy" can be defined as improvements in scores that represent a return to a desirable range—especially for biophysiologic outcomes such as blood pressure or cholesterol levels. Thresholds for these outcomes are available in clinical guidelines.

A third way to conceptualize clinical significance is not linked to change scores explicitly. Tubach and colleagues (Tubach et al., 2006; Tubach et al., 2007) argued that patients are more interested in "feeling good" than in simply "feeling better." In their view, a clinically significant state occurs when patients achieve an outcome that they perceive as important and meaningful. Tubach et al. called their benchmark the **patient acceptable symptom state (PASS)**. The PASS approach is discussed in greater detail in Polit and Yang (2015).

The fourth way of conceptualizing clinical significance dominates medical fields. In a paper cited hundreds of times in the medical literature, Jaeschke and colleagues (1989) offered the following definition: "The minimal clinically important difference (MCID) can be defined as the smallest difference in score in the domain of interest which patients perceive as beneficial and which would

mandate, in the absence of troublesome side effects and excessive cost, a change in the patient's management" (p. 408). Although these researchers, and many after them, have referred to the conceptual threshold for clinical significance as a minimal important *difference* (MID) or *minimal clinically important difference* (MCID), we follow the COSMIN group in using the term **minimal important change (MIC)** (De Vet et al., 2011) because the focus is on individual change scores (not differences between groups). We focus on methods that have been proposed for operationalizing this benchmark.

Operationalizing Clinical Significance: Establishing the Minimal Important Change Benchmark

To our knowledge, the definition of the MIC offered by Jaeschke and colleagues (1989) has never been fully operationalized. For example, patients have often been involved in helping researchers to link change scores on a focal measure to a criterion for change, but it is usually the researchers, not the patients, who decide on the cutpoint for what is deemed "meaningful" or "important." Side effects and costs are not typically taken into consideration in the thresholds. And "clinical" input on what amount of change in a score would result in a change in patient management is seldom sought. Thus, although the Jaeschke et al. definition regarding change score benchmarks has been cited extensively, researchers have gone in many different directions in translating and quantifying it. Nevertheless, the focus on *patient input* to establish the MIC has had a profound effect on establishing benchmarks for patient-reported outcomes (PROs).

The MIC benchmark is usually operationalized as a value for the amount of change score points on a PRO that an individual patient must achieve in order to be credited with having a clinically important change, although sometimes the benchmark is a percentage change. Sometimes two MICs are established for a measure: one MIC denoting the threshold for clinically significant improvement, and a second MIC as the threshold for clinically significant deterioration.

Dozens of methods have been used to derive MICs for widely used health care measures—and the developers of many new multi-item scales now make efforts to estimate the MIC as part of the psychometric assessment of their instrument. The methods of setting the interpretive MIC benchmark mainly fall into three categories.

A traditional approach to setting a benchmark for health outcomes is to obtain input from a panel of health care experts—often called a *consensus panel*. For example, the Initiative on Methods, Measurement, and Pain Assessment in Clinical Trials (IMMPACT) convened a special panel on clinical significance, and one recommendation of the consensus review was that a 30% improvement in self-reported pain intensity (e.g., on a visual analog scale) be considered the benchmark for positive clinical change (Dworkin et al., 2005).

The COSMIN group has advocated for a different approach. They defined the MIC as "the smallest change in score in the construct to be measured which patients perceive as important" (De Vet et al., 2011, p. 245). Even this definition has led to different interpretations: Some researchers have emphasized the "minimal" or "smallest" aspect in looking at a change score, and others have emphasized the "important" aspect. This divergence can be best explained with an illustration.

A widely used method of establishing the MIC value is called an *anchor-based approach*. This approach requires administering the focal measure on two occasions to a sample of people in which change is expected for at least some people. At the second administration, information about an "anchor" is also obtained. The anchor is a criterion for establishing the MIC benchmark on the focal scale. The anchor often is a single-item **global rating scale** (GRS), such as we described in Chapter 14 in our discussion of the criterion approach to responsiveness. Indeed, we can use the same example as the one shown in Figure 14.3, which illustrated a 7-point GRS for assessing the responsiveness of a composite physical function scale. We show in Figure 20.3 the mean scores on our physical functioning scale for each response category on the GRS. If we wanted to operationalize the MIC in a manner that emphasized the *smallest* noticeable improvement in score ("a little better"), we might conclude that the MIC was 2.17. In this case, any change in a person's score of 3 or better would be interpreted as clinically significant. Other researchers, however, have argued that "minimal change" is an insufficient criterion. They would use as their anchor the GRS rating of "much better" to establish the MIC for their scale. In that case, the MIC in this example would be 3.89, and a person's change would be deemed

Please rate the changes you have experienced in the past three months with regard to *your ability to perform regular activities of daily living*, such as standing up from a sitting position or taking a bath or shower:

GRS Rating	Mean Change Score on Composite Physical Function Scale (Posttest – Baseline)
1. Very much better	5.50
2. Much better	**3.89**
3. A little better	**2.17**
4. No change	0.75
5. A little worse	-1.89
6. Much worse	-4.03
7. Very much worse	-5.98

Highlighted categories indicate possible MIC thresholds.

FIGURE 20.3 Example of a global rating scale anchor used to establish a minimal important change (MIC) for improvement on a physical function scale.

clinically significant only if their change score on the focal scale was 4 points or higher. Other statistical approaches can also be used to establish an MIC using anchor-based methods, notably the use of a receiver operating characteristic (ROC) curve analysis.

Note that despite the widespread endorsement of using patients' input in defining clinical significance for PROs, it is almost always the researcher, not the patient, who defines what is "minimally important." When reading about the MIC, or when using a previously obtained MIC value in a study to assess clinical significance, it is crucial to understand how the researcher defined "minimally important."

➲ TIP: The anchor used as the criterion for the MIC needed not be based on patients' self-reports of change on a GRS. For example, the anchor for a physical functioning scale could be based on performance tests or on a clinician's assessment of physical functioning.

Calculating an MIC using an anchor-based approach requires a lot of work, and it also requires a careful research design with a large sample of people whose changes over time are expected to vary. Using an anchor-based approach, an MIC must be established for every new scale; moreover, the MIC value is population-specific. The MIC on a measure of pain intensity might be different for a population experiencing chronic pain than for a population recovering from surgery—and in a group with chronic pain, a separate threshold might be needed for both improvement and deterioration.

These complexities have led to a third approach to operationalizing the MIC—one that uses the distributional characteristics of a measure. Distribution methods are based on the statistical characteristics of a sample, and they express the MIC as a standardized metric. The most frequently used metric is based on Cohen's (1988) effect size index, operationalized at the individual level in terms of a fraction of the standard deviation (SD). Most often, the MIC using this approach is set to a threshold

of 0.5—that is, one half a standard deviation based on the distribution of baseline scores (Norman et al., 2003, 2004). Norman and colleagues found that there was "remarkable" consistency supporting a threshold equivalent to an SD of 0.5. They argued that this consistency was unlikely to be a coincidence but rather could be tied to theory and evidence on the psychology of human discrimination. They thus concluded that a change of 0.5 SD in baseline scores is a defensible benchmark for interpreting an individual change score as important.

This distributional approach does not directly yield an MIC threshold value in change score units, but this value can be easily computed. For example, if the baseline SD for a scale were 6.0, then the MIC using the 0.5 SD criterion would be 3.0. This value, like any MIC, can be used as the benchmark to classify individual patients as having or not having experienced clinically meaningful change.

An alternative distribution-based method is to establish the value of the MIC based on measurement error (see Chapter 14). In particular, a number of researchers have suggested using the standard error of measurement (SEM) to establish the threshold. Norman and colleagues (2003) pointed out that for measures with a test–retest reliability of .75, the 0.5 SD threshold is exactly equivalent to 1 SEM.

There is no consensus on which approach to calculating the MIC yields the most helpful benchmark of clinical significance, but many people agree that none of the approaches is ideal. The anchor-based approach is preferred by the COSMIN group, but it adds more work to the burdensome effort of constructing and evaluating new scales. It has also been argued that a single GRS is a poor choice for the anchor because a single item is unreliable and responses to it are subject to recall biases. Other anchors are, of course, feasible, but GRSs are widely used.

MICs based on distribution approaches are appealing because they are easy to compute, but it is often difficult to communicate what such an MIC represents. A persistent criticism of distribution methods is that they yield values that are not linked to any clinical yardstick—they do not embody any notion of "meaningfulness" or "importance." Another problem with MICs based on *SD*s is that the value is dependent on the heterogeneity of the population under study. Those who have suggested distribution-based MICs often emphasize that they are a reasonable starting point or "an approximate rule of thumb in the absence of more specific information" (Norman et al., 2003, p. 590).

Because both the anchor-based and the distribution-based approaches have potential problems, some researchers use combined approaches, as briefly discussed next.

Triangulation of Methods for the Minimal Important Change

Because there is no "gold standard" approach to setting the MIC, some experts argue that it is advantageous to triangulate information from more than one approach (e.g., Revicki et al., 2008). Many approaches to triangulation have been adopted. For example, some researchers have combined information from multiple anchors, including anchors reflecting both patients' and clinicians' perspectives. Most efforts at triangulation involve using both a distribution method, such as 1 SEM, plus an anchor-based method. This particular type of triangulation has the merit of enhancing the likelihood that a change score value is not only clinically meaningful but also "real."

An example of triangulation comes from the field of respiratory medicine. Patel and colleagues (2013) sought to establish the MIC for King's Brief Interstitial Lung Disease Questionnaire (K-BILD). These researchers used two distribution methods (1 SEM and 0.3 *SD*), a clinical anchor (a forced vital capacity [FVC] change of at least 7% from baseline), and patients' responses on four global rating scales. Integrating all information, the researchers established the MIC on the K-BILD at 8 points.

Procedures for Clinical Significance Inquiries

Nurse researchers who wish to assess the clinical significance of their results for individual participants, using some of the procedures described in this chapter, should begin by coming to conclusions about how they wish to conceptualize clini-cal significance. This is most easily illustrated in the context of intervention research. As noted by Kazdin (1999), clinical significance can have many meanings, and so the researcher must be clear at the outset about treatment goals. Is the goal to have patients achieve *real change*? Return to *normal functioning*? Achieve a *favorable state*? Or experience change at a level that is *minimally important*?

If researchers decide in advance how they want to approach clinical significance, they will be in a better position to operationalize it when they plan their studies. For example, if "return to normal functioning" is the treatment goal, the researchers should investigate whether there are measures of key outcomes for which normative information is readily available. If depression, for instance, is an outcome, then a researcher interested in assessing clinically significant changes in depression should select a depression scale with published norms or recommended cutpoints. If, on the other hand, the treatment goal is for patients to achieve important improvements, then researchers should search the literature for MIC values for their outcome measures. Hundreds of psychometric articles report MIC values for health scales. MIC values are population specific, so it is important to identify MIC thresholds that are appropriate for study participants. By looking for MIC information before the study is underway, researchers may be in a better position to select between alternative measures of a construct.

Triangulation is sometimes adopted by those who wish to *use* existing benchmarks of clinical significance in addition to those who undertake research to establish them. For example, Fleet and colleagues (2014) studied the effect of a subcutaneous administration of fentanyl in childbirth on the women's changes in pain scores, as measured on a 100-cm visual analog scale (VAS) for pain. Based on findings from four earlier studies, all of which had used an anchor-based approach to establishing the MIC on a VAS for pain, Fleet et al. concluded that 78% of the women in their sample had a clinically significant reduction in pain. In the four earlier studies, the MIC for pain reduction had been established at values ranging from 0.9 to 1.3 cm, and so Fleet and colleagues (some of whom were nurses) used a reduction of 1.2 cm as their benchmark for clinically significant improvement.

TIP: The Toolkit in the *Resource Manual* provides a few examples of MIC values that have been proposed for several health measures. We emphasize that these MICs are illustrative, as a means of showing that MIC information can be found in the literature. We found these examples by searching in PubMed, using as search terms the name of a construct (e.g., depression) or a scale (e.g., Beck Depression Inventory), combined with the terms "minimal important" OR "minimum important" OR "minimum clinically important."

Many measures that are widely used by nurse researchers have not, however, been subjected to analysis for establishing an MIC—which in itself suggests avenues for new research. When no MIC benchmark has been established for an outcome of interest, nurse researchers may have to adopt a distribution-based approach to estimating it.

Responder Analysis

Many researchers (including some nurse researchers) have used the MIC to interpret group-level findings. The MIC is, however, an index that concerns *individual* changes, not group differences. Experts have warned that it is not appropriate to interpret mean differences in relation to the MIC (Guyatt et al., 2002; Wyrwich et al., 2013). For example, if the MIC on an important outcome has been reported as 4.0, this value should not be used to interpret the mean difference between two groups in terms of the clinical significance. If the mean group difference were found to be 3.0, for instance, it would be inappropriate to conclude that the results were not clinically significant. A mean difference of 3.0 almost certainly implies that a sizeable percentage of the participants achieved a meaningful benefit—that is, an improvement of 4 points or more.

MIC thresholds can, however, be used to create new outcomes that facilitate the interpretation of group differences, such as in a clinical trial. Once the MIC is established, researchers can classify all people in the study in terms of their having attained or not attained the threshold. That is, study participants can be classified as *responders* or *nonresponders* to treatment based on an established threshold of meaningful change. Then, researchers can undertake a **responder analysis** that compares the percentage of responders in the study groups (e.g., those in the intervention and those in the control group). A distinct advantage of a responder analysis is that it is easy to understand and can facilitate comparisons across trials or across different outcomes in a trial.

TIP: A responder analysis is an excellent strategy with implications for evidence-based practice. By classifying people as responders and nonresponders, researchers can go on to examine who did and did not respond at clinically significant levels and explore their characteristics and treatment experiences.

CRITIQUING INTERPRETATIONS

Researchers offer their interpretation of the findings and discuss what the findings might imply for nursing in the discussion section of research reports. When critiquing a study, your own interpretation and inferences can be contrasted against those of the researchers.

As a reviewer, you should be wary if a discussion section fails to point out any limitations. Researchers are in the best position to detect and assess the impact of sampling deficiencies, practical constraints, data quality problems, and so on, and it is a professional responsibility to alert readers to these difficulties. Moreover, when researchers note methodologic shortcomings, readers have some confidence that these limitations were considered in interpreting the results. Of course, researchers are unlikely to note all relevant

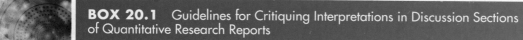

BOX 20.1 Guidelines for Critiquing Interpretations in Discussion Sections of Quantitative Research Reports

INTERPRETATION OF THE FINDINGS

1. Are all important results discussed?
2. Did the researchers discuss the limitations of the study and their possible effects on the credibility of the research evidence? In discussing limitations, were key threats to the study's validity and possible biases noted? Did the interpretations take limitations into account?
3. What types of evidence were offered in support of the interpretation, and was that evidence persuasive? If results were "mixed," were possible explanations offered? Were results interpreted in light of findings from other studies?
4. Were any supplementary analyses undertaken to facilitate interpretation? If not, should they have been?
5. Did the researchers make any unwarranted causal inferences? Were alternative explanations for the findings considered? Were the rationales for rejecting these alternatives convincing?
6. Did the interpretation take into account the precision of the results and/or the magnitude of effects?
7. Did the researchers discuss the generalizability of the findings? Did they draw any unwarranted conclusions about generalizability?

IMPLICATIONS OF THE FINDINGS AND RECOMMENDATIONS

8. Did the researchers discuss the study's implications for clinical practice, nursing theory, or future nursing research? Did they make specific recommendations?
9. If yes, are the stated implications appropriate, given the study's limitations and the magnitude of the effects—as well as evidence from other studies? Are there important implications that the report neglected to include?

CLINICAL SIGNIFICANCE

10. Did the researchers mention clinical significance? Did they make a distinction between statistical and clinical significance?
11. If yes, was clinical significance interpreted in terms of group-level information (e.g., effect sizes) or individual-level results? If the latter, how was clinical significance operationalized?

---

shortcomings of their own work. The task of reviewers is to develop independent interpretations and assessments of limitations, to challenge conclusions that do not appear to be warranted by the results, and to consider how the study's evidence could have been enhanced.

In addition to comparing your interpretation with that of the researchers, your critique should also draw conclusions about the stated implications of the study. Some researchers make grandiose claims or offer unfounded recommendations on the basis of modest results.

We have discussed the issue of clinical significance at some length in this chapter—a new topic in this edition of this book. The conceptualization and operationalization of clinical significance have not received much attention in nursing, and so studies that do not mention clinical significance should not be faulted for this omission. We hope that nurse researchers will pay more attention to this issue in the years ahead.

Some guidelines for evaluating researchers' interpretation and implications are offered in Box 20.1.

RESEARCH EXAMPLE

We conclude this chapter with an example of a study that involved an examination of clinical significance.

Study: Neurobehavioral effects of aspartame consumption (Lindseth et al., 2014)

Statement of Purpose: The purpose of this study was to examine the effects of consuming diets with higher amounts of aspartame (25 mg/kg body weight/day) versus lower amounts of aspartame (10 mg/kg body weight/day) on neurobehavioral outcomes.

Method: The researchers used a randomized crossover design to assess the effects of aspartame amounts. Study participants were 28 healthy adults, university students, who consumed study-prepared diets. Participants were randomized to orderings of the aspartame protocol (i.e., some received the high-aspartame diet first, others received the low amount first). Participants were blinded to which diet they were receiving. They consumed one of the diets for an 8-day period, followed by a 2-week washout period. Then they consumed the alternative diet for another 8 days. At the end of each 8-day session, measurements were made for neurobehavioral outcomes, including cognition (working memory and spatial visualization), depression, and mood (irritability).

Analyses: Within-subjects tests (paired *t*-tests, repeated-measures ANOVA) were used to test the statistical significance of differences in outcomes for the two dietary protocols, with alpha set at .05. In terms of clinical significance, a participant was considered to have a clinically significant neurobehavioral effect if his or her score was 2+ standard deviations outside the mean score for normal functioning. Thus, change or difference scores for participants were not computed. Rather, each measurement was assessed for any departure from a normative state—a criterion similar to that proposed as part of the J-T approach.

Results: Statistically significant differences, favoring the low-aspartame diet, were observed for three neurobehavioral outcomes: spatial orientation, depression, and irritability. Despite the fact that the participants were healthy adult students, a few of them experienced clinically significant outcomes in the high-aspartame condition. For example, four participants had clinically significant cognitive impairment (two with working memory deficits and two others with spatial orientation impairment) after 8 days of consuming the high-aspartame diet. Three other participants (different from the four with cognitive impairment) had clinically relevant levels of depression at the end of the high-aspartame condition. No scores on any outcome were clinically significant after 8 days with the low-aspartame diet.

Discussion: The researchers devoted a large section of their discussion section to the issue of *corroboration*, which we mentioned in connection with effects to interpret the credibility of study results. They pointed out ways in which their findings were consistent with (or diverged from) other studies on the effects of aspartame. In keeping with the researchers' use of a strong experimental design, they concluded that there was a causal relationship between high amounts of aspartame consumption and negative neurobehavioral effects: "A high dose of aspartame caused more irritability and depression than a low-aspartame dose consumed by the same participants, supporting earlier study findings by Walton et al. (1993)" (p. 191). The researchers also commented on the clinical significance findings: "Additionally, three participants in our study scored in the clinically depressed category while consuming the high-aspartame diet, despite no previous histories of depression" (p. 191). The researchers concluded their discussion section with remarks about the limitations of their study, which included problems of generalizability: "Limitations of our study included the small homogeneous sample, which may make it difficult to apply our conclusions to other study populations. Also, our sample size of 28 participants resulted in statistical power of .72, which is on the lower end of the acceptable range. A washout period before the baseline assessments and using food diaries during the between-treatment washout period to verify that aspartame was not consumed would have strengthened the design" (p. 191).

SUMMARY POINTS

- The interpretation of quantitative research **results** (the outcomes of the statistical analyses) typically involves consideration of (1) the credibility of the results, (2) precision of estimates of effects, (3) magnitude of effects, (4) underlying meaning of the results, (5) generalizability of results, and (6) implications for future research, theory development, and nursing practice.

- Inference is central to interpretation. Methodologic decisions made by researchers affect the inferences that can be made about the correspondence between study results and "truth in the real world." A cautious outlook is appropriate in drawing conclusions about the credibility and meaning of study results.

- An assessment of a study's credibility can involve various approaches, one of which involves evaluating the degree of congruence between abstract constructs or idealized methods on the one hand, and the proxies actually used on the other. Credibility assessments can also involve a careful assessment of study rigor through an analysis of validity threats and biases that could undermine the accuracy of the results. Corroboration (replication) of results is another approach in a credibility assessment.

- Broadly speaking, **clinical significance** refers to the practical importance of research results—that is, whether the effects are genuine and palpable in the daily lives of patients or in the management of their health. Clinical significance has not received great attention in nursing research.

- Clinical significance for group-level results is often inferred on the basis of such statistics as effect size indexes, confidence intervals, and number-needed-to-treat. However, clinical significance is most often discussed in terms of effects for individual patients—especially, whether they have achieved a clinically meaningful change.

- Definitions and operationalizations of clinical significance for individuals typically involve a **benchmark** or threshold that designates a meaningful amount of change. At the conceptual level, clinical significance has been defined in terms of whether a change in the attribute is real, whether a patient in a dysfunctional state returns to normal functioning, whether a patient has achieved a symptom state that is acceptable to them, and whether the amount of change in an attribute can be considered minimally important.

- The efforts to operationalize clinical significance in medical fields have mostly focused on the last definition. The goal is such efforts is to determine a benchmark (change score value) on a health measure that can be considered a **minimal important change (MIC)**, also called a *minimal important difference (MID)*.

- The MIC benchmark is a value for the amount of change score points that an individual patient must achieve in order to be credited with having a clinically important change.

- The primary methods of establishing the MIC for a measure are (a) through a consensus panel, (b) using an **anchor-based approach** that often involves linking changes on a focal measure to a criterion for meaningful change, and (c) using a **distribution-based method** that bases the MIC on the distributional characteristics of the sample (e.g., 0.5 *SD* of a baseline distribution, or 1 standard error of measurement). Triangulation of approaches is increasingly common.

- MICs cannot legitimately be used to interpret group means or differences in means. However, the MIC can be used to ascertain whether each person in a sample has or has not achieved a change greater than the MIC, and then a **responder analysis** can be undertaken to compare the percentage of responders in different study groups.

STUDY ACTIVITIES

Chapter 20 of the *Resource Manual for Nursing Research*: *Generating and Assessing Evidence for Nursing Practice*, *10th edition*, offers exercises and study suggestions for reinforcing concepts presented in this chapter. In addition, the following study questions can be addressed:

1. Read an article in a recent nursing research journal. Write out a brief interpretation of the

results based on the report's "Results" section and then compare your interpretation with that of the researchers.

2. Use the critiquing guidelines in Box 20.1 to critique the study used as the research example at the end of the chapter (Lindseth et al., 2014), referring to the full study as necessary.

STUDIES CITED IN CHAPTER 20

Al-Gamal, E., & Yorke, J. (2014). Perceived breathlessness and psychological distress among patients with chronic obstructive pulmonary disease and their spouses. *Nursing and Health Sciences*, 16, 103–111.

Bevan, D., Wittkowski, A., & Wells, A. (2013). A multiple-baseline study of the effects associated with metacognitive therapy in postpartum depression. *Journal of Midwifery & Women's Health*, 58, 69–75.

Bruner, S., Corbett, C., Gates, B., & Dupler, A. (2012). Clinical significance as it relates to evidence-based practice. *International Journal of Nursing Knowledge*, 23, 62–74.

Cohen, J. (1988). *Statistical power analysis for the behavioral sciences* (2nd ed.). Hillsdale, NJ: Lawrence Erlbaum Associates.

De Vet, H. C. W., Terwee, C., Mokkink, L. B., & Knol, D. L. (2011). *Measurement in medicine: A practical guide*. Cambridge, United Kingdom: Cambridge University Press.

Dotson, M. J., Dave, D., Cazier, J., & Spaulding, T. (2014). An empirical analysis of nurse retention: What keeps RNs in nursing? *Journal of Nursing Administration*, 44, 111–116.

Dworkin, R. H., Turk, D., Farrar, J., Haythornethwaite, J., Jensen, P., Katz, N., . . . Witter, J. (2005). Core outcome measures for chronic pain clinical trials: IMMPACT recommendations. *Pain*, 113, 9-19.

Dysvik, E., Kvaløy, J. T., & Natvig, G. K. (2011). The effectiveness of an improved multidisciplinary pain management programme: A 6- and 12-month follow-up study. *Journal of Advanced Nursing*, 68, 1061–1072.

Fethney, J. (2010). Statistical and clinical significance, and how to use confidence intervals to help interpret both. *Australian Critical Care*, 23, 93–97.

Fleet, J., Jones, M., & Belan, I. (2014). Subcutaneous administration of fentanyl in childbirth: An observational study on the clinical effectiveness of fentanyl for mother and neonate. *Midwifery*, 30, 36–42.

Froman, R. D., & Owen, S. (2014). Why you want to avoid being a causist. *Research in Nursing & Health*, 37, 171–173.

Gaskin, C., & Happell, B. (2014). Power, effects, confidence, and significance: An investigation of statistical practices in nursing research. *International Journal of Nursing Studies*, 51, 795–806.

Griffin, R., Polit, D., & Byrne, M. (2007). Stereotyping and nurses' recommendations for treating pain in hospitalized children. *Research in Nursing & Health*, 30, 655–666.

Guyatt, G. H., Osoba, D., Wu, A., Wyrwich, K., & Norman, G. R. (2002). Methods to explain the clinical significance of health status measures. *Mayo Clinic Proceedings*, 77, 371–383.

Hayat, M. J. (2010). Understanding statistical significance. *Nursing Research*, 59, 219–223.

*Jacobson, N. S., & Truax, P. (1991). Clinical significance: A statistical approach to defining meaningful change in psychotherapy research. *Journal of Consulting and Clinical Psychology*, 59, 12–19.

Jaeschke, R., Singer, J., & Guyatt, G. H. (1989). Measurement of health status: Ascertaining the minimal clinically important difference. *Controlled Clinical Trials*, 10, 407–415.

Kazdin, A. E. (1999). The meanings and measurement of clinical significance. *Journal of Consulting and Clinical Psychology*, 67, 332–339.

*Lavender, T., Bedwell, C., Roberts, S., Hart, A., Turner, M., Carter, L., & Cork, M. (2013). Randomized, controlled trial evaluating a baby wash product on skin barrier function in healthy, term neonates. *Journal of Obstetric, Gynecologic, & Neonatal Nursing*, 42, 203–214.

LeFort, S. M. (1993). The statistical versus clinical significance debate. *Image: The Journal of Nursing Scholarship*, 25, 57–62.

Lindseth, G. N., Coolahan, S., Petros, T., & Lindseth, P. (2014). Neurobehavioral effects of aspartame consumption. *Research in Nursing & Health*, 37, 185–193.

Mann, B. J., Gosens, T., & Lyman, S. (2012). Quantifying clinically significant change: A brief review of methods and presentation of a hybrid approach. *The American Journal of Sports Medicine*, 40, 2385–2393.

Ngai, F. W., & Ngu, S. F. (2014). Family sense of coherence and family adaptation among childbearing couples. *Journal of Nursing Scholarship*, 46, 82–90.

Norman, G. R., Sloan, J., & Wyrwich, K. W. (2003). Interpretation of changes in health-related quality of life: The remarkable universality of half a standard deviation. *Medical Care*, 41, 582–592.

Norman, G. R., Sloan, J., & Wyrwich, K. W. (2004). The truly remarkable universality of half a standard deviation: Confirmation through another look. *Expert Review of Pharmacoeconomics & Outcomes Research*, 4, 581–586.

Patel, A., Siegert, R., Keir, G., Bajwah, S., Barker, R., Maher, T., . . . Birring, S. (2013). The minimal important difference of the King's Brief Interstitial Lung Disease Questionnaire (K-BILD) and forced vital capacity in interstitial lung disease. *Respiratory Medicine*, 107, 1438–1443.

Polit, D. F., & Yang, F. M. (2015). *Measurement and the measurement of change: A primer for health professionals*. Philadelphia: Wolters Kluwer.

Revicki, D., Hays, R., Cella, D., & Sloan, J. (2008). Recommended methods for determining responsiveness and minimally important differences for patient-reported outcomes. *Journal of Clinical Epidemiology*, 61, 102–109.

Sackett, D. L., Straus, S. E., Richardson, W. S., Rosenberg, W., & Haynes, R. B. (2000). *Evidence-based medicine: How to practice and teach EBM* (2nd ed.). Edinburgh, Scotland: Churchill Livingstone.

Shadish, W. R., Cook, T. D., & Campbell, D. T. (2002). *Experimental and quasi-experimental designs for generalized causal inference.* Boston: Houghton Mifflin.

Tubach, F., Dougados, M., Falissard, B., Baron, G., Logeart, I., & Ravaud, P. (2006). Feeling good rather than feeling better matters more to patients. *Arthritis & Rheumatism, 55,* 526–530.

*Tubach, F., Ravaud, P., Beaton, D., Boers, M., Bombardier, C., Felson, D., . . . Dougados, M. (2007). Minimal clinically important improvement and patient acceptable symptom state for subjective outcome measures in rheumatic disorders. *Journal of Rheumatology, 34,* 1139–1193.

*Tunes da Silva, G. T., Logan, B., & Klein, J. (2009). Methods for equivalence and noninferiority testing. *Biology of Blood and Marrow Transplantation, 15,* 120–127.

Watt, S., Sword, W., Sheehan, D., Foster, G., Thabane, L., Krueger, P., & Landy, C. (2012). The effect of delivery method on breastfeeding initiation from the Ontario Mother and Infant Study (TOMIS). *Journal of Obstetric, Gynecologic, & Neonatal Nursing, 41,* 728–737.

Wyrwich, K. W., Norquist, J., Lenderking, W., & Acaster, S. (2013). Methods for interpreting change over time in patient-reported outcome measures. *Quality of Life Research, 22,* 475–483.

A link to this open-access journal article is provided in the Toolkit for this chapter in the accompanying Resource Manual. ✖

PART 4

DESIGNING AND CONDUCTING QUALITATIVE STUDIES TO GENERATE EVIDENCE FOR NURSING

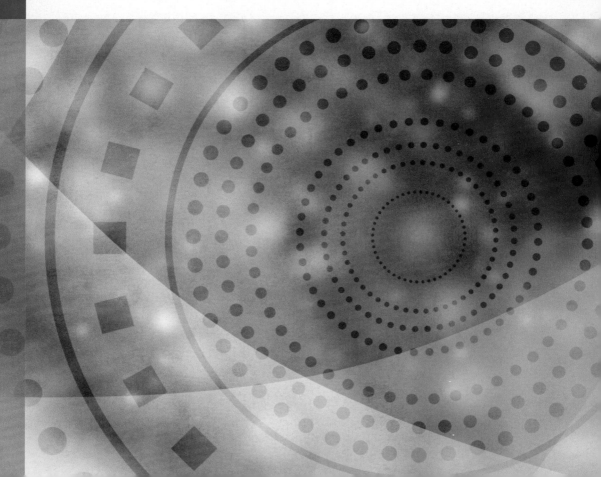

21 | Qualitative Research Design and Approaches

THE DESIGN OF QUALITATIVE STUDIES

Quantitative researchers specify a research design before collecting their data and rarely depart from that design once the study is underway. In qualitative research, by contrast, the design typically evolves over the course of the study. Qualitative studies use an **emergent design** that takes shape as researchers make ongoing decisions reflecting what they have already learned. An emergent design is not the result of laziness on the part of qualitative researchers but rather a reflection of their desire to have the inquiry based on the realities and viewpoints of participants—realities and viewpoints that are not known at the outset (Lincoln & Guba, 1985).

Characteristics of Qualitative Research Design

Qualitative inquiry has been used in many different disciplines, and each has developed methods for addressing particular types of questions. However, some characteristics of qualitative research design tend to apply across disciplines. In general, qualitative design:

- Is flexible, capable of adjusting to new information during the course of data collection
- Tends to be holistic, aimed at an understanding of the whole
- Often involves merging various data collection strategies (i.e., triangulation)
- Requires researchers to become intensely involved

- Relies on ongoing analysis of the data to formulate subsequent strategies and to determine when data collection is done

Qualitative researchers often put together a complex array of data, derived from a variety of sources and using a variety of methods. This process has sometimes been described as **bricolage**, and the qualitative researcher has been referred to as a *bricoleur*, a person who "is adept at performing a large number of diverse tasks, ranging from interviewing to intensive reflection and introspection" (Denzin & Lincoln, 2011, p. 5).

Qualitative Design and Planning

Although design decisions are not specified in advance, qualitative researchers typically do advance planning that supports their flexibility in pursuing an emergent design. In the total absence of planning, design choices might actually be constrained. For example, researchers might anticipate a 6-month period for data collection but may need to be prepared (financially and emotionally) to spend even longer periods of time in the field to pursue data collection opportunities that could not have been foreseen. In other words, qualitative researchers plan for broad contingencies that may be expected to pose decision opportunities once the study has begun. Advance planning is especially useful with regard to the following:

- Selecting a broad framework or tradition (described in the next section) to guide design decisions

- Determining the maximum amount of time available for the study, given costs and other constraints
- Developing a broad data collection strategy and identifying opportunities for enhancing trustworthiness (e.g., through triangulation)
- Collecting relevant site materials (e.g., maps, organizational charts, resource directories)
- Identifying the types of equipment that could aid in the collection and analysis of data in the field (e.g., audio and video recording equipment, computers or tablets)
- Identifying personal biases, views, and presuppositions vis-à-vis the phenomenon or the study site, as well as ideologic stances (reflexivity)

Thus, qualitative researchers need to plan for a variety of circumstances, but decisions about how to deal with them must be resolved when the social context is better understood. By allowing for and anticipating an evolution of strategies, qualitative researchers seek to make their research design responsive to the situation and to the phenomenon under study.

> **TIP:** In planning their qualitative studies, nurse researchers should reflect on how the findings might be useful to practicing nurses and seek opportunities to enhance the EBP-potential of the research.

Qualitative Design Features

In Chapter 8, we discussed three design features that are relevant to qualitative research—comparisons, settings, and time frames. Here we briefly review these features as a reminder of aspects of qualitative design that should be kept in mind in undertaking qualitative research.

Qualitative researchers seldom explicitly plan a comparative study (e.g., comparing children who have or do not have cancer). Nevertheless, patterns emerging in the data often suggest that certain comparisons are relevant and illuminating. Indeed, as Morse (2004) noted in an editorial in *Qualitative Health Research*, "All description requires comparisons" (p. 1323). Inevitably in coding qualitative

information and in evaluating whether categories are saturated, there is a need to compare "this" to "that." Morse pointed out that qualitative comparisons are often not dichotomous: "Life is usually on a continuum" (p. 1324). Of course, comparisons sometimes *are* planned in qualitative studies (e.g., a comparison of nurses and patients' perspectives about a phenomenon). Moreover, qualitative researchers can sometimes plan for the *possibility* of comparisons by selecting a richly diverse group of people as participants.

Example of Comparisons in a Qualitative Study: Lloyd and colleagues (2014) studied women's experiences after a radical vaginal trachelectomy for early stage cervical cancer. Twelve women with varying backgrounds participated in in-depth interviews. The researchers found considerable diversity in the women's experiences, and the researchers noted that "similarities and differences were searched for in the interview transcripts" (p. 364). They found, for example, that single women felt vulnerable in forming new relationships.

In terms of research settings, qualitative researchers usually collect their data in real-world, naturalistic settings. And, whereas quantitative researchers usually strive to collect data in one type of setting to maintain constancy in environmental conditions (e.g., conducting all interviews in participants' homes), qualitative researchers may deliberately strive to study phenomena in a variety of natural contexts.

With regard to time frames, qualitative research can be either cross-sectional, with one data collection point, or longitudinal, with multiple data collection points over an extended time period, to observe the evolution of some phenomenon. Sometimes qualitative researchers plan in advance for a longitudinal design, but sometimes a decision to study a phenomenon longitudinally may be made after preliminary analysis of the data.

Example of a Longitudinal Qualitative Study: Darcy and colleagues (2014) studied young children's experiences in striving for an ordinary life after a cancer diagnosis. Children and their parents were interviewed at 6 months and 1 year post-diagnosis.

Causality and Qualitative Research

In evidence hierarchies that rank evidence in terms of its ability to support causal inferences (e.g., Figure 2.1), qualitative inquiry is usually near the base—a fact that has led some to criticize the EBP movement. The issue of causality, which has been controversial throughout the history of science, is especially contentious in qualitative research.

Some qualitative researchers think that causality is not an appropriate construct within the constructivist paradigm. For example, Lincoln and Guba (1985) devoted an entire chapter of their book to a critique of causality and argued that it should be replaced with a concept that they called *mutual shaping*. According to their view of mutual and simultaneous shaping, "Everything influences everything else, in the here and now. Many elements are implicated in any given action, and each element interacts with all of the others in ways that change them all while simultaneously resulting in something that we . . . label as outcomes or effects" (p. 151).

Others, however, believe that causal explanation is not only a legitimate pursuit in qualitative research but also that qualitative methods are especially well-suited to understanding causal relationships. For example, Maxwell (2012) argued that qualitative research is important for causal explanations, noting that they "depend on the in-depth understanding of meanings, contexts, and processes that qualitative research can provide" (p. 655).

In attempting to not only describe but also to explain phenomena, qualitative researchers who undertake in-depth studies will inevitably reveal patterns and processes suggesting causal interpretations. These interpretations can be (and often are) subjected to more systematic testing using more controlled methods of inquiry.

OVERVIEW OF QUALITATIVE RESEARCH TRADITIONS

Despite some features common to many qualitative research designs, there is nevertheless a wide variety of approaches—but no readily agreed-upon classification system for these approaches. One system, as noted in Chapter 3, is to categorize qualitative research according to disciplinary traditions. These traditions vary in their conceptualization of what types of questions are important to ask and in the methods they consider appropriate for answering them. This section provides an overview of several qualitative research traditions, some of which are described in greater detail later in the chapter.

The research traditions that have provided a theoretical underpinning for qualitative studies come primarily from the disciplines of anthropology, psychology, and sociology. As shown in Table 21.1, each discipline has tended to focus on one or two broad domains of inquiry.

The discipline of anthropology is concerned with human cultures. **Ethnography** is the primary research tradition in anthropology. Ethnographers study cultural patterns and experiences in a holistic fashion. **Ethnoscience** (sometimes referred to as **cognitive anthropology**) focuses on the cognitive world of a culture, with particular emphasis on the semantic rules and shared meanings that shape behavior. Cognitive anthropologists assume that a group's cultural knowledge is reflected in its language.

Example of an Ethnoscientific Study: Kirshbaum and colleagues (2013) used an ethnoscience framework to examine the perceptions and experiences of fatigue held by patients attending a hospice in England. Their study suggested that symptom experience is socially constructed.

Phenomenology has its disciplinary roots in both philosophy and psychology. As noted in Chapter 3, phenomenology focuses on the meaning of lived experiences of humans. A closely related research tradition is **hermeneutics**, which uses lived experiences as a tool for better understanding the social, cultural, political, or historical context in which those experiences occur. Hermeneutic inquiry almost always focuses on meaning and interpretation—how socially and historically conditioned individuals interpret the world within their given context.

The discipline of psychology has several other qualitative research traditions that focus on *behavior*.

TABLE 21.1 • Overview of Qualitative Research Traditions

DISCIPLINE	DOMAIN	RESEARCH TRADITION	AREA OF INQUIRY
Anthropology	Culture	Ethnography Ethnoscience (cognitive anthropology)	Holistic view of a culture Mapping of the cognitive world of a culture; a culture's shared meanings, semantic rules
Psychology/ philosophy	Lived experience	Phenomenology Hermeneutics	Experiences of individuals within their lifeworld Interpretations and meanings of individuals' experiences
Psychology	Behavior and events	Ethology Ecological psychology	Behavior observed over time in natural context Behavior as influenced by the environment
Sociology	Social settings	Grounded theory Ethnomethodology Semiotics	Social structural processes within a social setting Manner by which shared agreement is achieved in social settings Manner by which people make sense of social interactions
Sociolinguistics	Human communication	Discourse analysis	Forms and rules of conversation
History	Past behavior, events, and conditions	Historical analysis	Description and interpretation of historical events

Human **ethology**, sometimes described as the biology of human behavior, studies behavior as it evolves in its natural context. Human ethologists use primarily observational methods in an attempt to discover universal behavioral structures. Warnock and Allen (2003) have urged nurse researchers to consider using ethologic methods and used neonatal pain to illustrate how ethology can be used to develop nursing knowledge and midrange theory.

Example of an Ethologic Study: Spiers (2006) used ethologic methods to study pain-related interactions between patients and home-care nurses. Spiers analyzed micropatterns of videotaped communication in the patients' homes over multiple home-nurse visits.

Ecologic psychology focuses on the influence of the environment on human behavior and attempts to identify principles that explain the interdependence of humans and their environmental context. Viewed from an ecologic context, people are affected by (and affect) a multilayered set of systems, including family, peer group, and neighborhood as well as the more indirect effects of health care and social services systems, and the larger cultural belief and value systems of the society in which individuals live.

Example of an Ecologic Study: Hudson and colleagues (2014) used an ecologic framework to study factors influencing hospital admissions and ED visits among children with complex chronic conditions.

Both parents and health care providers described risk factors and protective factors on multiple ecologic levels.

Sociologists study the social world in which we live and have developed several research traditions of importance to qualitative researchers. The *grounded theory* tradition involves efforts to describe and understand key social psychological and structural processes in social settings.

Ethnomethodology seeks to discover how people make sense of their everyday activities and interpret their social worlds so as to behave in socially acceptable ways. Within this tradition, researchers attempt to understand a group's norms and assumptions that are so deeply ingrained that members no longer think about the underlying reasons for their behaviors.

Example of an Ethnomethodologic Study: Lobar (2014) used an ethnomethodologic approach to examine perceptions of parents and caregivers of children diagnosed with autistic spectrum disorders. The focus was on the participants' actions, norms, understandings, and assumptions related to adjustment to the illness.

Symbolic interaction (or *interactionism*) is a sociologic tradition with roots in American pragmatism and is sometimes associated with grounded theory research. As noted in Chapter 6, symbolic interaction focuses on the manner in which people make sense of social interactions and the interpretations they attach to social symbols, such as language. Symbolic interactionists sometimes use **semiotics**, which is the study of signs and their meanings. A sign is any entity or object that carries information (e.g., a diagram, map, or picture).

Example of a Semiotic Analysis: Short and co-researchers (2013) used a semiotic framework to analyze cardiac rehabilitation patients' narratives concerning their experience with an innovative music therapy.

The domain of inquiry for sociolinguists is human communication. The tradition referred to as **discourse analysis** (sometimes called *conversation analysis*) seeks to understand the rules, mechanisms, and structure of conversations and texts. Discourse analysts seek to understand the action that a given kind of talk "performs." The data for discourse analysis often are transcripts from naturally occurring conversations, such as those between nurses and their patients. In discourse analysis, the texts are situated in their social, cultural, political, and historical context.

Example of a Discourse Analysis: Using discourse analysis methods, DeSouza (2014) analyzed group conversations among migrant fathers in New Zealand concerning their decision to have a child. Fathers drew on two key discourses to understand how they made reproductive decisions (as a financial decision and as a natural process).

Finally, **historical research**—the systematic collection and critical evaluation of data relating to past occurrences—is a tradition that relies primarily on qualitative data. Nurses have used historical research methods to examine a wide range of phenomena in both the recent and more distant past. An overview of the methods associated with historical research is provided on the Supplement to this chapter on thePoint°.

Researchers in each of these traditions have developed methodologic strategies for the design and conduct of relevant studies. Thus, once a researcher has identified what aspect of the human experience is of greatest interest, there is typically a wealth of advice available about methods likely to be productive in designing and undertaking the study.

TIP: Sometimes a research report identifies more than one tradition as having provided the framework for a qualitative inquiry (e.g., a phenomenologic study using the grounded theory method). Such "method slurring" (Baker et al., 1992) has been criticized because each research tradition has different intellectual assumptions and methodologic prescriptions. However, as noted by Nepal (2010), echoing some of the sentiments expressed in an editorial by Janice Morse (2009), mixed qualitative methods may be viable when "the researcher has ascertained, from the beginning . . ., that the research questions cannot be answered in their entirety unless and until there are two different qualitative methods used" (p. 281).

ETHNOGRAPHY

Ethnography involves the description and interpretation of cultural behavior. Ethnographies are a blend of a process and a product, fieldwork, and a written text. Fieldwork is how the ethnographer comes to understand a culture, and the ethnographic text is how that culture is communicated and portrayed. Because culture is, in itself, not visible or tangible, it must be constructed through ethnographic writing. Culture is inferred from the words, actions, and products of members of a group.

Ethnographic research is sometimes concerned with broadly defined cultures (e.g., an Afghan village culture) in a **macroethnography**. Ethnographies often focus on more narrowly defined cultures in a **microethnography** or **focused ethnography** (Cruz & Higginbottom, 2013). Microethnographies are exhaustive, fine-grained studies of either small units in a group or culture (e.g., the culture of homeless shelters) or of specific activities in an organizational unit (e.g., how nurses communicate with children in an emergency department). An underlying assumption of the ethnographer is that every human group eventually evolves a culture that guides the members' view of the world and the way they structure their experiences.

Example of a Focused Ethnography: Higginbottom and colleagues (2014) conducted a focused ethnography to examine the health and social care needs of Somali refugees with visual impairment living in the United Kingdom.

Ethnographers seek to learn from members of a cultural group—to understand their worldview. Ethnographic researchers sometimes refer to "emic" and "etic" perspectives (terms from linguistics, i.e., phon*emic* versus phon*etic*). An **emic perspective** is the way the members of the culture envision their world—it is the insiders' view.

The emic is the local language, concepts, or means of expression used by members of the group under study to characterize their experiences. The **etic perspective** is the outsiders' interpretation of the experiences of that culture; it is the language used by those doing the research to refer to the same phenomena. Ethnographers strive to acquire an emic perspective of a culture. Moreover, they strive to reveal **tacit knowledge** about the culture that is so deeply embedded in cultural experiences that members do not talk about it or may not even be consciously aware of it.

Ethnographic research typically is labor-intensive, requiring long periods (months or even years) in the field. The study of a culture requires a certain level of intimacy with members of the cultural group, and such intimacy can be developed only over time and by working directly with those members as active participants. The concept of **researcher as instrument** is frequently used by anthropologists to describe the significant role ethnographers play in analyzing and interpreting a culture.

Three broad types of information usually are sought by ethnographers: cultural behavior (what members of the culture do), cultural artifacts (what people make and use), and cultural speech (what people say). This implies that ethnographers rely on a wide variety of data sources, including observations, in-depth interviews, records, charts, and physical evidence such as photographs, diaries, and letters. Ethnographers often use a **participant observation** strategy in which they make observations of the culture while participating in its activities. Ethnographers observe people day after day in their natural environments to observe behavior in a wide array of circumstances. Ethnographers also enlist the help of **key informants** to help them understand and interpret the events and activities being observed.

Some ethnographers undertake an **egocentric network analysis**, which focuses on the pattern of relationships and networks of individuals. Each person has his or her own network of relationships that are presumed to contribute to the person's behaviors and attitudes. In studying these networks, researchers develop lists of a person's network members (called *alters*) and seek to understand the scope and nature of interrelationships and social supports. Network data from such efforts are often quantified and analyzed statistically. Egocentric network analysis is used to understand features of personal networks and has been used to explain such phenomena as longevity, coping with crisis, and risk taking.

Example of an Egocentric Network Analysis: Chaichanawirote and Higgins (2013) studied the social support networks of independent-living older adults using an egocentric network analysis.

The product of ethnographic research usually is a rich and holistic description of the culture. Ethnographers also make interpretations of the culture, describing normative behavioral and social patterns. Among health care researchers, ethnography provides access to the health beliefs and health practices of a culture or subculture. Ethnographic inquiry can thus help to facilitate understanding of behaviors affecting health and illness.

In addition to written reports about ethnographic findings, ethnographers have recently used their research as the basis for performance ethnographies. A **performance ethnography** has been described as a scripted and staged reenactment of ethnographically derived notes that reflect an interpretation of the culture. Denzin and Lincoln (2011), in the fourth edition of their widely acclaimed *Handbook of Qualitative Research*, stated an expectation of a continued performance "turn" in qualitative inquiry. C. A. Smith and Gallo (2007) have described how applications of performance ethnography can be used in nursing.

A rich array of ethnographic methods have been developed and cannot be fully explicated in this general textbook, but more information may be found in Fetterman (2010) and Wolcott (2008). Three variants of ethnographic research (ethnonursing research, institutional ethnography, and autoethnography) are described here, and a fourth (critical ethnography) is described later in this chapter.

Ethnonursing Research

Many nurse researchers have undertaken ethnographic studies. Leininger coined the phrase **ethnonursing research**, which she defined as "the study

and analysis of the local or indigenous people's viewpoints, beliefs, and practices about nursing care behavior and processes of designated cultures" (1985, p. 38). In conducting an ethnonursing study, investigators use a broad theoretical framework to guide the research, such as Leininger's Theory of Culture Care Diversity and Universality (Leininger & McFarland, 2006; McFarland & Wehbe-Alamah, 2015).

McFarland and Wehbe-Alamah (2015) described a number of enablers to support researchers' efforts in conducting ethnonursing research. *Enablers* are ways to discover complex phenomena like human care. Some of her enablers include the Stranger-Friend Model, Observation-Participation-Reflection Model, and Acculturation Enabler Guide. The stranger-friend enabler guides researchers in mapping their progress and becoming more aware of their feelings, behaviors, and responses as they transition from stranger to trusted friend. The phases of Leininger's observation-participation-reflection enabler go from (1) primary observation and active listening, (2) primary observation with limited participation, (3) primary participation with continuing observations, to (4) primary reflection and reconfirmation of results with informants. The acculturation enabler guide was designed to aid researchers in assessing the degree of acculturation of a person or group with regard to the specific culture under study.

Example of an Ethnonursing Study: Moss (2014) conducted an ethnonursing study to discover and understand the health care beliefs and practices of rural mestizo Ecuadorians.

Institutional Ethnography

A type of ethnographic approach called **institutional ethnography** was pioneered by Dorothy Smith, a Canadian sociologist (1999). Institutional ethnography has been used in such fields as nursing, social work, and community health to study the organization of professional services, examined from the perspective of those who are clients or frontline workers. Institutional ethnography seeks to understand the social determinants of people's everyday experiences, especially institutional work processes. The focus in institutional ethnography is on social organization and institutional processes, and so research findings have the potential to play a role in organizational change.

In institutional ethnography, a person's actions in the social world are labeled as "social relations." Relations of *ruling* occur when social relations involve powerful coordination in people's lives and day-to-day activities. Where individuals are situated in the social location within an institution dictates relations of ruling. Each individual's standpoint has implications for how their activities are organized within social relations. For example, a person's standpoint in an institution influences the problems that may present themselves.

Institutional ethnographers study the complexities of social and ruling relations. Central to D. E. Smith's (1999) method of institutional ethnography is her focus on how knowledge or information is circulated through texts, which are central to ruling relations. Texts can include, for example, an organization's reports, statistical analysis, and organizational forms. Rankin (2013) emphasized that an important step in an institutional ethnography is to decide on a standpoint within the organization of social relations. It will be from that standpoint that the researcher will study how activities are socially organized. The research question focuses on "How does it happen?"

Example of Institutional Ethnography: Rankin (2015) conducted an institutional ethnography to explore technologic advances designed as managerial improvement strategies to coordinate nurses' work. The research focused on discrepancies that arise between different organizational standpoints. Using data from observations and interviews with nurses, nurse managers, patients, and families, Rankin, referencing the "rhetoric" of patient and family centered care, concluded that nurses' work is "overwhelmed with the imperative to discharge patients" (p. 526).

Autoethnography

Ethnographers are often "outsiders" to the culture under study. A type of ethnography that involves self-scrutiny (including study of groups or cultures to which researchers belong) is **autoethnography**, but other terms such as *insider research* and *peer research* also have been used. Autoethnography offers numerous advantages, the most obvious being ease of access, ease of recruitment, and the ability to get particularly candid, in-depth data based on preestablished trust and rapport. Another potential advantage is the researcher's ability to detect subtle nuances that an outsider might miss or take months to uncover. A potential limitation, however, is the researcher's inability to be objective about group (or self) processes, which can result in unsuspected myopia about important but sensitive issues. Autoethnography demands that researchers maintain consciousness of their role and monitor their internal state and their interactions with others during the study. Various methodologic strategies have been developed for autoethnographic work (Ellis & Bochner, 2000). Peterson (2015) has argued for greater use of autoethnography in nursing research.

Example of an Autoethnography: Whybrow (2013) described an autoethnography that explored the experiences of mental health nurses providing psychiatric liaison to British forces deployed to combat zones.

PHENOMENOLOGY

Phenomenology, rooted in a philosophical tradition developed by Husserl and Heidegger, is an approach to understanding people's everyday life experiences.

Phenomenologic researchers ask, "What is the *essence* of this phenomenon as experienced by these people and what does it *mean*?" Phenomenologists assume there is an *essence*—an essential invariant structure—that can be understood, in much the same way that ethnographers assume that cultures exist. Essence is what makes a phenomenon what it is, and without which, it would not be what it is. Phenomenologists investigate subjective phenomena in the belief that critical truths about reality are grounded in people's lived experiences. The phenomenologic approach is especially useful when a phenomenon has been poorly defined or conceptualized. The topics appropriate to phenomenology are ones that are fundamental to the life experiences of humans.

Phenomenologists believe that lived experience gives meaning to each person's perception of a particular phenomenon. The goal of phenomenologic inquiry is to understand lived experience and the perceptions to which it gives rise. Four aspects of lived experience of interest to phenomenologists are *lived space*, or spatiality; *lived body*, or corporeality; *lived time*, or temporality; and *lived human relation*, or relationality.

Phenomenologists view human existence as meaningful and interesting because of people's consciousness of that existence. The phrase **being-in-the-world** (or *embodiment*) is a concept that acknowledges people's physical ties to their world—they think, see, hear, feel, and are conscious through their bodies' interaction with the world.

In phenomenologic studies, in-depth conversations are the main data source, with researchers and informants as co-participants. Researchers help informants to describe lived experiences without leading the discussion. Through in-depth conversations, researchers strive to gain entrance into the informants' world, to have full access to their experiences as lived. Multiple interviews or conversations are sometimes needed. Typically, phenomenologic studies involve a small number of study participants—often 10 or fewer. For some phenomenologic researchers, the inquiry includes not only gathering information from informants but also efforts to experience the phenomenon through participation, observation, and introspective reflection.

Phenomenologists share their insights in rich, vivid reports. A phenomenologic text describing study results should help readers "see" something in a different way that enriches their understanding of experiences. Van Manen (1997) warned that if a phenomenologic text is flat and boring, it "loses power to break through the taken-for-granted dimensions of everyday life" (p. 346). A wealth of resources is available on phenomenologic methods. Interested readers may wish to consult such classic sources as Giorgi (1985, 2005), Colaizzi (1973), or Van Manen (2002).

There are several variants and methodologic interpretations of phenomenology. The two main schools of thought are descriptive phenomenology and interpretive phenomenology (hermeneutics). Lopez and Willis (2004) provided a useful discussion about the need to differentiate the two and laid out underlying philosophical assumptions in nursing studies.

Descriptive Phenomenology

Descriptive phenomenology was developed by Husserl (1962), who was primarily interested in the question: What do we know as persons? His philosophy emphasized descriptions of human experience. Descriptive phenomenologists insist on the careful description of ordinary conscious experience of everyday life—a description of "things" as people experience them. These "things" include hearing, seeing, believing, feeling, remembering, deciding, evaluating, and acting.

Descriptive phenomenologic studies often involve the following four steps: bracketing, intuiting, analyzing, and describing. **Bracketing** is the process of identifying and holding in abeyance preconceived beliefs and opinions about the phenomenon under study. Bracketing can never be achieved totally, but researchers strive to bracket out the world and any presuppositions in an effort to confront the data in pure form. Bracketing is an iterative process that involves preparing, evaluating, and providing systematic ongoing feedback about the effectiveness of the bracketing. Phenomenologic researchers (as well as other qualitative researchers) often maintain a **reflexive journal** in their efforts to bracket. Ahern (1999) provided 10 tips to help qualitative researchers with bracketing through notes in a reflexive journal:

1. Make note of interests that, as a researcher, you may take for granted.
2. Clarify your personal values and identify areas in which you know you are biased.
3. Identify areas of possible role conflict.
4. Recognize gatekeepers' interest and make note of the degree to which they are favorably or unfavorably disposed toward your research.
5. Identify any feelings you have that may indicate a lack of neutrality.

6. Describe new or surprising findings in collecting and analyzing data.
7. Reflect on and profit from methodologic problems that occur during your research.
8. After data analysis is complete, reflect on how you write up your findings.
9. Reflect on whether the literature review is truly supporting your findings, or whether it is expressing the similar cultural background that you have.
10. Consider whether you can address any bias in your data collection or analysis by interviewing a participant a second time or reanalyzing the transcript in question.

Intuiting, the second step in descriptive phenomenology, occurs when researchers remain open to the meanings attributed to the phenomenon by those who have experienced it. Phenomenologic researchers then proceed to the analysis phase (i.e., extracting significant statements, categorizing, and making sense of the essential meanings of the phenomenon). Chapter 24 provides further information regarding the analysis of data collected in phenomenologic studies. Finally, the descriptive phase occurs when researchers come to understand and define the phenomenon.

Example of a Descriptive Phenomenologic Study: Yun and colleagues (2014) used a descriptive phenomenologic approach to study the sexuality experiences of older community-dwelling widows in Korea. In describing efforts to bracket preconceptions, the researchers noted that personal thoughts and feelings were summarized and recorded at the end of each interview session.

Interpretive Phenomenology

Heidegger, a student of Husserl, moved away from his professor's philosophy into **interpretive phenomenology** or hermeneutics. To Heidegger (1962), the critical question is: What is *being*? He stressed interpreting and understanding—not just describing—human experience. His premise is that the lived experience is inherently an interpretive process. Heidegger argued that hermeneutics is a basic characteristic of human existence. Indeed, the term hermeneutics refers to the art and philosophy

of interpreting the meaning of an object (such as a *text*, work of art, and so on). The goals of interpretive phenomenologic research are to enter another's world and to discover the practical wisdom, possibilities, and understandings found there.

Gadamer (1976), another influential interpretive phenomenologist, described the interpretive process as a circular relationship known as the **hermeneutic circle** where one understands the whole of a text (e.g., a transcribed interview) in terms of its parts and the parts in terms of the whole. In his view, researchers enter into a dialogue with the text, in which the researcher continually questions its meaning.

One distinction between descriptive and interpretive phenomenology is that in an interpretive phenomenologic study, bracketing does not necessarily occur. For Heidegger, it was impossible to bracket one's being-in-the-world. Hermeneutics presupposes prior understanding on the part of the researcher. Gearing (2004), who developed a typology of bracketing, described one type as *reflexive bracketing*—in which researchers attempt to identify internal suppositions to facilitate greater transparency but without bracketing them out—as a tool for hermeneutical inquiry. Interpretive phenomenologists ideally approach each interview text with openness—they must be open to hearing what the text is saying. As Heidegger (1971) stated, "We never come to thoughts. They come to us" (p. 6).

Example of an Interpretive Phenomenologic Study: Johnson and Bibbo (2014) used an interpretive phenomenologic approach in their study of how older adults in nursing homes constructed the meaning of *home* following the transition from community dwelling to a nursing home.

Interpretive phenomenologists, like descriptive phenomenologists, rely primarily on in-depth interviews with individuals who have experienced the phenomenon of interest, but they may go beyond a traditional approach to gathering and analyzing data. For example, interpretive phenomenologists sometimes augment their understandings of the phenomenon through an analysis of supplementary texts, such as novels, poetry, or other artistic expressions—or they use such materials in their conversations with study participants. Guidance in undertaking a hermeneutic phenomenologic nursing study is offered by Cohen and colleagues (2000).

In several recent health studies, researchers have cited the work of a group of psychological phenomenologists, who have described an approach called **interpretive phenomenologic analysis** or **IPA** (J. A. Smith, Flowers, & Larkin, 2009). The focus of IPA is on the subjective experiences of persons—their *lifeworld*. Studying individuals' experiences requires interpretation on the part of the researcher and the participant because it is not possible to directly access a person's lifeworld. There are three key principles to IPA: (1) It investigates the phenomenon of experience of a person, (2) it requires intense interpretation and engagement with the data obtained from the person, and (3) it is examined in detail.

The Parse Phenomenologic-Hermeneutic Research Method

Many nurse researchers use an approach that has been formulated by Rosemary Parse (2014) based on her Humanbecoming Paradigm. Parse's approach has elements of both phenomenology and

hermeneutics. The aim of Parse's research method is to uncover the meaning of universal living experiences by studying descriptions of people's experiences. The data are interpreted through the lens of Parse's paradigm. Parse's research methods consist of three processes: dialogic engagement, extraction-synthesis, and heuristic interpretation (Parse, 2001).

Dialogic engagement, the first process, is the data-gathering process. Parse stressed that this is not an interview but a unique dialogue where the researcher is a true presence with the participant, who is asked to talk about the experience under study. The second process calls for *extraction-synthesis* during which the descriptions are moved out of the participant's language into the language of science, a higher level of abstraction. The six steps in her extraction-synthesis process include the following:

a. Constructing a story that captures core ideas about the phenomenon from each person's dialogue.

b. Extracting and synthesizing *essences* from participants' descriptions. Essences are succinct expressions of the core ideas about the phenomenon.

c. Synthesizing and extracting essences as conceptualized in the researcher's language at a higher level of abstraction.

d. Formulating the language art from each participant's essences. A proposition is a nondirectional statement conceptualized by joining core ideas of the essences that arise from the participant's description in the researcher's language.

e. Extracting and synthesizing *core concepts* from the language art of all participants. Core concepts are ideas that capture the central meaning of the propositions.

f. Synthesizing a *structure* of the living experience from the core concepts. A structure involves a conceptualization in which the researcher joins the core concepts.

Heuristic interpretation, the third and final process, entails structural transposition, conceptual integration, metaphorical emergings, and artistic expression. By means of structural transposition, the structure of the description of the experience is moved to a higher level of abstraction. The structure of the experience is connected with the concepts of Parse's Humanbecoming Paradigm through conceptual integration. Metaphorical emergings entail identifying metaphors in the participants' descriptions that help illuminate the meaning of their experiences. Lastly, in artistic expression, the researchers' own choice of an artform is used to embody their transfiguring moments.

Example of Parse's Phenomenologic Method: Condon (2014) used Parse's method to investigate the lived experience of feeling overwhelmed. Participants in the study were adults from a general population. Descriptions were arrived at through dialogic engagement.

GROUNDED THEORY

Grounded theory, an important method for the study of nursing phenomena, has contributed to the development of many middle-range nursing theories. Grounded theory was formulated in the 1960s as a systematic method of qualitative inquiry by two sociologists, Glaser and Strauss (1967). An early grounded theory study (Glaser & Strauss, 1965) focused on dying in hospitals.

Grounded theory tries to account for actions in a substantive area from the perspective of those involved. Grounded theory researchers seek to understand actions by focusing on the main concern or problem that the individuals' behavior is designed to address (Glaser, 1998). The manner in which people resolve this main concern is called the **core variable**. One type of core variable is called a **basic social process (BSP)**. The goal of grounded theory is to discover this main concern and the basic social process that explains how people continually resolve it. The main concern must be discovered from the data.

Conceptualization is a key aspect of grounded theory (Glaser, 2003). Grounded theory researchers generate emergent conceptual categories and their properties and integrate them into a substantive theory grounded in the data. Through this conceptual process, the generated grounded theory represents an abstraction based on participants' actions and their meanings. The grounded theorist uncovers and names latent patterns (categories) from the participants' accounts. Glaser (2003) emphasized

that concepts transcend time, place, and person. "In grounded theory, behavior is a pattern that a person engages in; it is not the person. People are not categorized, behavior is" (p. 53).

Grounded theory methods constitute an entire approach to the conduct of field research. For example, a study that follows Glaser and Strauss's method does not begin with a focused research problem; the problem emerges from the data. In a grounded theory study, both the research problem and the process used to resolve it are discovered.

A fundamental feature of grounded theory research is that data collection, data analysis, and sampling of participants occur simultaneously. The grounded theory process is recursive: Researchers collect data, categorize them, describe the emerging central phenomenon, and then recycle earlier steps. In-depth interviews and observation are the most common data sources in grounded theory studies, but other data sources such as documents may also be used.

A procedure called **constant comparison** is used to develop and refine theoretically relevant categories. Categories elicited from the data are constantly compared with data obtained earlier so that commonalities and variations can be determined. As data collection proceeds, the inquiry becomes increasingly focused on emerging theoretical concerns. Data analysis in a grounded theory framework is described in greater depth in Chapter 24.

Example of a Grounded Theory Study: Morse and co-researchers (2014) used grounded theory methods to explicate the emotional experiences of women undergoing breast cancer diagnosis and were awaiting the results of breast biopsy. The basic social psychological process, preserving self, is the outcome of enduring. The study was the basis for developing a middle-range theory: Awaiting Diagnosis: Enduring for Preserving Self.

Like most theories, a grounded theory is modifiable as the researcher (or other researchers) collect new data. Modification is an ongoing process and is the method by which theoretical completeness is enhanced (Glaser, 2001). As more data are found and more qualitative studies are published in the substantive area, the grounded theory can be modified to accommodate new or different dimensions.

Example of a Modification of a Grounded Theory Study: Beck (2012) modified her 1993 grounded theory study, "Teetering on the Edge," which was a substantive theory of postpartum depression. After Beck's original study had been conducted, 27 additional qualitative studies of postpartum depression in women from other cultures had been published. The results from these 27 transcultural studies were compared with the findings from the original grounded theory. Maximizing differences among comparative groups is a powerful method for enhancing theoretical properties and extending the theory.

TIP: Glaser and Strauss (1967) distinguished two types of grounded theory: substantive and formal. **Substantive theory** is grounded in data on a specific substantive area, such as postpartum depression. It can serve as a springboard for **formal grounded theory**, which is at a higher level of conceptualization and is abstract of time, place, and persons. The goal of formal grounded theory is not to discover a new core variable but to develop a theory that goes beyond the substantive grounded theory and extends the general implications of the core variable. Kearney (1998) likened formal grounded theory to ready-to-wear clothing, in contrast to substantive grounded theory which is personally tailored.

Alternate Views of Grounded Theory

In 1990, Strauss and Corbin published what was to become a controversial book, *Basics of Qualitative Research: Grounded Theory Procedures and Techniques*. The authors stated that the book's purpose was to provide beginning grounded theory researchers with basic procedures for building theory at the substantive level.

Glaser, however, disagreed with some of the procedures advocated by Strauss (his original co-author) and Corbin (a nurse researcher). Glaser published a rebuttal in 1992, *Emergence versus Forcing: Basics of Grounded Theory Analysis*. Glaser believed that Strauss and Corbin developed a method that is not grounded theory but rather what he called "full conceptual description." According

to Glaser, the purpose of grounded theory is to generate concepts and theories about their relationships that explain, account for, and interpret variation in behavior in the substantive area under study. *Conceptual description*, in contrast, is aimed at describing the full range of behavior of what is occurring in the substantive area, "irrespective of relevance and accounting for variation in behavior" (Glaser, 1992, p. 19). In their latest edition, Corbin and Strauss (2015) stated that their method reflects Strauss's approach to doing grounded theory which is based on the philosophies of pragmatism and interactionism.

Nurse researchers have conducted grounded theory studies using both the original Glaser and Strauss's and the Strauss and Corbin's approaches. Heath and Cowley (2004) provide a comparison of the two approaches. We describe differences between the two in greater detail in Chapter 24.

Example of Strauss and Corbin's Grounded Theory Methods: In their study of older adults' experiences of pain associated with leg ulceration, Taverner and colleagues (2014) used Corbin and Strauss's grounded theory approach. The emergent grounded theory centered on a core category that the researcher named "The journey to chronic pain."

Constructivist Grounded Theory

Strauss and Glaser had different training and backgrounds. Strauss, trained at the University of Chicago, had a background in symbolic interactionism and pragmatist philosophy. Glaser, by contrast, came from a tradition of positivism and quantitative methods at Columbia University. In one of Glaser's (2005) later publications, in which he discussed the takeover of grounded theory by symbolic interaction, he argued that "grounded theory is a general inductive method possessed by no discipline or theoretical perspective or data type" (p. 141).

In recent years, an approach called **constructivist grounded theory** has emerged. A leading advocate is sociologist Kathy Charmaz, who has sought to bring the Chicago School antecedents of grounded theory into the forefront again. She has called for returning to the pragmatist foundation which "assumes that interaction is inherently dynamic and interpretive and addresses how people create, enact, and change meanings and actions" (Charmaz, 2014, p. 9). Charmaz views Glaser and Strauss's (and Strauss and Corbin's) versions of grounded theory as being based in the positivist tradition. Her position is that what is missing from their objective grounded theory method is the researcher's influence on the data collected and analyzed and interactions between the researcher and participants.

Charmaz uses the term *constructivist* "to acknowledge subjectivity and the researcher's involvement in the construction and interpretation of data" (2014, p. 14). In her approach, the developed grounded theory is seen as an interpretation. The data collected and analyzed are acknowledged to be constructed from shared experiences and relationships between the researcher and the participants. Charmaz's view is that "we start with the assumption that social reality is multiple, processual, and constructed, then we must take the researcher's position, privileges, perspective, and interactions into account as an inherent part of the research reality" (2014, p. 13). Reflexivity of both the researcher's own interpretations and the interpretations of the participants is important. Data and analyses are viewed as social constructions. Higginbottom and Lauridsen (2014) have described how Charmaz's approach is similar to and different from original grounded theory.

Example of a Constructivist Grounded Theory: MacDonald and co-researchers (2014) used constructivist grounded theory methods to explore current patient involvement in medication administration safety, from the perspective of both patients and nurses. The researchers wanted to understand factors that foster or impede the voice of the patient.

⮊ **TIP:** Beginning qualitative researchers should be aware that a grounded theory study is a much lengthier and more complex process than a phenomenologic study. This may be an important consideration if there are constraints in the amount of time you can devote to a study.

OTHER TYPES OF QUALITATIVE RESEARCH

Qualitative studies often can be characterized in terms of the disciplinary research traditions discussed in the previous section. However, several other important types of qualitative research also deserve mention. This section discusses qualitative research that is not associated with any particular discipline.

Case Studies

Case studies are in-depth investigations of a single entity (or small number of entities), which could be an individual, family, institution, community, or other social unit. In a case study, researchers obtain a wealth of descriptive information and may examine relationships among different phenomena, or may examine trends over time. Case study researchers attempt to analyze and understand issues that are important to the history, development, or circumstances of the entity under study.

One way to think of a case study is to consider what is at center stage. In most studies, whether qualitative or quantitative, a certain phenomenon or variable (or set of variables) is the core of the inquiry. In a case study, the *case* itself is central. As befits an intensive analysis, the focus of case studies is typically on understanding *why* an individual thinks, behaves, or develops in a particular manner rather than on *what* his or her status, progress, or actions are. It is not unusual for probing research of this type to require detailed study over a considerable period. Data are often collected that relate not only to the person's present state but also to past experiences and situational factors relevant to the problem being examined.

Yin (2014) has described four basic types of designs for case studies: single-case, holistic; single-case, embedded; multiple-case, holistic; and multiple-case, embedded. A **single-case study** is an appropriate design when (1) it is a critical case in testing a well-formulated theory, (2) it represents an extreme or unique case, (3) it is a representative or typical case, (4) it is a revelatory case, and (5) it is a longitudinal case. A **multiple-case design** is a study that involves more than a single case. Single and multiple case studies can be either holistic or embedded. In a **holistic design**, the global nature of a case—be it an individual, community, or organization—is examined. An **embedded design** involves multiple units of analysis. A wide variety of data can be used in case studies, including data from interviews, observations, documents, and artifacts.

A distinction is sometimes drawn between an intrinsic and instrumental case study (Stake, 1995). In an *intrinsic case study*, researchers do not have to select the case. For instance, an evaluation of the process of implementing an innovation is often a case study of a particular institution; the "case" is a given. In an *instrumental case study*, researchers begin with a research question or problem and seek out a case that offers illumination. The aim of such a case study is to use the case to understand a phenomenon of interest. In such a situation, a case is usually selected not because it is typical but rather because it can maximize what can be learned about the phenomenon.

Although understanding a particular case is the central concern of case studies, they are sometimes a useful way to explore phenomena that have not been rigorously researched. The information obtained in case studies can be used to develop hypotheses to be tested more rigorously in subsequent research. The intensive probing that characterizes case studies often leads to insights concerning previously unsuspected relationships. Furthermore, case studies may serve the important role of clarifying concepts or of elucidating ways to capture them.

⊃ TIP: Case study research is not a distinct methodology (Sandelowski, 2011). Many ethnographies focus on a specific "case," as do many historical studies. Although case studies typically involve the collection of in-depth qualitative information, some case studies are quantitative and use statistical methods to analyze data. And some case studies used mixed methods (i.e., both qualitative and quantitative approaches).

The greatest strength of case studies is the depth that is possible when a limited number of individuals, institutions, or groups is being investigated.

Case studies provide researchers with opportunities of having an intimate knowledge of a person's condition, thoughts, actions (past and present), intentions, and environment. On the other hand, this same strength is a potential weakness because researchers' familiarity with the person or group may make objectivity more difficult. Perhaps the biggest concern about case studies is generalizability: If researchers discover important relationships, it is difficult to know whether the same relationships would occur with others. However, case studies can often play a critical role in challenging generalizations based on other types of research.

It is important to recognize that case study *research* is not simply anecdotal descriptions of a particular incident or patient, such as a case report. Case study research is a disciplined process and typically requires a long period of data collection. Excellent resources for further reading on case studies are the writings of Yin (2014), Stake (2005), and Flyvbjerg (2011).

Example of a Case Study: McKenna and colleagues (2014) conducted a case study with the aim of providing a rich description of service delivery in a secure inpatient mental health service in Australia. Data were gathered by interviewing several stakeholder groups, and discrepancies in the perceptions of stakeholders were examined.

Narrative Analyses

Narrative analysis focuses on *story* as the object of inquiry to examine how individuals make sense of events in their lives. Narratives are viewed as a type of "cultural envelope" into which people pour their experiences (Riessman, 1991). What distinguishes narrative analysis from other types of qualitative research designs is its focus on the broad contours of a narrative; stories are not fractured and dissected. The broad underlying premise of narrative research is that people most effectively make sense of their world—and communicate these meanings—by constructing, reconstructing, and narrating stories. Individuals construct stories when they wish to understand specific events and situations that require linking an inner world of desire and motive to an external world of observable actions. Narrative analysts explore *form* as well as content, asking, "Why was the story told that way?" (Riessman, 2008).

A number of approaches can be used to analyze stories. The choice depends on the fit between the structural approach and the types of narrative to be analyzed. One popular approach is that of Labov and Waletzky (1967), who view narratives as a social phenomenon. Their structural approach proposes that a complete narrative consists of the following six components: the abstract (summary), orientation (time, place, individuals), complicating action (sequence of events), evaluation (significance of the action), result or resolution (what occurred at the end), and coda (perspective returned back to the present). As a social phenomenon, narratives vary by social context (hospital, home, and so on), and evaluative data extracted from the narratives vary by the social context in which they were collected.

Example of a Narrative Analysis, Labov and Waletzky's Approach: P. Montgomery and colleagues (2009) conducted a narrative analysis of "my husband" stories narrated by women with postpartum depression. They used a modified Labov-Waletzky approach in their analysis of interview data from 27 Canadian women.

Burke's (1969) **pentadic dramatism** is another approach to narrative analysis. For Burke, there are five key elements of a story: act, scene, agent, agency, and purpose. Analysis of a story "will offer some kind of answers to these five questions: what was done (act), when or where it was done (scene), who did it (agent), how he did it (agency), and why (purpose)" (p. xv). The five terms of Burke's pentad are meant to be understood paired together as ratios such as act: agent, act: scene, agent: agency, and purpose: agent. The analysis focuses on the internal relationships and tensions of these five terms to each other. Each pairing in the pentad provides a different way of directing the researcher's attention. What drives the narrative analysis is not just the interaction of the pentadic terms but an imbalance between two or more terms. Bruner (1991) modified Burke's pentad with the addition of a sixth term that he called Trouble with a capital T. Bruner included this sixth element to provide more focus in narrative analysis on Burke's imbalance between the terms in his pentad.

Example of a Narrative Analysis, Burke's Approach: Tobin, Murphy-Lawless, and Beck (an author of this textbook) (2014) conducted a narrative analysis of asylum-seeking women's experience of childbirth in Ireland. Twenty-two mothers participated in unstructured interviews lasting from 40 minutes to 1½ hours. Burke's pentad of terms was used to analyze these narratives and revealed numerous accounts of scene/agent and act/agency imbalances in the women's experiences. Their narratives highlighted the lack of communication, connection, and culturally competent care.

Another approach is that of Riessman (1993, 2008), whose method of thematic narrative analysis involves protecting each story as a whole and not fragmenting them. Each story is analyzed separately for themes. Then all the stories are compared to identify common themes for a *mega story*. Specific stories can be chosen by the researcher to illustrate common themes. The narrative analyst remains focused on the content of the stories rather than how or why the stories are told. Riessman (1993) represented five levels of experience in the research process for narrative analysts:

1. Attending: Participants create personal meaning by actively thinking about reality in new ways. Participants reflect and remember their experiences; they compose their own realities.
2. Telling: Participants "re-present" the events of an experience. They share the event by recounting characters, significant events, and their interpretation of the experience. The interviewer takes part in the narrative by listening to the story and asking questions (to clarify/further understand the story). As participants tell their story, they are also creating a vision of themselves.
3. Transcribing: Participants' stories are typically captured through video or audio recording. The analyst then creates a written narrative text representing the conversation.
4. Analyzing: The researcher analyzes each individual transcript. Similarities are noted, and a "mega story" is created by defining critical

moments within narratives and making meaning out of each story. The analyst also makes decisions about form, order, and style of presentation of the narratives.

5. Reading: The final level of experience in the research process is reading. Drafts are commonly shared with colleagues. The researcher frequently incorporates this editorial feedback into a final report that reflects the researcher's interpretation of the narrative.

Example of a Narrative Analysis, Riessman's Approach: McKelvey (2014) used Riessman's method of narrative analysis in her study of the postpartum experiences of nonbirth lesbian mothers. The study involved the analysis of 10 mothers' narratives describing their unique stories of their first year of motherhood.

Descriptive Qualitative Studies

Many qualitative researchers acknowledge a link to one of the research traditions discussed in this chapter. Many other qualitative studies, however, claim no particular disciplinary or methodologic roots. The researchers may simply indicate that they have conducted a qualitative study or a naturalistic inquiry, or they may say that they have done a *content analysis* of their qualitative data (i.e., an analysis of themes and patterns that emerge in the narrative content). We refer to the many qualitative studies that do not have a formal name as **descriptive qualitative studies**.

Sandelowski (2000), in a widely read article, noted that in doing such descriptive qualitative studies, researchers tend not to penetrate their data in any interpretive depth. These studies present comprehensive summaries of a phenomenon or of events. Qualitative descriptive designs tend to be eclectic and they often borrow or adapt methodologic techniques from other qualitative traditions, such as constant comparison.

In a more recent article, Sandelowski (2010) warned researchers not to call their studies *qualitative description* "after the fact to give a name to poorly conceived and conducted studies" (p. 80). She noted that qualitative descriptive studies produce findings closer to the data ("data-near") than

studies within such traditions as phenomenology or grounded theory, but that good qualitative descriptions are still interpretive products. She recognized that her article published in 2000 had provided justification for studies that primarily reproduce raw data, and stated that she "never intended to communicate . . . that qualitative description removes the researcher's obligation to do any analyzing or interpreting at all" (p. 79). Rather than being a distinct methodologic classification, qualitative description is perhaps viewed as a "distributed residual category" (p. 82) that signals a "confederacy" of diverse groups of qualitative researchers.

TIP: In their study of international differences in nursing research, Polit and Beck (2009) analyzed data from about 450 qualitative studies published in eight nursing journals over a 2-year period. More than half were descriptive, without naming a specific tradition. The tradition with the highest representation was phenomenologic, accounting for 20% of the qualitative studies.

Example of a Descriptive Qualitative Study: Beacham and Deatrick (2015) undertook a descriptive qualitative study to describe the perspectives of children with chronic health conditions—how they perceived their condition, its management, and its implications for their future.

Sally Thorne (2008) recently expanded qualitative description into a realm she called **interpretive description**. Her book outlined an approach that extends "beyond mere description and into the domain of the 'so what' that drives all applied disciplines" (p. 33) such as nursing. While acknowledging that her approach is neither novel nor distinctive, Thorne noted that it emphasizes the importance of having a disciplinary conceptual frame (such as nursing): "Interpretive description becomes a conceptual maneuver whereby a solid and substantive logic derived from the disciplinary orientation justifies the application of specific techniques and procedures outside of their conventional context" (p. 35). An important thrust of her approach is that it requires integrity of purpose from an actual practice goal, and it therefore seeks to generate new insights that can help shape applications of qualitative evidence to practice.

Thorne (2013) has acknowledged that she developed interpretive description to free qualitative nurse researchers from the constraints of qualitative methodologies. She noted that "the nursing disciplinary mind never truly accepts standardization; it always seeks to ensure that there is room for necessary variation" (p. 296). Interpretive description holds no attachment to any one qualitative method but rather it uses the wealth of research techniques available. Thorne offered examples of typical research questions for interpretive description, such as, "What are the common ways in which patients' experience . . .?" (p. 298).

Example of an Interpretive Descriptive Study: McArthur and colleagues (2014) conducted an interpretive descriptive study to identify enablers and barriers influencing middle-aged women's adherence to regular exercise.

RESEARCH WITH IDEOLOGIC PERSPECTIVES

Some qualitative researchers conduct inquiries within an ideologic framework typically to draw attention to social problems or the needs of certain groups and to effect change. These approaches, which are sometimes described as being within a **transformative paradigm** (Mertens, 2007), represent important investigative avenues and are briefly described in this section.

Critical Theory

Critical theory originated with a group of Marxist-oriented German scholars in the 1920s, referred to as the Frankfurt School. Essentially, a critical researcher is concerned with a critique of society and with envisioning new possibilities.

Critical social science is typically action-oriented. Its broad aim is to integrate theory and practice such that people become aware of contradictions and disparities in their beliefs and social practices and

become inspired to change them. Critical researchers reject the idea of an objective and disinterested inquirer and are oriented toward a transformation process. An important feature of critical theory is that it calls for inquiries that foster enlightened self-knowledge and sociopolitical action. Critical theory also involves a self-reflective aspect. To prevent a critical theory of society from becoming yet another self-serving ideology, critical theorists must account for their own transformative effects.

The design of critical research often begins with a thorough analysis of aspects of the problem. For example, critical researchers might analyze and critique taken-for-granted assumptions that underlie the problem, the language used to depict the situation, or the biases of prior researchers studying the problem. Critical researchers often triangulate multiple methodologies and emphasize multiple perspectives (e.g., alternative racial or social class perspectives) on problems. They typically interact with study participants in ways that emphasize participants' expertise. Some of the features that distinguish more traditional qualitative research and critical research are summarized in Table 21.2.

Critical theory has been applied in a number of disciplines and has played an especially important role in ethnography. **Critical ethnography** focuses on raising consciousness and aiding emancipatory goals in the hope of effecting social change. Critical ethnographers address the historical, social, political, and economic dimensions of cultures and their value-laden agendas. An assumption in critical ethnographic research is that actions and thoughts are mediated by power relationships (Hammersley, 1992). Critical ethnographers attempt to increase the political dimensions of cultural research and undermine oppressive systems—there is an explicit political purpose. Cook (2005) has argued that critical ethnography is especially well suited to health promotion research because both are concerned with enabling people to take control of their own situation.

Carspecken (1996) developed a five-stage approach to critical ethnography that has been found useful in nursing studies (e.g., Hardcastle et al., 2006) and in health promotion research. Madison (2012) also provides guidance about critical theory methodology.

TABLE 21.2 • Comparison of Traditional Qualitative Research and Critical Research

ISSUE	TRADITIONAL QUALITATIVE RESEARCH	CRITICAL RESEARCH
Research aims	Understanding; reconstruction of multiple constructions	Critique; transformation; consciousness raising; advocacy
View of knowledge	Transactional/subjective; knowledge is created in interaction between investigator and participants	Transactional/subjective; value-mediated and value-dependent; importance of historical insights
Methods	Dialectic: truth is arrived at logically through conversations	Dialectic and didactic: dialogue designed to transform naivety and misinformation
Evaluative criteria for inquiry quality	Authenticity; trustworthiness	Historical situatedness of the inquiry; erosion of ignorance; stimulus for change
Researcher's role	Facilitator of multivoice reconstruction	Transformative agent; advocate; activist

Example of a Critical Ethnography: Baumbusch and Phinney (2014) conducted a critical ethnography of highly *involved* families with family members in long-term residential care. The study took place over a 2-year period in two Canadian facilities. The main themes were "Hands On," "Hands Off," "Surveillance," and "Interlopers."

Feminist Research

Feminist research is similar to critical theory research, but the focus is on gender domination and discrimination within patriarchal societies. Like critical researchers, feminist researchers seek to establish collaborative and nonexploitative relationships with their informants, to place themselves within the study to avoid objectification, and to conduct research that is transformative.

Gender is the organizing construct in feminist research, and investigators seek to understand how gender and a gendered social order have shaped women's lives and their consciousness. The aim is to ameliorate the "invisibility and distortion of female experience in ways relevant to ending women's unequal social position" (Lather, 1991, p. 71).

Although feminist researchers agree on the importance of focusing on women's diverse situations and the relationships that frame those situations, there are many variants of feminist inquiry. Three broad models (within each of which there is diversity) have been identified: (1) *feminist empiricism*, whose adherents usually work within fairly standard norms of qualitative inquiry but who seek to portray more accurate pictures of the social realities of women's lives; (2) *feminist standpoint research*, which holds that inquiry ought to begin in and be tested against the lived everyday sociopolitical experiences of women and that women's views are particular and privileged; and (3) *feminist postmodernism*, which stresses that "truth" is a destructive illusion and views the world as endless stories, texts, and narratives. In nursing and health care, feminist empiricism and feminist standpoint research have been most prevalent.

The scope of feminist research ranges from studies of the subjective views of individual women to studies of social movements, structures, and broad policies that affect (and often exclude) women. Olesen (2000), a sociologist who studied nurses' career patterns and definitions of success, has noted that some of the best feminist research on women's subjective experiences has been done in the area of women's health.

Feminist research methods typically include in-depth, interactive, and collaborative individual or group interviews that offer the possibility of reciprocally educational encounters. Feminists usually seek to negotiate the meanings of the results with those participating in the study and to be self-reflective about what they themselves are experiencing and learning.

Feminist research, like other research that has an ideologic perspective, has raised the bar for the conduct of ethical research. With the emphasis on trust, empathy, and nonexploitative relationships, proponents of these newer modes of inquiry view any type of deception or manipulation as abhorrent. Those interested in feminist methodologies may wish to consult the writings of Hesse-Biber (2014) or Brisolara et al. (2014).

Example of Feminist Research: Using feminist methods and theory in a narrative analysis, E. Montgomery and colleagues (2015) studied the maternity care experiences of women who had been sexually abused during their childhood.

Participatory Action Research

A type of research known as participatory action research is closely allied to both critical research and feminist research. **Participatory action research** (PAR), one of several types of *action research* that originated in the 1940s with social psychologist Kurt Lewin, is based on a recognition that the production of knowledge can be political and can be used to exert power. Action researchers typically work with groups or communities that are vulnerable to the control or oppression of a dominant group or culture.

Participatory action research is, as the name implies, participatory. Researchers and study participants collaborate in defining the problem, selecting research methods, analyzing the data, and deciding on the use to which findings are put. The aim of PAR is to produce not only knowledge but also action and consciousness raising as well. Researchers seek to empower people through the process of constructing and using knowledge. The PAR tradition has as its starting point a concern for the powerlessness of the group under study. Thus, a key objective is to produce an impetus that is directly used to make improvements through education and sociopolitical action.

In PAR, research methods take second place to emergent processes of collaboration and dialogue that can motivate, increase self-esteem, and generate community solidarity. "Data-gathering" strategies are not only the traditional methods of interview and observation (including both qualitative and quantitative approaches) but may include storytelling, sociodrama, drawing and painting, plays and skits, and other activities designed to encourage people to find creative ways to explore their lives, tell their stories, and recognize their own strengths. Koch and Kralik (2006) offer a useful resource for learning more about PAR.

Example of Participatory Action Research: Sherwood and Kendall (2013) conducted a PAR project that focused on the well-being of Aboriginal women in prison in Australia. The researchers used PAR because they sought to adopt a "decolonising research methodology inclusive of enduring community and stakeholder dialogue and consultation" (p. 83).

CRITIQUING QUALITATIVE DESIGNS

Evaluating a qualitative design is often difficult. Qualitative researchers do not always document design decisions and are even less likely to describe the process by which such decisions were made. Researchers often do, however, indicate whether the study was conducted within a specific qualitative tradition, and this information can be used to come to some conclusions. For example, if a report indicated that the researcher conducted 2 months of fieldwork for an ethnographic study, there would be reason to suspect that insufficient time had been spent in the field to obtain an emic perspective of

BOX 21.1 Guidelines for Critiquing Qualitative Designs

1. Was a research tradition for the qualitative study identified? If none was identified, can one be inferred? If more than one was identified, is this justifiable or does it suggest "method slurring"?
2. Is the research question congruent with a qualitative approach and with the specific research tradition (i.e., is the domain of inquiry for the study congruent with the domain encompassed by the tradition)? Are the data sources, research methods, and analytic approach congruent with the research tradition?
3. How well was the research design described? Were design decisions explained and justified? Does it appear that the researcher made all design decisions up-front, or did the design emerge during data collection, allowing researchers to capitalize on early information?
4. Is the design appropriate, given the research question? Does the design lend itself to a thorough, in-depth, intensive examination of the phenomenon of interest? What design elements might have strengthened the study (e.g., a longitudinal perspective rather than a cross-sectional one)?
5. Did the researcher spend a sufficient amount of time doing fieldwork or collecting the research data?
6. Was there evidence of reflexivity in the design?
7. Was the study undertaken with an ideologic perspective? If so, is there evidence that ideologic methods and goals were achieved (e.g., Was there evidence of full collaboration between researchers and participants? Did the research have the power to be transformative, or is there evidence that a transformative process occurred?)?

the culture under study. Ethnographic studies may also be critiqued if their only source of information was from interviews rather than from a broader range of data sources, particularly observations.

In a grounded theory study, look for evidence about when the data were collected and analyzed. If all the data were collected before analysis, you might question whether constant comparison was used correctly. Glaser and Strauss (1967) offered four properties on which a grounded theory should be evaluated: fitness, understanding, generality, and control. The theory should fit the substantive area for which the data were collected. A grounded theory should increase the understanding of persons working in that substantive area. Also, the categories in the grounded theory should be abstract enough to allow the theory to be a general guide to changing situations—but not so abstract to decrease their sensitizing features. Lastly, the substantive theory must allow individuals who apply it to have some control in daily situations.

In critiquing a phenomenologic study, you should first determine if the study is descriptive or interpretive. This will help you to assess how closely the researcher kept to the basic tenets of that qualitative research tradition. For example, in a descriptive phenomenologic study, did the researcher bracket? When critiquing phenomenologic studies, in addition to critiquing the methodology, you should also look at the power of the studies to show and present the meaning of the phenomena being studied. Van Manen (1997) called for phenomenologic researchers to address five textual features in their reports: lived thoroughness (placing the phenomenon concretely in the lifeworld), evocation (phenomenon is vividly brought into presence), intensification (give key phrases their full value), tone (let the text speak to the reader), and epiphany (sudden grasp of the meaning).

The guidelines in Box 21.1 are designed to assist you in critiquing the designs of qualitative studies.

RESEARCH EXAMPLES

Nurse researchers have conducted studies in all of the qualitative research traditions described in this chapter, and several actual examples have been cited. In the following sections, we present more detailed descriptions of three qualitative nursing studies.

Research Example of an Ethnography

Study: The need to nurse the nurse: Emotional labor in neonatal intensive care (Cricco-Lizza, 2014)

Statement of Purpose: The purpose of this study was to describe the emotional labor and coping strategies of nurses working in a neonatal intensive care unit (NICU). *Emotional labor* is the labor in which a person suppresses his or her own feelings and maintains an outward appearance that can enhance a good frame of mind and a sense of safety in others. Earlier research had found that NICU nurses play key roles in mitigating parental distress, but "it is not known how nurses navigate the emotional labor of their everyday work" (p. 615).

Setting: The research was conducted in a level-4 NICU in a children's hospital in the northeastern United States.

Method: An ethnographic approach was used, with field-work conducted over a 14-month period. From the NICU staff, 114 participated as general informants who provided a "wide-angle picture of their everyday practices, emotions and coping strategies" (p. 616). More detailed information was obtained from 18 key informants. Cricco-Lizza also engaged in prolonged immersion in the NICU during 14 months of participant observation. Fieldwork, conducted in 1- to 2-hour sessions on varying days and shifts, involved observing nurses' behaviors during interactions with babies, families, nurses, and other staff throughout the course of activities in the unit. Cricco-Lizza observed and informally interviewed the general informants an average of 3.5 times each, and she recorded detailed field notes immediately after each session. Formal 1-hour interviews with the key informants were tape recorded and then transcribed. In these interviews, the researcher asked the nurses open-ended questions about their work and their feelings about their role as a NICU nurse.

Key Findings: Cricco-Lizza found that the emotional labor of nurses was "underrecognized in the day-to-day care in the NICU. Emotional labor was hidden behind the calm, capable deportment of the nurses and was a tacit part of the NICU culture" (p. 617). The nurses' emotional labor was not recognized, supported, or rewarded. The author described how her findings could contribute to the development of interventions to "nurse the nurse."

Research Example of a Phenomenologic Study

Study: Subsequent pregnancy after having a baby who was hospitalized in the NICU (Funaba et al., 2014)

Statement of Purpose: The purpose of this descriptive phenomenologic study was to understand the experiences of mothers who had a baby hospitalized in the NICU and then subsequently decided to have another pregnancy.

Sample: Study participants were recruited from a sample of 159 Japanese women who had previously participated in a study of mothers who had a child admitted to the NICU. Thirteen of these women had a subsequent child, and of these 12 agreed to participate in the new study.

Method: Data were collected 18 months to 6 years after the birth of the subsequent child. Mothers were interviewed in 1-hour semistructured interviews on at least two occasions. Five of the mothers were interviewed three or four times because "more time was needed to confirm the meaning of the mothers' words" (p. 307). The interviews were conducted either in the mothers' homes or in a private room at the researchers' university, whichever was most convenient for the mothers. The interview began with the question, "Tell me your experience of how you decided on a subsequent pregnancy after your child was hospitalized in the NICU." All interviews were audio recorded and transcribed. The data were analyzed using a descriptive phenomenologic method developed by Colaizzi, which we describe in Chapter 24.

Key Findings: The data analysis revealed five themes: (1) delaying pregnancy, (2) unwavering view about having subsequent children, (3) changing values regarding pregnancy and childbirth, (4) relief of anxiety and fear about repeated hospitalization in the NICU, and (5) preparedness to accept the outcome of pregnancy. The researchers noted that their findings have implications for family-centered care.

Research Example of a Grounded Theory Study

Study: Preserving the self: The process of decision making about hereditary breast cancer and ovarian cancer risk reduction (Howard et al., 2011)

Statement of Purpose: The purpose of the study was to understand how women make decisions about strategies to reduce the risk of hereditary breast and ovarian cancer (HBOC), such as cancer screening and risk-reducing surgeries.

Method: The researchers used a constructivist grounded theory approach to understanding women's decision-making processes. Participants were recruited through a hereditary cancer program. Women were eligible for the study if they were older than 18 and tested positive for *BRCA1/2* mutations in genetic testing. The researchers initially invited all eligible women to participate, but as the study progressed, they used preliminary findings to recruit women who might best refine conceptualizations. Data saturation was achieved with a total of 22 participants. In-depth interviews, lasting 45 to 90 minutes, were audiotaped and subsequently transcribed for analysis. Early interviews covered broad questions about decision making and changes in decisions over time. Later in the study, the questions became more focused to explore certain issues in greater depth and to verify emerging findings. Four women, whose decision experiences varied, were interviewed for a second time to obtain clarification and feedback about preliminary findings. The analysis of the data was guided by theories of relational autonomy and gender: "Using gender as an analytic tool helped us explore the role of femininity in decision making in the context of HBOC . . . It also enabled us to examine the influence of gendered roles in relation to family, friends, and health professionals on HBOC decision making" (p. 505).

Key Findings: The main concern in this study was making a decision about risk-reducing strategies, and the analysis suggested that the overarching decision-making process entailed *preserving the self*. The process was shaped by various contextual conditions, including characteristics of health services, gendered roles, the nature of the risk-reducing strategies to be considered, and the women's perceptions of their proximity to cancer. These contextual conditions contributed to different decision-making approaches and five distinct decision-making styles: "snap" decision making, intuitive decision making, deliberate decision making, deferred decision making, and "if-then" decision making. The researchers concluded that the findings provide insights that could inform the provision of decisional support to *BRCA1/2* carriers.

SUMMARY POINTS

- Qualitative research involves an **emergent design**—a design that emerges in the field as the study unfolds. Although qualitative design is flexible, qualitative researchers plan for broad contingencies that pose decision opportunities for study design in the field.
- As *bricoleurs*, qualitative researchers tend to be creative and intuitive, putting together an array of data drawn from many sources to develop a holistic understanding of a phenomenon.
- Qualitative research traditions have their roots in anthropology (e.g., **ethnography** and **ethnoscience**), philosophy (**phenomenology** and **hermeneutics**), psychology (**etiology** and **ecologic** psychology), sociology (**grounded theory**, **ethnomethodology**, and **semiotics**), sociolinguistics (**discourse analysis**), and history (**historical research**).
- Ethnography focuses on the culture of a group of people and relies on extensive fieldwork that usually includes **participant observation** and in-depth interviews with **key informants**. Ethnographers strive to acquire an **emic** (insider's) perspective of a culture rather than an **etic** (outsider's) perspective.
- Ethnographers use the concept of **researcher as instrument** to describe the researcher's significant role in analyzing and interpreting a culture. The product of ethnographic research is typically a holistic written description of the culture, but sometimes the products are **performance ethnographies** (interpretive scripts that can be performed).
- Nurses sometimes refer to their ethnographic studies as **ethnonursing research**. Other types of ethnographic work include **institutional ethnographies** (which focus on the organization of professional services from the perspective of the frontline workers or clients) and **autoethnographies** or *insider research* (which focus on the group or culture to which the researcher belongs).

- Phenomenology seeks to discover the *essence* and *meaning* of a phenomenon as it is experienced by people, mainly through in-depth interviews with people who have had the relevant experience.

- In **descriptive phenomenology,** which seeks to describe lived experiences, researchers strive to **bracket** out preconceived views and to **intuit** the essence of the phenomenon by remaining open to meanings attributed to it by those who have experienced it. **Interpretive phenomenology (hermeneutics)** focuses on interpreting the meaning of experiences rather than just describing them. In an approach called **interpretive phenomenologic analysis (IPA)**, researchers focus on people's subjective experiences (their *lifeworlds*).

- **Grounded theory** aims to discover theoretical concepts grounded in the data. Grounded theory researchers try to account for people's actions by focusing on the main concern that the behavior is designed to resolve. The manner in which people resolve this main concern is the **core variable**. The goal of grounded theory is to discover this main concern and the **basic social process (BSP)** that explains how people resolve it.

- Grounded theory uses **constant comparison**: Categories elicited from the data are constantly compared with data obtained earlier.

- A controversy among grounded theory researchers concerns whether to follow the original Glaser and Strauss's procedures or to use the adapted procedures of Strauss and Corbin; Glaser argued that the latter approach does not result in *grounded theories* but rather in *conceptual descriptions*.

- More recently, Charmaz's **constructivist grounded theory** has emerged as a method that emphasizes interpretive aspects in which the grounded theory is constructed from shared experiences and relationships between the researcher and study participants.

- **Case studies** are intensive investigations of a single entity or a small number of entities, such as individuals, groups, organizations, or communities; such studies usually involve collect-ing data over an extended period. Case study designs can be **single** or **multiple**, and **holistic** or **embedded**.

- **Narrative analysis** focuses on *story* in studies in which the purpose is to explore how people make sense of events in their lives. Several different structural approaches can be used to analyze narrative data, including, for example, Burke's **pentadic dramatism**.

- **Descriptive qualitative studies** do not fit into any disciplinary tradition. Such studies may be referred to as qualitative studies, naturalistic inquiries, or as qualitative content analyses. Qualitative description has been expanded into a realm called **interpretive description,** which emphasizes the importance of having a disciplinary conceptual frame, such as nursing.

- Research is sometimes conducted within an ideologic perspective, and such research tends to rely primarily on qualitative research.

- **Critical theory** entails a critique of existing social structures; critical researchers strive to conduct inquiries that involve collaboration with participants and foster enlightened self-knowledge and transformation. **Critical ethnography** applies the principles of critical theory to the study of cultures.

- **Feminist research**, like critical research, is designed to be transformative; the focus is on how gender domination and discrimination shape women's lives and their consciousness.

- **Participatory action research** (PAR) produces knowledge through close collaboration with groups or communities that are vulnerable to control or oppression by a dominant social group; in PAR research, methods take second place to emergent processes that can motivate people and generate community solidarity.

STUDY ACTIVITIES

Chapter 21 of the *Resource Manual for Nursing Research: Generating and Assessing Evidence for Nursing Practice, 10th edition*, offers exercises and study suggestions for reinforcing concepts presented in this chapter. In addition, the following study questions can be addressed:

1. Which of the following topics is best suited to a phenomenologic inquiry? To an ethnography? To a grounded theory study? Provide a rationale for each response.

   a. The passage through menarche among Haitian refugees
   b. The process of coping among AIDS patients
   c. The experience of having a child with leukemia
   d. Rituals relating to dying among nursing home residents
   e. The experience of waiting for service in a hospital emergency department
   f. Decision-making processes among nurses regarding do-not-resuscitate orders

2. Apply the questions in Box 21.1 to one of the three studies described at the end of the chapter, referring as necessary to the full research report for additional information. Also, do you think this study could have been undertaken with a critical or feminist perspective? Why or why not?

STUDIES CITED IN CHAPTER 21

Ahern, K. J. (1999). Ten tips for reflexive bracketing. *Qualitative Health Research*, 9, 407–411.

*Al Omari, O., & Wynaden, D. (2014). The psychosocial experience of adolescents with haematological malignancies in Jordan: An interpretive phenomenological analysis study. *Scientific World Journal*, 274036.

Baker, C., Wuest, J., & Stern, P. N. (1992). Method slurring: The grounded theory/phenomenology example. *Journal of Advanced Nursing*, 17, 1355–1360.

Baumbusch, J., & Phinney, A. (2014). Invisible hands: The role of highly involved families in long-term residential care. *Journal of Family Nursing*, 20, 73–97.

Beacham, B., & Deatrick, J. (2015). Children with chronic conditions: Perspectives on condition management. *Journal of Pediatric Nursing*, 30, 25–35.

Beck, C. T. (2012). Exemplar: Teetering on the edge: A continually emerging substantive theory of postpartum depression. In P. Munhall (Ed.), *Nursing research: A qualitative perspective* (5th ed., pp. 225–256). Sudbury, MA: Jones & Bartlett.

Brisolara, S., Seigart, S., & SenGupta, S. (Eds.). (2014). *Feminist evaluation and research: Theory and practice*. New York: Guilford Press.

Bruner, J. (1991). *Acts of meaning*. Cambridge, MA: Harvard University Press.

Burke, K. (1969). *A grammar of motives*. Berkeley, CA: University of California Press.

Carspecken, P. F. (1996). *Critical ethnography in educational research*. New York: Routledge.

Chaichanawirote, U., & Higgins, P. (2013). The complexity of older adults' social support networks. *Research in Gerontological Nursing*, 6, 275–282.

Charmaz, K. (2014). *Constructing grounded theory: A practical guide through qualitative analysis* (2nd ed.). Thousand Oaks, CA: Sage.

Cohen, M. Z., Kahn, D., & Steeves, R. (2000). *Hermeneutic phenomenological research: A practical guide for nurse researchers*. Thousand Oaks, CA: Sage.

Colaizzi, P. F. (1973). *Reflection and research in psychology*. Dubuque, IA: Kendall/Hunt.

Condon, B. B. (2014). The living experience of feeling overwhelmed: A Parse research study. *Nursing Science Quarterly*, 27, 216–225.

Cook, K. E. (2005). Using critical ethnography to explore issues in health promotion. *Qualitative Health Research*, 15(1), 129–138.

Corbin, J., & Strauss, A. (2015). *Basics of qualitative research: Techniques and procedures for developing grounded theory* (4th ed.). Thousand Oaks, CA: Sage.

Cricco-Lizza, R. (2014). The need to nurse the nurse: Emotional labor in neonatal intensive care. *Qualitative Health Research*, 24, 615–628.

Cruz, E. V., & Higginbottom, G. (2013). The use of focused ethnography in nursing research. *Nurse Researcher*, 20, 36–43.

Darcy, L., Björk, M., Enskär, K., & Knutsson, S. (2014). The process of striving for an ordinary, everyday life, in children living with cancer, at six months and one year post diagnosis. *European Journal of Oncology Nursing*, 18, 605–612.

Denzin, N. K., & Lincoln, Y. S. (Eds.). (2011). *Handbook of qualitative research* (4th ed.). Thousand Oaks, CA: Sage.

DeSouza, R. N. (2014). "This child is a planned baby": Skilled migrant fathers and reproductive decision-making. *Journal of Advanced Nursing*, 70, 2663–2672.

Ellis, C., & Bochner, A. P. (2000). Autoethnography, personal narrative, reflexivity. In N. K. Denzin & Y. S. Lincoln (Eds.), *Handbook of qualitative research* (2nd ed., pp. 733–768). Thousand Oaks, CA: Sage.

Fetterman, D. M. (2010). *Ethnography: Step by step* (3rd ed.). Thousand Oaks, CA: Sage.

Flyvbjerg, B. (2011). Case study. In N. Denzin & Y. Lincoln (Eds.), *The Sage handbook of qualitative research* (4th ed., pp. 301–316). Thousand Oaks, CA: Sage.

Funaba, Y., Yokoo, K., Ozawa, M., Fujimoto, S., Kido, Y., & Fukuhara, R. (2014). Subsequent pregnancy after having a baby who was hospitalized in the NICU. *MCN: American Journal of Maternal & Child Nursing, 39*, 306–312.

Gadamer, H. G. (1976). *Philosophical hermeneutics* (D. E. Linge, Ed. & Trans.). Berkeley, CA: University of California Press.

Gearing, R. E. (2004). Bracketing in research: A typology. *Qualitative Health Research, 14*, 1429–1452.

Giorgi, A. (1985). *Phenomenology and psychological research.* Pittsburgh, PA: Duquesne University Press.

Giorgi, A. (2005). The phenomenological movement and research in the human sciences. *Nursing Science Quarterly, 18*, 75–82.

Glaser, B. (1992). *Emergence versus forcing: Basics of grounded theory analysis.* Mill Valley, CA: Sociology Press.

Glaser, B. (1998). *Doing grounded theory: Issues and discussions.* Mill Valley, CA: Sociology Press.

Glaser, B. (2001). *The grounded theory perspective: Conceptualization contrasted with description.* Mill Valley, CA: Sociology Press.

Glaser, B. (2003). *The grounded theory perspective II: Description's remodeling of grounded theory methodology.* Mill Valley, CA: Sociology Press.

Glaser, B. (2005). *The grounded theory perspective III: Theoretical coding.* Mill Valley, CA: Sociology Press.

Glaser, B., & Strauss, A. (1965). *Awareness of dying.* Chicago: Aldine.

Glaser, B. G., & Strauss, A. (1967). *The discovery of grounded theory: Strategies for qualitative research.* New York: Aldine de Gruyter.

Hammersley, M. (1992). *What's wrong with ethnography? Methodological explorations.* London, United Kingdom: Routledge.

Hardcastle, M., Usher, K., & Holmes, C. (2006). Carspecken's five-stage critical qualitative research method: An application to nursing research. *Qualitative Health Research, 16*, 151–161.

Heath, H., & Cowley, S. (2004). Developing a grounded theory approach: A comparison of Glaser and Strauss. *International Journal of Nursing Studies, 41*, 141–150.

Heidegger, M. (1962). *Being and time.* New York: Harper & Row.

Heidegger, M. (1971). *Poetry, language, thought.* New York: Harper & Row.

Hesse-Biber, S. (Ed.). (2014). *Feminist research practice: A primer* (2nd ed.). Thousand Oaks, CA: Sage.

Higginbottom, G., & Lauridsen, E. (2014). The roots and development of constructivist grounded theory. *Nurse Researcher, 21*, 8–13.

Higginbottom, G. M., Rivers, K., & Story, R. (2014). Health and social care needs of Somali refugees with visual impairment living in the United Kingdom: A focused ethnography. *Journal of Transcultural Nursing, 25*, 192–201.

Howard, A. F., Balneaves, L., Bottorff, J., & Rodney, P. (2011). Preserving the self: The process of decision making about hereditary breast cancer and ovarian cancer risk reduction. *Qualitative Health Research, 21*, 502–519.

Hudson, S., Newman, S., Hester, W., Magwood, G., Mueller, M., & Laken, M. (2014). Factors influencing hospital admissions and emergency department visits among children with complex chronic conditions. *Issues in Comprehensive Pediatric Nursing, 37*, 61–80.

Husserl, E. (1962). *Ideas: General introduction to pure phenomenology.* New York: Macmillan.

Johnson, R. A., & Bibbo, J. (2014). Relocation decisions and constructing the meaning of home: A phenomenological study of the transition into a nursing home. *Journal of Aging Studies, 30*, 56–63.

Kearney, M. H. (1998). Ready-to-wear: Discovering grounded formal theory. *Research in Nursing & Health, 21*, 179–186.

Kirshbaum, M. N., Olson, K., Pongthavornkamol, K., & Graffigna, G. (2013). Understanding the meaning of fatigue at the end of life: An ethnoscience approach. *European Journal of Oncology Nursing, 17*, 146–153.

Koch, T., & Kralik, D. (2006). *Participatory action research in healthcare.* Chichester, United Kingdom: Wiley-Blackwell.

Labov, W., & Waletzky, J. (1967). Narrative analysis: Oral versions of personal experience. In J. Helm (Ed.), *Essays on the verbal and visual arts* (pp. 12–44). Seattle, WA: University of Washington Press.

Lather, P. (1991). *Getting smart: Feminist research and pedagogy with/in the postmodern.* New York: Routledge.

Lauterbach, S. S. (2007). Meanings in mothers' experience with infant death: Three phenomenological inquiries: In another world; five years later; and what forever means. In P. L. Munhall (Ed.), *Nursing research: A qualitative perspective* (4th ed., pp. 211–238). Sudbury, MA: Jones & Bartlett.

Leininger, M. M. (Ed.). (1985). *Qualitative research methods in nursing.* New York: Grune & Stratton.

Leininger, M. M., & McFarland, M. (2006). *Culture care diversity and universality: A worldwide nursing theory* (2nd ed.). Sudbury, MA: Jones & Bartlett.

Lincoln, Y. S., & Guba, E. G. (1985). *Naturalistic inquiry.* Newbury Park, CA: Sage.

Lloyd, P., Briggs, E., Kane, N., & Jeyarajah, A. (2014). Women's experiences after a radical trachelectomy for early stage cervical cancer: A descriptive phenomenological study. *European Journal of Oncology Nursing, 18*, 362–371.

Lobar, S. L. (2014). Family adjustment across cultural groups in autistic spectrum disorder. *Advances in Nursing Science, 37*, 174–186.

Lopez, K. A., & Willis, D. G. (2004). Descriptive versus interpretive phenomenology: Their contributions to nursing knowledge. *Qualitative Health Research, 14*, 726–735.

MacDonald, M., Heilermann, M. S., MacKinnon, N., Lang, A., Gregory, S., Gurnham, M., & Fillatre, T. (2014). Confirming delivery: Understanding the role of the hospitalized patient in medication administration safety. *Qualitative Health Research, 24*, 536–550.

Madison, D. S. (2012). *Critical ethnography: Methods, ethics, and performance* (2nd ed.). Thousand Oaks, CA: Sage.

Maxwell, J. (2012). The importance of qualitative research for causal explanation in education. *Qualitative Inquiry, 18*, 655–661.

*McArthur, D., Dumas, A., Woodend, K., Beach, S., & Stacey, D. (2014). Factors influencing adherence to regular exercise in middle-aged women: A qualitative study to inform clinical practice. *BMC Women's Health, 14*, 49.

McFarland, M. R., & Wehbe-Alamah, H. B. (2015). *Leininger's culture care and diversity and universality: A worldwide nursing theory.* Burlington, MA: Jones & Bartlett Learning.

McKelvey, M. M. (2014). The other mother: A narrative analysis of the postpartum experiences of nonbirth lesbian mothers. *Advances in Nursing Science, 37*, 101–116.

McKenna, B., Furness, T., Dhital, D., Park, M., & Connally, F. (2014). Recovery-oriented care in a secure mental health setting: "Striving for a good life." *Journal of Forensic Nursing, 10*, 63–69.

Mertens, D. M. (2007). Transformative paradigm: Mixed methods and social justice. *Journal of Mixed Methods Research, 1*, 212–225.

Montgomery, E., Pope, C., & Rogers, J. (2015). A feminist narrative study of the maternity care experiences of women who were sexually abused in childhood. *Midwifery, 31*, 54–60.

*Montgomery, P., Bailey, P., Johnson-Purdon, S., Snelling, S., & Kauppi, C. (2009). Women with postpartum depression: "My husband" stories. *BMC Nursing, 8*, 8.

Morse, J. M. (2004). Qualitative comparison: Appropriateness, equivalence, and fit. *Qualitative Health Research, 14*, 1323–1325.

Morse, J. M. (2009). Mixing qualitative methods. *Qualitative Health Research, 19*, 1523–1524.

*Morse, J. M., Pooler, C., Vann-Ward, T., Maddox, L. J., Olausson, J. M., Roche-Dean, M., . . . Martz, K. (2014). Awaiting diagnosis of breast cancer: Strategies of enduring for preserving self. *Oncology Nursing Forum, 41*, 350–359.

Moss, J. A. (2014). Discovering the healthcare beliefs and practices of rural mestizo Ecuadorians: An ethnonursing study. *Investigación y educación en enfermería, 32*, 326–336.

Nepal, V. (2010). On mixing qualitative methods. *Qualitative Health Research, 20*, 281.

Olesen, V. (2000). Feminisms and qualitative research at and into the millennium. In N. K. Denzin & Y. S. Lincoln (Eds.), *Handbook of qualitative research* (2nd ed., pp. 215–255). Thousand Oaks, CA: Sage.

Parse, R. R. (2001). *Qualitative inquiry: The path of science.* Sudbury, MA: Jones & Bartlett.

Parse, R. R. (2014). *The humanbecoming paradigm: A transformational worldview.* Pittsburgh, PA: Discovery International.

Peterson, A. L. (2015). A case for the use of autoethnography in nursing research. *Journal of Advanced Nursing, 71*, 226–233.

Polit, D., & Beck, C. T. (2009). International differences in nursing research, 2005–2006. *Journal of Nursing Scholarship, 41*, 44–53.

Rankin, J. M. (2013). Institutional ethnography. In C. T. Beck (Ed.), *Routledge international handbook of qualitative nursing research* (pp. 242–255). New York: Routledge.

Rankin, J. M. (2015). The rhetoric of patient and family centred care: An institutional ethnography into what actually happens. *Journal of Advanced Nursing, 71*, 526–534.

Riessman, C. K. (1991). Beyond reductionism: Narrative genres in divorce accounts. *Journal of Narrative and Life History, 1*, 41–68.

Riessman, C. K. (1993). *Narrative analysis.* Newbury Park, CA: Sage.

Riessman, C. K. (2008). *Narrative methods for the human sciences.* Thousand Oaks, CA: Sage.

Sandelowski, M. (2000). Whatever happened to qualitative description? *Research in Nursing & Health, 23*, 334–340.

Sandelowski, M. (2010). What's in a name? Qualitative description revisited. *Research in Nursing & Health, 33*, 77–84.

Sandelowski, M. (2011). "Casing" the research case study. *Research in Nursing & Health, 34*, 153–159.

Sherwood, J., & Kendall, S. (2013). Reframing spaces by building relationships: Community collaborative participatory action research with Aboriginal mothers in prison. *Contemporary Nurse, 46*, 83–94.

Short, A., Gibb, H., Fildes, J., & Holmes, C. (2013). Exploring the role of music therapy in cardiac rehabilitation after cardiac surgery: A qualitative study using the Bonny method of guided imagery and music. *Journal of Cardiovascular Nursing, 28*, E74–E81.

Smith, C. A., & Gallo, A. (2007). Applications of performance ethnography in nursing. *Qualitative Health Research, 17*, 521–528.

Smith, D. E. (1999). *Writing the social: Critique, theory, and investigation.* Toronto, Canada: University of Toronto Press.

Smith, J. A., Flowers, P., & Larkin, M. (2009). *Interpretive phenomenological analysis: Theory, method and research.* Los Angeles, CA: Sage.

Spiers, J. (2006). Expressing and responding to pain and stoicism in home-care nurse-patient interactions. *Scandinavian Journal of Caring Science, 20*, 293–301.

Stake, R. (1995). *The art of case study research.* Thousand Oaks, CA: Sage.

Stake, R. E. (2005). Qualitative case studies. In N. Denzin & Y. Lincoln (Eds.), *The Sage handbook of qualitative research* (3rd ed., pp. 443–466). Thousand Oaks, CA: Sage.

Strauss, A., & Corbin, J. (1990). *Basics of qualitative research: Grounded theory procedures and techniques.* Newbury Park, CA: Sage.

Taverner, T., Closs, S., & Briggs, M. (2014). The journey to chronic pain: A grounded theory of older adults' experiences of pain associated with leg ulceration. *Pain Management Nursing, 15*, 186–198.

Thorne, S. (2008). *Interpretive description.* Walnut Creek, CA: Left Coast Press.

Thorne, S. (2013). Interpretive description. In C. T. Beck (Ed.), *Routledge international handbook of qualitative nursing research* (pp. 295–306). New York: Routledge.

Tobin, C., Murphy-Lawless, J., & Beck, C. T. (2014). Childbirth in exile: Asylum seeking women's experience of childbirth in Ireland. *Midwifery, 30*, 831–838.

Van Manen, M. (1997). From meaning to method. *Qualitative Health Research, 7*, 345–369.

Van Manen, M. (2002). *Writing in the dark: Phenomenological studies in interpretive inquiry.* Ontario, Canada: Althouse Press.

Warnock, F. F., & Allen, M. (2003). Ethological methods to develop nursing knowledge. *Research in Nursing & Health, 26,* 74–84.

Whybrow, D. (2013). Psychiatric nursing liaison in a combat zone: An autoethnography. *Journal of Psychiatric and Mental Health Nursing, 20,* 896–901.

Wolcott, H. F. (2008). *Ethnography: A way of seeing* (2nd ed.). Plymouth, United Kingdom: AltaMira Press.

Yin, R. (2014). *Case study research: Design and methods* (5th ed.). Thousand Oaks, CA: Sage.

Yun, O., Kim, M., & Chiung, S. E. (2014). The sexuality experience of older widows in Korea. *Qualitative Health Research, 24,* 474–483.

A link to this open-access journal article is provided in the Toolkit for this chapter in the accompanying Resource Manual. ✖

22 | Sampling in Qualitative Research

In Chapter 12, we presented technical terms and concepts relating to sampling in quantitative research. Sampling in qualitative studies is quite different. Qualitative studies almost always use small, nonrandom samples. This does not mean that qualitative researchers are unconcerned with the quality of their samples but rather that they use different considerations in selecting participants. This chapter describes sampling approaches used by qualitative researchers.

THE LOGIC OF QUALITATIVE SAMPLING

Quantitative research is concerned with measuring attributes and relationships in a population, and therefore, a representative sample is desired to ensure that the measurements accurately reflect and can be generalized to the population. The aim of most qualitative studies is to discover *meaning* and to uncover multiple realities, not to generalize to a target population.

Qualitative researchers begin with the following types of sampling question in mind: Who would be an information-rich data source for my study? Whom should I talk to or observe to maximize my understanding of the phenomenon? A critical first step in qualitative sampling is selecting settings with high potential for information richness. As the study progresses, new sampling questions emerge, such as the following: Who can confirm my understandings? Challenge or modify my understandings? Enrich my understandings? Thus, as with the overall design in qualitative studies, sampling often is emergent and capitalizes on early learning to guide subsequent direction.

> **TIP:** Individuals are not always the *unit of analysis* in qualitative studies. Glaser and Strauss (1967) have noted that "incidents" or experiences are sometimes the basis for analysis. An information-rich informant may contribute dozens of incidents (e.g., of patients who fell), and so even a small number of informants can generate a large sample for analysis.

Qualitative researchers do not articulate an explicit population to whom results are intended to be generalized, but they do establish the kinds of people who are eligible to participate in their research. A prime criterion is whether a person has experienced the phenomenon (or culture) that is under study. Practical issues, such as costs, accessibility, health constraints, and researcher–participant language compatibility, also affect who can be included in the sample.

Example of Eligibility Criteria in a Qualitative Study: In their grounded theory study, Roberts and Bowers (2015) explored how residents of nursing homes develop relationships with peers and staff. Residents of two nursing homes were eligible if they spoke fluent English, could carry on a conversation, and understood the consent process. Residents who had a legal guardian or an activated health care power of attorney due to mental incapacity were excluded.

TYPES OF QUALITATIVE SAMPLING

Several different approaches to sampling in qualitative research are reviewed in this section. Despite differences, however, a few key features that characterize most sampling strategies have been distilled from an analysis of the qualitative literature (Curtis et al., 2000).

- Participants are not selected randomly. A random sample is not considered the best method of selecting people who will make good informants, that is, people who are knowledgeable, articulate, reflective, and willing to talk at length with researchers.
- Samples tend to be small and studied intensively, with each participant providing a wealth of data. Typically, qualitative studies involve fewer (and sometimes much fewer) than 50 participants.
- Sample members are not wholly prespecified; their selection is emergent.
- Sample selection is driven to a great extent by conceptual requirements rather than by a desire for representativeness.

Convenience Sampling

Qualitative researchers often begin with a convenience sample, which is sometimes referred to in qualitative studies as a *volunteer sample*. Volunteer samples are especially likely to be used when researchers need to have potential participants come forward and identify themselves. For example, if we wanted to study the experiences of people with frequent nightmares, we might have difficulty readily identifying potential participants. In such a situation, we might recruit sample members by placing a notice on a bulletin board, in a newspaper, or on Internet sites, requesting people with frequent nightmares to contact us. In this situation, we would be less interested in obtaining a representative sample of people with nightmares than in obtaining a diverse group representing various experiences with nightmares.

Sampling by convenience is easy and efficient, but it is not a preferred sampling approach, even in qualitative studies. The key in qualitative studies is to extract the greatest possible information from the few cases in the sample, and a convenience sample may not provide the most information-rich sources. However, a convenience sample may be an economical and easy way to begin the sampling process, relying on other methods as data are collected.

Convenience sampling may also work well with participants who need to be recruited from a particular clinical setting or from a specific organization. Thorne (2008), however, advised that in such situations, the researcher should carefully reflect on and understand any peculiarities of the study context. In essence, researchers must consider whether participants' narrations reflect the experience of the health care or organizational setting to a greater extent than the experience of the phenomenon under study.

> **Example of a Convenience Sample:** Senden and colleagues (2015) studied how older patients and their family caregivers experience receiving a cancer diagnosis and treatment, and how their experiences mutually influence each other. A convenience sample of older people diagnosed with cancer at a Belgian university hospital was recruited for the study.

Snowball Sampling

Qualitative researchers, like quantitative researchers, sometimes use snowball (or *chain*) sampling, asking early informants to refer other study participants. Snowball sampling has distinct advantages over convenience sampling from a broad population or community group. The first is that it may be more cost-efficient and practical. Researchers may spend less time screening people to determine if they are appropriate for the study, for example. Furthermore, with an introduction from the referring person, researchers may have an easier time establishing a trusting relationship with new participants. Finally, researchers can more readily specify the characteristics that they want new participants to have. For example, in the study of people with nightmares, we could ask early respondents if they knew anyone else who had the same problem *and* who was articulate. We could also ask for referrals to people who would add other dimensions to the sample, such as people who vary in age, race, socioeconomic status, and so on.

A weakness of this approach is that the eventual sample might be restricted to a rather small network of acquaintances. Moreover, the quality of the referrals may be affected by whether the referring sample members trusted the researcher and truly wanted to cooperate.

TIP: Researchers should be careful about protecting the rights of the individuals whom early participants refer. It is wise to suggest that early informants first check with the potential referrals to make sure they are interested in participating before their names are shared with the researcher. This is especially true if the study focuses on sensitive issues (e.g., suicide attempts).

Example of Snowball Sampling: Higginbottom and colleagues (2015) conducted a focused ethnography of the communication challenges of immigrant women in rural Canada with regard to maternity care. A sample of 31 immigrant women were recruited, relying in part on referrals from women already in the sample as well as gatekeepers in the community.

Purposive Sampling

Qualitative sampling may begin with volunteer informants and may be supplemented with new participants through snowballing, but many qualitative studies eventually evolve to a purposive (or *purposeful*) sampling strategy—that is, selecting cases that will most benefit the study.

More than a dozen purposive sampling strategies have been identified (Patton, 2002). We briefly describe many of these strategies to illustrate the diverse approaches qualitative researchers have used to meet the conceptual and substantive needs of their research. As an organizing structure, we have adapted the typology of purposive sampling proposed by Teddlie and Tashakkori (2009).

TIP: Researchers themselves do not necessarily refer to their sampling plans with the labels suggested by Patton (2002) or as categorized by Teddlie and Tashakkori (2009).

Sampling for Representativeness or Comparative Value

The first broad category of purposive sampling involves two general goals: (1) sampling to find examples that are representative or typical of a broader group on some dimension of interest or (2) sampling to set up the possibility of comparisons or replications across different types of cases on a dimension of interest.

Maximum variation sampling is perhaps the most widely used method of purposive sampling. It involves purposefully selecting persons (or settings) with variation on dimensions of interest. By selecting participants with diverse perspectives and backgrounds, researchers invite enrichments of and challenges to emerging conceptualizations. Maximum variation sampling might involve ensuring that people with diverse backgrounds are represented in the sample (ensuring that there are men and women, poor and affluent people, and so on). It might also involve deliberate attempts to include people with different viewpoints about the phenomenon under study. For example, researchers might use snowballing to ask early participants for referrals to people who hold different points of view. One major advantage of maximum variation sampling is that any common patterns emerging despite the diversity of the sample are of particular value in capturing core experiences.

Maximum variation sampling is often an emergent approach: Information from initial participants helps to guide the subsequent selection of a diverse group of participants. However, there may be an advantage to having some up-front insights into the dimensions of variation that will likely prove productive. The factors that affect the health or wellness experience under scrutiny can often be anticipated or identified in advance, and having a mental list of such factors can be useful in ensuring sufficient diversity in the sample.

Example of Maximum Variation Sampling: Kurth and colleagues (2014) studied the views and practices of first-time and experienced mothers regarding their response to infant crying in the first 3 months after birth. The study involved two interviews and observation of 15 mothers, sampled so as to maximize variation in terms of their parity and education.

At the other end of the spectrum, **homogeneous sampling** deliberately reduces variation and permits a more focused inquiry. Researchers may use this approach if they wish to understand a particular group of people especially well. Homogeneous sampling is often used to select people for group interviews.

Example of Homogeneous Sampling: Ko and co-researchers (2014) explored how Taiwanese patients with chronic schizophrenia live with their illness experiences. Using purposeful homogeneous sampling, they recruited 15 participants, all of whom lived in the community, were not experiencing acute psychosis, and were between the ages of 30 and 64 years.

Typical case sampling involves selecting cases that illustrate or highlight what is typical, average, normal, or representative. Identifying typical cases can help the researcher understand key aspects of a phenomenon as they are manifested under ordinary circumstances. The data resulting from this sampling strategy can be used to create a qualitative profile illustrating typical manifestations of the phenomenon being studied. Such profiles can be especially helpful to those not familiar with the social setting or culture.

Example of Typical Case Sampling: Olli and colleagues (2014) conducted a case study in Finland of the "habilitation" nursing of children with developmental disabilities. The researchers selected a ward that had a good staffing level and had nurses that used many different habilitation methods. An observation was undertaken to include the entire hospital stay of one child, who was selected through typical case sampling: a preschool-aged child with the most common diagnosis on the ward (mixed specific development disorders).

Typical case sampling can be expanded by selecting a **stratified purposive sample** of average, above average, and below average cases. This strategy approaches maximum variation sampling but is typically done along a single dimension (e.g., income or illness severity). In this approach, each "stratum" would comprise a fairly homogeneous sample.

Example of Stratified Purposive Sampling: Walker (2013) explored minority caregivers' perceptions of the emotional responses of their children to asthma. Walker used stratified purposive sampling to select four Latina and four African American caregivers who were participants in the Asthma in Central Texas Study.

Extreme (deviant) case sampling provides opportunities for learning from the most unusual and extreme informants—cases that at least on the surface seem like "exceptions to the rule" (e.g., outstanding successes and notable failures). The assumption underlying this approach is that extreme cases are rich in information because they are special in some way. In some circumstances, more can be learned by intensively studying extreme cases, but extreme cases can also distort understanding of a phenomenon. Most often, this approach is a supplement to other sampling strategies—the extremes are sought out to develop a richer or more nuanced understanding of the phenomenon under study.

Example of Extreme Case Sampling: In a longitudinal descriptive study, Tan and co-researchers (2012) studied the bereavement experience of parents whose infants died in acute care settings with a complex chronic condition. Extreme case sampling, with variation on race, social class, and prenatal diagnosis, was used to select seven cases.

Intensity sampling is similar to extreme case sampling but with less emphasis on the extremes. Intensity samples involve information-rich cases that manifest the phenomenon of interest intensely but not as extreme or potentially distorting manifestations. Thus, the goal in intensity sampling is to select rich cases that offer *strong* examples of the phenomenon. Intensity sampling is well suited as an adjunct method of sampling. For example, a researcher could collect data from 20 or so participants, using (for example) maximum variation or typical case sampling. Then, a subset set of intense cases could be sampled for more in-depth questioning or analysis.

Reputational case sampling, a variant of purposive sampling not included in Patton's (2002) list, involves selecting cases based on a recommendation of an expert or key informant. This approach, most often used in ethnographies, is useful when researchers have little information about how best to proceed with sampling and must rely on recommendations from others.

Many of the sampling strategies discussed thus far require that researchers have some knowledge about the context in which the study is taking place. For example, to choose extreme cases, typical cases, or homogeneous cases, researchers must have information about the range of variation of the phenomenon and how it manifests itself. Early participants may be helpful in implementing these sampling strategies.

TIP: Quantitative researchers design sampling plans that avoid sampling biases, but Morse (2003) has argued that "biasphobia" can undermine good qualitative research. She noted that the goal of sampling should be to actively and purposefully pursue the *best*, rather than the average, case. Her advice was to start with excellent examples of the phenomenon being studied, and then—once the phenomenon is better understood and there is a sense of what to look for—to examine "weaker instances and average occurrences" of the phenomenon.

Sampling Special or Unique Cases

The second broad category of purposive sampling involves selecting special or unique cases. In these approaches, individual cases or a specific group of cases is the focus of the investigation. Several of these approaches are especially likely to be used in case study research.

Critical case sampling involves selecting important cases regarding the phenomenon of interest. With this approach, researchers look for the particularly good story that illuminates critical aspects of the phenomenon and then intensely explore that story. To identify critical cases, the researcher must be able to identify the factors that make a case critical.

Example of Critical Case Sampling: Speraw (2009) explored the concept of personhood and its relationship to health care delivery in the context of a case study of a 16-year-old girl disfigured by multiple cancer treatments. The case study was part of a larger phenomenologic study of children and adolescents with disabilities or special needs. Speraw wrote that "Kelly's case is selected for presentation here both because of the striking clarity in description of life experience and its unique and articulate emphasis on the dilemmas associated with striving to express the fullness of humanity" (p. 736).

Criterion sampling involves selecting cases that meet a predetermined criterion of importance. For example, in studying patient satisfaction with nursing care, researchers might sample only those patients whose responses to questions upon discharge expressed a complaint about some aspect of nursing care. Criterion sampling is another approach that has the potential for identifying and understanding cases that are fertile with experiential information on the phenomenon of interest.

Example of Criterion Sampling: Hamilton and colleagues (2013) explored how religious songs were used to cope with stressful life events among older African Americans. Criterion sampling guided their selection of 65 participants with known religious affiliations.

Yin (2014), whose work on case study research is widely cited, described **revelatory case sampling**. This approach involves identifying and gaining access to a single case representing a phenomenon that was previously inaccessible to research scrutiny.

Example of Revelatory Case Sampling: Beck (2009) used revelatory case sampling to choose the participant for the single, holistic case study of an adult survivor of child sexual abuse and her breastfeeding experience.

A final type of special-case sampling is **sampling of politically important cases**. This approach is used to select or search for politically sensitive cases (or sites) for analysis. Sometimes, politically salient cases or sites can enhance the visibility of a study or increase the likelihood that it has an impact. The approach sometimes is used to select *out* politically sensitive locales or individuals to avoid attracting unwanted attention.

Sampling Sequentially

Several of the purposive strategies already described can be combined in a single study. For example, extreme case sampling could occur after an initial strategy such as maximum variation sampling. The strategies in this third broad category of purposive sampling involve a gradual, and often planned, sequence of sampling. One such strategy, theory-based or theoretical sampling, is discussed separately in the next section.

A type of sampling called **opportunistic sampling** (or *emergent sampling*) involves adding new cases to a sample based on changes in research circumstances as data are being collected, or in response to new leads and opportunities that may develop in the field. As the researcher gains greater knowledge of a setting or a phenomenon, on-the-spot sampling decisions can take advantage of unfolding events. This approach, although seldom labeled as opportunistic sampling, is used often in qualitative research because of its flexible and emergent nature.

Sampling confirming and disconfirming cases tends to be used toward the end of data collection. This approach involves testing ideas and assessing the viability of emergent findings and conceptualizations with new data. **Confirming cases** are additional cases that fit researchers' conceptualizations and offer enhanced credibility, richness, and depth to the analysis and conclusions. **Disconfirming cases** (or **negative cases**) are examples that do not fit and serve to challenge researchers' interpretations. These negative cases may simply be "exceptions that prove the rule," but they may be exceptions that disconfirm earlier insights and suggest rival explanations about the phenomenon. These cases can bring to light how the original conceptualization needs to be revised or expanded.

Example of Sampling Negative Cases:
Matthew-Maich and colleagues (2013) explored the processes and strategies used by frontline leaders

to support the uptake of best practice breastfeeding guidelines by nurses in maternity care practice settings. The researchers used several approaches to sampling 58 health professionals and 54 clients. They noted that they undertook negative case interviewing "whenever gaps or inconsistencies were noted in the data codes or categories" (p. 1761).

> **TIP:** Some qualitative researchers appear to call their sample *purposive* simply because they "purposely" selected people who have experienced the phenomenon of interest. However, exposure to the phenomenon is an eligibility criterion—the group of interest comprises people with that exposure. If the researcher then recruits *any* person with the desired experience, the sample is selected by convenience, not purposively. Purposive sampling implies an intent to choose *particular* exemplars or *types* of people who can best enhance the researcher's understanding of the phenomenon.

Theoretical Sampling

Patton (2002) described **theoretical sampling** (or *theory-based sampling*) as a strategy involving the selection of "incidents, slices of life, time periods, or people on the basis of their potential manifestation or representation of important theoretical constructs" (p. 238). Although Patton categorized this type of sampling as purposive sampling, we devote a separate subsection to this sampling strategy because of its importance in grounded theory.

> **TIP:** In Patton's (2002) scheme, theory-based sampling is viewed as a focused approach that could be based on an *a priori* theory that is being examined qualitatively, and so it is a different approach to linking sampling decisions to theoretical constructs than is found in grounded theory studies.

Glaser (1978) defined theoretical sampling as "the process of data collection for generating theory whereby the analyst jointly collects, codes, and analyzes his data and decides what data to collect next and where to find them, in order to develop his theory as it emerges" (p. 36). The process of theoretical sampling is guided by the developing grounded theory. Theoretical sampling is not envisioned as a single, unidirectional line. This complex sampling technique requires researchers to be involved with multiple lines and directions as they go back and forth between data and categories in the emerging theory.

Glaser stressed that theoretical sampling is not the same as purposive sampling. Theoretical sampling's purpose is to discover categories and their properties and to offer interrelationships that occur in the substantive theory. "The basic question in theoretical sampling is: what groups or subgroups does one turn to next in data collection?" (Glaser, 1978, p. 36). These groups are not chosen before the research begins but only as they are needed for their theoretical relevance for developing further emerging categories.

Example of a Theoretical Sampling: Beck (2002) used theoretical sampling in her grounded theory study of mothering twins during the first year of life. A specific example of theoretical sampling concerned what the mothers kept referring to as the "blur period"—the first few months of caring for the twins. Initially, Beck interviewed mothers whose twins were around 1 year of age. Her rationale was that these mothers would be able to reflect back over the entire first year of mothering the multiples. When these mothers referred to the "blur period," Beck asked them to describe this period more fully. The mothers said they could not provide many details about this period because "it was such a blur!" Beck then chose to interview mothers whose twins were 3 months of age or younger to ensure that mothers were still immersed in the "blur period" and would be able to provide rich detail about what this phase of mothering twins was like.

⟳ TIP: No matter what type of qualitative sampling you use, you should keep a journal or notebook to jot down ideas and reminders regarding the sampling process (e.g., who you should interview next). Memos to yourself will help you remember valuable ideas about your sample.

SAMPLE SIZE IN QUALITATIVE RESEARCH

There are no fixed rules for sample size in qualitative research. In qualitative studies, sample size should be based on informational needs. Hence, a guiding principle is **data saturation**—that is, sampling to the point at which no new information is obtained and redundancy is achieved. The goal is to generate enough in-depth data that can illuminate the patterns, categories, and dimensions of the phenomenon under study. Redundancy, and hence sample size, can be affected by the purpose of the inquiry, the quality of the informants, and the type of sampling strategy used. For example, a larger sample is likely to be needed with maximum variation sampling than with typical case sampling.

Morse (2000) noted that the number of participants needed to reach saturation depends on a number of factors. One factor concerns the scope of the research question: The broader the scope, the more participants will likely be needed. A broader scope may mean not only more interviews with people who have experienced the phenomenon but also a search for supplementary data sources. Researchers should consider this issue of scope and its implications for data needs before embarking on a study.

Data quality can also affect sample size. If participants are good informants who are able to reflect on their experiences and communicate effectively, saturation can be achieved with a relatively small sample. For this reason, convenience sampling may require more cases to achieve saturation than purposive or theoretical sampling.

Another issue that can affect sample size is the sensitivity of the phenomenon being studied. If the topic is one that is deeply personal or perhaps embarrassing, participants may be more reluctant to fully share their thoughts. Thus, to obtain sufficient data for a deep understanding of sensitive or controversial phenomena, more data may be required.

Greater amounts of data can be created by increasing the sample size, but sometimes depth and richness in the data can be achieved by longer, more intense interviews (or observations), or by going back to the same participants more than once. Multiple interviews often has the advantage of not only generating more data but also yielding better quality data if participants are more forth-coming in later sessions because of increased trust.

Morse (2000) noted that sample size can also be affected by the availability of what she called *shadowed data*. These are data provided by participants who are able to discuss not only their own experiences but also the experiences of others. Morse noted that shadowed data can provide researchers "with some idea of the range of experiences and the domain of the phenomena beyond the single participant's personal experience" (p. 4). Such shadowed data can help inform decisions relevant to purposive and theoretical sampling.

The skills and experience of the researcher also can affect sample size. Researchers with strong interviewing or observational skills often require fewer participants because they are more successful in putting participants at ease, encouraging candor, and soliciting important revelations. Thus, students who are just starting out on a qualitative project are likely to require a larger sample size to achieve data saturation than their more experienced mentors.

One final suggestion that may be especially important for beginning researchers is to "test" whether data saturation has been achieved. Essentially, this involves adding one or two cases after achieving informational redundancy to ensure that no new information emerges.

Example of Data Saturation: Roudsari and co-researchers (2013) conducted a grounded theory study to explore the process of decision making relating to family planning among Iranian women of reproductive age. A sample of 28 women and 17 other informants (e.g., the women's husbands, family health providers) participated. The authors noted that "theoretical saturation was achieved after conducting 39 interviews and was confirmed after completing 6 more interviews with women" (p. 410).

➔ **TIP:** Sample size estimation can create practical dilemmas if you are seeking approval or funding for a project. Patton (2002) recommended that, in a proposal, researchers should specify *minimum* samples that would reasonably be adequate for understanding the phenomenon. Additional cases can then be added, as necessary, to achieve saturation.

SAMPLING IN THE THREE MAIN QUALITATIVE TRADITIONS

There are similarities among the various qualitative traditions with regard to sampling: Samples are small, probability sampling is not used, and final sampling decisions usually take place during data collection. However, there are some differences as well.

Sampling in Ethnography

Ethnographers may begin by adopting a "big net" approach—that is, mingling with and having conversations with as many members of the culture under study as possible. Although they may converse with many people (often 50 or more), they often rely heavily on a smaller number of key informants. *Key informants* (or *cultural consultants*) are individuals who are highly knowledgeable about the culture or organization and who develop special, ongoing relationships with the researcher. These key informants are often the researcher's main link to the "inside."

Key informants are chosen purposively, guided by the ethnographer's informed judgments. Developing a pool of potential key informants often depends on ethnographers' prior knowledge to construct a relevant framework. For example, an ethnographer might make decisions about different types of key informants to seek out based on roles (e.g., physicians, nurse practitioners) or on some other substantively meaningful distinction. Once a pool of potential key informants is developed, the primary considerations for final selection are their level of knowledge about the culture and their willingness to collaborate with the ethnographer in revealing and interpreting the culture.

➔ **TIP:** Be careful not to choose key informants too quickly. The first participants who want to be key informants may be "deviant" members of the culture being studied. If ethnographers align themselves with marginal members of the culture, this may prevent gaining access to other valuable informants (Bernard, 2011).

Sampling in ethnography typically involves more than selecting informants because observation and other means of data collection play an important role in helping researchers understand a culture. Ethnographers have to decide not only *whom* to sample but *what* to sample as well. For example, ethnographers have to make decisions about observing *events* and *activities*, about examining *records* and *artifacts*, and about exploring *places* that provide clues about the culture. Key informants can play an important role in helping ethnographers decide what to sample.

Sampling in Phenomenologic Studies

Phenomenologists tend to rely on very small samples—often 10 or fewer participants. There is one guiding principle in selecting the sample for a phenomenologic study: All participants must have experienced the phenomenon and must be able to articulate what it is like to have lived that experience. Although phenomenologic researchers seek participants who have had the targeted experiences, they also want to explore diversity of individual experiences. Thus, they may specifically look for people with demographic or other differences who have shared a common experience.

Example of a Sample in a Phenomenologic Study: Using a hermeneutic phenomenologic approach, Saab and colleagues (2014) studied the lived experience of Lebanese men who were survivors of testicular cancer. A purposive sample of eight men aged 18-50 who were in remission for at least 3 years was recruited. The researchers deliberately sought "a heterogeneous sample in terms of age, marital and socioeconomic status, time since diagnosis, and type of treatment" (p. 204).

Sampling in Grounded Theory Studies

Grounded theory research is typically done with samples of about 20 to 30 people, using theoretical sampling. The goal in a grounded theory study is to select informants who can best contribute to the evolving theory. Sampling, data collection, data analysis, and theory construction occur concurrently. Study participants are selected serially and

contingently (i.e., contingent on the emerging conceptualization). Sampling might evolve as follows:

1. The researcher begins with a general notion of where and with whom to start. The first few cases may be solicited purposively, by convenience, or through snowballing.
2. In the early part of the study, a strategy such as maximum variation sampling might be used to gain insights into the range and complexity of the phenomenon under study.
3. The sample is adjusted in an ongoing fashion. Emerging conceptualizations help to inform the sampling process.
4. Sampling continues until saturation is achieved.
5. Final sampling may include a search for confirming and disconfirming cases to test, refine, and strengthen the theory.

Draucker and colleagues (2007) have provided particularly useful guidance with regard to actual implementation of theoretical sampling, based on strategies used in their study of responses to sexual violence. Their article included a model for a "theoretical sampling guide."

Example of a Sample in a Grounded Theory Study: Jeffers and colleagues (2014) studied the concerns and coping strategies of women on Northern Ireland with hereditary breast and ovarian cancer who undergo genetic testing for BRCA1/2. The researchers recruited adult women who had tested positive for a BRCA mutation through a regional genetics service. The first group of 11 women had received a positive BRCA result within 6 to 24 months prior to study entry. A second group of 15 women who had received their test result 1 month earlier was included in a longitudinal component. As part of their approach to theoretical sampling, the researchers asked: To which groups should we turn next? "Relatives and health professionals were approached to elaborate and refine existing categories and further develop and substantiate the theory" (p. 412).

SAMPLING AND GENERALIZABILITY IN QUALITATIVE RESEARCH

Qualitative research, perhaps because of its richly diverse disciplinary and philosophical roots, is beleaguered by many dilemmas and debates. Several important controversies concern the issue of study integrity and validity, which we discuss in Chapter 25. We focus in this chapter on the controversial issue of generalizability because of its relevance to sampling strategies.

Qualitative researchers seldom worry explicitly about the issue of generalizability. The goal of most qualitative studies is to provide a contextualized understanding of human experience through the intensive study of a few cases. Sampling decisions are not guided by a desire to generalize to a target population. Qualitative researchers are not in agreement, however, about the importance or attainability of generalizability. At one extreme are those who challenge the possibility of generalizability in any type of research. In this view, knowledge is to be found in the particulars. Generalization requires extrapolation that can never be fully justified because findings are never free from context. On the other hand, some believe that in-depth qualitative inquiry is particularly well suited for revealing higher level concepts that are not unique to a particular person or setting (Glaser, 2002; Misco, 2007). It might also be argued that the rich, highly detailed nature of qualitative findings make them especially suitable for extrapolation.

Many who have written about generalizability in qualitative research take a middle ground and attempt to find a balance between the generalizable and the particular through "reasonable extrapolation" (Patton, 2002, p. 489). A position that we think is sensible has been advanced by leading thinkers in both quantitative research (Lee Cronbach) and qualitative research (Egon Guba), both of whom asserted that any generalization represents a *working hypothesis*. Cronbach (1975) noted, "When we give proper weight to local conditions, any generalization is a working hypothesis, not a conclusion" (p. 125). Guba (1978) concurred, writing that "in the spirit of naturalistic inquiry [the researcher] should regard each possible generalization only as a working hypothesis, to be tested again in the next encounter and again in the encounter after that" (p. 70).

In the current evidence-based practice environment, the issue of the applicability of research findings beyond the particular people who took part in a study is a critical one. Indeed, Groleau and colleagues (2009), in discussing generalizability, have argued that an important goal of qualitative studies is to shape the opinion of decision makers whose actions affect people's health and well-being. They noted that "it is not qualitative data itself that must have a direct impact on decision makers but the insights they foster in relation to the problem under investigation" (p. 418).

Firestone (1993) developed a useful typology depicting three models of generalizability. The first model is extrapolating from a sample to a population, the model that guides most sampling designs in quantitative research, as discussed in Chapter 12. The second model is analytic or conceptual generalization, and the third is case-to-case translation, which is more often referred to as transferability—both of which have relevance for qualitative research. In **analytic generalization**, the goal is to generalize from the particulars to a broader theory. Case-to-case translation (**transferability**) involves judgments about whether findings from an inquiry can be extrapolated to a different setting or group of people. **Thick description**—richly thorough depictions of research settings and the sample of study participants (or events)—is needed in qualitative reports to support transferability. Analytic generalization and transferability are described more fully in the Supplement to this chapter on thePoint®. Ⓢ

CRITIQUING SAMPLING PLANS

Qualitative researchers do not always describe in much detail their method of identifying, recruiting, and selecting participants. Yet, readers will have difficulty drawing conclusions about the study findings without knowing something about researchers' sampling strategies. Indeed, there have been increased demands for making sampling decisions and processes in qualitative research more "public" (Onwuegbuzie & Leech, 2007). To facilitate transferability, qualitative reports should ideally describe the following:

- The type of sampling approach used (e.g., snowball, purposive, theoretical), together with an indication of how variation was dealt with (e.g., in

maximum variation sampling, the dimensions chosen for diversification)
- Eligibility criteria for inclusion in the study
- The nature of the setting or community
- The time period during which data were collected
- The number of participants, and a rationale for the sample size, such as an explicit statement that data saturation was achieved
- The main characteristics of participants (e.g., age, gender, length of illness, and so forth)

Inadequate description of the researcher's sampling strategy can be an impediment to assessing whether the strategy was productive. Moreover, if the description is vague, it will be difficult for readers to come to a conclusion about whether the evidence can be applied in their clinical practice. Thus, in critiquing a report, you should see whether the researcher provided an adequately rich description of the sample and the context in which the study was carried out so that someone interested in transferring the findings could make an informed decision.

Various writers have proposed criteria for evaluating sampling in qualitative studies. Morse (1991), for example, advocated two criteria: adequacy and appropriateness. *Adequacy* refers to the sufficiency and quality of the data the sample yielded. An adequate sample provides data without any "thin" spots. When the researcher has truly obtained data saturation, informational adequacy has been achieved, and the resulting description or theory is richly textured and complete.

Appropriateness concerns the methods used to select a sample. An appropriate sample is one resulting from the identification and use of participants who can best supply information according to the conceptual requirements of the study. Researchers should use a strategy that yields the fullest possible understanding of the phenomenon of interest. A sampling approach that excludes negative cases or that fails to include participants with unusual experiences may not meet the information needs of the study.

Curtis and colleagues (2000) proposed six criteria for evaluating qualitative sampling strategies. These criteria are as relevant for a self-evaluation by qualitative researchers themselves as for a critique by readers. First, the sampling strategy should be relevant to the tradition, conceptual framework,

and research question addressed by the research. Second, the sample should yield rich information on the phenomenon under study. Third, the sample should enhance the analytic generalizability of the findings. Fourth, the sample should produce believable descriptions, in the sense of being true to real life. Fifth, the sampling strategy should be ethical. Finally, the sampling plan should be feasible in terms of resources, time, and researcher's skills—and in terms of the researcher's or participants' ability to cope with the data collection process.

Some specific questions that can be used to critique sampling in a qualitative study are presented in Box 22.1.

BOX 22.1 Guidelines for Critiquing Qualitative Sampling Designs

1. Was the setting or context adequately described? Is the setting appropriate for the research question?
2. Were the sample selection procedures clearly delineated? What type of sampling strategy was used?
3. Were the eligibility criteria for the study specified? How were participants recruited into the study? Did the recruitment strategy yield information-rich participants?
4. Given the information needs of the study—and, if applicable, its qualitative tradition—was the sampling approach appropriate? Are dimensions of the phenomenon under study adequately represented?
5. Is the sample size adequate and appropriate for the qualitative tradition of the study? Did the researcher indicate that saturation had been achieved?
6. Do the findings suggest a richly textured and comprehensive set of data without any apparent "holes" or thin areas? Did the sample contribute sufficiently to analytic generalization?
7. Were key characteristics of the sample described (e.g., age, gender)? Was a rich description of participants and context provided, allowing for an assessment of the transferability of the findings?

⚫⚪⚫⚪⚫⚪⚫⚪⚫⚪⚫⚪⚫⚪⚫⚪⚫⚪⚫

RESEARCH EXAMPLE

Examples of various approaches to sampling in qualitative research have been presented throughout this chapter. In this section, we describe in some detail the sampling plan used in an ethnographic study.

Study: Information sharing with rural family caregivers during care transitions of hip fracture patients (Elliott et al., 2014)

Purpose: The researchers sought to understand family caregivers' experience of communication and information-sharing in health care transitions following surgery in patients with hip fracture and to identify facilitators and barriers of effective information sharing among patients, family caregivers, and health care providers.

Method: The study, part of a larger Canadian study of care transitions for hip-fracture patients, used a focused ethnographic approach. The goal was to examine practices in everyday, real-life settings and to gain an understanding of participants' experiences as they transitioned to different types of care (e.g., another hospital, rehabilitation, long-term care). The study setting was a hospital in southwest Ontario as well as postsurgical care settings. Data were collected primarily through in-depth interviews at each care setting through the recovery journey and observations at key junctures in the patient's care. Medical documents relevant to participants' care and transfers within and between health care settings were also collected and analyzed.

Sampling Strategy: English-speaking patients, care providers, and family members were recruited. Patients were included if they were over the age of 65 and were undergoing surgery for a hip fracture. In selecting 11 patients (8 women, 3 men) as informants, efforts were made to ensure a variety of participants. Eight family members who were identified as being involved in the care of the patient were included. At each point of care transition, health care providers involved in the patient's admission or discharge were recruited. A total of 24 health care providers were interviewed, including both those who were directly involved in the patient's care and some who could, as key informants, provide information relating to the policies or procedures of a care setting. In terms of

observations, several types of events were sampled for observation, including rehabilitation exercise sessions and discharges. Sixty-five hours of observation time were recorded.

Key Findings: The report provided thick description about the patients and their transition experiences. For example, a table identified all transitions that the 11 patients experienced (e.g., participant 4 transitioned from a retirement home, to a rural hospital, to another rural hospital, to long-term care, back to the first rural hospital, and then back to long-term care). In their analysis, the researchers found that trust was a key issue: When caregivers began to trust the health care providers, they were more comfortable asking questions and soliciting advice from the patients' care providers. But trust was often absent, and the caregivers were often disappointed with care providers' failure to share information.

⚫⚪⚫⚪⚫⚪⚫⚪⚫⚪⚫⚪⚫⚪⚫⚪⚫⚪⚫

SUMMARY POINTS

- Qualitative researchers use the conceptual demands of the study to select articulate and reflective informants with certain types of experience in an emergent way, typically capitalizing on early learning to guide subsequent sampling decisions. Qualitative samples tend to be small, nonrandom, and intensively studied.
- Sampling in qualitative inquiry may begin with a convenience (or *volunteer*) sample. Snowball (*chain*) sampling may also be used.
- Qualitative researchers often use **purposive sampling** to select data sources that enhance information richness. Various purposive sampling strategies have been used by qualitative researchers and can be loosely categorized as (1) sampling for representativeness or comparative value, (2) sampling special or unique cases, or (3) sampling sequentially.
- An important purposive strategy in the first category is **maximum variation sampling**, which entails purposely selecting cases with a range of variation. Other strategies used for comparative purposes or representativeness include **homogeneous sampling** (deliberately reducing

variation), **typical case sampling** (selecting cases that illustrate what is typical), **extreme case sampling** (selecting the most unusual or extreme cases), **intensity sampling** (selecting cases that are intense but not extreme), **stratified purposeful sampling** (selecting cases within defined strata), and **reputational case sampling** (selecting cases based on a recommendation of an expert or key informant).

• Purposive sampling in the "special cases" category include **critical case sampling** (selecting cases that are especially important or illustrative), **criterion sampling** (studying cases that meet a predetermined criterion of importance), **revelatory case sampling** (identifying and gaining access to a case representing a phenomenon that was previously inaccessible to research scrutiny), and **sampling politically important cases** (searching for and selecting or deselecting politically sensitive cases or sites).

• Although many qualitative sampling strategies unfold while in the field, purposive sampling in the "sequential" category involve deliberative emergent efforts and include **theoretical sampling** (selecting cases on the basis of their representation of important constructs) and **opportunistic sampling** (adding new cases based on changes in research circumstances or in response to new leads that develop in the field). Another important sequential strategy is **sampling confirming and disconfirming cases**—that is, selecting cases that enrich or challenge the researchers' conceptualizations.

• A guiding sample size principle is **data saturation**—sampling to the point at which no new information is obtained and redundancy is achieved. Factors affecting sample size include data quality, researcher skills and experience, and scope and sensitivity of the problem.

• Ethnographers make numerous sampling decisions, including not only *whom* to sample but also *what* to sample (e.g., activities, events, documents, artifacts); sampling decision making is often aided by *key informants* who serve as guides and interpreters of the culture.

• Phenomenologists typically work with a small sample of people (often 10 or fewer) who meet the criterion of having lived the experience under study.

• Grounded theory researchers typically use **theoretical sampling** in which sampling decisions are guided in an ongoing fashion by the emerging theory. Samples of about 20 to 30 people are typical in grounded theory studies.

• Generalizability in qualitative research is a controversial issue, with some writers claiming it to be unattainable because of the highly contextualized nature of qualitative findings. Yet most qualitative researchers strive to have their findings be relevant and meaningful beyond the confines of their particular study participants and settings.

• Two models of generalizability have relevance for qualitative research. In **analytic generalization**, researchers strive to generalize from particulars to broader conceptualizations and theories. **Transferability** involves judgments about whether findings from an inquiry can be extrapolated to a different setting or group of people. **Thick description**—richly thorough depictions of research settings and participant—is needed in qualitative reports to support transferability.

⬤⬤⬤⬤⬤⬤⬤⬤⬤⬤⬤⬤⬤⬤⬤⬤⬤⬤⬤⬤⬤⬤

STUDY ACTIVITIES

Chapter 22 of the *Resource Manual for Nursing Research*: *Generating and Assessing Evidence for Nursing Practice*, *10th edition*, offers exercises and study suggestions for reinforcing concepts presented in this chapter. In addition, the following study questions can be addressed:

1. Read a qualitative study involving a patient population that is personally relevant or interesting to you. Was the description of the sample and setting sufficiently detailed to allow you to draw conclusions about the similarity of your own setting and patients to those described in the study?

2. Answer relevant questions from Box 22.1 with regard to the grounded theory study by Jeffers and colleagues (2014), briefly described in this chapter.

STUDIES CITED IN CHAPTER 22

Beck, C. T. (2002). Releasing the pause button: Mothering multiples during the first year of life. *Qualitative Health Research, 12,* 593–608.

Beck, C. T. (2009). An adult survivor of child sexual abuse and her breastfeeding experience: A case study. *MCN: The American Journal of Maternal/Child Nursing, 34,* 91–97.

Bernard, H. R. (2011). *Research methods in anthropology: Qualitative and quantitative approaches* (5th ed.). Lanham, MD: AltaMira Press.

Cronbach, L. (1975). Beyond the two disciplines of scientific psychology. *American Psychologist, 30,* 116–127.

Curtis, S., Gesler, W., Smith, G., & Washburn, S. (2000). Approaches to sampling and case selection in qualitative research. *Social Science & Medicine, 50,* 1001–1014.

Draucker, C., Martsoff, D., Ross, R., & Rusk, T. (2007). Theoretical sampling and category development in grounded theory. *Qualitative Health Research, 17,* 1137–1148.

*Elliott, J., Forbes, D., Chesworth, B., Ceci, C., & Stolee, P. (2014). Information sharing with rural family caregivers during care transitions of hip fracture patients. *International Journal of Integrated Care, 14,* e018.

*Firestone, W. A. (1993). Alternative arguments for generalizing from data as applied to qualitative research. *Educational Researcher, 22,* 16–23.

Glaser, B. (1978). *Theoretical sensitivity.* Mill Valley, CA: Sociology Press.

Glaser, B. (2002). Conceptualisation: On theory and theorizing using grounded theory. In A. Bron & M. Schemmenn (Eds.), *Social science theories and adult education research* (pp. 313–335). Münster, Germany: Lit Verlag.

Glaser, B. G., & Strauss, A. (1967). *The discovery of grounded theory: Strategies for qualitative research.* New York: Aldine de Gruyter.

Groleau, D., Zelkowitz, P., & Cabral, I. (2009). Enhancing generalizability: Moving from an intimate to a political voice. *Qualitative Health Research, 19,* 416–426.

Guba, E. (1978). *Toward a methodology of naturalistic inquiry in educational evaluations.* Los Angeles: University of California, Center for the Study of Evaluation.

Hamilton, J., Sandelowski, M., Moore, A., Agarwal, M., & Koenig, H. (2013). "You need a song to bring you through": The use of religious songs to manage stressful life events. *The Gerontologist, 53,* 26–38.

Higginbottom, G., Safipour, J., Yohani, S., O'Brien, B., Mumtaz, Z., & Paton, P. (2015). An ethnographic study of communication challenges in maternity care for immigrant women in rural Alberta. *Midwifery, 31,* 297–304.

Jeffers, L., Morrison, P., McCaughan, E., & Fitzsimons, D. (2014). Maximising survival: The main concern of women with hereditary breast and ovarian cancer who undergo genetic testing for BRCA1/2. *European Journal of Oncology Nursing, 18,* 411–418.

Ko, C. J., Smith, P., Liao, H., & Chiang, H. (2014). Searching for reintegration: Life experiences of people with schizophrenia. *Journal of Clinical Nursing, 23,* 394–401.

Kurth, E., Kennedy, H., Zemp Stutz, E., Kesselring, A., Fornaro, I., & Spichiger, E. (2014). Responding to a crying infant-you do not learn overnight: A phenomenological study. *Midwifery, 30,* 742–749.

Matthew-Maich, N., Ploeg, J., Jack, S., & Dobbins, M. (2013). Leading on the frontlines with passion and persistence: A necessary condition for Breastfeeding Best Practice Guideline uptake. *Journal of Clinical Nursing, 22,* 1759–1770.

*Misco, T. (2007). The frustrations of reader generalizability and grounded theory: Alternative considerations for transferability. *Journal of Research Practice, 3,* 1–11.

Morse, J. M. (1991). Strategies for sampling. In J. M. Morse (Ed.), *Qualitative nursing research: A contemporary dialogue* (pp. 127–145). Newbury Park, CA: Sage.

Morse, J. M. (2000). Determining sample size. *Qualitative Health Research, 10,* 3–5.

Morse, J. M. (2003). Biasphobia. *Qualitative Health Research, 13,* 891–892.

*Olli, J., Vehkakoski, T., & Salanterä, S. (2014). The habilitation nursing of children with development disabilities—Beyond traditional nursing practices and principles? *International Journal of Qualitative Studies on Health and Well-being, 9,* 10.

*Onwuegbuzie, A., & Leech, N. (2007). Sampling designs in qualitative research: Making the sampling process more public. *The Qualitative Report, 12,* 238–254.

Patton, M. Q. (2002). *Qualitative evaluation and research methods* (3rd ed.). Thousand Oaks, CA: Sage.

Roberts, T., & Bowers, B. (2015). How nursing home residents develop relationships with peers and staff: A grounded theory study. *International Journal of Nursing Studies, 52,* 57–67.

*Roudsari, R. L., Khadivzadeh, T., & Bahrami, M. (2013). A grounded theory approach to understand the process of decision making on fertility control methods in urban society of Mashad, Iran. *Iranian Journal of Nursing & Midwifery Research, 18,* 408–415.

Saab, M., Noureddine, S., Aub-Saad Huijer, H., & DeJong, J. (2014). Surviving testicular cancer: The Lebanese lived experience. *Nursing Research, 63,* 203–210.

Senden, C., Vandecasteele, T., Vandenberghe, E., Versluys, K., Piers, R., Gyrpdonck, M., & Van den Noortgate, N. (2015). The interaction between lived experiences of older patients and their family caregivers confronted with a cancer diagnosis and treatment. *International Journal of Nursing Studies, 52,* 197–206.

Speraw, S. (2009). "Talk to me—I'm human": The story of a girl, her personhood, and the failures of health care. *Qualitative Health Research, 19,* 732–743.

*Tan, J. S., Docherty, S., Barfield, R., & Brandon, D. (2012). Addressing parental bereavement support needs at the end of life for infants with complex chronic conditions. *Journal of Palliative Medicine, 15*, 579–584.

Teddlie, C., & Tashakkori, A. (2009). *Foundations of mixed methods research.* Thousand Oaks, CA: Sage.

Thorne, S. (2008). *Interpretive description.* Walnut Creek, CA: Left Coast Press.

Walker, V. G. (2013). Minority caregivers' emotional responses and perceptions of the emotional responses of their chil-

dren to asthma: Comparing boys and girls. *Issues in Mental Health Nursing, 34*, 325–334.

Yin, R. (2014). *Case study research: Design and methods* (5th ed.). Thousand Oaks, CA: Sage.

***A link to this open-access journal article is provided in the Toolkit for this chapter in the accompanying* Resource Manual.**

Data Collection in Qualitative Research

This chapter provides an overview of unstructured data collection approaches and strategies used in qualitative research, with a focus on self-reports and observations.

DATA COLLECTION ISSUES IN QUALITATIVE STUDIES

In qualitative studies, data collection usually is more fluid than in quantitative research, and decisions about what to collect evolve in the field. For example, as researchers gather and digest information, they may realize that it would be fruitful to pursue an unanticipated line of questioning. Even while allowing for and profiting from this flexibility, however, qualitative researchers make several up-front decisions about data collection and need to be prepared for problematic situations that may arise in the field. Creativity for workable solutions and new strategies is often needed.

Types of Data for Qualitative Studies

Qualitative researchers typically go into the field knowing the most likely sources of data, while not ruling out other possible data sources that might come to light as data collection progresses. The primary method of collecting qualitative data is by interviewing study participants. Observation is a part of many qualitative studies as well. Physiologic data are rarely collected in a constructivist inquiry,

except perhaps to describe participants' characteristics or to ascertain eligibility for the study.

Table 23.1 compares the types of data used by researchers in the three main qualitative traditions as well as other aspects of the data collection process for each tradition. As noted in Chapter 21, ethnographers typically collect a wide array of data, with observation and interviews being the primary methods. Ethnographers also gather or examine products of the culture under study, such as documents, records, artifacts, photographs, and so on. Phenomenologists and grounded theory researchers rely primarily on in-depth interviews, although observation and documents also play a role in grounded theory studies.

The research tradition also has implications for how the researcher as "self" is used (Lipson, 1991). Phenomenologic researchers use "self" to collect rich descriptions of human experiences and to develop relationships with a small number of people in intensive interviews. Grounded theorists use themselves not only to collect data but also to process the data and generate categories for the emerging theory. Ethnographers use themselves as observers who collect data not only through interviews but also through active participation in field settings.

Field Issues in Qualitative Studies

The collection of qualitative data in the field often gives rise to several important issues, which are particularly salient in ethnographies. Ethnographic researchers must deal with such issues as

TABLE 23.1 • Comparison of Data Collection Issues in Three Qualitative Traditions

ISSUE	ETHNOGRAPHY	PHENOMENOLOGY	GROUNDED THEORY
Types of data	Primarily observation and interviews, plus artifacts, documents, photographs, genealogies, maps, social network diagrams	Primarily in-depth interviews, sometimes diaries, other written materials	Primarily individual interviews, sometimes group interviews, observation, participant journals, documents
Unit of data collection	Cultural systems	Individuals	Individuals
Data collection points	Mainly longitudinal	Mainly cross-sectional	Cross-sectional or longitudinal
Length of time for data collection	Typically long, many months or years	Typically moderate	Typically moderate
Data recording	Field notes, logs, interview notes/recordings	Interview notes/recordings	Interview notes/recordings, memoing, observational notes
Salient field issues	Gaining entrée, reactivity, determining a role, learning how to participate, encouraging candor and other interview logistics, loss of objectivity, premature exit, reflexivity	Bracketing one's views, building rapport, encouraging candor, listening while preparing what to ask next, keeping "on track," handling emotionality	Building rapport, encouraging candor, listening while preparing what to ask next, keeping "on track," handling emotionality

gaining entrée, negotiating for space and privacy for interviewing and recording data, deciding on an appropriate role (i.e., the extent to which they will actually participate in the culture's activities), and taking care not to exit from the field prematurely. Ethnographers also need to be able to cope with culture shock and should have a high tolerance for uncertainty and ambiguity. Other field issues apply to most qualitative research.

Gaining Trust

Researchers who do qualitative research must, to an even greater extent than quantitative researchers, gain and maintain a high level of trust with participants. Researchers need to develop strategies in the field to establish credibility among those being studied. This may be a delicate balancing act because re-

searchers must try to "be like" the people being studied while at the same time keeping a certain distance. "Being like" participants means that researchers should be sensitive to such issues as styles of dress, modes of speech, customs, and schedules. In ethnographic research, it is important not to take sides on any controversial issue and not to appear too strongly affiliated with a particular subgroup of the culture—especially with leaders or prominent members of the culture. It is often impossible to gain the trust of the group if researchers appear close to those in power.

The Pace of Data Collection

In qualitative studies, data collection is often an intense and exhausting experience, especially if the phenomenon being studied concerns an illness experience or other stressful life event (e.g., domestic violence). Collecting high-grade qualitative data requires deep concentration and energy. The process can be an emotional strain for which researchers need to prepare. One way to deal with this is to collect data at a pace that minimizes stress. For example, it may be prudent to limit interviewing to no more than one a day and to engage in emotionally releasing activities (e.g., exercising) between interviews. It may also be helpful to debrief about any feelings of distress with a co-researcher, colleague, or advisor.

Emotional Involvement with Participants

Qualitative researchers need to guard against getting too emotionally involved with participants, a pitfall that has been called "**going native.**" Researchers who get too close to participants run several risks, including compromising their ability to collect meaningful and trustworthy data, and becoming overwhelmed with participants' suffering. It is important, of course, to be supportive and to listen carefully to people's concerns, but it usually is not advisable to intervene and try to solve participants' problems, or to share personal problems with them. If participants need help, it is better to give advice about where they can get it than to give it directly.

Reflexivity

As noted in Chapter 8, reflexivity is an important concept in qualitative data collection. Reflexivity refers to researchers' awareness of themselves as part of the data they are collecting. Researchers need to be conscious of the part they play in their own study and reflect on their own behavior and how it can affect the data they obtain.

Example of Reflexivity: Rix and colleagues (2014) described the complex layers of reflexivity required for "white nurses" serving, and doing research with, Aboriginal people in Australia. In their study of Aboriginal people's experience of being hemodialysis recipients, the researchers instituted three layers of reflexivity: examining self within the research, examining interpersonal relationships with participants, and examining health systems.

Recording and Storing Qualitative Data

In addition to thinking about the types of data to be gathered, qualitative researchers need to plan ahead for how data will be recorded and stored. Interview data can be recorded by taking detailed notes of what participants say, or by audio or video recording. To ensure that interview data are participants' actual verbatim responses, we strongly recommend that qualitative interviews be recorded and subsequently transcribed rather than relying on interviewer notes. Notes tend to be incomplete and may be biased by the interviewer's memory or personal views. Moreover, note taking can distract researchers, whose main job is to listen intently and direct the flow of questioning based on what has already been said.

TIP: In addition to traditional audiotaping equipment, new technologies are emerging to facilitate recording in the field. For example, digital voice recorders with transcription capabilities allow researchers to record and transfer voice data to a personal computer using a USB interface. Some digital voice recorders come bundled with voice recognition software (see Chapter 24). A recent innovation is the *smartpen*—a ballpoint pen with an embedded computer and digital audio recorder—that can record up to 200 hours of audio. When used with *digital paper*, the smartpen records written material for uploading to a computer and synchronizes the notes with any material that was audio recorded. Many researchers use their smartphones to record interviews.

Environmental distractions are a common pitfall in recording interviews. A quiet setting without disruptions is ideal but is not always possible. The second author of this book (Beck) has conducted many challenging interviews. As one example, a mother of three children was interviewed in her home about her experience with postpartum depression. The interview was scheduled during the toddlers' normal naptime, but when Beck arrived, the toddlers had already taken their nap. The television was on to occupy the toddlers, but they kept trying to play with the tape recorder. The 6-week-old baby was fussy, crying through most of the interview. The background noise level on the tape made accurate transcription difficult.

When observations are made, detailed observational notes must be maintained, unless it is possible to videotape. Observational notes should be made shortly after an observational session, usually onto a computer file. Whatever method is used to record observations, researchers need to go into the field with the equipment or supplies needed to record their data, and be sure that the equipment is functioning properly.

Grounded theory researchers write *analytic memos* that document researchers' ideas about how the theory is developing (e.g., how some themes are interrelated). These memos can vary in length from a sentence to multiple pages. Montgomery and Bailey (2007) offer some guidance and examples of grounded theory notes and memos.

If assistants are used to collect the data, qualitative researchers need to be as concerned as quantitative researchers about hiring appropriate staff and training them to collect high-quality data. In particular, the data collectors must be trained to elicit rich and vivid descriptions. Qualitative interviewers need to be good listeners; they need to hear all that is being said rather than trying to anticipate what is coming next. A good data collector must have both self-awareness and an awareness of participants (e.g., by paying attention to nonverbal behavior). Qualitative data collectors must be able to create an atmosphere that safely allows for the sharing of experiences and feelings. Respect and authentic caring for participants are critical.

➲ TIP: In qualitative studies, data are often collected by a single researcher working alone, in which case self-training and self-preparation are important. When a team of researchers works together on a qualitative study, attention needs to be paid to team issues related to fieldwork—and to group decision making and planning in general (Hall et al., 2005).

QUALITATIVE SELF-REPORT TECHNIQUES

Unstructured or loosely structured self-report methods provide narrative data for qualitative analysis. Most qualitative self-report data are collected through interviews rather than by questionnaire.

Types of Qualitative Self-Reports

Researchers use various approaches in collecting qualitative self-report data. The main methods are described here.

Unstructured Interviews

Researchers who do not have a preconceived view of the content or flow of information to be gathered may conduct completely **unstructured interviews**. Unstructured interviews are conversational and interactive and are the mode of choice when researchers do not have a clear idea of what it is they do not know. Researchers using unstructured interviews do not have a set of prepared questions because they do not yet know what to ask or even where to begin—they let participants tell their stories, with little interruption. Phenomenologic, grounded theory, and ethnographic studies often involve unstructured interviews.

Researchers using a completely unstructured approach often begin by informally asking a broad question (sometimes called a **grand tour question**) relating to the research topic, such as, "What happened when you first learned you had AIDS?" Subsequent questions are more focused and are guided by responses to the broad question. Some respondents may request direction after the initial broad question is posed, perhaps asking, "Where should I begin?" Respondents should be encouraged to begin wherever they wish.

Van Manen (1990) provided suggestions for guiding a phenomenologic interview in a manner likely to produce rich descriptions of the experience under study:

- "Describe the experience from the inside, as it were; almost like a state of mind: the feelings, the mood, the emotions, etc.
- Focus on a particular example or incident of the object of experience: describe specific events, an adventure, a happening, a particular experience.
- Try to focus on an example of the experience which stands out for its vividness, or as it was the first time.
- Attend to how the body feels, how things smell(ed), how they sound(ed), etc." (pp. 64–65).

Kahn (2000), discussing unstructured interviews in hermeneutic phenomenologic studies, recommended interviews that resemble conversations. If the experience under study is an ongoing one, Kahn suggested obtaining as much detail as possible about the participant's daily life. For example, a question that can be used is, "Pick a normal day for you and tell me what happened" (p. 62). If the experience being studied is primarily in the past, then Kahn advocated a retrospective approach. The interviewer would begin with a general question such as, "What does this experience mean to you?" (p. 63), and would then probe for more detail until the experience is thoroughly described.

Example of Unstructured Interviews: Yousefi and co-researchers (2014) studied the experiences and decision-making processes of Iranian families with regard to the organ donation of a family member with brain death. In unstructured interviews lasting up to 4 hours, the researchers first asked, "Can you introduce yourself?" (p. 325). Then, participants were asked to explain their experience of giving consent concerning their deceased family member's organ donation.

In grounded theory, questioning changes as the theory is developed. At the outset, interviews are similar to open-ended conversations using unstructured interviews. Glaser and Strauss (1967) suggested researchers initially should just sit back and listen to participants' stories. Later, as the theory emerges, researchers ask more direct questions related to categories in the grounded theory. The more direct questions can be answered rather quickly, and so the interviews tend to get shorter as the grounded theory develops.

Ethnographic interviews are also unstructured. Spradley (1979) describes three types of question used to guide interviews: descriptive, structural, and contrast questions. *Descriptive questions* ask participants to describe their experiences in their own language and are the backbone of ethnographic interviews. *Structural questions* are more focused and help to develop the range of terms in a category or domain. Last are *contrast questions*, which are asked to distinguish differences in the meaning of terms and symbols.

Example of Ethnographic Interviewing: Using Spradley's developmental research sequence, Davies (2010) conducted an ethnographic study with parents of children in pain with Down syndrome. An example of a descriptive question was "Can you describe a time when your child was in pain?" An example of a structural question was "What words, gestures, or signs does your child use to express pain?" An example of a contrast question was "What is the difference between administering acetaminophen and making your child comfortable?" (p. 261).

Semistructured Interviews

Researchers sometimes want to be sure that a specific set of topics is covered in their qualitative interviews. They know what they want to ask but cannot predict what the answers will be. Their role in the process is somewhat structured, whereas the participants is not. In such **focused** or **semistructured interviews**, researchers prepare a written **topic guide**, which is a list of areas or questions to be covered with each participant. The interviewer's job is to encourage participants to talk freely about all the topics on the guide and to tell stories in their own words. This technique ensures that researchers will obtain all the information required and gives people the freedom to provide as many illustrations and explanations as they wish.

In preparing the topic guide, questions should be ordered in a logical sequence—perhaps chronologically or perhaps from the general to the specific. Interviewers need to be attentive, however, because respondents often volunteer information about questions that are later on the list. The topic guide might include suggestions for *probes* designed to elicit more detailed information. Examples of such probes include, "What happened next?" and "When that happened, how did you feel?" Questions that require one- or two-word responses, such as "yes" or "no," should be avoided. Questions should give people an opportunity to provide rich, detailed information about the phenomenon under study.

Example of Semistructured Interviews: Mao and colleagues (2014) conducted an ethnographic study to explore the personal and social determinants that play a key role in sustaining smoking practices among rural people in China. The topic guide for interviews with members of 22 families covered four areas: (1) smoking practices in the homes, (2) knowledge about tobacco risks and attitudes toward smoking, (3) opinions about why people continue to smoke, and (4) strategies used to restrict smoking in the home.

> **TIP:** Bevan (2014) has suggested an approach to interviewing that introduces "phenomenologic structure." He described three types of interview structure: contextualization, apprehending the phenomenon, and clarifying the phenomenon, and provided examples of questions for each type of structure.

Focus Group Interviews

Focus group interviews have become popular in the study of health problems. In a focus group interview, a group of people (usually five or more) is assembled for a discussion. The interviewer (or **moderator**) guides the discussion according to a written set of questions or topics to be covered, as in a semistructured interview. Focus group sessions are carefully planned discussions that take advantage of group dynamics for accessing rich information in an economical manner.

Typically, the people selected are a fairly homogeneous group to promote a comfortable group dynamic. People usually feel more at ease expressing their views when they share a similar background with other group members. Thus, if the overall sample is diverse, it is best to organize separate focus groups for people with similar characteristics (e.g., in terms of age or gender).

Several writers have suggested that the optimal group size for focus groups is 6 to 12 people, but Côté-Arsenault and Morrison-Beedy (1999) advocated smaller groups of about five participants when the topic is emotionally charged or sensitive.

> **TIP:** In recruiting group members, it is usually wise to recruit one or two more people than is considered optimal because of the risk of no-shows. Monetary incentives can help reduce this risk. It is also important to call recruits the night before the session to remind them of the appointment and confirm attendance.

Moderators play a critical role in the success of focus group interviews. At the start of a focus group session, moderators establish some ground rules with the participants. For example, they might advise participants to please speak one at a time, to be respectful of each other, and to maintain the confidentiality of what is said in the focus group. Moderators must take care to solicit input from all group members and not let a few vocal people dominate the discussion. Researchers other than the moderator should be present to take detailed observational notes about each session.

A major advantage of a group format is that it is efficient—researchers obtain the viewpoints of many people in a short time. Moreover, focus groups capitalize on the fact that members react to what is being said by others, thereby potentially leading to deeper expressions of opinion. Focus group interviews are also usually stimulating to respondents, but one problem is that some people are uncomfortable about expressing their views in front of a group. Another concern is that the dynamics of the session may foster a group culture that could inhibit individual expression as "group think" takes hold. Studies of focus groups suggest that they are similar to individual interviews in terms of number and quality of ideas generated (Kidd & Parshall, 2000), but some critics have worried about whether data from focus groups are as "natural" as data obtained from individual interviews (Morgan, 2001).

Key to an effective focus group is the researcher's *questioning route*, that is, the series of questions used to guide the interview. A typical 2-hour focus group session should include about 12 questions. Krueger and Casey (2015) provide these guidelines for developing a good questioning route:

1. Brainstorm.
2. Sequence the questioning. Arrange general questions first and then more specific questions. Ask positive questions before negative ones.
3. Phrase the questions. Use open-ended questions. Ask participants to think back and reflect on their personal experiences. Avoid asking "why" questions. Keep questions simple and make your questions sound conversational. Be careful about giving examples.
4. Estimate the time for each question. Consider the following when estimating time: the complexity of the questions, the category of questions, level of participant's expertise, the size of the focus group, and the amount of discussion you want related to the question.
5. Obtain feedback from others.
6. Revise the questions.
7. Test the questions.

Focus groups have been used by researchers in many qualitative research traditions and can play an important role in feminist, critical theory, and participatory action research. Nurse researchers have offered excellent guidance on studies with focus groups (e.g., Côté-Arsenault & Morrison-Beedy, 2005; Morrison-Beedy et al., 2001), and books on how to do focus group research are available (e.g., Carey & Asbury, 2012; Krueger & Casey, 2015). The Toolkit in the accompanying *Resource Manual* also has additional resources on focus groups. ⊗

Example of Focus Group Interviews: Kieft and co-researchers (2014) studied the perceptions of Dutch nurses with regard to how their work and their work environments contribute to patients' experiences of care. The data were collected in four focus groups with six to seven nurses in each. Separate focus groups were convened for nurses in mental health care, hospital care, home care, and nursing home care. The topic list included questions such as "Which elements in daily nursing practice influence patient experiences?"

Joint Interviews

Nurse researchers are sometimes interested in phenomena that involve interpersonal relationships or that require understanding the perspective of more than one person. For example, the phenomenon might be the grief that mothers *and* fathers experience on losing a child, or the experiences of AIDS patients *and* their caretakers. In such cases, it can be productive to conduct **joint (dyadic) interviews** in which two or more people are simultaneously questioned, using either an unstructured or semistructured format. Unlike focus group interviews, which typically involve group members who do not know each other, joint interviews involve respondents who are intimately related.

Joint interviews usually supplement rather than replace individual interviews because there are things that cannot readily be discussed in front of the other party (e.g., criticisms of the other person's behavior). Joint interviews can be especially helpful, however, when researchers want to *observe* the dynamics between two key actors. Morris (2001) raised important issues to consider in the conduct of joint interviews.

Example of Joint Interviews: Chen and Habermann (2013) explored how couples living with advanced multiple sclerosis (MS) approach planning for health changes together. Ten couples were interviewed—10 patients with advanced MS and their spouses. Participants were interviewed in their homes using a semistructured interview guide.

Diaries and Journals

Personal **diaries** have long been used as a source of data in historical research. It is also possible to generate new data for a nonhistorical study by asking study participants to maintain a diary or journal over a specified period—or by asking them to share a diary they wrote. Diaries can be useful in providing an intimate and detailed description of a person's everyday life.

The diaries may be completely unstructured; for example, individuals who have undergone organ transplantation could be asked simply to spend 10 to 15 minutes a day jotting down their thoughts and feelings. Frequently, however, participants are requested to make entries into a diary regarding a specific aspect of their experience, sometimes in a semistructured format (e.g., about their appetite or sleeping). Nurse researchers have used health diaries to collect information about how people prevent illness, maintain health, experience morbidity, and treat health problems.

Although diaries are a useful means of learning about ongoing experiences, one limitation is that they can be used only by people with adequate literacy skills, although there are examples of studies in which diary entries were audiorecorded rather than written out. Diaries also require a high level of participant cooperation.

Example of Diaries: Curtis and colleagues (2014) explored subjective responses to stress among Irish women with breast cancer. Thirty women with newly diagnosed breast cancer maintained diaries during their participation in a clinical trial. They were asked to write regularly about their experiences, thoughts, and feelings since their diagnosis. A facilitator reminded them weekly about the diaries over the course of a 5-week intervention but gave no further instructions.

Photo Elicitation Interviews

Photo elicitation involves an interview stimulated and guided by photographic images. This procedure, most often used in ethnographies, is a method that can break down barriers between researchers and study participants and promote a collaborative discussion (Frith & Harcourt, 2007). The photographs sometimes are ones that researchers have made of the participants' world, through which researchers can gain insights into a new culture. Participants may need to be continually reassured that their taken-for-granted explanations of the photos are providing new and useful information.

Photo elicitation can also be used with photos that participants have in their homes, although in such case researchers have less time to frame useful questions, and no opportunity to select the photos that will be the stimulus for discussion. Researchers have also used the technique of asking participants to take photographs themselves and then interpret them, a method called **photovoice** that is often used in participatory action research. Oliffe and colleagues (2008) offered useful suggestions for a four-part strategy of analyzing participant-produced photographs.

Example of Photovoice: Olausson and co-researchers (2014) explored nurses' lived experiences of ICU bed spaces as a place for the care of critically ill patients in Sweden. Fourteen nurses in three hospitals were asked to take photographs of the bed space, capturing what was important to them in providing care. In-depth interviews relating to the photographs lasted about 1 hour.

Self-Report Narratives on the Internet

In addition to the possibility of soliciting narrative data on the Internet through structured or semi-structured "interview" methods (as we describe in the next section), a potentially rich data source for qualitative researchers involves narrative self-reports available directly on the Internet. For example, researchers can enter into long conversations with other users in a chat room.

Some data that can be analyzed qualitatively are simply "out there," as when a researcher enters a chat room or blog site (or compiles tweets) and analyzes the content of existing, unsolicited messages. As pointed out by Keim-Malpass et al. (2014), the Internet is a rich source of interactive and socially mediated data, giving rise to *Internet ethnography*. Interest has focused, in particular, on illness blogs as a means of studying illness experiences.

Using the Internet to access narrative data has obvious advantages. This approach is economical and allows researchers to obtain information from geographically dispersed and perhaps remote Internet users (Fitzpatrick & Montgomery, 2004). However, a number of ethical concerns have been raised, and authenticity and other methodologic challenges need to be considered (Heilferty, 2011; Kralik et al., 2006; Robinson, 2001).

Example of an Analysis of Blogs: Asenhed and colleagues (2014) studied the process of first-time fatherhood among men whose partner was pregnant. The study involved the analysis of Internet blogs by 11 expectant fathers living in Sweden.

Other Unstructured Self-Reports

Although we have described that primary means of collecting in-depth data for qualitative studies, many other forms of unstructured self-reports have been developed. Examples include the following:

- **Life history interviews**, which are individual interviews directed at documenting a person's life story, or an aspect of it that has developed over the life course
- **Oral histories**, a method often used by historical researchers to gather personal recollections about events or issues
- The **critical incidents technique**, a method of gathering in-depth information regarding specific incidents witnessed by study participants
- The **think-aloud method**, which involves obtaining real-time narrative data about how a person solves a problem or makes a decision

These methods are briefly described, and some examples are provided, on the Supplement to this chapter on thePoint®.

Gathering Qualitative Self-Report Data through Interviews

The purpose of gathering narrative self-report data is to enable researchers to construct reality in a way that is consistent with the constructions of the people being studied. This goal requires researchers to take steps to overcome communication barriers and to enhance the flow of meaning. Asking good questions and eliciting good narrative data are far more difficult than appears. This section offers some suggestions about gathering qualitative self-report data through in-depth interviews. Further suggestions are offered by Fontana and Frey (2003), Rubin and Rubin (2012), and Gubrium et al. (2012).

Locating the Interview

Researchers must decide where the interviews will take place. For one-on-one interviews, in-home interviews are often preferred because interviewers can then observe the participants' world and take observational notes. When in-home interviews are not desired by participants (e.g., if they prefer more privacy), it is wise to identify alternative suggestions, such as an office, coffee shop, and so on. The important thing is to select places that offer privacy, that protect insofar as possible against interruptions, and that are adequate for recording the interview. It is sometimes useful to let participants select the setting, but in some cases, the setting will be dictated by circumstances, as when interviews take place while participants are hospitalized.

The setting for focus group sessions should be selected carefully and, ideally, should be a neutral one. Churches, hospitals, or other settings that are strongly identified with particular values or expected behaviors may not be suitable, depending on the topic. The location should be comfortable, accessible, easy to find, and acoustically amenable to audio recording.

Most qualitative interviews are conducted in person, but new technologies have opened up other options. For example, videoconferencing makes it possible to conduct face-to-face interviews with participants remotely. Videoconferencing is advantageous from the perspective of having both a visual and auditory record of the interview.

Example of Video Interviews: Karlsson and colleagues (2012) used video-recorded interviews in their study of patients' experiences of receiving mechanical ventilation while conscious. The video camera was placed in front of the patient, beside the bed, so that facial expressions could be captured. The video interviews lasted between 3 and 16 minutes with an average time of 10 minutes.

A particularly important option is to conduct interviews using Skype or other synchronous online services, which have become widely available. Janghorban and colleagues (2014) have noted that such services can be used for both individual interviews and small focus group interviews. Such technologies are especially useful for gathering data from geographically dispersed participants or from people living in rural areas, without the financial burdens typically associated with such participants. Also, virtual focus groups open the door for including people who are unable or unwilling to participate in traditional focus groups that meet physically in a room. Liamputtong (2011) has described the many advantages of virtual focus groups. For example, in addition to being relatively inexpensive, participants' inhibitions are often lessened, anonymity can be enhanced, and pressures to conform can be reduced.

Study participants can also be "interviewed" asynchronously (not in real time) via e-mails, and asynchronous methods have also been used with focus groups. A distinct advantage of e-mail interviewing is that participants' narratives are already typed, thus avoiding the expense of transcribing taped interviews. Mann and Steward (2001) have offered advice about Internet interviewing.

Example of Internet Interviewing: Beck (the second author of this textbook) and Watson are currently conducting a phenomenologic study via the Internet about women's experiences of posttraumatic growth following a traumatic childbirth. A recruitment notice is posted on the website of Trauma and Birth Stress, a charitable trust in New Zealand, dedicated to supporting women who have experienced birth trauma. Women who are interested in participating e-contact Beck. Each woman is asked to respond to the following statement: "Please describe for us in as much detail as you can remember your experiences of any positive changes in your beliefs or life as a result of your traumatic childbirth. Any specific examples you can share about your posttraumatic growth will be extremely valuable in helping to educate clinicians so that they can provide better care to mothers who have experienced a traumatic childbirth."

➜ TIP: In an Internet environment, researchers need to devote time and effort to crafting individual e-mail responses to make sure all participants feel valued and understand that their narratives made a contribution to the study.

In-depth telephone interviews are also possible but are relatively rare. Novick (2008) has speculated about a bias against telephone interviews among qualitative researchers. The argument against telephone interviews concerns the absence of visual cues—although that is also true in asynchronous Internet interviews.

Preparing for In-Depth Interviews

Although qualitative interviews are conversational, this does not mean that they are entered into casually. The conversations are purposeful ones that require advance preparation. For example, careful thought should be given to the wording of questions. To the extent possible, the wording should make sense to respondents and reflect their worldview. Researchers and respondents should, for example, have a common vocabulary. If the researcher is studying a different culture or a group that uses distinctive terms or slang, efforts should be made before data collection begins to understand those terms and their nuances.

Researchers usually prepare for the interview by developing, mentally or in writing, the broad questions to be asked (or the initial questions, in unstructured interviews). Sometimes it is useful to do a practice interview with a stand-in respondent. If there are sensitive questions, it is a good idea to ask them late in the interview after rapport has been established.

> **TIP:** Memorize central questions if you have written them out, so that you will be able to maintain eye contact with participants.

It is important to decide in advance how to present yourself—as a researcher, a nurse, an ordinary person like participants, a humble "learner," and so on. An advantage of assuming the nurse role is that people often trust nurses. Yet, people may be overly deferent if nurses are perceived as better educated or more knowledgeable than they are. Moreover, participants may use the interview as an opportunity to ask health questions or to solicit opinions about particular health practitioners. Jack (2008) provided some guidelines to support nurse researchers in their reflection on this role conflict in qualitative interviewing.

For interviews done in the field, researchers must anticipate needs for equipment and supplies. Preparing a checklist of all such items is helpful. The checklist typically would include recording equipment, batteries or chargers, consent and demographic forms, notepads, and pens. Other possibilities include laptop computers or tablets, incentive payments, cookies or donuts to help break the ice, and distracting toys or books if children will be home. It may be necessary to bring proper identification to assure participants of the legitimacy of the visit. And, if the topic under study is likely to elicit emotional narratives, tissues should be readily at hand.

> **TIP:** It is wise to use high-quality equipment to ensure proper recording. For example, for recording interviews, make sure that the microphone is adequately sensitive for the acoustics of the environment, or use lapel microphones for both respondents and interviewers.

Conducting the Interview

Qualitative interviews are typically long, sometimes lasting hours. Researchers often find that the respondents' construction of their experience begins to emerge after lengthy, in-depth dialogues. Interviewers must prepare respondents for the interview by putting them at ease. Part of this process involves sharing pertinent information about the study (e.g., about confidentiality), and another part is using the first few minutes for ice-breaking exchanges of conversation before actual questioning begins. Up-front "small talk" can help to overcome stage fright, which can occur for both interviewers and respondents. Participants may be particularly nervous when interviews are being recorded. They typically forget about the recorder after the interview is underway, so the first few minutes should be used to help both parties "settle in."

Study participants will not share much information with interviewers they do not trust. Close rapport with respondents provides access to richer information and to intimate details of their stories. Interviewer personality plays a role in developing rapport: Good interviewers are usually congenial people who have the ability to see the situation from the respondent's perspective. Nonverbal communication can be critical in conveying concern and interest. Facial expressions, nods, and so on, help to set the tone for the interview. Gaglio and colleagues (2006) offered some insights concerning the development of rapport in primary care settings.

The most critical interviewing skill for in-depth interviews is being a good listener. It is especially important not to interrupt respondents, to "lead" them, to offer advice or opinions, or to counsel them. The interviewer's job is to listen intently to the respondents' stories. Only by attending carefully to what respondents are saying can interviewers develop appropriate follow-up questions. Even when a topic guide is used, interviewers must not let the flow of dialogue be bound by those questions.

> **TIP:** In-depth interviewers must be comfortable with pauses and silences and should let participants set the pace. Interviewers can encourage respondents with nonspecific prompts, such as "Mmhm."

Interviewers need to be prepared for strong emotions, such as anger, fear, or grief, to surface. Narrative disclosures can "bring it all back" for respondents, which can be a cathartic or therapeutic experience if interviewers create an atmosphere of concern and caring—but it can also be stressful.

Interviewers may need to manage potential crises during the interviews (MacDonald & Greggans, 2008). One frequent problem is the failed or improper recording of the interview. Thus, even when interviews are recorded, notes should be taken immediately after the interview to ensure the highest possible reliability of data and to prevent total information loss. Interruptions (usually the telephone) and other distractions are another common problem when interviewing in participants' homes. If respondents are willing, telephones can be controlled by unplugging them or turning them off in the case of cell phones. Interruptions by personal intrusions of friends or family members may be more difficult to manage. In some cases, the interview may need

to be terminated and rescheduled—for example, when a woman is discussing domestic violence and the perpetrator enters and stays in the room.

Interviewers should strive for positive closure to interviews. The last questions in in-depth interviews should usually be along these lines: "Is there anything else you would like to tell me?" or "Are there any other questions that you think I should have asked you?" Such probes can often elicit a wealth of important information. In closing, interviewers normally ask respondents whether they would mind being contacted again, in the event that additional questions come to mind after reflecting on the information, or in case interpretations of the information need to be verified.

> **TIP:** It is usually unwise to schedule back-to-back interviews. It is important not to rush or cut short the first interview to be on time for the next one, and you may be too emotionally drained to do a second interview in 1 day. It is also important to have an opportunity to write out notes, impressions, and analytic ideas, and it is best to do this when an interview is fresh in your mind.

Postinterview Procedures

Recorded interviews should be listened to and checked for audibility and completeness soon after the interview is over. If there have been problems with the recording, the interview should be reconstructed in as much detail as possible. Listening to the interview may also suggest possible follow-up questions that could be asked if respondents are recontacted. Morse and Field (1995) recommend that interviewers listen to the recordings objectively and critique their own interviewing style, so that improvements can be made in subsequent interviews.

Steps also need to be taken to ensure that interview transcriptions are done with rigor. It is prudent to hire experienced transcribers, to check the quality of initial transcriptions, and to give the transcribers feedback. Transcribers can sometimes unwittingly change the meaning of text by misspelling words, omitting words, or not adequately entering information about pauses, laughter, crying, or speech volume (see the Supplement to Chapter 24 **S** for more information about transcriptions). Transcriptionists, like interviewers, can be affected by hearing heart-wrenching interviews. Researchers may need to warn transcriptionists about upcoming interviews that are particularly stressful and allow transcribers the opportunity to talk about their reaction to interviews (Lalor et al., 2006).

> ➔ **TIP:** Transcriptions can be the most expensive part of a study. It generally takes about 4-5 hours of transcription time for every hour of interviewing. New and improved voice recognition computer software may help with transcribing interviews.

Evaluation of Qualitative Self-Report Approaches

In-depth interviews are an extremely flexible approach to gathering data and, in many research contexts, offer distinct advantages. In clinical situations, for example, it is often appropriate to let people talk freely about their problems and concerns, allowing them to take much of the initiative in directing the flow of information. Unstructured self-reports may allow investigators to ascertain what the basic issues or problems are, how sensitive or controversial the topic is, how individuals conceptualize and talk about the problems, and what range of opinions or behaviors exist relevant to the topic. In-depth interviews may also help elucidate the underlying meaning of a pattern or relationship repeatedly observed in more structured research. On the other hand, qualitative methods are extremely time-consuming and demanding of researchers' skills in gathering, analyzing, and interpreting the resulting data.

UNSTRUCTURED OBSERVATION

Qualitative researchers sometimes collect loosely structured observational data, often as an important supplement to self-report data. The aim of their research is to understand the behaviors and experiences of people as they actually occur in naturalistic settings.

Unstructured observational data are most often gathered in field settings through **participant observation**. Participant observers participate in the functioning of the social group under investigation and strive to observe, ask questions, and record information within the contexts and structures that are relevant to group members. Participant observation is characterized by prolonged periods of social interaction between researchers and participants, in the participants' sociopolitical and cultural milieu.

Example of Participant Observation: In their focused ethnography, Gustafsson and colleagues (2013) explored the everyday work undertaken by Swedish case managers of older persons with multiple morbidities. Nine case managers were interviewed and observed (125 hours of observation). Participant observations "were performed as part of the case managers' everyday work, during their weekly follow-up meetings and during reflective meetings" (p. 4).

Not all qualitative observational research is *participant* observation (i.e., with observations occurring from *within* the group under study). Some unstructured observations involve watching and recording behaviors without the observers participating in activities.

Example of Unstructured Nonparticipant Observation: Leach and Mayo (2013) conducted a grounded theory study of the effectiveness of rapid response teams from team members' perspectives. In addition to interviews with 17 informants, the researchers observed nine events that involved a rapid response team and that occurred on different days of the week.

Nevertheless, if a key research objective is to learn how group interactions and activities give meaning to human behaviors and experiences, then participant observation is an appropriate method. The members of any group or culture are influenced by assumptions they take for granted, and observers can, through active participation as members, gain access to these assumptions. Participant observation is most often used by ethnographers, grounded theory researchers, and researchers with ideologic perspectives.

The Observer–Participant Role in Participant Observation

The role that observers play in the groups under study is important because the observers' social position determines what they are likely to see. That is, the behaviors that are likely to be available for observation depend on observers' position in a network of relations.

McFarland and Wehbe-Alamah (2015), in describing Leininger's methods, depicted a participant observer's role as evolving through a four-phase sequence:

1. Primarily observation and active listening
2. Primarily observation with limited participation
3. Primarily participation with continued observation
4. Primary reflection and reconfirmation of findings with informants

In the initial phase, researchers observe and listen to those under study to obtain a broad view of the situation. This phase allows both observers and the observed to "size up" each other, to become acquainted, and to become comfortable interacting. This first phase involves "learning the ropes." In the next phase, observation is enhanced by a modest degree of participation. By participating in the group's activities, researchers can study not only people's behaviors but also people's reactions to them. In phase 3, researchers become more active participants, learning by the actual experience of doing rather than just by watching and listening. In phase 4, researchers reflect on what transpired and how people interacted with and reacted to them.

Junker (1960) described a somewhat different continuum that does not assume an evolving process: complete participant, participant as observer, observer as participant, and complete observer. Complete participants conceal their identity as researchers, entering the group ostensibly as regular members. For example, a nurse researcher might accept a job as a clinical nurse with the express intent of studying, in a concealed fashion, some aspect of the clinical environment. At the other extreme, complete observers do not attempt participation in the group's activities but rather make observations as outsiders. At both extremes, observers may have difficulty asking probing questions—albeit for different reasons.

Complete participants may arouse suspicion if they make inquiries not congruent with a total participant role, and complete observers may not have personal access to, or the trust of, those being observed. Most observational fieldwork lies in between these two extremes and usually shifts over time.

Example of Participant Observer Roles:
Dupuis-Blanchard and colleagues (2009) conducted an ethnographic study about social engagement in elders relocated to senior-designated apartments. Here is what they said about their participant observation: ". . . The researcher observed the senior-designated apartment building's environment for day-to-day transactions . . ., followed by the observation of events in the environment. In a low-key manner, the researcher tried to become part of the subculture being studied . . . by engaging in participant observation of older adults during specific events or activities to identify attributes and behaviors of the culture" (p. 1189).

➔ **TIP:** Being a fully participating member of a group does not *necessarily* offer the best perspective for studying a phenomenon—just as being an actor in a play does not offer the most advantageous view of the performance.

Getting Started

Observers must overcome at least two initial hurdles: gaining entrée into the social group or culture under study, and establishing rapport and developing trust within the social group. Without gaining entrée, the study cannot proceed; but without the group's trust, researchers could be restricted to "front stage" knowledge (Leininger, 1985), that is, information distorted by the group's protective facades. The observer's goal is to "get backstage"—to learn about the realities of the group's experiences and behaviors. This section discusses some practical and interpersonal aspects of getting started in the field.

Gaining an Overview

Before fieldwork begins, or in the earliest stage of fieldwork, it is usually useful to gather some written or pictorial descriptive information that provides an overview of the setting. In an institutional setting, for example, it is helpful to obtain a floor plan, an organizational chart, an annual report, and so on. Then, a preliminary personal tour of the setting should be undertaken to gain familiarity with its ambiance and to note major activities, social groupings, and transactions.

In community studies, ethnographers sometimes conduct a **windshield survey** (or *windshield tour*), which involves an intensive exploration (sometimes in an automobile, and hence the name) to "map" important features of the community under study. Such community mapping can include documenting community resources (e.g., churches, businesses, public transportation, community centers), community liabilities (e.g., vacant lots, empty stores, dilapidated buildings), and social and environmental characteristics (e.g., condition of streets and buildings, traffic patterns, types of signs, children playing in public places). A protocol for a windshield survey is included in the Toolkit of the accompanying *Resource Manual*.

Example of a Windshield Survey: Parra-Medina and Messias (2011) undertook an assessment of community assets and resources, and community members' experiences and values, with regard to participation in leisure physical activity among Mexican-origin women. One data source was windshield tours in two Latino communities.

Establishing Rapport

After gaining entrée into a setting and obtaining permissions and suggestions from gatekeepers, the next step is to enter the field. In some cases, it may be possible just to "blend in" or ease into a social group, but often researchers walk into a "head-turning" situation in which there is considerable curiosity because they stand out as strangers. Participant observers often find that, for their own comfort level and also for that of participants, it is best to have a brief, simple explanation about their presence. Except in rare cases, deception is neither necessary nor recommended, but vagueness has many advantages. People rarely want to know *exactly* what researchers are studying; they simply want an introduction and enough information to satisfy their curiosity and erase suspicions about the researchers' ulterior motives.

After initial introductions with members of the group, it is usually best to keep a fairly low profile. At the beginning, researchers are not yet familiar with the customs, language, and norms of the group, and it is critical to learn these things. Politeness and friendliness are essential, but ardent socializing is not appropriate at the early stages of fieldwork.

➲ TIP: Your initial job is to listen intently and learn what it takes to fit into the group, that is, what you need to do to become accepted as a member. To the extent possible, you should downplay any expertise you might have because you do not want to distance yourself from participants. Your overall goal is to gain people's trust and to move relationships to a deeper level.

As rapport is developed and trust is established, researchers can play a more active participatory role and collect observational data in earnest.

Gathering Unstructured Observational Data

Participant observers typically place few restrictions on the nature of the data collected, in keeping with the goal of minimizing observer-imposed meanings and structure. Nevertheless, participant observers often have a broad plan for the types of information to be gathered. Among aspects likely to be considered relevant are the following:

1. *The physical setting*. What are key features of the setting? What is the context within which human behavior unfolds? What behaviors and characteristics are promoted (or constrained) by the physical environment?
2. *The participants*. What are the characteristics of the people being observed? How many people are there? What are their roles? Who is given free access to the setting—who "belongs"? What brings these people together?
3. *Activities and interactions*. What are people doing and saying? Is there a discernible progression of activities? How do people interact with one another? How—and how often—do

they communicate? What type of emotions do they show during their interactions? How are participants interconnected to one another or to activities underway?

4. *Frequency and duration.* When did the activity or event begin, and when is it scheduled to end? How much time has elapsed? Is the activity a recurring one, and if so, how regularly does it recur? How typical of such activities is the one that is under observation?

5. *Precipitating factors.* Why is the event or interaction happening? What contributes to how the event or interaction unfolds?

6. *Organization.* How is the event or interaction organized? How are relationships structured? What norms or rules are in operation?

7. *Intangible factors.* What did *not* happen (especially if it ought to have happened)? Are participants saying one thing verbally but communicating different messages nonverbally? What types of things were disruptive to the activity or situation?

Clearly, this is far more information than can be absorbed in a single session (and not all categories may be relevant to the research question). However, this framework provides a starting point for thinking about observational possibilities while in the field. (This list of features amenable to in-depth observation is included in the Toolkit 🛠 as a Word document.)

TIP: When we enter a social setting in our everyday lives, we unconsciously process many of the questions on this list. Usually, however, we do not consciously *attend* to our observations and impressions in any systematic way and are not careful about making note of the details that contribute to our impressions. This is precisely what participant observers must learn to do.

Spradley (1980) distinguished three levels of observation that typically occur during fieldwork. The first level, **descriptive observation**, tends to be broad and helps observers figure out what is going on. During these descriptive observations,

researchers make every attempt to observe as much as possible. Later in the inquiry, observers do **focused observations** on more carefully selected events and interactions. Based on the research aims and on what has been learned from descriptive observations, participant observers begin to focus more sharply on key aspects of the setting. From these focused observations, they may develop a system for organizing observations, such as a taxonomy or category system. **Selective observations** are the most highly focused and are undertaken to facilitate comparisons between categories or activities. Spradley describes these levels as analogous to a funnel, with an increasingly narrow and more systematic focus.

While in the field, participant observers have to decide how to sample observations and select observational locations. **Single positioning** means staying in a single location for a period to observe behaviors and transactions in that location. **Multiple positioning** involves moving around the site to observe behaviors from different locations. **Mobile positioning** involves following a person throughout a given activity or period. It is usually useful to use a combination of positioning approaches in selecting observational locations.

Because participant observers cannot spend a lifetime in one site and because they cannot be in more than one place at a time, observation is almost always supplemented with information from unstructured interviews or conversations. For example, key informants may be asked to describe what went on in a meeting that the observer was unable to attend or to describe events that occurred before the observer entered the field. In such a case, the informant functions as the observer's observer.

Recording Observations

Participant observers may be tempted to put more emphasis on the *participation* and *observation* parts of their research than on the recording of those activities. Without systematic recording of observational data, however, the project will flounder. Observational information cannot be trusted to memory; it must be diligently recorded as soon after the observations as possible.

Types of Observational Records

The most common forms of record keeping in participant observation are logs and field notes, but photographs and videorecordings may also be used. A **log** (or **field diary**) is a daily record of events and conversations in the field. A log is a chronologic listing of how researchers have spent their time and can be used for planning, for keeping track of expenses, and for reviewing what work has already been completed. Box 23.1 presents an example of a log entry from Beck's (2002) study of mothers of multiples (i.e., twins).

Field notes are broader, more analytic, and more interpretive than a simple listing of occurrences. Field notes represent the participant observer's efforts to record information and also to synthesize and understand the data.

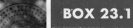 **TIP:** Field notes are important in many types of studies, not just in studies involving participant observation. For example, field notes are critical in grounded theory studies, process evaluations, and in inquiries relating to intervention fidelity.

The Content of Field Notes

Participant observers' field notes contain a narrative account of what is happening in the field; they serve as the data for analysis. Most "field" notes are not written while observers are literally in the field but rather are written after an observational session in the field has been completed.

Field notes are usually lengthy and time-consuming to prepare. Observers need to discipline themselves to provide a wealth of detail, the meaning and importance of which may not emerge for weeks. Descriptions of what has transpired must include enough contextual information about time, place, and actors to portray the situation fully. *Thick description* is the goal for participation observers' field notes (as it is in describing a completed qualitative study).

TIP: Especially in the early stages of fieldwork, a general rule of thumb is this: When in doubt, write it down.

Field notes are both descriptive and reflective. **Descriptive notes** (or **observational notes**) are objective descriptions of observed events and conversations; information about actions, dialogue, and context are recorded as completely and objectively as possible. Sometimes descriptive notes are recorded on loosely structured forms analogous to topic guides to ensure that key information is captured.

BOX 23.1 Example of a Log Entry: Mothering Multiples Grounded Theory Study

Log entry for Mothers of Multiples Support Group Meeting (Beck, 2002)
July 15, 1999 10–11:30 AM

This is my fourth meeting that I have attended. Nine mothers came this morning with their twins. One other woman attended. She was pregnant with twins. She came to the support group for advice from the other mothers regarding such issues as what type of stroller to buy, etc. All the moms sat on the floor with their infants placed on blankets on the floor next to them. Toddlers and older children played together off to the side with a box of toys. I sat next to a mom new to the group with her twin 4-month-old girls. I helped her hold and feed one of the twins. On my other side was a mom who had signed up at the last meeting to participate in my study. I hadn't called her yet to set up an appointment. She asked how my research was going. We then set up an appointment for next Thursday at 10 AM at her home for me to interview her. The new mother that I sat next to also was eager to participate in the study. In fact, she said we could do the interview right after the meeting ends today, but I couldn't due to another meeting. We scheduled an interview appointment for next Thursday at 1 PM. I also set up a third appointment for an interview for next week with I.K. for Monday at 1 PM. She had participated in an earlier study of mine. She came right over to me this morning at the support group meeting.

Reflective notes, which document the researcher's personal experiences, reflections, and progress while in the field, can serve several purposes:

- **Methodologic notes** are reflections about observational strategies. Sometimes observers do things that do not "work," and methodologic notes document thoughts about new approaches or about why a strategy was especially effective. Methodologic notes also can provide instructions or reminders about how subsequent observations will be made.
- **Theoretical notes** (or **analytical notes**) document researchers' thoughts about how to make sense of what is going on. These notes serve as a starting point for subsequent analysis.
- **Personal notes** are comments about researchers' own feelings in the field. Almost inevitably, field experiences give rise to personal emotions and challenge researchers' assumptions. It is essential to reflect on such feelings because there is no other way to know whether the feelings are influencing what is being observed or what is being done in the participant role. Personal notes can also contain reflections relating to ethical dilemmas.

Box 23.2 presents examples of various types of field notes from Beck's (2002) study of mothering multiples.

Reflective notes are typically not integrated into the descriptive notes but are kept separately as parallel notes; they may be maintained in a journal or series of self-memos. Strauss and Corbin (1990) argue that these reflective memos or journals help researchers to achieve analytic distance from the actual data and therefore play a critical role in the project's success.

➔ **TIP:** Personal notes should begin even before entering the field. By recording your feelings, assumptions, and expectations, you will have a baseline against which to compare feelings and experiences that emerge in the field.

The Process of Writing Field Notes

The success of participant observation depends on the quality of the field notes, and timing is important to quality. Field notes should be written as soon as possible after an observation is made. The longer the interval between an observation and field note preparation, the greater the risk of forgetting or distorting the data. If the delay is long, intricate details will be lost; moreover, memory of what was observed may be biased by things that happened subsequently.

➔ **TIP:** Be sure not to talk to anyone about your observation before you have had a chance to write up the observational notes. Such discussions could color what you record.

Participant observers cannot usually write their field notes while they are in the field, in part because this would distract them from their job of being keen observers, and also because it would undermine their role as ordinary group members. Researchers must develop the skill of making detailed mental notes that can later be committed to a permanent record. In addition, observers usually try to jot down unobtrusively a phrase or sentence that will later serve as a reminder of an event, conversation, or impression. Many experienced field-workers use the tactic of frequent trips to the bathroom to record these **jottings**, either in a small notebook or onto a recording device. With the widespread use of cell phones, researchers can also excuse themselves to make a call and "phone in" their jottings. Observers use jottings and mental recordings to develop more extensive field notes.

➔ **TIP:** It is important to schedule enough time to record field notes after an observation. An hour of observation can take 3 or 4 hours to record, so advance planning is essential. Try to find a quiet place for recording field notes, preferably a location where you can work undisturbed for several hours. Most researchers record field notes onto computers or tablets.

BOX 23.2 Example of Field Notes: Mothering Multiples Grounded Theory Study

Observational Notes: O.L. attended the mothers of multiples support group again this month but she looked worn out today. She wasn't as bubbly as she had been at the March meeting. She explained why she wasn't doing as well this month. She and her husband had just found out that their house has lead-based paint in it. Both twins do have increased lead levels. She and her husband are in the process of buying a new home.

Theoretical Notes: So far, all the mothers have stressed the need for routine in order to survive the first year of caring for twins. Mothers, however, have varying definitions of routine. I.R. had the firmest routine with her twins. B.L. is more flexible with her routine, i.e., the twins are always fed at the same time but aren't put down for naps or bed at night at the same time. Whenever one of the twins wants to go to sleep is fine with her. B.L. does have a daily routine in regards to housework. For example, when the twins are down in the morning for a nap, she makes their bottles up for the day (14 bottles total).

Methodologic Notes: The first sign-up sheet I passed around at the Mothers of Multiples Support Group for women to sign up to participate in interviews for my grounded theory study only consisted of two columns: one for the mother's name and one for her telephone number. I need to revise this sign-up sheet to include extra columns for the age of the multiples, the town where the mother lives, and older siblings and their ages. My plan is to start interviewing mothers with multiples around 1 year of age so that the moms can reflect back over the process of mothering their infants for the first 12 months of their lives.

Right now, I have no idea of the ages of the infants of the mothers who signed up to be interviewed. I will need to call the nurse in charge of this support group to find out the ages.

Personal Notes: Today was an especially challenging interview. The mom had picked the early afternoon for me to come to her home to interview her because that is the time her 2-year-old son would be napping. When I arrived at her house, her 2-year-old ran up to me and said hi. The mom explained that he had taken an earlier nap that day and that he would be up during the interview. So in the living room with us during our interview were her two twin daughters (3 months old) swinging in the swings and her 2-year-old son. One of the twins was quite cranky for the first half hour of the interview. During the interview, the 2-year-old sat on my lap and looked at the two books I had brought as a little present. If I didn't keep him occupied with the books, he would keep trying to reach for the microphone of the tape recorder.

From Beck, C.T. (2002). Releasing the pause button: Mothering twins during the first year of life. *Qualitative Health Research, 12*, 593–608.

Observational field notes need to be as complete and detailed as possible. This means that hundreds of pages of field notes typically will be created, and so systems need to be developed for managing them. For example, each entry should have the date and time the observation was made, the location, and the name of the observer (if several are working as a team). It is useful to give observational sessions a name that will trigger a memory (e.g., "Emotional Outburst by a Patient with Ovarian Cancer").

Thought also needs to be given to how to record participants' dialogue. The goal is to record conversations as accurately as possible, but it is not always possible to make verbatim recordings if researchers are trying to maintain a stance as regular participating group members. Procedures need to be developed to distinguish different levels of accuracy in recording dialogue (e.g., by using quotation marks and italics for true verbatim recordings, and a different designation for paraphrasings).

➔ **TIP:** Observation, participation, and record keeping are exhausting, labor-intensive activities. It is important to establish the proper pace of these activities to ensure the highest possible quality notes for analysis.

Evaluation of Participant Observation

Participant observation can provide a deeper and richer understanding of human behaviors and social situations than is possible with structured procedures. Participant observation is particularly valuable for its ability to "get inside" a situation and provide understanding of its complexities. Furthermore, this approach is inherently flexible and therefore gives observers the freedom to reconceptualize problems after becoming more familiar with the situation. Participant observation is a good method for answering questions about phenomena that are difficult for insiders to explain because these phenomena are taken for granted.

Like all research methods, however, participant observation faces potential problems. Observer bias and observer influence are prominent risks. Observers may lose objectivity in viewing and recording observations; they may also inappropriately sample events and situations to be observed. Once researchers begin to participate in a group's activities, the possibility of emotional involvement becomes a salient concern. Researchers in their member role may fail to attend to scientifically relevant aspects of the situation or may develop a myopic view on issues of importance to the group. Participant observation may thus be an unsuitable approach when the risk of identification is strong. Another important issue concerns the ethical dilemmas that often emerge in participant observation studies. Finally, the success of participant observation depends on the observer's observational and interpersonal skills—skills that may be difficult to cultivate.

On the whole, participant observation and other unstructured observational methods are extremely profitable for in-depth research in which researchers wish to develop a comprehensive description and conceptualization of phenomena within a social setting or culture.

➔ **TIP:** Although this chapter emphasized the two most frequently used methods of collecting unstructured data (self-reports and observation), we encourage you to think about other data sources, such as documents. Miller and Alvarado (2005) offer useful suggestions for incorporating documents into qualitative nursing research.

CRITIQUING THE COLLECTION OF UNSTRUCTURED DATA

It is usually not easy to critique the decisions that researchers have made in collecting qualitative data because details about those decisions are seldom spelled out in research reports. In particular, there is often scant information about participant observation. It is not uncommon for a report to simply say that the researcher undertook participant observation, without descriptions of how much time was spent in the field, what exactly was observed, how observations were recorded, and what level of participation was involved. In fact, we suspect that many projects described as having used a participant observation approach were unstructured observations with little actual participation. Thus, one aspect of a critique is likely to involve an appraisal of how much information the research report provided about the data collection methods used. Even though space constraints in journals make it impossible for researchers to fully elaborate their methods, researchers have a responsibility to communicate basic information about their approach so that readers can assess the quality of evidence that the study yields. Researchers should provide examples of questions asked and types of observations made.

As we discuss more fully in Chapter 25, triangulation of methods provides important opportunities for qualitative researchers to enhance the quality of their data. Thus, an important issue to consider in evaluating unstructured data is whether the types and amount of data collected are sufficiently rich to support an in-depth, holistic understanding of the phenomena under study. Box 23.3 ✪ provides

BOX 23.3 Guidelines for Critiquing Unstructured Data Collection Methods

1. Was the collection of unstructured data appropriate to the study aims?
2. Given the research question and the characteristics of study participants, did the researcher use the best method of capturing study phenomena (i.e., self-reports, observation)? Should supplementary data collection methods have been used to enrich the data available for analysis?
3. If self-report methods were used, did the researcher make good decisions about the specific method used to solicit information (e.g., focus group interviews, semistructured interviews, and so on)? Was the modality of obtaining the data appropriate (e.g., in-person interviews, telephone interviews, Internet questioning)?
4. If a topic guide was used, did the report present examples of specific questions? Were the questions appropriate and comprehensive? Did the wording minimize the risk of biases? Did the wording encourage full and rich responses?
5. Were interviews recorded and transcribed? If interviews were not recorded, what steps were taken to ensure the accuracy of the data?
6. Were self-report data gathered in a manner that promoted high-quality responses (e.g., in terms of privacy, efforts to put respondents at ease)? Who collected the data, and were they adequately prepared for the task?
7. If observational methods were used, did the report adequately describe what the observations entailed? What did the researcher actually observe, in what types of setting did the observations occur, and how often and over how long a period were observations made? Were decisions about positioning described? Were risks of observational bias addressed?
8. What role did the researcher assume in terms of being an observer and a participant? Was this role appropriate?
9. How were observational data recorded? Did the recording method maximize data quality?

guidelines for critiquing the collection of unstructured data.

RESEARCH EXAMPLE

This section provides an example of a qualitative study that collected a rich variety of unstructured data.

Study: Canadian adolescents' perspectives of cancer risks: A qualitative study (Woodgate et al., 2014)

Statement of Purpose: The purpose of this study was to extend knowledge about Canadian adolescents' perspectives of cancer and cancer prevention, including how they conceptualize and understand cancer risk. The goal was to gain an understanding of how best to develop meaningful health promotion and cancer prevention programs for adolescents.

Design: The researchers used an ethnographic approach that involved the use of multiple data collec-

tion methods. A purposive sample of 75 adolescents was recruited, with efforts to "maximize variation in demographic . . . and cancer experiences" (p. 3). Recruitment and analysis occurred concurrently, and recruitment ended when saturation was achieved. The study took place over a 3-year period.

Data Collection: Two face-to-face interviews were planned for each adolescent, with the second one scheduled 4–5 weeks after the first. The second interview was intended to ensure "thick description" and to provide an opportunity for follow-up questions that helped to clarify issues identified in the initial interview. Each interview, lasting between 60 and 90 minutes, was digitally recorded and transcribed. For the first interview, the topic guide included general questions about cancer risk and prevention (e.g., "How do people get cancer?). Photovoice methods were also introduced. The participants were given cameras and were asked to take pictures of what they felt depicted cancer, cancer risks, and cancer prevention over a period of a month. Then, in the second interview, the adolescents were asked to describe what the photos meant to them. They were guided by such questions as, "How does this [picture] relate to cancer?" (p. 4). Finally, four focus group interviews were conducted with adolescents who were previously interviewed "to complement existing findings and gather new group-based knowledge on cancer risks" (p. 4). Field notes were maintained to describe verbal and nonverbal behaviors of participants after both individual and focus group interviews.

Key Findings: The adolescents conceptualized cancer risk in terms of specific risk factors; lifestyle factors (e.g., smoking) were prominent. They rationalized risky health behaviors using a variety of cognitive strategies that helped to make cancer risks more acceptable to them. However, they did believe that it was possible for individuals to delay getting cancer by making the right choices.

SUMMARY POINTS

- Qualitative studies typically adopt flexible data collection plans that evolve as the study progresses. Self-reports are the most frequently used type of data in qualitative studies, followed by observation. Ethnographies are likely to combine these two data sources with others such as the products of the culture (e.g., photographs, documents, artifacts).

- Qualitative researchers often confront such fieldwork issues as gaining participants' trust, pacing data collection to avoid being overwhelmed by the intensity of data, avoiding emotional involvement with participants ("**going native**"), and maintaining reflexivity (awareness of the part they play in the study and possible effects on their data).

- Qualitative researchers need to plan in advance for how their data will be recorded and stored. If technical equipment is used (e.g., audio recorders, video recorders), care must be taken to select high-quality equipment that functions properly in the field.

- Unstructured and loosely structured self-reports, which offer respondents and interviewers lati-

tude in their questions and answers, yield rich narrative data for qualitative analysis.

- Methods of collecting qualitative self-report data include the following: (1) **unstructured interviews**, which are conversational discussions on the topic of interest; (2) **semistructured** (or **focused**) **interviews**, in which interviewers are guided by a **topic guide** of questions to be asked; (3) **focus group interviews**, which involve discussions with small, homogeneous groups; (4) **joint interviews**, which involve simultaneously talking with members of a dyad; (5) **diaries** and journals, in which respondents maintain ongoing records about some aspects of their lives; (6) **photo elicitation interviews**, which are stimulated and guided by photographic images; and (7) narrative communications available on the Internet. Additional methods include **life histories**, **oral histories**, **critical incident interviews**, and **think-aloud methods**.

- In preparing for in-depth interviews, researchers learn about the language and customs of participants, formulate broad questions, make decisions about how to present themselves, develop ideas about interview settings, and take stock of equipment needs.

- Most qualitative interviews take place in face-to-face situations, but technologic advances are making remote synchronous interviewing possible (e.g., via Skype).

- Conducting good in-depth interviews requires considerable skill in putting people at ease, developing trust, listening intently, and managing possible crises in the field.

- Qualitative researchers sometimes collect unstructured observational data, often through **participant observation**. Participant observers obtain information about the dynamics of social groups or cultures within members' own frame of reference.

- In the initial phase of participant observation studies, researchers are primarily observers gaining an understanding of the site, sometimes including *windshield surveys*. Researchers later become more active participants.

- Observations tend to become more focused over time, ranging from **descriptive observation** (broad observations) to **focused observation** of more carefully selected events or interactions, and then to **selective observations** designed to facilitate comparisons.

- Participant observers usually select events to be observed through a combination of **single positioning** (observing from a fixed location), **multiple positioning** (moving around the site to observe in different locations), and **mobile positioning** (following a person around a site).
- **Logs** of daily events and **field notes** are the major methods of recording unstructured observational data. Field notes are both descriptive and reflective.
- Descriptive notes (or **observational notes**) are detailed, objective accounts of what transpired in an observational session. Observers strive for detailed, thick description.
- **Reflective notes** include **methodologic notes** that document observers' thoughts about their strategies, **theoretical notes** (or **analytic notes**) that represent ongoing efforts to make sense of the data, and **personal notes** that document observers' feelings and experiences.
- In-depth unstructured data collection methods tend to yield data of considerable richness and are useful in gaining an understanding about little-researched phenomena, but they are time-consuming and yield a volume of data that are challenging to analyze.

STUDY ACTIVITIES

Chapter 23 of the *Resource Manual for Nursing Research: Generating and Assessing Evidence for Nursing Practice, 10th edition,* offers exercises and study suggestions for reinforcing concepts presented in this chapter. In addition, the following study questions can be addressed:

1. Identify which qualitative self-report methods might be appropriate for the following research problems and provide a rationale:
   a. What are the coping strategies of parents whose child has a brain tumor?
   b. How do nurses in emergency departments make decisions about their activities?
   c. What are the health beliefs and practices of Filipino immigrants in the United States?
   d. What is it like to experience having a family member undergo open heart surgery?
2. Suppose you were interested in observing fathers' behavior in the delivery room during the birth of their first child. Identify the observer–observed relationship that you would recommend adopting for such a study and defend your recommendation. What are the possible drawbacks of your approach, and how might you deal with them?
3. Apply relevant questions in Box 23.3 to the research example at the end of the chapter (Woodgate et al., 2014), referring to the full open-access journal article as necessary.

STUDIES CITED IN CHAPTER 23

Asenhed, L., Kilstam, J., Alehagen, S., & Baggens, C. (2014). Becoming a father is an emotional roller coaster—An analysis of first-time fathers' blogs. *Journal of Clinical Nursing, 23,* 1309–1317.

Beck, C. T. (2002). Releasing the pause button: Mothering twins during the first year of life. *Qualitative Health Research, 12,* 593–608.

Bevan, M. T. (2014). A method of phenomenological interviewing. *Qualitative Health Research, 24,* 136–144.

Carey, M. A., & Asbury, J. (2012). *Focus group research.* Walnut Creek, CA: Left Coast Press.

*Chen, H., & Habermann, B. (2013). Ready or not: Planning for health declines in couples with advanced multiple sclerosis. *Journal of Neuroscience Nursing, 45,* 38–43.

Côté-Arsenault, D., & Morrison-Beedy, D. (1999). Practical advice for planning and conducting focus groups. *Nursing Research, 48,* 280–283.

Côté-Arsenault, D., & Morrison-Beedy, D. (2005). Maintaining your focus in focus groups: Avoiding common mistakes. *Research in Nursing & Health, 28,* 172–179.

Curtis, R., Groarke, A., McSharry, J., & Kerin, M. (2014). Experience of breast cancer: Burden, benefit, or both? *Cancer Nursing, 37,* E21–E30.

Davies, R. B. (2010). Pain in children with Down syndrome: Assessment and intervention by parents. *Pain Management Nursing, 11,* 259–267.

Dupuis-Blanchard, S., Neufeld, A., & Strang, V. (2009). The significance of social engagement in relocated older adults. *Qualitative Health Research, 19,* 1186–1195.

Fitzpatrick, J. J., & Montgomery, K. S. (2004). *Internet for nursing research: A guide to strategies, skills, and resources.* New York: Springer.

Fontana, A., & Frey, J. H. (2003). The interview: From structured questions to negotiated text. In N. K. Denzin & Y. S. Lincoln (Eds.), *Collecting and interpreting qualitative materials* (pp. 61–106). Thousand Oaks, CA: Sage.

Frith, H., & Harcourt, D. (2007). Using photographs to capture women's experiences with chemotherapy: Reflecting on the method. *Qualitative Health Research, 17,* 1340–1350.

Gaglio, B., Nelson, C., & King, D. (2006). The role of rapport: Lessons learned from conducting research in a primary care setting. *Qualitative Health Research, 16,* 723–734.

Glaser, B. G., & Strauss, A. (1967). *The discovery of grounded theory: Strategies for qualitative research.* New York: Aldine de Gruyter.

Gubrium, J. F., Holstein, J. A., Marvasti, A., & McKinney, K. (Eds.). (2012). *The Sage handbook of interview research: The complexity of the craft* (2nd ed.). Thousand Oaks, CA: Sage.

*Gustafsson, M., Kristensson, J., Holst, G., Willman, A., & Bohman, D. (2013). Case managers for older persons with multi-morbidity and their everyday work—A focused ethnography. *BMC Health Services Research, 13,* 496.

Hall, W. A., Long, B., Bermbach, N., Jordan, S., & Patterson, K. (2005). Qualitative teamwork issues and strategies: Coordination through mutual adjustment. *Qualitative Health Research, 15,* 394–410.

Heilferty, C. M. (2011). Ethical considerations in the study of online illness narratives: A qualitative review. *Journal of Advanced Nursing, 67,* 945–953.

*Jack, S. (2008). Guidelines to support nurse-researchers reflect on role conflict in qualitative interviewing. *The Open Nursing Journal, 2,* 58–62.

*Janghorban, R., Latifinejad Roudsair, R., & Taghipour, A. (2014). Skype interviewing: The new generation of online synchronous interview in qualitative research. *International Journal of Qualitative Studies on Health and Well-being, 9,* 24152.

Junker, B. H. (1960). *Field work: An introduction to the social sciences.* Chicago: University of Chicago Press.

Kahn, D. L. (2000). How to conduct research. In M. Z. Cohen, D. L. Kahn, & R. H. Steeves (Eds.), *Hermeneutic phenomenological research* (pp. 57–70). Thousand Oaks, CA: Sage.

Karlsson, V., Lindahl, B., & Bergbom, I. (2012). Patients' statements and experiences concerning receiving mechanical ventilation: A prospective video-recorded study. *Nursing Inquiry, 19,* 247–258.

Keim-Malpass, J., Steeves, R., & Kennedy, C. (2014). Internet ethnography: A review of methodological considerations for studying online illness blogs. *International Journal of Nursing Studies, 51,* 1686–1692.

Kidd, P. S., & Parshall, M. B. (2000). Getting the focus and the group: Enhancing analytic rigor in focus group research. *Qualitative Health Research, 10,* 293–308.

*Kieft, R., de Brouwer, B., Francke, A., & Delnoij, D. (2014). How nurses and their work environment affect patient experiences of the quality of care. *BMC Health Services, 14,* 249.

Kralik, D., Proce, K., Warren, J., & Koch, T. (2006). Issues in data generation using email group conversations for nursing research. *Journal of Advanced Nursing, 53,* 213–220.

Krueger, R., & Casey, M. (2015). *Focus groups: A practical guide for applied research* (5th ed.). Thousand Oaks, CA: Sage.

Lalor, J. G., Begley, C., & Devane, D. (2006). Exploring painful experiences: Impact of emotional narratives on members of a qualitative research team. *Journal of Advanced Nursing, 56,* 607–616.

*Leach, L., & Mayo, A. (2013). Rapid response teams: Qualitative analysis of their effectiveness. *American Journal of Critical Care, 22,* 198–210.

Leininger, M. M. (Ed.). (1985). *Qualitative research methods in nursing.* New York: Grune & Stratton.

Liamputtong, P. (2011). *Focus group methodology: Principles and practice.* Los Angeles, CA: Sage.

Lipson, J. G. (1991). The use of self in ethnographic research. In J. M. Morse (Ed.), *Qualitative nursing research: A contemporary dialog* (pp. 73–89). Newbury Park, CA: Sage.

MacDonald, K., & Greggans, A. (2008). Dealing with chaos and complexity: The reality of interviewing children and families in their own homes. *Journal of Clinical Nursing, 17,* 3123–3130.

Mann, C., & Steward, F. (2001). Internet interviewing. In J. F. Gubrium & J. A. Holstein (Eds.), *Handbook of interview research: Context and method* (pp. 603–627). Thousand Oaks, CA: Sage.

*Mao, A., Yang, T., Bottorff, J., & Sarbit, G. (2014). Personal and social determinants sustaining smoking practices in rural China. *International Journal for Equity in Health,12,* 12.

McFarland, M. R., & Wehbe-Alamah, H. B. (2015). *Leininger's culture care diversity and universality: A worldwide nursing theory.* Burlington, MA: Jones & Bartlett Learning.

Miller, F., & Alvarado, K. (2005). Incorporating documents into qualitative nursing research. *Journal of Nursing Scholarship, 37,* 348–353.

Montgomery, P., & Bailey, P. (2007). Field notes and theoretical memos in grounded theory. *Western Journal of Nursing Research, 29,* 65–79.

Morgan, D. L. (2001). Focus group interviewing. In J. F. Gubrium & J. A. Holstein (Eds.), *Handbook of interview research: Context and method* (2nd ed., pp. 141–159). Thousand Oaks, CA: Sage.

Morris, S. M. (2001). Joint and individual interviewing in the context of cancer. *Qualitative Health Research, 11,* 553–567.

Morrison-Beedy, D., Côté-Arsenault, D., & Feinstein, N. (2001). Maximizing results with focus groups. *Applied Nursing Research, 14,* 48–53.

Morse, J. M., & Field, P. A. (1995). *Qualitative research methods for health professionals* (2nd ed.). Thousand Oaks, CA: Sage.

Novick, G. (2008). Is there a bias against telephone interviews in qualitative research? *Research in Nursing & Health, 31,* 391–298.

Olausson, S., Ekebergh, M., & Österberg, S. (2014). Nurses' lived experiences of intensive care unit bed spaces as a place of care: A phenomenological study. *Nursing in Critical Care, 19*, 126–134.

Oliffe, J., Bottorff, J., Kelly, M., & Halpin, M. (2008). Analyzing participant produced photographs from an ethnographic study of fatherhood and smoking. *Research in Nursing & Health, 31*, 529–539.

*Parra-Medina, D., & Messias, D. K. H. (2011). Promotion of physical activity among Mexican-origin women in Texas and South Carolina: An examination of social, cultural, economic, and environmental factors. *Quest, 63*,100–117.

*Rix, E. F., Barclay, L., & Wilson, S. (2014). Can a white nurse get it? "Reflexive practice" and the non-indigenous clinician/researcher working with Aboriginal people. *Rural and Remote Health, 14*, 2679.

Robinson, K. M. (2001). Unsolicited narratives from the Internet: A rich source of qualitative data. *Qualitative Health Research, 11*, 706–714.

Rubin, H., & Rubin, I. S. (2012). *Qualitative interviewing: The art of hearing data* (3rd ed.). Thousand Oaks, CA: Sage.

Spradley, J. (1979). *The ethnographic interview*. New York: Holt, Rinehart & Winston.

Spradley, J. P. (1980). *Participant observation*. New York: Holt, Rinehart & Winston.

Strauss, A., & Corbin, J. (1990). *Basics of qualitative research: Grounded theory procedures and techniques*. Newbury Park, CA: Sage.

Van Manen, M. (1990). *Researching lived experience: Human science for an action sensitive pedagogy*. Ontario, Canada: Althouse Press.

*Woodgate, R. L., Safipour, J., & Tailor, K. (2014). Canadian adolescents' perspectives of cancer risk: A qualitative study. *Health Promotion International*. Advance online publication. doi:10.1093/heapro/dau011

*Yousefi, H., Roshani, A., & Nazari, F. (2014). Experiences of the families concerning organ donation of a family member with brain death. *Iranian Journal of Nursing and Midwifery Research, 19*, 323–330.

A link to this open-access journal article is provided in the Toolkit for this chapter in the accompanying Resource Manual. 🔗

24 | Qualitative Data Analysis

Qualitative data take the form of such narrative materials as verbatim dialogue between an interviewer and a respondent, field notes of participant observers, and diaries kept by study participants. This chapter describes methods for analyzing such qualitative data.

INTRODUCTION TO QUALITATIVE ANALYSIS

The purpose of data analysis is to organize, provide structure to, and elicit meaning from data. In qualitative studies, data collection and data analysis often occur concurrently rather than after all data are collected. The search for important themes and concepts begins from the moment data collection gets underway.

Qualitative analysis is a labor-intensive activity that requires creativity, conceptual sensitivity, and sheer hard work. First, we discuss some general considerations relating to qualitative analysis.

Qualitative Analysis Challenges

Qualitative data analysis is a particularly challenging enterprise. There are no universal rules for analyzing qualitative data, and the absence of standard procedures makes it hard to explain how to do such analyses. It is also difficult for researchers to describe how their analysis was done in a report and to present findings in a way that their validity is apparent. Procedures described in the next chapter are

important tools for enhancing the trustworthiness of the analysis.

A second challenge of qualitative analysis is the enormous amount of work required. Qualitative analysts must organize and make sense of pages and pages of narrative materials. In a study by one of us (Polit), the data consisted of transcribed interviews with 100 poor women discussing life stressors and health problems. The transcriptions ranged from 30 to 50 pages, resulting in more than 3,000 pages that had to be read, reread, analyzed, and interpreted.

Another challenge comes in reducing data for reporting purposes. Quantitative results can often be summarized in a few tables. Qualitative researchers, by contrast, must balance the need to be concise with the need to maintain the richness and evidentiary value of their data.

TIP: Qualitative analyses are more difficult to *do* than quantitative ones, but qualitative findings are easier to understand than quantitative ones because the stories are told in everyday language. Qualitative analyses are often harder to evaluate critically than quantitative analyses, however, because readers cannot know if researchers adequately captured thematic patterns in the data.

The Qualitative Analysis Process

The analysis of qualitative data is an active and interactive process. Qualitative researchers typically scrutinize their data carefully and deliberatively, often reading the data over and over in search of meaning and understanding. Insights and theories cannot emerge until researchers become completely familiar with their data. Morse and Field (1995) noted that qualitative analysis is a "process of fitting data together, of making the invisible obvious, of linking and attributing consequences to antecedents. It is a process of conjecture and verification, of correction and modification, of suggestion and defense" (p. 126).

QUALITATIVE DATA MANAGEMENT AND ORGANIZATION

Qualitative analysis is supported by several tasks that help to manage the mass of narrative data.

Transcribing Qualitative Data

Audio-recorded interviews and field notes are major data sources in qualitative studies. Verbatim transcription of the recordings is a critical step in preparing for data analysis, and researchers need to ensure that transcriptions are accurate and that they validly reflect the interview experience. Researchers should begin data analysis with the best possible quality data, which requires careful training of transcribers, ongoing feedback, and continuous efforts to verify accuracy. The Supplement to this chapter on thePoint® offers guidance on transcribing qualitative data.

Developing a Coding Scheme

Qualitative analysis begins with data organization. Researchers must be able to gain access to parts of the data, without having repeatedly to reread the data set in its entirety. This phase of data analysis is essentially reductionist—data must be converted to smaller, more manageable units that can be retrieved and reviewed.

The most widely used procedure is to develop a coding scheme and then to code data. A preliminary coding system (called a *template*) is sometimes drafted before data collection, but more typically, qualitative analysts develop categories based on a scrutiny of actual data. There are no straightforward or easy guidelines for this task. Developing a high-quality coding scheme involves a careful reading of the data, with an eye to identifying underlying concepts and clusters of concepts. The nature of the codes may vary in level of detail or specificity as well as in level of abstraction.

Researchers whose aims are primarily descriptive tend to use codes that are fairly concrete. For example, the coding scheme may focus on differentiating various types of actions or events.

Example of a Descriptive Coding Scheme: Ersek and Jablonski (2014) studied the adoption of evidence-based pain practices in nursing homes. Data from focus group interviews with staff were coded into broad categories of facilitators and barriers within Donabedian's schema of structure, process, and outcome. For example, categories of barriers in the process group included provider mistrust, lack of time, and staff and family knowledge and attitudes.

Studies that are designed to develop a theory are more likely to involve abstract, conceptual categories. In creating conceptual categories, researchers must break the data into segments, closely examine them, and compare them to other segments for similarities and dissimilarities to determine what the meaning of those phenomena are. (This is part of the *constant comparison* process espoused in grounded theory research.) The researcher asks questions such as the following about discrete events, incidents, or statements:

What is this?
What is going on?
What does it stand for?
What else is like this?
What is this distinct from?

Important concepts that emerge from close examination of the data are then given a label that forms the basis for a category. These labels are necessarily abstractions, but they should be sufficiently graphic that the nature of the material to which they refer is clear—and, often, provocative.

Example of a Conceptual Coding Scheme:
Box 24.1 shows the category scheme developed by
Beck and Watson (2010) to code data from their Internet interviews on subsequent childbirth following a
previous traumatic birth. The coding scheme included
four major categories with subcodes. For example,
an excerpt that described how a mother felt that
this subsequent birth was healing because she felt
respected during this labor and delivery would be
coded 3A, the category for "treated with respect."

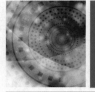

BOX 24.1 Beck and
Watson's (2010) Coding
Scheme for the Subsequent
Childbirth after a Previous
Traumatic Birth

TIP: A good coding scheme is critical to a
thoughtful analysis, and so a substantial sample
of the data should be read before the scheme is
drafted. To the extent possible, you should read
materials that vary along key dimensions to capture a range of content. The dimensions might
be informant characteristics (e.g., men versus
women) or aspects of the data collection experience (e.g., data from different interview contexts). Saldaña (2013) offers useful suggestions
on categorizing and coding qualitative data.

Coding Qualitative Data

Once a coding scheme has been developed, the data
are read in their entirety and coded for correspondence to the categories—a task that is seldom easy.
Researchers may have difficulty deciding the most
appropriate code or may not fully comprehend the
underlying meaning of some data segments. It may
take a second or third reading of the material to
grasp its nuances.

Researchers often discover during coding that the
initial categories were incomplete. It is common for
categories to emerge that were not initially identified.
When this happens, it is risky to assume that the category was absent in materials that have already been
coded. A concept might not be identified as salient
until it has emerged a few times. In such a case, it
would be necessary to reread all previously coded material to have a truly complete grasp of that category.

Another issue is that narrative materials usually
are not linear. For example, paragraphs from transcribed interviews may contain elements relating
to three or four different categories, embedded in a
complex fashion.

**THEME 1: RIDING THE TURBULENT WAVE
OF PANIC DURING PREGNANCY**

A. Reactions to learning of pregnancy
B. Denial during the first trimester
C. Heightened state of anxiety
D. Panic attacks as delivery date gets closer
E. Feeling numb toward the baby

**THEME 2: STRATEGIZING: ATTEMPTS TO
RECLAIM THEIR BODY AND COMPLETE
THE JOURNEY TO MOTHERHOOD**

A. Spending time nurturing self by exercising,
   going to yoga classes, and swimming
B. Keeping a journal throughout pregnancy
C. Turning to doulas for support during labor
D. Reading avidly to understand the birth process
E. Engaging in birth art exercises
F. Opening up to health care providers about
   their previous birth trauma
G. Sharing with partners about their fears
H. Learned relaxation techniques

**THEME 3: BRINGING REVERENCE
TO THE BIRTHING PROCESS AND
EMPOWERING WOMEN**

A. Treated with respect
B. Pain relief taken seriously
C. Communicated with labor and delivery staff
D. Reclaimed their body
E. Strong sense of control
F. Birth plan was honored by labor and
   delivery staff
G. Mourned what they missed out with prior birth
H. Healing subsequent birth but it can never
   change the past

**THEME 4: STILL ELUSIVE: THE LONGED
FOR HEALING BIRTH EXPERIENCE**

A. Failed again as a woman
B. Better than first traumatic birth but not healing
C. Hopes of a healing home birth dashed

Excerpt	Codes
"After 3 months of denying the fact that I was going to have to go through birth	1B
again I decided that I would treat my next labor and delivery as a healing and	
empowering experience. I wanted to get myself as physically ready for labor as	
possible so I focused on getting my body strong and my mind strong, too. I took	2A
antenatal yoga which helped me bond with my unborn son. I did stretching exercises	
and put an exercise plan in place. We hired a doula so I would have more support	2C
this time around in labor. I read many books and kept a journal so I could be fully	2B, 2D
informed about my choices for labor and delivery. I learned relaxation techniques to	
help me with all the anxiety I felt throughout the 9 long months of my pregnancy."	1C, 2H

FIGURE 24.1 Coded excerpt from Beck and Watson's (2010) study on subsequent childbirth after a previous traumatic birth.

Example of a Multitopic Segment: An example of a multitopic segment of an interview from Beck and Watson's (2010) phenomenologic study of subsequent childbirth after a previous birth trauma is shown in Figure 24.1. The codes in the margin represent codes from the scheme presented in Box 24.1.

It is sometimes recommended that a single person code the entire data set to ensure the highest possible coding consistency across interviews or observations, but team coding is recommended by others (e.g., de Casterlé et al., 2012). It may be prudent to have at least a portion of the interviews coded by two or more people early in the coding process to evaluate and enhance reliability.

Example of Teamwork in Coding: Hansen and colleagues (2012) studied life-sustaining treatment decisions in the ICU from the perspective of patients, family members, and ICU staff. Four researchers read transcripts and developed a codebook. Coding was also done by all four, in two dyadic pairs: "Members of a pair coded individually and then met with their coding partners weekly to discuss coding and come to consensus on discrepancies" (p. 522). Both pairs of coders met weekly as a group to review and audit the emerging findings.

TIP: It is wise to develop a codebook—written documentation describing the exact definition of the various categories used to code the

data. Good qualitative codebooks usually include one or more actual excerpts that typify materials coded in each category. The Toolkit section of the accompanying *Resource Manual* includes an example of a codebook from Beck's work.

Manual Methods of Organizing Qualitative Data

Traditional manual methods of organizing qualitative data are becoming less common as a result of the widespread use of software that can perform indexing functions. Here, we briefly describe some manual methods of data management; the next section describes computer methods.

Qualitative researchers sometimes use a file card system, placing significant statements from interviews on a file card of its own. The file cards are then sorted into piles representing themes. Some researchers use different-colored file cards for each person's data.

Before the advent of computer software for managing qualitative data, a typical procedure was to develop **conceptual files**. In this approach, researchers create a physical file folder for each category and insert material relating to that category into the file. Researchers first go through all the data, writing relevant codes in the margins, as in Figure 24.1. Then they cut up a copy of the material by category area and place the excerpts into the file for that category. All of the content on a particular topic then can be retrieved by going to the applicable file folder.

Creating such files is cumbersome, especially when segments of the narrative materials have multiple codes, as in Figure 24.1. For example, there would need to be seven copies of the paragraph, corresponding to the seven codes. Researchers must also provide enough context that the cut-up material can be understood (e.g., including material preceding or following the directly relevant materials). Finally, researchers must usually include pertinent administrative information. For example, for interview data, each excerpt would need to include the ID number for the participant so that researchers could, if necessary, obtain additional information from the master copy.

Computer Programs for Managing Qualitative Data

Computer-assisted qualitative data analysis software (CAQDAS) removes the work of cutting up pages of narrative material. These programs allow researchers to enter the entire data file onto the computer, code each portion of the narrative, and then retrieve and display text for specified codes for analysis. The software can also be used to examine relationships between codes. Software cannot, however, *do* the coding, and it cannot tell researchers how to analyze the data. Researchers must continue to be analysts and critical thinkers.

Dozens of CAQDAS have been developed. The main types of software packages that are available to handle and manage qualitative data include text retrievers, code and retrieve, theory building, concept maps and diagrams, and data conversion/collection (Lewins & Silver, 2014). *Text retrievers* are programs that help researchers locate text and terms in databases and documents. *Code-and-retrieve packages* permit researchers to code text.

More sophisticated *theory building software*, the most frequently used type of CAQDAS, permits researchers to examine relationships between concepts, develop hierarchies of codes, diagram, and create hyperlinks to create nonhierarchical networks. Examples of theory building packages

include ATLAS.ti, HyperRESEARCH, MAXQDA, and NVivo10. NVivo10, software from Qualitative Solutions and Research (QSR), combines the best of two earlier packages (NVivo and NUD*IST). NVivo10 helps researchers find patterns in their data and explore hunches and enables them to display and analyze relationships in the data.

Software for *concept mapping* permits researchers to construct more sophisticated diagrams than theory building software. Concept maps are a means for organizing and representing knowledge (Novak & Cañas, 2006). Concept maps include concepts (enclosed in circles or boxes) and relationships between them (indicated by connecting lines). CmapTools, an example of concept mapping software, is available at no cost.

Data conversion/collection software, such as voice recognition software, converts audio into text. Such software may be attractive because of the time and expense needed to transcribe audio-recorded interviews—although a study by Johnson (2011) suggests that the time savings may not be enormous. Voice recognition software is designed for a single user. The software must be "trained" to recognize the voice of the user, typically an *oral transcriptionist*.

Voice recognition programs are available from a number of vendors. Their performance is variable and depends on such factors as the capability of the computer on which the software is installed, the quality of the microphone, and the amount of background noise. One disadvantage is voice recognition software's inability to automatically punctuate. The oral transcriptionist must specifically state the punctuation, such as "period" and "comma." Oral transcriptionists also still need to edit the text to correct errors.

MacLean et al. (2004) used voice recognition software to transcribe their interviews in their research on health promotion initiatives and discussed some problems they encountered. For instance, the voice recognition program consistently misinterpreted common homonyms like "here" and "hear" and "to," "too," and "two," resulting in inaccuracies in the transcript. Thus, the time-saving advantages in using voice recognition software may be modest.

Computer programs offer many advantages for managing qualitative data, but some people prefer manual methods because they allow researchers to get closer to the data. Others have raised objections to having a process that is basically cognitive turned into an activity that is mechanical. Despite concerns, many researchers have switched to computerized data management. Proponents insist that it frees up their time and permits them to pay greater attention to important conceptual issues. CAQDAS is constantly revised and upgraded so it is important to stay current on this topic.

→ TIP: Articles that describe the application of qualitative data analysis software are helpful to read before starting your own project. For example, Bringer and colleagues (2004) described in detail their use of the software program NVivo in a grounded theory study. A number of print screens from their analysis are included in the article as illustrations.

Example of Using Computers to Manage Qualitative Data: Hendson and colleagues (2015) studied the perspectives of health care providers from multiple disciplines regarding the provision of culturally competent care to new immigrant families in the neonatal intensive care unit. NVivo software was used to manage the transcribed data from focus group interviews with 58 health care staff.

ANALYTIC PROCEDURES

Data *management* in qualitative research is reductionist in nature: It involves converting masses of data into smaller, manageable segments. By contrast, qualitative data *analysis* is constructionist: It involves putting segments together into meaningful conceptual patterns. Qualitative analysis involves discovering pervasive ideas and searching for general concepts (*analytic generalization*) through an inductive process. Although there are various approaches to qualitative data analysis, some elements are common to several of them—and yet, it is also true that qualitative analysis is eclectic

and nonprescriptive. We begin with describing some general analytic strategies.

An Overview of Qualitative Analysis

The analysis of qualitative materials typically begins with a search for broad categories and then themes. In their thorough review of how the term *theme* is used among qualitative researchers, DeSantis and Ugarriza (2000) offered this definition: "A **theme** is an abstract entity that brings meaning and identity to a current experience and its variant manifestations. As such, a theme captures and unifies the nature or basis of the experience into a meaningful whole" (p. 362).

Thematic analysis often relies on what Spradley (1979) called the similarity principle and the contrast principle. The *similarity principle* involves looking for units of information with similar content, symbols, or meanings. The *contrast principle* guides efforts to find out how content or symbols differ from other content or symbols—that is, to identify what is distinctive about emerging themes or categories.

During analysis, qualitative researchers must distinguish between ideas that apply to all (or many) people, and aspects of the experience that are unique to particular participants. Ayres and colleagues (2003) argued cogently for the importance of doing both across-case analysis and within-case analysis. The analysis of individual cases "enables the researcher to understand those aspects of experience that occur not as individual 'units of meaning' but as part of the pattern formed by the confluence of meanings within individual accounts" (p. 873). Themes that have explanatory or conceptual power both in individual cases and across the sample have the best potential for analytic generalization. Ayres and colleagues illustrated how within-case and across-case analyses were integrated in three nursing studies.

Themes emerge from the data. They often develop within categories of data but may also cut across them. For example, in Beck and Watson's (2010) study on subsequent childbirth after a previous traumatic birth (Box 24.1), one theme that emerged was bringing reverence to the birthing process and empowering women, which included codes 3E (strong sense of control) and 3G (mourned what they missed out with the prior birth).

Thematic analysis involves not only discovering commonalities across participants but also seeking natural variation. Themes are never universal. Researchers must attend not only to what themes arise but also to how they are patterned. Does the theme apply only to certain types of people? In certain contexts? At certain periods? What are the conditions that precede the observed phenomenon, and what are the apparent consequences of it? In other words, the qualitative analyst must be sensitive to *relationships* within the data.

Researchers' search for themes and patterns sometimes can be facilitated by charting devices that enable them to summarize the evolution of behaviors, events, and processes. For example, for qualitative studies that focus on dynamic experiences—such as decision making—it is sometimes useful to develop flowcharts or timelines that highlight time sequences, major decision points and events, and factors affecting the decisions. Another device, in research on families, is the creation of a *genogram*, which is a family tree depicting internal family structure.

Example of a Genogram: In their study of families caring for a child with a progressive neurodegenerative disease, Rallison and Raffin-Bouchal (2013) gathered data from 27 family members of six families. Families participated in developing a genogram, which the researchers found "useful as an engagement tool to provide rich data about the family" (p. 196).

Two-dimensional matrices to array thematic material is another frequently used method of displaying thematic material (Miles & Huberman, 2014). Traditionally, each row of a matrix is allocated to individual participants, and columns are used to enter either raw data or themes. Although matrices can be done by hand, computer spreadsheets enhance opportunities for sorting the data in various ways.

Identifying key categories and themes is seldom a tidy, linear process—iteration is almost always necessary. That is, researchers derive themes from the narrative materials, go back to the materials with the themes in mind to see if the materials really do fit, and then refine the themes as necessary. Sometimes apparent insights early in the process have to be abandoned.

Example of Abandoning an Early Conceptualization: In their study of the experiences of family caregivers of relatives with dementia, Strang and colleagues (2006) commented as follows: "We coded data categories in stages with each stage representing a higher level of conceptual complexity . . . the interplay within the caregiver dyad reminded us of *dancing*. As the analysis progressed, the dance metaphor failed to fully represent the increasingly complex nature of the interactions between caregiver and the family member with dementia. We abandoned it completely" (p. 32).

Some qualitative researchers—especially phenomenologists—use metaphors as an analytic strategy, as the preceding example suggests. A **metaphor** is a symbolic comparison, using figurative language to evoke a visual analogy. Metaphors can be a powerfully expressive tool for qualitative analysts. As a literary device, metaphors can permit greater insight and understanding in qualitative analysis and can help link together parts to the whole. Thorne and Darbyshire (2005) have, however, criticized the overuse of metaphors. In their view, metaphoric allusions can be a compelling approach to articulating human experience, but they can run the risk of "supplanting creative insight with hackneyed cliché masquerading as profundity" (p. 1111). Carpenter (2008) also warned that when researchers mix metaphors, fail to follow through with metaphors, or use metaphors that do not fit, they can misrepresent the data.

Example of a Metaphor: Kisch and colleagues (2014) explored the experiences of having a sibling donor for allogeneic hematopoietic stem cell transplantation. The researchers identified the main theme as the metaphor "Being in no man's land" to characterize the patients' complex situations.

TIP: It is also possible to do an analysis of the metaphors that study participants themselves use. For example, Cheryl Beck, one of the authors of this textbook, is currently conducting a metaphorical analysis of mothers' descriptions of posttraumatic stress disorder (PTSD) due to traumatic childbirth. Some of the metaphors used by the mothers to describe PTSD include ticking time bomb, invisible wall, a video on constant replay, a robot, and a thief.

A further step involves validation. In this phase, the concern is whether the themes accurately represent the perspectives of the participants. Several validation procedures are discussed in Chapter 25. If more than one researcher is working on the study, sessions in which the themes are reviewed and specific cases discussed can be productive. Such investigator triangulation cannot ensure thematic integrity, but it can minimize idiosyncratic biases.

In validating and refining themes, some researchers introduce **quasi-statistics**—a tabulation of the frequency with which certain themes or insights are supported by the data. The frequencies cannot be interpreted in the same way as frequencies generated in survey studies because of imprecision in the enumeration of the themes, but, as Becker (1970) pointed out, "Quasi-statistics may allow the investigator to dispose of certain troublesome null hypotheses. A simple frequency count of the number of times a given phenomenon appears may make untenable the null hypothesis that the phenomenon is infrequent" (p. 81).

Sandelowski (2001) expressed her belief that numbers are underutilized in qualitative research because of two myths: first, that real qualitative researchers *do not* count, and second, that qualitative researchers *cannot* count. Numbers can be helpful in highlighting the complexity and work of qualitative research. Numbers may also be useful in documenting and testing interpretations and conclusions and in describing events and experiences (although Sandelowski warned of the pitfalls of overcounting). We discuss this issue at greater length in the chapter on mixed methods research (Chapter 26).

Example of Tabulating Data: Bradbury-Jones and colleagues (2013) explored public health nurses' assessment of oral health in preschool children, through in-depth interviews with 16 Scottish nurses. After their thematic analysis, the researchers calculated how many public health nurses cited each major theme or subtheme "to provide an impression of the salience of a theme" (p. 5). For example, 13 nurses reported asking about teeth brushing; 6 asked about recent dental care.

In the final analysis stage, researchers strive to weave thematic pieces together into an integrated whole. The various themes need to be interrelated to provide an overall structure (such as a theory or integrated description) to the data. The integration task is a difficult one because it demands creativity and intellectual rigor if it is to be successful.

In the sections that follow, we discuss analytic procedures used by ethnographers, phenomenologists, and grounded theory researchers. We begin by first discussing a general approach that is often used by qualitative researchers who conduct descriptive qualitative studies not based in a specific tradition, that is, content analysis.

TIP: Given the nonprescriptive nature of content analysis—and all qualitative analysis—it might be said that it is a process best learned by *doing* it.

Qualitative Content Analysis

Content analysis is a family of analytic approaches ranging from intuitive and impressionistic analyses to systematic and fairly strict textual analyses. Indeed, quantitative researchers sometimes perform a content analysis—for example, by counting words or phrases and formally testing hypotheses.

Qualitative content analysis is the analysis of the content of narrative data to identify prominent themes and patterns among the themes. Patton (2002) defined qualitative content analysis as "any qualitative data reduction and sense-making effort that takes a volume of qualitative material and attempts to identify core consistencies and meaning" (p. 453). Thus, a central feature of content analysis is that it is a way to *condense* a voluminous number of words of a text into smaller content categories.

Qualitative content analysis involves breaking down data into smaller units. The literature on content analysis often includes references to *meaning units*. Graneheim and Lundman (2004) defined a meaning unit as "words, sentences or paragraphs containing aspects related to each other through their content and context" (p. 106). A meaning unit, essentially, is the smallest segment of a text that contains a recognizable piece of information.

The labels attached to meaning units are the codes (sometimes referred to as *tags*). Codes are heuristic devices; "labelling a condensed meaning unit with a code allows the data to be thought about in new and different ways" (Graneheim & Lundman, 2004, p. 107). The success of a content analysis is highly dependent on the integrity of the coding process. Codes are, in turn, the basis for developing categories. In what is sometimes referred to as "secondary coding," the creation of categories involves gathering meaning units together that capture the substance of a topic—that is, that fit into a cluster (Krippendorff, 2013).

Graneheim and Lundman (2004) offered a good example of how data were coded and categorized in a study of people living with diabetes. Here is an excerpt from an interview that was considered a meaning unit: "There is a curious feeling in the head in some way, empty in some way." The code attached to this meaning unit was "emptiness in the head." In turn, this code was categorized in a subcategory of "Unfamiliar bodily sensations," which was one of three subcategories in the broad category called "Sensations."

Content analysts often make the distinction between manifest and latent content. *Manifest content* is what the text actually says—its visible components. In purely descriptive studies, qualitative researchers may decide to focus mainly on summarizing the manifest content communicated in the text. More often, however, content analysts also analyze what the text talks *about*, which involves interpretation of the meaning of its *latent content*. Interpretations vary in depth and level of abstraction and are usually the basis for themes. In Graneheim and Lundman's (2004) example, data coded in the category of "Sensations," together with data from two other categories, were subsumed under the theme "Lack of control and struggle for regaining control."

Hsieh and Shannon (2005) offered a good discussion of three different approaches to content analysis, based on the degree of involvement of inductive reasoning. In "conventional" content analysis (often referred to as *inductive content analysis*), the study starts with data and the codes emerge and are defined during data analysis. In "directed" content analysis, researchers begin with a theory or earlier relevant findings, and codes are defined before data analysis and then expanded during the analysis. Thus, directed content analysis typically combines a deductive and

an inductive approach to coding. This approach is often used to validate or extend a theory or conceptual model. In "summative" content analysis, keywords are the starting point; keywords are identified before data analysis (e.g., from a literature review) as well as during data analysis (manifest content). This third approach has aspects that seem quantitative in nature at the outset (e.g., counting manifest content), but it seeks to explore words and indicators in an inductive manner as the process unfolds.

⊘ TIP: Elo and Kyngäs (2007) present a good figure illustrating and distinguishing processes in inductive and deductive approaches to content analysis.

Example of a Content Analysis: Nilsson and colleagues (2013) used a conventional content analysis in their study of factors influencing positive birth experiences of first-time mothers. The data were written narratives about the experiences of 14 Swedish mothers. The authors specifically noted their intent to focus on the narratives' latent content. Meaning units were categorized into three categories (To trust the body and to face the pain, Interaction between body and mind in giving birth, and Consistency of support). In their analysis, an overall theme emerged: To be empowered to increase the chances for a positive birth experience.

Ethnographic Analysis

Analysis begins from the moment ethnographers set foot in the field. Ethnographers are continually looking for *patterns* in the behavior and thoughts of participants, comparing one pattern against another, and analyzing many patterns simultaneously (Fetterman, 2010). As they analyze patterns of everyday life, ethnographers acquire a deeper understanding of the culture being studied. Maps, flowcharts, and organizational charts are useful tools that help to crystallize and illustrate the data. Matrices (two-dimensional displays) can also help to highlight a comparison graphically, to cross-reference categories, and to discover emerging patterns.

Spradley's (1979) research sequence can be used for data analysis in ethnographies. His method is based on the premise that language is the primary means that relates cultural meaning in a culture. The task of ethnographers is to describe cultural symbols and to identify their coding rules. His sequence of 12 steps, which includes data collection and data analysis, is as follows:

1. Locating an informant
2. Interviewing an informant
3. Making an ethnographic record
4. Asking descriptive questions
5. Analyzing ethnographic interviews
6. Making a domain analysis
7. Asking structural questions
8. Making a taxonomic analysis
9. Asking contrast questions
10. Making a componential analysis
11. Discovering cultural themes
12. Writing the ethnography

Thus, in Spradley's (1979) method, there are four levels of data analysis, the first of which is **domain analysis**. Domains, which are units of cultural knowledge, are broad categories that encompass smaller ones. During this first level of data analysis, ethnographers identify relational patterns among terms in the domains that are used by members of the culture. The ethnographer focuses on the cultural meaning of terms and symbols (objects and events) used in a culture and their interrelationships.

In **taxonomic analysis**, the second level of data analysis, ethnographers decide how many domains the analysis will encompass. Will only one or two domains be analyzed in depth, or will a number of domains be studied less intensively? After making this decision, a **taxonomy**—a system of classifying and organizing terms—is developed to illustrate the internal organization of a domain and the relationship among the subcategories of the domain.

In **componential analysis**, relationships among terms in the domains are examined. The ethnographer analyzes data for similarities and differences among cultural terms in a domain. Finally, in **theme analysis**, cultural themes are uncovered. Domains are connected in cultural themes, which help to provide a holistic view of the culture being studied. The discovery of cultural meaning is the outcome.

Example Using Spradley's Method: Davies (2010) followed Spradley's 12-step sequence in a study of parental assessment and intervention for pain for their children with Down syndrome. In step 11, discovering cultural themes, Davies identified four themes. For example, one theme was identifying differences in pain expressions between the child and siblings.

Other approaches to ethnographic analysis have been developed. For example, in Leininger's ethnonursing research method, as described in McFarland and Wehbe-Alamah (2015), ethnographers follow a four-phase ethnonursing data analysis guide. In the first phase, ethnographers collect, describe, and record data. The second phase involves identifying and categorizing descriptors. In phase 3, data are analyzed to discover repetitive patterns in their context. The fourth and final phase involves abstracting major themes and presenting findings.

Example Using Leininger's Method: Raymond and Omeri (2015) studied the culture care for Mauritian immigrant childbearing families living in New South Wales, Australia. Using Leininger's four phases of ethnonursing inquiry, the researchers identified five dominant themes: care as extended family and friendship support, care as best professional and/or folk practices, self-care as responsibility, care as enabling and empowerment, and care as maintenance of a hygienic and supportive environment.

Phenomenologic Analysis

Many qualitative analysts use what might be called "fracturing" strategies that break down the data and rearrange them into categories that facilitate comparisons across cases (e.g., grounded theory researchers). Phenomenologists often prefer holistic, "contextualizing" strategies that involve interpreting the narrative data within the context of a "whole text."

Three frequently used methods for descriptive phenomenology are the methods of Colaizzi (1978), Giorgi (1985), and Van Kaam (1966), all of whom are from the Duquesne school of phenomenology, based on Husserl's philosophy.

Phenomenologic analysis using all three methods involves a search for common patterns, but there are some important differences among these approaches, as summarized in Table 24.1. The basic

TABLE 24.1 • Comparison of Three Phenomenologic Analytic Methods

COLAIZZI (1978)	GIORGI (1985)	VAN KAAM (1966)
1. Read all protocols to acquire a feeling for them.	1. Read the entire set of protocols to get a sense of the whole.	1. List and group preliminarily the descriptive expressions that must be agreed upon by expert judges. Final listing presents percentages of these categories in that particular sample.
2. Review each protocol and extract significant statements.	2. Discriminate units from participants' description of phenomenon being studied.	2. Reduce the concrete, vague, and overlapping expressions of the participants to more descriptive terms. (Intersubjective agreement among judges needed.)
3. Spell out the meaning of each significant statement (i.e., formulate meanings).	3. Articulate the psychological insight in each of the meaning units.	3. Eliminate elements not inherent in the phenomenon being studied or that represent blending of two related phenomena.
4. Organize the formulated meanings into clusters of themes. a. Refer these clusters back to the original protocols to validate them. b. Note discrepancies among or between the various clusters, avoiding the temptation of ignoring data or themes that do not fit.	4. Synthesize all of the transformed meaning units into a consistent statement regarding participants' experiences (referred to as the "structure of the experience"); can be expressed on a specific or general level.	4. Write a hypothetical identification and description of the phenomenon being studied.
5. Integrate results into an exhaustive description of the phenomenon under study.		5. Apply hypothetical description to randomly selected cases from the sample. If necessary, revise the hypothesized description, which must then be tested again on a new random sample.
6. Formulate an exhaustive description of the phenomenon under study in as unequivocal a statement of identification as possible.		6. Consider the hypothesized identification as a valid identification and description once preceding operations have been carried out successfully.
7. Ask participants about the findings thus far as a final validating step.		

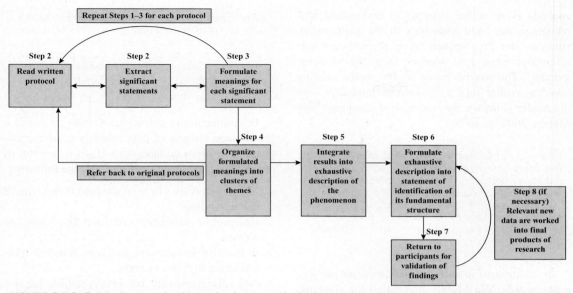

FIGURE 24.2 Colaizzi's procedural steps in phenomenologic data analysis (Reprinted with permission from Beck, C. T. [2009]. The arm: There is no escaping the reality for mothers of children with obstetric brachial plexus injuries. *Nursing Research*, 58, 237–245.)

outcome of all three methods is the description of the meaning of an experience, often through the identification of essential themes. Colaizzi's (1978) method, however, is the only one that calls for a validation of results by returning to study participants. Figure 24.2 provides an illustration of the steps involved in data analysis using Colaizzi's approach. Giorgi's (1985) analysis relies solely on researchers. His view is that it is inappropriate to return to participants to validate findings or to use external judges to review the analysis. Van Kaam's (1966) method requires that intersubjective agreement be reached with other expert judges.

Example of a Study Using Colaizzi's Method:
Rashotte and colleagues (2014) studied the daily experience of adolescents living with sensor-augmented pump therapy (SAPT) for type 1 diabetes. Seven adolescents and nine parents were interviewed and transcripts were subjected to analysis using Colaizzi's method. The overarching theme was *seeking harmony*, reflecting the adolescents' and parents' daily struggles. Four themes reflected the struggle to find harmony: struggling with hopes and expectations for SAPT, being ready for SAPT, living the burdens of continuous glucose monitoring, and creating partnerships.

A second school of phenomenology is the Utrecht School. Phenomenologists using this approach combine characteristics of descriptive and interpretive phenomenology. Van Manen's (1990) method is an example of this approach, in which researchers try to grasp the essential meaning of the experience being studied. According to Van Manen, thematic aspects of experience can be uncovered or isolated from participants' descriptions of the experience by three methods: (1) the holistic approach, (2) the selective (highlighting) approach, and (3) the detailed (line-by-line) approach. In the **holistic approach**, researchers view the text as a whole and try to capture its meanings. In the **selective approach**, researchers highlight or pull out statements or phrases that seem essential to the experience under study. In the **detailed approach**, researchers analyze every sentence. Once themes have been identified, they become the objects of reflection and interpretation through follow-up interviews with participants. Through this process, essential themes are discovered.

Van Manen (2006) stressed that this phenomenologic method cannot be separated from the practice of writing. Writing up the results of qualitative analysis is an active struggle to understand and recognize the lived meanings of the phenomena studied. The text written by a phenomenologic researcher must lead readers to a "questioning wonder." The words chosen by the writer need to take the reader into a "wondrous landscape" as the reader is drawn into the textual meaning (Van Manen, 2002, p. 1675).

Example of a Study Using Van Manen's Method: Rasmussen and Delmar (2014) provided a detailed description of their use of Van Manen's methods in the study of patient dignity as perceived by surgical patients in a Danish hospital. Holistic, selective, and detailed analyses were undertaken to reveal the basic theme: *to be an important person.*

In addition to identifying themes from participants' words, Van Manen also called for gleaning thematic descriptions from artistic sources. Van Manen urged qualitative researchers to keep in mind that literature, music, painting, and other art forms can provide a wealth of experiential information that can increase insights as the phenomenologist tries to grasp the essential meaning of the experience being studied. Experiential descriptions in literature and art help challenge and stretch phenomenologists' interpretive sensibilities.

A third school of phenomenology is an interpretive approach called Heideggerian hermeneutics. As noted in Chapter 21, a key notion in a hermeneutic study is the *hermeneutic circle*. The circle signifies a methodologic process in which, to reach understanding, there is continual movement between the parts and the whole of the text being analyzed. Gadamer (1975) stressed that, to interpret a text, researchers cannot separate themselves from the meanings of the text and must strive to understand possibilities that the text can reveal. Ricoeur (1981) broadened this notion of text to include not just the written text but any human action or situation.

Example of Gadamerian Hermeneutics: Smythe and colleagues (2014) explored the nature of high-quality postnatal care through a "hermeneutic unpacking" of the notion of *tact*, drawing on the philosophical writings of Heidegger and Gadamer.

In their analysis of extracts from interviews with nine mothers, six midwives, and four nurses who provided postnatal care in New Zealand, the researchers "examined moments of practice to discern what happened in the interplay that could be tact in action" (p. 165).

Diekelmann and colleagues (1989) proposed a seven-stage process of data analysis in hermeneutics that involves collaborative effort by a team of researchers. The seven stages include the following:

1. All the interviews or texts are read for an overall understanding.
2. Interpretive summaries of each interview are written.
3. A team of researchers analyzes selected transcribed interviews or texts.
4. Any disagreements on interpretation are resolved by going back to the text.
5. Common meanings are identified by comparing and contrasting the text.
6. Relationships among themes emerge.
7. A draft of the themes with exemplars from texts is presented to the team. Responses or suggestions are incorporated into the final draft.

According to Diekelmann and colleagues (1989), the discovery in step 6 of a **constitutive pattern**—a pattern that expresses the relationships among relational themes and is present in all the interviews or texts—forms the highest level of hermeneutical analysis. A situation is constitutive when it gives actual content to a person's self-understanding or to a person's way of being in the world.

Example of a Diekelmann's Hermeneutical Analysis: Papadatou et al. (2015) used Diekelmann's method to explore the experiences of infertile women in Greece who achieved a pregnancy through use of sperm, oocyte, or embryo donation or surrogate motherhood. Each member of the research team independently coded every interview and identified recurrent themes. The constitutive pattern of "journeying through hope and despair" was discovered.

Benner (1994) offered another analytic approach for hermeneutic phenomenology. Her interpretive analysis consists of three interrelated processes: the search for paradigm cases, thematic analysis, and analysis of exemplars. **Paradigm cases** are "strong instances of concerns or ways of being in the world" (Benner, 1994, p. 113). Paradigm cases are used early in the analytic process as a strategy for gaining understanding. Thematic analysis is done to compare and contrast similarities across cases. Paradigm cases and thematic analysis can be enhanced by *exemplars* that illuminate aspects of a paradigm case or theme. The presentation of paradigm cases and exemplars in reports allows readers to play a role in consensual validation of the results by deciding whether the cases support the researchers' conclusions. Crist and Tanner (2003) provide some explicit guidance for a hermeneutical interpretive process that includes features of both Benner's and Diekelmann's approaches.

Example Using Benner's Hermeneutical Analysis: Palacios and colleagues (2012) conducted an interpretive phenomenologic study of the embodied meanings of early childbearing among American Indian women. They used Benner's triadic approach in their analysis, which included paradigm cases, thematic analysis, and exemplars. Three themes were discovered that reflected mourning a lost childhood, seeking fulfillment, and embodying responsibility.

Grounded Theory Analysis

Grounded theory methods emerged in the 1960s in connection with Glaser and Strauss's (1967) research program on dying in hospitals. The two co-originators eventually split and developed divergent schools of thought, which have been called the "Glaserian" and "Straussian" versions of grounded theory (Walker & Myrick, 2006). The division between the two mainly concerns the manner in which the data are analyzed.

Glaser and Strauss's Grounded Theory Method

Grounded theory in both systems of analysis uses the *constant comparative* method of analysis. This method involves a comparison of elements present in one data source (e.g., in one interview) with those in another to determine if they are similar. The process continues until the content of each source has been compared to the content in all sources. In this fashion, commonalities are identified.

The concept of fit is an important element in Glaserian grounded theory analysis. By **fit**, Glaser meant that the developing categories of the substantive theory must fit the data. Fit enables the researcher to determine if data can be placed in the same category or if they can be related to one another. However, Glaser (1992) warned qualitative researchers not to force an analytic fit, noting that "if you torture data enough it will give up!" (p. 123). Forcing a fit hinders the development of a relevant theory. *Fit* is also an important issue when a grounded theory is applied in new contexts: The theory must closely "fit" the substantive area where it will be used (Glaser & Strauss, 1967).

Coding in the Glaserian approach is used to conceptualize data into patterns. The substance of the topic under study is conceptualized through **substantive codes**, while **theoretical codes** provide insights into how substantive codes relate to each other. Substantive codes are either open or selective. **Open coding**, used in the first stage of the constant comparative analysis, captures what is going on in the data. Open codes may be the actual words used by the participants. Through open coding, data are broken down into incidents, and their similarities and differences are examined. During open coding, researchers ask "What category or property of a category does this incident indicate?" (Glaser, 1978, p. 57).

There are three levels of open coding that vary in degree of abstraction. **Level I codes** (or *in vivo codes*) are derived directly from the language of the substantive area and have vivid imagery. Table 24.2 presents five level I codes from Beck's (2002) grounded theory study on mothering twins, and interview excerpts associated with those codes. (A figure showing Beck's hierarchy of codes, from level I to one of her level III codes, is shown in the Toolkit of the accompanying *Resource Manual*.)

Researchers constantly compare new level I codes to previously identified ones and then condense them into broader **level II codes**. For example, in Table 24.2, Beck's five level I codes were

TABLE 24.2 • Collapsing Level I Codes into the Level II Code of *"Reaping the Blessings"* (Beck, 2002)

QUOTE	LEVEL I CODE
I enjoy just watching the twins interact so much. Especially now that they are mobile. They are not walking yet but they are crawling. I will tell you they are already playing. Like one will go around the corner and kind of peek around and they play hide and seek. They crawl after each other.	Enjoying Twins
With twins it's amazing. She was sick and she had a fever. He was the one acting sick. She didn't seem like she was sick at all. He was. We watched him for like 6–8 hours. We gave her the medicine and he started calming down. Like WOW! That is so weird. Cause you read about it but it's like, Oh come on! You know that doesn't really happen and it does. It's really neat to see.	Amazing
These days it's really neat cause you go to the store or you go out and people are like "Oh, they are twins, how nice." And I say, "Yeah they are. Look, look at my kids."	Getting Attention
I just feel blessed to have two. I just feel like I am twice as lucky as a mom who has one baby. I mean that's the best part. It's just that instead of having one baby to watch grow and change and develop and become a toddler and school-age child you have two.	Feeling Blessed
It's very exciting. It's interesting and it's fun to see them and how the twin bond really is. There really is a twin bond. You read about it and you hear about it but until you experience it, you just don't understand. One time they were both crying and they were fed. They were changed and burped. There was nothing wrong. I couldn't figure out what was wrong. So I said to myself, "I am just going to put them together and close the door." I put them in my bed together and they patty-caked their hands and put their noses together and just looked at each other and went right to sleep.	Twin Bonding

collapsed into the level II code, "Reaping the Blessings." **Level III codes** (or theoretical constructs) are the most abstract. These constructs "add scope beyond local meanings" (Glaser, 1978, p.70) to the generated theory. Collapsing level II codes aids in identifying constructs.

Open coding ends when the core category is discovered, and then selective coding begins. The **core category** is a pattern of behavior that is relevant and/or problematic for participants. In **selective coding** (which can also have three levels of abstraction), researchers code only those data that are related to the core variable. One kind of core variable is a **basic social process (BSP)** that evolves over time in two or more phases. All BSPs are core variables, but not all core variables have to be BSPs.

Glaser (1978) provided nine criteria to help researchers decide on a core category:

1. It must be central, meaning that it is related to many categories.
2. It must reoccur frequently in the data.
3. It takes more time to saturate than other categories.
4. It relates meaningfully and easily to other categories.
5. It has clear and grabbing implications for formal theory.
6. It has considerable carry-through.

7. It is completely variable.
8. It is a dimension of the problem.
9. It can be any kind of theoretical code.

Theoretical codes help grounded theorists to weave the broken pieces of data back together. Theoretical codes have the power "to grab," which Glaser (2005) called "theoretical code capture" (p. 74). Theoretical codes provide a grounded theory with greater explanatory power because they enhance the abstract meaning of the relationships among categories. Glaser (1978) first proposed 18 families of theoretical codes that researchers can use to conceptualize how substantive codes relate to each other (Box 24.2). Recently, Glaser (2005) identified many new possibilities for theoretical codes, offering examples from biochemistry (bias random walk), economics (amplifying causal looping), and political science (conjectural causation). The larger the array of theoretical codes available, the less tendency a researcher will have to force on the developing theory a pet or favorite theoretical code (Glaser, 2005).

Throughout coding and analysis, grounded theory analysts document their ideas about the data, categories, and emerging conceptual scheme in **memos**. Memos preserve ideas that may initially not seem productive but may later prove valuable once further developed. Memos also encourage researchers to reflect on and describe patterns in the data, relationships between categories, and emergent conceptualizations.

➔ **TIP:** Glaser (1978) offered guidelines for preparing effective memos to generate substantive theory, including the following:

- Keep memos separate from data.
- Stop coding when an idea for a memo occurs, so as not to lose the thought.
- A memo can be brought on by forcing it, by beginning to write about a code.
- Memos can be modified as growth and realizations occur.
- In writing memos, do not focus on persons; talk conceptually about substantive codes.

BOX 24.2 Families of Theoretical Codes for Grounded Theory Analysis

1. The six Cs: causes, contexts, contingencies, consequences, covariances, and conditions
2. Process: stages, phases, passages, transitions
3. Degree: intensity, range, grades, continuum
4. Dimension: elements, parts, sections
5. Type: kinds, styles, forms
6. Strategy: tactics, techniques, maneuverings
7. Interaction: mutual effects, interdependence, reciprocity
8. Identity–self: self-image, self-worth, self-concept
9. Cutting point: boundaries, critical junctures, turning points
10. Means–goal: purpose, end, products
11. Cultural: social values, beliefs
12. Consensus: agreements, uniformities, conformity
13. Mainline: socialization, recruiting, social order
14. Theoretical: density, integration, clarity, fit, relevance
15. Ordering/elaboration: structural ordering, temporal ordering, conceptual ordering
16. Unit: group, organization, collective
17. Reading: hypotheses, concepts, problems
18. Models: pictorial models of a theory

Adapted from Glaser, B. G. (1978). *Theoretical sensitivity*. Mill Valley, CA: Sociological Press.

- When you have two ideas, write each idea up as a separate memo to prevent confusion.
- Always remain flexible with memoing approaches.

The Toolkit in the *Resource Manual* includes an example of a memo from Beck's work.

Glaser's grounded theory method is concerned with the *generation* of categories and hypotheses rather than testing them. The product of the typical grounded theory analysis is a theoretical model that endeavors to generate "a theory of continually resolving the main concern, which explains most of the behavior in an area of interest" (Glaser, 2001, p. 103). Once the basic problem or central concern emerges, the grounded theorist goes on to discover the process these participants experience in coping with or resolving this problem.

Example of Glaser and Strauss's Grounded Theory Analysis: Figure 24.3 presents Beck's (2002) model from a grounded theory study in which "Releasing the Pause Button" was conceptualized as the core category and process through which mothers of twins progressed as they attempted to resume their lives after giving birth. According to this model, the process involves four phases: Draining Power, Pausing own Life, Striving to Reset, and Resuming own Life. Beck used 10 coding families in her theoretical coding for the Releasing the Pause Button process. The family *cutting point* provides an illustration. Three months seemed to be the turning point for mothers, when life started to become more manageable. Here is an excerpt that Beck coded as a cutting point: "Three months came around and the twins sort of slept through the night and it made a huge, huge difference."

Although Glaser and Straus cautioned against consulting the literature before a theoretical framework is stabilized, they also viewed grounded theory as an "ever modifying process" (Glaser, 1978, p. 5) that could benefit from scrutiny of other work. Glaser discussed the evolution of grounded theories through the process of **emergent fit** to prevent individual substantive theories from being "respected little islands of knowledge" (p. 148). As Glaser pointed out, generating grounded theory does not necessarily require discovering all new categories or ignoring ones previously identified in the literature: "The task is, rather, to develop an emergent fit between the data and a pre-existent category that might work. Therefore, as in the refitting of a generated category as data emerge, so must an extant category be carefully fitted as data emerge to be sure it works. In the bargain, like the generated category, it may be modified to fit and work. In this sense, the extant category was not merely borrowed but earned its way into the emerging theory" (p. 4). Through constant comparison, researchers can compare concepts emerging from the data with similar concepts from existing theory or research to assess which parts have emergent fit with the theory being generated.

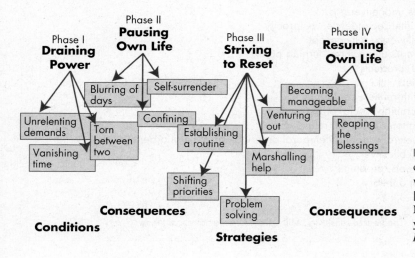

FIGURE 24.3 Beck's (2002) model of mothering twins. (Reprinted with permission from Beck, C. T. [2002]. Releasing the pause button: Mothering twins during the first year of life. *Qualitative Health Research, 12*, 593–608.)

Strauss and Corbin's Approach

The Strauss and Corbin's approach to grounded theory analysis, most recently described in Corbin and Strauss (2015), differs from the original Glaser and Strauss's method with regard to method, processes, and outcomes. Table 24.3 summarizes major analytic differences between these two grounded theory analysis methods.

Glaser (1978) stressed that to generate a grounded theory, the basic problem must emerge from the data—it must be discovered. The theory is, from the very start, grounded in the data rather than starting with a preconceived problem. Strauss and Corbin, however, stated that the research itself is only one of four possible sources of a research problem. Research problems can, for example, come from the literature, a researcher's personal and professional experience, an advisor or mentor, or a pilot project.

The Corbin and Strauss's method involves two types of coding: open and axial coding. In **open coding**, data are broken down into parts and concepts identified for interpreted meaning of the raw data. In **axial coding**, the analyst codes for context. Here the analyst is "locating and linking action-interaction within a framework of subconcepts that give it meaning and enable it to explain what interactions are occurring, and why and what consequences real or anticipated are happening" (Corbin & Strauss, 2015, p. 156).

The *paradigm* is used as an analytic strategy to help integrate structure and process. The basic components of the paradigm include conditions, actions–interactions, and consequences or outcomes. Corbin and Strauss suggested the conditional/consequential matrix as an analytic strategy for considering the range of possible conditions and consequences that can enter into the context.

The first step in integrating the findings is to decide on the **central category** (sometimes called the *core category*), which is the main theme of the research. Recommended techniques to facilitate identifying the central category are writing the storyline, using diagrams, and reviewing and organizing memos. The outcome of the Strauss and Corbin's approach is, as Glaser (1992) termed it, a full conceptual description. The original grounded theory method (Glaser & Strauss, 1967), by contrast, generates a theory that explains how a basic social problem that emerged from the data is processed in a social setting.

TABLE 24.3 • Comparison of Glaser's and Corbin and Strauss's Methods

	GLASER	CORBIN AND STRAUSS
Initial data analysis	Breaking down and conceptualizing data involves comparison of incident to incident so patterns emerge	Breaking down and conceptualizing data includes taking apart a single sentence, observation, and incident
Types of coding	Open, selective, theoretical	Open and axial
Connections between categories	18 coding families plus theoretical codes from many different fields of study	Paradigm (conditions, actions–interactions, and consequences or outcomes) and the conditional/consequential matrix
Outcome	Emergent theory (discovery)	Conceptual description (verification)

Example of Strauss and Corbin's Grounded Theory Analysis: Lawler and colleagues (2015) sought to understand the process of transitioning to motherhood for women with a disability. Their data from interviews with 22 women were analyzed using Strauss and Corbin's method of open and axial coding: "The data were broken down, examined, compared, conceptualized and categorized so that the data could be interpreted, concepts and categories selected. Once the categories and subcategories were sufficiently reinforced the data were reconstructed in different ways through the linking of categories and subcategories . . . Categories were then integrated to refine the evolving theory" (p. 1675).

Constructivist Grounded Theory Approach

The constructivist approach to grounded theory is not dissimilar to a Glaserian approach. According to Charmaz (2014), in constructivist grounded theory, the "coding generates the bones of your analysis. Theoretical centrality and integration will assemble these bones into a working skeleton" (p. 113). Charmaz offered guidelines for types of coding: word-by-word coding, line-by-line coding, and coding incident to incident.

Charmaz distinguished *initial coding* and *focused coding*. In initial coding, the pieces of data (e.g., words, lines, segments, incidents) are studied so the researcher begins to learn what the participants view as problematic. In focused coding, the analysis is directed toward using the most significant codes from the initial coding. Decisions are made by the researcher on which codes are most important for further analysis, which are then theoretically coded.

Example of a Constructivist Grounded Theory Analysis: Hoare and colleagues (2012) provide an in-depth description of how Charmaz's approach was used to code and analyze data in a study of information use by practice nurses.

Analysis of Focus Group Data

Focus group interviews yield rich and complex data that pose special analytic challenges. Indeed, there is little consensus about analyzing data from focus groups, despite their widespread use.

Focus group interviews are especially difficult to transcribe, partly because of technical problems. For example, it is difficult to place microphones so that the voices of all group members are picked up with equal clarity, particularly because participants tend to speak at different volumes. An additional issue is the inevitability that several participants will speak at once, making it impossible for transcriptionists to discern everything being said.

A controversial issue in the analysis of focus group data is whether the unit of analysis is the group or individual participants. Some writers (e.g., Morrison-Beedy et al., 2001) maintain that the group is the proper unit of analysis. Analysis of group-level data involves a scrutiny of themes, interactions, and sequences within and between groups. Others, however (e.g., Carey & Smith, 1994; Kidd & Parshall, 2000), have argued that analysis should occur at both the group and individual level. Those who insist on only group-level analysis argue that what individuals say in focus groups cannot be treated as personal disclosures because they are inevitably influenced by the dynamics of the group. However, even in personal interviews individual responses are shaped by social processes, and analysis of individual-level data (independent of group) is thought by some analysts to add important insights.

Carey and Smith (1994) advocated a third level of analysis—namely, the analysis of individual responses *in relation* to group context (e.g., whether a participant's view is in accord with or in contrast to majority opinion). Duggleby (2005) observed that two methods for analyzing focus group interaction data have been suggested—first, describing interactions as a means of interpreting the findings, and second, incorporating the group interaction data directly into the transcripts. She proposed a third alternative: a *congruent methodologic approach* that analyzes interaction data in the same manner as group or individual data.

For those who wish to analyze data from individual participants, it is essential to maintain information about what each person said—a task that is not possible if researchers rely solely on audio recordings. Video recordings, as supplements to audio recordings, are sometimes used to identify who said what in focus group sessions. More frequently, however, researchers have members of the research team in attendance at the sessions, and their job is to take detailed field notes about the order of speakers and about significant nonverbal behavior, such as pounding or clenching of fists, crying, aggressive body language, and so on.

Example of Integrating Focus Group Interview and Observational Data: Morrison-Beedy and colleagues (2001) provided several examples of integrating data across sources from their focus group research. For example, one verbatim quote was, "It was no big deal." This was supplemented with data from the field notes that the woman's eyes were cast downward as she said this, and that the words were delivered sarcastically. The complete transcript for this entry, which included researcher interpretation in brackets, was as follows: "'It was no big deal.' (said sarcastically, with eyes looking downward). [It really was a very big deal to her, but others had not acknowledged that.]" (p. 52).

Because of group dynamics, focus group analysts must be sensitive to both the thematic content of these interviews, and also to how, when, and why themes are developed. Some of the issues that could be central to focus group analysis are the following:

- Does an issue raised in a focus group constitute a *theme* or merely a strongly held viewpoint of one or two members?
- Do the same issues or themes arise in more than one group?
- If there are group differences, why might this be the case—were participants different in characteristics and experiences, or did group processes affect the discussions?
- Are some issues sufficiently salient that not only are they discussed in response to specific questions posed by the moderator but also spontaneously emerge at multiple points in the session?
- Do group members find certain issues both interesting *and* important?

Some focus group analysts, such as Kidd and Parshall (2000), use quantitative methods as adjuncts to their qualitative analysis. Using qualitative analysis software, they conduct such analyses as assessing similarities and differences between groups, determining coding frequencies to aid pattern detection, examining codes in relation to participant

characteristics, and examining how much dialogue individual members contributed. They use such methods not so that interpretation can be based on frequencies but so that they can better understand context and identify issues that require further critical scrutiny and interpretation.

Also, **sociograms** can be used to understand the flow of conversation as it goes around the members of the focus group. In a sociogram, the structure of interpersonal relations in a focus group is plotted on a chart. Weighted arrows can illustrate the number of times the conversation goes from one person to another (Drahota & Dewey, 2008).

INTERPRETATION OF QUALITATIVE FINDINGS

Interpretation and analysis of qualitative data occur virtually simultaneously in an iterative process. That is, researchers interpret the data as they read and reread them, categorize and code them, inductively develop a thematic analysis, and integrate the themes into a unified whole.

It is difficult to provide guidance about the process of interpretation in qualitative studies, but there is considerable agreement that the ability to "make meaning" from qualitative texts depends on researchers' immersion in and closeness to the data. **Incubation** is the process of *living* the data, a process in which researchers must try to understand their meanings, find their essential patterns, and draw legitimate, insightful conclusions. Another key ingredient in interpretation and meaning making is researchers' self-awareness and the ability to reflect on their own worldview and perspectives—that is, reflexivity.

Creativity also plays an important role in uncovering meaning in the data. Chandler, in writing about the transition from *saturation* to *illumination* wrote that, "Strategies for creativity take time and require incubation for new ideas to percolate. Insight into the incubation of data is critical to the final theoretical revelations" (Chandler in Hunter et al., 2002, p. 396). Thus, researchers need to give themselves sufficient time to achieve the *aha* that comes with making meaning beyond the facts.

Efforts to validate the analysis are necessarily efforts to validate interpretations as well. Prudent qualitative researchers hold their interpretations up for closer scrutiny—self-scrutiny as well as review by peers and outside reviewers. For both qualitative and quantitative researchers, it is important to consider possible alternative explanations or meanings.

Example of Seeking Alternative Explanations: James and colleagues (2009) studied family carers' experiences of hospital encounters between informal and professional care at the end of life. Their hermeneutic study followed Gadamer's analytic approach to identifying meanings and patterns in the data as a continuous movement between the whole and the parts. The researchers noted that "preliminary interpretations were called into question using counterarguments based on different theories" (p. 260).

In drawing conclusions, qualitative researchers are increasingly considering the transferability of the findings and the potential uses to which the qualitative evidence can be put. Like quantitative researchers, qualitative researchers need to give thought to the implications of their study findings for future research and for nursing practice.

CRITIQUING QUALITATIVE ANALYSIS

Evaluating a qualitative analysis in a report is not easy to do, even for experienced researchers. The main problem is that readers do not have access to the information they would need to determine whether researchers exercised good judgment and critical insight in coding the narrative materials, developing a thematic analysis, and integrating materials into a meaningful whole. Researchers are seldom able to include more than a handful of examples of actual data in a journal article. Moreover, the process they used to abstract meaning from the data is difficult to describe and illustrate.

In a critique of qualitative analysis, a primary task usually is assessing whether researchers took sufficient steps to validate inferences and conclusions. A major focus of a critique, then, is whether the researchers adequately documented the analytic

process. The report should provide information about the approach used to analyze the data. For example, a report for a grounded theory study should indicate whether the researchers used the Glaser and Strauss, Strauss and Corbin, or constructivist method.

Critiquing analytic decisions is substantially less clear-cut in a qualitative than in a quantitative study. For example, it would be inappropriate to critique a phenomenologic analysis for following Giorgi's approach rather than Colaizzi's approach. Both are respected methods of conducting a phenomenologic study—although phenomenologists themselves may have cogent reasons for preferring one approach over the other.

One aspect of a qualitative analysis that *can* be critiqued, however, is whether the researchers documented that they have used one approach consistently and have been faithful to the integrity of its procedures. Thus, for example, if researchers say they are using the Glaser and Strauss's approach to grounded theory analysis, they should not also include elements from the Strauss and Corbin's method. An even more serious problem occurs when, as sometimes happens, the researchers "muddle" traditions. For example, researchers who describe their study as a grounded theory study should not present *themes* because grounded theory analysis does not yield themes. Furthermore, researchers who attempt to blend elements from two traditions may not have a clear grasp of the analytic precepts of either one. For example, a researcher who claims to have undertaken an ethnography using a grounded theory approach to analysis may not be well-informed about the underlying goals and philosophies of these two traditions.

Some further guidelines that may be helpful in evaluating qualitative analyses are presented in Box 24.3. ⊗

● ●
RESEARCH EXAMPLES

We have illustrated different analytic approaches through examples of studies throughout this chapter. Here, we present more detailed descriptions of two qualitative nursing studies.

BOX 24.3 Guidelines for Critiquing Qualitative Analyses and Interpretations

1. Was the data analysis approach appropriate for the research design, the qualitative tradition, and nature of the data?
2. Was the coding/category scheme described? If so, does the scheme appear logical and complete? Does there seem to be unnecessary overlap or redundancy in the categories?
3. Were manual methods used to index and organize the data, or was a computer program used?
4. Did the report adequately describe the process by which the actual analysis was performed? Did the report indicate whose approach to data analysis was used (e.g., Glaserian or Straussian or constructivist, in grounded theory studies)? Was this method consistently and appropriately applied?
5. What major themes or processes emerged? If excerpts from the data were provided, do the themes appear to capture the meaning of the narratives—that is, does it appear that the researcher adequately interpreted the data and conceptualized the themes or categories? Is the analysis parsimonious—could two or more themes be collapsed into a broader and perhaps more useful conceptualization?
6. What evidence did the report provide that the analysis is accurate and appropriate? Were data displayed in a manner that allows you to verify the researcher's conclusions?
7. Was a conceptual map, model, or diagram effectively displayed to communicate important processes?
8. Was a metaphor used to communicate key elements of the analysis? Did the metaphor offer an insightful view of the findings, or did it seem contrived?
9. Was the context of the phenomenon adequately described? Did the report give you a clear picture of the social or emotional world of study participants?
10. Did the analysis yield a meaningful and insightful picture of the phenomenon under study? Is the resulting theory or description trivial or obvious?

Example of a Phenomenologic Analysis

Study: Caregivers' experiences seeking hospice care for loved ones with dementia (Lewis, 2014)

Statement of Purpose: The purpose of this study was to explore the essence of caregivers' experiences in seeking formal end-of-life support.

Method: In this descriptive phenomenologic study, Lewis conducted in-depth interviews with 11 caregivers regarding 14 patients. Participants were asked to respond to the following statement: "Please describe for me your experiences seeking formal end-of-life care, and in particular hospice care, for your loved one" (p. 1224). Interviews, which were between 15 and 70 minutes in length, were audio recorded and transcribed.

Analysis: Colaizzi's method was used to analyze (manually) the data from these interviews. Lewis extracted significant statements and then formulated meanings from them. For example, the significant statement: "She had been out at the hospital because she had,

um, congestive heart failure. And actually a doctor there that knew my sister said. 'Oh, she should be on hospice'" was changed to the following formulated meaning: "When her mother was in the hospital with congestive heart failure, a doctor there who knew her sister said that her mother should be on hospice" (p. 1224). Themes were identified and then an exhaustive description was developed. Lewis went back to two participants to validate her exhaustive description. No modifications to her analysis were necessary based on these participants' feedback.

Key Findings: Caregivers' experiences of seeking hospice care for loved ones with dementia were categorized into five themes: (1) Setting the stage for heartbreak: A time of loss and despair; (2) Reaching the boiling point: A change in mentality; (3) Getting through the front lines: No one was there; (4) Settling for less: Too little, too late; and (5) Welcoming death: Grateful for the end.

Example of a Grounded Theory Analysis

Study: Trialing to pain control: A grounded theory (McDonald, 2014)

Statement of Purpose: The purpose of this study was to examine the basic social psychological process of managing inadequately relieved pain in adults.

Method: This study used classic (Glaserian) grounded theory methods. The researcher collected new data through in-depth interviews with four experts in pain management and four community-living adults with current pain problems. The experts were asked to respond to prompts such as, "Tell me how you talk to your patients about pain management and pain problems" (p. 108). The patients were asked to respond to prompts such as, "Tell me about your personal experience in talking with your doctor(s) or nurse(s) about your pain" (p. 108). McDonald also incorporated data from an earlier study of 23 older adults with osteoarthritis pain and their five primary care physicians. The combined data set included interview data from individual and patient perspectives on pain management as well as transcripts of audio recordings of patient–practitioner interactions during ambulatory medical visits.

Analysis: Data were analyzed using constant comparison. McDonald began her analysis by open coding all interview and medical visit transcripts, reviewing the data line by line, and noting content that concerned pain management. McDonald generated memos that described concepts and relationships among concepts. Once the core variable was identified, selective coding began. For theoretical coding, McDonald used the consensus family of codes and basic six Cs (see Box 24.2). McDonald further explained, "As data were analyzed and memos reviewed, the basic problem and the core variable used to resolve the problem were identified. Coding continued, moving back and forth between the data and memo generation, and progressed . . . until a clear process for managing pain was identified" (p. 108). McDonald provided illustrations of coding for the concept of *trialing*. For example, an excerpt from an interview was: "And he'll go from one thing to the next to the next for the patient until he finds something that works for them" (p. 109). This was coded as "Being open to revising" in the category "Initiating trialing."

Key Findings: The basic problem was the perception of running out of options for treating the pain. Trialing, which consisted of four phases, was the process used to resolve the problem. McDonald presented a conceptual model that showed how the four phases (finding the right practitioner, initiating the trial, adjusting treatments, and continued monitoring) were interconnected in the pain management process.

SUMMARY POINTS

- Qualitative analysis is a challenging, labor-intensive activity, with few standardized rules.
- The first major step in analyzing qualitative data is to organize and index materials for easy retrieval, typically by coding the content of the data according to a coding scheme.
- Traditionally, researchers organized their data by developing **conceptual files**—physical files in which coded excerpts of data relevant to specific categories are placed. Computer programs are now widely used to perform indexing functions and to facilitate analysis.
- The actual analysis of data usually begins with a search for categories and **themes**, which involves the discovery not only of commonalities across participants but also of natural variation and patterns in the data. Some qualitative analysts use **metaphors** or figurative comparisons to evoke a visual and symbolic analogy.
- The next analytic step often involves validating the thematic analysis. Some researchers use **quasi-statistics**, which involves a tabulation of the frequency with which certain themes or relations are supported by the data.
- In a final analytic step, analysts weave thematic strands together into an integrated picture of the phenomenon under investigation.
- Researchers whose focus is qualitative description may say that they used **qualitative content analysis** as their analytic method. Content analysis can vary in terms of an emphasis on *manifest content* or *latent content* and in the role of induction.

- In ethnographies, analysis begins as the researcher enters the field. Ethnographers continually search for *patterns* in the behavior and expressions of study participants.
- One approach to analyzing ethnographic data is Spradley's method, which involves four levels of data analysis: **domain analysis** (identifying *domains*, or units of cultural knowledge), **taxonomic analysis** (selecting key domains and constructing **taxonomies** or systems of classification), **componential analysis** (comparing and contrasting terms in a domain), and a **theme analysis** (uncovering cultural themes).
- Leininger's ethnonursing method involves four phases: collecting and recording data, categorizing descriptors, searching for repetitive patterns, and abstracting major themes.
- There are numerous approaches to phenomenologic analysis, including the descriptive methods of Colaizzi, Giorgi, and Van Kaam, in which the goal is to find common patterns of experiences shared by particular instances.
- In Van Manen's approach, which involves efforts to grasp the essential meaning of the experience being studied, researchers search for themes, using either a **holistic approach** (viewing text as a whole), **selective approach** (pulling out key statements and phrases), or **detailed approach** (analyzing every sentence).
- Central to analyzing data in a hermeneutic study is the notion of the **hermeneutic circle**, which signifies a methodologic process in which there is continual movement between the parts and the whole of the text under analysis.
- Hermeneutics has several choices for data analysis. Diekelmann's team approach calls for the discovery of a **constitutive pattern** that expresses the relationships among themes. Benner's approach consists of three processes: searching for **paradigm cases**, thematic analysis, and analysis of *exemplars*.
- Grounded theory uses the **constant comparative** method of data analysis, which involves identifying characteristics in one piece of data and comparing them with those of others to assess similarity. Developing categories in a substantive theory must **fit** the data and not be forced.

- One approach to grounded theory is the Glaser and Strauss's (Glaserian) method, in which there are two broad types of codes: **substantive codes** (in which the empirical substance of the topic is conceptualized) and **theoretical codes** (in which relationships among the substantive codes are conceptualized).
- Substantive coding involves **open coding** to capture what is going on in the data, and then **selective coding**, in which only variables relating to a core category are coded. The **core category**, a behavior pattern that has relevance for participants, is sometimes a **basic social process (BSP)** that involves an evolving process of coping or adaptation.
- In the Glaser and Strauss's method, open codes begin with **level I (in vivo) codes**, which are collapsed into a higher level of abstraction in **level II codes**. Level II codes are then used to formulate **level III codes**, which are theoretical constructs.
- Through constant comparison, the researcher compares concepts emerging from the data with similar concepts from existing theory or research to explore which parts have **emergent fit** with the theory being generated.
- Strauss and Corbin's method is an alternative grounded theory method whose outcome is a full preconceived conceptual description. This approach to grounded theory analysis involves two types of coding: open (in which categories are generated) and **axial coding** (where categories are linked with subcategories and integrated).
- A controversy in the analysis of focus group data is whether the unit of analysis is the group or individual participants—some analysts examine the data at both levels. A third analytic option is the analysis of group interactions.

STUDY ACTIVITIES

Chapter 24 of the *Resource Manual for Nursing Research: Generating and Assessing Evidence for Nursing Practice, 10th edition,* offers exercises and study suggestions for reinforcing concepts presented in this chapter. In addition, the following study questions can be addressed:

1. Read a qualitative nursing study. If a different investigator had gone into the field to study the same problem, how likely is it that the conclusions would have been the same? How transferable are the researcher's findings? What did the researcher learn that he or she would probably not have learned with a more structured and quantified approach?

2. Apply relevant questions in Box 24.3 to one of the two research examples at the end of the chapter, referring to the full journal article as necessary.

STUDIES CITED IN CHAPTER 24

Ayres, L., Kavanagh, K., & Knafl, K. (2003). Within-case and across-case approaches to qualitative data analysis. *Qualitative Health Research, 13*, 871–883.

Beck, C. T. (2002). Releasing the pause button: Mothering twins during the first year of life. *Qualitative Health Research, 12*, 593–608.

Beck, C. T. (2009). The arm: There is no escaping the reality for mothers of children with obstetric brachial plexus injuries. *Nursing Research, 58*, 237–245.

Beck, C. T., & Watson, S. (2010). Subsequent childbirth after a previous traumatic birth. *Nursing Research, 59*, 241–249.

Becker, H. S. (1970). *Sociological work*. Chicago: Aldine.

Benner, P. (1994). The tradition and skill of interpretive phenomenology in studying health, illness, and caring practices. In P. Benner (Ed.), *Interpretive phenomenology* (pp. 99–127). Thousand Oaks, CA: Sage.

*Bradbury-Jones, C., Innes, N., Evans, D., Ballantyne, F., & Taylor, J. (2013). Dental neglect as a marker of broader neglect: A qualitative investigation of public health nurses' assessments of oral health in preschool children. *BMC Public Health, 13*, 370.

*Bringer, J. D., Johnston, L. H., & Brackenridge, C. H. (2004). Maximizing transparency in a doctoral thesis: The complexities of writing about the use of QRS*NVIVO within a grounded theory study. *Qualitative Research, 4*, 247–265.

Carey, M. A., & Smith, M. W. (1994). Capturing the group effect in focus groups: A special concern in analysis. *Qualitative Health Research, 4*, 123–127.

Carpenter, J. (2008). Metaphors in qualitative research: Shedding light or casting shadows. *Research in Nursing & Health, 31*, 274–282.

Charmaz, K. (2014). *Constructing grounded theory* (2nd ed.). Thousand Oaks, CA: Sage.

Colaizzi, P. F. (1978). Psychological research as the phenomenologist views it. In R. Valle & M. King (Eds.), *Existential phenomenological alternative for psychology*. New York: Oxford University Press.

Corbin, J., & Strauss, A. (2015). *Basics of qualitative research: Techniques and procedures for developing grounded theory*. Thousand Oaks, CA: Sage.

Crist, J. D., & Tanner, C. A. (2003). Interpretation/analysis methods in hermeneutic interpretive phenomenology. *Nursing Research, 52*, 202–205.

Davies, R. B. (2010). Pain in children with Down syndrome: Assessment and intervention by parents. *Pain Management Nursing, 11*, 259–267.

de Casterlé, B. D., Gastmans, C., Bryon, E., & Denier, Y. (2012). QUAGOL: A guide for qualitative data analysis. *International Journal of Nursing Studies, 49*, 360–371.

Diekelmann, N. L., Allen, D., & Tanner, C. (1989). *The NLN criteria for appraisal of baccalaureate programs: A critical hermeneutic analysis*. New York: National League for Nursing Press.

DeSantis, L., & Ugarriza, D. N. (2000). The concept of theme as used in qualitative nursing research. *Western Journal of Nursing Research, 22*, 351–372.

Drahota, A., & Dewey, A. (2008). The sociogram: A useful tool in the analysis of focus groups. *Nursing Research, 57*, 293–297.

Duggleby, W. (2005). What about focus group interaction data? *Qualitative Health Research, 15*, 832–840.

Elo, S., & Kyngäs, H. (2007). The qualitative content analysis process. *Journal of Advanced Nursing, 62*, 107–115.

*Ersek, M., & Jablonski, A. (2014). A mixed-method approach to investigating the adoption of evidence-based pain practices in nursing homes. *Journal of Gerontological Nursing, 40*, 52–60.

Fetterman, D. M. (2010). *Ethnography: Step by step* (3rd ed.). Thousand Oaks, CA: Sage.

Gadamer, H. G. (1975). *Truth and method*. London, United Kingdom: Sheed and Ward.

Giorgi, A. (1985). *Phenomenology and psychological research*. Pittsburgh, PA: Duquesne University Press.

Glaser, B. (1978). *Theoretical sensitivity*. Mill Valley, CA: Sociology Press.

Glaser, B. (1992). *Emergence versus forcing: Basics of grounded theory analysis*. Mill Valley, CA: Sociology Press.

Glaser, B. (2001). *The grounded theory perspective: Conceptualization contrasted with description*. Mill Valley, CA: Sociology Press.

Glaser, B. (2005). *The grounded theory perspective III: Theoretical coding*. Mill Valley, CA: Sociology Press.

Glaser, B. G., & Strauss, A. (1967). *The discovery of grounded theory: Strategies for qualitative research*. New York: Aldine de Gruyter.

*Graneheim, U., & Lundman, B. (2004). Qualitative content analysis in nursing research: Concepts, procedures and measures to achieve trustworthiness. *Nurse Education Today, 24*, 105–112.

*Hansen, L., Press, N., Rosenkranz, M., Baggs, J., Gray, E., Kendall, J., . . . Chestnut, M. (2012). Life-sustaining treatment decisions in the ICU for patients with ESLD. *Research in Nursing & Health, 35,* 518–532.

Hendson, L., Reis, M., & Nicholas, D. (2015). Health care providers' perspectives of providing culturally competent care in the NICU. *Journal of Obstetric, Gynecologic, & Neonatal Nursing, 44,* 17–27.

Hoare, K., Mills, J., & Francis, K. (2012). Sifting, sorting, and saturating data in a grounded theory study of information use by practice nurses: A worked example. *International Journal of Nursing Practice, 18,* 582–588.

*Hsieh, H., & Shannon, S. (2005). Three approaches to qualitative content analysis. *Qualitative Health Research, 15,* 1277–1288.

Hunter, A., Lusardi, P., Zucker, D., Jacelon, C., & Chandler, G. (2002). Making meaning: The creative component in qualitative research. *Qualitative Health Research, 12,* 388–398.

James, I., Andershed, B., & Ternestedt, B. (2009). The encounter between informal and professional care at the end of life. *Qualitative Health Research, 19,* 258–271.

Johnson, B. E. (2011). The speed and accuracy of voice recognition software-assisted transcription versus the listen-and-type method: A research note. *Qualitative Research, 11,* 91–97.

Kidd, P. S., & Parshall, M. B. (2000). Getting the focus and the group: Enhancing analytic rigor in focus group research. *Qualitative Health Research, 10,* 293–308.

Kisch, A., Bolmsjö, I., Lenhoff, S., & Bengtsson, M. (2014). Having a sibling as donor: Patients' experiences immediately before allogeneic hematopoietic stem cell transplantation. *European Journal of Oncology Nursing, 18,* 436–442.

Krippendorff, K. (2013). *Content analysis: An introduction to its methodology* (3rd ed.). Thousand Oaks, CA: Sage.

Lawler, D., Begley, C., & Lalor, J. (2015). (Re)constructing myself: The process of transition to motherhood for women with a disability. *Journal of Advanced Nursing, 71*(7), 1672–1683.

Lewins, A., & Silver, C. (2014). *Using software in qualitative research* (2nd ed.). Thousand Oaks, CA: Sage.

Lewis, L. F. (2014). Caregivers' experiences seeking hospice care for loved ones with dementia. *Qualitative Health Research, 24,* 1221–1231.

MacLean, L., Meyer, M., & Estable, A. (2004). Improving accuracy of transcripts in qualitative research. *Qualitative Health Research, 14,* 113–123.

McDonald, D. D. (2014). Trialing to pain control: A grounded theory. *Research in Nursing & Health, 37,* 107–116.

McFarland, M. R., & Wehbe-Alamah, H. B. (2015). *Leininger's culture care diversity and universality: A worldwide nursing theory.* Burlington, MA: Jones & Bartlett Learning.

Miles, M., & Huberman, M. (2014). *Qualitative data analysis: An expanded sourcebook* (3rd ed.). Thousand Oaks, CA: Sage.

Morrison-Beedy, D., Côté-Arsenault, D., & Feinstein, N. (2001). Maximizing results with focus groups. *Applied Nursing Research, 14,* 48–53.

Morse, J. M., & Field, P. A. (1995). *Qualitative research methods for health professionals* (2nd ed.). Thousand Oaks, CA: Sage.

Nilsson, A., Rasmussen, B., & Edvardsson, D. (2013). Falling behind: A substantive theory of care for older people with cognitive impairment in acute settings. *Journal of Clinical Nursing, 22,* 1682–1691.

*Novak, J., & Cañas, A. (2006). *The theory underlying concept maps and how to construct them* (IHMC CmapTools Technical Report 2006-01). Pensacola, FL: Institute for Human and Machine Cognition.

*Palacios, J., Chesla, C., Kennedy, H., & Strickland, J. (2012). Embodied meanings of early childbearing among American Indian women: A turning point. *Journal of Midwifery & Women's Health, 57,* 502–508.

Papadatou, D., Papaligoura, Z. G., & Bellali, T. (2015). From infertility to successful third-party reproductions: The trajectory of Greek women. *Qualitative Heath Research.* Advance online publication. doi:10.1177/1049732314566322

Patton, M. Q. (2002). *Qualitative research and evaluation methods.* Thousand Oaks, CA: Sage.

Rallison, L., & Raffin-Bouchal, S. (2013). Living in the in-between: Families caring for a child with progressive neurodegenerative illness. *Qualitative Health Research, 23,* 194–206.

Rashotte, J., Tousignant, K., Richarson, C., Fotherfill-Bourbonnais, F., Nakhla, M., Olivier, P., & Lawson, M. (2014). Living with sensor-augmented pump therapy in type 1 diabetes: Adolescents' and parents' search for harmony. *Canadian Journal of Diabetes, 38*(4), 256–262.

*Rasmussen, T. S., & Delmar, C. (2014). Dignity as an empirical lifeworld construction—In the field of surgery in Denmark. *International Journal of Qualitative Studies on Health and Well-being, 9,* 24849.

Raymond, L. M., & Omeri, A. (2015). Transcultural midwifery: Culture care for Mauritian immigrant childbearing families living in New South Wales, Australia. In M. R. McFarland & H. B. Wehbe-Alamah (Eds.), *Leininger's culture care diversity and universality: A worldwide nursing theory* (pp. 183–254). Burlington, MA: Jones & Bartlett Learning.

Ricoeur, P. (1981). *Hermeneutics and the social sciences* (J. Thompson, Trans. & Ed.). New York: Cambridge University Press.

Saldaña, J. (2013). *The coding manual for qualitative researchers* (2nd ed.). Thousand Oaks, CA: Sage.

Sandelowski, M. (2001). Real qualitative researchers do not count: The use of numbers in qualitative research. *Research in Nursing & Health, 24,* 230–240.

Smythe, E., Payne, D., Wilson, S., Paddy, A., & Heard, K. (2014). Revealing tact with postnatal care. *Qualitative Health Research, 24,* 163–167.

Spradley, J. (1979). *The ethnographic interview.* New York: Holt, Rinehart & Winston.

Strang, V., Koop, P., Dupuis-Blanchard, S., Nordstrom, M., & Thompson, B. (2006). Family caregivers and transition to long-term care. *Clinical Nursing Research, 15,* 27–45.

Thorne, S., & Darbyshire, P. (2005). Land mines in the field: A modest proposal for improving the craft of qualitative health research. *Qualitative Health Research, 15,* 1105–1113.

Van Kaam, A. (1966). *Existential foundations of psychology.* Pittsburgh, PA: Duquesne University Press.

Van Manen, M. (1990). *Researching lived experience: Human science for an action sensitive pedagogy*. Ontario, Canada: Althouse Press.

Van Manen, M. (2002). *Writing in the dark: Phenomenological studies in interpretive inquiry*. Ontario, Canada: Althouse Press.

Van Manen, M. (2006). Writing qualitatively or the demands of writing. *Qualitative Health Research, 16*, 713–722.

Walker, D., & Myrick, F. (2006). Grounded theory: An exploration of process and procedure. *Qualitative Health Research, 16*, 547–559.

Wuest, J., & Hodgins, M. J. (2011). Reflections on methodological approaches and conceptual contributions in a program of caregiving research: Development and testing of Wuest's theory of family caregiving. *Qualitative Health Research, 21*, 151–161.

A link to this open-access journal article is provided in the Toolkit for this chapter in the accompanying Resource Manual. ✖

25 | Trustworthiness and Integrity in Qualitative Research

Integrity in qualitative research is an all-encompassing issue that begins as questions are formulated and continues through writing the report. The issues discussed in this chapter are critical for those learning to do qualitative research.

PERSPECTIVES ON QUALITY IN QUALITATIVE RESEARCH

Qualitative researchers agree on the importance of doing high-quality research, yet few issues in qualitative inquiry have generated more controversy than efforts to define what is meant by "high-quality." We provide an overview of this debate to help you identify a position that is compatible with your philosophical and methodologic views.

Debates about Rigor and Validity

One contentious issue in the debate about quality concerns the use of terms such as *rigor* and *validity*. These terms are shunned by some because of their association with the positivist paradigm—they are not seen as appropriate goals for the constructivist or critical paradigms. Those who advocate different criteria and terms for evaluating quality in qualitative research argue that the philosophical underpinnings and goals in the various paradigms are fundamentally different and so require different terminology. For these critics, the concept of rigor does not fit into an interpretive approach that values

insight and creativity (e.g., Denzin & Lincoln, 2000). As Sandelowski (1993a) put it, "We can preserve or kill the spirit of qualitative work; we can soften our notion of rigor to include the . . . soulfulness (and) imagination . . . we associate with more artistic endeavors, or we can further harden it by the uncritical application of rules. The choice is ours: rigor or rigor mortis" (p. 8).

Others defend using the term *validity*. Whittemore and colleagues (2001), for example, argued that validity is an appropriate term in all paradigms, noting that the dictionary definition of validity (the quality of being sound, just, and well-founded) lends itself equally to qualitative and quantitative research. Morse and colleagues (2002) posited that "the broad and abstract concepts of reliability and validity can be applied to all research because the goal of finding plausible and credible outcome explanations is central to all research" (p. 3). Another, more pragmatic, argument favoring the use of "mainstream" terms like validity and rigor is precisely that they *are* mainstream. In a world dominated by quantitative researchers whose quality criteria are used to make funding decisions, it may be useful to use recognizable terms and criteria.

Sparkes (2001) contended that the debate over validity is not a simple dichotomy and suggested that there are four possible perspectives on the issue. The first, which he called the *replication perspective*, is that validity is an appropriate criterion for assessing quality in both qualitative and quantitative studies, although qualitative researchers use different procedures to achieve it. Those who adopt a *parallel perspective* maintain that a separate set of evaluative criteria needs to be developed for qualitative inquiry. This perspective resulted in the development of standards for the **trustworthiness** of qualitative research that parallel the standards of reliability and validity in quantitative research (Lincoln & Guba, 1985). The third perspective in Sparke's typology is the *diversification of meanings perspective*, which is characterized by efforts to establish new forms of validity that do not have reference points in traditional quantitative research. As one example, Lather (1986) discussed *catalytic validity* in connection with critical and feminist research as the degree to which the research process energizes study participants and alters their consciousness. The final perspective in Sparke's typology was what he called the *letting-go-of-validity perspective*, which involves a total abandonment of the concept of validity. Wolcott (1994), an ethnographer, represented this perspective in his discussion of the absurdity of validity. Yet, as Wolcott (1995) himself noted, validity can be dismissed, but the issue itself will not go away: "Qualitative researchers need to understand what the debate is about and *have* a position; they do not have to resolve the issue itself" (p. 170).

Generic versus Specific Standards

Another issue in the controversy about quality criteria for qualitative studies concerns whether there should be a generic set of standards or specific standards for different types of study—for example, for ethnographers and grounded theory researchers. Many writers have endorsed the notion that research conducted within different traditions must attend to different concerns and that techniques for enhancing and demonstrating research integrity vary. Watson and Girard (2004), for example, proposed that quality standards must be "congruent with the philosophical underpinnings supporting the research tradition endorsed" (p. 875). Many writers have offered standards for specific forms of qualitative inquiry, such as grounded theory (Chiovitti & Piran, 2003); phenomenology and hermeneutics (De Witt & Ploeg, 2006; Whitehead, 2004); ethnography (Hammersley, 1992; LeCompte & Goetz, 1982);

descriptive qualitative research (Milne & Oberle, 2005); and critical research (Lather, 1986).

Some writers believe, however, that certain quality criteria are fairly universal within the constructivist paradigm. In their synthesis of criteria for developing evidence of validity in qualitative studies, Whittemore and associates (2001) proposed four primary criteria that they viewed as essential to all qualitative inquiry.

Standards for Conduct versus Assessment of Qualitative Research

Yet another issue concerns whose point of view is being considered in the quality standards. Morse and colleagues (2002) contended that many of the established standards are relevant for *assessment* by readers rather than as guides to conducting high-quality qualitative research. They believe that Lincoln and Guba's criteria—often considered the gold standard—are best described as *post hoc* tools that reviewers can use to evaluate trustworthiness of a completed study: "While strategies of trustworthiness may be useful in attempting to *evaluate* rigor, they do not in themselves *ensure* rigor" (p. 9).

As an example of how the viewpoint of evaluators has been given prominence, one suggested indicator of integrity is **researcher credibility**—that is, the faith that can be put in the researcher (Patton, 1999, 2002). Such an indicator might affect readers' confidence in the integrity of the inquiry, but it clearly is not a *strategy* that researchers can adopt to make their study more rigorous.

Morse and colleagues (2002) have emphasized the importance of verification strategies that researchers can use throughout the inquiry "so that reliability and validity are actively attained, rather than proclaimed by external reviewers on the completion of the project" (p. 9). In their view, responsibility for ensuring rigor should rest with researchers, not with external judges. They advocated a proactive stance involving self-scrutiny and verification. Morse (2006) noted that "good qualitative inquiry must be verified reflexively in each step of the analysis. This means that it is self-correcting" (p. 6).

From the point of view of qualitative researchers, the ongoing question must be: How can I be confident that my account is an accurate and insightful representation? From the point of view of a critical reader, the question is: How can I trust that the researcher has offered an accurate and insightful representation?

Terminology Proliferation and Confusion

The result of all these controversies is that there is no common vocabulary for quality criteria in qualitative research—nor, for that matter, for quality goals. Terms such as *goodness*, *integrity*, *truth value*, *rigor*, and *trustworthiness* abound, and for each proposed descriptor, several critics refute the term as an appropriate name for an overall goal.

Establishing a consensus on what the quality criteria for qualitative inquiry should be, and what they should be named, remains elusive, and it is unlikely that a consensus will be achieved in the near future, if ever. Some feel that the ongoing debate is healthy, but others feel that "the situation is confusing and has resulted in a deteriorating ability to actually discern rigor" (Morse et al., 2002, p. 5).

Given the lack of consensus, and the heated arguments supporting and contesting various frameworks, it is difficult to offer definitive guidance. We present information about *criteria* from two frameworks in the section that follows and then describe *strategies* for diminishing threats to integrity in qualitative research. We recommend that these frameworks and strategies be viewed as points of departure for explorations on how to make a qualitative study as rigorous/trustworthy/insightful/valid as possible.

FRAMEWORKS OF QUALITY CRITERIA

Although not without critics, the quality criteria most often cited by qualitative researchers are those proposed by Lincoln and Guba (1985) and later augmented by Guba and Lincoln (1994). A second framework is a synthesis proposed of 10 quality guidelines, as proposed by Whittemore and colleagues (2001).

In thinking about criteria for qualitative inquiry, attention needs to be paid to both "art" and "science" and to interpretation and description. Creativity and insightfulness need to be encouraged and sustained but not at the expense of scientific

excellence. And the quest for rigor cannot sacrifice inspiration and elegant abstractions, or else the results are likely to be "perfectly healthy but dead" (Morse, 2006, p. 6). Good qualitative work is both descriptively sound and explicit and interpretively rich and innovative.

Lincoln and Guba's Framework

Lincoln and Guba (1985) suggested four criteria for developing the *trustworthiness* of a qualitative inquiry: credibility, dependability, confirmability, and transferability. These four criteria represent parallels to the positivists' criteria of internal validity, reliability, objectivity, and external validity, respectively. This framework provided the platform on which much of the current controversy on rigor emerged. Responding to numerous criticisms and to their own evolving conceptualizations, a fifth criterion that is more distinctively within the constructivist paradigm was added: authenticity (Guba & Lincoln, 1994).

Credibility

Credibility is viewed by Lincoln and Guba as an overriding goal of qualitative research and is a criterion identified in several qualitative frameworks. **Credibility** refers to confidence in the truth of the data and interpretations of them. Qualitative researchers must strive to establish confidence in the truth of the findings for the particular participants and contexts in the research. Lincoln and Guba pointed out that credibility involves two aspects: first, carrying out the study in a way that enhances the believability of the findings, and second, taking steps to *demonstrate* credibility in research reports.

Dependability

The second criterion in the Lincoln–Guba framework is **dependability**, which refers to the stability (reliability) of data over time and conditions. The dependability question is: Would the findings of an inquiry be repeated if it were replicated with the same (or similar) participants in the same (or similar) context? Credibility cannot be attained in the absence of dependability.

Confirmability

Confirmability refers to objectivity, that is, the potential for congruence between two or more independent people about the data's accuracy, relevance, or meaning. Confirmability concerns establishing that the data represent the information participants provided and that the interpretations of those data are not invented by the inquirer. For this criterion to be achieved, findings must reflect the participants' voices and the conditions of the inquiry, and not the researcher's biases or perspectives.

Transferability

Transferability refers to the potential for extrapolation, that is, the extent to which findings can be transferred to or have applicability in other settings or groups. As Lincoln and Guba (1985) noted, the investigator's responsibility is to provide sufficient descriptive data so that consumers can evaluate the applicability of the data to other contexts: "Thus the naturalist cannot specify the external validity of an inquiry; he or she can provide only the thick description necessary to enable someone interested in making a transfer to reach a conclusion about whether transfer can be contemplated as a possibility" (p. 316).

→ **TIP:** You may run across the term *fittingness*, a term Guba and Lincoln used earlier to refer to the degree to which research findings have meaning to others in similar situations. In later work, however, they used the term *transferability*. Similarly, they used the term *auditability*, a concept that was later refined and called *dependability*.

Authenticity

Authenticity refers to the extent to which researchers fairly and faithfully show a range of realities. Authenticity emerges in a report when it conveys the feeling tone of participants' lives as they are lived. A text has authenticity if it invites readers into a vicarious experience of the lives being described and enables readers to develop a heightened sensitivity to the issues being depicted. When a text achieves authenticity, readers are better able to understand the lives being portrayed "in the round," with some sense of the mood, feeling, experience, language, and context of those lives.

Whittemore and Colleagues' Framework

Whittemore and colleagues (2001), in their synthesis of quality criteria from 10 prominent frameworks (including that of Lincoln and Guba), used the term *validity* as the overarching goal. In their view, four primary criteria are essential to all qualitative inquiry, and six secondary criteria provide supplementary benchmarks of validity that are not relevant to every study. Researchers must decide, based on the goals of their research, the optimal weight that should be given to each criterion.

The four primary criteria in the Whittemore et al. (2001) framework are credibility and authenticity (overlapping the Lincoln and Guba framework) and criticality and integrity. **Criticality** refers to the researcher's critical appraisal of all decisions made throughout the research process. **Integrity** is demonstrated by ongoing self-reflection and self-scrutiny to ensure that interpretations are valid and grounded in the data. Criticality and integrity are interrelated and sometimes considered jointly (e.g., Milne & Oberle, 2005).

→ **TIP:** The six secondary criteria in the Whittemore et al. (2001) framework are explicitness, vividness, creativity, thoroughness, congruence, and sensitivity. These are described in the Supplement to this chapter on thePoint®. 🔊

STRATEGIES TO ENHANCE QUALITY IN QUALITATIVE INQUIRY

The criteria for establishing integrity in a qualitative study are challenging—regardless of the names people attach to them. Various strategies have been proposed to address these challenges, and this section describes many of them.

Many quality-enhancing strategies simultaneously address multiple criteria. For this reason, we have not organized strategies according to quality criteria—for example, identifying strategies specifically to enhance *credibility*. Instead, we have organized strategies according to different phases of an inquiry, namely, data collection, coding and analysis, and report preparation. This organization is imperfect due to the nonlinear and iterative nature of research activities in qualitative studies, and so we acknowledge that some activities described under one aspect of a study are likely to have relevance under another.

Table 25.1 suggests how various quality-enhancement strategies map onto the criteria in the Lincoln and Guba (1985) framework and the four primary criteria in the Whittemore et al. (2001) framework.

Quality-Enhancement Strategies in Collecting Data

Several strategies that qualitative researchers use to enrich and strengthen their studies have been mentioned in previous chapters and will not be elaborated here. For example, intensive listening during an interview, careful probing to obtain rich and comprehensive data, audio-recording interviews for transcription, and monitoring transcription accuracy are all strategies to enhance data quality, as are methods to gain people's trust during fieldwork (Chapter 23). In this section, we focus on additional strategies used primarily during the collection of qualitative data.

Prolonged Engagement and Persistent Observation

An important step in establishing credibility is **prolonged engagement** (Lincoln & Guba, 1985)—the investment of sufficient time collecting data to have an in-depth understanding of the people under study, to test for misinformation and distortions, and to ensure saturation of key categories. Prolonged engagement is also essential for building trust and rapport with informants, which in turn makes it more likely that rich, detailed information will be obtained. In planning a qualitative study, researchers must ensure that they have adequate time and resources to stay engaged in fieldwork for a sufficiently long period.

TIP: *Premature closure* can undermine qualitative data quality (Thorne & Darbyshire, 2005). Without a commitment to prolonged engagement, researchers may make a claim of saturation simply because they have reached a convenient stopping point.

Example of Prolonged Engagement:
Zakerihamidi and colleagues (2015) conducted a focused ethnographic study of pregnant women's perceptions of vaginal delivery versus cesarean section in Iran. The lead researcher had "long-term involvement with the participants during data collection" (p. 43). It was noted that "the researcher fully immersed herself in the culture related to the selection of the mode of delivery . . . She attended health care centers and clinics . . . for long periods" (p. 42).

High-quality data collection in qualitative inquiries also involves **persistent observation**, which concerns the salience of the data being gathered and recorded. Persistent observation refers to the researchers' focus on the characteristics or aspects of a situation or a conversation that are relevant to the phenomena being studied. As Lincoln and Guba (1985) noted, "If prolonged engagement provides scope, persistent observation provides depth" (p. 304).

Example of Persistent Observation:
Ward-Griffin and colleagues (2012) conducted a critical ethnography of the management of dementia home care resources in Ontario. They made detailed observations and conducted multiple interviews with persons with dementia, family caregivers, in-home providers, and case managers in nine dementia care networks over a 19-month period.

Reflexivity Strategies

As noted in Chapter 8, *reflexivity* involves attending systematically and continually to the context of knowledge construction—and, in particular, to the researcher's effect on the collection, analysis, and interpretation of data. Reflexivity involves awareness that the researcher as an individual brings to the inquiry a unique background, set of values, and a social and professional identity that can affect the research process.

The most widely used strategy for maintaining reflexivity and delimiting subjectivity is to maintain a reflexive journal or diary, which we discussed in Chapter 21 in connection with bracketing in phenomenologic inquiry. Reflexive notes can be used to record, from the outset of the study and in an ongoing fashion, thoughts about the impact of previous

TABLE 25.1 • Quality-Enhancement Strategies in Relation to Quality Criteria for Qualitative Inquiry

STRATEGY	CRITERIA: GUBA & LINCOLN[a]			SHARED CRITERIA		CRITERIA: WHITTEMORE et al. (Primary)[b]	
Throughout the Inquiry	Depend-ability	Confirm-ability	Transfer-ability	Credi-bility	Authen-ticity	Criticality	Integrity
Reflexivity/reflexive journaling				X	X		X
Careful documentation, audit trail	X	X				X	X
Data Generation							
Prolonged engagement				X	X		
Persistent observation				X	X		X
Comprehensive field notes			X	X			X
Theoretically driven sampling				X			
Audio recording and verbatim transcription				X	X		
Triangulation (data, method)	X			X			
Saturation of data			X	X			
Member checking	X			X		X	
Data Coding/Analysis							
Transcription rigor				X		X	
Intercoder checks; development of a codebook		X		X		X	
Quasi-statistics				X		X	
Triangulation (investigator, theory, analysis)		X		X		X	
Search for confirming evidence		X	X	X		X	
Search for disconfirming evidence/negative case analysis				X		X	X
Peer review/debriefing		X		X		X	
Inquiry audit	X	X				X	X
Presentation of Findings							
Documentation of quality-enhancement efforts				X			X
Thick, vivid description			X	X	X		
Impactful, evocative writing					X		
Disclosure of researcher credentials, background				X			
Documentation of reflexivity				X			X

[a]The criteria from the Guba and Lincoln framework (Guba & Lincoln, 1994) include dependability, confirmability, transferability, credibility, and authenticity; the last two criteria are identical to two primary criteria in the Whittemore et al. (2001) framework.
[b]The primary criteria from the Whittemore et al. (2001) framework include, in addition to credibility and authenticity, criticality and integrity.

life experiences and previous readings about the phenomenon on the inquiry. Through self-interrogation and reflection, researchers seek to be well positioned to probe deeply and to grasp the experience, process, or culture under study through the lens of participants. Some argue that systematic efforts like maintaining a journal are not merely a means of constraining subjectivity—recognition of one's own perspectives can be exploited as an interpretive advantage because ultimately findings are co-created by participants and respondents (Jootun et al., 2009).

Other reflexive strategies can be used. For example, researchers sometimes begin a study by being interviewed themselves with regard to the phenomenon under study. This approach only makes sense if the researcher has experienced that phenomenon.

Example of a Self-Interview: Zinsli and Smythe (2009) explored the experience of humanitarian disaster nursing. Participants were New Zealand nurses who had been on international relief/disaster missions. The authors wrote that the lead researcher "has himself been on several Red Cross missions. He was interviewed by a colleague early in the study for the purpose of revealing his own experiences and prejudices" (p. 235).

Other researchers ask a colleague to conduct a "bracketing interview" (or co-researchers interview each other). In such an interview, a person who is knowledgeable about reflexivity and about the study phenomenon queries the researcher about his or her a priori assumptions and perspectives.

Example of a Bracketing Interview: Champlin (2009) studied caretaking relationships between informal caretakers and mentally ill persons. A nurse with a background in phenomenology interviewed Champlin, asking such questions as "How do you expect that the participants will describe their experiences?" and "What have patients' families said to you in the past that made you interested in this experience?" (p. 1527). The interview was audio recorded and analyzed and revealed several assumptions and expectations.

Further guidance with regard to reflexivity is available in an article by Bradbury-Jones (2007) and in an edited volume of papers by Finlay and Gough (2003).

TIP: Although reflexivity is usually considered a desirable attribute in qualitative inquiry, some writers have cautioned researchers not to become so reflexive that creativity is stifled (McGhee et al., 2007). Glaser (2001) also warned against "reflexivity paralysis," (p. 47) referring to a possibly damaging compulsion to locate the inquiry within a particular theoretical context.

Data and Method Triangulation

As previously noted, triangulation refers to the use of multiple referents to draw conclusions about what constitutes truth and has been compared to convergent validation. The aim of triangulation is to "overcome the intrinsic bias that comes from single-method, single-observer, and single-theory studies" (Denzin, 1989, p. 313). Patton (1999) also advocated triangulation, arguing that "no single method ever adequately solves the problem of rival explanation" (p. 1192). Triangulation can also help to capture a more complete and contextualized portrait of key phenomena. Denzin (1989) identified four types of triangulation (data triangulation, investigator triangulation, method triangulation, and theory triangulation), two of which we describe here because they relate to data collection.

Data triangulation involves the use of multiple data sources for the purpose of validating conclusions and can take several forms. **Time triangulation** involves collecting data on the same phenomenon multiple times. Time triangulation can involve gathering data at different times of the day or at different times in the year. This concept is similar to test–retest reliability assessment—the point is not to study a phenomenon longitudinally to assess change but to assess congruence of the phenomenon across time. **Space triangulation** involves collecting data on the same phenomenon in multiple sites to test for cross-site consistency. Finally, **person triangulation** involves collecting data from different types or levels of people (e.g., individuals, their family members, clinical staff), with the aim of validating data through multiple perspectives on the phenomenon.

Method triangulation involves using multiple methods of data collection about the same phenomenon. In qualitative studies, researchers often use a rich blend of unstructured data collection methods (e.g., interviews, observations, documents) to develop a comprehensive understanding of a phenomenon. Multiple data collection methods provide an opportunity to evaluate the extent to which a consistent and coherent picture of the phenomenon emerges.

Comprehensive and Vivid Recording of Information

In addition to taking steps to record interview data accurately, researchers need to prepare thoughtful field notes that are rich with descriptions of what transpired in the field. Even if interviews are the primary data source, researchers should record descriptions of the participants' demeanor and behaviors during the interactions and should thoroughly describe the interview context.

Other record-keeping activities are also important. A log of decisions needs to be maintained, and reflexive journals should be maintained regularly with rich detail. Thoroughness helps readers and reviewers to develop confidence in the data.

Researchers sometimes specifically develop an **audit trail**, that is, a systematic collection of

materials and documentation that would allow an independent auditor to come to conclusions about the data. Six classes of records are useful in creating an adequate audit trail: (1) the raw data (e.g., interview transcripts), (2) data reduction and analysis products (e.g., theoretical notes, working hypotheses), (3) process notes (e.g., methodologic notes), (4) materials relating to researchers' intentions and dispositions (e.g., reflexive notes), (5) instrument development information (e.g., pilot forms), and (6) data reconstruction products (e.g., drafts of the final report).

TIP: Diligence in maintaining information does not in and of itself ensure the validity of the inquiry. Morse and colleagues (2002) pointed out that "audit trails may be kept as proof of the decisions made throughout the project, but they do not identify the quality of those decisions, the rationale behind those decisions, or the responsiveness and sensitivity of the investigator to data" (pp. 6–7).

Member Checking

Lincoln and Guba considered member checking a particularly important technique for establishing the credibility of qualitative data. In a **member check**, researchers provide feedback to participants about emerging interpretations and obtain participants' reactions. The argument is that if researchers' interpretations are good representations of participants' realities, participants should be able to confirm their accuracy.

Member checking can be carried out in an ongoing way as data are being collected (e.g., through deliberate probing to ensure that participants' meanings were understood) and more formally after data have been analyzed. Member checks are sometimes done in writing. For example, researchers can ask participants to review and comment on interpretive notes, thematic summaries, or drafts of the research report. Member checks are more typically done in face-to-face discussions with individual participants or small groups of participants.

> **TIP:** For focus group studies, it is usually recommended that member checking occur *in situ*. That is, moderators develop a summary of major themes or viewpoints in real time and present that summary to focus group participants at the end of the session for their feedback. Rich data often emerge from participants' reactions to those summaries.

Despite the potential contribution that member checking can make to a study's credibility, several issues need to be kept in mind. First, not all participants are willing to engage in this process. Some—especially if the topic is emotionally charged—may feel they have attained closure once they have shared their experiences. Further discussion might not be welcomed. Others may decline involvement in member checking because they are afraid it might arouse suspicions of their families.

> **TIP:** If member checking is used as a validation strategy, participants should be encouraged to provide critical feedback about factual errors or interpretive deficiencies. In writing about the study, it is important to be explicit about how member checking was done and what role it played as a validation strategy. Readers cannot develop much confidence in the study simply by learning that "member checking was done."

Another issue is that member checks can lead to misleading conclusions of credibility if participants "share some common myth or front, or conspire to mislead or cover up" (Lincoln & Guba, 1985, p. 315). Also, some participants might fail to disagree with researchers' interpretations either out of politeness or in the belief that researchers

are "smarter" or more knowledgeable than they themselves are. Thorne and Darbyshire (2005), in fact, caution against what they irreverently called *Adulatory Validity*, which they described as "the epistemological pat on the back for a job well done, or just possibly it might be part of a mutual stroking ritual that satisfies the agendas of both researcher and researched" (p. 1110). They noted that member checking tends to privilege interpretations that place study participants in the most favorable light.

Thorne and Darbyshire are not alone in their concerns about member checking as a validation strategy. Indeed, few strategies for enhancing data quality are as controversial as member checking. Morse (1999), for example, disputed the idea that participants have more analytic and interpretive authority than the researcher. Giorgi (1989) also argued that asking participants to evaluate the researcher's psychological interpretation of their own descriptions exceeds the role of participants. Morse and colleagues (2002), as well as Sandelowski (1993b), have worried that because study results have been synthesized, decontextualized, and abstracted across various participants, individual participants may not recognize their own experiences or perspectives in a member check. Even more scathingly, some critics view member checking as antithetical to the epistemology of qualitative inquiry. Smith (1993), in particular, criticized the philosophical contradictions inherent in this strategy, arguing that it is inconsistent with inquiry that purports to reveal multiple realities and multiple ways of knowing.

> **TIP:** Researchers sometimes invite participants to review their own interview transcripts for accuracy and clarification. Hagens and colleagues (2009) carefully assessed this technique in terms of improvements to rigor in a study that involved interviews with 51 key informants. They found that the review added little to the accuracy of the transcript and in some cases resulted in biases when some participants wanted to remove valuable material.

Example of Member Checking: Fenstermacher (2014) conducted a grounded theory study of the experience of perinatal bereavement in black adolescents. After the data were analyzed and a grounded theory was developed, the researcher asked two participants, "Do these results ring true for you?" Participants responded that the researcher was "right on target" and "got it exactly right" (p. 137).

Quality-Enhancement Strategies Relating to Coding and Analysis

Excellent qualitative inquiry is likely to involve the concurrent collection and analysis of data, and so several strategies described in the preceding section are also relevant to promoting analytic integrity. Member checking, for example, can occur in an ongoing fashion during data collection but typically involves participants' review of preliminary findings. Also, we discussed in Chapter 24 some strategies for analytic rigor (e.g., intensive and multiple readings of texts) and validation (e.g., use of quasi-statistics). In this section, we introduce a few other strategies that relate to the coding, analysis, and interpretation of qualitative data.

Investigator and Theory Triangulation

The overall purpose of triangulation is to converge on the truth. Triangulation offers opportunities to sort out "true" information from irrelevant or idiosyncratic information by using multiple perspectives. Several types of triangulation are pertinent during analysis. **Investigator triangulation** refers to the use of two or more researchers to make coding, analysis, and interpretation decisions. The premise is that investigators can reduce the risk of biased decisions and idiosyncratic interpretations through collaboration.

Investigator triangulation, conceptually similar to interrater reliability in quantitative studies, is often used in coding qualitative data. Coding consistency depends on having clearly defined categories and decision rules that are documented in a codebook or coding dictionary. Researchers sometimes formally compare two or more independent category schemes or a subset of independent coding decisions. Some advice on developing a codebook and assessing coding

reliability is offered by Fonteyn et al. (2008) and Burla et al. (2008).

Example of Independent Coding: Aujoulat and co-researchers (2014) studied the challenges of self-care for young liver transplant recipients. In-depth interviews were conducted with 18 patients (ages 16-30) and with several parental caregivers. Initial coding of transcripts was undertaken by two researchers, who met regularly to discuss emerging categories.

Collaboration can also be used at the analysis stage. If investigators bring to the analysis task a complementary blend of methodologic, disciplinary, and clinical expertise, the analysis and interpretation can potentially benefit from divergent perspectives. In Aujoulat and colleagues' (2014) study of young liver transplant recipients, emerging themes were discussed in four "focus group" meetings with the multidisciplinary team of researchers.

> **TIP:** In focus group studies, immediate post-session debriefings are recommended. In such debriefings—which should be tape-recorded—team members who were present during the session meet to discuss issues and themes. They also should share their views about group dynamics, such as coercive group members, censoring of controversial opinions, individual conformity to group viewpoints, and discrepancies between verbal and nonverbal behavior.

With **theory triangulation**, researchers use competing theories or hypotheses in analyzing and interpreting the data. Qualitative researchers who develop alternative hypotheses while still in the field can test the validity of each because the flexible design of qualitative studies provides ongoing opportunities to direct the inquiry. Theory triangulation can help researchers to rule out rival hypotheses and to prevent premature conceptualizations.

Although Denzin's (1989) seminal work discussed four types of triangulation, other types have been suggested. For example, Kimchi and colleagues (1991) described **analysis triangulation** (i.e., using two or more analytic techniques to analyze the same set of data). This approach offers another opportunity to validate the meanings inherent in a qualitative data set. Analysis triangulation can also involve using multiple units of analysis (e.g., individuals, dyads, families).

> **➲ TIP:** Farmer and colleagues (2006) provided a useful description of the triangulation protocol they used in the Canadian Heart Health Dissemination Project that illustrates how triangulation was operationalized.

Searching for Confirming Evidence

Member checking with participants, as already noted, is one approach to validating the findings. Another verification strategy is to seek external evidence from other studies or from sources such as artistic or literary representations of the phenomenon. Another possibility, and one that has implications for transferability, is to have people from other sites, or even other disciplines, review preliminary findings.

> **Example of Confirming Evidence:** Doornbos and colleagues (2013) sought to identify mental health concerns of women in three urban, impoverished neighborhoods. Focus group interviews were conducted with 61 women living in those neighborhoods. The researchers returned to the communities "for a presentation of the preliminary results and solicitation of feedback from community members in an effort to confirm the accuracy, relevance, and meaning of the data" (p. 82).

Searching for Disconfirming Evidence and Competing Explanations

A powerful verification procedure that occurs at the intersection of data collection and data analysis involves a systematic search for data that will challenge an emerging categorization or explanation. The search for disconfirming evidence occurs through purposive or theoretical sampling methods, as described in Chapter 22. Clearly, this strategy depends on concurrent data collection and data analysis: Researchers cannot look for disconfirming data unless they have a sense of what they need to know.

> **Example of Searching for Disconfirming Evidence:** Andersen and Owen (2014) conducted a grounded theory study to explain the process of quitting smoking cigarettes. The two investigators worked together to analyze transcripts from interviews with 16 participants: "We engaged in discussion of emerging categories, seeking out contradictory evidence" (p. 254).

Lincoln and Guba (1985) discussed the related activity of **negative case analysis**. This strategy is a process by which researchers search for cases that appear to disconfirm earlier hypotheses and then revise their interpretations as necessary. The goal of this procedure is to continuously refine a hypothesis or theory until it accounts for *all* cases.

> **Example of a Negative Case Analysis:** Begley and colleagues (2015) studied whether clinical specialists in Ireland were fulfilling role expectations in terms of involvement with research and EBP activities. After collecting the data (interviews and 184 hours of observation), the team came together to develop themes. The team searched for examples of negative cases "that might disprove, or validate, emerging findings" (p. 104).

Patton (1999) similarly encouraged a systematic exploration for rival themes and explanations during the analysis: "Failure to find strong supporting evidence for alternative ways of presenting the data or contrary explanations helps increase confidence in the original, principal explanation generated by the analyst" (p. 1191). This strategy can be addressed both inductively and logically. Inductively, the strategy involves seeking other ways of organizing the data that might lead to different conclusions and interpretations. Logically, it means conceptualizing other logical possibilities and then searching for evidence that could support those competing explanations.

> **Example of Search for Rival Explanations:** In the previously cited study of smoking cessation, Andersen and Owen (2014) noted that "potential relationships among categories were examined for competing explanations to enhance credibility of findings" (p. 254).

Peer Review and Debriefing

Another quality-enhancement strategy involves external review. **Peer debriefing** involves sessions with peers to review and explore various aspects of the inquiry. Peer debriefing exposes researchers to the searching questions of others who are experienced in either the methods of qualitative inquiry, the phenomenon being studied, or both.

In a peer debriefing session, researchers might present written or oral summaries of the data, emergent categories and themes, and interpretations of the data. In some cases, taped interviews might be played or transcripts might be given to reviewers to read. Peer debriefers might be asked to address questions such as the following:

• Is there evidence of researcher bias? Have the researchers been sufficiently reflexive?

• Do the gathered data adequately portray the phenomenon?

• Are there any apparent errors of fact?

• Are there possible errors of interpretation? Are there competing interpretations? More comprehensive or parsimonious interpretations?

• Have all important themes been identified?

• Are the themes and interpretations knit together into a cogent and creative conceptualization of the phenomenon?

Example of Peer Review: Cricco-Lizza (2014), whose study of the emotional labor of NICU nurses was summarized in Chapter 21, described efforts to verify her findings "I sought peer review through an ongoing process with oral and written critique from pre- and post-doctoral students and faculty at my university research center" (p. 617).

Inquiry Audits

A similar, but more formal, approach is to undertake an **inquiry audit**, which involves scrutiny of the data and supporting documents by an external reviewer. Such an audit requires careful documentation of all aspects of the inquiry, as previously discussed. Once the audit trail materials are assembled, the inquiry auditor proceeds to audit, in a fashion analogous to a financial audit, the trustworthiness of the data and the meanings attached to them. Although such auditing is complex, it can serve as a tool for persuading others that qualitative findings are worthy of confidence. Relatively few comprehensive inquiry audits have been reported in the literature, but some studies report partial audits. Rodgers and Cowles (1993) and Erwin and colleagues (2005) provide useful information about inquiry audits.

Example of an Inquiry Audit: Rotegård and colleagues (2012) studied cancer patients' experiences and perceptions of their personal strengths through their illness and recovery in four focus group interviews with 26 participants. A partial audit was undertaken by having an external researcher review a sample of transcripts and interpretations.

Quality-Enhancement Strategies Relating to Presentation

The strategies discussed thus far are steps that researchers can undertake to convince *themselves* that their study has integrity and credibility. This section describes some issues relating to convincing *others* of the high quality of the inquiry.

Disclosure of Quality Enhancement Strategies

A large part of demonstrating integrity to others involves providing a good description of the quality-enhancement activities that were undertaken. Many research reports fail to include information that would give readers confidence in the integrity of the research. Some qualitative reports do not address the subject of rigor, integrity, or trustworthiness at all, while others pay lip service to such concerns, simply noting, for example, that member checking was done. Just as clinicians seek *evidence* supporting health care decisions, readers of reports need evidence that the findings are believable and true. Readers can draw meaningful conclusions about study quality only if they are provided with sufficient information about quality-enhancement strategies. The research example at the end of this chapter is exemplary with regard to the information provided to readers.

> **TIP:** Avoid stating that your quality-enhancement strategies *ensured* validity or rigor. Strategies are used to *enhance* or *promote* rigor, but nothing ensures it.

Thick and Contextualized Description

Thick description, as noted in previous chapters, refers to a rich, thorough, and vivid description of the research context, the people who participated in the study, and the experiences and processes observed during the inquiry. Transferability cannot occur unless investigators provide detailed information to permit judgments about contextual similarity. Lucid and textured descriptions, with the judicious inclusion of verbatim quotes from study participants, also contribute to the authenticity and vividness of a qualitative study.

⬆ TIP: Sandelowski (2004) cautioned that " . . . the phrase *thick description* likely ought not to appear in write-ups of qualitative research at all, as it is among those qualitative research words that should be seen but not written" (p. 215).

In high-quality qualitative studies, descriptions typically need to go beyond a faithful and thorough rendering of information. Powerful description often has an evocative quality and the capacity for emotional impact. Qualitative researchers must be careful, however, not to misrepresent their findings by sharing only the most dramatic or poignant stories. Thorne and Darbyshire (2005) cautioned against "lachrymal validity," a criterion for evaluating research based on the extent to which the report can wring tears from its readers. At the same time, they noted that the opposite problem with some reports is that they are "bloodless." Bloodless findings are characterized by a tendency of some researchers to "play it safe in writing up the research, reporting the obvious (possibly in the most thinly 'salami-sliced' 'findings' articles), failing to apply any inductive analytic spin to the sequence, structure, or form of the findings" (p. 1109).

Researcher Credibility

In qualitative studies, researchers *are* the data-collecting instruments—as well as creators of the analytic process. Therefore, researcher qualifications, experience, and reflexivity are relevant in establishing confidence in the findings. Patton (2002) argued that trustworthiness is enhanced if the report contains information about the researchers and their credentials. In addition, the report may need to make clear the personal connections researchers had to the people, topic, or community under study. For example, it is relevant for a reader of a report on AIDS patients' coping to know that the researcher is HIV-positive. Patton recommended that researchers report "any personal and professional information that may have affected data collection, analysis and interpretation—either negatively or positively . . . " (p. 566).

Example of Researcher Credibility: Kindell and colleagues (2014) explored the experience of living with semantic dementia, using a case study design. Kindell was described as a speech and language therapist with 21 years of experience specializing in dementia care. She conducted all interviews, and her experience was described as a "sensitizing experience [that] served as a resource for facilitating their stories" (p. 403). A co-author was a community mental health nurse who had worked in dementia care for more than 25 years.

DEVELOPING A QUALITY-MINDED OUTLOOK

Conducting high-quality qualitative research is not just about methods and strategies—that is, it is not just about what researchers *do*. It is also about who the researchers *are*—that is, about their outlook, self-demands, and ingenuity. As Morse and colleagues (2002) succinctly put it, "Research is only as good as the investigator" (p. 10). Attributes that good qualitative researchers must possess are difficult to teach, but it is important to know what those attributes are so they can be cultivated. We express several important attributes as *commitments* to which researchers can aspire.

1. **Commitment to Transparency.** Good qualitative inquiry cannot be a secretive enterprise that masks decisions, biases, and limitations from outside scrutiny. Conscientious qualitative researchers maintain the records needed to document and justify decisions. A commitment to transparency also means seeking opportunities to have decisions reviewed by others. To the extent

possible, researchers should seek opportunities to demonstrate transparency in their writing, including how themes and categories were formulated from the initial participant data.

2. **Commitment to Thoroughness and Diligence.** Meticulousness is essential to high-quality research. Researchers who are not thorough run the risk of having thin, unsaturated data that undermine rich description of phenomena. The concept of *replication* within the study is crucial: There must be sufficient, and redundant, data to account for all aspects of the phenomenon (Morse et al., 2002). In good qualitative research, investigators must commit to reading and rereading their data, returning repeatedly to check whether their interpretations are true to their data. Thoroughness also implies that researchers will seek opportunities to challenge early conceptualizations and to find sources of corroborating evidence both internally (i.e., within the study data) and externally (e.g., in the literature).

3. **Commitment to Verification.** Confidence in the data, and in the analysis and interpretation of those data, is possible only when researchers are committed to instituting verification and self-correcting procedures throughout the study. Morse and colleagues (2002) wrote at length about the importance of verification, noting that verification is "the process of checking, confirming, making sure, and being certain" (p. 9). A strong commitment to verification strengthens methodologic coherence and helps to promote the likelihood that errors and missteps are corrected before they undermine the enterprise.

4. **Commitment to Reflexivity.** While there is not always agreement about the forms that self-reflection will assume, there is widespread agreement that qualitative researchers need to devote time and energy to analyzing and documenting their presuppositions, biases, and ongoing emotions. Reflexivity involves a continuous self-scrutiny and asking, "How might my previous experiences, values, background, and prejudices be shaping my methods, my analysis, and my interpretations?"

5. **Commitment to Participant-Driven Inquiry.** In good qualitative research, the inquiry is driven forward by the participants, not the researcher. Researchers must continuously remain responsive to the flow and content of interactions with, and observations of, their informants. Participants shape the scope and breadth of questioning, and they help to guide sampling decisions. The analysis and interpretation must give voice to those who participated in the inquiry.

6. **Commitment to Insightful Interpretation.** Morse (2006) has written that *insight* is a major process in qualitative inquiry but has been neglected and overlooked as a topic of discussion—perhaps because it is not easily acquired. Morse argued that researchers must be *ready* for insight—they must have considerable knowledge about their data and be able to link them meaningfully to relevant literature. Immersion in one's own data—and having good-quality data—are essential. Morse also noted, however, that qualitative researchers need to give themselves "*permission* to use insight and the confidence to do it well" (p. 3). Relatedly, Morse and colleagues (2002) urged researchers to *think theoretically*, which "requires macro-micro perspectives, inching forward without making cognitive leaps, constantly checking and rechecking, and building a solid foundation" (p. 13).

CRITIQUING OVERALL QUALITY IN QUALITATIVE STUDIES

For qualitative research to be judged trustworthy, investigators must *earn* their readers' trust. Many qualitative reports do not provide much information about the researchers' efforts to enhance trustworthiness, but there appears to be a trend toward greater forthrightness about quality issues. In a world that is very conscious about the quality of research evidence, qualitative researchers need to be proactive in doing high-quality research and sharing their quality-enhancement efforts with readers.

Part of the difficulty that qualitative researchers face in demonstrating trustworthiness and authen-

BOX 25.1 Guidelines for Evaluating Quality and Integrity in Qualitative Studies

1. Did the report discuss efforts to enhance or evaluate the quality of the data and the overall inquiry? If so, is the description sufficiently detailed and clear? If not, was there other information that allows you to draw inferences about the quality of the data, the analysis, and the interpretations?
2. Which specific techniques (if any) did the researcher use to enhance the quality of the inquiry? Were these strategies used judiciously and to good effect?
3. What quality-enhancement strategies were not used? Would supplementary strategies have strengthened your confidence in the study and its evidence?
4. Given the efforts to enhance data quality, what can you conclude about the study's integrity, rigor, or trustworthiness?

ticity is that page constraints in journals impose conflicting demands. It takes a precious amount of space to report quality-enhancement strategies adequately and convincingly. Using space for such documentation means that there is less space for the thick description of context and the rich verbatim accounts that are also necessary in high-quality qualitative research. As Pyett (2003) has noted, qualitative research is often characterized by the need for critical compromises. It is well to keep such compromises in mind in critiquing qualitative research reports.

Some guidelines that may be helpful in evaluating qualitative studies are presented in Box 25.1. Some additional questions that could be useful in evaluating the quality of qualitative reports are presented in the Supplement.

RESEARCH EXAMPLE

Study: Staff and students' perceptions and experiences of teaching and assessment in clinical skills laboratories: Interview findings from a multiple case study (Houghton et al., 2012); Rigour in qualitative case-study research (Houghton et al., 2013)

Statement of the Purpose: The purpose of this study was to examine nursing students' experiences in clinical practice and their perceptions of the teaching strategies in clinical skills laboratory.

Method: In this multiple case study, data were collected by semistructured interviews with 43 students in five study sites, nonparticipant observations, and documentary analysis. Data were analyzed using Morse's framework, which consists of the following four stages: comprehension, synthesis, theorizing, and recontextualization. Additional analytic strategies (e.g., memoing, distilling and ordering, and developing propositions) were also employed. NVivo 8 was used to manage the data.

Quality-Enhancement Strategies: The researchers provided detailed information about their efforts to enhance the trustworthiness of their study. With regard to *credibility*, the researchers used the following strategies: prolonged engagement and persistent observation, triangulation, peer debriefing, and member checking. Regarding prolonged engagement and persistent observation, nonparticipant observations were conducted over a 12-hour shift in each of the five study site hospitals. During the last observations, the researchers did not find new concepts emerging, which helped to confirm saturation. In terms of triangulation, the researchers used multiple sources of qualitative data. For example, observations were made to identify factors that helped or hindered nursing students in using the skills they had learned in the skills laboratory. Then, the nursing students were interviewed to describe their perceptions of these factors. Using both observation and the participants' interviews confirmed the congruence of the findings. Peer debriefing was used with an expert qualitative researcher to assess whether the expert agreed with coding decisions. The expert coded three interview transcripts and found that the codes were consistent with that of the research team. In terms of member checking, nursing students were asked to review the transcription of their interview, and none of the participants expressed any concerns. In addressing *dependability* and *confirmability*, the researchers used both an audit trail and reflexivity. Query tools in NVivo allowed the researchers to have an audit trail and help prevent excessive emphasis on isolated findings. A reflective diary helped to illustrate the transparency of decisions made in the study. The researchers provided an excerpt from their reflective diary about the development of one of the final themes of creating a bridge to the real world of practice. Finally, the researchers provided thick description to address *transferability*. Direct quotes from the nursing students were provided to illustrate the themes. Also, the researchers presented field notes to show how the themes developed from the data.

Key Findings: Findings from the study revealed the importance of having an educational setting that mirrors clinical reality. The need for effective links between the hospital setting and the educational institution in order to develop a pathway for practice was emphasized.

SUMMARY POINTS

- Several controversies surround the issue of *quality* in qualitative studies, one of which involves terminology. Some have argued that terms such as *rigor* and *validity* are quantitative terms that are unsuitable goals in qualitative inquiry, but others think that these terms are appropriate.
- Other controversies involve what criteria to use as indicators of rigor or integrity, whether there should be generic or study-specific criteria, and what strategies to use to address the quality criteria.
- The most often used framework of quality criteria is that of Lincoln and Guba, who identified five criteria for evaluating the **trustworthiness** of the inquiry: credibility, dependability, confirmability, transferability, and (added to their framework at a later date) authenticity.
- **Credibility**, which refers to confidence in the truth value of the findings, is sometimes said

to be the qualitative equivalent of internal validity. **Dependability** refers to the stability of data over time and conditions and is somewhat analogous to reliability in quantitative studies. **Confirmability** refers to the objectivity or neutrality of the data. **Transferability**, the analog of external validity, is the extent to which findings from the data can be transferred to other settings or groups. **Authenticity** refers to the extent to which researchers fairly and faithfully show a range of different realities and convey the feeling tone of lives as they are lived.

- An alternative framework, representing a synthesis of 10 qualitative validity schemes (Whittemore et al., 2001), proposed four primary criteria (credibility, authenticity, criticality, and integrity) and six secondary criteria (explicitness, vividness, creativity, thoroughness, congruence, and sensitivity). The primary criteria can be applied to any qualitative inquiry.
- **Criticality** refers to the researcher's critical appraisal of every research decision. **Integrity** is demonstrated by ongoing self-scrutiny to enhance the likelihood that interpretations are valid and grounded in the data.
- Strategies for enhancing the quality of qualitative data as they are being collected include **prolonged engagement**, which strives for adequate scope of data coverage; **persistent observation**, which is aimed at achieving adequate depth; reflexivity; comprehensive and vivid recording of information (including maintenance of an **audit trail** of key decisions); triangulation; and member checking.
- **Triangulation** is the process of using multiple referents to draw conclusions about what constitutes the truth. During data collection, key forms of triangulation include **data triangulation** (using multiple data sources to validate conclusions) and **method triangulation** (using multiple methods, such as interviews and observations, to collect data about the same phenomenon).
- **Member checks** involve asking participants to review and react to study data and emerging themes and conceptualizations. Member checking is among the most controversial methods of addressing quality issues in qualitative inquiry.

- Strategies for enhancing quality during the coding and analysis of qualitative data include **investigator triangulation** (independent coding and analysis of at least a portion of the data by two or more researchers), **theory triangulation** (use of competing theories or hypotheses in the analysis and interpretation of data), searching for confirming and disconfirming evidence, searching for rival explanations and undertaking a **negative case analysis** (revising interpretations to account for cases that appear to disconfirm early conclusions), external validation through **peer debriefings** (exposing the inquiry to the searching questions of peers), and launching a formal **inquiry audit** (a formal scrutiny of the research process and audit trail documents by an independent external auditor).
- Strategies to convince qualitative report readers of high quality include disclosure of key quality-enhancement strategies, using *thick description* to vividly portray contextualized information about participants and the central phenomenon, and making efforts to be transparent about researcher credentials and reflexivity so that **researcher credibility** can be assessed.
- Doing high-quality qualitative research is not just about *method* and what the researchers *do*—it is also about who they *are*. To become an outstanding qualitative researcher, there must be a commitment to transparency, thoroughness, verification, reflexivity, participant-driven inquiry, and insightful and artful interpretation.

STUDY ACTIVITIES

Chapter 25 of the *Resource Manual for Nursing Research: Generating and Assessing Evidence for Nursing Practice*, *10th edition*, offers exercises and study suggestions for reinforcing concepts presented in this chapter. In addition, the following study questions can be addressed:

1. You have been asked to be a peer reviewer for a team of nurse researchers who are conducting a phenomenologic study of the experiences of physical abuse during pregnancy. What specific questions would you ask the team during debriefing, and what documents would you want the researchers to share?
2. Apply relevant questions in Box 25.1 to the research example at the end of the chapter, referring to the full journal article as necessary.

STUDIES CITED IN CHAPTER 25

Andersen, J. S., & Owen, D. (2014). Helping relationships for smoking cessation. *Nursing Research*, *63*, 252–259.

Aujoulat, I., Janssen, M., Libion, F., Charles, A., Struyf, C., Smets, F., . . . Reding, R. (2014). Internalizing motivation to self-care: A multifaceted challenge for young liver transplant recipients. *Qualitative Health Research*, *24*, 357–365.

Begley, C., Elliott, N., Lalor, J., & Higgins, A. (2015). Perceived outcomes of research and audit activities of clinical specialists in Ireland. *Clinical Nurse Specialist*, *29*, 100–111.

Bradbury-Jones, C. (2007). Enhancing rigour in qualitative health research: Exploring subjectivity through Peshkin's I's. *Journal of Advanced Nursing*, *59*, 290–298.

Burla, L., Knierim, B., Barth, J., Liewald, K., Duetz, M., & Abel, T. (2008). From text to codings: Intercoder reliability assessment in qualitative content analysis. *Nursing Research*, *57*, 113–117.

Champlin, B. (2009). Being there for another with serious mental illness. *Qualitative Health Research*, *19*, 1525–1535.

Chiovitti, R., & Piran, N. (2003). Rigour and grounded theory research. *Journal of Advanced Nursing*, *44*, 427–435.

Cricco-Lizza, R. (2014). The need to nurse the nurse: Emotional labor in neonatal intensive care. *Qualitative Health Research*, *24*, 615–628.

De Witt, L., & Ploeg, J. (2006). Critical appraisal of rigour in interpretive phenomenological nursing research. *Journal of Advanced Nursing*, *55*, 215–229.

Denzin, N. K. (1989). *The research act* (3rd ed.). New York: McGraw-Hill.

Denzin, N. K., & Lincoln, Y. S. (Eds.). (2000). *Handbook of qualitative research* (2nd ed.). Thousand Oaks, CA: Sage.

Doornbos, M. M., Zandee, G., DeGroot, J., & Warpinski, M. (2013). Desired mental health resources for urban, ethnically diverse, impoverished women struggling with anxiety and depression. *Qualitative Health Research*, *23*, 78–92.

Erwin, E., Meyer, A., & McClain, N. (2005). Use of an audit in violence prevention research. *Qualitative Health Research*, *15*, 707–718.

Farmer, T., Robinson, K., Elliott, S., & Eyles, J. (2006). Developing and implementing a triangulation protocol for qualitative health research. *Qualitative Health Research*, *16*, 377–394.

Fenstermacher, K. H. (2014). Enduring to gain new perspectives: A grounded theory study of the experience of bereavement in black adolescents. *Research in Nursing & Health*, *37*, 135–143.

Finlay, L., & Gough, B. (Eds.). (2003). *Reflexivity: A practical guide for researchers in health and social sciences*. Oxford, United Kingdom: Blackwell Science.

Fonteyn, M., Vettese, M., Lancaster, D., & Bauer-Wu, S. (2008). Developing a codebook to guide content analysis of expressive writing transcripts. *Applied Nursing Research*, *21*, 165–168.

Garrino, L., Picco, E., Finiguerra, I., Rossi, D., Simone, P., & Roccatello, D. (2015). Living with and treating rare diseases: Experiences of patients and professional health care providers. *Qualitative Health Research*, *25*, 636–651.

Giorgi, A. (1989). Some theoretical and practical issues regarding the psychological and phenomenological method. *Saybrook Review*, *7*, 71–85.

Glaser, B. (2001). *The grounded theory perspective: Conceptualization contrasted with description*. Mill Valley, CA: Sociology Press.

Guba, E., & Lincoln, Y. (1994). Competing paradigms in qualitative research. In N. Denzin & Y. Lincoln (Eds.), *Handbook of qualitative research* (pp. 105–117). Thousand Oaks, CA: Sage.

*Hagens, C., Dobrow, M., & Chafe, R. (2009). Interviewee transcript review: Assessing the impact on qualitative research. *BMC Medical Research Methodology*, *9*, 47.

Hammersley, M. (1992). *What's wrong with ethnography? Methodological explorations*. London, United Kingdom: Routledge.

Houghton, C., Casey, D., Shaw, D., & Murphy, K. (2012). Staff and students' perceptions and experiences of teaching and assessment in clinical skills laboratories: Interview findings from a multiple case study. *Nurse Education Today*, *32*, e29–e34.

Houghton, C., Casey, D., Shaw, D., & Murphy, K. (2013). Rigour in qualitative case-study research. *Nurse Researcher*, *20*, 12–17.

Jootun, D., McGhee, G., & Marland, G. (2009). Reflexivity: Promoting rigour in qualitative research. *Nursing Standard*, *23*, 42–46.

Kimchi, J., Polivka, B., & Stevenson, J. S. (1991). Triangulation: Operational definitions. *Nursing Research*, *40*, 364–366.

Kindell, J., Sage, K., Wilkinson, R., & Keady, J. (2014). Living with semantic dementia: A case study of one family's experience. *Qualitative Health Research*, *24*, 401–411.

*Konradsen, H., Lillebaek, T., Wilcke, T., & Lomborg, K. (2014). Being publicly diagnosed: A grounded theory study of Danish patients with tuberculosis. *International Journal of Qualitative Studies on Health and Well-being*, *9*, 23644.

Lather, P. (1986). Issues of validity in openly ideological research: Between a rock and a hard place. *Interchange*, *17*, 63–84.

LeCompte, M., & Goetz, J. (1982). Problems of reliability and validity in ethnographic research. *Review of Educational Research*, *52*, 31–60.

Lincoln, Y. S., & Guba, E. G. (1985). *Naturalistic inquiry*. Newbury Park, CA: Sage.

McGhee, G., Marland, G., & Atkinson, J. (2007). Grounded theory research: Literature reviewing and reflexivity. *Journal of Advanced Nursing*, *60*, 334–342.

Mill, J., Harrowing, J., Rae, T., Richter, S., Minnie, K., Mbalinda, S., & Hepburn-Brown, C. (2013). Stigma in AIDS nursing care in sub-Saharan Africa and the Caribbean. *Qualitative Health Research*, *23*, 1066–1078.

Milne, J., & Oberle, K. (2005). Enhancing rigor in qualitative description. *Journal of Wound, Ostomy, and Continence Nursing*, *32*, 413–420.

Morse, J. M. (1999). Myth # 93: Reliability and validity are not relevant to qualitative inquiry. *Qualitative Health Research*, *9*, 717–718.

*Morse, J. M. (2006). Insight, inference, evidence, and verification: Creating a legitimate discipline. *International Journal of Qualitative Methods*, *5*(1).

*Morse, J. M., Barrett, M., Mayan, M., Olson, K., & Spiers, J. (2002). Verification strategies for establishing reliability and validity in qualitative research. *International Journal of Qualitative Methods*, *1*(2).

*Patton, M. (1999). Enhancing the quality and credibility of qualitative analysis. *Health Services Research*, *34*, 1189–1208.

Patton, M. Q. (2002). *Qualitative evaluation and research methods* (3rd ed.). Thousand Oaks, CA: Sage.

Pyett, P. M. (2003). Validation of qualitative research "in the real world." *Qualitative Health Research*, *13*, 1170–1179.

Rodgers, B. L., & Cowles, K. V. (1993). The qualitative research audit trail: A complex collection of documentation. *Research in Nursing and Health*, *16*, 219–226.

Rotegård, A., Fagermoen, M., & Ruland, C. (2012). Cancer patients' experiences of their personal strengths through illness and recovery. *Cancer Nursing*, *35*, E8–E17.

Sandelowski, M. (1993a). Rigor or rigor mortis: The problem of rigor in qualitative research revisited. *Advances in Nursing Science*, *16*, 1–8.

Sandelowski, M. (1993b). Theory unmasked: The uses and guises of theory in qualitative research. *Research in Nursing & Health*, *16*, 213–218.

Sandelowski, M. (2004). Counting cats in Zanzibar. *Research in Nursing & Health*, *27*, 215–216.

Smith, J. (1993). *After the demise of empiricism: The problem of judging social and educational inquiry*. Norwood, NJ: Ablex.

Sparkes, A. (2001). Myth 94: Qualitative health researchers will agree about validity. *Qualitative Health Research*, *11*, 538–552.

Thorne, S., & Darbyshire, P. (2005). Land mines in the field: A modest proposal for improving the craft of qualitative health research. *Qualitative Health Research*, *15*, 1105–1113.

*Ward-Griffin, C., Hall, J., DeForge, R., St-Amant, O., McWilliam, C., Oudshoorn, A., . . . Klosek, M. (2012). Dementia home care resources: How are we managing? *Journal of Aging Research*, *2012*, 590724.

Watson, L., & Girard, F. (2004). Establishing integrity and avoiding methodological misunderstanding. *Qualitative Health Research, 14,* 875–881.

Whitehead, L. (2004). Enhancing the quality of hermeneutic research. *Journal of Advanced Nursing, 45,* 512–518.

Whittemore, R., Chase, S. K., & Mandle, C. L. (2001). Validity in qualitative research. *Qualitative Health Research, 11,* 522–537.

Wolcott, H. (1994). *Transforming qualitative data.* London, United Kingdom: Sage.

Wolcott, H. (1995). *The art of fieldwork.* London, United Kingdom: Sage.

*Zakerihamidi, M., Roudsari, L., & Khoei, E. (2015). Vaginal delivery vs. cesarean section: A focused ethnographic study of women's perceptions in the north of Iran. *International Journal of Community Based Nursing & Midwifery, 3,* 39–50.

Zinsli, G., & Smythe, E. (2009). International humanitarian nursing work: Facing differences and embracing sameness. *Journal of Transcultural Nursing, 20,* 234–241.

A link to this open-access journal article is provided in the Toolkit for this chapter in the accompanying Resource Manual. ✪

PART 5

DESIGNING AND CONDUCTING MIXED METHODS STUDIES TO GENERATE EVIDENCE FOR NURSING

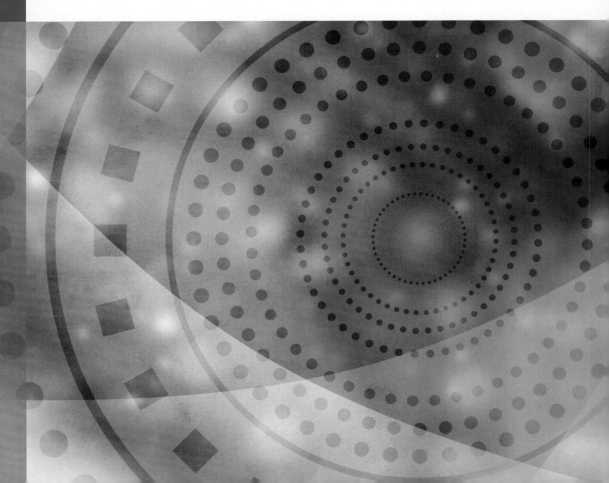

26 | Basics of Mixed Methods Research

OVERVIEW OF MIXED METHODS RESEARCH

A methodologic trend that has been gaining momentum is the planned integration of qualitative and quantitative data within single studies or a coordinated series of studies. **Mixed methods research** in the health sciences has been called "a quiet revolution" (O'Cathain, 2009). A decade ago, there was little guidance on conducting mixed methods research. Now there are abundant resources in the form of handbooks and textbooks (e.g., Andrew & Halcomb, 2009; Creswell, 2015; Creswell & Plano Clark, 2011; Morse & Niehaus, 2009; Tashakkori & Teddlie, 2010; Teddlie & Tashakkori, 2009) as well as many examples of mixed methods studies in the nursing and health care literature.

This chapter presents basic information about mixed methods research in nursing, and the next two discuss the use of mixed methods in developing and testing nursing interventions. To streamline these chapters, we will use the acronym MM in referring to mixed methods research.

Definition of Mixed Methods Research

The concept of combining qualitative and quantitative data in a study is straightforward, but definitions of MM research are not. This is partly because, in some sense, most studies could be considered MM if the definition is too broad. For example, if a grounded theory researcher asks structured demographic questions about age and education at the end of an in-depth interview, does that count as mixed methods? Or, if a survey asks a broad open-ended question at the end of a questionnaire (e.g., "Is there anything else you would like to add?"), is that MM research? We do not consider such inquiries as MM research.

We use the definition offered in the first issue of *Journal of Mixed Methods Research*, which is that MM research is "research in which the investigator collects and analyzes data, *integrates* the findings, and *draws inferences* using both qualitative and quantitative approaches or methods in a single study or program of inquiry" (Tashakkori & Creswell, 2007, p. 4). MM research at its best involves not just the collection of qualitative and quantitative data but also the *integration* of the two at some stage of the research process, giving rise to meta-inferences. A **meta-inference** is a conclusion generated by integrating inferences obtained from the results of the qualitative and quantitative strands of an MM study (Teddlie & Tashakkori, 2009).

TIP: There is widespread agreement that the term to use is *mixed methods research*, and not *multimethod research*, *triangulated research*, or *integrated research*, terms that were used in the literature in the 1990s.

Rationale for Mixed Methods Studies

The dichotomy between quantitative and qualitative data represents a key methodologic distinction in the behavioral and health sciences. Some have argued that the paradigms that underpin qualitative and quantitative research are fundamentally incompatible. Many people, however, now believe that many areas of inquiry can be enriched through the judicious triangulation of qualitative and quantitative data. The advantages of mixed methods include the following:

- *Complementarity*. Qualitative and quantitative approaches are complementary; they represent words and numbers, the two fundamental languages of human communication. By using mixed methods, researchers can allow each to do what it does best, possibly avoiding the limitations of a single approach—although Sandelowski (2014) has noted that "strength and weakness are not attributes of research approaches but rather of judgments researchers make about them" (p. 4).
- *Practicality*. Given the complexity of phenomena, it is practical to use whatever methodologic tools are best suited to addressing pressing research questions and to not have one's hands tied by rigid adherence to a single approach. MM researchers often ask questions that cannot be answered with a single approach.
- *Incrementality*. Progress on a topic tends to be incremental, relying on feedback loops. Qualitative findings can generate hypotheses to be tested quantitatively, and quantitative findings sometimes need clarification through in-depth probing. It can be productive to build such a loop into a study design, simultaneously addressing exploratory and confirmatory questions.
- *Enhanced validity*. When a hypothesis or model is supported by complementary types of data, researchers can be more confident about the validity of their results. The triangulation of methods can provide opportunities for testing alternative interpretations of the data and for examining the extent to which the context helped to shape the results.
- *Collaboration*. Mixed methods research provides opportunity and encouragement for collaboration between qualitative and quantitative researchers working on similar problems.

Paradigm Issues and Mixed Methods Studies

Although MM research has been around for decades, specific methodologic developments and broad acceptance are recent phenomena. Mixed methods approaches emerged from the ashes of the so-called *paradigm wars* involving philosophical and methodologic debates between the post-positivist and constructivist camps that raged during the 1970s and 1980s. MM research gained momentum at the turn of the 21st century, in what some have called the *third methodologic movement* (Tashakkori & Teddlie, 2003) or the *third research community* (Teddlie & Tashakkori, 2009).

Discussions about an appropriate paradigmatic stance for MM research abound. Viewpoints range from those claiming the irrelevance of paradigms to those advocating multiple paradigms. The paradigm called **pragmatism** is most often associated with MM research. Pragmatism provides a basis for a stance that has been stated as the "dictatorship of the research question" (Tashakkori & Teddlie, 2003, p. 21). Pragmatist researchers consider that it is the research question that should drive the inquiry and that the question is more important than the methods used. They reject a forced choice between the traditional post-positivists' and constructivists' modes of inquiry. In the pragmatist paradigm, both induction and deduction are important, theory generation and theory verification can be accomplished, and a pluralistic view is encouraged. Pragmatism is, as the name suggests, practical: Whatever works best to arrive at good evidence is appropriate.

Practical Issues and Mixed Methods Studies

Mixed methods studies have become attractive to graduate students and seasoned researchers alike, but the decision to pursue such a study should not be made lightly. The researcher's skills should be critically evaluated in deciding whether to undertake an MM study because the researcher must be competent in both qualitative and quantitative methods. Although a team approach is a useful way to proceed because experts in both approaches can make contributions, all members of a team should be methodologically bilingual and have basic understanding of varied approaches.

> **TIP:** In dissertation MM research, the judicious selection of advisers with a mix of methodologic skills is imperative. Keep in mind, however, that advisers from different backgrounds may have conflicting views about the merit of your strategies and the emphasis given to different aspects of your study.

Mixed methods research can be expensive. Although funding agencies increasingly are looking favorably on MM studies, it is obviously costly to collect, analyze, and integrate two or more types of data. Relatedly, mixed methods studies are often time-consuming. Inevitably, the use of multiple methods requires more time than if only a single method were used. It is wise to develop a realistic timeline before embarking on an MM inquiry.

GETTING STARTED ON A MIXED METHODS STUDY

In this chapter, we discuss many aspects of mixed methods research, with particular emphasis on research design and the analysis of MM data. We begin, however, by considering the kinds of problems and questions that lend themselves to MM research.

Purposes and Applications of Mixed Methods Research

Creswell and Plano Clark (2011) identified six broad types of research situations that are especially well suited to MM research:

1. The concepts are new and poorly understood and there is a need for qualitative exploration before more formal, structured methods can be used.
2. Neither a qualitative nor a quantitative approach, by itself, is adequate in addressing the complexity of the research problem.

3. The findings from one approach can be greatly enhanced with a second source of data.
4. The quantitative results are puzzling and difficult to interpret, and qualitative data can help to explain the results.
5. A particular theoretical perspective might require both qualitative and quantitative data.
6. A multiphase project is needed to attain key objectives, such as the development and assessment of an intervention.

As this list suggests, mixed methods research can be used in various situations. Some specific applications are noteworthy because MM research has made important contributions in these areas.

Instrument Development
Instrumentation is a good example of the first situation. Researchers sometimes collect qualitative data as a basis for developing structured instruments for research or clinical applications. The questions for a formal instrument are sometimes derived from clinical experience or prior research. When a construct is new, however, these mechanisms may be inadequate to capture its full dimensionality. Thus, researchers sometimes gather qualitative data as the basis for generating items for quantitative instruments that are then rigorously tested, as described in Chapter 15.

> **Example of Instrumentation:** Beck and Gable (2000) developed the Postpartum Depression Screening Scale for screening new mothers. Scale items were based on in-depth interviews of mothers suffering from postpartum depression in three qualitative studies. As an example of how an item was developed from mothers' words, the quote "I was extremely obsessive with my thoughts. They would never stop. I could not control them" was developed into the item: I could not control the thoughts that kept coming into my mind (Beck & Gable, 2001).

Intervention Development
Qualitative research is playing an increasingly important role in the development of promising nursing interventions and in efforts to assess their efficacy. There is growing recognition that the development of effective interventions must take clients' perspective into account. Intervention research

is increasingly likely to be MM research, a topic we address in the next chapter.

> **Example of Intervention Research:** Zoffmann and Kirkevold (2012) described how their grounded theory studies on barriers to empowerment among patients with diabetes led to the development of a problem-solving intervention called Guided Self-Determination (GSD). The intervention was subsequently evaluated in a randomized controlled trial.

Hypothesis Generation and Testing

In-depth qualitative studies are often fertile with insights about constructs or relationships among them. These insights then can be tested and confirmed with larger samples in quantitative studies. This often happens in separate investigations. One problem, however, is that it usually takes years to do a study and publish results, which means that considerable time may elapse between the qualitative insights and the formal testing of hypotheses based on those insights. A researcher can undertake a coordinated set of MM studies that has hypothesis generation and testing as an explicit goal.

> **Example of Hypothesis Generation/Testing:** Elstad and co-researchers (2011) undertook a mixed methods study of how individuals with lower urinary tract symptoms (LUTS) use fluid manipulation to self-manage their symptoms. Quantitative data came from a random sample of over 5,000 adults participating in a community health survey. Qualitative data came from in-depth interviews and focus group interviews with 152 of the survey participants who had LUTS. Themes from the qualitative data were used as the basis for hypotheses that were then tested statistically using the quantitative data.

Explication

Qualitative data are sometimes used to explicate the *meaning* of quantitative descriptions or relationships. Quantitative methods can demonstrate that variables are systematically related but may fail to provide insights about *why* they are related. Such explications can corroborate statistical findings and guide the interpretation of results. Qualitative data can provide more global and dynamic views of the phenomena under study.

> **Example of Explicating Relationships with Qualitative Data:** Edinburgh and co-researchers (2014) undertook a mixed methods study of multiple-perpetrator rape among girls evaluated at a Child Advocacy Center. Quantitative data from records were used to understand differences in the circumstances of girls raped by a single perpetrator versus multiple perpetrators (e.g., higher incidence of alcohol use). In-depth forensic interviews with 32 multiple-perpetrator victims revealed that alcohol was a common weapon used by offenders, resulting in the victims having trouble remembering details of the rape.

Theory Building, Testing, and Refinement

An ambitious application of MM research is in the area of theory exploration and construction. A theory gains acceptance as it escapes disconfirmation, and the use of multiple methods provides good opportunity for potential disconfirmation of a theory. If the theory can survive these assaults, it can provide a stronger base for the organization of clinical and intellectual work.

> **Example of Theory Exploration:** Granger and colleagues (2013) used mixed methods in a study designed to explore key constructs in the Meaning-Response theory for understanding medication adherence in patients with chronic heart failure. Ten patients completed guided interviews related to six theoretical concepts and also completed standardized measures of medication-related beliefs, behaviors, and symptoms.

Research Questions for Mixed Methods Research

In many mixed methods studies, the research questions are the driving force behind the scope of the inquiry. Investigators in MM studies typically pose questions that can *only* be addressed (or that can *best* be addressed) with more than one type of data.

In mixed methods research, there is typically an overarching goal, but there are inevitably at least two research questions, each of which requires a different type of data and approach. For example, MM researchers may simultaneously ask exploratory (qualitative) questions and confirmatory (quantitative) questions. In a mixed methods study, researchers can examine causal *effects* in a

TABLE 26.1 • Examples of Mixed Methods Question Combinations

TYPE OF RESEARCH	EXAMPLE OF A QUANTITATIVE QUESTION	EXAMPLE OF A QUALITATIVE QUESTION
Clinical trial	Are boomerang pillows more effective than straight pillows in improving the respiratory capacity of hospitalized patients?	Why did some patients complain about the boomerang pillows? How did the pillows feel?
Evaluation	How effective and cost-effective is a nurse-managed special care unit compared with traditional intensive care units?	How accepting were other health care workers of the special unit, and what problems of implementation ensued?
Outcomes research	What effect do alternative levels of nursing intensity have on the functional ability of elderly residents in long-term care facilities?	How do elderly long-term care residents interact with nurses in environments with different nursing intensity?
Survey	How prevalent is asthma among inner-city children, and what are the risk factors for this disease?	How is asthma experienced by inner-city children and their parents?
Ethnography	What percentage of women in rural Appalachia seek and obtain prenatal care, and what are their birth outcomes?	How do women in rural Appalachia view their pregnancies and how do they prepare for childbirth?
Case study	How have the demographic characteristics of the caseload of St. Jude's Homeless Shelter changed over a 10-year period?	How are social, health, and psychological services integrated in St. Jude's Homeless Shelter?

quantitative component but can also shed light on causal *mechanisms* in a qualitative component.

Throughout this book, we have identified various designs and approaches, some qualitative and some quantitative. Table 26.1 has examples of questions that can be addressed in an MM study for several types of study, illustrating diverse opportunities for integrating multiple types of data in a study. As the questions in Table 26.1 suggest, qualitative questions are likely to concern processes, experiences, and feelings, and quantitative questions often involve descriptive prevalence, relationships among variables, and causal connections.

In addition to such questions, MM studies benefit from having a specific MM question relating to the mixing or linking of qualitative and quantitative data (Creswell & Plano Clark, 2011). Examples include such questions as, To what extent do the two types of

data confirm each other? and How does one type of data help to explain the results from the other type?

> **TIP:** Creswell and Plano Clark's (2011) book includes a table with a series of mixed methods questions (pp. 166–167). An adapted version of this table (and of a similar table in their first edition) is included in the Toolkit section of the accompanying *Resource Manual*. Also, Plano Clark and Badiee (2010) provide guidance on framing research questions in MM research.

MIXED METHODS DESIGNS

Mixed methods designs have been developing over the past two decades and are continuing to evolve as greater thought is given to devising fruitful approaches—and as greater experience in conducting MM research occurs. At the moment, over a dozen design typologies have been developed by mixed methods scholars, so it is challenging to discuss this important topic.

We begin by describing some important design considerations, then present methods of portraying designs through a notation system and through diagrams, and finally, present the design typology offered by Creswell (2015). We note, however, that no typology will ever encompasses every possible MM design, because a hallmark of the MM approach is that it permits creativity and an emergent approach to design. Typologies and nomenclatures for designs are useful primarily because of their value in communicating an approach to others in proposals, IRB applications, and research articles. The designs we cover in this chapter are ones that have been adopted in many studies, but other possibilities exist for structuring an MM study.

Key Decisions in Mixed Methods Designs

In designing an MM study, researchers make several important decisions. One is whether to even *have* a fixed design at the outset. Novice researchers are likely to benefit by having a "roadmap" to follow, but seasoned researchers may prefer the flexibility of allowing answers from an initial *strand* (e.g., the qualitative component) guide them in subsequent strands (e.g., the quantitative component). Other key design decisions concern sequencing, prioritization, and integration.

Sequencing in Mixed Methods Designs

There are three main options for sequencing components of a mixed methods study: Qualitative data are collected first, quantitative data are collected first, or both types are collected simultaneously (or at approximately the same time). When the two types of data are not collected at the same time, the approach is called **sequential**. When the data are collected at the same time, the approach usually is called **concurrent**, although the terms *simultaneous* and *parallel* have also been used. Concurrent designs occur in a single phase, whereas sequen-

tial designs unfold in two or more distinct phases. In well-conceived sequential designs, the analysis and interpretation in one phase often informs the collection and analysis of data in the second. Another possibility is *multiphase timing*, which occurs when researchers launch a multiphase project that includes several sequential and/or concurrent substudies over a program of study.

Prioritization in Mixed Methods Designs

Researchers usually decide which approach—qualitative or quantitative—to emphasize in an MM study. One option is that the two components are given equal, or roughly equal, weight. Often, however, one approach is given priority. The distinction is sometimes referred to as *equal status* versus *dominant status*.

Several factors may affect the priority decision. The first concerns the researcher's worldview, an issue raised in Morse's (1991) seminal paper. Researchers' philosophical orientation (positivist or constructivist) leads them to tackle research problems for which one approach is dominant, and the other is viewed as a useful supplementary data source. The dominant approach should be the one that is best suited to addressing the overall study goals.

Although giving equal priority to the qualitative and quantitative strands of a study may in some cases be attractive, practical considerations may influence the weighting decision. If resources are limited, or if the researcher's skills are stronger in qualitative or quantitative methods, these issues will probably result in an MM study in which one approach has dominant status. The other factor to consider is the audience for the research. If the target audience—be that an adviser, funder, journal editor, or a broader research community—is unaccustomed to qualitative or quantitative research, then the prioritization decision may need to take that into account.

Integration in Mixed Methods Designs

A third key design decision concerns how the qualitative and quantitative methods will be combined and integrated. It can be argued that MM research can only achieve its full potential for providing enhanced insights when integration of strands occurs.

Creswell and Plano Clark (2011) have suggested that there are several basic strategies for integration decisions. First, the data types can be mixed during the interpretation of the qualitative and quantitative findings. Second, *merging* can occur during data analysis, through a combined analysis. Third, integration can occur during data collection by using a strategy of *connecting* in which the results from one strand influence data collection in a subsequent strand.

Notation and Diagramming in Mixed Methods Designs

Morse (1991), a prominent nurse researcher, made a critical contribution to the MM literature by proposing a notation system that has been adopted by virtually all writers across disciplines. Her notation system concerns the sequencing and prioritization decisions and is thus useful in quickly summarizing major features of an MM design.

In Morse's notation system, priority is designated by upper case and lower case letters: QUAL/quan designate a mixed methods study in which the dominant approach is qualitative, while QUAN/qual designates the reverse. If neither approach is dominant (i.e., both are equal), the notation stipulates QUAL/QUAN. Sequencing is indicated by the symbols + or →. The arrow designates a sequential approach. For example, QUAN → qual is the notation for a primarily quantitative MM study in which qualitative data collection occurs in Phase II. When both approaches occur concurrently, a plus sign is used (e.g., QUAL + quan).

Figure 26.1 illustrates several possible permutations of design options that can be illustrated with the notation system. Several options have been named as specific designs by Creswell (2015) and are discussed in the next section.

In addition to the notation system, MM designs can be visually diagrammed. Such diagrams can be useful in illustrating processes to reviewers and can also provide guidance to researchers themselves. Figure 26.2 illustrates a basic diagram for an instrument development study in which qual data informed the development of QUAN instruments in a qual → QUAN design. Additional information can

PRIORITY	SEQUENCE/TIMING	
	CONCURRENT	SEQUENTIAL
EQUAL	A1. QUAL + QUAN (Convergent Design[a])	B1. QUAN → QUAL QUAL → QUAN
DOMINANT	A2. QUAN + qual QUAL + quan	B2. QUAN → qual quan → QUAL (Explanatory Design[a]) B3. QUAL → quan qual → QUAN (Exploratory Design[a])

[a]Design names are based on Creswell (2015).

FIGURE 26.1 Mixed methods design matrix.

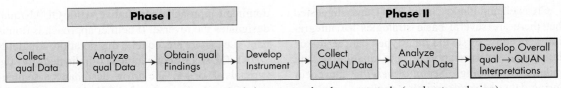

FIGURE 26.2 Visual diagram of a mixed methods instrument development study (exploratory design).

be added under the boxes in the diagram to provide richer detail. For example, under the first box (Collect qual Data), there might be greater detail, such as, "Conduct focus group interviews."

The diagram in Figure 26.2 is a simplified version of what happens in MM instrument development research. In many carefully designed instrument development studies, there are more than two phases. For example, there is often a content validation effort involving the collection of data from a panel of experts (Chapter 15). Such a design might have the following notation: qual → qual+quan → QUAN. In this scheme, the middle term represents qualitative and quantitative feedback from content validity experts.

TIP: Creswell and Plano Clark (2011) offer 10 guidelines for drawing visual diagrams of MM studies (Figure 4.1, p. 111). Their book also includes dozens of such visual diagrams that can be used as models.

Specific Mixed Methods Designs

Although numerous design typologies have been developed by different MM methodologists, we focus on the typology proposed by Creswell (2015). He identified three designs that are basic designs, which we briefly describe in this section. We emphasize, however, that these designs are just points of departure for designing mixed methods inquiries: Typologies should not be used to force what should be a fluid and creative process into oversimplified boxes (Guest, 2013). Many advanced designs exist, including ones that are multiphase (progressing in multiple phases with various quan/qual combinations in each phase) and ones that are multilevels (gathering different combinations of qual/

quan data from multiple levels in an organizational system).

Convergent Design

The purpose of the **convergent design** (sometimes called a *triangulation design*) is to obtain different, but complementary, data about the central phenomenon under study—that is, to triangulate data sources. In this design, qualitative and quantitative data are collected simultaneously and with equal priority. The notation for a convergent design is QUAL + QUAN (Box A1, Figure 26.1). The goal of this design is to converge on "the truth" about a problem or phenomenon. The researcher's job is to link the two data sets, often at the interpretation stage of the project.

The convergent design has several variants. The most conventional is the *parallel databases variant* (Creswell & Plano Clark, 2011). In this variant, QUAN data are collected and analyzed in parallel with the collection and analysis of QUAL data. The results of the two separate analyses are compared and contrasted, leading to an overall interpretation of both sets of results. The goal of the convergence model is to develop internally confirmed conclusions about a single phenomenon.

Another variant is called the *data transformation variant*. This design also involves the separate but concurrent collection of QUAL and QUAN data, followed by QUAL and QUAN analysis. A novel step in this model involves transforming the QUAL data into quan data (or the QUAN data into qual data) and then comparing and interrelating the data sets. Data conversions are described later in this chapter.

A major advantage of convergent designs is that they are efficient because both types of data are collected simultaneously. A major drawback, however, is that these designs, which give equal weight to

QUAL and QUAN data, are difficult for a single researcher working alone to do. Another potential problem can arise if the data from the two strands are not congruent.

Explanatory Sequential Designs

Explanatory designs are sequential designs with quantitative data collected in the first phase, followed by qualitative data collected in the second phase. Either the qualitative or the quantitative data can be given a stronger priority in explanatory designs. That is, the design can be either QUAN → qual or quan → QUAL (B2 in Figure 26.1), although the former sequence is more typical.

In explanatory designs, data from the second phase are used to build on or explain the data from the initial phase. A QUAN → qual design is especially suitable when the quantitative results are surprising (e.g., unanticipated nonsignificant results or significant serendipitous results), when results are complicated and tricky to interpret, or when the sample has numerous outliers that are difficult to explain.

Creswell and Plano Clark (2011) described two variants of the explanatory design. In the *follow-up explanations variant*, the researcher collects qual data that can best help to explain the initial QUAN findings. The primary emphasis is on the quantitative aspects of the study, and the analysis involves connecting data between the two phases. This model is one that is often attractive to researchers who are primarily quantitative oriented but who recognize that their study can be enriched by adding a qualitative component.

The second variant is the *participant selection variant* in which the first-stage quan data are in service of the second-phase QUAL component. In this model, information about the characteristics of a large group, as identified in the first phase, is used

to purposefully select participants in the second dominant phase—for example, using extreme case sampling or stratified purposive sampling (Chapter 22).

➔ TIP: In describing a design in a proposal or a report, it is probably best to combine words and notation. A citation should be provided for specifically named designs. For example, the following might summarize a design: "A sequential, qualitative-dominant (quan → QUAL) explanatory design (Creswell, 2015), will be adopted in the proposed research." A visual diagram would be a good supplement if space allows.

Advantages of explanatory designs are that they are straightforward and easy to describe and can be done by a single researcher. Another attractive feature, given page constraints in journals, is that the results can often be summarized in two separate papers. On the other hand, explanatory designs can be time-consuming—the second phase cannot begin until data from the first phase are analyzed. Another potential problem is that it may be difficult to secure up-front approval from ethical review boards for the second phase because the details of the Phase II study design are seldom known in advance.

Exploratory Sequential Designs

Exploratory designs are also sequential MM designs, but qualitative data are collected in the first phase. The design has its central premise the need for initial in-depth exploration of a phenomenon. Findings from the initial phase are then used in a second, quantitative phase. Usually the first phase focuses on detailed exploration of a little-researched phenomenon, and the second phase is focused on measuring it or classifying it. In an exploratory design, either the qualitative phase can be dominant (QUAL → quan) or the quantitative phase can be dominant (qual → QUAN), as shown in B3 of Figure 26.1.

Creswell and Plano Clark (2011) described two variants of an exploratory design. The first is the *instrument development model*, which is used when data from the qual phase are used in the development of QUAN instruments. This model, depicted graphically in Figure 26.2, has been used by many nurse researchers. In some cases, however, researchers extend an exploratory design, into what Creswell and Plano Clark described as a multiphase design.

> **Example of an Exploratory Design Extended to Multiple Phases:** Czuber-Dochan and colleagues (2014) developed and tested a patient self-assessment scale to measure inflammatory bowel disease fatigue. A five-phase sequential mixed method design was used, beginning with a qual phase to explore patients' experience of fatigue and its impact on their lives. This was followed by four qual-QUAN phases to develop and refine the scale and evaluate its psychometric properties.

In the second variant of an exploratory design, the *theory development variant*, the researcher identifies important constructs and develops a theory, taxonomy, or classification system grounded in the in-depth data gathered during the QUAL phase. Then the quan phase is used to test or explore the taxonomy or theory with a broader group. This is the model used when formal hypotheses generated in the initial phase are tested in a subsequent phase.

The advantages and disadvantages of an explanatory MM design also apply to exploratory MM designs. Separate phases make the inquiry easy to explain, implement, and report. Yet such a project can be time-consuming, and it may be difficult to get up-front approval from ethics review committees because the second phase methods

usually depend on what transpires in the first phase.

Other Mixed Methods Designs

Many MM designs do not have explicit names in the Creswell (2015) or Creswell and Plano Clark (2011) system. In Figure 26.1 (A2), for example, we see that concurrent dominant QUAN + qual and QUAL + quan designs do not have names. Nor do sequential nondominant designs (QUAN → QUAL and QUAL → QUAN) have a label (B1 in Figure 26.1). In fact, many design options are possible, and the basic designs are often the building blocks for more complex and creative ones.

Creswell (2015) specifically mentioned several "advanced" designs. One is the *intervention design* using multiple methods and intricately related components that unfold over time. This type of MM research is described in the next chapter. *Social justice* (or *transformative*) *designs* are mixed methods designs within a critical framework.

> **TIP:** Creswell and Plano Clark (2011) described a design called the *embedded design*—a term that is sometimes used in nursing studies. However, Creswell (2015) subsequently stopped referencing this design. An embedded design is one in which a second type of data is totally subservient to the other type of data. Creswell now sees embedding as an analytic strategy rather than as a design type.

Mixed methods can also be applied in within-paradigm research. Morse (2012) has argued that a qualitative-qualitative study is a legitimate form of inquiry, using either a concurrent or sequential design. One of the qualitative methods is a "complete" method (e.g., grounded theory, phenomenology), and the other is a supplemental component (e.g., QUAL + qual or qual → QUAL). The supplementary component does not involve a complete qualitative method but rather some research strategy such as a type of interview or an observational technique. The supplementary strategy is not complete enough to stand on its own. As an example, the core component could be a complete phenomenologic inquiry, and the supplementary component could involve nonparticipant observation. Here is another actual example:

> **Example of a QUAL + qual Design:** Wills and Morse (2007) conducted a QUAL-qual mixed methods study to describe responses of Chinese elderly living in Edmonton, Canada, during the severe acute respiratory syndrome (SARS) pandemic, and their use of Western and/or traditional Chinese medicine. Grounded theory was the core method, and ethnographic strategies were used to inform the cultural aspects of this research.

➲ **TIP:** MM designs are often portrayed as cross-sectional, even when they are sequential—that is, the goal in sequential designs usually is not to understand how a phenomenon unfolds over time. Plano Clark and colleagues (2014) have presented a conceptualization of longitudinal mixed methods designs.

Selecting a Mixed Methods Design

The most critical issue in selecting a design is its appropriateness for the research questions. Having a *name* for a design is far less important than having a solid rationale for structuring a study in a certain way. Yet, practical issues are also relevant in designing a study. For example, few researchers are equally skillful in qualitative and quantitative methods. This suggests three possibilities: (1) selecting a design in which your methodologic strengths are dominant, (2) working as a team with researchers whose strengths are complementary, or (3) strengthening your skills in your nondominant area. The first option is likely to be most realistic for many students. As noted previously, practical concerns such as resource availability and time constraints also play a role in choosing a design. Concurrent designs often require shorter time commitments, and QUAL dominant designs can often be less resource-intensive.

Morse (2003) advised researchers, in deciding on an MM design, to have a basic grasp of the project's *theoretical drive*. The theoretical drive may be *discovery*, which puts the main emphasis of a project on the inductive, QUAL aspects of the research. Alternatively, the theoretical drive can be

verification, which would give priority to the deductive QUAN aspects of the inquiry.

It is advisable to learn the details of a particular MM design before making a selection. In addition to reading methodologic writings of MM scholars, it is useful to examine the methods section of reports that have used a design you are considering. Teddlie and Tashakkori (2009) also advised that "you should look for the most appropriate or single best available research design, rather than the 'perfect fit.' You may have to combine existing designs, or create new designs, for your study" (p. 163).

SAMPLING AND DATA COLLECTION IN MIXED METHODS STUDIES

When a study design has been selected, an MM researcher can proceed to plan how best to collect the needed qualitative and quantitative data by developing a sampling and data collection plan. Sampling and data collection in MM studies are often a blend of approaches that we described in earlier chapters. A few special sampling and data collection issues for an MM study merit brief discussion.

Sampling in a Mixed Methods Study

Mixed methods researchers can combine sampling designs in various creative ways. The quantitative component is likely to rely on a sampling strategy that enhances the researcher's ability to generalize to a broader population. As noted in Chapter 12, probability samples are especially well suited to selecting a representative sample of participants, but researchers often must compromise, using such designs as consecutive samples or quota samples to enhance representativeness. For the qualitative strand of the project, MM researchers usually adopt purposive sampling methods (Chapter 22) to select information-rich cases who are good informants about the phenomenon of interest.

Sample sizes are often different in the qualitative and quantitative components, in ways one might expect—that is, larger samples for the quantitative component. Ideally, MM researchers should use power analyses to guide sample size decisions for the quantitative component, to diminish the risk of Type II errors in their statistical analyses.

The qualitative sample usually has fewer cases, and saturation is the principle most often used to make decisions about when sampling can stop.

A unique sampling issue in MM studies concerns whether the same people will be in both the qualitative and quantitative strands. The best strategy depends on the study purpose and the research design, but using overlapping samples can be advantageous. Having the same people in both parts of an MM study offers opportunities for convergence and for comparison between the two data sets.

Onwuegbuzie and Collins (2007) have categorized mixed methods sampling designs according to the *relationship* between the qualitative and quantitative components. The four relationships are identical, parallel, nested, or multilevel. An **identical** relationship occurs when exactly the same people are in both components of the study. This approach might occur if everyone in a survey or intervention study was asked a series of probing, open-ended questions—or if everyone in a primarily QUAL study was administered a formal instrument, such as a self-efficacy scale.

Example of Identical Sampling: Tocher (2014) studied postoperative pain expectations and experiences in patients undergoing open surgical repair of abdominal aortic aneurysm. A sample of 22 patients completed formal pain measurement before (pain expectations) and after (actual pain) surgery. All 22 patients also completed a semistructured interview that focused on their pain expectations and factors that might have contributed to those expectations.

In a **parallel** relationship, the samples in the two strands are completely different, although they are usually drawn from the same or a similar population. Like identical sampling, parallel sampling can occur in either concurrent or sequential designs and with any of the prioritization schemes.

Example of Parallel Sampling: In their sequential qual → QUAN study, VanDevanter and colleagues (2014) explored challenges of nurses' deployment to other New York City hospitals in the aftermath of a disaster, Hurricane Sandy. Initially, in-depth data were collected from a maximum variation sample of 20 nurses. Subsequently, an Internet-based survey was sent to all RNs employed at a New York Medical Center (N = 1,668).

In a **nested** relationship, the participants in the qualitative strand are a subset of the participants in the quantitative strand. Nested sampling is an especially common sampling approach in MM studies, especially in those with an explanatory design. Indeed, as discussed in the previous section, one of the variants of an explanatory design is geared to participant selection from the first phase for in-depth scrutiny in the second. If the intent of a qualitative component is to offer detail and elaboration about phenomena and relationships captured quantitatively, then a nested sample is likely to enrich the researcher's understanding. Mixed methods studies with an exploratory design, by contrast, often use completely different people in the two study phases. For example, the people who are interviewed in-depth about their experience with a phenomenon in an instrument development study are rarely used to test a new formal instrument in a later phase. In convergent designs, the relationship is more variable; the decision should ultimately be based on which approach best addresses overall study aims.

Example of Nested Sampling: Hall and colleagues (2014) studied women's views about the support they received for breastfeeding from nurses, midwives, and lactation consultants in southern Australia. A survey was distributed to mothers in clinics. A total of 175 women returned completed questionnaires. Nineteen women who participated in the survey also participated in follow-up focus group interviews.

Finally, a **multilevel** relationship involves selecting samples from different levels of a hierarchy. Usually this means sampling from different but related populations. (e.g., hospital administrators, clinical staff, and patients).

Example of Multilevel Sampling: Horne and co-researchers (2015) studied practices and experiences of mouth hygiene in stroke care units in the United Kingdom. Questionnaires about policies and practices were completed by senior nurses in 11 stroke units. Qualitative data were collected in two focus groups with 10 health care professionals and by in-depth interviews with five stroke survivors.

Kemper et al. (2003) noted that the overall mixed method sample should be capable of generating a thorough data set about the phenomenon under study. The sampling plan should allow for "credible explanations" (p. 276). Kemper and colleagues also pointed out that the sampling plan should be one that permits the conclusions from the study to be transferred/generalized to other settings or groups.

Data Collection in a Mixed Methods Study

Mixed methods researchers, by definition, collect and analyze both qualitative and quantitative data. All of the data collection methods discussed in Chapters 13 (structured methods) and 23 (unstructured methods) can be creatively combined in a mixed method study. Thus, possible sources of data for MM studies include group and individual interviews, psychosocial scales, observations, biophysiologic measures, records, diaries, cognitive tests, Internet postings, photographs, and physical artifacts. Johnson and Turner (2003) noted that MM studies can involve both *intramethod mixing* (e.g., structured and unstructured self-reports), and *intermethod mixing* (e.g., biophysiologic measures and in-depth interviews).

In selecting data collection methods for each strand of an MM study, a goal should be to use each method to address the research questions in a manner that enhances overall understanding of the problem. An important consideration concerns the methods' complementarity—that is, having the limitations of one method be offset by the strengths of the other. This in turn means that when MM researchers are devising their data collection strategies, they need to be fully aware of the strengths and weaknesses of each approach.

> ● TIP: Self-reports are the most common data source in both qualitative and quantitative nursing studies, and blending unstructured and structured self-report data is the most common approach in MM research as well.

In concurrent designs, decisions about data collection methods must be made up-front. In sequential designs, however, MM researchers often have an emergent approach, with the types of data to be collected in the second phase shaped to some extent by findings in the first phase. Sequential designs have rich potential for incremental findings that build on one another.

In planning a data collection strategy, MM researchers may need to consider whether one method could introduce bias in the other method. For example, do closed-ended questions about a phenomenon have an effect on how participants might think about the phenomenon when asked in an unstructured fashion (or vice versa)? In other words, researchers should give some thought to whether one of the methods is an "intervention" that could influence people's behavior or responses.

One final data collection issue concerns the possible need for additional data at the analysis and interpretation stage of a project. If findings from the qualitative and quantitative strands conflict, it is sometimes useful to collect supplementary data to shed light on and possibly resolve contradictions or inconsistencies.

ANALYSIS OF MIXED METHODS DATA

One of the greatest challenges in doing mixed methods research concerns how best to analyze the qualitative and quantitative data in a manner that integrates the results and interpretation. It is not uncommon, unfortunately, for the two strands of data to be analyzed and reported separately, without any integration of the findings.

The real benefits of MM research cannot be realized if there is no attempt to merge results from the two strands and to develop interpretations and practice recommendations based on integrated understandings. As eloquently noted by Sandelowski (2003), a high-quality MM analysis merges measurement with meaning, graphs with graphical accounts, and tables with tableaux.

Students often want specific guidance about how to analyze their data, but there are no formulas or sets of rules for MM data analysis and integration. Decisions about how to blend the data sets hinge on a number of factors. A particularly important factor is the study's sampling plan. Many of the techniques discussed in this section are only appropriate for identical and nested samples—that is, for sampling plans in which both qualitative and quantitative data are obtained from the same people. Research design, especially the sequencing decision, also affects analytic choices.

This section describes a few analysis options for MM studies, but it is far from comprehensive. Additional resources should be consulted, such as the work of Bazely (2009a, 2009b), Creswell and Plano Clark (2011), Happ and colleagues (2006), and Onwuegbuzie and Teddlie (2003). Also, Mendlinger and Cwikel (2008) provided a useful illustration of how "spiraling" between qualitative and quantitative data contributed to an integration of their strands of data.

⮕ **TIP:** Brewer and Hunter (2006) recommended "a creative and at times even playful meshing of data-collecting methods to encourage serendipity and openness to new ideas" (p. 69). Creativity, however, is difficult to describe in a proposal. It is probably best to identify a few strategies that seem fruitful a priori but to pursue others that seem productive during the analysis process.

Decisions in Analyzing Mixed Methods Data

Before pursuing a specific analytic strategy, MM researchers should make several broad preliminary decisions that will affect how they proceed. Our list here is not exhaustive but is meant to encourage preanalytic thinking about important issues.

1. *What is the overall goal of the study?* In selecting analytic strategies, the overall purpose of the study should be kept firmly in mind. For example, is the purpose primarily descriptive, exploratory, or explanatory? It is also important to consider the purpose in terms of evidence-based practice goals: How best can the data be analyzed to yield high-quality evidence for practicing nurses?
2. *Will integration occur at the analysis stage or the interpretation stage?* Sometimes interpretive integration is the only path possible—for example,

when parallel sampling of different people in the two strands has been used—but in other cases, researchers choose the point of integration. An observation by many whose integration happens during analysis is that "this was the key to unfolding the complex relationships in the topic of the study" (Bazely, 2009b, p. 205).

3. *What will be the unit of analysis?* Often the unit is individual participants, but other options include events (Happ et al., 2006) or subgroups of people. If the MM design involves a multilevel model, the levels are usually the unit of primary interest.
4. *Is the focus of the study more case-oriented or more construct-oriented?* Case-oriented research, more common in QUAL-dominant research, focuses on the complexity of a phenomenon within its context and examines patterns within cases. Construct-oriented research is more conceptual and theory-centered and involves the exploration of a phenomenon with the goal of explicating key constructs.
5. *Will either type of data be converted or transformed?* Sometimes researchers convert their qualitative data into quantitative data, and vice versa. We discuss such strategies later in this section and also in the Supplement to this chapter on thePoint®. Ⓢ
6. *Will direct comparisons be made between the qualitative and quantitative data—and, if so, at what level will the comparisons be made?* In nested and identical sampling designs, comparisons can be made at the individual level—for example, comparing each participant's score on a health promotion scale with how he or she described lifestyle and activities in in-depth interviews. Comparisons can also be made between subgroups—for example, how high scorers on the health promotion scale differ from low scorers in terms of themes that emerge in the qualitative analysis. Finally, overall comparisons are possible—for example, is the picture of the salience of health promotion consistent in the qualitative and quantitative data sets? This latter type of comparison, at a minimum, is essential if the MM research question involves congruence or complementarity between the strands.
7. *Will integration involve the use of specialized software?* Tremendous advances have been made

with regard to software for integration in MM studies. A software package called QDA Miner has been identified as useful (Silver, 2014). Bazely (2003, 2009a) has offered suggestions for how quantitative data can be transferred to a qualitative program and vice versa. Qualitative data analysis software such as NVivo and MAXQDA are especially useful, and statistical packages such as SPSS now has text analyses software than can categorize text responses and combine them with other quantitative variables. Even if specialized software for combining qualitative and quantitative data is not used, MM researchers can use basic spreadsheets to good advantage.

The next few sections describe a few specific strategies that mixed methods researchers use to integrate their qualitative and quantitative strands of data. We begin with interpretive integration, followed by several strategies for analytic integration: data conversion, meta-matrixes, and mixed method displays. These strategies are not mutually exclusive and several can be effectively combined in an MM study.

Interpretive Integration

Many, and perhaps most, mixed methods researchers who make efforts to integrate the different strands do so at the point of interpretation rather than during analysis.

Mixed Methods Designs and Interpretive Integration

Interpretive integration is especially common in concurrent MM designs. In this approach, quantitative data are analyzed using statistical techniques and qualitative data are analyzed using qualitative analysis methods, both according to standards of excellence for each method. Findings from the two separate analyses are then drawn together in an effort to synthesize the results and to develop an overall interpretation. The focus is on *comparing* the two types of findings, which can involve the creation of matrices—a method we describe in a later section. Often, however, the integration is simply at a narrative level and is summarized in the discussion section of reports.

Interpretive integration can also occur in sequential designs—although such integration is often what Bazely (2009a) called "integration 'on

the way'" (p. 92) rather than formal integration at the end of the study. That is, the analysis of one data strand is interpreted and used to inform the design and analysis of the second. An overall interpretive integration of the two strands may occur but often does not.

Creswell and Plano Clark (2011) noted that in sequential designs, a focus of the first-stage analysis is selecting results to use as a basis for scrutiny in the next phase. For example, in explanatory designs, the QUAN data are analyzed with an eye toward selecting cases or lines of questioning for the second qual phase. Options include selecting outliers or extreme cases, selecting negative cases, focusing on significant or nonsignificant results for more intensive follow-up, or identifying comparison groups based on key constructs. In exploratory designs, the QUAL results may suggest themes to examine (e.g., in an instrument development study) or hypotheses to test in the quan phase.

Bazely (2009a) has described what she called **iterative analysis**, which involves ongoing interpretive feedback loops. Iterative analysis involves "taking what is learned in one stage of a project into a further stage to inform that data collection or analysis, and then on again for refinement or development through one or more subsequent iterations" (p. 109). She offered as an example a study in which a researcher developed a formal instrument based on themes from in-depth phenomenologic interviews. The factor analytic results from psychometric testing of the scale were then taken back to the phenomenologic data for further thematic exploration.

Nature of Results from Interpretive Integration

Interpretive integration, which focuses on comparisons between the two strands, can result in convergent results, divergent results, or nuanced (qualifying) results. Most researchers consider that an ideal situation occurs when findings from each strand are consistent and shed complementary perspectives on the phenomenon of interest. Yet, many MM scholars have pointed out the critical role that divergent results can play in advancing knowledge. As Greene (2007) noted, "Convergence, consistency, and corroboration are overrated in social inquiry. The interactive mixed methods analyst looks just as keenly for instances of divergence and dissonance, as these may represent important nodes for further and highly generative analytic work" (p. 144).

Moffatt and colleagues (2006) suggested possible steps to take when MM findings conflict. Their study involved quantitative data from 126 participants in a clinical trial and in-depth data from a purposive sample of 25 of them. The quantitative results suggested that the intervention (which was designed to improve health and social outcomes for older people) was not successful, yet the qualitative data suggested wide-ranging improvements. The researchers suggested six ways of further exploring the discrepancy: (1) treating the methods as fundamentally different, (2) examining rigor in the respective strands, (3) exploring data set comparability, (4) collecting additional data, (5) exploring intervention processes, and (6) exploring whether the outcomes of the two components were really matched.

Although many MM scholars discuss convergence-divergence of results as a dichotomy, in fact, it is often the case that interpretive integration leads to a nuanced portrayal of the phenomenon because results are neither precisely convergent nor divergent. Thus, although the MM research question often being addressed in interpretive integration is "To what extent do the quantitative and qualitative data converge?" (Creswell & Plano Clark, 2011, p. 166). Another important question might be: How do the findings from one strand qualify, delimit, or temper findings from the other?

An example comes from an MM study of one of this book's authors, whose convergent design involved a survey of 4,000 low-income women and ethnographic interviews with 67 women from a parallel sample (Polit et al., 2000). The analyses focused on hunger and food insecurity, and in both samples, about half the women were food insecure—results that appeared convergent. Yet, the in-depth interviews revealed that the term "food secure" in low-income urban families may be a misleading label: Mothers in the qualitative sample had to *struggle* enormously to be food secure, piecing together with great effort "numerous strategies to make sure that there was an adequate amount of

food for themselves and their children" (p. 22). This led the authors to hypothesize that *food security* is achieved in a different manner and is experienced differently among poor and middle-class families—and is perhaps a totally different phenomenon.

Example of Interpretive Integration: Cleaver and co-researchers (2014) used a convergent design to understand the attitudes of emergency care staff toward young people who self-harm. Quantitative data came from a survey of 143 staff members from accident and emergency units and an ambulance service. In-depth interviews were conducted with seven nurses and five ambulance staff. Findings from the two strands were compared and contrasted, and the interpretation took both data sets into account. Data from both strands revealed the presence of ambivalence and ambiguity in attitudes toward young people who self-harm.

Converting Quantitative and Qualitative Data

A technique that can be used in analytic and interpretive integration in mixed methods research involves converting data of one type into data of another type. Qualitative data are sometimes converted into numeric codes that can be analyzed quantitatively (**quantitizing**). It is also possible to transform quantitative data into qualitative information (**qualitizing**).

Although some qualitative researchers believe that quantitizing is inappropriate, Sandelowski (2001) argued that some amount of quantitizing is almost inevitable. She noted that every time qualitative researchers use terms such as *a few*, *some*, *many*, or *most*, they are implicitly conveying quantitative information about the frequency of occurrence of a theme or pattern. In addition to being inevitable, quantification of qualitative data can sometimes offer distinct benefits. Sandelowski described how this strategy can be used to achieve two important goals:

- *Generating meaning from qualitative data.* If qualitative data are displayed in a quantitative fashion (e.g., by displaying frequencies of certain phenomena), *patterns* sometimes emerge with greater clarity than they might have if the researchers had simply relied on their impressions. Tabular displays can also reveal unsuspected patterns that can help in the development of hypotheses.

- *Documenting and confirming conclusions.* The use of numbers can assure people that researchers' conclusions are valid. Researchers can be more confident that the data are fully accounted for if they can document the extent to which emerging patterns were observed—or *not* observed. Sandelowski noted that quantitizing can address some pitfalls of qualitative analysis, which include giving too much weight to dramatic or vivid accounts, giving too little weight to disconfirming cases, and smoothing out variation, to clean up some of the "messiness" of human experience.

In a more recent article, Sandelowski and her colleagues (2009) noted that quantitizing can also serve the critical function of encouraging researchers to think about and interact with their data. They noted that quantitizing, "when used creatively, critically, and reflexively, can show the complexity of qualitative data and, thereby the 'multivariate nature' of the experiential worlds researchers seek to understand" (p. 219). Such higher level understanding of a phenomenon is an overarching goal of many MM studies.

Procedures for qualitizing quantitative data and quantitizing qualitative data are described in the Supplement to this chapter on thePoint®. 🅢

Constructing Meta-Matrices

A widely used approach to analytic integration involves the use of matrices, which is a good method for identifying patterns and making comparisons across data sources. Matrices are a method that has been advocated for qualitative data analysis (Miles et al., 2014), and the concept has gained popularity among MM researchers.

In a **meta-matrix**, researchers array information from qualitative and quantitative data sources. In a typical case-by-variable meta-matrix, the rows correspond to cases, that is, to individual participants. Then, for each participant, data from multiple data sources are entered in the columns, so that the analyst can see at a glance such information as scores on psychosocial, comments from open-ended dialogue with participants (e.g., verbatim narratives),

hospital record data (e.g., physiologic information), and the researchers' own notes. A third dimension can be added if, for example, there are multiple sources of data relating to multiple constructs (e.g., depression, pain). A third dimension can also be used if the qualitative and quantitative data have been collected longitudinally.

Patterns of regularities, as well as anomalies, often come to light through detailed inspection of meta-matrices. Their key advantage is that they allow for fuller exploration of all sources of data simultaneously. The construction of a meta-matrix also allows researchers to explore whether statistical conclusions are supported by the qualitative data for individual study participants, and vice versa.

A simplified example of a meta-matrix is presented in Figure 26.3. This example shows only five cases and a handful of variables/constructs, but it illustrates how diverse information can be displayed to facilitate inferences about patterns and relationships. It also suggests, however, that such meta-matrices may not be productive with large samples—although one strategy is to have separate matrices for distinct subgroups within a large sample (e.g., in our example, those with high versus low levels of fatigue). Meta-matrix data such as those portrayed in Figure 26.3 can easily be entered into spreadsheet software and some qualitative software packages. Software has important advantages over manual methods—in particular, the ability to sort and re-sort the data to identify patterns.

Meta-matrices can also be used to integrate data and findings after some level of analysis has been accomplished. For example, Figure 26.4 shows a meta-matrix summarizing themes identified from in-depth interviews, according to different subgroups defined on the basis of a response to a structured question about using sleep medication.

Example of a Study Using a Meta-Matrix: Campesino and colleagues (2012) used mixed methods to explore women's perceptions of breast cancer care delivery, including treatment choices. The qualitative data were content analyzed, and then both quantitative and qualitative data were triangulated using matrix analysis techniques. The authors noted that the resulting data display facilitated the examination of qualitative findings for key subgroups (e.g., those with and without insurance).

Case	Pseudonym	Age	Sex	Average Hours of Sleep Daily	Current Fatigue Level Rating[a]	Use of Sleep Medication[b]	Fatigue Narrative
1	Anna	57	F	6.0	9	1	I *never* sleep through the night. I usually don't have much trouble falling asleep, but I just can't *stay* asleep. There is never a day when I don't wake up exhausted.
2	Jonathan	45	M	5.5	5	1	I've never really needed all that much sleep. Ever since I was in college, I get by with just a few hours and I feel just fine.
3	Claire	49	F	8.0	2	1	I'm a good sleeper, I can fall asleep anywhere, anytime. So, I get what I need.
4	Rosalind	51	F	7.0	7	2	I sleep just fine, but my husband is an insomniac, and a pain in my neck. When he's awake, he wants me awake, too!
5	Michael	54	M	7.5	6	3	I like my shut-eye. I can't concentrate if I don't get enough. I do what I have to, which usually means going to bed before anyone else and taking sleeping pills.

[a]Rating scale anchors: 0 = extremely energetic, 10 = totally exhausted
[b]Use of medication codes: 1 = Never, 2 = Occasionally, 3 = Regularly

FIGURE 26.3 Fictitious example of a meta-matrix with raw qualitative data.

Displaying Data in Mixed Methods Analysis

Meta-matrixes are an important tool for displaying data from multiple sources, but other visual methods exist as well. These display techniques serve a similar function—helping MM analysts to recognize patterns and conceptualize higher order constructs.

Happ and colleagues' (2006) article is a useful resource for thinking about visual displays in mixed

Use of Sleep Medication	Themes from In-Depth Interviews		
	The Role of Others	**Health Issues**	**Patterns of Sleep**
Never (*n* = 12)	• No one in household with sleeping problems • No pets in household	• No special health problems • Avoids *all* medication	• Never a problem falling asleep • Lifelong history of being good sleeper • Despite problems, averse to sleeping aids
Occasionally (*n* = 13)	• Spouse sleeping problems • Teens coming home late • Pet disturbances	• Stressful job • On a diet causing jitters • Anxiety about upcoming medical procedures/tests	• Problem staying asleep, not falling asleep • Sleeping only a problem if under stress • Frequent napping
Regularly (*n* = 7)	• Spouse works late or irregular shift • Infant in household • Severely ill family member	• Recent hospitalization • Diagnosed with life-threatening illness • Severely depressed	• Problems arise if medications not taken • Daily battles with insomnia

FIGURE 26.4 Fictitious example of a summary meta-matrix.

methods research. Their paper included examples of using bar charts to show frequencies of quantitized qualitative data. Another type of display was what Happ and colleagues called a *modified stem leaf plot*. In their example from a study of health locus of control in lung transplant recipients, behaviors that were considered "internality behaviors" from unstructured data sources were listed on one side, and the identification numbers of the lung transplant recipients who exhibited those behaviors were listed on the right. The result was a representation of the qualitative data in a quantitative manner that "provided a visual sense of the proportion of recipients who exhibited the internality behaviors" (p. S46). The display prompted further analyses about commonalities and differences among recipients' behaviors.

Another clever use of visualization involved the construction of a scatterplot. The values along the vertical axis were internality scores, those along the horizontal axis were externality scores. The scatterplot space was divided into quadrants (e.g., high internality, high externality) that corresponded to four profiles of health locus of control beliefs. The identification numbers of individual participants were then plotted in the two-dimensional space. This visual display allowed the researchers to more clearly identify clusterings and "outliers" that were difficult to identify from quantitative analysis alone. Further advice regarding visual displays of information from mixed methods analyses is provided by Onwuegbuzie and Dickinson (2008).

Clearly, data analysis in mixed methods research is ripe with opportunities for creative blending and juxtaposition of data visually, verbally, and statistically.

Meta-Inferences in Mixed Methods Research

It has been argued that the most important step in mixed methods studies is when the integrated findings from the qualitative and quantitative components are incorporated into an overall conceptualization that effectively answers the overarching mixed methods question (Teddlie & Tashakkori, 2009). To achieve this, *active* interpretation and exploration of the results are required.

In arriving at meta-inferences in an MM study, researchers must actively engage in meaning making. Teddlie and Tashakkori (2009) suggested that researchers must consider the quality of the inputs (i.e., the quality of the design, the data, the analytic procedures), and the process of meaning making through systematic linking and interpreting of results. Interpretation can be enhanced by allowing the two strands of a study to "talk to each other" in a meaningful, reflexive, and thought-provoking way.

Teddlie and Tashakkori (2009) offered several guidelines for making appropriate inferences at the interpretive stage of an MM study. Their "golden rule" is especially noteworthy: "*Know thy participants*" (p. 289). Mixed methods research offers great potential for getting a rounded picture of the complex lives of human participants.

QUALITY CRITERIA IN MIXED METHODS RESEARCH

It can be argued that mixed methods research offers particularly good opportunities to assess the overall "goodness" of the data. As we noted in Chapter 25, triangulation is a technique that can be used to develop evidence about the trustworthiness and validity of the findings. Triangulation often occurs at the data, investigator, analysis, and theoretical level in MM research.

Mixed methods scholars who have proposed standards for evaluating the quality of MM studies often avoid terms like *validity* (associated with quantitative quality criteria) and *trustworthiness* (associated with qualitative criteria). It is too early in the development of MM methodology to know what terms will be adopted, but one prominent team of scholars have proposed the terms *inference quality* and *inference transferability* (Teddlie & Tashakkori, 2003, 2009).

Inference quality is an overarching criterion for evaluating the quality of conclusions and interpretations made on the basis of mixed methods findings. Inference quality incorporates notions of both *internal validity* and *statistical conclusion validity* within a quantitative framework and *credibility* within a qualitative framework. Inference quality essentially refers to the believability and accuracy

BOX 26.1 Guidelines for Critiquing Mixed Methods Studies

1. Did the researcher state an overarching mixed methods objective that required the integration of qualitative and quantitative approaches? In addition to individual questions that formed the basis for the qualitative or quantitative components, was there an explicit mixed methods question about how the findings from the two strands relate to one another?

2. Did the researcher identify the research design? Was mixed methods design notation (or a visual diagram) used to communicate key aspects of the design? If a design was not specified, can you infer what the design was? Was it concurrent or sequential? Which strand (if either) was given priority?

3. Is the design appropriate for the research questions or study objective? Does the design for each component match the requirement for addressing its corresponding question? (*design suitability*)[a]

4. Do the components of the design fit together in a seamless manner? Are the strands linked logically? Were procedures implemented to enhance rigor and trustworthiness of the various components? (*within-design consistency*)

5. What sampling strategy was used (identical, parallel, nested, multilevel), and was this strategy appropriate? Were the setting, context, and participants adequately described, and are they appropriate for the research question?

6. How were study data gathered? Did the researcher take advantage of opportunities to triangulate data sources? In sequential designs, did the second-phase data collection (and sampling) flow from the analysis of data from the initial phase?

7. Overall, were the design components and sampling/data collection strategies implemented with the care and rigor needed to fully capture the complex nature of the target phenomenon? (*design fidelity*)

8. Did integration of the strands occur? Was integration at the interpretive or analytic level? Was adequate integration achieved? Do the combined findings suggest richly textured and comprehensive data sets from the respective strands?

9. What specific analytic techniques were used to achieve analytic integration (e.g., was data conversion or meta-matrices used)? Were these techniques adequate? Were visual displays of the data used effectively?

10. Were the analytic or interpretive steps appropriate and sufficient to answer the qualitative questions and to achieve integration? (*analytic adequacy*)

11. Are the researcher's meta-inferences consistent with the individual findings? Are the inferences consistent with each other? (*interpretive consistency*)

12. Are the researchers' interpretations consistent with the current state of evidence and theory? (*theoretical consistency*) What was done to assess agreement among team members, peers, or participants regarding the interpretations? Are the inferences consistent with participants' constructions? (*interpretive agreement*)

13. Are inferences and interpretations credible and more plausible than other possible interpretations of the findings? (*interpretive distinctiveness*)

14. Do the meta-inferences adequately encompass and integrate inferences from each strand? If the findings from each strand are conflicting or qualifying, were theoretical explanations for the discrepancies offered, and are they plausible? (*integrative efficacy*)

15. Do the meta-inferences adequately address the stated goals of the study? (*interpretive correspondence*)

[a]The terms in parentheses correspond to criteria identified by Teddlie and Tashakkori (2009). The questions corresponding to the criteria were adapted from ones they included in their Table 12.5 (pp. 301–302).

of the inductively and deductively derived conclusions from an MM study.

Inference transferability, another umbrella term, encompasses the quantitative term *external validity* and the qualitative term *transferability*. Inference transferability is the degree to which the mixed methods conclusions can be applied to other similar people, context, settings, time periods, and theoretical representations of the phenomenon.

Although mixed methods research offers opportunities for triangulation and corroboration, it can be challenging to achieve and demonstrate strong inference quality because there are three sets of standards that apply: Inferences derived from the quantitative component must be judged in terms of standard validity criteria, inferences from the qualitative component must be judged in terms of trustworthiness standards, and the meta-inferences from the two integrated strands must also be evaluated for their soundness. For the first two, methods of enhancing validity and trustworthiness that we have proposed in earlier chapters are relevant in strengthening the quality of MM research.

Teddlie and Tashakkori (2009) have proposed an *integrative framework for inference quality*. This framework, which incorporates many of the standards from both qualitative and quantitative approaches, encompasses two broad families of criteria for evaluating quality: *design quality* and *interpretive rigor*. These criteria, which can serve as guides for MM researchers as well as for those evaluating an MM report, are briefly described in the next section.

CRITIQUING MIXED METHODS RESEARCH

Individual components of mixed methods studies can be critiqued using guidelines we have offered throughout this book. Key critiquing questions for quantitative studies (Box 5.2) and qualitative studies (Box 5.3) were presented in Chapter 5.

Box 26.1 ❌ offers supplementary questions that are explicitly about the integration of methods in MM studies. Many of these questions were derived from Teddlie and Tashakkori's (2009) integrative framework for inference quality that encompasses

design quality and interpretive rigor. Their criteria with regard to *design quality* are design suitability, design fidelity, within-design consistency, and analytic adequacy. Criteria with regard to *interpretive rigor* are interpretive consistency, theoretical consistency, interpretive agreement, interpretive distinctiveness, integrative efficacy, and interpretive correspondence. These criteria are shown in parentheses next to the relevant questions in Box 26.1. The overarching consideration in MM studies is whether true integration occurred and contributed to strong meta-inferences about the phenomenon under scrutiny.

It is worth noting that several critiquing frameworks for evaluating mixed methods study have been proposed. Heyvaert and colleagues (2013) have developed an overview of several critical appraisal frameworks developed to evaluate mixed methods research.

➲ **TIP:** In evaluating the strengths and weaknesses of mono-method (qualitative or quantitative) studies, it is worth asking whether a mixed methods approach would have enhanced the conclusions.

●●●●●●●●●●●●●●●●●●●●●●

RESEARCH EXAMPLE OF A MIXED METHODS STUDY

Study: A mixed methods study of secondary traumatic stress in certified nurse-midwives: Shaken belief in the birth process (Beck et al., 2015)

Statement of Purpose: The purpose of this study was to examine secondary traumatic stress (STS) among certified nurse-midwives (CNMs) exposed to traumatized patients during childbirth. The researchers asked four research questions: (1) What are the prevalence and severity of STS in CNMs due to exposure to traumatic birth? (2) What is the relationship of CNMs' demographic characteristics to STS? (3) What are the experiences of CNMs who attend at traumatic births? and (4) How do the quantitative and qualitative sets of results develop a more complete picture of STS in CNMs?

Methods: A convergent design (QUAL + QUAN) was used, that is, independent strands of data were collected in a single phase. CNMs who had attended at least one traumatic birth were invited to participate in a survey. A total of 473 CNMs completed the quantitative portion—a questionnaire that included demographic and background questions and the 17-item STS Scale. Data for the qualitative strand, obtained from a nested sample of 246 survey participants, came from responses to the following: "Please describe in as much detail as you can remember your experience of attending one or more traumatic births. Please describe all of your thoughts, feelings, and perceptions until you have no more to write. Specific examples of points you are making are extremely valuable. If attending traumatic births has impacted your midwifery practice, please describe this impact" (p. 17).

Data Analysis and Integration: Beck et al. provided a good description and a useful diagram, depicting their analytic procedures. Statistical methods were used to answer research questions 1 and 2. For example, correlation procedures were used to look at the relationship between CNMs' background characteristics and their STS Scale scores. Question 3 was addressed by means of a content analysis of the qualitative data on the CNMs' actual experiences. Some segments of the qualitative data were also quantitized, that is, converted to codes signifying the presence or absence of narrative material relating to four variables: whether they had bonded with the mother or couple, whether they experienced litigation, whether they had been new to midwifery when the traumatic birth occurred, and whether the traumatic births had impacted their practice. These quantitized data were then merged into a matrix with other quantitative data. Themes were cross-tabulated with information about CNMs' characteristics and reported symptoms. The merged results were then integrated into an overall interpretation.

Key Findings: In this sample, 29% of the CNMs reported high to severe STS; 36% screened positive for PTSD due to attending traumatic births. The most often mentioned types of traumatic births were fetal demise/neonatal death, shoulder dystocia, and infant resuscitation. Six themes were identified in the content analysis of qualitative data (e.g., protecting my patients: agonizing sense of powerlessness and helplessness; shaken belief in the birth process: impacting

midwifery practice). More than half of the participants said that their practice had been impacted. For example, 22% reported having lost faith in the natural birth process, and 8% left midwifery altogether. Having both quantitative and qualitative findings allowed the researchers to paint a more complete picture of STS in CNMs. The quantitative results from the STS Scale revealed the previously unknown high percentage of CNMs experiencing STS. The addition of the qualitative results, however, provided an insider's glimpse to what it is like to walk a mile in the shoes of CNMs as they struggle with STS. For example, one of the items on the STS Scale that was rated the highest by CNMs was "I had trouble sleeping." Here is an excerpt from the qualitative data that brought this scale item to life: "The baby must have been dead for 5 days or so as the skin was peeling badly and blistered. Between the slime of the meconium and the skin issues it was hard to grip the head to help deliver the rest of the body. I felt like I was pulling off skin and worried I would pull off the head. For weeks I could not get pictures of that dead baby girl out of my mind. I had difficulty sleeping due to the nightmares" (p. 21).

SUMMARY POINTS

- **Mixed methods (MM) research** involves the collection, analysis, and integration of both qualitative and quantitative data within a study or coordinated set of studies, often with an overarching goal of achieving both discovery and verification.
- Mixed methods research has numerous advantages, including the complementarity of qualitative and quantitative data and the practicality of using methods that best address a question. MM research has many applications, including the development and testing of instruments, theories, and interventions.
- The paradigm often associated with MM research is **pragmatism**, which has as a major tenet "the dictatorship of the research question."
- Mixed methods studies involve asking at least two questions that require different types of data, but high-quality MM research also asks

integrative questions that focus on linking the two *strands*.

- Key decisions in designing an MM study involve how to sequence the components, which strand (if either) will be given priority, and how to integrate the two strands.
- In terms of sequencing, MM designs are either **concurrent designs** (both strands occurring in one simultaneous phase) or **sequential designs** (one strand occurring prior to and informing the second strand).
- Notation for MM research often designates both *priority*—all capital letters for the dominant strand and all lower case letters for the nondominant strand—and sequence. An arrow is used for sequential designs, and a "+" is used for concurrent designs. QUAL → quan, for example, is a sequential, qualitative-dominant design.
- Specific MM designs in the Creswell taxonomy include the **convergent design** (QUAL + QUAN), **explanatory design** (QUAN → qual or quan → QUAL), and **exploratory design** (QUAL → quan or qual → QUAN). In reality, complex MM designs are often adopted in a creative, emergent fashion.
- Sampling strategies can be described as **identical** (the same participants are in both strands), **nested** (some participants from one strand are in the other strand), **parallel** (participants are either in one strand or the other, drawn from a similar population), or **multilevel** (participants are not the same and are drawn from different populations at different levels in a hierarchy).
- Data collection in MM research can involve all methods of structured and unstructured data. In sequential designs, decisions about data collection for the second phase are based on findings from the first phase.
- Data analysis in MM research should involve integration of the strands to arrive at **meta-inferences** about the phenomenon under study. Integration often occurs at the interpretive level, after separate analyses have been completed. A focus in such integrations is often to assess congruence and to explore complementarity.

- Methods of integration of qualitative and quantitative data during analysis include *data conversions*, such as **qualitizing** quantitative data or **quantitizing** qualitative data, and the use of **meta-matrices** in which both qualitative and quantitative data are arrayed in a spreadsheet-type matrix.
- Criteria that have been proposed for enhancing the integrity of MM studies include **inference quality** (the believability and accuracy of inductively and deductively derived conclusions) and **inference transferability** (the degree to which conclusions can be applied to other similar people or contexts.
- Two families of criteria in Teddlie and Tashakkori's integrative framework for inference quality are *design quality* and *interpretive rigor*.

STUDY ACTIVITIES

Chapter 26 of the *Resource Manual for Nursing Research: Generating and Assessing Evidence for Nursing Practice, 10th edition*, offers exercises and study suggestions for reinforcing concepts presented in this chapter. In addition, the following study questions can be addressed:

1. Look at the list of questions in Table 26.1. Add to the list of questions for other types of research design.
2. Use the criteria in Box 26.1 to assess the study described at the end of the chapter, referring to the original article for full details.

STUDIES CITED IN CHAPTER 26

Andrew, S., & Halcomb, E. (Eds.). (2009). *Mixed methods research for nursing and the health sciences*. Oxford, United Kingdom: Blackwell-Wiley.

Bazely, P. (2003). Computerized data analysis for mixed methods research. In A. Tashakkori & C. Teddlie (Eds.), *Handbook of mixed methods in social and behavioral research* (pp. 385–422). Thousand Oaks, CA: Sage.

Bazely, P. (2009a). Analysing mixed methods data. In S. Andrew & E. Halcomb (Eds.), *Mixed methods research for nursing and the health sciences* (pp. 84–117). Oxford, United Kingdom: Blackwell-Wiley.

Bazely, P. (2009b). Integrating data analyses in mixed methods research. *Journal of Mixed Methods Research, 3,* 203–207.

Beck, C. T., & Gable, R. K (2000). Postpartum Depression Screening Scale: Development and psychometric testing. *Nursing Research, 49,* 272–282.

Beck, C. T., & Gable, R. K. (2001). Ensuring content validity: An illustration of the process. *Journal of Nursing Measurement, 9,* 201–215.

Beck, C. T., LoGuidice, J., & Gable, R. (2015). A mixed methods study of secondary traumatic stress in certified nurse-midwives: Shaken belief in the birth process. *Journal of Midwifery & Women's Health, 60,* 16–23.

Brewer, J., & Hunter, A. (2006). *Foundations of multi-method research: Synthesizing styles.* Thousand Oaks, CA: Sage.

*Campesino, M., Koithan, M., Ruiz, E., Glover, J., Juarez, G., Choi, M., & Krouse, R. (2012). Surgical treatment differences among Latina and African American breast cancer survivors. *Oncology Nursing Forum, 39,* E324–E331.

*Catallo, C., Jack, S. M., Ciliska, S., & Macmillan, H. L. (2013). Mixing a grounded theory approach with a randomized controlled trial related to intimate partner violence: What challenges arise for mixed methods research? *Nursing Research and Practice, 2013,* 798213.

Cleaver, K., Meerabeau, L., & Maras, P. (2014). Attitudes towards young people who self-harm: Age, an influencing factor. *Journal of Advanced Nursing, 70,* 2884–2896.

Creswell, J. W. (2015). *A concise introduction to mixed methods research.* Thousand Oaks, CA: Sage.

Creswell, J. W., & Plano Clark, V. L. (2011). *Designing and conducting mixed methods research* (2nd ed.). Thousand Oaks, CA: Sage.

*Czuber-Dochan, W., Norton, C., Bassett, P., Berliner, S., Bredin, F., Darvell, M., . . . Terry, H. (2014). Development and psychometric testing of inflammatory bowel disease fatigue (IBD-F) patient self-assessment scale. *Journal of Crohn's & Colitis, 8,* 1398–1406.

Edinburgh, L., Pape-Blabolil, J., Harpin, S., & Sawwyc, E. (2014). Multiple perpetrator rape among girls evaluated at a hospital-based Child Advocacy Center: Seven years of reviewed cases. *Child Abuse & Neglect, 38,* 1540–1551.

*Elstad, E., Maserejian, N., McKinlay, J., & Tennstedt, S. (2011). Fluid manipulation among individuals with lower urinary tract symptoms: A mixed methods study. *Journal of Clinical Nursing, 20,* 156–165.

Granger, B. B., McBroom, K., Bosworth, H., Hernandez, A., & Ekman, I. (2013). The meanings associated with medicines in heart failure patients. *European Journal of Cardiovascular Nursing, 12,* 276–283.

Greene, J. C. (2007). *Mixing methods in social inquiry.* San Francisco, CA: Jossey-Bass.

Guest, G. (2013). Describing mixed methods research: An alternative to typologies. *Journal of Mixed Methods Research, 7,* 141–151.

Hall, H., McLelland, G., Gilmour, C., & Cant, R. (2014). "It's those first few weeks": Women's views about breastfeeding support in an Australian outer metropolitan region. *Women and Birth, 27,* 259–265.

Happ, M., Dabbs, A., Tate, J., Hricik, A., & Erlen, J. (2006). Exemplars of mixed methods data combination and analysis. *Nursing Research, 55,* S43–S49.

Heyvaert, M., Hannes, K., Maes, B., & Onghena, P. (2013). Critical appraisal of mixed methods studies. *Journal of Mixed Methods Research, 7,* 302–327.

Horne, M., McCracken, G., Walls, A., Tyrrell, P., & Smith, C. (2015). Organisation, practice and experiences of mouth hygiene in stroke unit care: A mixed methods study. *Journal of Clinical Nursing, 24,* 728–738.

Johnson, B., & Turner, L. (2003). Data collection strategies in mixed methods research. In A. Tashakkori & C. Teddlie (Eds.), *Handbook of mixed methods in social and behavioral research* (pp. 297–319). Thousand Oaks, CA: Sage.

Kemper, E., Stringfield, S., & Teddlie, C. (2003). Mixed methods sampling strategies in social science research. In A. Tashakkori & C. Teddlie (Eds.), *Handbook of mixed methods in social and behavioral research* (pp. 273–296). Thousand Oaks, CA: Sage.

Mendlinger, S., & Cwikel, J. (2008). Spiraling between qualitative and quantitative data on women's health behaviors: A double helix model for mixed methods. *Quantitative Health Research, 18,* 280–293.

Miles, M., Huberman, M., & Saldaña, J. (2014). *Qualitative data analysis: A methods source book* (3rd ed.). Thousand Oaks, CA: Sage.

*Moffatt, S., White, M., Mackintosh, J., & Howel, D. (2006). Using quantitative and qualitative data in health services research—What happens when mixed method findings conflict? *BMC Health Services Research, 6,* 28.

Morse, J. M. (1991). Approaches to qualitative-quantitative methodological triangulation. *Nursing Research, 40,* 120–123.

Morse, J. M. (2003). Principles of mixed methods and multimethod research design. In A. Tashakkori & C. Teddlie (Eds.), *Handbook of mixed methods in social and behavioral research* (pp. 189–208). Thousand Oaks, CA: Sage.

Morse, J. M. (2012). Simultaneous and sequential qualitative mixed method designs. In P. L. Munhall (Ed.), *Nursing research: A qualitative perspective* (pp. 553–569). Sudbury, MA: Jones & Bartlett Learning.

Morse, J. M., & Niehaus, L. (2009). *Mixed method design: Principles and procedures.* Walnut Creek, CA: Left Coast Press.

O'Cathain, A. (2009). Mixed methods research in the health sciences: A quiet revolution. *Journal of Mixed Methods Research, 3,* 3–6.

*Onwuegbuzie, A., & Collins, K. (2007). A typology of mixed methods sampling designs in social science research. *The Qualitative Report, 12*(2), 281–316.

*Onwuegbuzie, A. J., & Dickinson, W. (2008). Mixed methods analysis and information visualization: Graphical display for effective communication of research results. *The Qualitative Report, 13,* 204–225.

Onwuegbuzie, A., & Teddlie, C. (2003). A framework for analyzing data in mixed methods research. In A. Tashakkori & C. Teddlie (Eds.), *Handbook of mixed methods in social and behavioral research* (pp. 351–384). Thousand Oaks, CA: Sage.

Plano Clark, V. L., Anderson, N., Wertz, J., Zhou, Y., Schumacher, K., & Miaskowski, C. (2014). Conceptualizing longitudinal mixed methods designs: A methodological review of health sciences research. *Journal of Mixed Methods Research.* Advance online publication. doi:10.1177/1558689814543563

Plano Clark, V., & Badiee, M. (2010). Research questions in mixed methods research. In A. Tashakkori & C. Teddlie (Eds.), *Sage handbook of mixed methods in social and behavioral science* (pp. 275–304). Thousand Oaks, CA: Sage.

*Polit, D. F., London, A., & Martinez, J. (2000). *Food security and hunger in poor, mother-headed families in four U. S. cities.* New York: Manpower Demonstration Research Corporation.

Sandelowski, M. (2001). Real qualitative researchers do not count: The use of numbers in qualitative research. *Research in Nursing & Health, 24,* 230–240.

Sandelowski, M. (2003). Tables or tableaux? The challenges of writing and reading mixed methods studies. In A. Tashakkori & C. Teddlie (Eds.), *Handbook of mixed methods in social and behavioral research* (pp. 321–350). Thousand Oaks, CA: Sage.

Sandelowski, M. (2014). Unmixing mixed-methods research. *Research in Nursing & Health, 37,* 3–8.

*Sandelowski, M., Voils, C., & Knafl, G. (2009). On quantitizing. *Journal of Mixed Methods Research, 3,* 208–222.

Silver, C. (2014). QDA Miner (with WordStat and SimStat). *Journal of Mixed Methods Research.* Advance online publication. doi:10.1177/1558689814538833

Tashakkori, A., & Creswell, J. (2007). The new era of mixed methods. *Journal of Mixed Methods Research, 1,* 3–7.

Tashakkori, A., & Teddlie, C. (Eds.). (2003). *Handbook of mixed methods in social and behavioral research.* Thousand Oaks, CA: Sage.

Tashakkori, A., & Teddlie, C. (Eds.). (2010). *Handbook of mixed methods in social and behavioral research* (2nd ed.). Thousand Oaks, CA: Sage.

Teddlie, C., & Tashakkori, A. (2003). Major issues and controversies in the use of mixed methods in the social and behavioral sciences. In A. Tashakkori & C. Teddlie (Eds.), *Handbook of mixed methods in social and behavioral research* (pp. 3–50). Thousand Oaks, CA: Sage.

Teddlie, C., & Tashakkori, A. (2009). *Foundations of mixed methods research.* Thousand Oaks, CA: Sage.

Tocher, J. M. (2014). Expectations and experiences of open abdominal aortic aneurysm repair patients: A mixed methods study. *Journal of Clinical Nursing, 23,* 421–428.

VanDevanter, N., Kovner, C., Raveis, V., McCollum, M., & Keller, R. (2014). Challenges of nurses' deployment to other New York City hospitals in the aftermath of Hurricane Sandy. *Journal of Urban Health, 91,* 603–614.

Wills, B. S. H., & Morse, J. M. (2007). Responses of Chinese elderly to the threat of severe acute respiratory syndrome (SARS) in a Canadian community. *Public Health Nursing, 25,* 57–68.

Wittenberg-Lyles, E., Washington, K., Oliver, D. P., Shaunfield, S., Gage, L. A., Mooney, M., & Lewis, A. (2015). "It is the 'starting over' part that is so hard": Using an online support group to support hospice bereavement. *Palliative and Supportive Care, 13,* 351–357.

Zoffmann, V., & Kirkevold, M. (2012). Realizing empowerment in difficult diabetes care: A guided self-determination intervention. *Qualitative Health Research, 22,* 103–118.

A link to this open-access journal article is provided in the Toolkit for this chapter in the accompanying Resource Manual. ⊗

27 Developing Complex Nursing Interventions Using Mixed Methods Research

This chapter discusses research-based efforts to develop innovative nursing interventions. Historically, there has been much more guidance on how to test and evaluate interventions than on how to develop them, but that situation is changing. There is a growing recognition that new interventions should be based on research evidence and on strong conceptualizations of the problem. Such endeavors benefit from mixed methods designs.

NURSING INTERVENTION RESEARCH

The term *intervention research* is increasingly being used by nurse researchers to describe a research approach characterized not only by its research methods but also by a distinctive *process* of developing, implementing, testing, and disseminating interventions (e.g., Richards & Rahm Hallberg, 2015; Sidani & Braden, 1998, 2011). Naylor (2003) defined **nursing intervention research** as "as studies either questioning existing care practices or testing innovations in care that are shaped by nursing's values and goals, guided by a strong theoretical basis, informed by recent advances in science, and designed to improve the quality of care and health of individuals, families, communities, and society" (p. 382).

Some nursing interventions are fairly simple and do not require extensive development. For example, Burrai and colleagues (2014) undertook a randomized controlled trial (RCT) to test the effect of live saxophone music on pain, mood, blood pressure, and oxygen saturation in patients with cancer. The intervention was relatively simple—one 30-minute session of music therapy—and the researchers did not "develop" the intervention; rather, they developed a protocol for its implementation. Many nursing interventions that are currently being tested, however, are complex and created by nurses themselves, usually within a focused program of research involving an integrated series of studies.

Complex Interventions

The term **complex intervention** has become a buzzword in research circles and has been the topic of several articles in the nursing literature (e.g., Corry et al., 2013; Fredericks & Yau, 2014; Seers, 2007). We begin, then, by discussing what the term means.

The Medical Research Council (MRC) in the United Kingdom proposed an influential framework for developing and testing complex interventions, and we describe that framework in the next section. According to the MRC report, complexity in an intervention can arise along several dimensions, including the following:

- The number of different components within the intervention ("bundling") and interactions between the components

- The number of different behaviors required by those delivering or receiving the intervention and the difficulty level of those behaviors
- The number of different groups or organizational levels targeted by the intervention
- The number and diversity of intervention outcomes targeted
- The degree to which the intervention can be tailored to individual patients (Craig et al., 2008a, 2008b).

Other dimensions can also contribute to complexity. For example, interventions that unfold in multiple sessions over 3 months are likely to be more complex than those that can be administered in one 30-minute session. Another complexity dimension concerns the number of different types of *intervention agents* needed to implement it (e.g., nurses, family members, other health care staff). A content analysis of 207 researchers' descriptions of complex interventions described complexity in terms of intervention design, implementation, context, outcomes, and evaluation challenges (Datta & Petticrew, 2013).

Complexity in interventions clearly exists along a continuum rather than as a dichotomy. There is no single point at which a simple intervention becomes complex. There is a wide range of possible complexities, and many nursing interventions are complex along more than one dimension identified in the MRC report. The more complex the intervention, the stronger is the need for an intervention framework.

⊃ **TIP:** Complex interventions are likely to be needed when complex problems are being treated, when a conceptual framework suggests multiple mediating forces, and when prior research suggests that simple interventions are ineffective.

Frameworks for Developing and Testing Complex Interventions

Proponents of using a framework to guide the intervention development and testing process are critical of the simplistic and atheoretical approach that has often been used with nursing interventions. The recommended process for intervention research involves an in-depth understanding of the problem and the target population, careful integration of diverse evidence, and the use of a guiding intervention theory. The recommendations call for a systematic, progressive sequence that places evidence-based developmental work at a premium.

Several intervention frameworks for health interventions have been proposed, and they have many similarities. One such framework is for the development of health promotion programs (Bartholomew et al., 2011). The most prominent framework to date, however, is the MRC framework, which was first described in the literature in 2000 (Campbell et al., 2000; MRC, 2000) and has been cited in hundreds of intervention reports in the health care literature.

Figure 27.1 shows that the original MRC framework was conceptualized as a five-phase process

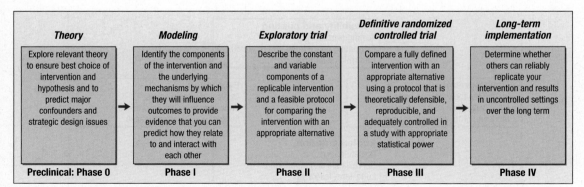

Theory	*Modeling*	*Exploratory trial*	*Definitive randomized controlled trial*	*Long-term implementation*
Explore relevant theory to ensure best choice of intervention and hypothesis and to predict major confounders and strategic design issues	Identify the components of the intervention and the underlying mechanisms by which they will influence outcomes to provide evidence that you can predict how they relate to and interact with each other	Describe the constant and variable components of a replicable intervention and a feasible protocol for comparing the intervention with an appropriate alternative	Compare a fully defined intervention with an appropriate alternative using a protocol that is theoretically defensible, reproducible, and adequately controlled in a study with appropriate statistical power	Determine whether others can reliably replicate your intervention and results in uncontrolled settings over the long term
Preclinical: Phase 0	**Phase I**	**Phase II**	**Phase III**	**Phase IV**

FIGURE 27.1 Medical Research Council's original framework for developing and testing complex health care interventions. (Adapted from Campbell, M., Fitzpatrick, R., Haines, A., Kinmouth, A., Sandercrock, P., Spiegelhalter, D., & Tryer, P. [2000]. Framework for design and evaluation of complex interventions to improve health. *BMJ, 321*, 694–696.)

in which a continuum of evidence is pursued. In Phase 0, which corresponds to what was called the *preclinical phase*, the focus is on developing a theoretical rationale for the intervention. Phase I, the *modeling phase*, involves achieving an understanding of the underlying mechanisms by which the components of the intervention will work in influencing the outcomes of interest. In practice, Phases 0 and I are often combined. In Phase II, the intervention protocol is piloted in an exploratory trial. Phase III corresponds to a full, rigorous test of the intervention's effects using a randomized design. As noted in Chapter 11, this phase is often referred to as efficacy research, with a focus on understanding possible intervention effects under controlled conditions. Phase IV of the first MRC framework involves tests of whether the intervention can be reliably replicated under more usual conditions (effectiveness research).

The original MRC framework is similar in some regards to the four-phase sequence delineated by the National Institutes of Health for clinical trials, as described in Chapter 11. Another four-phase model developed by nurses in the Netherlands emphasized the importance of strong development work and pilot testing (van Meijel et al., 2004).

In 2008, the MRC published a revised framework, which reflects suggestions made by many critics who thought the process outlined in the original was too linear. Figure 27.2 shows that the new MRC framework consists of a set of four interconnected "elements" of the intervention development and evaluation process: (1) development, (2) feasibility and piloting, (3) evaluation, and (4) implementation. Although these elements are not connected in a linear, nor even in a cyclical fashion, Craig and colleagues (2008a) noted that it is often "useful to think in terms of stages" (p. 8), and so we have organized much of this chapter in terms of four broad "phases" corresponding to the MRC elements. The central focus of this chapter, however, is on the initial development phase.

Key Features of Complex Intervention Research

In the past decade, considerable effort has been put into fleshing out (and using) the MRC guidance. It has become clear that certain features of intervention research are critical to success. Here we identify a few key features.

First, in both the old and new MRC framework, there is strong support for mixed methods research. In moving from a problem to be solved to the rigorous testing of a proposed intervention, a wide variety of questions need to be answered. As we discussed in the previous chapter, different types of question call for diverse methodologic strategies. Borglin (2015) has recently described the value of mixed methods in intervention research.

Second, intervention research is undertaken in the context of coordinated teamwork, and efforts to develop high-quality complex interventions are often multidisciplinary. Nurses can productively collaborate

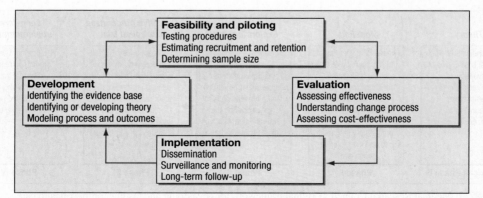

FIGURE 27.2 Medical Research Council's revised framework for developing and testing complex health care interventions (Craig et al., 2008a, 2008b).

with other health professionals (e.g., physicians, physical therapists, psychologists, nutritionists) on thorny problems requiring a multifaceted solution.

Another key feature of intervention research is that it requires many years of work. The MRC framework calls for a sequence of activities that involves a long investment of time to "get it right." Commentators have begun to note that there is a lot of *research waste*—research that gets little or no *return on investment*—because some researchers do not ask the right questions, do not take into account what is already known, use weak research methods, or fail to disseminate their work promptly and effectively (e.g., Chalmers & Glasziou, 2009; Chalmers et al., 2014). Research on complex interventions benefits from being embedded in an ongoing, dedicated program of research (Rahm Hallberg, 2015). Coordinated efforts to understand

a problem, integrate relevant evidence, develop and test an intervention, and promote its wider adoption are strategies for reducing research waste.

Finally, there is growing recognition that patient and public involvement (PPI) is important throughout the process of developing and testing complex interventions (Richards, 2015a). The literature on complex interventions is filled with cautions about potential challenges and pitfalls. Many of the pitfalls concern resistance on the part of patients (Table 27.1), family members or caretakers, and health care staff in the settings where interventions get tested (Table 27.2). Thus, in embarking on the pathway of complex intervention research, it is important to understand that a lot of things *can* go wrong, and so strategies should be designed to prevent them from happening to the extent possible. That is why skillful foundational work during the

TABLE 27.1 • Common "Pitfalls" in Intervention Research: Clients and Study Participants[a]

PITFALL	CAUSES/CONTRIBUTORS
Clients who do not want to receive the intervention or participate in research	Poor "match" between clients' goals and researchers' goals; lack of trust; language barriers; resistance by family gatekeepers; insufficient time; practical constraints (e.g., child care, transportation); health problems; lack of incentive; concerns about privacy invasion
Clients who do not want to be randomized	Lack of trust; fear of experimentation; strong preference for one treatment condition or the other; resistance to not being "in control"
Clients who do not adhere to protocols (e.g., poor attendance, lack of attention)	Lack of incentive; lack of time or competing demands; concerns about the intervention; scheduling conflicts; material not engaging or understandable; agents not sufficiently persuasive; poor communication about scheduling
Participants who drop out of the study	Lack of incentive; perceived irrelevance of outcome measures; competing demands; health problems (or death); transportation or child care problems; intervention material not engaging or understandable; boredom with treatment or with data collection; concerns about inadequate attention (control group)
Inadequate enactment of intervention behaviors in real-life settings (e.g., at home)	Lack of incentive; competing demands; lack of conviction about intervention efficacy; inadequate support for continuation; inadequate "rehearsal" of behaviors; resistance to changing normal routines; family or peer opposition

[a]Pitfalls and contributing factors were compiled from various sources, including Rowlands et al. (2005), Whittemore and Grey (2002), and Pruitt and Privette (2001).

TABLE 27.2 • Common "Pitfalls" in Intervention Research: Agents Delivering the Intervention[a]

PITFALL	CAUSES/CONTRIBUTORS
Staff who do not want to recruit participants	Low perceived salience of problem; misgivings about the intervention or about research in general; inadequate time; lack of interest; inadequate incentive to cooperate
Intervention agents who do not adhere to protocols (includes deliberate non-adherence, inadvertent nonadherence, and noncompetent delivery)	Inadequate time; lack of interest; low salience of problem; commitment to the status quo; inadequate training; inadequate incentive to change
Intervention agents who offer intervention to control group members ("contamination")	Commitment to or belief in efficacy of intervention; confusion or inadequate training; inability to "forget" intervention protocols when caring for nonintervention patients
Administrative or organizational issues	Staff turnover; policy changes

[a]Pitfalls and contributing factors were compiled from various sources, including Buckwalter et al. (2009), Kearney and Simonelli (2006), Mahoney et al. (2006), and McGuire et al. (2000).

development phase is so crucial, including efforts to understand the perspectives of patients and other stakeholders.

⮞ **TIP:** Despite the challenges, the time is ripe for designing nursing interventions. A prominent nurse researcher asked her audience during a keynote address at a nursing research society: "If you are not doing nursing intervention research, why not? If not now, when?" (Conn, 2005, p. 249). Another research team in Europe (Richards et al., 2014) urged nurse researchers to pursue skills in developing, testing, evaluating, and reporting complex nursing interventions.

Ideal Features of a Nursing Intervention

Nursing interventions are developed to lead to improvements in health outcomes. Before embarking on an intervention development project, nurse researchers should carefully consider the relative importance of achieving certain overall goals.

Box 27.1 identifies features that may be considered "ideal" for nursing interventions—although

in any situation, some features would be more important than others. In some cases, the desirable features compete with one another—for example, cost and efficacy often involve trade-offs. Indeed, most of the ideals could plausibly be achieved if cost were not an issue.

Yet, practical issues *are* important considerations. Especially in this time of heightened consciousness about health care costs, an intervention should be one that has potential to be cost-effective. In designing new ways to address health needs, nurse researchers should give up-front thought to whether the intervention is feasible from a resource perspective in real-world settings. As noted by Richards (2015b), "We should consider the 'implementability' of our complex interventions from the moment we begin the process of design, testing, and evaluation" (p. 333). Some of the ideals in Box 27.1 may need to be relaxed in the face of cost constraints, but this should be a conscious decision and not left to serendipity.

One ideal feature that should never be relaxed, of course, is the first one on the list—having an intervention that addresses a pressing problem. When such problems arise in clinical settings, other ideals

BOX 27.1 Features of an "Ideal" Nursing Intervention

An ideal clinical intervention would be:

- **Salient**—addresses a pressing problem
- **Efficacious**—leads to improved client outcomes
- **Safe**—avoids any adverse outcomes, burdens, or stress
- **Conceptually sound**—has a theoretical underpinning
- **Cost-effective**—is affordable and has economic benefits to clients or society
- **Feasible**—can be implemented in real-world settings and integrated into current models of care
- **Developmentally appropriate**—is suitable for the age group for whom it is intended
- **Culturally sensitive**—demonstrates sensitivity to various groups
- **Accessible**—can be easily accessed by the people for whom it is intended
- **Acceptable**—is viewed positively by clients and other stakeholders, including family members, nurses, physicians, administrators, policy makers
- **Adaptable**—can be tailored to local contexts
- **Readily disseminated**—can be sufficiently described and packaged for adoption in other locales

such as acceptability and feasibility are likely to be more easily attained.

PHASE 1: INTERVENTION DEVELOPMENT

The best current practice is to develop interventions in a systematic fashion, using (or creating) good evidence and an appropriate theory of how the intervention would achieve desired effects. In other words, interventions should be evidence-based from the start, and this can require extensive and diverse types of foundational work.

Each phase in the intervention development and testing process can be thought of as having three aspects: (1) key *issues* that must be addressed during this stage, (2) *actions* and strategies that can be brought to bear on those issues, and (3) the *products* that pave the way for movement onto the next phase. Table 27.3 summarizes issues, actions, and products for intervention development in Phase 1.

TABLE 27.3 • Key Issues, Activities, and Products of Phase 1 Developmental Work for Nursing Interventions

KEY ISSUES	MAJOR ACTIVITIES	PRODUCTS AND OUTCOMES
• Conceptualization of the problem • Articulation of an evidence base for the intervention • Conceptualization of solutions, strategies, and outcomes • Construct validation of the intervention • Identification of potential pitfalls within the implementation context • Cultivation of relationships	• Critical synthesis of relevant literature • Concept and theory development • Exploratory and descriptive research • Consultation with experts; content validation • Brainstorming with colleagues, team building, partnerships with stakeholders • Modeling and designing the intervention	• An intervention theory • Preliminary specification of the content, intensity, dose, timing, setting, and delivery method of the intervention • Preliminary identification of key outcomes • Strategies to overcome pitfalls in implementing and testing the intervention • A design for a pilot study • A plan for sponsorship of the pilot study

Key Issues in Intervention Development

Conceptualization and in-depth understanding of the problem are key issues during Phase 1. The starting point is the problem itself, which must be understood in the context where the intervention will be implemented. In Chapter 5, we discussed how those doing a literature review must "own" the literature. When it comes to intervention development, researchers must "own" the problem. A thorough understanding of the target group—their needs, fears, preferences, constraints, and circumstances—is part of that ownership. It is only through such understanding that researchers can know whether key pitfalls (Table 27.1) are relevant in their own situation. Ownership of the problem also requires a thorough grasp of existing evidence on similar interventions.

Thorough knowledge of the intended beneficiaries can also clarify how far from the "ideal" (Box 27.1) preliminary intervention plans are likely to be. Awareness of patient preferences, for example, could provide insight into how acceptable an intervention would be (Sidani et al., 2006). Moreover, patient preference and needs are sometimes incorporated into the design of tailored or individualized interventions (Lauver et al., 2002).

Another development issue involves identifying key *stakeholders*—people who have a stake in the intervention—and getting them "on board." Interventions sometimes fail because researchers have not developed the relationships needed to ensure that the intervention will be given a fair test. Who the key stakeholders are varies from project to project. In addition to the target group, stakeholders might include family members, advocates, community leaders, service providers in multiple disciplines, intervention agents, health care administrators, support staff in intervention settings, and content experts. Buckwalter and colleagues (2009) advised, "Investigators should think broadly about whose support could affect their ability to conduct the planned research" (p. 118).

Relationship building can contribute to the content of the intervention itself because stakeholders can offer insight into the scope and depth of the problem. Relationships with stakeholders are also important because researchers must figure out not only *what* to deliver but also *how* to deliver it in a manner that will gain the support of administrators and health care staff, appeal to the target group, enhance recruitment and retention of participants, and strengthen intervention fidelity in later phases.

Activities and Strategies in Intervention Development

Developmental issues can be addressed through a variety of activities, several of which are discussed in this section. The vital importance of adequate development cannot be overemphasized.

Synthesizing Existing Evidence

As shown in Figure 27.2, development work includes "identifying the evidence base," and thus, development work often begins with intensive and extensive scrutiny of the literature. In intervention studies, the literature needs to be searched for guidance about the content and mechanisms of the intervention—for its active ingredients. Systematic reviews may be available for evidence about the efficacy of specific strategies, but it may also be necessary to undertake a new or updated systematic review (see Chapter 29).

Researchers' efforts to understand the problem and possible solutions are an important, but not exhaustive, part of a literature review effort. Table 27.4 provides examples of other questions that should be addressed through a scrutiny of existing evidence during the intervention development phase, including evidence from any relevant systematic reviews of qualitative and mixed methods studies. When relevant literature is thin or nonexistent, other sources to address remaining uncertainties need to be pursued.

Example of a Literature Review in Nursing Intervention Research: Kirkevold and colleagues (2012) described the development of a complex intervention designed to promote psychosocial well-being following a stroke. They undertook a detailed analysis of relevant quantitative and qualitative research. They examined existing systematic reviews regarding the psychosocial challenges experienced by stroke survivors, and they completed a synthesis of qualitative research on the trajectory of stroke rehabilitation and recovery.

TABLE 27.4 • Examples of Literature Review Questions for Designing an Evidence-Based Intervention

ISSUE	QUESTIONS FOR WHICH EVIDENCE CAN BE SOUGHT IN A LITERATURE REVIEW
Conceptualizing the problem	What is known about the nature and causes of this problem and possible solutions? What theories help to explain the problem? What are key mediators in the pathway between the causes or contributing factors and the outcomes?
Focusing the target group	What have been the targets of efforts to address the problem—individuals? families? health care providers? health care systems? What populations appear to be most amenable to the intervention?
Developing intervention content and components	What is the content of other similar interventions? Is the presence of certain types of components linked to better outcomes? Are interventions generic or individualized?
Selecting outcomes and assessment strategies	What behaviors or outcomes have been targeted by similar interventions? Have the interventions had significant effects on these outcomes? Have they affected key mediators? What assessment approaches and measures have been used with other similar interventions?
Making decisions about dose	How intense have other similar interventions been? Has dose been found to be related to outcomes?
Making decisions about timing of intervention	When are interventions of this type typically delivered? Is timing related to outcomes?
Making decision about mode of delivery	How have similar interventions been delivered? in face-to-face situations (group or individual delivery)? by telephone? Internet? video? Is there evidence that different delivery modes are especially effective?
Making decisions about timing of outcome measurement	When have data for this type of intervention typically been collected? Does the literature suggest that effects deteriorate? Or, are there delayed effects?
Making decisions about settings and agents	Where (in what types of settings) have interventions of this type been delivered? Do impacts vary by type of setting? Who usually delivers them? Do outcomes vary by type of agent?
Assessing acceptability of the intervention	Is there evidence of strong (or weak) rates of participation in interventions of this type? Have recruitment or retention problems been reported?
Assessing cultural appropriateness	Is there evidence that cultural issues affect implementation of similar interventions? Is there cultural variation in outcomes?

Exploratory and Descriptive Research

Most researchers find that evidence from the literature is insufficient to satisfactorily address the questions suggested in Table 27.4. Almost inevitably, the developmental phase involves exploratory and descriptive research, usually using mixed methods. Qualitative studies are virtually essential to the success of well-founded intervention development efforts, a position articulated in all the intervention frameworks described earlier.

As previously noted, efforts to design acceptable and efficacious interventions require understanding clients' perspectives. Examples of the kinds of questions that could be pursued in exploratory research with clients include, What is it like to have this problem? Who is in greatest need of an intervention? What are clients' goals—what do *they* want as an intervention outcome? (Additional exploratory research questions are available in the Supplement to this chapter on thePoint⬢.) Answers to questions such as these could help to shape the intervention and make it more effective, tolerable, and appropriate for the group for whom the intervention is designed.

Exploratory research with other stakeholders can also be valuable. Many of the pitfalls of intervention research involve lack of cooperation, support, or trust among key stakeholders, including intervention agents. Stakeholders should be engaged in the development process to the extent possible. Stakeholders who have had experience working with the target group often can contribute to the development of effective intervention strategies.

Exploratory work can also be undertaken to better understand the context within which an intervention would unfold (McGuire et al., 2000). For example, it may be important to understand issues such as staff turnover, staff morale, nurse workload, and nurse autonomy. An analysis of context may be especially important when introducing interventions into highly unstable environments (Buckwalter et al., 2009). Van Meijel and colleagues (2004) also recommended undertaking a "current practice analysis" to understand the status quo of how the problem under scrutiny is being addressed.

The nursing literature has hundreds of examples of descriptive or exploratory studies done as part of intervention development. Research strategies run the gamut of those discussed in this book, such as focus group interviews, needs assessment surveys, in-depth or critical-incident interviews, records reviews, and observations in clinical settings. It is not unusual for researchers to conduct three or four small descriptive studies during the development phase of an intervention project.

Example of Exploratory Research for a Nursing Intervention: Gray and colleagues (2013) developed a community-based intervention designed to improve the quality of life in people with colorectal cancer. During the development phase, the researchers conducted several qualitative substudies to help in the design and refinement of the intervention protocol. One involved in-depth interviews with 28 patients with colorectal cancer to identify symptoms and activities of importance to them and to understand their goals. Also, semistructured interviews were conducted with 16 cancer specialists and 14 primary care professionals.

➔ **TIP:** Morden and colleagues (2015) provide a compelling argument about the importance of qualitative research in informing the development and implementation of complex interventions.

Consultation with Experts

Experts in the content area of the problem or with the target population can play a crucial role during the development of an intervention. Expert consultants are especially useful if the evidence base is thin and resources for undertaking exploratory research are limited. Many of the questions in Table 27.4 that are not answered by evidence in the research literature or from new descriptive studies are good candidates for discussion with experts.

➔ **TIP:** In selecting expert consultants, think in an interdisciplinary fashion. For example, the use of a cultural consultant may be valuable to assess the cultural sensitivity and appropriateness of some interventions. A developmental psychologist could help assess developmental suitability.

Often, experts are asked to review preliminary intervention protocols, to corroborate their utility, and to solicit suggestions for strengthening them. Curiously, this process is less often formalized than the process for reviewing new measurement scales. Procedures used to assess the *content validity* of new instruments using an expert panel (Chapter 15) can also be used to review draft intervention protocols. Indeed, if the intervention is intended for use in diverse settings or contexts, content validation is likely to be a valuable approach.

> **Example of Content Validation of a Nursing Intervention:** Lu and Haase (2011) used an interdisciplinary panel of six scientists and clinicians to assess the content validity of the Daily Enhancement of Meaningful Activity (DEMA) program, an intervention for mild cognitive impairment patient–spouse dyads.

Brainstorming and Team Building

Development work is often interpersonal in nature and involves cultivating relationships. At the team level, this involves putting together an enthusiastic and committed project team with diverse clinical, research, and dissemination skills. (If development work is undertaken for a dissertation, the "team" includes the dissertation committee, so members of this committee should be chosen carefully.)

Ideally, frequent brainstorming sessions occur during the development period to discuss evidence summaries, conceptual maps, descriptive findings, expert feedback, and preliminary protocols. Technologic advances such as videoconferencing make it possible to include team members from different locations. The team may include ongoing involvement of key stakeholders as participating partners in the development and testing of an intervention.

TIP: In addition to seeking information about the stakeholders' perspectives on the problem through in-depth research, it is wise to develop mechanisms for ongoing communication and collaboration. For example, it can be useful to form an advisory group of stakeholders and to have a project-specific website or Facebook page.

Intervention Theory Development

A critical activity in the development phase is to delineate a strong conceptual basis for the intervention (Craig et al., 2008a, 2008b; MRC, 2000). An **intervention theory** guides what must be done to achieve desired outcomes and provides a theoretical rationale for why an intervention should "work." The theory indicates, based on the best available knowledge, the nature of the clinical intervention and factors that would mediate the effects of clinical procedures on expected outcomes.

The intervention theory can be an existing one that has been well-validated. Examples of theories that have been used in nursing intervention studies include Social Cognitive Theory, the Health Promotion Model, the Transtheoretical Model, the Health Belief Model, and the Theory of Planned Behavior (see Chapter 6). These theories provide guidance on how to fashion an intervention because they propose mechanisms to explain human behavior and behavior change. Abraham and colleagues (2015) offer perspectives on the theoretical basis of behavior change interventions.

Intervention theories can also be developed from qualitatively derived theory, a point made most eloquently by Morse (2006). Morse and colleagues (2000) developed a strategy called qualitative outcome analysis (QOA), which is a process for extending the findings of a qualitative study by identifying intervention strategies related to the phenomenon of concern.

Researchers may find it productive to develop their own evidence-based model that purports to explain the link between the causes of a problem and outcomes of concern. An example concerning humor as an intervention was presented in Chapter 6. A conceptual map, such as the one presented in Figure 6.2, can be a useful visual tool for articulating the intervention theory and can serve as a "road map" for designing and testing the intervention and the counterfactual (control condition). Sidani and Braden (1998) have offered useful guidance about components of an intervention theory.

Example of a Qualitatively Derived Intervention Theory: Harvey Chochinov and other researchers (including nurse researchers) developed a theory of dignity based on in-depth interviews with hospice patients. The theory formed the basis for an intervention (Dignity Therapy) to promote dignity and reduce stress at the end of life. Hall and colleagues (2009) conducted a pilot test of the acceptability, feasibility, and potential effectiveness of the intervention. Hall and colleagues (2012) also evaluated Dignity Therapy for older people in care homes and undertook further qualitative research as part of the trial (Hall et al., 2013).

Modeling and Designing the Intervention

The MRC framework (Figure 27.2) includes "modeling processes and outcomes" as a component of intervention development. Modeling involves synthesizing the information gleaned during the development phase (Figure 27.3), constructing components of the intervention, and visualizing the pathways that patients will take in going through the intervention. As described by Sermeus (2015), the aim of modeling is to unravel the "black box" between intervention components and desired outcomes.

An evidence-based intervention theory lays the groundwork for proceeding with the modeling task and developing intervention content. The model for the intervention should describe the active components and explain how they are expected to work on the outcomes of interest. It should also describe how the active components relate to each other.

Intervention content can often be adapted from other similar interventions or from clinical practice guidelines. In addition to content, however, the research team needs to make many decisions about

the intervention's ingredients. We have hinted at these decisions in Table 27.4, but here we offer more explicit information.

1. **Dose and Intensity.** The treatment must be sufficiently powerful to achieve a desired, measurable effect on outcomes of interest but cannot be so powerful that it is cost-prohibitive or burdensome to clients. Among the dose-related issues that need to be decided are the *potency* or *intensity* of the treatment (How much content is appropriate, and will it be given individually or in groups?), the *amount* of dose per session, the *frequency* of administering doses (number of sessions), and the *duration* of the intervention over time. It may be important to consider whether "boosters" are needed to maintain effects.

2. **Timing.** In some cases, it is important to decide when, relative to other events, the intervention will be delivered. The question is, When is the optimal point (in terms of an illness or recovery trajectory, individual development, or severity of a problem) to administer the intervention? Ideally, the intervention theory would suggest the most advantageous timing.

3. **Outcomes.** A major decision concerns the outcomes that will be targeted. Thought should be given to selecting outcomes that are nursing sensitive and important to clients. One issue is whether the focus will be on proximal outcomes or more distal ones. *Proximal outcomes* are immediate and directly connected to the intervention—and thus, usually most sensitive to intervention effects. For example, knowledge gains from a teaching component of an intervention are proximal. *Distal outcomes* are potentially more important ones but more difficult to affect (e.g., behavior change). Consideration should also be given to the information needs of people making decisions about using the intervention—what outcomes would affect uptake by administrators or policy makers? Timing of outcome measurement is also important. For example, do knowledge gains decay? Do behavior changes accumulate over time? The timing of measuring outcomes is important because effect size is not constant—the goal is to decide when the *peak response* to an intervention will occur.

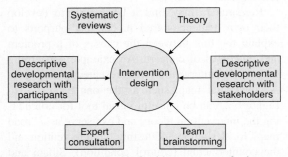

FIGURE 27.3 Synthesis of evidence sources for intervention development.

4. **Setting.** Another design decision involves the setting for the intervention. Settings can vary in terms of ease of implementation and costs. In deciding about settings (and sites), researchers need to think about the type of setting that will be acceptable and accessible to clients, offer good potential for impacts, provide needed resources or supports, and be cost-effective.

5. **Agents.** Researchers must decide who will deliver the intervention and how intervention agents will be trained. In many cases, the agents will be nurses, but nurses are not necessarily the best choice. For example, some clients might feel more comfortable if the interventionists were community members or patients who have experienced a similar illness or problem (i.e., peers).

6. **Delivery Mode.** With technologic innovations occurring regularly, options for delivering interventions—or components of interventions—have broadened tremendously. Among the possibilities are face-to-face delivery, video or audio recordings, print materials, telephone or texting contacts, e-mail transmissions, Internet discussion boards, and social networking sites. Care should be taken to match any technologic delivery methods to the needs of the clients and to the requirements of the content. The latest technology is not always the optimal. Conn et al. (2001) noted that there should be clarity about whether the intervention being tested is the content, the delivery mode, or both. When both the content and the delivery mode are new, a factorial design that varies mode on one dimension and receipt of content on the other might be a good design strategy for testing the intervention's efficacy.

7. **Individualization.** Another decision concerns the extent to which the intervention will be tailored to the needs and circumstances of a particular group (e.g., older adults) or individualized to particular clients. When individual information is used to guide content, the intervention is inherently more complex than a one-size-fits-all treatment but may be more effective and attractive to participants (Lauver et al., 2002).

These various decisions ideally would be evidence-based, using synthesized evidence from various sources. The development work should provide the basis for the intervention to be piloted in the next phase. As noted by the authors of the MRC framework, "the intervention must be developed to the point where it can reasonably be expected to have a worthwhile effect" (Craig et al., 2008b, p. 980).

Products of Phase 1 Development

Phase 1 typically results in several products (Table 27.3). These include an intervention theory and conceptual map, preliminary intervention components and protocols, and strategies for addressing potential implementation pitfalls. Hopefully, the research team will have documented the development work and major decisions in an ongoing fashion. Detailed written information about the theory, the intervention components and strategies, and expected outcomes will be valuable for writing reports about the intervention and for making funding requests.

> ⊗ **TIP:** A matrix can often be useful in summarizing *key decisions* in one column, and *supporting evidence* for those decisions in another. Such a matrix is a good communication tool for discussing decisions with others. A worksheet for such a matrix is included in the Toolkit for this chapter in the *Resource Manual*.

If the evidence synthesis provides support for moving forward with a pilot test of the intervention, another product of Phase 1 work will be a full design for a pilot study, usually in the form of a research proposal (proposal development is discussed in Chapter 31).

OTHER PHASES OF INTERVENTION RESEARCH

Other phases of intervention research include feasibility and pilot testing, a rigorous evaluation to test and confirm efficacy, and implementation of the intervention (should it prove to be effective) into real-world settings with ongoing monitoring and longer term follow-up. These other phases are briefly described next.

Phase 2: Pilot Testing an Intervention

The second phase of intervention research is a pilot test of the newly developed intervention. Key issues in this phase are *feasibility* (Can the intervention be implemented as conceptualized?), *acceptability* (Do recipients and other key stakeholders find the intervention relevant and appropriate?), and *promise* (Is it plausible that the intervention will result in desired effects on key outcomes?). The central *activities* of Phase 2 are undertaking the pilot study and analyzing pilot data. An important *product* of a pilot study is documentation of the results and the "lessons learned." Although each pilot test yields its own context-specific and intervention-specific lessons, some "lessons" are recurrent. In particular, you should expect the reality of the pilot to be different from what is on paper. Assuming that the intervention proves feasible and promising, Phase 2 products include a formal intervention protocol for testing in a Phase 3 clinical trial as well as ancillary products such as training manuals and finalized outcome measures. Another product is a formal plan for a Phase 3 evaluation, often in the form of a grant application. Chapter 28 discusses pilot testing in greater detail.

Example of a Mixed Methods Pilot Intervention Study: Barley and colleagues (2014) developed a personalized care intervention for coronary heart disease patients who report depression and chest pain, after doing extensive developmental work (e.g., Barley et al., 2012; Simmonds et al., 2013). The 6-month nurse-led intervention was pilot tested with 81 patients. The researchers concluded that the intervention was feasible and acceptable.

Phase 3: Evaluation of the Intervention

The third phase of an intervention study is to undertake a full test of the intervention, typically using a randomized design. Many important issues of a Phase 3 evaluation were discussed in Chapter 10, which outlined various threats to the validity of a rigorous quantitative study and presented some strategies to address those threats. Whereas construct validity is particularly salient in the development phase of an intervention project, internal validity and statistical conclusion validity are key issues during the evaluation.

Although a major goal of Phase 3 is to assess the *efficacy* of the intervention, it is perhaps better to think of the trial as ongoing development rather than as simply "confirmatory." Even with a strong pilot study, problems and issues will usually emerge in the full test. As part of a process evaluation (Chapter 11), problems should be identified, and researchers should make recommendations for how the intervention could be improved or how its implementation could be made smoother.

Both qualitative and quantitative data should be gathered during the evaluation. Quantitative data are essential for providing evidence about the intervention's effects on outcomes, but many pressing questions simply cannot be answered with quantitative data alone. Some of the benefits of obtaining qualitative data during Phase 3 include the following:

1. **Intervention Fidelity.** Mixed methods research is often needed to inform judgments about whether the intervention was faithfully implemented. If intervention effects are modest, one possibility is that it was not implemented according to plan and so the protocols or training materials might need "tweaking" (see Chapter 10).

2. **Intervention Clarification.** A qualitative component in a clinical trial can help to clarify the nature and course of the intervention in its natural context. It is useful to understand how intervention recipients and other stakeholders "actually experience the intervention in real time and in real life" (Sandelowski, 1996, p. 362).

3. **Variation in Effects.** Intervention effects represent averages. For individual participants, the effects might be much greater than the average, while for others the intervention might have no benefit. Sometimes subgroup analyses can be done quantitatively, but these are productive only if the dimension along which variation occurs is a measurable attribute about which hypotheses have been developed in advance. A qualitative study of participants who experienced the intervention differently could illuminate how to target the intervention more effectively in the future or how to improve it to reach a more diverse audience.

Example of Exploring Variation: Burke and colleagues (2009) conducted in-depth interviews with (and obtained diary data from) 15 people who completed a behavioral weight loss treatment. They explored variation in how people self-monitored their diet during the treatment. Three categories of self-monitoring were identified: well-disciplined (those with high adherence), those "missing the connection" (those with moderate adherence), and diminished support (those with poor adherence).

4. **Clinical Significance.** Quantitative results from a randomized trial indicate whether the results are statistically significant, and methods have been developed to quantitatively assess clinical significance as well (see Chapter 20). Qualitative information could shed additional light—clinically relevant effects sometimes can be discerned qualitatively even when treatment effects are not statistically significant.

5. **Interpretation.** Quantitative results indicate *whether* an intervention had beneficial effects—but do not explain *why* effects occurred. A strong conceptual framework offers a theoretical rationale for explaining the results but may not tell the whole story if the effects were weaker than expected, if they were observed for some outcomes but not for others, or even if they were consistent with expectations but represent *nonspecific effects*—that is, effects resulting from factors not specified in the intervention theory (Donovan et al., 2009). Moreover, even if there are specific theory-driven intervention effects, it is inevitable that people will pose "black box" questions about what is *driving* the results. Such questions often stem from practical concerns, reflecting a desire to streamline successful interventions when resources are tight.

Example of Interpreting Results: Berg and co-researchers (2014) conducted a trial to test the effectiveness of a complex cardiac rehabilitation intervention for patients with implantable cardioverter defibrillators. Nearly 200 patients were randomized in the Phase 3 trial, and intervention effects were found with regard to peak oxygen uptake, general health, and mental health. The researchers embedded a qualitative component involving in-depth interviews with 10 patients, and the qualitative findings helped them explain the mechanisms of the effects.

6. **Visibility.** Quantitative results do not have much "sex appeal." As astutely pointed out by Sandelowski (1996), qualitative research embedded in intervention studies can enhance the power of the study findings: " . . . Storied accounts of scientific work are often the more compelling and culturally resonant way to communicate research results to diverse audiences, including patient groups and policy-makers" (p. 361).

A Phase 3 evaluation, then, includes both an analysis of intervention effectiveness and a process evaluation that provides rich information about the roll-out of the intervention and the processes of change that occurred. One final evaluation component is crucial to the intervention's potential for widespread adoption: a cost–benefit analysis. Interventions are unlikely to be integrated into health care systems if their costs outweigh any benefits, and so the evaluation team should seek to understand economic implications. Payne and Thompson (2015) provide an overview of economic evaluations of complex interventions.

The primary product of Phase 3 is a report summarizing the evaluation results. Often, single papers are insufficient for providing the full range of information about the project, particularly if a mixed methods approach was used. Ideally, one report would integrate findings from the qualitative and quantitative components and offer recommendations for further adoption of the intervention.

TIP: Several writers have observed recently that interventions are inadequately described in research reports (e.g., Conn & Groves, 2011; Richards et al., 2014). Although journal constraints may limit a full elaboration of interventions, detailed descriptions should be prepared so they can be shared with others through correspondence. Further advice is offered in Chapter 30.

Phase 4: Implementation

In the MRC framework, the final phase of intervention research is the *implementation* of a complex intervention that has been found to have beneficial effects and favorable economic results. Implementation involves embedding a new and promising intervention into routine health and nursing services. The process of implementation is sometimes referred to as *normalization*.

Increasingly, researchers have come to recognize that their work does not end with the publication of a research report on the findings from a Phase 3 trial. A whole new field of *implementation science* has burgeoned in efforts to help researchers plan for undertaking implementation research. Several conceptual models and frameworks have been devised to guide the implementation process. One widely used framework is called **normalization process theory** (May, 2013; May & Finch, 2009). It is beyond the scope of this book to describe the "how to's" of implementation science, but interested readers can find several chapters devoted to this topic in Richards and Rahm Hallberg (2015).

MIXED METHODS DESIGNS FOR INTERVENTION RESEARCH

The full cycle of research activity in developing and testing complex interventions addresses myriad questions that can only be answered using a rich blend of research methods—that is, using mixed methods. Creswell (2015) identified as a possible advanced mixed methods design what he called the *intervention design*, which involves *embedding* qualitative data into a trial before, during, or after the experimental treatment has been implemented. Creswell's design is totally consistent with the MRC's intervention framework.

Visual diagrams for two possible two-stage mixed methods designs are presented in Figure 27.4. The notation in the top panel would be qual → QUAN + qual, and that in the bottom panel would be QUAN + qual → qual. Models such as these can work reasonably well for interventions that are closer to the "simple" end of the simple → complex continuum. They might also be appropriate for a small-scale study (such as a dissertation project) in which the main QUAN component is essentially a pilot study.

For complex interventions such as those described in the MRC framework, it is better to think of a separate design structure for each phase because each has its own purpose, research questions, design, sampling plan, and data collection strategy. For the project overall, QUAN typically has priority with qual playing a secondary role. Yet, foundational work in the development phase often involves QUAL-dominant research.

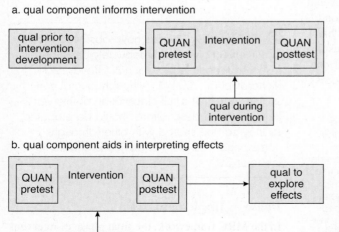

a. qual component informs intervention

b. qual component aids in interpreting effects

FIGURE 27.4 Mixed methods designs for a two-phase intervention project. (Adapted from Creswell, J. W., & Plano Clark, V. L. [2011]. *Designing and conducting mixed methods research* [2nd ed.]. Thousand Oaks, CA: Sage.)

Nursing Intervention Diagram

Phase 1 Development	Phase 2 Pilot Study	Phase 3 Controlled Trial
QUAL + quan or QUAL + QUAN or QUAL → quan or QUAL → qual	QUAN + qual or QUAN + QUAL or QUAN → qual or QUAN → QUAN	QUAN + qual or QUAN + qual → qual or QUAN → qual

FIGURE 27.5 Possible methods designs for a three-phase nursing intervention project.

Figure 27.5 shows some of the design possibilities for a three-phase intervention project, and many others are possible. For the project overall, the design is inherently sequential, but within each phase, the design could be either sequential or concurrent. Both qualitative and quantitative approaches are often used in each phase, although there may be no need to collect quantitative data during Phase 1 if there is a strong existing evidence base.

It is difficult to offer guidance on which of the myriad design possibilities to adopt because many factors influence which is most appropriate. Fewer design components may be required for simpler interventions, for "mainstream" target populations, for studies in a familiar site, and for studies of adaptations to well-tested interventions. Also, resources may force researchers to forego components they would have liked to include. The design for the Phase 3 trial is also likely to be affected by which of the six goals for qualitative inquiry (as described in the previous section) is most salient. For example, if the researchers want to understand variation in intervention effects, the design likely would be a QUAN→ qual sequential one. If the desire to monitor intervention fidelity is the primary objective of including a qualitative component, a QUAN + qual design would be needed.

Sampling designs, as discussed in Chapter 26, are also likely to differ in the three phases. During Phase 1, a multilevel sampling approach is often used to gather in-depth QUAL data from different populations—for example, from patients, family members, and health care staff. In Phases 2 and 3, by contrast, sampling is likely to be either identical or nested—although multilevel sampling may also be useful for understanding intervention fidelity.

In summary, researchers can be creative in developing an overall design that matches their needs, circumstances, and budgets. Inevitably, however, strong research for developing and testing complex interventions will rely on a mixed methods design.

CRITIQUING INTERVENTION RESEARCH

Many chapters of this book offer guidelines for evaluating methodologic aspects of the studies that would be included in an intervention project. For example, guidelines in Chapters 9 and 10 would be useful for critiquing the Phase 3 design. Qualitative components could be evaluated using guidelines in Chapters 21 through 25. Additionally, the previous chapter included critiquing suggestions for mixed methods research.

Box 27.2 offers a few additional questions on intervention issues, with many of them focusing on intervention development. An overarching question might be: How close did the researchers get to an "ideal" intervention, in terms of criteria identified in Box 27.1? Of course, being able to answer this overall question and many of the questions in Box 27.2 will depend on the care taken in documenting the full effort. Most often, aspects of the development and testing are reported in separate articles, but the team should strive to prepare a summary report that integrates qualitative and quantitative findings from all phases and that offers evidence-based recommendations for how to proceed with implementing the intervention in everyday practice settings.

BOX 27.2 Guidelines for Critiquing Aspects of Intervention Projects

1. On a simple-to-complex continuum, where would you locate the intervention? If the intervention is complex, along which dimensions is complexity found (e.g., number of components, complexity of behaviors required, number of intervention sessions, time required, and so on)?
2. Is there an intervention theory, and is it adequate? Was there an explanation of how the theory was selected, adapted, or developed?
3. What strategies were used to identify and create evidence in support of intervention development? Was a systematic review performed? Were expert consultants involved? Were descriptive or exploratory studies undertaken? Overall, was developmental work adequate?
4. What efforts were made to validate the intervention and its protocols?
5. Was there a pilot study? Was pilot work sufficient for a decision to move forward with a full clinical trial?
6. For the overall project and for individual phases, was a mixed methods approach used? Which design was adopted, and is the design appropriate for the goals of different phases of the project?
7. What *was* the intervention? Was it described in sufficient detail in terms of content, target population, dose, outcomes, timing, individualization, intervention agents, and so on?
8. Did the final report integrate key findings from the various strands of research? Did the report offer recommendations for replication, extension, or adaptation of the intervention, or for use in different settings or with different populations?

RESEARCH EXAMPLE OF A MIXED METHODS INTERVENTION PROJECT

Study: The development and testing of a proactive care program (U-CARE) to maintain physical functioning of frail older people in primary care in the Netherlands

Statement of Purpose: The overall purpose of this research was to develop and test the efficacy of a theory-based complex intervention to preserve physical functioning and enhance the quality of life of frail older people. The development process and details of the intervention were described "to allow its replication" (Bleijenberg et al., 2013a, p. 230). The researchers followed the MRC framework for complex interventions.

Phase 1: The developmental work for this project unfolded over several years. The study team, which included nurses and physicians with clinical experience in primary care, did a thorough literature review. The researchers also reviewed numerous clinical guidelines. After studying the existing evidence, the researchers concluded that the most promising elements for an intervention were based on those in the Chronic Care Model, which provided the theoretical framework. The emerging U-CARE program

was developed to comprise three steps: a frailty assessment to identify frail patients, a comprehensive geriatric assessment of frail patients at home, and then an individualized care plan with evidence-based interventions. The researchers also explored measures to use in the intervention, such as an assessment tool for measuring frailty (e.g., Drubbel et al., 2014). The "face validity" of the intervention and the assessment procedures were discussed with a panel of experienced nurses in 10 meetings. The research team also sought input from other geriatric experts, and a few adaptations to care plans were made based on their recommendations. The content of U-CARE was also "assessed and approved by a panel of five independent older people" (p. 233), who met twice.

Phase 2: Small pilot and feasibility studies of the U-CARE program were undertaken, involving the collection of both quantitative and qualitative data. In terms of feasibility, a mixed methods approach (QUAN → qual) was used to gather information from a sample of 32 general practitioners and 21 practice nurses. The study explored the participants' expectations and experiences with regard to a proactive and structured care program for frail elders (Bleijenberg et al., 2013b). This revealed several potential barriers, but participants affirmed the feasibility of such an approach in primary practices. The researchers also undertook a small-scale 6-week pilot test of the intervention with 30 patients. Patient outcomes were not formally assessed, but the nurses who delivered the pilot intervention reported gains in their own knowledge and their understanding of patients' needs.

Phase 3: A full-scale mixed methods evaluation of U-CARE, using a three-armed cluster randomized design, is currently underway in 39 clusters of general practices in the Netherlands (Bleijenberg et al., 2012). More than 3,000 patients are expected to be randomized. Prior to undertaking the full trial, 21 nurses with experience working with older people were recruited and trained, and careful attention was paid to matters of intervention fidelity. The primary outcome of the trial is level of activities of daily living (ADL). Secondary outcomes include quality of life, mortality, nursing home admission, emergency department visits, and caregiver burden. Outcome data are being collected at baseline and at 6-month and 12-month follow-ups. (The researchers have undertaken some analyses of the baseline data to explore factors associated with participants' ADL disabilities [Laan et al., 2013]). Qualitative data will also be gathered to explore patients' satisfaction with the U-CARE program. Finally, a cost-effectiveness analysis will be undertaken.

SUMMARY POINTS

- **Nursing intervention research** refers to a distinctive *process* of developing, implementing, testing, and disseminating nursing interventions—particularly complex interventions.
- *Complexity* in **complex interventions** can arise along several dimensions, including number of components, number of outcomes targeted, number and complexity of behaviors required, and the time needed for the full intervention to be delivered.
- Several frameworks for developing and testing complex interventions have been proposed. The most widely cited one is the **Medical Research Council (MRC) framework** (United Kingdom), which was published in 2000 and then revised in 2008.
- Most frameworks emphasize the critical importance of strong development efforts at the outset,

followed by pilot tests of the intervention, and then a rigorous controlled trial to assess efficacy. The frameworks are idealized models; the process is rarely linear. Virtually all frameworks for intervention development and testing call for mixed methods (MM) research.

- Conceptualization and in-depth understanding of the problem and the target population are key issues during Phase 1 development work. An important product during Phase 1 is a carefully conceived **intervention theory** from which the design of the intervention flows. The theory indicates what inputs are needed to effect improvements on specific outcomes.
- In addition to theory, resources for creating an evidence-based intervention and intervention strategies during Phase 1 development include systematic reviews, descriptive research with the target population or key stakeholders, consultation with experts, and discussions with a dedicated and diverse team.
- In developing an intervention, researchers must make decisions about not only the *content* of the intervention but also about dose and intensity, timing of the intervention, outcomes to target and when to measure them, intervention setting, intervention agents, mode of delivery, and individualization.
- In a Phase 2 pilot study, the preliminary intervention is tested for feasibility and preliminary effectiveness. Pilots often include supplementary qualitative components to understand the experience of being in the intervention and problems with recruitment and retention.
- A mixed methods approach can strengthen the test of the intervention during the Phase 3 controlled trial. The inclusion of qualitative components can shed light on intervention fidelity, variation in effects, clinical significance, and interpretive ambiguities.
- Mixed methods are appropriate (and beneficial) in all phases of an intervention project. Broadly speaking, the design is sequential, but each phase can involve the use of various mixed methods designs. In Phase 1, QUAL often has priority, while in Phases 2 and 3, QUAN is usually dominant.

STUDY ACTIVITIES

Chapter 27 of the *Resource Manual for Nursing Research: Generating and Assessing Evidence for Nursing Practice, 10th edition*, offers exercises and study suggestions for reinforcing concepts presented in this chapter. In addition, the following study questions can be addressed:

1. Review the research example of a randomized controlled trial described at the end of Chapter 10 ("Investigation of standard care versus sham Reiki placebo versus actual Reiki therapy to enhance comfort and well-being in a chemotherapy infusion center," Catlin & Taylor-Ford, 2011). Suggest how the study could potentially be enhanced using a QUAN → qual design. What mixed methods questions would be addressed by your proposed enhancement?

2. For the same study as in Question 1 (Catlin & Taylor-Ford, 2011), would you describe the intervention as complex? Why or why not?

STUDIES CITED IN CHAPTER 27

Abraham, C., Denford, S., Smith, J., Dean, S., Greaves, C., Lloyd, J., . . . Wyatt, K. (2015). Designing interventions to change health-related behaviour. In D. Richards & I. Rahm Hallberg (Eds.), *Complex interventions in health: An overview of research methods* (pp. 103–110). Oxford, United Kingdom: Routledge.

*Barley, E., Haddad, M., Simmonds, R., Fortune, Z., Walters, P., Murray, J., . . . Tylee, A. (2012). The UPBEAT depression and coronary heart disease programme: Using the UK Medical Research Council framework to design a nurse-led complex intervention for use in primary care. *BMC Family Practice, 13,* 119.

*Barley, E., Walters, P., Haddad, M., Phillips, R., Achilla, E., McCrone, P., . . . Tylee, A. (2014). The UPBEAT nurse-delivered personalized care intervention for people with coronary heart disease who report current chest pain and depression: A randomised controlled pilot study. *PLOS One, 9,* e98704.

Bartholomew, L. K., Parcel, G. S., Kok, G., Gottlieb, N., & Fernandez, M. (2011). *Planning health promotion programs: An intervention mapping approach* (3rd ed.). San Francisco, CA: Jossey-Bass.

Berg, S. K., Moons, P., Christensen, A., Zwisler, A., Pedersen, P., & Pedersen, P. (2014). Clinical effects and implications of cardiac rehabilitation for implantable cardioverter defibrillator patients: A mixed-methods approach embedding data from the Copenhagen Outpatient ProgrammE-implantable cardioverter defibrillator randomized clinical trial with qualitative data. *Journal of Cardiovascular Nursing, 30,* 420–427.

*Bleijenberg, N., Drubbel, I., ten Dam, V., Numans, M., Schuurmans, M., & deWit, N. (2012). Proactive and integrated primary care for frail older people: Design and methodological challenges of the Utrecht primary care PROactive frailty intervention trial (U-PROFIT). *BMC Geriatrics, 12,* 16.

Bleijenberg, N., ten Dam, V., Drubbel, I., Numans, M., deWit, N., & Schuurmans, M. (2013a). Development of a proactive care program (U-CARE) to preserve physical functioning of frail older people in primary care. *Journal of Nursing Scholarship, 45,* 230–237.

Bleijenberg, N., ten Dam, V., Steunenberg, B., Drubbel, I., Numans, M., deWit, N., & Schuurmans, M. (2013b). Exploring the expectations, needs and experiences of general practitioners and nurses toward a proactive and structured care programme for frail older patients: A mixed methods study. *Journal of Advanced Nursing, 69,* 2262–2273.

Borglin, G. (2015). The value of mixed methods for researching complex interventions. In D. Richards & I. Rahm Hallberg (Eds.), *Complex interventions in health: An overview of research methods* (pp. 29–45). Oxford, United Kingdom: Routledge.

*Buckwalter, K., Grey, M., Bowers, B., McCarthy, A., Gross, D., Funk, M., & Beck, C. (2009). Intervention research in highly unstable environments. *Research in Nursing & Health, 32,* 110–121.

*Burke, L., Swigart, V., Warziski Turk, M., Derro, N., & Ewing, L. (2009). Experiences of self-monitoring: Successes and struggles during treatment for weight loss. *Qualitative Health Research, 19,* 815–828.

Burrai, F., Micheluzzi, V., & Bugani, V. (2014). Effects of live sax on various physiological parameters, pain level, and mood level in cancer patients: A randomized controlled trial. *Holistic Nursing Practice, 28,* 201–311.

*Campbell, M., Fitzpatrick, R., Haines, A., Kinmouth, A., Sandercrock, P., Spiegelhalter, D., & Tryer, P. (2000). Framework for design and evaluation of complex interventions to improve health. *BMJ, 321,* 694–696.

Chalmers, I., & Glasziou, P. (2009). Avoidable waste in the production and reporting of research evidence. *The Lancet, 374,* 86–89.

Chalmers, I., Bracken, M., Djulbegovic, B., Garattini, S., Grant, J., Gulmezoglu, A., . . . Oliver, S. (2014). How to increase value and reduce waste when research priorities are set. *The Lancet, 383,* 156–165.

Conn, V. S. (2005). Nursing intervention research. *Western Journal of Nursing Research, 27,* 249–251.

*Conn, V. S., & Groves, P. (2011). Protecting the power of interventions through proper reporting. *Nursing Outlook, 59,* 318–325.

Conn, V. S., Rantz, M. J., Wipke-Tevis, D. D., & Maas, M. L. (2001). Designing effective nursing interventions. *Research in Nursing & Health, 24*, 433–442.

Corry, M., Clarke, M., While, A., & Lalor, J. (2013). Developing complex interventions for nursing: A critical review of key guidelines. *Journal of Clinical Nursing, 22*, 2366–2386.

*Craig, P., Dieppe, P., Macintyre, S., Michie, S., Nazareth, I., & Petticrew, M. (2008a). *Developing and evaluating complex interventions: New guidance.* London, United Kingdom: Medical Research Council.

*Craig, P., Dieppe, P., Macintyre, S., Michie, S., Nazareth, I., & Petticrew, M. (2008b). Developing and evaluating complex interventions: The new Medical Research Council guidance. *BMJ, 337*, 979–983.

Creswell, J. W. (2015). *A concise introduction to mixed methods research.* Thousand Oaks, CA: Sage.

Creswell, J. W., & Plano Clark, V. L. (2011). *Designing and conducting mixed methods research* (2nd ed.). Thousand Oaks, CA: Sage.

*Datta, J., & Petticrew, M. (2013). Challenges to evaluating complex interventions: A content analysis of published papers. *BMC Public Health, 13*, 568.

*Donovan, H., Kwekkeboom, K., Rosenzweig, M., & Ward, S. (2009). Nonspecific effects in psychoeducational intervention research. *Western Journal of Nursing Research, 31*, 983–998.

*Drubbel, I., Numans, M., Kranenburg, G., Bleijenberg, N., deWit, N., & Schuurmans, M. (2014). Screening for frailty in primary care: A systematic review of the psychometric properties of the frailty index in community-dwelling older people. *BMC Geriatrics, 14*, 27.

Fredericks, S. M., & Yau, T. (2014). Preparing for a randomized controlled trial: Strategies to optimize the design of an individualized cardiovascular surgical patient education intervention. *Applied Nursing Research, 27*, 137–140.

*Gray, N., Allan, J., Murchie, P., Browne, S., Hall, S., Hubbard, G., . . . Campbell, N. (2013). Developing a community-based intervention to improve quality of life in people with colorectal cancer: A complex intervention development study. *BMJ Open, 3*(4).

*Hall, S., Chochinov, H., Harding, R., Murray, S., Richardson, A., & Higginson, I. (2009). A phase II randomised controlled trial assessing the feasibility, acceptability and potential effectiveness of dignity therapy for older people in care homes. *BMC Geriatrics, 9*, 9.

Hall, S., Goddard, C., Opio, D., Speck, P., & Higginson, I. (2012). Feasibility, acceptability and potential effectiveness of dignity therapy for older people in care homes. *Palliative Medicine, 26*, 703–712.

Hall, S., Goddard, C., Speck, P., & Higginson, I. (2013). "It makes me feel that I'm still relevant": A qualitative study of the views of nursing home residents on dignity therapy and taking part in a phase II randomised controlled trial of palliative care psychotherapy. *Palliative Medicine, 27*, 358–366.

Kearney, M., & Simonelli, M. (2006). Intervention fidelity: Lessons learned from an unsuccessful pilot study. *Applied Nursing Research, 19*, 163–166.

Kirkevold, M., Bronken, B., Martinsen, R., & Kvigne, K. (2012). Promoting psychosocial well-being following a stroke: Developing a theoretically and empirically sound complex intervention. *International Journal of Nursing Studies, 49*, 386–397.

*Laan, W., Bleijenberg, N., Drubbel, I., Numans, M., de Wit, N., & Schuurmans, M. (2013). Factors associated with increasing functional decline in multimorbid independently living older people. *Maturitas, 75*, 276–281.

Lauver, D. R., Ward, S. E., Heidrich, S. M., Keller, M. L., Bowers, B. J., Brennan, P. F., . . . Wells, T. J. (2002). Patient-centered interventions. *Research in Nursing & Health, 25*, 246–255.

*Lu, Y. Y., & Haase, J. (2011). Content validity and acceptability of the daily enhancement of meaningful activity program intervention for mild cognitive impairment patient-spouse dyads. *Journal of Neuroscience Nursing, 43*, 317–328.

Mahoney, E., Trudeau, S., Penyack, S., & MacLeod, C. (2006). Challenges to intervention implementation: Lessons learned in the bathing persons with Alzheimer's disease at home study. *Nursing Research, 55*, S10–S16.

*May, C. (2013). Towards a general theory of implementation. *Implementation Science, 8*, 8–18.

May, C., & Finch, T. (2009). Implementing, embedding, and integrating practice: An outline of normalization process theory. *Sociology: Journal of the British Sociological Association, 43*, 535–554.

McGuire, D., DeLoney, V., Yeager, K., Owen, D., Peterson, D., Lin, L., & Webster, J. (2000). Maintaining study validity in a changing clinical environment. *Nursing Research, 49*, 231–235.

Medical Research Council. (2000). *A framework for development and evaluation of RCTs for complex interventions to improve health.* London, United Kingdom: Author.

Morden, A., Ong, B., Brooks, L., Jinks, C., Porcheret, M., Edwards, J., & Dziedzic, K. (2015). Introducing evidence through research "push": Using theory and qualitative methods. *Qualitative Health Research.* Advance online publication. doi:10.1177/1049732315570120

Morse, J. M. (2006). The scope of qualitative derived clinical interventions. *Qualitative Health Research, 16*, 591–593.

Morse, J., Penrod, J., & Hupcey, J. (2000). Qualitative outcome analysis: Evaluating nursing interventions for complex clinical phenomena. *Journal of Nursing Scholarship, 32*, 125–130.

Naylor, M. D. (2003). Nursing intervention research and quality of care. *Nursing Research, 52*, 380–385.

Payne, K., & Thompson, A. J. (2015). Economic evaluations of complex interventions. In D. Richards & I. Rahm Hallberg (Eds.), *Complex interventions in health: An overview of research methods* (pp. 326–333). Oxford, United Kingdom: Routledge.

Pruitt, R. H., & Privette, A. B. (2001). Planning strategies for the avoidance of pitfalls in intervention research. *Journal of Advanced Nursing, 35*, 514–520.

Rahm Hallberg, I. (2015). Knowledge for health care practice. In D. Richards & I. Rahm Hallberg (Eds.), *Complex interventions in health: An overview of research methods* (pp. 16–28). Oxford, United Kingdom: Routledge.

Richards, D. A. (2015a). The critical importance of patient and public involvement for research into complex interventions.

In D. Richards & I. Rahm Hallberg (Eds.), *Complex interventions in health: An overview of research methods* (pp. 46–50). Oxford, United Kingdom: Routledge.

Richards, D. A. (2015b). A few final thoughts. In D. Richards & I. Rahm Hallberg (Eds.), *Complex interventions in health: An overview of research methods* (pp. 326–333). Oxford, United Kingdom: Routledge.

Richards, D. A., Coulthard, V., & Borglin, G. (2014). The state of European nursing research: Dead, alive, or chronically diseased? *Worldviews on Evidence-Based Nursing, 11,* 147–155.

Richards, D. A., & Rahm Hallberg, I. (Eds.). (2015). *Complex interventions in health: An overview of research methods.* Oxford, United Kingdom: Routledge.

*Rowlands, G., Sims, J., & Kerry, S. (2005). A lesson learned: The importance of modeling in randomized controlled trials for complex interventions in primary care. *Family Practice, 22,* 132–139.

Sandelowski, M. (1996). Using qualitative methods in intervention studies. *Research in Nursing & Health, 19,* 359–365.

Seers, K. (2007). Evaluating complex interventions. *Worldviews on Evidence-Based Nursing, 4,* 67.

Sermeus, W. (2015). Modelling process and outcomes in complex interventions. In D. Richards & I. Rahm Hallberg (Eds.), *Complex interventions in health: An overview of research methods* (pp. 111–126). Oxford, United Kingdom: Routledge.

Sidani, S., & Braden, C. J. (1998). *Evaluating nursing interventions: A theory driven approach.* Thousand Oaks, CA: Sage.

Sidani, S., & Braden, C. J. (2011). *Design, evaluation, and translation of nursing interventions.* New York: Wiley-Blackwell.

Sidani, S., Epstein, D., & Miranda, J. (2006). Eliciting patient treatment preferences: A strategy to integrate evidence-based and patient-centered care. *Worldviews of Evidence-Based Nursing, 3,* 116–123.

*Simmonds, R., Tylee, A., Walters, P., & Rose, D. (2013). Patients' perceptions of depression and coronary heart disease: A qualitative UPBEAT-UK study. *BMC Family Practice, 14,* 38.

Thompson, C. (2004). Fortuitous phenomena: On complexity, pragmatic randomised controlled trials, and knowledge for evidence-based practice. *Worldviews on Evidence-Based Nursing, 1,* 9–17.

van Meijel, B., Gamel. C., van Swieten-Duijfjes, B., & Grypdonck, M. (2004). The development of evidence-based nursing interventions. *Journal of Advanced Nursing, 48,* 84–92.

Whittemore, R., & Grey, M. (2002). The systematic development of nursing interventions. *Journal of Nursing Scholarship, 34,* 115–120.

***A link to this open-access journal article is provided in the Toolkit for this chapter in the accompanying* Resource Manual.** ✖

In the Medical Research Council's (MRC) framework for complex interventions, as described in Chapter 27, mixed methods are used as part of the development of a preliminary intervention. The next phase is devoted to assessing whether the intervention, and initial ideas about rigorously testing it, makes sense—that is, whether it is feasible, acceptable, and shows promise of positive effects.

There is considerable agreement in the health care literature that pilot studies are often poorly designed and reported. Until recently, there was little direction on how to plan and conduct pilot work. Indeed, in their often cited "tutorial" on pilot studies, Thabane and colleagues (2010) stated with regard to coverage of pilot work in research methods textbooks, "We are not aware of any textbook that dedicates a chapter on this issue" (p. 2). We are attempting to remedy this situation by devoting this chapter to a discussion of feasibility assessments and pilot tests of interventions. Many other resources that offer excellent and cutting-edge advice for conducting pilot work have become available (e.g., Arain et al., 2010; Lancaster et al., 2004; Moore et al., 2011; Richards & Rahm Hallberg, 2015).

⬁ **TIP:** Wisdom relating to the value of piloting and planning can be seen in many cultures. For example, a 10th century bowl with a Kufic inscription on display in the Metropolitan Museum of Art in New York bears a relevant Iranian proverb: "Planning before work protects you from regret." Another relevant proverb comes from Africa: "Only a fool tests the depth of a river with both feet."

BASIC ISSUES IN PILOTING INTERVENTIONS

This section lays the groundwork for some specific suggestions for conducting successful pilot work, the focus of which is to address *uncertainties* about the intervention or the planned evaluation.

Definition of Pilot Tests and Feasibility Assessments

The term *pilot study* has been defined in dozens of ways in the research literature, with no clear consensus. Often, the terms pilot study and feasibility study are used interchangeably. Recently, however, some experts are drawing a distinction between the two (e.g., Arain et al., 2010; Richards & Rahm Hallberg, 2015). The distinction is consistent with the feedback loops and iterative nature of intervention development envisioned in the revised MRC framework (Craig et al., 2008a, 2008b).

In the United Kingdom, the National Institute for Health Research Evaluation, Trials and Studies Coordinating Centre (NETSCC) has offered distinct guidelines for feasibility studies and pilot studies. A **feasibility study** is research completed prior to a main intervention study to test specific and discrete aspects of an emerging intervention or the anticipated trial. For example, a feasibility study might assess whether a 10-week intervention is feasible and acceptable or whether a shorter intervention would be preferable. Or, a feasibility study might be undertaken to assess whether a sufficient number of sites could be enlisted to participate in a multisite trial. Feasibility studies help to build the foundation for a trial—and sometimes for a pilot trial. Feasibility studies do not focus on the outcome of interest but rather examine other important parameters that are integral to the conduct of a full intervention trial. Feasibility studies typically do not use a randomized design.

Pilot studies are considered small-scale versions of a full trial. Thabane and colleagues (2010) defined a pilot study as an investigation designed to test the feasibility of, and to support refinements of, the protocols, methods, and procedures to be used in a larger scale trial of an intervention. Feasibility is also a major issue in a pilot study, but the emphasis is on assessing the feasibility of an entire set of procedures for a randomized assessment, including recruitment (participants' willingness to be randomized), protocol implementation, data collection procedures, outcome measurement, blinding, and the ability to avoid contamination across treatment groups. Thus, according to the NETSCC definition, a pilot study for a full trial typically requires a randomized design. Taylor and colleagues (2015) offer guidelines for when a pilot or feasibility study requires randomization.

As the distinction between feasibility and pilot study suggests, it might be necessary for researchers to undertake both a feasibility assessment and a pilot trial for some complex interventions. Lessons learned in an early feasibility assessment might, for example, lead to further development work, as suggested in the revised MRC framework (Figure 27.2). In other cases, especially if there is a strong evidence base and a well-conceived intervention theory for the intervention, a single pilot study might suffice.

The distinction between a feasibility and a pilot study is an important one for the researchers doing them—for example, a study should be properly labeled in seeking funding or in publishing findings. However, to streamline our presentation in this chapter, we will for the most part describe activities under a general rubric of *pilot work*. In some cases, the activities would be undertaken in a small-scale feasibility study, whereas in others, they would be part of a more rigorous pilot trial. We note that pilot work is sometimes undertaken for nonintervention studies (e.g., for a large-scale survey), but in this chapter, we focus on intervention research.

➔ TIP: In the medical literature, some writers distinguish between an internal and external pilot. An *external pilot* is a stand-alone study, the findings from which inform the design and implementation of a full RCT. An *internal pilot* is an early phase of a large trial, the findings from which are typically used to make adjustments to sample size projections. In this chapter, we primarily discuss stand-alone (external) pilot work.

Overall Purpose of Pilot Work

The overall purpose of pilot work is simply this: to avoid a costly fiasco. Fully powered RCTs are extremely expensive. Without adequate piloting, a full-scale trial can result in wasted resources and erroneous conclusions. A strong pilot can enhance the likelihood that a full test will be methodologically and conceptually sound, ethical, and informative. As mentioned in Chapter 27, there is growing concern about waste and inefficiency in health care research (Chalmers et al., 2014; Treweek & Born, 2014), and pilots represent an important tool in combatting these problems in a responsible manner. Large-scale trials typically cannot get funded unless adequate pilot work has been undertaken.

➔ TIP: Tens of thousands of studies in the health care literature are described as "pilots," and many are inappropriately labeled—they are often simply small or exploratory studies. As noted by Moore and colleagues (2011), the term *pilot* is "liberally applied to projects with little or no funding" (p. 1). The term should not be used unless there is an explicit goal of learning how best to design and implement a more rigorous study.

Recent guidance on pilot work has emphasized an important point that is often not appreciated by those conducting pilots: *The purpose of a pilot is not to test hypotheses about the efficacy of the intervention.* That is, a goal should *not* be to test the effectiveness of an intervention on key outcomes— and if statistical hypothesis tests are used in pilot work, they should be interpreted cautiously (Arain et al., 2010; Thabane et al., 2010). As pointed out by Arnold and colleagues (2009), "conducting analyses to glean information about efficacy from pilot trials is tempting but dangerous" (p. S73). Given the small sample size of most pilots, hypothesis tests are almost invariably underpowered. As a consequence, effect size estimates in pilots are notoriously unreliable. We discuss this issue again later in the chapter.

➲ TIP: Moore and colleagues (2011) bemoaned the cycle of nonproductive work than can ensue when young researchers undertake a pilot, find nonsignificant results, abandon their ideas, and then pursue another topic. When hypothesis testing is a major objective of a pilot, disappointment is common and results are often unreported.

Lessons from Pilot Work

As mentioned in the previous chapter, an important product of pilot work is the description of the "lessons learned." Almost inevitably, the pilot will reveal that the intervention did not play out in "real life" the way it was intended "on paper."

A review of published reports on lessons learned in pilot studies reveals that some lessons are recurrent—which in theory should make them easier to avoid. The following are among the most frequently mentioned lessons from pilot intervention studies:

- Fewer people meet the eligibility criteria than anticipated.
- Recruitment of participants is more difficult and takes longer than anticipated.
- Materials intended for direct use by participants (e.g., pamphlets, educational materials) need to be simplified.

- Participant burden, especially with regard to data collection, needs to be reduced.
- Effect sizes tend to be larger in the pilot than in the main trial.
- Key ingredients of the intervention should be front-loaded—that is, delivered early—because greater attention and higher attendance occurs early.
- When there is a control condition, diffusion and contamination are recurrent problems.
- Even expert interventionists need to be trained (and this includes the researchers themselves).
- Relationships with others need to be continuously nurtured.

Researchers who undertake pilot work should keep these lessons in mind and try to design their study in such a way that frequently occurring problems are avoided.

Example of an Important Lesson Learned in Pilot Work: Beebe (2007) provided a good example of how her pilot study of an exercise intervention for outpatients with schizophrenia revealed an unexpected need. She and her co-researchers found that some of their study participants lacked appropriate footwear for the intervention, and so they learned the need to plan for "the provision of footwear in the budgets for future projects" (p. 216).

OBJECTIVES AND CRITERIA IN PILOT WORK

Writers who offer advice about the conduct of feasibility and pilot studies almost invariably encourage researchers to carefully articulate explicit objectives. Vagueness in delineating what exactly needs to be known in pilot work is likely to result in gaps in the lessons that need to be learned.

For any given pilot study, the specific objectives can be wide-ranging. Thabane and colleagues (2010) organized pilot objectives into four broad categories: process, resources, management, and scientific. We use this organization to suggest some objectives that are good targets for pilot work. Of course, our examples are not exhaustive, but hopefully they will suggest ideas for how pilot work can inform decisions about a full trial of an intervention.

Process-Related Objectives

Process-related objectives focus on the feasibility of planned procedures for launching and maintaining the study. These include such issues as eligibility criteria, recruitment, retention, comprehension, adherence, acceptability, and human subjects concerns. Each objective can be addressed by gathering data to answer a variety of questions, examples of which are suggested in Table 28.1. As the table indicates, process-related objectives are often best addressed by collecting both qualitative and quantitative data. Pilot and feasibility assessments are a good way of investigating potential problems in putting an intervention into place—and exploring ways to remedy those problems.

Although preliminary answers to some of the questions in Table 28.1 are sometimes obtained during intervention development, those answers often need to be confirmed. For example, there may be a big difference between patients saying they *would be* interested in an intervention, and *agreeing* to actually participate. Moreover, a person might be willing to participate in an intervention but may *not* be willing to be randomized to a control group condition. Or, even if a person is willing and interested, motivation may wane over the course of a multisession intervention. Thus, development work alone cannot answer important questions about feasibility of an intervention implemented in real-world settings.

Pilot work can be useful in revealing the adequacy of the initial eligibility criteria and in suggesting how eligibility criteria affect recruitment, retention, and protocol adherence. Defining the eligibility criteria must take numerous concerns into account, including substantive ones (Should some people be excluded because they might not benefit?), ethical ones (Might certain people be harmed?), methodologic ones (Can eligibility criteria be readily measured? Will the criteria result in an adequate pool for the full-scale trial?), and scientific ones (Will eligibility criteria constrain the generalizability of the findings?). Pilot data can be used to fine-tune decisions about eligibility and about the length of time needed to recruit a sufficiently large sample.

→ TIP: Unfounded optimism about the size of the pool of eligibles is common—indeed, it is so common that it has been given a name: *Lasagna's law* (van der Wouden et al., 2007).

A particularly important process issue concerns recruitment—not only of study participants but also of sites and research staff. If a multisite trial is envisioned for the full RCT, feasibility of enlisting cooperative sites should be explored early. It is not just an issue of getting enough sites to achieve an adequate sample size but also of making sure that there are sites that represent the diversity of the target population of participants. Also, if exploration of sites suggests a very high rate of refusals, researchers might want to explore what factors led to refusals by site administrators—especially if those factors are relevant for the eventual uptake of the intervention, should the RCT reveal promising results. For example, if concerns about staff time are a key consideration, the intervention may have little hope of being translated on a large scale.

Recruitment of participants is a perennial problem in clinical trials, and recruitment is becoming increasingly more challenging. A review of funded trials in the United Kingdom revealed that fewer than one out of three clinical trials successfully recruited the targeted number of participants (Campbell et al., 2007). Quantitative data from the pilot work will answer questions about the feasibility of recruiting a sufficient number for a full trial, but qualitative data may suggest how key barriers can be eliminated or how additional recruitment techniques could be pursued. Treweek (2015) provides useful advice about participant recruitment.

Poor retention of participants in the study and low protocol adherence (on the part of participants or intervention agents) are two other problems that are strong candidates for scrutiny in pilot work. Attrition can reduce the final sample size for analyses and can also lead to biases in estimating the intervention's potential benefits. High attrition, low adherence to protocols, and low levels of satisfaction suggest that an intervention is not yet ready for a full RCT.

TABLE 28.1 • Examples of Process-Related Objectives and Questions for Pilot Work

OBJECTIVE	QUESTIONS (QUANTITATIVE)	QUESTIONS (QUALITATIVE)
Recruitment: To assess the feasibility of recruiting an adequate number of study participants	• How many people were screened for eligibility each week/month? • What percentage of eligible people agreed to participate (and what percentage actually did participate)? • What percentage of eligibles had a strong preference for treatment condition? • How many eligibles enrolled each week/month? • What were the characteristics of those who did versus those who did not agree to participate? • How long did it take to recruit the needed sample?	• Why did eligibles decline to participate? What would make the intervention (or study participation) more appealing? Was randomization a factor in their decision? • What barriers exist in the research sites regarding successful recruitment? • Did certain recruitment strategies work well? Work poorly?
Eligibility criteria: To assess the adequacy of the eligibility criteria	• How many eligible people were there in each site? What proportion of all clients/patients were eligible? • Which eligibility criterion was associated with the biggest loss of potential participants? • Was attrition from the pilot associated with a particular eligibility criterion?	• Were procedures for identifying eligibles clear and manageable? • Would loosening or tightening the eligibility criteria be acceptable to some stakeholders (e.g., family members)? Would it affect ease of recruitment?
Retention: To assess the ability to retain an adequate proportion of participants	• What percentage of initial study participants remained in the study as they moved through the trial? • Were there differences in attrition by study group (intervention vs. control)? • What were the characteristics of those who remained and those who did not? • At what point did attrition occur?	• Why did participants decide to withdraw from the study? • What barriers exist in the research sites regarding successful retention?
Protocol adherence: To assess the degree to which participants adhere to protocols	• What percentage of participants got the full "dose" of the intervention? What "dose" of the intervention did the typical participant get? • What are the characteristics of those who adhered and those who did not? • Were there particular components for which adherence was especially poor?	• Why did participants not adhere to the intervention protocol (or not adhere to particular components)? • What barriers exist in the research sites regarding successful adherence?

(table continues on page 628)

TABLE 28.1 • Examples of Process-Related Objectives and Questions for Pilot Work (continued)

OBJECTIVE	QUESTIONS (QUANTITATIVE)	QUESTIONS (QUALITATIVE)
Acceptability: To assess the extent to which the intervention/research is acceptable to recipients and key stakeholders	• How satisfied were recipients (or other stakeholders) with the intervention or with specific components of the intervention? • What percentage of recipients were allocated to their preferred treatment condition? • To what extent did recipients feel overburdened by the data collection demands?	• What did recipients/stakeholders like and dislike about the intervention? What changes to the intervention protocol would make it more acceptable? • What did recipients most dislike about research aspects (e.g., the amount of time needed, the frequency of data collection)?
Human subjects: To assess the adequacy of human protections	Were there any breaches of human protections (e.g., privacy, confidentiality)?	Did participants feel that they their rights and privacy were adequately protected?

Human subjects issues also can be explored during the pilot phase. In particular, researchers need to be vigilant during a pilot regarding any unanticipated human subjects protection transgressions that would need to be remedied before a main trial could be undertaken. Pilots are also a good place to get feedback about the consent process. Several commentators have pointed out the absence of any special guidelines for the ethical conduct of pilot studies. There is some agreement, however, that researchers have an obligation to disclose the feasibility nature of pilot studies during informed consent procedures (Arain et al., 2010; Thabane et al., 2010).

Example of Pilot Work Addressing Process Objectives: Villegas and colleagues (2014) described the development and feasibility testing of an Internet-based intervention designed to prevent sexually transmitted diseases and HIV among Chilean women. The feasibility objectives concerned protocol adherence (percentage of participation in the Internet modules), retention in the study (percentage of completing follow-up questionnaires), and acceptability (satisfaction with various aspects of the intervention, measured with a 9-item scale).

Resource-Related Objectives

Pilots are often a useful way to get a handle on the resources that would be needed in a full-scale trial.

Resource objectives typically concern questions about the following aspects of a study:

• Monetary costs
• Time demands
• Institutional capacity
• Personnel requirements and availability
• Other resource needs such as equipment, technology, and lab facilities

Tickle-Degnen (2013) provided some good examples of resource-related questions asked in a pilot study of a self-management intervention for patients with Parkinson's disease. Here are a few of them: Do we have the capacity to handle the desired number of participants? Do we have phone and communication technology capacity to stay in touch with and coordinate participants? Do we have institutional willingness and capacity to carry through with project-related tasks and to support investigator time and effort? Some additional questions relating to resource objectives are suggested in a table (analogous to Table 28.1 for process-type objectives) in the Supplement to this chapter on thePoint®. 🅢

A full-scale RCT of a complex intervention costs many thousands of dollars. A pilot study can help researchers develop a realistic budget for such a trial. It can also shed light on whether the costs of the intervention are likely to be commensurate with the benefits. Even at an early stage, researchers should consider whether it is realistic to pursue a costly trial for an intervention that is unlikely to be translated into real-world settings because of prohibitive costs or modest benefits.

> **Example of Pilot Work and Resource Objectives:** Watson and co-researchers (2015) pilot tested a brief intervention delivered by an occupational health nurse to reduce alcohol-related harm in the workplace. A total of 57 employees who agreed to participate were randomized to either the intervention or a control group. The cost of the intervention was calculated, and net savings per person in terms of health and other care costs were estimated.

Management-Related Objectives

Another category of objectives for pilot work are ones that concern the ability for the research team to manage the effort and for research staff to work productively as a team. Pilot work can help to identify management "glitches" that should be addressed before moving on to a full-scale trial. The management-related objectives in pilot work include assessing feasibility in terms of the following:

• Viability of the site or sites
• Motivation and competence of project staff
• Adequacy of reporting, monitoring, technologic, and other systems
• Ability to manage or nurture interpersonal relationships

In articles that have described "lessons learned" from pilot work, a recurrent theme is that interpersonal relationships can create problems. These can be the result of tensions among staff, between staff and management, and between staff and study participants or their family members. Researchers have found that it is often useful to give various stakeholders a sense of ownership and an opportunity to make suggestions or air complaints.

In the previously mentioned paper on pilot work for a self-management intervention for patients with Parkinson's disease, Tickle-Degnen (2013) addressed various feasibility questions relating to management objectives. For example, what are

the challenges and strengths of the investigators' administrative capacity to

• Manage the planned RCT?
• Design systems to document participant progress through the trial?
• Enter data and perform quality checks?
• Manage the ethical aspects of the trial?

Some additional examples of questions relating to management objectives are presented in Table 2 of the Supplement to this chapter on thePoint®. 🌐

Scientific-Related Objectives: Substantive Issues

In Thabane and colleagues' (2010) system of classifying pilot objectives, the fourth category concerned scientific objectives. For this crucial class of objectives, we discuss two subcategories separately. The first set of scientific objectives are ones that are substantive in nature—that is, they concern the intervention itself. The second set of scientific objectives are methodologic ones that relate to the feasibility of rigorously testing the intervention. In this section, we discuss substantive scientific objectives for pilot work.

Intervention Attributes

A pilot test provides an opportunity to make judgments about whether the decisions made during the development phase regarding intervention content, dose, timing, setting, sequencing, and so on, were sensible ones (Feeley & Cossette, 2015). A pilot study is an ideal time to make final revisions to the intervention protocols, based on feedback from participants and intervention staff and such other indicators as attendance and feedback about satisfaction. Table 3 in the Supplement to this chapter provides some examples of questions relating to the objective of assessing attributes of the intervention during a pilot. 🌐

Safety and Tolerability

Assessing the safety of patients in trials of a new intervention and the tolerability of the intervention are crucial objectives of many pilot studies. Unfortunately, it is widely acknowledged that pilots do a poor job of providing reliable safety and tolerability data because of their small sample size. For example, in a pilot with 30 patients, zero adverse events does not necessarily mean that there are no safety risks.

Leon and colleagues (2011) advised that group-specific adverse events rates in pilots should be reported, with 95% confidence intervals. They further recommended that when no adverse event is observed, the *rule of three* should be used to estimate the upper bound of the 95% CI. This "rule" uses as the upper bound the value of $3/n$. Thus, if there are 30 participants per group, and zero adverse events are observed in the intervention group, the 95% CI for the adverse event rate for that group would be estimated as 0% to 10%. Such a calculation, which suggest the possibility that 1 out of 10 participants could experience an adverse event, illustrates the tenuous nature of pilot data on safety and tolerability.

Nevertheless, it is important to monitor safety and tolerability if the intervention is one that has potential for adverse events—even relatively minor ones, such as fatigue or dizziness. Moreover, as noted by Leon et al. (2011), pilots are useful for testing the adequacy of safety monitoring systems. Pilots may also suggest the desirability of requiring permissions to participate in the trial from participants' physicians. Feedback from participants about perceptions of safety and tolerability are also very useful for evaluating potential safety problems. Some specific questions about safety and tolerability assessments are included in the chapter Supplement. (S)

Example of Pilot Work and Safety Assessment: Bloom and colleagues (2014) developed and pilot tested an online safety planning intervention for pregnant abused women. Given the intervention's emphasis on the women's safety, the safety of study participants was carefully monitored. For example, research staff attempted to contact all women who enrolled for the study but did not complete baseline forms to ascertain if safety issues relating to enrollment had emerged. Among those who participated, no adverse events related to the study were reported.

Intervention Efficacy

Most pilot studies are undertaken with the objective of gaining preliminary evidence of the intervention's potential to be efficacious. As previously

noted, hypothesis testing is not considered appropriate in pilot tests because of the high risk of making a Type II error—that is, falsely concluding that the intervention is not more beneficial than the control treatment, even when it was.

Effect size (ES) estimates provide information about the potential of an intervention to achieve beneficial effects on key outcomes, but extreme caution is needed in interpreting the ES results. We illustrate the problem by presenting some information about 95% confidence intervals around ES estimates (d) of different magnitude for various sample sizes that are common in pilot studies (Table 28.2). As a reminder, the effect size d is computed by dividing the difference between two group means (i.e., intervention and control group postintervention means on an outcome) by the pooled standard deviation. For example, suppose that in a pilot study with 40 participants (20 per group), we calculated d for the primary outcome to be .50, which is considered a moderately strong ES. As Table 28.2 indicates, in this scenario, there is a 95% probability that the *true* effect size lies somewhere between −.13 (i.e., the intervention is mildly detrimental) and 1.13 (i.e., the intervention is extremely beneficial). Increasing the sample size decreases the width of the estimated range and thus offers stronger evidence of the intervention's potential effectiveness. For example, with a sample size of 100 pilot participants (50 per group), the 95% CI for a d of .50 ranges from .10 (mildly favorable) to .90 (strongly favorable). The pilot effect size should at last be encouraging; for example, a d of .04 is unlikely to instill confidence about the intervention's benefits. (As we discuss later, a 95% CI is considered by some experts to be too stringent for pilot work, although it is the conventional standard.)

Because the objective in a pilot is to obtain preliminary (and not definitive) evidence of the intervention's potential benefits, researchers should use supplementary means of drawing conclusions about an intervention's effects. In particular, in-depth interviews with program participants and intervention agents concerning their perceptions of benefits or disappointments are an important means of illuminating statistical results. For example,

TABLE 28.2 • 95% Confidence Intervals* around *d*, for Various *N*s and *d*s Assuming Two Groups of Equal Size

d	N = 20 10 PER GROUP	N = 30 15 PER GROUP	N = 40 20 PER GROUP	N = 50 25 PER GROUP	N = 60 30 PER GROUP	N = 100 50 PER GROUP
.20	−.69 to 1.09	−.53 to .93	−.43 to .83	−.37 to .77	−.32 to .72	−.20 to .60
.30	−.59 to 1.19	−.43 to 1.03	−.33 to .93	−.27 to .87	−.22 to .82	−.10 to .70
.40	−.49 to 1.29	−.33 to 1.13	−.23 to 1.03	−.17 to .97	−.12 to .92	0.0 to .80
.50	−.39 to 1.39	−.23 to 1.23	−.13 to 1.13	−.07 to 1.07	−.02 to 1.02	.10 to .90
.60	−.29 to 1.49	−.13 to 1.33	−.03 to 1.23	.03 to 1.17	.08 to 1.12	.20 to 1.00
.70	−.19 to 1.59	−.03 to 1.43	.07 to 1.33	.13 to 1.27	.18 to 1.22	.30 to 1.10

*Approximation of 95% CI using formula provided in Leon et al. (2011): $d \pm (4 \div \sqrt{N})$.

the plausibility of weak beneficial effects (based on the lower limit of the confidence limit) can sometimes be put in doubt through a fuller understanding of how an intervention was valued by those who participated. If there is a consistent pattern of positive ES estimates for several key outcomes, and if there is corroborating qualitative data, researchers may be well poised to conclude that intervention efficacy is promising.

Example of Pilot Work and Effect Size Estimates: Ward and Brown (2015) conducted two pilot studies of a culturally adapted depression intervention for African American adults. In the first pilot study, 73% of participants completed the full intervention, and the estimated effect on a measure of depressive symptoms was .38. In the second pilot, 66% fully completed the intervention, and the effect size was estimated to be high for men (1.01) and moderate for women (.41).

⮕ **TIP:** It is important to remember that every major change made to the intervention based on pilot work (e.g., to the intervention content or dose) may put into question the legitimacy of the pilot effect size as an estimate of what would be obtained in a full trial. Modifications to the intervention that strengthen the potential effects of an intervention are desirable.

Clinical Significance

Another possible objective for pilot work is an assessment of the likelihood that the intervention will be clinically significant. At the group level, ES estimates are often used to draw conclusions about clinical significance of positive effects, as discussed in Chapter 20. This means that the researchers should establish in advance the size of the effect that would be regarded as clinically significant. For example, the criterion could be based on a consensus reached by an advisory panel of experts. Arnold and colleagues (2009) advised that an intervention can be declared to have potential efficacy if the 95% CI around the estimated effect size includes a predesignated minimal for clinical significance. However, given the width of 95% CIs when the sample is small, this may be too liberal a standard. For example, with a sample of 50 pilot participants (25 per group), and a criterion of .50 for a clinically significant *d*, even an obtained *d* of 0.0 would meet this criterion (95% CI = −.57 to .57). Thus, it might be more prudent for the advisory group to establish not only the criterion for clinical significance but also the acceptable range. For example, if the criterion were .50, experts might set the lower bound at .20.

As described in Chapter 20, there is another approach to considering clinical significance. If the primary outcome is one with an established minimal important change benchmark, the percentage of participants who have achieved a clinically significant change can be computed. Evidence of clinical significance would then be provided by a demonstration that a sizable percentage of intervention recipients had meaningful improvement.

Scientific-Related Objectives: Methodologic Issues

Scientific objectives encompass not only substantive concerns about the intervention but also methodologic concerns about the feasibility of undertaking a rigorous controlled trial. This section focuses on pilot objectives relating to the methods of testing a new intervention.

Research Design

Preliminary evidence about feasibility can be obtained in feasibility studies using fairly simple designs, such as a one-group pretest–posttest design. However, for a pilot study, the design ideally should be a trial run of the full-scale test. It is precisely because of the need to be confident that an RCT of the full trial is feasible that experts recommend that a pilot study use a randomized design rather than a quasi-experimental one (e.g., Conn et al., 2010; Lancaster et al., 2004; Thabane et al., 2010). As noted by Leon and colleagues (2011), the inclusion of a randomized control group in a pilot study "allows for a more realistic examination of recruitment, randomization, implementation of intervention, blinded assessment procedures, and retention" (p. 627).

Various aspects of the study design should be evaluated in a pilot study, including the actual procedures for randomization, allocation concealment, and blinding. A crucial issue in randomized trials is whether there has been any contamination between the treatment groups. Pilot trials also provide a good opportunity to assess whether any co-interventions could inflate intervention benefits (if those in the intervention receive them) or dilute benefits (if control group members receive them). Some questions about the viability of various design features, as well as other methodologic objectives, are provided in Table 4 of the chapter Supplement on thePoint®. Ⓢ

Intervention Fidelity

Pilots offer researchers the opportunity to examine whether the intervention agents can successfully implement the intervention as planned. In addition, pilots offer an opportunity to assess the adequacy of intervention fidelity procedures. As with other objectives, both quantitative and qualitative data play an important role in helping researchers understand how successful the implementation of the intervention was and identify barriers to full enactment of the intervention protocols. Quantitative data can be used to calculate actual rates of achieving fidelity, and qualitative data can help researchers understand factors that made fidelity difficult to accomplish.

Example of Pilot Work and Intervention Fidelity: Resnick and colleagues (2014) pilot tested an intervention to improve the health-related behaviors of senior housing residents. The researchers implemented a strong intervention fidelity plan. For example, there was an ongoing review of the interventionists' adherence to the theory of self-efficacy–based interventions. An observer monitored every class to assess the lay trainer's adherence to exercise protocols and the intervention nurse's adherence to motivational protocols. The researchers concluded that there was sufficient evidence of intervention fidelity in terms of training for, delivery of, and receipt of the intervention.

Data Collection Protocols and Instruments

Researchers make many decisions about data collection instruments and procedures for intervention studies, and a pilot trial offers researchers an opportunity to assess those decisions. Data quality and participant burden are two key areas of inquiry. A pilot provides an opportunity to examine patterns of missing data, to evaluate internal consistency of any scales, to assess comprehension, to explore variability in responses, and to estimate how much time is required to administer the package of instruments. Given the evidence that people often drop out of studies because of a burdensome schedule of data collection, it is important to understand the practicability of the data collection methods. A lengthy data collection instrument is not only risky in terms of attrition but also has cost implications for data collection staff, data entry, and analysis. The pilot might lead researchers to eliminate one or more outcome, to select shorter instruments, or to alter the schedule for measuring outcomes. Van Teijlingen and Hundley (2001) have offered some explicit advice about pilot testing instruments for use in a full-scale study.

> **Example of Pilot Work and Data Collection:** In the previously mentioned pilot study of an exercise intervention for patients with schizophrenia, Beebe (2007) conducted *exit interviews* with study participants. She learned that two outcomes that were important to the participants had not been measured in the pilot: flexibility and energy levels.

It should be noted that instruments for measuring outcomes should not be developed and evaluated for reliability, validity, and responsiveness in the context of a pilot trial of an intervention, because such evaluations require large samples. Researchers should select instruments with prior evidence of high quality, and then these instruments can be assessed for their adequacy in the context of the pilot.

Sample Size

An objective that is among the most commonly cited reasons for conducting a pilot study is to inform sample size decisions for the main trial. However, performing a power analysis using ES estimates from a pilot is risky because, as we have seen, pilot ES estimates are not reliable.

Using the pilot study ES estimate to calculate sample size for a full trial can result in both types of errors in statistical decision making. A large pilot effect size (e.g., $d = .80$) could reflect an inflated positive result, and possibly a Type I error. In turn, this inflated value would likely result in an underpowered full-scale trial because the sample size projection based on a large ES estimate would be too small. On the other hand, pilot ES estimates can result in a Type II error if the estimate is unduly small. This could lead to a decision to abandon a potentially promising intervention.

→ TIP: Vickers (2003) found that many trials published in four major medical journals were considerably underpowered when sample size

needs were estimated on the basis of a pilot trial. He found, for example, that about one out of four of the full-scale trials needed five times as many participants as had been estimated. There is also some evidence that pilot work might result in abandoning a project. For example, Polit (2006) found that of 21 pilot intervention studies published in nursing journals in 1998 or 1999, only four subsequently led to a full-scale trial by 2005.

Several approaches to this dilemma have been proposed. One is to calculate confidence intervals around the ES estimate and then use the lower limit of the CI in the power calculations. However, because the 95% CI results in a range that is unreasonably large with small pilot samples (Table 28.2), less conservative CIs have been suggested, such as an 80% CI (Lancaster et al., 2004) or a 68% CI (Hertzog, 2008).

Let us consider an example. Suppose that in a pilot study with 30 participants (15 per group), we calculated the pilot ES as $d = .50$. As shown in Table 28.2, the 95% CI around .50 for this sample size ranges from $-.23$ to 1.23. However, the 80% CI around a d of .50 ranges from $-.03$ to .97, and the 68% CI ranges from .12 to .88. Using the lower limit as our estimate for d—that is, .12—the needed sample size for the final trial would be over 1,000 subjects per group for power = .80 and alpha = .05 for a two-tailed test.

In many cases, researchers can draw on additional evidence to support their sample size projections. For example, if there were consistent evidence from earlier trials of similar interventions that group differences on the primary outcome would favor the intervention group, we might be willing to use a one-tailed test. This would result in a needed sample size of about 850 per group for the main trial for a d of .12.

Additional avenues for deriving sample size estimates can be pursued when there is evidence from previous similar intervention trials. To continue with our example of $d = .50$ from our pilot, suppose there were three prior RCTs of a similar intervention. In these trials, the values of d were .26, .34, and .42 for the same primary outcome (e.g., pain). We could argue that triangulating the evidence provides the best basis for estimating sample size requirements for a full-scale RCT. We might choose to use $d = .26$ (because it is the most conservative of four estimates), or we might elect to use $d = .34$ (if the study with that ES was the most rigorous), or we might use $d = .38$ (the average of the four trials, including our own pilot). (Essentially, this is analogous to conducting a crude mini meta-analysis.) For a two-tailed test, these decisions would result in projected sample size needs of 233, 136, and 109, respectively, per group. If we had simply used our $d = .50$, our projected sample size needs would have been 63 per group, which very well could have resulted in an underpowered full trial and a Type II error with nonsignificant results. On the other hand, if we had used $d = .12$ (the lower bound of the 68% CI around .50), we likely would not have pursued a full trial because it would have required a total sample size of over 2,000 participants.

A supplementary strategy is to factor in clinical significance in the power calculations (Kraemer et al., 2006). The rationale is that if the intervention cannot achieve benefits that are minimally significant clinically, it may not matter that the trial is underpowered. Thus, in our example, suppose the judgment of the research team or an advisory group of experts is that the effect size would need to be at least .40 to be clinically significant. In other words, there is a consensus that an ES of .40 is the threshold below which clinicians are unlikely to be interested in the intervention. If we used $d = .40$, the estimated sample size for the full trial would be about 100 per group for a two-group design. Based on our pilot results, an ES of .40 is plausibly attainable because it falls well within a 95% CI for a d of .50. And its attainability is supported by the results from another trial of a similar intervention in which $d = .42$ was obtained.

In short, the most defensible strategy for sample size calculation is to consider a totality of evidence to estimate the size of the effect that is plausibly attainable and clinically meaningful in a main test. More detailed and sophisticated guidance is provided by Ukoumunne and colleagues (2015).

Criteria and Pilot Objectives

We have presented a plethora of objectives as potentially relevant in pilot work for interventions. Clearly, no pilot or feasibility study can address all of the objectives we described. It is crucial to identify the key objectives of the pilot work in advance, however, because important design and data collection decisions for the pilot depend on what the objectives are.

We recommend that researchers select pilot objectives based on several considerations. First, choose objectives for which information is genuinely lacking—that is, objectives that address key *uncertainties*. You may already have a good estimate of how much attrition to expect, for example, based on your own previous work with the target population or based on attrition rates in other similar trials. Second, select objectives that impinge most significantly on the feasibility of a full-scale trial. For example, if you cannot recruit a sufficient number of participants, a large trial may be impossible, so assessing and enhancing recruitment would be important objectives. Lastly, focus on objectives about which funders will be particularly vigilant. These might include recruitment and efficacy, for example, and might also include resource requirements.

The importance of articulating key pilot objectives stems from the fact that pilot work should lead to a decision about "next steps." Essentially, there are three options. One decision would be to proceed to a full clinical trial. A second decision would be to make revisions to the intervention protocols, the methodologic protocols, or the procedural processes. The decision to make changes might lead to further Phase I (developmental) work and perhaps to a second pilot, if the needed revisions are major. A third decision would be to abandon the entire effort because of poor prospects of feasibility or acceptability, or lack of adequate evidence that the intervention could be effective.

How do researchers make the critical decision about what course to take next? The answer lies not only in articulating objectives but also in stating in advance the criteria for making decisions—a course of action strongly advocated by pilot study experts (e.g., Arain et al., 2010; Arnold et al., 2009;

Thabane et al., 2010). Prior to launching the pilot, the research team should formulate threshold criteria for claiming the feasibility of a full-scale RCT.

Table 28.3 provides some examples of pilot objectives and criteria for concluding that the pilot confirmed the feasibility of a full trial. As these examples suggest, the criteria are quantitative and can be expressed either as raw numbers or as rates. For example, the second and third entries in this table concern the objective of assessing recruitment in the pilot. In the second objective, the benchmark for success involves having a certain percentage of all eligible people agreeing to participate in the pilot (in this example, 60%). In the third objective, on the other hand, recruitment success is defined as getting a specific number of eligible people to agree to participate in the pilot study sites each week.

The criteria will have to be based on the judgment of the research team, but those judgments ideally would be informed by evidence gathered during the development phase (e.g., during in-depth discussions with the target population or based on recruitment rates from other similar trials). The criteria should achieve a degree of balance between what is ideal (e.g., 100% recruitment success) and what is realistic. Proposed criteria can be evaluated by an advisory group of experts and stakeholders. We emphasize that the criteria included in Table 28.3 are only *examples*—they should not be adopted literally without considering the actual context of pilot work, including the nature of the intervention, site, and target population.

Clearly, decision making is facilitated when criteria for the pilot's success are articulated. In the recruitment example, if only 30% of eligible patients agreed to participate in the pilot trial, the next step probably should not be to move forward to a full trial. Exploratory (qualitative) inquiry might help to reveal why the recruitment effort went awry. Perhaps different recruitment techniques are needed, perhaps the intervention or the research is too burdensome, or perhaps the eligibility criteria need to be adjusted. Without criteria for a pilot's success, researchers may be tempted to overinterpret their pilot data in the desired direction—that is, to move forward to a full trial before it is wise to do so.

Most often, researchers who establish criteria look for opportunities to take corrective actions. The decision about "next steps" is likely to depend on how many criteria are not met and the degree of deficiency in meeting them. For example, a 30% recruitment rate when 60% or higher was the benchmark might lead to abandoning the project, but a 50% recruitment rate might lead to making adjustments to enhance recruitment. If identified problems cannot readily be rectified, then researchers might be forced to "go back to the drawing board" in efforts to solve a clinical problem.

The decision to move forward to a full trial should be a carefully considered one. In preparing a proposal to fund a rigorous RCT, the research team should be persuaded that (1) the intervention and the research methods have been found to be feasible, (2) any pitfalls for a rigorous test have been identified and solutions to potential problems have been identified, (3) there is preliminary evidence that the intervention will be effective, and (4) important stakeholders are "on board."

Example of Stakeholder Issues: Bird and her colleagues (2011) described experiences from an evaluation of a complex rehabilitation intervention for patients undergoing stem cell transplantation. The intervention had not been rigorously piloted, and several problems were identified in the course of the actual trial. One problem was resistance to the trial by staff, one of whom commented that "the trial killed the intervention" (p. 5).

THE DESIGN AND METHODS OF PILOT AND FEASIBILITY STUDIES

In this section, we offer comments and recommendations relating to the design and conduct of pilot work.

Research Design in Pilot Work

As previously noted, we strongly encourage using a randomized design for a pilot trial, especially if the plan is to use the pilot as the basis for requesting funding for a full-scale trial. To the extent possible, all of the design features for the full

TABLE 28.3 • Examples of Pilot Objectives and Criteria for Success

OBJECTIVE	CRITERION	MEASUREMENT
To assess the willingness of the site to screen prospective participants for eligibility	At least 50 patients per month will be screened for eligibility	Number of patients screened per month (and, possibly, number of patients not screened)
To assess the feasibility of recruiting study participants	60% of eligible people will agree to participate	Number agreeing to participate, divided by all eligibles
To assess the feasibility of recruiting study participants	At least 3 participants per week will be successfully recruited at each study site	Number of people agreeing to participate per site
To assess the willingness of people to sign consent forms and be randomized	95% of people who agree to participate will be randomized to a treatment group	Number randomized, divided by number originally agreeing to participate
To assess the initiation of the intervention in a timely manner	90% of the people randomized to the intervention group will begin within 7 days of randomization	Number beginning the intervention within 7 days of randomization, divided by total number randomized
To assess adherence to the intervention	80% of those in the intervention group will complete at least 8 of the 10 intervention sessions	Number completing 8+ sessions, divided by the number randomized to the intervention
To assess the efficiency of the data collection protocols	90% of participants will complete the data collection package in ≤30 minutes	Number completing package within 30 minutes, divided by all completing the package
To assess trial retention rates	80% of participants in both study groups will complete 3-month follow-up instruments	Number of people in each group completing 3-month follow-ups, divided by number randomized to each group
To assess the intervention's acceptability	75% of participants will say they are "satisfied" or "completely satisfied" with the intervention	Number of patients who are satisfied, divided by number of intervention participants
To assess the preliminary efficacy of the intervention	Lower limit of the 68% CI around the value of d will be at least .20	The value of d, minus the value for a 68% confidence interval
To assess the clinical significance of the intervention	40% of those in the intervention group will have a reduction of 8+ cm on a VAS for pain (the MIC) at 3 months post-baseline	Number in the intervention group whose follow-up VAS pain score is ≥8 cm lower than that at baseline, divided by the number randomized to the intervention group

CI, confidence interval; VAS, Visual Analog Scale; MIC, minimal important change.

trial should be tested, including the control group strategy, procedures for blinding, outcome measures, and the schedule of data collection. Arnold and colleagues (2009) have suggested that it might be constructive to conduct a pilot trial in multiple sites. A multisite pilot "has the advantage of ensuring that the protocol can be implemented outside of experienced, well-resourced centers" (p. S70) and also gives project managers experience in multisite supervision.

In a feasibility study, simpler designs are usually sufficient. Simple descriptive designs may suffice—for example, if a major goal is to assess the number of eligible or to estimate how many sites could be recruited. One-group designs are often used to assess aspects of the intervention itself, such as whether the content is adequate or whether participants find the intervention acceptable.

It is highly advantageous to use mixed methods (MM) designs in pilot work because feasibility questions concern not only whether key objectives can be met but also about why they might have fallen short—and how to make modifications to remedy problems that emerged. Thus, in many cases, the appropriate design for a pilot trial will be either concurrent MM designs (e.g., QUAN + qual or QUAN + QUAL) or sequential ones (e.g., QUAN → qual or QUAN → QUAL). The qual component of pilot studies is likely to assume greater importance if the QUAN component suggest feasibility problems. Qualitative data are especially important for clarifying *why* an aspect of the pilot was unsuccessful and for suggesting ways to fix potential problems.

Example of a Research Design for a Pilot Study: Sin and colleagues (2013) provided a detailed description of their design for a planned pilot trial to test an online, multicomponent intervention for siblings of patients with an episode of psychosis (an intervention that was designed using the MRC framework). Their plan is to recruit and randomize 120 eligible siblings and assign them to one of four groups (three treatment groups, one control group) using a permuted block randomization scheme carried out by a centralized service to ensure allocation concealment. The mixed method QUAN → qual design includes follow-up interviews with a subsample of participants in all treatment groups to explore their experiences with the intervention.

Sampling in Pilot Work

The sample used in pilot work should be drawn from the same population as the population for the main trial. This means that the eligibility criteria should be the same—although these criteria might be adjusted during the course of the pilot if researchers run into unanticipated problems.

The sample size for pilot studies is typically small. Hertzog (2008) examined pilot studies that had been funded by the National Institute of Nursing Research between 2002 and 2004 and found that for the studies with two-group designs, the median number of total participants was about 50. Arain and colleagues (2010) reported that for 26 reports of pilot studies published in 2007-2008 in seven top-tier medical journals, the median total sample size was 76.

Conventional power calculations are not appropriate for pilot studies because the study purpose is not to test hypotheses about intervention outcomes. However, several experts have suggested that researchers could use confidence intervals to estimate the sample size needed to establish feasibility (e.g., Arnold et al., 2009; Hertzog, 2008; Thabane et al., 2010). For example, suppose we decided *a priori* that a full-scale trial would be feasible if the rate of attrition from the study was no more than 20% at a 3-month follow-up. Based on evidence from other similar trials (or Phase I development work), we predict that the *actual* rate of attrition will be 12%. If we used a confidence interval of 95% around the expected attrition rate of 12%, we would need a total sample size of 64 for the upper bound of the confidence interval not to exceed the criterion of 20% attrition (95% CI around 12% = 4% to 20% for $N = 64$). If we relaxed our standard to a less stringent 90% CI for the same scenario, the needed total sample size would be 46 (90% CI around 12% = 4% to 20% for $N = 46$).

The ideal sample size for a pilot will vary from study to study because of differences in objectives and populations. Hertzog (2008), however, has recommended a pilot size of at least 30-40 per group if funding for the pilot is being sought.

Data Collection in Pilot Work

The data collection plan for pilots is typically complex because the pilot data serve two purposes: to test the viability of the instruments that would be used in the main trial and to address the various objectives of the pilot itself.

In terms of the second purpose, the type of data to be collected depends on what the specific objectives are. For example, if one objective is to assess the acceptability of the intervention (Table 28.3), then a quantitative measure of patient satisfaction should probably be used. If an objective is to ascertain success in screening for eligibility, then forms for extracting information from records are required.

Detailed documentation about the trial and its progress should be maintained to help illuminate what went right and what went wrong. It is useful to keep a diary or journal to record impressions and observations about the pilot experience. Diary entries are probably best organized thematically rather than chronologically. For example, one organizational scheme might involve journal sections devoted to each pilot objective. Entries for each objective should be made at least weekly, if not daily.

Thought needs to be given to how best to "get inside" the workings of the pilot through the collection of in-depth data. This is likely to include unstructured observations of various intervention activities (e.g., recruitment, consent procedures, intervention sessions). Participants in both the intervention and control group could be asked to complete **exit interviews**. Focus group interviews could also be conducted with various stakeholders, including participants, family members, and pilot study staff.

Data Analysis in Pilot Work

The analysis of quantitative data from a pilot study should be driven by the pilot study objectives and therefore tends to involve mainly descriptive statistics. For example, the analysis might indicate what percentage of eligible people agreed to participate or were randomized. Means and standard deviations are likely to be computed (e.g., mean number of sessions completed, mean length of time to complete the data collection forms). ES estimates may also be computed. For obtaining preliminary evidence about clinical significance, some researchers compute the number needed to treat (NNT).

In most of these cases, it is a good idea to compute confidence intervals around estimates. An upfront decision should be made about the desired level of precision (e.g., 68%, 90%). These analyses should yield information that would be compared to the criteria established at the outset and then to a decision about how best to proceed.

It has been argued that researchers should pay more attention to individual results in pilot studies than to group averages. Shih and colleagues (2004), for example, suggest that the emphasis should be on testing whether *any* individual subject has experienced a beneficial effect and provided statistical guidance for such an approach. One approach is to assess whether, for each person, a reliable improvement has occurred (Chapter 14) or whether a clinically significant change has occurred in a *responder analysis* (Chapter 20). If the main outcomes are ones for which minimal important change (MIC) benchmarks have not been established, the research team, with input from experts, can decide how large an improvement is needed to be deemed meaningful.

The analysis of the quantitative data from pilots can be used to guide decisions about how to proceed based on a comparison of the results to the preestablished criteria. Thematic analysis of the qualitative can confirm the wisdom of that decision and can also help researchers make adjustments to improve the likelihood that a full trial will be successful in giving the intervention a fair test.

Example of Data Collection in a Pilot Trial: Lovell and colleagues (2014) assessed several feasibility objectives in their pilot test of culturally sensitive psychosocial interventions for underserved people with high levels of mental distress in primary care. They collected quantitative data on rates of referral, recruitment, uptake, and delivery of the intervention as well as on outcomes such as global distress, depression, anxiety, and quality of life. Additional semistructured interviews with consenting participants were conducted in patients' homes. The interviews resulted in rich data regarding participants' decision to participate, their access to the intervention venue, their perceptions of the intervention in terms of cultural fit and intervention content, and overall acceptability.

PRODUCTS OF PILOT WORK

Pilot work should result in several products. As previously noted, one product should be a compilation of "lessons learned," which ideally should be drafted and reviewed by the research team, advisory panel, and key stakeholders for accuracy and completeness. Other products may include the following:

- Revised protocols for the intervention and the research plan (or, if major revisions are needed, a plan for further descriptive and exploratory research)
- A finalized list of proposed outcomes
- A formal proposal for a full Phase III trial (or for another pilot) and a plan for seeking funding
- A written manuscript for publication in a professional journal

With regard to publishing findings from pilot studies, Arain and colleagues (2010) queried seven editors of top medical journals and asked about their policies for publishing pilot study results. Several editors responded that they do not encourage the publication of pilots because they do not consider them sufficiently rigorous. However, there has been much discussion recently about the desirability—and even the obligation—of publishing information from pilots (e.g., Beebe, 2007; Conn et al., 2010; Thabane et al., 2010).

Moore and colleagues (2011) lamented that some researchers fail to publish pilot results because they "didn't find anything" (p. 3). This may well be the conclusion of researchers who primarily focus on results from hypothesis tests of the intervention's efficacy, which are often negative. However, as we have discussed in this chapter, the main purpose of pilot work is *not* to test the statistical significance of outcomes but to assess the feasibility of a full-scale rigorous trial. Others are likely to be interested in the "lessons learned" from a pilot.

Even if a pilot trial suggests that the intervention has little hope of being effective, that knowledge should be shared. Others working on the same or a similar problem can benefit from learning about failures as well as successes. A related issue is the importance of including findings from pilots in meta-analyses and systematic reviews, especially if the pilot does not translate into a full trial. As we discuss in the next chapter, meta-analysts must struggle with the issue of *publication bias*—that is, the tendency to publish studies only when there are statistically significant results. Such a tendency does a disservice to evidence-based practitioners who are then using a biased subset of the evidence.

Several commentators have also noted that there is an ethical obligation to communicate the results from a pilot (e.g., Thabane et al., 2010; van Teijlingen et al., 2001). The argument is that participants have agreed to volunteer their time for an endeavor they believed would be helpful scientifically, and researchers fail to fulfill their end of the bargain if the findings are not shared. Moreover, precious research funds spent on pilots are wasted if the results are not published so that others can learn from what was done.

The quality of reporting of pilot studies has been criticized by many recent writers. Reports should clearly state the objectives of the pilot as well as the criteria used to make decisions about next steps. Given that the emerging advice on pilot testing is relatively new, researchers may have to "educate" reviewers and journal editors about the focus on feasibility objectives and not on hypothesis testing, citing the leading experts' advice about the risks of interpreting *p* values in pilots. We offer some further suggestions about reporting pilot work in the Supplement to Chapter 30 on disseminating research evidence.

➔ **TIP:** Researchers sometimes wonder if the data from an external pilot can be pooled with the data from a main study—in other words, treating the pilot participants as the early participants in the larger trial. This practice is considered acceptable only if there have been no changes in the intervention or study protocols and if the population is the same. This is not likely to be the case in most circumstances. Lancaster et al. (2004) discuss the biases that can result from the practice of pooling data from the pilot into a main trial.

CRITIQUING FEASIBILITY AND PILOT STUDIES

Reports of pilot studies should adhere to many of the guidelines described in earlier chapters. For example, the report should provide descriptions of sample characteristics, design elements, instruments, and so on. The intervention theory and development of the intervention should be described or a reference should be provided to any previously published papers on intervention development work. Readers should be able to draw their own conclusions about the potential feasibility and efficacy of the intervention, and so information about the key features of intervention itself needs to be included.

A critique of pilot work should focus on the researchers' description of the pilot objectives, the criteria used to make decisions about feasibility, and the methods associated with feasibility assessments. Of course, if objectives and criteria were not articulated, readers should be critical of these omissions. If objectives and criteria were stated, readers can assess their reasonableness and judge whether the methods used to assess them were adequate.

We have stressed that the small sample sizes of pilot trials make hypothesis testing for intervention efficacy a risky business. However, we hesitate to recommend that pilot studies be criticized for including such information. Many journals expect such analyses, and editors may reject manuscripts that do not include them. (Confidence intervals around the point estimates for outcomes or around ES estimates are preferred.) However, if a pilot study does report the results of hypothesis testing, the researchers should be cautious in their interpretation of the results. Whether the results are statistically significant or not, the researchers should warn readers that the results are preliminary, that the sample size precludes definitive conclusions, and that further research is likely warranted.

Box 28.1 ⚙ offers some questions that can be used to critique a report of a pilot study. The overarching question is whether the researchers were successful in securing the data needed to make a decision about what the next steps should be.

RESEARCH EXAMPLE OF A PILOT TRIAL

Study: Web-based symptom management for women with recurrent ovarian cancer: A pilot randomized controlled trial of the WRITE Symptoms intervention (Donovan et al., 2014)

Statement of Purpose: The overall purpose of this research was to pilot test the Written Representational Intervention To Ease Symptoms (WRITE Symptoms), an intervention designed for women with recurrent ovarian cancer.

Intervention: WRITE Symptoms is an educational intervention delivered through asynchronous web-based message boards between a participant and a nurse. It was based on the Representational Approach (RA) to patient education and was the first RA intervention using a web-based delivery mode. The approach included seven elements to be covered during the course of the intervention (e.g., identifying gaps and confusions, goal setting, and planning).

Objectives: A major objective of the pilot trial was to assess the "feasibility of conducting the study via message boards" (p. 218). Feasibility was assessed by examining participant retention and the time and number of postings from the date of the first message to the date of the last one. The researchers also addressed another process-type objective, the acceptability of the intervention. A third objective was a management-related one: to assess the usability of the web-based system. Finally, the researchers sought to obtain preliminary information about the intervention's efficacy in terms of symptom severity, distress, consequences, and controllability.

Design and Sample: A total of 271 women responded to various recruitment solicitations; 84 of the women met eligibility criteria, and of these, 68 eligible women (81%) completed consent forms. Actual study participants were 65 eligible women recruited from 25 states, who were randomized with equal allocation to either the intervention group or to a wait-list control group. Random assignments were generated using minimization techniques that used race/ethnicity as a stratifying factor. Quantitative data relating to intervention outcomes were collected online at baseline and 2 and 6 weeks after the intervention. Open-ended comments and suggestions were also solicited.

BOX 28.1 Guidelines for Critiquing Aspects of Pilot Work

1. Did the title and abstract of the paper describe the study as a pilot or feasibility study? Which term was used? Was the term "pilot" used appropriately—or was the study simply a small-scale or exploratory study with no mention of its role as part of a larger scale effort?
2. Did the report state the explicit objectives of the study? Were specific feasibility outcomes identified, and was a description of how they were measured provided?
3. If objectives were stated, were they ones that would provide important knowledge about the design and conduct of a full-scale trial? Were potentially important objectives ignored? Were too many objectives tested?
4. Did the researchers state what criteria would be used as a basis for decision making about "next steps"? If no, was there any discussion of how decisions might be made?
5. If there were explicit criteria for the pilot objectives, were the criteria reasonable ones? Were they too liberal or too harsh?
6. To what extent did the design mirror the likely design for a full-scale trial? If randomization was not used, was there an adequate justification?
7. How large was the pilot sample? Was the sample size adequate for addressing the study objectives?
8. Was the data collection plan adequate for measuring feasibility outcomes and for testing data collection protocols for a larger trial? Were both quantitative and qualitative data judiciously collected and blended to provide a strong portrayal of feasibility?
9. Were analyses mostly descriptive? Were confidence intervals around key variables reported? Was effectiveness tested for key outcomes using statistical hypothesis testing procedures? If so, was sufficient caution used in interpreting the results?
10. Did the report describe important lessons learned? Did the discussion section describe how the intervention or the trial methods might be altered on the basis of the pilot?
11. Overall, was pilot work sufficient for a decision to move forward with a full clinical trial?

Results: A total of 56 of the 65 study participants (88%) were retained in the study. The majority of participants assigned to the intervention (76%) completed all elements of the intervention, and only two women never posted to the message board. The mean length of participants' posts were 260 words, and the mean length of nurses' posts were 300 words. It took the nurse–participant dyads an average of 79 days to complete all elements of the intervention. Responses to questions on a satisfaction survey indicated that patients were very satisfied with the program. For example, the mean response to the item "I enjoyed participating in the symptom management program" was 6.35 on a 7-point satisfaction scale. On a scale that measured usability of the message boards, there was strong agreement that the website was easy to learn to use. Individual complaints concerned being timed out of the message board and needing to check and recheck the message board to see if a nurse had posted

a message. The researchers also reported evidence of "preliminary efficacy." Women in the intervention group reported significantly lower distress than those in the control group. Group differences were also encouraging (although not at conventional levels of statistical significance) for symptom severity.

Conclusions: The researchers concluded that the study "supports the feasibility, acceptability, and efficacy of web-based educational interventions" (p. 228). A larger RCT, with funding from the National Institute of Nursing Research, is currently underway.

SUMMARY POINTS

- Although the terms *feasibility study* and *pilot study* are sometimes used interchangeably in intervention research, an emerging trend is to distinguish the two. A **feasibility study** tests specific and discrete aspects of an emerging intervention, often using a fairly simple design. A **pilot study** is a small-scale version of a full trial, designed to assess an entire set of procedures for implementing and evaluating an intervention, and ideally involves a randomized design.

- Full-scale evaluations of new interventions are costly. The overall purpose of pilot work, then, is to avoid a costly failure.
- There is a growing consensus among experts in pilot study methods that the purpose of pilot work should *not* be to test hypotheses about the effectiveness of the intervention because sample sizes in pilots are too small to yield reliable estimates of effects.
- Pilot work can address a variety of *objectives*, and researchers should articulate their objectives at the outset. The objectives can focus on processes (e.g., recruitment, retention, acceptability), resources (e.g., monetary costs, time demands), management issues (e.g., system adequacy, interpersonal relationships), and scientific issues.
- Scientific objectives can concern inquiries about the substantive aspects of the intervention, such as intervention content and dose, safety, preliminary evidence of efficacy, and clinical significance.
- Preliminary effect size estimates are often computed, together with confidence intervals (CIs). Because only preliminary evidence of efficacy is sought in pilots, CIs that are not stringent (e.g., 68% CI) may be sufficient.
- Scientific objectives also concern the methodologic aspects of a trial, such as whether randomization can be undertaken. A major issue in many pilots is the estimation of the sample size that would be needed to adequately power a full trial. Using the effect size estimate from a pilot to estimate sample size needs directly is unwise because such an estimate often leads to Type II errors—that is, underpowered studies.
- Pilots are meant to inform the decision about whether to (1) move forward with a full trial,

(2) make revisions that require an additional pilot, or (3) abandon the project altogether. To make this decision, researchers should articulate *criteria* for each objective in advance and then assess the degree to which the criteria were met.

- Mixed methods designs are especially well suited for pilot work. Quantitative data can be used to assess whether feasibility criteria were met, and qualitative data can elucidate *why* they were not met, or how the intervention of study protocols could be improved.
- Sample sizes for pilots are typically small. Some experts recommend at least 30-40 subjects per group, especially if funding for the pilot is sought.
- A major product from pilot work is a description of "lessons learned" that inform the final protocols for a full trial. Another product, if the intervention has been found to be feasible, acceptable, and promising, is a proposal for a full-scale trial.
- Ideally, regardless of the outcome, the findings from pilot work will be published so that others can benefit from learning about both the successes and the failures.

STUDY ACTIVITIES

Chapter 28 of the *Resource Manual for Nursing Research: Generating and Assessing Evidence for Nursing Practice, 10th edition*, offers exercises and study suggestions for reinforcing concepts presented in this chapter. In addition, the following study questions can be addressed:

1. Find a pilot study published in a nursing journal in 2010 or earlier. Then search forward for a larger subsequent study. Did the pilot lead to a larger trial? If so, what major changes were made to the study design as a result of the pilot?
2. Use the critiquing guidelines in Box 28.1 to review the study by Donovan et al. (2014) described at the end of the chapter, referring to the full report as necessary.

STUDIES CITED IN CHAPTER 28

*Arain, M., Campbell, M., Cooper, C., & Lancaster, G. (2010). What is a pilot or feasibility study? A review of current practice and editorial policy. *BMC Medical Research Methodology*, *10*, 67.

Arnold, D., Burns, K., Adhikari, N., Kho, M., Meade, M., & Cook, D. (2009). The design and interpretation of pilot trials in clinical research in critical care. *Critical Care Medicine*, *37*, S69–S74.

Beebe, L. (2007). What can we learn from pilot studies? *Perspectives in Psychiatric Care*, *43*, 213–218.

*Bird, L., Arthur, A., & Cox, K. (2011). "Did the trial kill the intervention?" Experiences from the development, implementation and evaluation of a complex intervention. *BMC Medical Research Methodology*, *11*(24).

Bloom, T., Glass, N., Case, J., Wright, C., Nolte, K., & Parsons, L. (2014). Feasibility of an online safety planning intervention for rural and urban pregnant women. *Nursing Research*, *63*, 243–251.

*Campbell, M., Snowdon, C., Francis, D., Elbourne, D., McDonald, A., Knight, R., . . . Grant, A. (2007). Recruitment to randomised trials: Strategies for trial enrollment and participation study. *Health Technology Assessment*, *11*(48), iii, ix–105.

Chalmers, I., Bracken, M., Djulbegovic, B., Garattini, S., Grant, J., Gulmezoglu, A., . . . Oliver, S. (2014). How to increase value and reduce waste when research priorities are set. *The Lancet*, *383*, 156–165.

Conn, V. S., Algase, D., Rawl, S., Zerwic, J., & Wyman, J. (2010). Publishing pilot intervention work. *Western Journal of Nursing Research*, *32*, 994–1010.

*Craig, P., Dieppe, P., Macintyre, S., Michie, S., Nazareth, I., & Petticrew, M. (2008a). *Developing and evaluating complex interventions: New guidance.* London, United Kingdom: Medical Research Council.

*Craig, P., Dieppe, P., Macintyre, S., Michie, S., Nazareth, I., & Petticrew, M. (2008b). Developing and evaluating complex interventions: The new Medical Research Council guidance. *BMJ*, *337*, 979–983.

*Donovan, H. S., Ward, S., Serieka, S., Knapp, J., Sherwood, P., Bender, C., . . . Ingel, R. (2014). Web-based symptom management for women with recurrent ovarian cancer: A pilot randomized controlled trial of the WRITE Symptoms intervention. *Journal of Pain and Symptom Management*, *47*, 218–230.

Feeley, N., & Cossette, S. (2015). Testing the waters: Piloting a complex intervention. In D. Richards & I. Rahm Hallberg (Eds.), *Complex interventions in health: An overview of research methods* (pp. 166–174). Oxford, United Kingdom: Routledge.

Hertzog, M. A. (2008). Considerations in determining sample size for pilot studies. *Research in Nursing & Health*, *31*, 180–191.

Kraemer, H. C., Mintz, J., Noda, A., Tinklenberg, J., & Yesavage, J. (2006). Caution regarding the use of pilot studies to guide power calculations for study proposals. *Archives of General Psychiatry*, *63*, 484–489.

Lancaster, G., Dodd, S., & Williamson, P. (2004). Design and analysis of pilot studies: Recommendations for good practice. *Journal of Evaluation in Clinical Practice*, *10*, 307–312.

Leon, A., Davis, L., & Kraemer, H. (2011). The role and interpretation of pilot studies in clinical research. *Journal of Psychiatric Research*, *45*, 626–629.

*Lovell, K., Lamb, J., Gask, L., Bower, P., Waheed, W., Chew-Graham, C., . . . Dowrick, C. (2014). Development and evaluation of culturally sensitive psychosocial interventions for under-served people in primary care. *BMC Psychiatry*, *14*, 217.

*Moore, C., Carter, R., Nietert, P., & Stewart, P. (2011). Recommendations for planning pilot studies in clinical and translational research. *Clinical and Translational Science*, *4*, 332–337.

Polit, D. F. (2006). *Common misconceptions in nursing research.* Saratoga Springs, NY: Humanalysis.

Resnick, B., Hammersla, M., Michael, K., Galik, E., Klinedinst, J., & Demehin, M. (2014). Changing behavior in senior housing residents: Testing of phase I of the PRAISEDD-2 intervention. *Applied Nursing Research*, *27*, 162–169.

Richards, D. A., & Rahm Hallberg, I. (Eds.). (2015). *Complex interventions in health: An overview of research methods.* Oxford, United Kingdom: Routledge.

Shih, W. J., Ohman-Strickland, P., & Lin, Y. (2004). Analysis of data and early phase studies with small sample sizes. *Statistics in Medicine*, *23*, 1827–1842.

*Sin, J., Henderson, C., Pinfold, V., & Norman, I. (2013). The E-Sibling Project—Exploratory randomised controlled trial of an online multi-component psychoeducational intervention for siblings of individuals with first episode psychosis. *BMC Psychiatry*, *13*, 123.

Taylor, R., Ukoumunne, O., & Warren, F. (2015). How to use feasibility and pilot trials to test alternative methodologies and methodological procedures prior to a full-scale trial. In D. Richards & I. Rahm Hallberg (Eds.), *Complex interventions in health: An overview of research methods* (pp. 136–144). Oxford, United Kingdom: Routledge.

*Thabane, L., Ma, J., Chu, R., Cheng, J., Ismaila, A., Rios, L. P., . . . Goldsmith, C. H. (2010). A tutorial on pilot studies: The what, why and how. *BMC Medical Research Methodology*, *10*(1).

*Tickle-Degnen, L. (2013). Nuts and bolts of conducting feasibility studies. *American Journal of Occupational Therapy*, *67*, 171–176.

Treweek, S. (2015). Addressing issues in recruitment and retention using feasibility and pilot trials. In D. Richards & I. Rahm Hallberg (Eds.), *Complex interventions in health: An overview of research methods* (pp. 155–165). Oxford, United Kingdom: Routledge.

*Treweek, S., & Born, A. (2014). Clinical trial design: Increasing efficiency in evaluating new healthcare interventions. *Journal of Comparative Effectiveness Research*, *3*, 233–236.

Ukoumunne, O., Warren, F., Taylor, R., & Ewings, P. (2015). How to use feasibility studies to derive parameter estimates in order to power a full trial. In D. Richards & I. Rahm Hallberg (Eds.), *Complex interventions in health: An overview of research methods* (pp. 145–154). Oxford, United Kingdom: Routledge.

Van der Wouden, J., Blankenstein, A., Huibers, M., van der Windt, D., Stalman, W., & Verhagen, A. (2007). Survey among 78 studies showed that Lasagna's law holds in Dutch primary care research. *Journal of Clinical Epidemiology*, 60, 819–824.

*Van Teijlingen, E. R., & Hundley, V. (2001). The importance of pilot studies. *Social Research Update*, 35.

Van Teijlingen, E. R., Rennie, A., Hundley, V., & Graham, W. (2001). The importance of conducting and reporting pilot studies: The example of the Scottish Births Survey. *Journal of Advanced Nursing*, 34, 289–295.

Vickers, A. J. (2003). Underpowering in randomized trials reporting a sample size calculation. *Journal of Clinical Epidemiology*, 56, 717–720.

*Villegas, N., Santisteban, D., Cianelli, R., Ferrer, L., Ambrosia, T., Peragallo, N., & Lara, L. (2014). The development, feasibility and acceptability of an Internet-based STI-HIV prevention intervention for young Chilean women. *International Nursing Review*, 61, 55–63.

Ward, E., & Brown, R. (2015). A culturally adapted depression intervention for African Amerian adults experiencing depression: Oh Happy Day. *American Journal of Orthopsychiatry*, 85, 11–22.

Watson, H., Godfrey, C., McFadyen, A., McArthur, K., Stevenson, M., & Holloway, A. (2015). Screening and brief intervention delivery in the workplace to reduce alcohol-related harm: A pilot randomized controlled trial. *International Journal of Nursing Studies*, 52, 39–48.

***A link to this open-access journal article is provided in the Toolkit for this chapter in the accompanying* Resource Manual.** ⊗

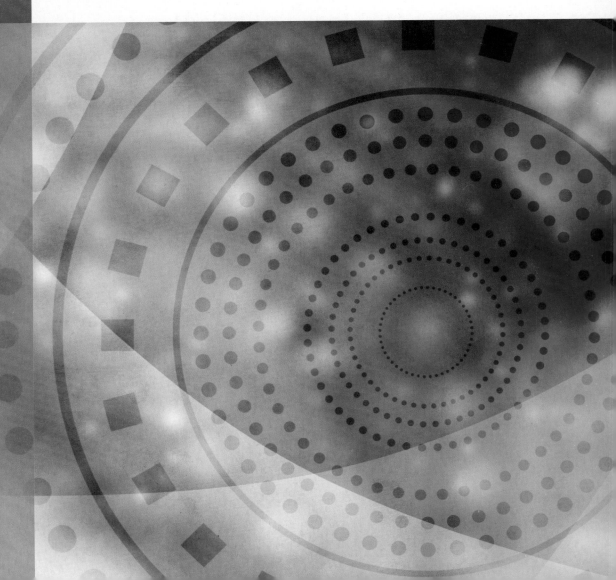

PART 6

BUILDING AN EVIDENCE BASE FOR NURSING PRACTICE

29 | Systematic Reviews of Research Evidence: Meta-Analysis, Metasynthesis, and Mixed Studies Review

In Chapter 5, we described major steps in conducting a literature review as an early step in designing and conducting a new study. This chapter also discusses reviews of existing evidence but focuses on the conduct and evaluation of systematic reviews, which in themselves are considered research.

RESEARCH INTEGRATION AND SYNTHESIS

A **systematic review** is a review that methodically integrates research evidence about a specific research question using careful sampling and data collection procedures that are spelled out in advance in a protocol. In a systematic review, reviewers use procedures that are, for the most part, reproducible and verifiable. Although subjectivity cannot be totally removed in a systematic review, the review process is disciplined and largely transparent, so that readers of the review can assess the conclusions. Systematic reviewers aim to avoid reaching erroneous conclusions that could arise from a biased review process or from a biased selection of studies included in the review.

Many consider systematic reviews a cornerstone of evidence-based practice (EBP) because EBP relies on meticulous integration of research evidence. The types of integrative activities we discuss in this

chapter are not just literature reviews but rather systematic inquiries that follow many of the same rules as those described in this book for **primary studies**, that is, original research investigations. What is distinctive about a systematic review, compared to a simple literature review, is the process of developing, testing, and adhering to a protocol with explicit rules for gathering the data—the research evidence—from studies that address a particular question.

Systematic reviews that integrate research evidence can take various forms and result in different products. Systematic reviews of evidence from quantitative studies—especially those that assess the effects of an intervention—are likely to use meta-analytic techniques. In a **meta-analysis**, reviewers use a common metric for combining evidence statistically. Most of the systematic reviews in the Cochrane Collaboration, for example, are meta-analyses. As we shall see, however, statistical integration is sometimes inappropriate. When evidence cannot be integrated statistically, a systematic review usually involves narrative integration.

Qualitative researchers also are developing techniques to integrate findings across studies. Many terms exist for such endeavors (e.g., metastudy, metamethod, metasummary, meta-ethnography, qualitative meta-analysis, formal grounded theory), but the one that appears to be emerging as the leading term among nurse researchers is *metasynthesis*.

means of refining the specific question for a systematic review. Although scoping studies have been defined in many ways (Davis et al., 2009), we refer here to scoping as a preliminary investigation that clarifies the range and nature of the evidence base. Unlike a systematic review, a scoping review addresses broad questions and uses flexible procedures and typically does not formally evaluate evidence quality. Such scoping reviews can provide background and suggest strategies for a full systematic review and can also indicate whether statistical integration (a meta-analysis) is feasible. Arksey and O'Malley (2005) have written an often-cited paper on the conduct of scoping reviews, and Daudt and colleagues (2013) elaborated on their framework.

Example of a Scoping Review: Yost and colleagues (2014) conducted a scoping review of knowledge translation strategies for enhancing evidence-informed decision making. They concluded that there were a sufficiently high number of studies to conduct a more focused systematic review by care settings, implementation strategies, or outcomes.

Designing the Meta-Analysis Study

Meta-analysts, like other researchers, make many decisions that affect the validity of their conclusions. Most decisions should be made in a conscious, planful manner *before the study is underway* and should be fully documented so they can be communicated to readers of the review. We identify a few major design decisions in this section. Some design options of a technical nature, however, can best be explained in our discussion of analytic procedures.

One up-front decision involves project organization. Systematic reviews are sometimes done by individuals, but it is preferable to have at least two reviewers. With multiple reviewers, the workload is shared and subjectivity is minimized. Reviewers should have substantive knowledge of the problem and sufficiently strong methodologic skills to evaluate study quality and undertake the analysis. Even with a knowledgeable team, clear guidelines are essential, just as they are in the collection of data for a primary study.

Sampling must also be planned. In a systematic review, the sample consists of the primary studies that have addressed the research question.

Reviewers make many decisions about the sample, including a specification of the exclusion or inclusion criteria for the search. Sampling criteria typically cover substantive, methodologic, and practical elements. Substantively, the criteria must stipulate specific variables. For example, if the review concerns the effectiveness of a nursing intervention, what outcomes (dependent variables) must the researchers have studied and what types of intervention are of specific interest? Another substantive issue concerns the study population—for example, will certain age groups of participants (e.g., children, the elderly) be excluded? Methodologically, the criteria might specify that (for example) only studies that used a randomized design will be included. From a practical standpoint, the criteria might exclude reports written in a language other than English, or reports published before a certain date. Of particular importance is the decision about whether both published and unpublished reports will be included in the review, a topic we discuss in the next section.

Example of Sampling Criteria: Beeckman and colleagues (2014) did a meta-analysis of evidence on three specific risk factors for pressure ulcer development: incontinence-associated dermatitis, incontinence, and moisture. Quantitative primary studies were included if they examined the relationship between the risk factors and the development of pressure ulcers; focused on patients aged 18 and older; and were written in English, French, or Dutch. Studies were excluded if there was insufficient data about the association between risk factors and pressure ulcers and if the design was a case study. Publications of any date were included in the review.

A related issue concerns the quality of the primary studies, a topic that has stirred debate. Researchers sometimes use quality as a sampling criterion, either directly or indirectly. Indirect screening can occur if, for example, a meta-analyst excludes studies that did not use a randomized design, or studies that were not published in a peer-reviewed journal. More directly, potential primary studies can be rated for quality, and excluded if the quality rating falls below a threshold. Alternatives to handling study quality are discussed in a later section. Suffice it to say, however, that evaluations of study quality are inevitably part of the review process. Thus, analysts need to decide how quality assessments will be made and what will be done with assessment information.

Another design issue concerns the **statistical heterogeneity** of results in primary studies. For each study, meta-analysts compute an index to summarize the strength and direction of relationship between an independent variable and a dependent variable. Just as there is inevitably variation *within* studies (not all people in a study have identical scores on outcome measures), so there is inevitably variation in effects *across* studies. If results are highly variable (e.g., results are conflicting across studies), a meta-analysis may be inappropriate. But if the results are modestly variable, an important design decision concerns steps that will be taken to explore the source of the variation. For example, the effects of an intervention might be systematically different for men and women (*clinical heterogeneity*). Or, the effects may be different if the period of follow-up is 6 months rather than 3 months (*methodologic heterogeneity*). If such effects are hypothesized, it is important to plan for subgroup analyses during the design phase of the project.

Design decisions are incorporated into a formal protocol that articulates the sampling criteria that will be applied, the search methods that will be used, and the information that will be extracted from the studies. The protocol and aspects of it (e.g., the search strategy) should be pilot tested before it is finalized.

Searching the Literature for Data

In Chapter 5, we discussed the importance of *owning* the research literature before preparing a written review. Ownership—becoming a leading authority on the research question under review—is even more important in a systematic review because of the pivotal role that such reviews play in EBP. Traditional strategies of searching for relevant studies, using electronic databases and ancestry/descendancy approaches that were described in Chapter 5, are rarely adequate without further retrieval efforts.

A decision that should be made before a search begins is whether the review will cover both published and unpublished results. There is some disagreement about whether reviewers should limit their sample to published studies or should cast as wide a net as possible and include **grey literature**—that is, studies with a more limited distribution, such as dissertations, conference presentations, and so on. Some people restrict their sample to published reports in peer-reviewed journals, arguing that the peer review system is an important, tried-and-true screen for findings worthy of consideration as evidence.

The limitations of excluding nonpublished findings, however, have been noted in the literature on systematic reviews (e.g., Ciliska & Guyatt, 2005; Conn et al., 2003). The primary issue is **publication bias**—the tendency for published studies to overrepresent statistically significant findings (this bias is sometimes called the *bias against the null hypothesis*). Explorations of this bias have revealed that the bias is widespread: Authors tend to refrain from submitting manuscripts with negative findings, reviewers and editors tend to reject such papers when they are submitted, and users of evidence tend to ignore the findings when they are published. The exclusion of grey literature in a systematic review can, however, lead to bias, particularly the overestimation of effects (Conn et al., 2003; Dwan et al., 2013).

We advocate retrieving as many relevant studies as possible because methodologic weaknesses in unpublished reports can be dealt with later. Aggressive search strategies are essential and may include, in addition to methods noted in Chapter 5, the following:

- *Handsearching* journals known to publish relevant content—that is, doing a manual search of the tables of contents of key journals
- Identifying and contacting key researchers in the field to see if they have done studies that have not (yet) been published, and asking them about other members of the *invisible college* and about their participation in relevant listservs or newsgroups
- Doing an "author search" of key researchers in the field in bibliographic databases and on the Internet
- Reviewing abstracts from conference proceedings, and networking with researchers at conferences; conference abstracts are often available

on the websites of the professional organizations sponsoring the conference.

• Searching for unpublished reports, such as dissertations and theses, government reports, and registries of studies in progress (e.g., in the United States, through the NIH RePORTER [http://projectreporter.nih.gov/reporter.cfm]).

• Contacting foundations, government agencies, or corporate sponsors of the type of research under study to get leads on work in progress or recently completed

Once potentially relevant studies are identified, they must be retrieved, which can be a labor-intensive process. Retrieved studies need to be carefully screened to determine if they do, in fact, meet the inclusion criteria. All decisions relating to exclusions (preferably made by at least two reviewers to ensure objectivity) should be well documented and justified.

Example of a Search Strategy from a Systematic Review: Fox and co-researchers (2013) did a meta-analysis of studies that assessed the effectiveness of early discharge planning in hospitalized older adults. Their comprehensive strategy included a search of over a dozen electronic databases, handsearching of several journals, and reference and citation searching. Teams of two reviewers independently screened abstracts for potential inclusion and disagreements were resolved by consensus or by a third reviewer.

TIP: The reports of studies that meet the sampling criteria do not always contain sufficient information for computing effect sizes. Be prepared to devote time and resources to communicating with researchers to obtain supplementary information.

Evaluating Study Quality

In systematic reviews, the evidence from primary studies should be evaluated to determine how much confidence to place in the findings, using criteria similar to those we have presented throughout this book. Strong studies should be given more weight than weaker ones in coming to conclusions about a body of evidence.

Evaluations of study quality sometimes involve quantitative ratings of each study in terms of the strength of evidence it yields. Literally, dozens of quality assessment scales that yield summary scores have been developed (Agency for Healthcare Research and Quality, 2002). One widely used scale was developed by Jadad and colleagues (1996). Despite the availability of many such instruments, overall scales are becoming somewhat less popular in meta-analyses. Quality criteria vary from instrument to instrument, and the result is that study quality can be rated differently with different assessment tools—or by different raters using the same tool. Moreover, there is a decided lack of transparency to users of the review when an overall scale score is used.

Because of these problems, the *Cochrane Handbook* (Higgins & Green, 2008) recommends against using a global scale. They recommend a *domain-based evaluation*, that is, a *component approach*, as opposed to a *scale approach*. Individual features are given a separate rating or code for each study, and the relationship between these features and effect size estimates can be analyzed. So, for example, a researcher might code for such design elements as whether randomization was used, whether subjects were blinded, the extent of attrition from the study, and so on. Decisions about such features need to be articulated in the review protocol so that the relevant information can be systematically extracted from reports. Cooper (2010) offers an excellent discussion about quality assessment in meta-analyses.

TIP: For systematic reviews of interventions, the *Cochrane Handbook* (Higgins & Green, 2008) includes a tool for assessing the risk of bias in six domains (Table 8.5).

Coding for quality elements in primary studies should be done by at least two qualified individuals. If there are disagreements between the coders, there should be a discussion until a consensus has been reached or, if necessary, a third person should be asked to help resolve the difference. Interrater reliability can be calculated to demonstrate to readers that rater agreement on study quality elements was adequate.

Example of a Quality Assessments: Bryanton et al. (2013) completed a Cochrane review of RCTs testing the effects of structured postnatal education for parents. They used the Cochrane domain approach to capture elements of trial quality. Both reviewers completed assessments, and disagreements were resolved by discussion.

Extracting and Encoding Data for Analysis

The next step in a systematic review is to extract relevant information about study characteristics, methods, and findings from each report. A data extraction form (either paper-and-pencil or computerized) must be developed, along with a coding manual to guide those who will be extracting and encoding information.

Basic data source information should be recorded for all studies. This includes such features as year of publication, country where data were collected, type of report (journal article, dissertation, etc.), and language in which the report was published. Supplementary information that may also be of interest includes whether the report was peer-reviewed, the impact factor of the journal (see Chapter 30), whether the study was funded (and by whom), and the year in which data were collected.

In terms of methodologic information that should be encoded, a critical element across all studies is sample size. Measurement issues may also be important. For example, there could be codes to designate the specific instruments used to operationalize outcome variables, and scale reliability information could be recorded. Other attributes that should be recorded vary by study question. In longitudinal studies, length of time between waves of data collection is important as well as rates of attrition. In intervention studies, design elements should be coded (e.g., whether there was randomization and blinding, whether intention-to-treat analysis was used). Features of the intervention also should be recorded, such as type of setting, length of intervention, and primary modality of the intervention. If a scale is used to rate the studies' methodologic quality, the scale score should be recorded.

Characteristics of the study participants must be encoded as well. A useful strategy is to record characteristics as percentages. For example, it is almost always possible to determine the percentage of the sample that was female. Other categorical characteristics that could be represented as percentages include race/ethnicity, educational level, and illness/treatment information (e.g., percentages of participants in different stages of cancer). Age should be recorded as mean age of sample members.

Finally, the findings must be encoded. Either effect sizes (discussed in the next section) need to be calculated and entered, or the data extraction form needs to record sufficient statistical information that the computer program can compute the indexes. Effect size information is often recorded for multiple outcomes and may also be recorded for different subgroups of study participants (e.g., effects for males versus females on the various outcomes).

Extraction and coding of information should be completed by two or more people, at least for a portion of the studies. This allows for an assessment of interrater agreement, which should be sufficiently high to persuade readers of the review that the recorded information is accurate.

Example of Intercoder Agreement: In Conn and colleagues' (2012) meta-analysis of the effects of physical activity interventions with healthy minority adults, all 77 primary studies were coded by two carefully trained and supervised coders, and effect size information was verified by a third coder. Following review, the coders achieved 100% consensus.

A basic data extraction form is provided in the Toolkit section of the accompanying *Resource Manual* as a Word document that can be adapted for use in simple meta-analyses. ✪ A paper-and-pencil form such as this one should be developed and pretested, but moving to a computerized platform is often attractive because data can be entered using pull-down menus and error detection is usually possible by establishing out-of-range values (e.g., it would be impossible to enter a publication date of 1016 in lieu of 2016). Guidance on developing coding forms is offered by Brown et al. (2003) and by Higgins and Green (2008).

Calculating Effects

Meta-analyses depend on the calculation of an index that encapsulates the relationship between the independent and dependent variables of interest in each study. Because effects are captured differently depending on the variables' level of measurement, there is no single formula for calculating an effect size. In nursing, the most common scenarios for meta-analysis involve comparisons of two groups on a continuous outcome (e.g., the body mass index or BMI), comparisons of two groups on a dichotomous outcome (e.g., obese versus non-obese), or correlations between two continuous variables (e.g., the correlation between BMI and scores on a depression scale). Other scenarios are described in the *Cochrane Handbook* (Higgins & Green, 2008).

The first scenario, comparison of group means, is especially common; for simplicity, most of our discussion focuses on this situation. When the outcomes across studies are on identical scales (e.g., measures of weight in pounds), the effect can be captured by simply subtracting the mean for one group from the mean for the other in each study. For example, if the mean weight in an intervention group were 182.0 pounds and that for a control group were 194.0 pounds, the effect would be −8.0. More typically, outcomes are measured on different scales. For example, postpartum depression might be measured by Beck's Postpartum Depression Screening Scale in one study and by the Edinburgh Postnatal Depression Scale in another. In such situations, mean differences across studies cannot be combined and averaged—we need an index that is neutral to the original metric used in the primary study. Cohen's *d*, described in Chapter 17, is the effect size (ES) index most often used. It may be recalled that the formula for *d* is the group difference in means, divided by the pooled standard deviation, or

$$d = \frac{\overline{X}_1 - \overline{X}_2}{SD_p}$$

where $\overline{X}_1$ is the mean of group 1, $\overline{X}_2$ is the mean of group 2, and SD_p is the pooled standard deviation. This effect size index transforms all effects to standard deviation units. That is, if *d* were .50, it means that the mean for one group was one half a standard deviation higher than that for the other group—regardless of the original measurement scale.

➲ **TIP:** The preferred term for the effect size *d* in Cochrane reviews is **standardized mean difference** or SMD. Lipsey and Wilson (2001) refer to *d*, as described here, as ES_{SM}, that is, the effect size for standardized means. Cooper (2010) uses both *d* and SMD interchangeably.

If meta-analysis software is used in the meta-analysis—as it often is—there is no need to calculate effect sizes manually. The relevant means and standard deviations would be entered. But what if this information is absent from the report, as is all too often the case? Fortunately, there are alternative formulas for calculating *d* from information in the primary study reports. For example, it is possible to derive the value of *d* when the report gives such information as the value of *t* or *F*, an exact probability value, or a 95% confidence interval around the mean group difference. (The Toolkit in the *Resource Manual* 💿 includes alternative formulas for computing *d*.) If none of this information is available in a report, the authors could be contacted for additional information.

When the outcomes in the primary studies are expressed as dichotomies, meta-analysts have a choice of effect size index, but the most usual are ones we discussed in earlier chapters—the relative risk (RR) index, the odds ratio (*OR*), and absolute risk reduction (ARR). Guidance on computing these indexes was provided in Table 16.6. The selection of a summary effect index depends on several criteria, such as mathematical properties, ease of interpretation, and consistency. As noted in the *Cochrane Handbook* (Higgins & Green, 2008), no single index is uniformly best. The odds ratio is, unfortunately, difficult for many users of systematic reviews to interpret. Nevertheless, it appears to be the most frequently used effect size index for dichotomous outcomes in the nursing literature.

For nonexperimental studies, a common statistic used to express the relationship between independent and dependent variables is Pearson's *r*. If the primary studies in a meta-analysis provide statistical information in the form of a correlation coefficient, the *r* itself serves as the indicator of the magnitude and direction of effect.

Meta-analysts sometimes face a situation in which findings are not all reported using the same level of measurement. For example, if the variable *weight* (a continuous variable) was our key outcome variable, some studies might present findings for weight as a dichotomous outcome (e.g., *obese* versus *not obese*). One approach is to do separate meta-analyses for differently expressed effects. Another is to re-express some of the effect indicators so that all effects can be pooled. For example, an odds ratio can be converted to *d*, as can a value of *r*—and vice versa. A large number of formulas for converting effect size information is presented in Appendix B of Lipsey and Wilson (2001).

➔ **TIP:** Our discussion of calculating effects sizes glosses over a number of complexities. Alternative methods may be needed for some studies, when the unit of analysis was not individual people, if a crossover design was used, when data were severely skewed, and so on. Those embarking on a meta-analysis project should seek additional guidance from books on meta-analysis or from statisticians.

Analyzing the Data

Meta-analysis is often described as a two-step analytic process. In the first step, a summary statistic that captures an effect is computed for each study, as just described. In the second step, a pooled effect estimate is computed as a **weighted average** of the effects for individual primary studies. A weighted average is defined as follows, with ES representing effect size estimates from each study:

$$\text{weighted average} = \frac{\text{sum of (ES} \times \text{weight for that ES)}}{\text{sum of the weights}}$$

The bigger the weight given to any study, the more that study will contribute to the weighted average. Thus, weights should reflect the amount of information that each study provides. One widely used approach is the **inverse variance method**, which uses the inverse of the variance of the effect size estimate (i.e., one divided by the square of its standard error) as the weight. Thus, larger studies, which have smaller standard errors, are given greater weight than smaller ones. The basic data needed for this type of analysis is the estimate of the effect size and its standard error, for each study.

Meta-analysts make many decisions at the point of analysis. In this brief overview, we present some basic information about the following analytic issues: identifying heterogeneity, deciding whether to use a fixed effects or random effects model, incorporating clinical and methodologic diversity into the analysis, and handling study quality. The issue of addressing possible publication biases is described in the Supplement to this chapter on thePoint®. 🅢

➔ **TIP:** The Cochrane Collaboration has developed its own software, the Review Manager (RevMan) software, which is currently distributed as copyrighted freeware. Macros are also available for doing meta-analyses within major software packages such as SPSS and SAS. Links to websites for other meta-analysis software are included in the Toolkit.

Identifying Heterogeneity. Heterogeneity of effects across studies may rule out the possibility that a meta-analysis can be done, but it also remains an issue for the analyst even when statistical pooling is justifiable. Unless it is obvious that effects are consistent in magnitude and direction based on perusal, heterogeneity should be formally tested.

Visual inspection of heterogeneity can most readily be accomplished by constructing a **forest plot**, which can be generated using meta-analytic software. A forest plot graphs the estimated effect size for each study, together with the 95% CI around each estimate. Figure 29.1 illustrates two forest plots for situations in which there is low heterogeneity (A) and high heterogeneity (B) for five studies in which the odds ratio was the effect size index. In Panel A, all effect size estimates favor the intervention group and are statistically significant for three of them (studies 2, 4, and 5), according to the 95% CI information. In Panel B, by contrast, results are "all over the map," with two studies

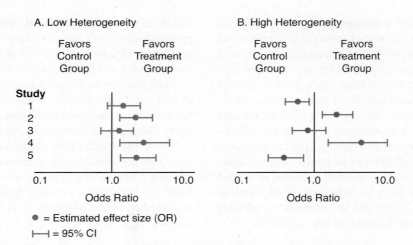

FIGURE 29.1 Two forest plots for five studies with low (**A**) and high (**B**) heterogeneity of effect size estimates.

favoring controls at significant levels (studies 1 and 5) and two favoring the treatment group (studies 2 and 4). A meta-analysis is not appropriate for the five studies in B.

Heterogeneity can be evaluated using a statistical procedure that tests the null hypothesis that heterogeneity across studies represents random fluctuations. The test—often a chi-squared test—yields a p value indicating the probability of obtaining ES differences as large as those observed if the null hypothesis were true. An alpha of .05 is usually used as the significance criterion but, because the test is underpowered when the meta-analysis involves a small number of studies, an α of .10 is sometimes considered an acceptable criterion.

Deciding on a Fixed Effect versus Random Effects Analysis. Two basic statistical models can be used in a meta-analysis, and the choice relates to heterogeneity. In a **fixed effects model**, the underlying assumption is that a single true effect size underlies all study results and that observed estimates vary only as a function of chance. The error term in a fixed effects model represents only within-study variation, and between-study variation is ignored.

A **random effects model**, by contrast, assumes that each study estimates *different*, yet related, true effects and that the various effects are normally distributed around a mean effect size value. A random

effects model takes both within- and between-study variation into account.

When there is little heterogeneity, both models yield nearly identical results. With extensive heterogeneity, however, the analyses yield different estimates of the average effect size. Moreover, when there is heterogeneity, the random effects model yields wider confidence intervals than the fixed effects model and is thus usually more conservative. But it is precisely when there *is* heterogeneity that the random effects model should be used.

Some argue that a random effects model is needed only when the test for heterogeneity is statistically significant, and others argue that a random effects model is almost always more tenable. A recommended approach is to perform a *sensitivity analysis*—a test of how sensitive the results of an analysis are to changes in the way the analysis was done. In this case, it would involve using both models to assess how the results are affected. If the results differ substantially, it is more prudent to use estimates from the random effects model.

TIP: In a set of studies with heterogeneous effects, a random effects model will award relatively more weight to small studies than such studies would receive in a fixed effects model. If effects from small studies are systematically different from those in larger ones, a random effects meta-analysis could yield biased results. One strategy is to perform another sensitivity analysis, running the analysis with and without small studies to see if results vary.

Examining Factors Affecting Heterogeneity. A random effects meta-analysis incorporates heterogeneity into the analysis but is intended primarily to address variation that cannot be explained. Many meta-analysts seek to understand determinants of effect size diversity through formal analyses. Such analyses should always be considered exploratory because they are inherently nonexperimental (observational). Consequently, causal interpretations are necessarily speculative. To be considered scientifically appropriate, explorations of heterogeneity should be specified before doing the review to minimize the risk of finding spurious associations.

Heterogeneity across studies could reflect systematic differences with regard to clinical or methodologic characteristics, and both can be explored. Clinical heterogeneity can result from participant differences (e.g., men and women) or in the way that the independent variable was operationalized. For example, in intervention studies, variation in effects could reflect who the agents were (e.g., nurses versus others), what the setting or delivery mode was, or how long the intervention lasted.

Methodologic heterogeneity could involve several study characteristics. Some could represent research design decisions, such as when the measurements were made (e.g., 3 months versus 6 months after an intervention), whether or not a randomized design was used, or whether other design features (e.g., blinding) were in place. Other methodologic variables could be after-the-fact "outcomes," such as a high versus low attrition rates.

Explorations of methodologic diversity focus primarily on the possibility that the studies suffer from different types or degrees of bias. Explorations of clinical diversity, on the other hand, are more substantively relevant: They examine the possibility that effects differ in relation to clinically relevant factors (e.g., Are effects larger for certain types of people?).

Two types of strategy can be used to explore *moderating effects* on effect size: subgroup analysis

and meta-regression. **Subgroup analyses** involve splitting the effect size information from studies into distinct categorical groups—for example, gender groups. Effects for studies with all-male (or predominantly male) samples could be compared to those for studies with all or predominantly female samples, using some threshold for "predominance" (e.g., 75% or more of participants). Of course, if it is possible to derive separate effect size estimates for males and females directly from study data, it is advantageous to do so, but this is seldom possible without contacting the researchers. The simplest procedure for comparing subgroup effects is to see whether there is any overlap in the confidence intervals around the effect size estimates for the groups.

Example of a Subgroup Analysis: Shin and colleagues (2015) did a meta-analysis of the effects of patient simulation in nursing education. Significant aggregate improvements in several domains were found for participants who received simulation education, compared to the control groups (pooled random effects SMD of 0.71). The researchers also tested effects for subgroups of studies based on a number of variables, such as what type of evaluation measures were used, what type of learner was included in the study, and the fidelity of the simulators.

When variables thought to influence study heterogeneity are continuous (e.g., "dose" of the intervention), or when there is a mix of continuous and categorical factors, then meta-regression might be appropriate. **Meta-regression** involves predicting the average effect size based on possible explanatory factors. As in ordinary regression, the statistical significance of regression coefficients indicates a nonrandom linear relationship between effect sizes and the associated explanatory variable.

Handling Study Quality. There are four basic strategies for dealing with the issue of study quality in a meta-analysis. One is to set a quality threshold for study inclusion. Exclusions could reflect requirements for certain methodologic features (e.g., only randomized studies) or for a sufficiently high score on a quality assessment scale. We prefer other alternatives that allow reviewers to summarize the full range of evidence in an area, but quality exclusions might in some cases be justified.

A second strategy is to undertake sensitivity analyses to determine whether the exclusion of lower quality studies changes the results of analyses based only on the most rigorous studies. Conn and colleagues (2003) have described as one option beginning the meta-analysis with high-quality studies and then sequentially adding studies of progressively lower quality to evaluate how robust the effect size estimates are to variation in quality.

Example of a Sensitivity Analysis for Study Quality: Mist and colleagues (2013) did a meta-analysis of the effects of complementary and alternative exercise for patients with fibromyalgia. They used a widely used measure of study quality, the Jadad instrument, to assign scores to the 16 studies in their meta-analysis. They analyzed their results in relation to the Jadad score and found greater heterogeneity of effects in the low-scoring studies.

Another approach is to consider quality as the basis for exploring heterogeneity of effects, the issue discussed in the previous section. For example, do randomized designs yield different average effect size estimates than quasi-experimental designs? Do effects vary as a function of the study's score on a quality assessment scale? Both individual study components and overall study quality can be used in subgroup analyses and meta-regressions.

Example of a Meta-Regression Including Study Quality: Park and colleagues (2013) did a meta-analysis of research on the relationship between depression and all-cause mortality among individuals with diabetes. They examined the effect of several moderator variables on study effect size, including age, gender, duration of follow-up, location (United States versus another country), and study quality, as assessed in a rating scale with scores than could range from 0 to 16.

A fourth strategy is to weight studies according to quality criteria. Most meta-analyses routinely give more weight to larger studies, but effect sizes can also be weighted by quality scores, thereby placing more weight on the estimates from rigorous studies. One persistent problem, however, is the previously mentioned issue of the validity of quality assessment scales and the unreliability of ratings. A mix of strategies, together with appropriate sensitivity analyses, is probably the most prudent approach to dealing with variation in study quality.

⮑ **TIP:** Quality information, using either a formal scale approach or a component approach, is important descriptively and should be reported in the review. For example, with a 25-point quality scale, the reviewers should report the mean scale score across primary studies, or the percentage of scoring above a threshold (e.g., 20 or higher). Many researchers who do not incorporate study quality into their actual analysis provide descriptive information about the quality of studies in the review sample.

Writing a Meta-Analytic Report

The final step in a systematic review project is to prepare a report to disseminate the findings. Typically, such reports follow much the same format as for a research report for a primary study, with an Introduction, Method section, Results section, and Discussion (see Chapter 30).

Particular care should be taken in preparing the Method section. Readers of the review need to be able to assess the validity of the review, and so methodologic and statistical decisions, and their rationales, should be described. If the reviewers decided that a meta-analysis was not justified, the rationale for this decision must be made clear. The *Cochrane Handbook* (Higgins & Green, 2008) offers excellent suggestions for preparing reports for a systematic review. There is also an explicit reporting guideline for meta-analyses of RCTs called **PRISMA** or Preferred Reporting Items for Systematic reviews and Meta-Analyses (Liberati et al., 2009; Moher et al., 2009) and another for meta-analyses of observational studies called **MOOSE** (Meta-analysis of Observational Studies in Epidemiology; Stroup et al., 2000). Our critiquing guidelines later in this chapter also suggest the types of information to include.

A thorough discussion section is also crucial in systematic reviews. The discussion should include an overall summary of the findings, noting the magnitude of average effects and the numbers of studies and participants involved. The discussion should present an assessment of the overall quality of the body of evidence and the consistency of findings across studies—as well as an interpretation of why there might be inconsistencies. Implications of the review should also be described, including a discussion of further research needed to improve the evidence base and the clinical implications of the review. It is important in reports of meta-analyses of interventions to emphasize that "insufficient evidence of effectiveness" is not the same as "evidence of no effectiveness" (Stoltz et al., 2009).

Tables and figures typically play a key role in reports of systematic reviews. Forest plots are often presented, showing effect size and 95% CI information for each study as well as for the overall pooled result. Typically, there is also a table showing the characteristics of studies included in the review. A template for such a table is included in the Toolkit of the accompanying *Resource Manual*. Also, the PRISMA guidelines call for the inclusion of a flowchart, analogous to a CONSORT flowchart (Chapter 30), that documents the identification, screening, and inclusion of studies in a systematic review.

Finally, full citations for the entire sample of studies included in the review should be provided in the bibliography. Often these are identified separately from other citations—for example, by noting them with asterisks.

METASYNTHESIS

The systematic integration of qualitative findings is a burgeoning field. As several commentators have noted, metasynthesis holds exciting promise for those concerned about the generalizability and transferability of findings from individual studies (Finfgeld-Connett, 2010; Polit & Beck, 2010). Metasyntheses, like meta-analyses, can play an important role in evidence-based practice.

Metasynthesis: Definition and Types

Terminology and approaches to qualitative synthesis are diverse and complex. Five leading thinkers on qualitative integration, acknowledging the diversity, used the term metasynthesis as an umbrella term,

with metasynthesis broadly representing "a family of methodologic approaches to developing new knowledge based on rigorous analysis of existing qualitative research findings" (Thorne et al., 2004, p. 1343).

Like other types of systematic reviews, metasyntheses are a systematic approach to reviewing and integrating findings from completed studies. Yet, just as there are many different approaches to doing qualitative research, there are diverse approaches to doing a metasynthesis and to defining what it is.

There is more agreement on what a metasynthesis is *not* than on what it *is*. **Metasynthesis** is not a literature review—that is, not the collating of research findings—nor is it a concept analysis. Many writers have followed the definition of metasynthesis offered by Schreiber and colleagues (1997): " . . . the bringing together and breaking down of findings, examining them, discovering the essential features and, in some way, combining phenomena into a transformed whole" (p. 314). Sandelowski (in Thorne et al., 2004) suggested that "metasyntheses are integrations that are more than the sum of parts, in that they offer novel interpretations of findings" (p. 1358). Most, but not all, methods of qualitative synthesis involve a transformational process.

Barnett-Page and Thomas (2009) identified 12 different approaches for synthesizing qualitative research. The approaches that appear to have been most attractive to nurse researchers are

- Meta-ethnography (Noblit & Hare, 1988)
- Metastudy (Paterson et al., 2001)
- Qualitative metasummary (Sandelowski & Barroso, 2007)
- Critical interpretive synthesis or CIS (Dixon-Woods et al., 2006)
- Grounded formal theory (Eaves, 2001)
- Thematic synthesis (Thomas & Harden, 2008)

As a means of characterizing and comparing the various approaches, Barnett-Page and Thomas (2009) used a system called *dimensions of difference* to distinguish them. One dimension concerned underlying epistemologic assumptions, which they felt explained the rationale for different approaches. Both Patterson's metastudy method and critical interpretive synthesis (CIS) were categorized as exemplars of *subjective idealism* in which "there is no shared reality independent of multiple alternative human constructions." Meta-ethnography and grounded formal theory were viewed as having an epistemologic stance described as *objective idealism*, "there is a world of collectively shared understandings." Thematic synthesis was categorized as *critical realism*, "knowledge of reality is mediated by our perceptions and beliefs" (p. 5).

Other dimensions of difference in the Barnett-Page and Thomas (2009) system were the degree of iteration, the type and degree of quality assessment in the process, the degree of focus on comparisons among primary studies, and the extent to which the aim is to "go beyond" the primary studies. With respect to the latter, all of the approaches most closely allied with nursing seek to push beyond the data in the original primary studies to a fresh interpretation of the phenomenon under review—although they go about this in different ways.

Alternative typologies of metasynthesis have been proposed. For example, Schreiber and colleagues (1997) suggested a typology that puts the role of theory at center stage. Their categorization includes three types linked to the purpose of the synthesis—theory building, theory explication, and description. *Theory-building metasyntheses* are inquiries that extend the level of theory beyond what could be achieved in individual studies. Both grounded formal theory and metastudy methods fall in this category. In *theory explication metasyntheses*, researchers "flesh out" and reconceptualize abstract concepts. Finally, *descriptive metasynthesis* involves a comprehensive analysis of a phenomenon based on a synthesis of qualitative findings; findings are not typically deconstructed and then reconstructed as they are in theory-related reviews.

The decision on which approach to use is likely to depend on several factors, including the nature of the problem and the philosophical leanings of the reviewers. For students, the decision is likely to be affected by the preferences and experience of their advisers.

⬆ TIP: Paterson (2013) identified more than 20 different variations of metasyntheses that have been developed over the past two decades.

She offers a framework to help researchers make a decision about which qualitative synthesis method works best for which questions they are asking. In her framework, there are four considerations: nature of the research, nature of the research team, nature of the researcher, and resources requirements. Paterson (2012) listed several questions that researchers need to consider in deciding on an approach.

Steps in a Metasynthesis

Many of the steps in a metasynthesis are similar to ones we described in connection with a meta-analysis, and so some details will not be repeated here. However, we point out a few distinctive issues relating to qualitative integration.

Formulating the Problem

In metasynthesis, researchers begin with a research question or a focus of investigation, and a key issue concerns the scope of the inquiry. Finfgeld (2003) recommended a strategy that balances breadth and utility. She advised that the scope be broad enough to fully capture the phenomenon of interest but sufficiently focused to yield findings that are meaningful to clinicians, other researchers, and public policy makers. Reviewers sometimes state a specific research question guiding the synthesis but more often declare their overall study purpose.

> **Example of a Statement of Purpose in a Metasynthesis:** O'Rourke and colleagues (2015) stated that the objective of their synthesis was "to comprehensively and systematically identify, appraise, and synthesize qualitative research findings that affect quality of life from the perspective of people with dementia" (p. 24).

Designing a Metasynthesis

Like a quantitative systematic review, a metasynthesis requires advance planning. Having a team of at least two researchers to design and implement the study is often advantageous, perhaps to an even greater extent than for a quantitative systematic review because of the subjective nature of interpretive efforts. Just as in a primary study, the design of a qualitative metasynthesis should involve efforts to enhance integrity and rigor, and investigator triangulation is one such strategy.

TIP: Meta-analyses often are undertaken by researchers who did not do one of the primary studies in the review. Metasyntheses, by contrast, are often completed by researchers whose area of interest has led them to do both original studies and metasyntheses on the same topic. Prior work in an area offers advantages in terms of researchers' ability to grasp subtle nuances and to think abstractly about a topic, but a disadvantage may be a certain degree of partiality about one's own work.

Metasynthesists, like meta-analysts, must make up-front decisions about sampling, and they face the same issue of deciding whether to include findings only from peer-reviewed journals in the analysis. One advantage of including alternative sources, in addition to wanting a more complete sample, is that journal articles are constrained in what can be reported because of space limitations. Finfgeld (2003) noted that in her metasynthesis on *courage*, she used dissertations even when a peer-reviewed journal article was available from the same study because the dissertation offered richer information.

An aspect of sampling that has been controversial in metasyntheses concerns whether to integrate studies that were based on different research traditions and methods. Some researchers have argued against combining studies from different epistemologic perspectives and have recommended separate analyses for different traditions. Others, however, advocate combining findings across traditions and methodologies. Which path to follow is likely to depend on the focus of the inquiry, its intent vis-à-vis theory development, and the nature of the available evidence.

Example of Sampling Decisions: Chen and Yeh (2015) conducted a metasynthesis of studies on the experiences of diabetics relating to self-monitoring of blood glucose. They searched for relevant studies from all qualitative traditions published between 2004 and 2013. Of the seven primary studies in their analysis, five were grounded theory studies, one was descriptive qualitative, and the third was a thematic network analysis.

Another sampling issue concerns decisions about the *type* of findings to include. Sandelowski and Barroso (2003a, 2007) describe a continuum of qualitative findings that involves how close the analysis is to the original data—that is, the extent to which the researcher *transforms* the data to yield findings. The continuum ranges from a category closest to the data that they called "no finding" (meaning that the data themselves are presented, without judgments or integrated discoveries) to a category farthest from the data that they called "interpretive explanation." The category scheme is intended to be neutral to the underlying method and research tradition. Sandelowski and Barroso argued that "no finding" studies are not research, and so metasynthesists may choose not to include them.

Searching the Literature for Data

It is generally more difficult to find qualitative than quantitative studies using mainstream approaches such as searching electronic databases. One factor contributing to this difficulty is that some databases do not index studies by methodology—although there have been many improvements in recent years. For example, "qualitative research" was added as a MeSH (Medical Subject Heading) term in MEDLINE in 2003. "Qualitative studies" is also used in the controlled vocabulary of CINAHL. Still, it is risky to rely totally on proper coding of studies for a metasynthesis. It may be wise to search for many different terms (e.g., "grounded theory," phenomenolog*, ethnograph*, "case study," and so on). Strategies for searching the grey literature, such as those suggested earlier, may also yield important sources. Barroso and colleagues (2003) have discussed strategies for finding qualitative primary studies for integration purposes. Further search guidance is offered by Wilczynski and colleagues (2007), Cooke et al. (2012), and the Cochrane Qualitative and Implementation Methods Group (http://cqim.cochrane.org/).

TIP: Sample sizes in nursing metasyntheses are highly variable, ranging from a very small number—for example, three primary studies in the meta-ethnography of Varcoe and colleagues

(2003)—to nearly 300 in Paterson's (2001) synthesis of qualitative studies on chronic illness. As with primary studies, one guideline for sampling adequacy is whether categories in the metasynthesis are saturated (Finfgeld, 2003).

Evaluating Study Quality

Formal evaluations of primary study quality are increasingly being undertaken by metasynthesists (Hannes & Macaitis, 2012) in some cases simply to describe the sample of studies in the review but in other cases to make sampling decisions. Many nurse researchers use the 10-question assessment tool from the Critical Appraisal Skills Programme (CASP) of the Centre for Evidence-Based Medicine in the United Kingdom. Sandelowski and Barroso (2007) offered a "reading guide" that can be used for a more detailed appraisal. The Primary Research Appraisal Tool, developed by Paterson and colleagues (2001), was designed to be used to screen primary studies for inclusion in a metasynthesis—although metastudy in its most recent form includes all relevant studies except those deemed not to be qualitative (Paterson, 2007). Hannes and colleagues (2010) have undertaken a comparative analysis of three online quality appraisal instruments (including the CASP tool) qualitative studies.

There is some disagreement about whether quality ought to be a criterion for eliminating studies for a metasynthesis. Sandelowski and Barroso (2003c), for example, advocated inclusiveness: "Excluding reports of qualitative studies because of inadequacies in reporting, or because of what some reviewers might perceive as methodologic mistakes, will result in the exclusion of reports with findings valuable to practice that are not necessarily invalidated by these errors" (p. 155). Finfgeld (2003) suggested that, at a minimum, studies included in the review must have used accepted qualitative methods and must have findings that are well supported by raw data—that is, quotes from participants.

Noblit and Hare (1988) advocated including all relevant studies but also suggested giving more weight to higher quality studies. A more systematic application of assessments in a metasynthesis is to use quality information in a sensitivity analysis that explores whether interpretations are altered when low-quality studies are removed (Thomas & Harden, 2008).

Example of a Sensitivity Analysis: Bridges and colleagues (2010) synthesized studies on the experiences of older people and relatives in acute care settings, using a thematic synthesis approach. Primary studies were appraised using the CASP criteria. A total of 42 primary studies and a previous synthesis were included in the review. A sensitivity analysis revealed that the findings and interpretations were robust to the removal of nine low-quality studies.

Extracting and Encoding Data for Analysis

Information about various features of the study need to be abstracted and coded as part of the project. Just as in quantitative integration, the metasynthesists usually record data source information (e.g., year of publication, country), characteristics of the sample (e.g., number of participants, mean age, gender distribution), and methodologic features (e.g., research tradition).

Most important, of course, information about the study findings must be extracted and recorded. Sandelowski and Barroso (2003b) have defined *findings* as the "data-based and integrated discoveries, conclusions, judgments, or pronouncements researchers offered regarding the events, experiences, or cases under investigation (i.e., their interpretations, no matter the extent of the data transformation involved)" (p. 228). Others characterize findings as the key themes, metaphors, categories, concepts, or phrases from each study.

As Sandelowski and Barroso (2002, 2003a) have noted, however, *finding* the findings is not always easy. For example, qualitative researchers intermingle data with interpretation, and findings from other studies with their own. Noblit and Hare (1988) advised that, just as primary study researchers must read and reread their data before they can proceed with a meaningful analysis, metasynthesists must read the primary studies multiple times to fully grasp the categories or metaphors being explicated. In essence, a metasynthesis becomes "another 'reading' of data, an opportunity to reflect on the data in new ways" (McCormick et al., 2003, p. 936).

Analyzing and Interpreting the Data

Strategies for metasynthesis diverge most markedly at the analysis stage. We briefly describe three approaches and advise you to consult more advanced resources for further guidance. Regardless of approach, metasynthesis is a complex interpretive task that involves "carefully peeling away the surface layers of studies to find their hearts and souls in a way that does the least damage to them" (Sandelowski et al., 1997, p. 370).

The Noblit and Hare Approach. Noblit and Hare's (1988) methods of integration, which they called meta-ethnography, have been influential among nurse researchers. Noblit and Hare argued that a meta-ethnography should be interpretive and not aggregative—that is, that the synthesis should focus on constructing interpretations rather than analyses. Their approach for synthesizing qualitative studies included seven phases that overlap and repeat as the metasynthesis progresses, the first three of which are preanalytic: (1) deciding on the phenomenon, (2) deciding which studies are relevant for the synthesis, and (3) reading and rereading each study. Phase 7 involves writing up the synthesis, but Phases 4 through 6 concern the analysis:

Phase 4: Deciding how the studies are related to each other. In this phase, the researcher makes a list of the key metaphors in each study and their relation to each other. Noblit and Hare used the term "metaphor" to refer to themes, perspectives, and/or concepts that emerged from the primary studies. Studies can be related in three ways: *reciprocal* (directly comparable), *refutational* (in opposition to each other), and in a line of argument rather than either reciprocal or refutational.

Phase 5: Translating the qualitative studies into one another. Noblit and Hare noted that "translations are especially unique syntheses because they protect the particular, respect holism, and enable comparison. An adequate translation maintains the central metaphors and/or concepts of each account in their relation to other key metaphors or concepts in that account" (p. 28). *Reciprocal translation analysis* (RTA) involves exploring and explaining similarities

and contradictions between studies and is not unlike a constant comparative process.

Phase 6: Synthesizing translations. Here, the challenge for the researcher is to make a whole into more than the individual parts imply. *Line-of-argument* (LOA) *synthesis* involves building up a new picture of the whole (e.g., a whole culture or phenomenon) from a scrutiny of its parts.

Atkins and colleagues (2008), noting that some aspects of meta-ethnography were not well-defined by Noblit and Hare, have offered further guidance on the analytic process. Also, Campbell and colleagues (2011) have prepared a useful open-access document that presents an evaluation of meta-ethnographic methods.

Example of Noblit and Hare's Approach: Toye and colleagues (2014b) used Noblit and Hare's approach in their metasynthesis of 32 studies on patients' experiences with chronic pelvic pain. Two team members read each paper and extracted and described key concepts. Concepts were then compared across studies and organized into categories with shared meaning. The researchers then developed a conceptual model, or line of argument, to explain conceptual categories. The overarching concept was struggling to construct chronic pelvic pain as "real." (In another publication, Toye et al. [2014a] described the challenges of undertaking a meta-ethnography.)

The Paterson, Thorne, Canam, and Jillings Approach. Paterson and colleagues' (2001) **metastudy method** of metasynthesis involves three components: metadata analysis, metamethod, and metatheory. These components often are conducted concurrently, and the metasynthesis results from the integration of findings from these three analytic components. Paterson and colleagues define **metadata analysis** as the study of results of reported research in a specific substantive area of investigation by means of analyzing the "processed data." **Metamethod** is the study of the methodologic rigor of the studies included in the metasynthesis. Lastly, **metatheory** refers to the analysis of the theoretical underpinnings on which the studies are grounded. Metastudy uses metatheory to describe and deconstruct theories that shape a body of inquiry. The end product of a metastudy is a metasynthesis that results from bringing back together the findings of these three components.

Example of Paterson's Approach: Bench and Day (2010) used the Paterson framework in their metasynthesis focusing on the specific problems faced by patients and relatives immediately following discharge from a critical care unit to another hospital unit.

The Sandelowski and Barroso Approach. The strategies developed by Sandelowski and Barroso (2007) reflect the results of a multi-year methodologic project. They developed the previously described continuum relating to how much data transformation occurred in a primary study. Further, they dichotomized studies based on level of synthesis and interpretation. Reports are described as *summaries* if the findings are descriptive synopses of the qualitative data, usually with lists and frequencies of topics and themes, without conceptual reframing. *Syntheses* are findings that are more interpretive and explanatory and that involve conceptual or metaphorical reframing. Sandelowski and Barroso have argued that only syntheses should be used in a metasynthesis.

Both summaries and syntheses can, however, be used in a **metasummary**, which can lay a good foundation for a metasynthesis. Sandelowski and Barroso (2003b) provided an example of a metasummary in which they used studies (including both summaries and syntheses) of mothering within the context of HIV infection. The first step, extracting findings, resulted in almost 800 complete sentences from the 45 reports they identified. The 800 sentences were then reduced to 93 thematic statements, or abstracted findings.

The next step in the metasummary was to calculate **manifest effect sizes**, that is, effect sizes calculated from the manifest content pertaining to motherhood within the context of HIV as represented in the 93 abstracted findings. Qualitative effect sizes are not to be confused with treatment effects: the " . . . calculation of effect sizes constitutes a quantitative transformation of qualitative data in the service of extracting more meaning from those data and verifying the presence of a pattern or theme" (Sandelowski & Barroso, 2003b, p. 231). They argued that by calculating effect sizes, integration can avoid the possibility of over- or under-weighting findings.

Two types of effect size can be created from abstracted findings. A **frequency effect size**, which indicates the magnitude of the findings, is the number of reports with unduplicated information that contain a given finding, divided by all unduplicated reports. For example, Sandelowski and Barroso (2003b) calculated an overall frequency effect size of 60% for the finding concerning a mother's struggle about whether or not to disclose her HIV status to her children. In other words, 60% of the 45 reports had a finding of this nature. Such effect size information can be calculated for subgroups of reports—for example, for published versus unpublished reports, for reports from different research traditions, and so on.

An **intensity effect size** indicates the concentration of findings *within* each report. It is calculated by dividing the number of different findings in a given report, divided by the total number of findings in all reports. As an example, one primary study, reported in a book, had 29 out of the 93 total findings for an intensity effect size of 31% for that study (Sandelowski & Barroso, 2003b).

Metasyntheses can build on metasummaries but require findings that are more interpretive, that is, from reports that are characterized as syntheses. The purpose of a metasynthesis is not to summarize but to offer novel interpretations of interpretive findings. Such interpretive integrations require metasynthesists to piece the individual syntheses together to craft a new coherent description or explanation of a target event or experience. An array of qualitative analytic methods can be used to achieve this goal, including, " . . . for example, constant comparison, taxonomic analysis, the reciprocal translation of in vivo concepts, and the use of imported concepts to frame data" (Sandelowski in Thorne et al., 2004, p. 1358).

> **TIP:** Rigor and integrity are important in metasyntheses, as in all research. Sandelowski and Barroso (2007) offered useful advice on how to optimize the validity of metasyntheses (Chapter 8).

Example of Sandelowski and Barroso's Approach: Fegran and colleagues (2014) conducted a metasynthesis to understand the experiences of adolescents and young adults with chronic diseases as they transferred from pediatric to adult care. Metasummary techniques were used to aggregate findings from 18 studies, and metasynthesis techniques were used to interpret the findings. Frequency effect sizes ranged from 11% to 89%, and intrastudy intensity effect size ranged from 15% to 100%. Four themes that illustrated the experience of loss of familiar surroundings and relationships were developed in the metasynthesis.

Writing a Metasynthesis Report

Metasynthesis reports are similar in many respects to meta-analytic reports—except that the results section contains the new interpretations rather than the quantitative findings. When a metasummary has been done, meta-findings would typically be presented in a table, a template for which is available in the Toolkit of the accompanying *Resource Manual*.

The method section of a metasynthesis report should contain a detailed description of the sampling criteria, the search procedures, study appraisal methods, and efforts made to enhance the integrity and rigor of the integration. The sample of selected studies should also be described. Key features of the sample of studies are often summarized in a table. A PRISMA-type flowchart highlighting sampling decisions and outcomes ideally should be included.

SYSTEMATIC MIXED STUDIES REVIEWS

The emergence of mixed methods research as a "third research community" (Chapter 26) has given rise to interest in systematic reviews that integrate findings from a broad methodologic array of studies. Such reviews are a relatively new endeavor, and so both terminology and approaches are still evolving. Pluye and colleagues (2009) used the term *mixed studies review* (MSR) but noted that many other names have been used, such as *mixed methods review* (Harden & Thomas, 2005) and *mixed research synthesis* (Sandelowski, et al., 2013; Sandelowski, et al., 2012). We use the term **systematic mixed**

studies review to refer to a systematic review that uses disciplined and auditable procedures to integrate and synthesize findings from qualitative, quantitative, and mixed methods studies.

As in mixed methods research, the "dictatorship of the research question" is a driving force behind mixed studies reviews. Harden and Thomas (2005), whose work at the EPPI Centre (Evidence for Policy and Practice Information) in London focused on health promotion interventions, noted that their reviews "were beginning to answer multiple questions" and that their reviews increasingly involved "more than one section in which the results of studies are brought together" (p. 261). As a result, they began to develop strategies for doing systematic mixed studies reviews.

Margarete Sandelowski has been in the forefront of such development in the United States. She and her colleagues (2007) astutely noted that "the research synthesis enterprise, in general, and the mixed research synthesis, in particular, entail *comparability work* [emphasis added] whereby reviewers impose similarity and difference on the studies to be reviewed" (p. 236). In other words, part of the reviewers' job in any synthesis project is to manage difference, and this takes on particular prominence when there are major differences in goals, epistemologic assumptions, and methodologic approaches. Comparability work is what allows "the previously incompatible and uncommon to be compared" (p. 238).

Sandelowski et al. (2006) described three models of mixed studies review that vary in terms of both approach and goals. In a *segregated design*, two separate syntheses are undertaken, one of qualitative findings and the other of quantitative findings, and then the mixed methods synthesis integrates the two. They viewed this approach as appropriate when qualitative and quantitative findings are regarded as complementing each other, as opposed to confirming or refuting each other. Complementarity is observed when the qualitative and quantitative research has addressed different but connected questions.

The segregated design model characterizes many mixed studies reviews and is similar to the approach described by Harden and Thomas (2005), who noted that this model "preserves the integrity of findings of different types of studies" (p. 268). This design has been found to be especially useful in integrating information about both effectiveness and context/processes in intervention research. Harden and Thomas provided a good example of their integration of findings on interventions to promote the inclusion of fruits and vegetables in children's diets. They combined findings from a meta-analysis of intervention effects with those from a metasynthesis of findings about barriers to and facilitators of children's healthy eating to address such questions as these: "Which interventions match recommendations derived from children's views and experiences? Which recommendations have yet to be addressed by soundly evaluated interventions? and Do those interventions that match recommendations show bigger effect sizes and/or explain heterogeneity?" (p. 264).

The second model is an *integrated design* (Sandelowski et al., 2006), which can be used when qualitative and quantitative findings in an area of inquiry are perceived as able to confirm, extend, or refute each other. In an integrated design, studies are grouped not by method but by findings viewed as answering the same research question. The analytic approach may involve transforming the findings (quantitizing qualitative findings or qualitizing quantitative findings) to enable them to be combined. A variant of this model is to use a *Bayesian synthesis*, as exemplified in a study in which Sandelowski participated (Voils et al., 2009).

A third model is a *contingent design* (Sandelowski et al., 2006) that involves a coordinated and sequential series of syntheses. In such a design, the findings from the systematic synthesis to address one research question is used to address a second research question—which may lead to yet another synthesis addressing a different question. Some of the mixed studies reviews as described in the *Cochrane Handbook* (Higgins & Green, 2008) might use such a design. For example, a qualitative synthesis can precede a meta-analysis and may help to define key outcomes or key variables for an analysis of heterogeneity for the meta-analysis.

As with all types of systematic review, mixed studies reviews face several issues of contention. One issue concerns how best to evaluate quality

(see Pluye et al., 2009) and what role appraisals should play in the reviews. Another issues concerns the specific analytic approaches that are likely to be productive. Techniques such as textual narrative, thematic synthesis, and critical interpretive synthesis (an adaptation of meta-ethnography) have been described (Flemming, 2010; Lucas et al., 2007). It seems likely that guidance (and debate) on how best to conduct mixed studies reviews will continue in the years ahead and that such reviews will play an important role in evidence-based practice.

Example of a Systematic Mixed Studies Review: Soininen and colleagues (2014) undertook a systematic mixed studies review of psychiatric inpatients' perceptions of coercion. Their paper outlined the main methodologic challenges they faced in doing the review.

CRITIQUING SYSTEMATIC REVIEWS

Like all studies, systematic reviews should be thoroughly critiqued before the findings are deemed trustworthy and relevant to clinicians. Box 29.1 offers guidelines for evaluating systematic reviews. Although these guidelines are fairly broad, not all questions apply equally well to all types of systematic reviews. In particular, we have distinguished questions about analysis separately for meta-analyses and metasyntheses. The list of questions in Box 29.1 is not necessarily comprehensive. Supplementary questions might be needed for particular types of review—for example, for mixed studies reviews. The PRISMA guidelines are an additional resource for checking on whether a review included sufficient information.

In drawing conclusions about a research synthesis, a major issue concerns the nature of the decisions the researcher made. Sampling decisions, approaches to handling quality of the primary studies, and analytic approaches should be carefully evaluated to assess the soundness of the reviewers' conclusions. Another aspect, however, is drawing inferences about how you might use the evidence in clinical practice. It is not the reviewers' job, for example, to consider such issues as barriers to

BOX 29.1 Guidelines for Critiquing Systematic Reviews

THE PROBLEM

- Did the report clearly state the research problem and/or research questions? Is the scope of the project appropriate?
- Is the topic of the review important for nursing?
- Were concepts, variables, or phenomena adequately defined?
- Was the integration approach adequately described, and was the approach appropriate?

SEARCH STRATEGY

- Did the report clearly describe criteria for selecting primary studies, and are those criteria reasonable?
- Were the bibliographic databases used by the reviewers identified, and are they appropriate and comprehensive? Were key words identified, and are they exhaustive?
- Did the reviewers use adequate supplementary efforts to identify relevant studies?
- Was a PRISMA-type flowchart included to summarize the search strategy and results?

THE SAMPLE

- Were inclusion and exclusion criteria clearly articulated, and were they defensible?
- Did the search strategy yield a strong and comprehensive sample of studies? Were strengths and limitations of the sample identified?
- If an original report was lacking key information, did reviewers attempt to contact the original researchers for additional information—or did the study have to be excluded?
- If studies were excluded for reasons other than insufficient information, did the reviewers provide a rationale for the decision?

QUALITY APPRAISAL

- Did the reviewers appraise the quality of the primary studies? Did they use a defensible and well-defined set of criteria, or a respected quality appraisal scale?
- Did two or more people do the appraisals, and was interrater agreement reported?
- Was the appraisal information used in a well-defined and defensible manner in the selection of studies, or in the analysis of results?

DATA EXTRACTION

- Was adequate information extracted about methodologic and administrative aspects of the study? Was adequate information about sample characteristics extracted?
- Was sufficient information extracted about study findings?
- Were steps taken to enhance the integrity of the data set (e.g., were two or more people used to extract and record information for analysis)?

DATA ANALYSIS—GENERAL

- Did the reviewers explain their method of pooling and integrating the data?
- Was the analysis of data thorough and credible?
- Were tables, figures, and text used effectively to summarize findings?

(box continues on page 668)

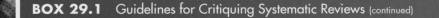

BOX 29.1 Guidelines for Critiquing Systematic Reviews (continued)

DATA ANALYSIS—QUANTITATIVE

- If a meta-analysis was not performed, was there adequate justification for using a narrative integration method? If a meta-analysis *was* performed, was this justifiable?
- For meta-analyses, were appropriate procedures followed for computing effect size estimates for all relevant outcomes?
- Was heterogeneity of effects adequately dealt with? Was the decision to use a random effects model or a fixed effects model sound? Were appropriate subgroup analyses undertaken—or was the absence of subgroup analyses justified?
- Was the issue of publication bias adequately addressed?

DATA ANALYSIS—QUALITATIVE

- In a metasynthesis, did the reviewers describe the techniques they used to compare the findings of each study, and did they explain their method of interpreting their data?
- If a metasummary was undertaken, did the abstracted findings seem appropriate and convincing? Were appropriate methods used to compute effect sizes? Was information presented effectively?
- In a metasynthesis, did the synthesis achieve a fuller understanding of the phenomenon to advance knowledge? Do the interpretations seem well grounded? Was there a sufficient amount of data included to support the interpretations?

CONCLUSIONS

- Did the reviewers draw reasonable conclusions about the quality, quantity, and consistency of evidence relating to the research question?
- Were limitations of the review/synthesis noted?
- Were implications for nursing practice and further research clearly stated?

�	All systematic reviews
▢	Systematic reviews of quantitative studies
▢	Metasyntheses

making use of the evidence, acceptability of an innovation, costs and benefits of change in various settings, and so on. These are issues for practicing nurses seeking to maximize the effectiveness of their actions and decisions.

●●●●●●●●●●●●●●●●●●●●●●●
RESEARCH EXAMPLES

We conclude this chapter with a description of two systematic reviews. Two reports (a meta-analysis

and a metasynthesis) appear in their entirety in the accompanying *Resource Manual*.

Example 1: A Meta-Analysis

Study: Breastfeeding and the risk of ovarian cancer: A meta-analysis (Feng et al., 2014)

Purpose: The purpose of the meta-analysis was to integrate research evidence concerning possible association between breastfeeding and ovarian cancer and whether duration of breastfeeding decreases the risk.

Eligibility Criteria: A study was considered eligible for the meta-analysis if it met the following criteria: (1) the study design was either a cohort study or a case-control study, (2) the sample included women who had breastfed and those who had exclusively formula-fed, and (3) the analysis involved the calculation of odds ratios (ORs) with 95% confidence intervals for ovarian cancer incidence for women who had breastfed compared to those who had not. The reports were limited to those written in English, but there was no restriction based on publication date.

Search Strategy: A search was undertaken in the MEDLINE and EMBASE databases, using "breastfeeding," "lactation," and "ovarian cancer" as search terms. Ancestry searching was also conducted, and the search was supplemented by reviewing relevant conference proceedings.

Sample: The analysis was based on a sample of 19 eligible studies. Initially, 76 citations were identified in the electronic search, 60 of which were excluded based on failure to meet eligibility criteria. Three studies were added on the basis of further searching. The studies included 4 cohort studies and 15 case-control studies. The sample for the main analysis included 469,095 women who had or had not breastfed, including 9,438 women with ovarian cancer.

Data Extraction: A formal extraction protocol was developed for data extraction. The data that were abstracted included publication year, study design, year of ovarian cancer diagnosis, length of follow-up, duration of breastfeeding, sample size in the two groups, and effect size information. The quality of the studies was assessed using a formal 8-item scale, with scores that could range from 0 to 9. Two reviewers independently rated the study quality, and disagreements were resolved by a third reviewer. The quality rating of the included studies ranged from 6 to 8, and thus, most studies were considered of high quality.

Effect Size Calculation: The odds ratio (*OR*) was used as the effect size index. The majority of studies in the review (15 of the 19) provided *OR* estimates that were adjusted for major confounders: smoking, body mass index, hysterectomy status, use of menopausal hormone therapy, age of menarche, age at menopause, and family history of ovarian cancer.

Statistical Analyses: The researchers found evidence of significant statistical heterogeneity. This analysis led to the decision to use a random effects model for their main analysis, in which the *OR*s were weighted by the sample size of included studies. However, they also used a fixed effects model in a sensitivity analysis. A subgroup analysis was conducted for the two study designs (cohort versus case-control), and publication bias was assessed. The researchers also examined the dose-response relationship between breastfeeding duration, when this information was provided, and ovarian cancer risk.

Key Findings: The pooled ovarian cancer incidence was 1.5% in women who breastfed, compared to 4.3% among women who did not. The overall *OR* for risk of ovarian cancer among women who breastfed was .66 (95% CI 0.57-0.76), as shown in a forest plot. This association was observed in both cohort and case-control studies. The analysts also found a significant association between breastfeeding duration and ovarian cancer risk. They found a sharp decrease in ovarian cancer risk when breastfeeding lasted 8-10 months. The researchers found no evidence of publication bias.

Discussion: The researchers concluded that their results support guidelines for breastfeeding duration of at least 6 months from the American College of Obstetricians and Gynecologists. They pointed out that such breastfeeding practices are not typical in most modern cultures.

Example 2: A Metasynthesis

Study: Parents' experiences and expectations of care in pregnancy after stillbirth or neonatal death: A metasynthesis (Mills et al., 2014)

Purpose: The purpose of the metasynthesis was to synthesize qualitative studies on parents' experiences of maternity care in pregnancy after stillbirth or neonatal death.

Eligibility Criteria: A study was included if it used a qualitative approach, was published in English, and described parents' care experiences in pregnancy after perinatal loss. The researchers placed no limits based on publication date, country of origin, or research tradition. Studies were excluded if they failed to meet a quality criterion.

Search Strategy: A systematic search strategy was developed during a preliminary scoping review. Search terms were formulated based on a PICO framework and supplementary methods. A search of several electronic databases was undertaken (CINAHL, MEDLINE, EMBASE, PsychInfo, British Nursing Index, and ProQuest). The researchers presented a figure that showed the details of their search strategy in CINAHL. The search was undertaken in December 2011 and repeated in March 2013. An ancestry search was also conducted, using the reference lists of eligible studies.

Quality Appraisal: The researchers used an existing quality appraisal tool that graded studies from A to D. Two authors did independent ratings. Studies with a grade of "D" were automatically excluded. Those graded "C" were discussed by the research team for possible inclusion.

Sample: The report presented a PRISMA-type flowchart showing the researchers' sampling decisions. Of the 991 studies initially identified by title, 174 abstracts were screened, and then 45 full papers were examined for eligibility. Some were rejected after full reading (22) or as a result of critical appraisal (9). In all, 14 papers were included in the analysis. Most studies focused primarily on women's experiences.

Data Analysis: The metasynthesis was based on Noblit and Hare's approach. Two reviewers independently read and reread each paper to identify and understand key concepts and themes. Initial findings were compared with analysis from previous papers and repeated across the 14 studies. Synthesis was completed in two phases. First, the researchers sought similarities in themes and concepts across the studies (reciprocal findings). Then they searched for any conflict in findings with the emerging theory (refutational analysis). Finally, the similarities and differences were drawn together to develop a line of argument.

Key Findings: Three main themes were identified: (1) co-existence of emotions, (2) helpful and unhelpful coping activities, and (3) seeking reassurance through interactions. Each of these main themes had several subthemes, which were summarized in a table that also showed the relevant studies for each subtheme. For example, for the first theme relating to emotions, there were three subthemes: profound ongoing grief and anxiety, isolation from friends and family, and maintaining hope.

Discussion: The reviewers concluded that their findings have important implications for professionals providing maternity care for families who have experienced perinatal bereavement. They encouraged efforts to develop interventions to reduce psychological morbidity in this population.

SUMMARY POINTS

- Evidence-based practice relies on rigorous integration of research evidence on a topic through systematic reviews. A **systematic review** methodically integrates research evidence about a specific research question using carefully developed sampling and data collection procedures that are spelled out in advanced in a protocol.
- Systematic reviews of quantitative studies often involve statistical integration of findings through **meta-analysis**, a procedure whose advantages include objectivity, enhanced power, and precision; meta-analysis is not appropriate, however, for broad questions or when there is substantial inconsistency of findings.
- The steps in both quantitative and qualitative integration are similar and involve formulating the problem, designing the study (including establishing sampling criteria), searching the literature for a sample of **primary studies**, evaluating study quality, extracting and encoding data for analysis, analyzing the data, and reporting the findings.
- There is no consensus on whether systematic reviews should include the **grey literature**—that is, unpublished reports. In quantitative studies, a concern is that there is a *bias against the null hypothesis*, a **publication bias** stemming from the underrepresentation of nonsignificant findings in the published literature.
- In meta-analysis, findings from primary studies are represented by an **effect size** index that quantifies the magnitude and direction of relationship between variables (e.g., an intervention and its outcomes). Three common effect size indexes in nursing are d (the **standardized mean difference**), the odds ratio, and Pearson's r.

- Effects from individual studies are pooled to yield an estimate of the population effect size by calculating a **weighted average** of effects, often using the **inverse variance** as the weight—which gives greater weight to larger studies.
- **Statistical heterogeneity** (diversity in effects across studies) affects decisions about using a **fixed effects model** (which assumes a single true effect size) or a **random effects model** (which assumes a distribution of effects). Heterogeneity can be examined using a **forest plot**.
- Nonrandom heterogeneity (moderating effects) can be explored through **subgroup analyses** or **meta-regression**, in which the purpose is to identify clinical or methodologic features systematically related to variation in effects.
- Quality assessments (which may involve formal ratings of overall methodologic rigor) are sometimes used to exclude weak studies from reviews, but they can also be used to differentially weight studies or in *sensitivity analyses* to test whether including or excluding weaker studies changes conclusions.
- **Metasyntheses** are more than just summaries of prior qualitative findings; they involve a discovery of essential features of a body of findings and, typically, a transformation that yields new insights and interpretations.
- Numerous approaches to metasynthesis (and many terms related to qualitative integration) have been proposed. Metasynthesis methods that have been used by nurse researchers include meta-ethnography, metastudy, metasummary, critical interpretive synthesis (CIS), grounded formal theory, and thematic synthesis.
- The various metasynthesis approaches have been classified on various *dimensions of difference*, including epistemologic stance, extent of iteration, and degree of "going beyond" the primary studies. Another system classifies approaches according to the degree to which theory building and theory explication are achieved.
- One approach to qualitative integration, **meta-ethnography**, as proposed by Noblit and Hare,

involves listing key themes or metaphors across studies and then reciprocally translating them into each other; *refutational* and *line of argument syntheses* are two other types.
- Paterson and colleagues' metastudy method integrates three components: (1) **metadata analysis**, the study of results in a specific substantive area through analysis of the "processed data"; (2) **metamethod**, the study of the studies' methodologic rigor; and (3) **metatheory**, the analysis of the theoretical underpinnings on which the studies are grounded.
- Sandelowski and Barroso distinguish qualitative findings in terms of whether they are *summaries* (descriptive synopses) or *syntheses* (interpretive explanations of the data). Both summaries and syntheses can be used in a **metasummary**, which can lay the foundation for a metasynthesis.
- A metasummary involves developing a list of abstracted findings from the primary studies and calculating **manifest effect sizes**. A **frequency effect size** is the percentage of studies in a sample of studies that contain a given findings. An **intensity effect size** indicates the percentage of all findings that are contained within any given report.
- In the Sandelowski and Barroso approach, only studies described as *syntheses* can be used in a metasynthesis, which can use a variety of qualitative approaches to analysis and interpretations (e.g., constant comparison).
- Mixed methods research has contributed to the emergence of **systematic mixed studies reviews**, which refer to systematic reviews that use disciplined procedures to integrate and synthesize findings from qualitative, quantitative, and mixed methods studies.
- An explicit reporting guideline called **PRISMA** (Preferred Reporting Items for Systematic reviews and Meta-Analyses) is useful for writing up a systematic review of RCTs, and another called **MOOSE** (Meta-analysis of Observational Studies in Epidemiology) guides reporting of meta-analyses of observational studies.

STUDY ACTIVITIES

Chapter 29 of the accompanying *Resource Manual for Nursing Research: Generating and Assessing Evidence for Nursing Practice, 10th edition*, offers various exercises and study suggestions for reinforcing the concepts taught in this chapter. In addition, the following study questions can be addressed:

1. Discuss the similarities and differences between the term "effect size" in qualitative and quantitative integration.
2. Apply relevant questions in Box 29.1 to one of the research examples at the end of the chapter, referring to the full journal article as necessary.

STUDIES CITED IN CHAPTER 29

*Agency for Healthcare Research and Quality. (2002). *Systems to rate the strength of scientific evidence*. Washington, DC: Author.

Arksey, H., & O'Malley, L. (2005). Scoping studies: Toward a methodologic framework. *International Journal of Social Research Methodology*, 8, 19–32.

*Atkins, S., Lewin, S., Smith, H., Engel, M., Fretheim, A., & Volmink, J. (2008). Conducting a meta-ethnography of qualitative literature: Lessons learnt. *BMC Medical Research Methodology*, 8, 21.

*Barnett-Page, E., & Thomas, J. (2009). Methods for the synthesis of qualitative research: A critical review. *BMC Medical Research Methodology*, 9, 59.

Barroso, J., Gollop, C., Sandelowski, M., Meynell, J., Pearce, P., & Collins, L. (2003). The challenges of searching for and retrieving qualitative studies. *Western Journal of Nursing Research*, 25, 153–178.

Beeckman, D., Van Lancker, A., Van Hecke, A., & Verhaeghe, S. (2014). A systematic review and meta-analysis of incontinence-associated dermatitis, incontinence, and moisture as risk factors for pressure ulcer development. *Research in Nursing & Health*, 37, 204–218.

Bench, S., & Day, T. (2010). The user experience of critical care discharge: A meta-synthesis of qualitative research. *International Journal of Nursing Studies*, 47, 487–499.

Borenstein, M., Hedges, L., Higgins, J., & Rothstein, H. (2009). *Introduction to meta-analysis*. Chichester, United Kingdom: John Wiley & Sons.

Bridges, J., Flatley, M., & Meyer, J. (2010). Older people's and relatives' experiences in acute care settings: Systematic review and synthesis of qualitative studies. *International Journal of Nursing Studies*, 47, 89–107.

Brown, S., Upchurch, S., & Acton, G. (2003). A framework for developing a coding scheme for meta-analysis. *Western Journal of Nursing Research*, 25, 205–222.

Bryanton, J., Beck, C. T., & Montelpare, W. (2013). Postnatal parental education for optimizing infant general health and parent-infant relationships. *Cochrane Database of Systematic Reviews*, (11), CD004068.

*Campbell, R., Pound, P., Morgan, M., Daker-White, G., Britten, N., Pill, R., . . . Donovan, J. (2011). Evaluating meta-ethnography: Systematic analysis and synthesis of qualitative research. *Health Technology Assessment*, 15, 1–164.

Chen, C. M., & Yeh, M. C. (2015). The experiences of diabetics on self-monitoring of blood glucose: A qualitative metasynthesis. *Journal of Clinical Nursing*, 24, 614–626.

Ciliska, D., & Guyatt, G. (2005). Publication bias. In A. Di Censo, G. Guyatt, & D. Ciliska (Eds.), *Evidence-based nursing: A guide to clinical practice* (pp. 373–380). St. Louis, MO: Elsevier Mosby.

*Conn, V., Phillips, L., Ruppar, T., & Chase, J. (2012). Physical activity interventions with healthy minority adults: Meta-analysis of behavior and health outcomes. *Journal of Health Care for the Poor and Underserved*, 23, 59–80.

Conn, V., Valentine, J., Cooper, H., & Rantz, M. (2003). Grey literature in meta-analyses. *Nursing Research*, 52, 256–261.

Cooke, A., Smith, D., & Booth, A. (2012). Beyond PICO: The SPIDER tool for qualitative evidence synthesis. *Qualitative Health Research*, 22, 1435–1443.

Cooper, H. (2010). *Research synthesis and meta-analysis: A step-by-step approach* (4th ed.). Thousand Oaks, CA: Sage.

*Dal Molin, A., Allara, E., Montani, D., Milani, S., Frassati, C., Cossu, S., . . . Rasero, L. (2014). Flushing the central venous catheter: Is heparin necessary? *The Journal of Vascular Access*, 15, 241–248.

*Daudt, H., van Mossel, C., & Scott, S. (2013). Enhancing the scoping study methodology: A large, inter-professional team's experience with Arksey and O'Malley's framework. *BMC Medical Research Methodology*, 13, 48.

Davis, K., Drey, N., & Gould, D. (2009). What are scoping studies? A review of the nursing literature. *International Journal of Nursing Studies*, 46, 1386–1400.

*Dixon-Woods, M., Cavers, D., Agarwal, S., Annandale, E., Arthur, A., Harvey, J., . . . Sutton, A. (2006). Conducting a critical interpretive synthesis of the literature on access to healthcare by vulnerable groups. *BMC Medical Research Methodology*, 6, 35.

*Dwan, K., Gamble, C., Williamson, P. R., Kirkham, J. J., & Reporting Bias Group. (2013). Systematic review of the empirical evidence of study publication bias and outcome reporting bias: An updated review. *PLoS ONE*, 8, e66844.

Eaves, Y. D. (2001). A synthesis technique for grounded theory data analysis. *Journal of Advanced Nursing*, 35, 654–663.

Fegran, L., Hall, E., Uhrenfeldt, L., Aagaard, H., & Ludvigsen, M. (2014). Adolescents' and young adults' transition experiences when transferring from paediatric to adult care:

A qualitative metasynthesis. *International Journal of Nursing Studies, 51*, 123–135.

Feng, L. P., Chen, H. L., & Shen, M. Y. (2014). Breastfeeding and the risk of ovarian cancer: A meta-analysis. *Journal of Midwifery & Women's Health, 59*, 428–437.

Finfgeld, D. (2003). Metasynthesis: The state of the art—So far. *Qualitative Health Research, 13*, 893–904.

Finfgeld-Connett, D. (2010). Generalizability and transferability of meta-synthesis research findings. *Journal of Advanced Nursing, 66*, 246–254.

Flemming, K. (2010). Synthesis of quantitative and qualitative research: An example using critical interpretive synthesis. *Journal of Advanced Nursing, 66*, 201–217.

*Fox, M. T., Persaud, M., Maimets, I., Brooks, D., O'Brien, K., & Tregunno, D. (2013). Effectiveness of early discharge planning in acutely ill or injured hospitalized older adults: A systematic review and meta-analysis. *BMC Geriatrics, 13*, 70.

Hannes, K., & Lockwood, C. (2012). *Synthesizing qualitative research: Choosing the right approach*. Chichester, United Kingdom: Wiley-Blackwell.

Hannes, K., Lockwood, C., & Pearson, A. (2010). A comparative analysis of three online appraisal instruments' ability to assess validity in qualitative research. *Qualitative Health Research, 20*, 1736–1743.

Hannes, K., & Macaitis, K. (2012). A move to more systematic and transparent approaches in qualitative evidence synthesis: Update on a review of published papers. *Qualitative Research, 12*, 402–442.

Harden, A., & Thomas, J. (2005). Methodological issues in combining diverse study types in systematic reviews. *International Journal of Social Research Methodology, 8*, 257–271.

Higgins, J., & Green, S. (Eds.). (2008). *Cochrane handbook for systematic reviews of interventions*. Chichester, United Kingdom: Wiley-Blackwell.

Jadad, A. R., Moore, R., Carroll, D., Jenkinson, C., Reynolds, D., Gavaghan, D., & McQuay, H. (1996). Assessing the quality of reports of randomized controlled trials. *Controlled Clinical Trials, 17*, 1–12.

*Langbecker, D., & Janda, M. (2015). Systematic review of interventions to improve the provision of information for adults with primary brain tumors and their caregivers. *Frontiers in Oncology, 5*, 1–11.

*Liberati, A., Altman, D., Tetzlaff, J., Mulrow, C., Gøtzsche, P., Ioannidis, J., . . . Moher, D. (2009). The PRISMA statement for reporting systematic reviews and meta-analyses of studies that evaluate health care interventions: Explanation and elaboration. *Journal of Clinical Epidemiology, 62*, e1–e34.

Lipsey, M. W., & Wilson, D. B. (2001). *Practical meta-analysis*. Thousand Oaks, CA: Sage.

*Lucas, P., Baird, J., Arai, L., Law, C., & Roberts, H. (2007). Worked examples of alternative methods for the synthesis of qualitative and quantitative research in systematic reviews. *BMC Medical Research Methodology, 7*, 4.

McCormick, J., Rodney, P., & Varcoe, C. (2003). Reinterpretations across studies: An approach to meta-analysis. *Qualitative Health Research, 13*, 933–944.

Mills, T. S., Ricklesford, C., Cooke, A., Heazell, A., Whitworth, M., & Lavender, T. (2014). Parents' experiences and expectations of care in pregnancy after stillbirth or neonatal death: A metasynthesis. *BJOG, 121*, 943–950.

*Mist, S. D., Firestone, K., & Jones, K. (2013). Complementary and alternative exercise for fibromyalgia. *Journal of Pain Research, 6*, 247–260.

*Moher, D., Liberati, A., Tetzlaff, J., & Altman, D. (2009). Preferred reporting items for systematic reviews and meta-analyses: The PRISMA statement. *BMJ, 339*, b2535.

Noblit, G., & Hare, R. D. (1988). *Meta-ethnography: Synthesizing qualitative studies*. Newbury Park, CA: Sage.

O'Rourke, H., Duggleby, W., Fraser, K., & Jerke, L. (2015). Factors that affect quality of life from the perspective of people with dementia: A metasynthesis. *Journal of the American Geriatrics Society, 63*, 24–38.

*Park, M., Katon, W., & Wolf, F. (2013). Depression and risk of mortality in individuals with diabetes: A meta-analysis and systematic review. *General Hospital Psychiatry, 35*, 217–225.

Paterson, B. L. (2001). The shifting perspectives model of chronic illness. *Journal of Nursing Scholarship, 33*, 57–62.

Paterson, B. (2007). Coming out as ill: Understanding self-disclosure in chronic illness from a meta-synthesis of qualitative research. In C. Webb & B. Roe (Eds.), *Reviewing research evidence for nursing practice* (pp. 73–83). Oxford, United Kingdom: Blackwell.

Paterson, B. (2012). It looks great but how do I know if it fits? An introduction to meta-synthesis research. In K. Hannes & C. Lockwood (Eds.), *Synthesizing qualitative research: Choosing the right approach* (pp. 1–20). Chichester, United Kingdom: Wiley-Blackwell.

Paterson, B. (2013). Metasynthesis. In C. T. Beck (Ed.), *Routledge international handbook of qualitative nursing research* (pp. 331–346). New York: Routledge.

Paterson, B. L., Thorne, S. E., Canam, C., & Jillings, C. (2001). *Meta-study of qualitative health research*. Thousand Oaks, CA: Sage.

Pluye, P., Gagnon, M., Griffiths, F., & Johnson-Lafleur, J. (2009). A scoring system for appraising mixed methods research, and concomitantly appraising qualitative, quantitative and mixed methods primary studies in mixed studies review. *International Journal of Nursing Studies, 46*, 529–546.

Polit, D. F., & Beck, C. T. (2010). Generalization in quantitative and qualitative research: Myths and strategies. *International Journal of Nursing Studies, 47*, 1451–1458.

Sandelowski, M., & Barroso, J. (2002). Finding the findings in qualitative studies. *Journal of Nursing Scholarship, 34*, 213–219.

Sandelowski, M., & Barroso, J. (2003a). Classifying the findings in qualitative studies. *Qualitative Health Research, 13*, 905–923.

Sandelowski, M., & Barroso, J. (2003b). Creating metasummaries of qualitative findings. *Nursing Research, 52*, 226–233.

Sandelowski, M., & Barroso, J. (2003c). Toward a metasynthesis of qualitative findings on motherhood in HIV-positive women. *Research in Nursing & Health, 26*, 153–170.

Sandelowski, M., & Barroso, J. (2007). *Handbook for synthesizing qualitative research.* New York: Springer.

Sandelowski, M., Docherty, S., & Emden, C. (1997). Qualitative metasynthesis: Issues and techniques. *Research in Nursing & Health, 20,* 365–377.

*Sandelowski, M., Voils, C., & Barroso, J. (2006). Defining and designing mixed research synthesis studies. *Research in the Schools, 13,* 29.

*Sandelowski, M., Voils, C., & Barroso, J. (2007). Comparability work and the management of difference in research synthesis studies. *Social Science and Medicine, 64,* 236–247.

Sandelowski, M., Voils, C. I., Crandell, J. L., & Leeman, J. (2013). Synthesizing qualitative and quantitative research findings. In C. T. Beck (Ed.), *Routledge international handbook of qualitative nursing research* (pp. 347–356). New York: Routledge.

*Sandelowski, M., Voils, C., Leeman, J., & Crandell, J. (2012). Mapping the mixed methods—Mixed research synthesis terrain. *Journal of Mixed Methods Research, 6,* 317–331.

Schreiber, R., Crooks, D., & Stern, P. N. (1997). Qualitative meta-analysis. In J. M. Morse (Ed.), *Completing a qualitative project* (pp. 311–326). Thousand Oaks, CA: Sage.

Shin, S., Park, J., & Kim, J. (2015). Effectiveness of patient simulation in nursing education: Meta-analysis. *Nurse Education Today, 35,* 176–182.

*Soininen, P., Putkonen, H., Joffe, G., Korkeila, J., & Välimäki, M. (2014). Methodological and ethical challenges in studying patients' perceptions of coercion: A systematic mixed studies review. *BMC Psychiatry, 14,* 162.

Stoltz, P., Skärsäter, I., & Willman, A. (2009). "Insufficient evidence of effectiveness" is not "evidence of no effectiveness": Evaluating computer-based education for patients with severe mental illness. *Worldviews of Evidence-Based Nursing, 6,* 190–199.

Stroup, D., Berlin J., Morton, S., Olkin, I., Williamson, G., Rennie, D., . . . Thacker, S. (2000). Meta-analysis of observational studies in epidemiology: A proposal for reporting. Meta-analysis Of Observational Studies in Epidemiology (MOOSE). *Journal of the American Medical Association, 283,* 208–2012.

*Thomas, J., & Harden, A. (2008). Methods for the thematic synthesis of qualitative research in systematic reviews. *BMC Medical Research Methodology, 8,* 45.

Thorne, S., Jensen, L., Kearney, M., Noblit, G., & Sandelowski, M. (2004). Qualitative metasynthesis: Reflections on methodologic orientation and ideological agenda. *Qualitative Health Research, 14,* 1342–1365.

*Toye, F., Seers, K., Allcock, N., Briggs, M., Carr, E., & Barker, K. (2014a). Meta-ethnography 25 years on: Challenges and insights for synthesizing a large number of qualitative studies. *BMC Medical Research Methodology, 14,* 80.

Toye, F., Seers, K., & Barker, K. (2014b). A meta-ethnography of patients' experiences of chronic pelvic pain: Struggling to construct chronic pain as "real." *Journal of Advanced Nursing, 70,* 2713–2727.

Varcoe, C., Rodney, P., & McCormick, J. (2003). Health care relationships in context: An analysis of three ethnographies. *Qualitative Health Research, 13,* 957–973.

*Voils, C., Hasselblad, V., Crandell, J., Chang, Y., Lee, E., & Sandelowski, M. (2009). A Bayesian method for the synthesis of evidence from qualitative and quantitative reports: The example of antiretroviral medication adherence. *Journal of Health Services Research & Policy, 14,* 226–233.

Wilczynski, N., Marks, S., & Haynes, R. (2007). Search strategies for identifying qualitative studies in CINAHL. *Qualitative Health Research, 17,* 705–710.

*Yost, J., Thompson, D., Ganann, R., Aloweni, F., Newman, K., McKibbon, A., . . . Ciliska, D. (2014). Knowledge translation strategies for enhancing nurses' evidence-informed decision making. *Worldviews on Evidence-Based Nursing, 11,* 156–167.

***A link to this open-access journal article is provided in the Toolkit for this chapter in the accompanying* Resource Manual.** ✹

30 Disseminating Evidence: Reporting Research Findings

No study is complete until the findings have been shared with other health professionals. This chapter offers assistance on disseminating research results. Further guidance is offered in several books devoted to the topic of publishing research findings (e.g., Lang, 2010; Oermann & Hays, 2011; Wager, 2010).

GETTING STARTED ON DISSEMINATION

Researchers must consider various issues in developing a dissemination plan, as we discuss in this section.

Selecting a Communication Medium and Outlet

Researchers who want to communicate their findings to others can present them orally or in writing. Oral presentations (typically at professional conferences) can be a formal talk in front of an audience or integrated with visual material in a *poster session*. Major advantages of conference presentations are that they can be done soon after study completion (or even while it is in progress) and offer opportunities for dialogue among people interested in the same topic. Written reports, in addition to theses or dissertations, can take the form of journal articles published in traditional or open-access professional journals. A major advantage of journal articles,

especially ones that are open-access, is worldwide accessibility. Most of our advice in this chapter is relevant for most types of dissemination, but publication in journals is featured.

Knowing the Audience

Good research communication depends on providing information that can be understood, so researchers should think about the audience they are hoping to reach. Here are some questions to consider:

1. Will the audience be nurses only, or will it include professionals from other disciplines (e.g., physicians, psychologists, physical therapists)?
2. Will the audience be researchers, or will it include other professionals (clinicians, health care policy makers)?
3. Are clients (lay people) a possible audience?
4. Will the audience include people whose native language is not English?
5. Will reviewers, editors, and readers be experts in the field?

Researchers often have to write with multiple audiences in mind, which means writing clearly and avoiding technical jargon to the extent possible. It also means that researchers sometimes must develop a multipronged strategy—for example, publishing a report for nurse researchers in a journal such *Nursing Research* and then publishing a summary for clinicians in a publication of a specialty organization.

→ **TIP:** Oermann and colleagues (2006) provide some suggestions about presenting research results to clinical audiences.

Although writing for a broad audience may be a goal, it is also important to keep in mind the needs of the *main* intended audience. If consumers of a report are mostly clinical nurses, it is essential to emphasize what the findings mean for practice. If the audience is administrators or policy makers, explicit information should be included about how the findings relate to such outcomes as *cost* and *accessibility*. If other researchers are the primary audience, explicit information about methods, study limitations, and implications for future research is important.

Developing a Plan

Before preparing a report, researchers should have a plan. Part of that plan involves how best to coordinate the actual tasks of preparing a **manuscript** (i.e., an unpublished paper).

Deciding on Authorship

When a study has been completed by a team, division of labor and authorship must be addressed. The International Committee of Medical Journal Editors (ICMJE, 2013) advised that authorship credit should be based on (1) having made a substantial contribution to the study's conception and design, or to data acquisition, data analysis, and interpretation; (2) drafting or revising the manuscript critically for intellectual content; (3) approving the final version of the manuscript to be published; and (4) agreeing to be accountable for all aspects of the work.

The **lead author**, usually the first named author, has overall responsibility for the report. The lead author and coauthors should reach an agreement in advance about responsibilities for producing the manuscript. To avoid possible subsequent conflicts, they should also decide beforehand the order of authors' names. Ethically, it is most appropriate to list names in the order of authors' contribution to the work, not according to status. When contributions of coauthors are comparable, an alphabetical listing

is appropriate. The editorial board of the *Western Journal of Nursing Research* has prepared some guidelines for coauthorship (Conn et al., 2015), as has the editor of *Research in Nursing & Health* (Kearney, 2014).

Deciding on Content

In many studies, more data are collected than can be presented in one report, and multiple publications are thus possible. In such situations, an early decision involves what part of the findings to present in a given paper. If there are multiple research questions, more than one paper may be required to communicate results adequately. In mixed methods research, separate reports are sometimes needed to summarize qualitative and quantitative findings.

It is, however, inappropriate and even unethical to write several papers when one would suffice—a practice that has been called "salami slicing" (Baggs, 2008; Jackson et al., 2014). Each paper from a study should make an independent contribution. Editors, reviewers, and readers expect original work, so unnecessary overlap should be avoided. It is also unethical to submit essentially the same or similar paper to two journals simultaneously. Oermann and Hays (2011) offer guidelines regarding duplicate and redundant publications.

Assembling Materials

Planning also involves assembling materials needed to begin a draft, including information about manuscript requirements. Traditional and online journals issue guidelines for authors, and these guidelines should be retrieved and understood.

Other materials also need to assembled, including copies of the relevant literature, details about instruments used in the study, descriptions of the study sample, output of computer analyses, relevant analytic memos or reflexive notes, figures or photographs that illustrate some aspect of the study, and permissions to use copyrighted materials. Other important tools are style manuals that provide information about both grammar and language use (e.g., Strunk & White, 2014) as well as more specific information about writing professional and scientific papers (e.g., American Psychological Association, 2010; ICMJE, 2013).

⮕ TIP: For authors whose native language is not English but who plan to submit their work to an English-language journal, a review of the article by someone proficient in English is advisable. For authors from developing countries, assistance may be available through AuthorAID (http://www.authoraid.info/en/).

Finally, a written outline and a timeline should be developed, especially if there are multiple coauthors who have responsibility for different sections of the paper. The overall outline and individual assignments, together with due dates, should be developed collaboratively.

Writing Effectively

Many people have a hard time putting their ideas down on paper. It is beyond the scope of this book to teach good writing skills, but we can offer a few suggestions. One suggestion, quite simply is: *Do it*. Get in the habit of writing, even if it is only 15 minutes a day. *Writer's block* is probably responsible for thousands of unfinished (or never-started) manuscripts each year. So, just begin somewhere, and keep at it regularly—writing gets easier with practice.

Writing *well* is, of course, important, and several resources offer suggestions on how to write compelling sentences, select good words, and organize your ideas effectively (e.g., Zinsser, 2006). It is usually better to write a draft in its entirety and then go back later to rewrite awkward sentences, correct errors, reorganize, and generally polish it up.

In a survey of 63 nursing journal editors, Northam and colleagues (2010) found that the single most common reason for rejecting a manuscript was that it was poorly written. A frequently mentioned suggestion by these editors was to have others review the manuscript—and even to read it out loud to someone to see if it is understood.

⮕ TIP: It should go without saying that plagiarism should always be avoided. In some cases, this means not even "plagiarizing" yourself. Most journals now have powerful plagiarism detection software that will trigger an editorial response,

and in some cases, you may be asked to rewrite sentences that you "lifted" from your own prior publication.

CONTENT OF RESEARCH REPORTS

Research reports vary in terms of audience, purpose, and length. Theses or dissertations not only communicate research results but also document students' ability to perform scholarly work and therefore tend to be long. Journal articles, by contrast, are short because they compete for limited journal space and are read by busy professionals. Nevertheless, the general form and content of research reports are often similar. Chapter 3 summarized the content of major sections of research reports, and here we offer a few additional tips. Distinctions among various kinds of reports are described later in the chapter.

Quantitative Research Reports

Quantitative reports typically follow the **IMRAD format**, which involves organizing content into four sections—the **I**ntroduction, **M**ethod, **R**esults, **and D**iscussion. These sections, respectively, address the following questions:

* Why was the study done? (I)
* How was the study done? (M)
* What was learned? (R)
* What does it mean? (D)

The Introduction

The introduction acquaints readers with the research problem, its significance, and its context. The introduction sets the stage by describing existing literature, the study's conceptual framework, the problem, research questions, or hypotheses, and the study rationale. Although the introduction includes multiple components, it should be concise. A common critique of research manuscripts by reviewers is that the introduction is too long.

Introductions are often written in a funnel-shaped structure, beginning broadly to establish a framework for understanding the study and then narrowing to the specifics of what researchers sought to learn. The end point of the introduction should be a concise delineation of the research questions or hypotheses, which provides a good transition to the method section.

> **TIP:** An up-front, clearly stated problem statement is of immense value. The first paragraph should be written with special care because the goal is to grab readers' attention.

The introduction typically includes a summary of related research to provide a pertinent context. Except for dissertations, the literature review should be a brief summary, not an exhaustive review. The review should make clear what is already known, and what the deficiencies are, thus helping to clarify the contribution of the new study.

The introduction also should describe the study's theoretical or conceptual framework. The framework should be sufficiently explained so that readers who are unfamiliar with it can understand its main thrust. The introduction should include conceptual definitions of the concepts under investigation.

The various background strands need to be convincingly and cogently interwoven to persuade readers that, in fact, the new study holds promise for adding to evidence for nursing. The introduction, in other words, lays out the *argument* for new research.

> **TIP:** Many journal articles begin without an explicit heading labeled *Introduction*. In general, all the material before the method section is considered to be the introduction. Some introductions include subheadings such as *Literature Review* or *Hypotheses*.

The Method Section

To evaluate the quality of a study's evidence, readers need to know exactly what methods were used to address the research problem. In traditional dissertations, the method section should provide sufficient detail that another researcher could replicate the study. In journal articles and conference presen-

tations, the method section is condensed, but the degree of detail should permit readers to draw conclusions about the integrity of the findings. Faulty method sections are a leading cause of manuscript rejection by research journals. Your job in writing the method section of a quantitative report is to persuade readers that evidence from your study has sufficient validity to merit consideration.

> **TIP:** The method section is often subdivided into several parts, which helps readers to locate vital information. As an example, the method section might contain the following subsections: Research Design, Sample and Setting, Data Collection Instruments, Procedures, and Data Analysis.

The method section usually begins with the description of the research design and its rationale. The design is often given detailed coverage in clinical trials, with information about what specific design was adopted, how subjects were assigned to groups, and whether (and with whom) blinding was used. Reports for studies with multiple points of data collection should indicate the number of times data were collected and the amount of time elapsed between those points. In all types of quantitative studies, it is important to identify steps taken to control the research situation in general and confounding variables in particular. The method section also describes the steps taken to protect the rights of study participants.

Readers also need to know about study participants. This subsection (which may be labeled *Research Sample*, *Subjects*, or *Study Participants*) normally includes a list of eligibility criteria to clarify the population to whom results can be generalized. The method of sample selection and its rationale, recruitment techniques, and sample size should be indicated so readers can determine how representative subjects are of the target population. If a power analysis was undertaken to estimate sample size needs, this should be described. There should also be information about response rates and, if possible, about response bias (or attrition bias, if this is relevant). Basic characteristics of study participants (e.g., age, gender, health status) should also be described—although this is sometimes presented in the results section.

Data collection methods are another critical component of the method section and may be presented in a subsection labeled *Instruments*, *Measures*, or *Data Collection*. A description of study instruments, and a rationale for their use, should be provided. If instruments were constructed specifically for the project, the report should describe their development. Any special equipment that was used (e.g., to gather biophysiologic or observational data) should be described, including information about the manufacturer. The report should also indicate who collected the data (e.g., the authors, research assistants, staff nurses) and how they were trained. The report must also convince readers that the data collection methods were sound. Any information relating to data quality, and the procedures used to evaluate that quality, should be described.

In intervention research, there is usually a procedures subsection that includes information about the intervention. What exactly did the intervention entail? How was the intervention theory translated into components? How and by whom was the treatment administered, and how were they trained? What was the control group condition? How much time elapsed between the intervention and the measurement of the dependent variable? How was intervention fidelity monitored?

Analytic procedures are also described in the method section. It is usually sufficient to identify the statistical tests used; formulas or references for commonly used statistics such as analysis of variance are not necessary. For unusual procedures, or unusual applications of a common procedure, a technical reference justifying the approach should be noted. If confounding variables were controlled statistically, the specific variables controlled should be mentioned. The level of significance is typically set at .05 for two-tailed tests, which may or may not be explicitly stated; however, if a different significance level or one-tailed tests were used, this must be specified.

A recent development is that there are now explicit guidelines for reporting methodologic information for various types of studies, as shown in Table 30.1. The most well-known is the Consolidated Standards of Reporting Trials or **CONSORT guidelines**. These guidelines focus on reporting information about RCTs, and extensions have been developed for particular designs, such as cluster randomized trials. The CONSORT guidelines have been adopted by most major medical and nursing journals. The 2010 CONSORT guidelines include a checklist of 25 items to include in reports of RCTs (Moher et al., 2010).

The CONSORT guidelines, as well as other guidelines, recommend inclusion of a flowchart to track participants through a study, from eligibility screening through analysis of outcomes. Flowcharts should be as detailed as possible, within space constraints, about reasons for loss of subjects during the study. Figure 30.1 provides an example of such a flowchart for a randomized controlled trial (RCT). This chart summarizes withdrawals from the intervention as well as loss of participants during follow-up. It also shows that data for all subjects were analyzed in an intention-to-treat analysis, which is recommended in CONSORT (Polit & Gillespie, 2010).

Guidelines for various types of studies are regularly being updated or expanded. The EQUATOR Network (http://www.equator-network.org) is a useful resource for information on reporting guidelines and for tips on good reporting in health studies.

> **TIP:** The CONSORT 2010 checklist is included in the Toolkit of the *Resource Manual* that accompanies this book. Further information about the CONSORT guidelines is available at http://www.consort-statement.org, which includes an interactive checklist with detailed information about components in the checklist.

In response to commentaries regarding inadequacies in reporting details about intervention features (e.g., Conn et al., 2008; Glasziou et al., 2008), several relevant guidelines have emerged. The **CReDECI** guidelines (Möhler et al., 2012, 2015) offer criteria for reporting the phases researchers have undertaken in the development, piloting, and evaluation of complex interventions. CReDECI is useful for providing information about the *processes* of intervention research. The **TIDieR** guidelines (Hoffmann et al., 2014) offer a template

TABLE 30.1 • Reporting Guidelines for Various Types of Papers

TYPE OF STUDY	GUIDELINE
Parallel group randomized controlled trials (RCTs)	CONSORT: Consolidated Standards of Reporting Trials (Moher et al., 2010)
Pragmatic trials	CONSORT extension for pragmatic trials (Zwarenstein et al., 2008)
Trials of nonpharmacalogic interventions	CONSORT extension for nonpharmacologic treatments (Boutron et al., 2008)
Cluster randomized trials	CONSORT extension for cluster randomized trials (Campbell et al., 2012)
Noninferiority and equivalence trials	CONSORT extension for noninferiority and equivalence trials (Piaggio et al., 2012)
Processes of intervention research	CReDECI: Criteria for Reporting the Development and Evaluation of Complex Interventions (Möhler et al., 2012)
Features of an intervention	TIDieR: Template for Intervention Description and Replication (Hoffman et al., 2014)
Nonexperimental (observational) studies	STROBE: Strengthening the Reporting of Observational Studies in Epidemiology (von Elm et al., 2014)
Qualitative studies (focus groups and interview studies)	COREQ: Consolidated Criteria for Reporting Qualitative Research (Tong et al., 2007)
Meta-analyses of RCTs	PRISMA: Preferred Reporting Items for Systematic Reviews and Meta-Analyses (Moher et al., 2009)
Meta-analyses of non-RCTs	MOOSE: Meta-analysis of Observational Studies in Epidemiology (Stroup et al., 2000)
Synthesis of qualitative research	ENTREQ: Enhancing transparency in reporting the synthesis of qualitative research (Tong et al., 2012)
Studies of measurement reliability and agreement	GRRAS: Guidelines for Reporting Reliability and Agreement Studies (Kottner et al., 2011)
Diagnostic accuracy studies	STARD: Standards for Reporting of Diagnostic Accuracy (Bossuyt et al., 2004)
Health care quality improvement studies	SQUIRE: Standards for Quality Improvement Reporting Excellence (Ogrinc et al., 2008)
Evaluations of interventions using quasi-experimental designs	TREND: Transparent Reporting of Evaluations with Nonrandomized Designs (Des Jarlais et al., 2004)
Statistical reporting	SAMPL: Statistical Analysis and Methods in the Published Literature (Lang & Altman, 2013)
Clinical trial protocols	SPIRIT: Standard Protocol Items—Recommendations for Interventional Trials (Chan et al., 2013)

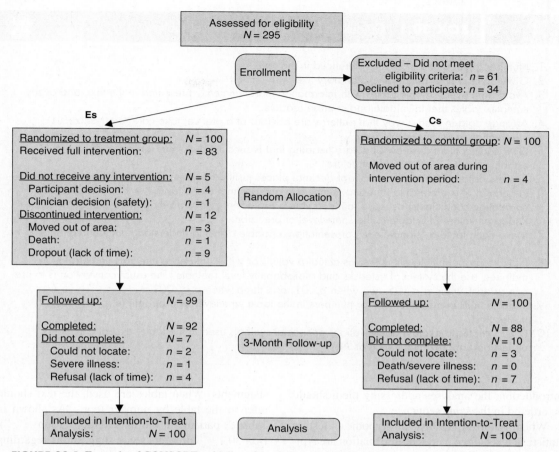

FIGURE 30.1 Example of CONSORT guidelines flowchart: progression of participants in an intervention study.

for a thorough description of interventions. Key elements of an intervention should always be summarized in a report of a trial, but a separate article describing the intervention in greater detail might be needed. Additional guidance on reporting on interventions is available in Mayo-Wilson et al. (2013) and Michie et al. (2013).

> **TIP:** An extension of the CONSORT reporting guidelines specific to pilot and feasibility studies is under development, but details were not available when this book went to press (Dolgin, 2013). The EQUATOR Network should be consulted for further updates.

The Results Section

Readers scrutinize the method section to know if the study was done with rigor, but the results section is the heart of the report. In a quantitative study, the results of the statistical analyses are summarized in a factual manner. Descriptive statistics are ordinarily presented first to provide an overview of study variables. If key research questions involve comparing groups with regard to dependent variables (e.g., in an experimental or case-control study), the results section often begins with information about the groups' comparability on baseline variables, so readers can evaluate selection bias.

Research results are usually ordered in terms of overall importance. If, however, research questions or hypotheses have been numbered in the

BOX 30.1 Guidelines for Preparing Statistical Tables

1. Number tables so they can be referenced in the text.
2. Give tables a brief but clear explanatory title.
3. Avoid both overly simple tables with information more efficiently presented in the text, and overly complex tables that intimidate and confuse readers.
4. Arrange data in such a way that patterns are obvious at a glance; take care to organize information in an intelligible way.
5. Give each column and row of data a heading that is succinct but clear; table headings should establish the logic of the table structure.
6. Express data values to the number of decimal places justified by the precision of the measurement. In general, it is preferable to report numbers to one decimal place (or to two decimal places for correlation coefficients) because rounded values are easier to absorb than more precise ones. Report all values in a table to the same level of precision.
7. Make each table a "stand-alone" presentation, capable of being understood without reference to the text.
8. Indicate probability levels, either as actual p values or with confidence intervals. In correlation matrixes, use the system of asterisks and a probability level footnote. The usual convention is to use one asterisk when $p < .05$, two when p, .01, and three when $p < .001$.
9. Indicate units of measurement for numbers in the table whenever appropriate (e.g., pounds, milligrams).
10. Use footnotes to explain abbreviations or special symbols used in the table, except commonly understood abbreviations such as N.

introduction, the analyses addressing them should be ordered in the same sequence.

When reporting results of hypothesis-testing statistical tests, three pieces of information are typically reported: the value of the calculated statistic, degrees of freedom, and the exact probability level. For instance, it might be stated, "Patients who were exposed to the intervention were significantly less likely to develop decubitus ulcers than patients in the control group ($\chi^2 = 8.23$, $df = 1$, $p = .008$)." However, the current publication manual of the American Psychological Association (2010) urges authors to report confidence intervals: "Because confidence intervals combine information on location and precision and can often be directly used to infer significance levels, they are, in general, the best reporting strategy" (p. 34). The manual also strongly encourages reporting effect sizes, which can facilitate meta-analyses.

When results from several statistical analyses are reported, they should be summarized in a **table**. Good tables, with precise headings, titles, and notes, are an important way to avoid dull, repetitious

statements. When tables are used, the text should refer to the table by number (e.g., "As shown in Table 2, patients in the intervention group . . . "). Box 30.1 ⊗ presents some suggestions regarding the construction of effective statistical tables, and the table templates in the Toolkit (Chapters 16–18) can help you create clear and concise tables. ⊗

➲ **TIP:** Do not simply repeat statistical information in text and tables. Tables should display information that would be monotonous to present in the text—and to display it in such a way that patterns among the numbers are more evident. The text can be used to highlight major findings.

Figures may also be used to summarize results. Figures that display the results in graphic form are used less as an economy than as a means of dramatizing important findings and relationships. Figures are especially helpful for displaying information on some phenomenon over time or for portraying conceptual or empirical models.

TIP: Research evidence does not constitute *proof* of anything, and so the report should never claim that the data proved, verified, confirmed, or demonstrated that hypotheses were correct or incorrect. Hypotheses are supported or unsupported, accepted or rejected.

The Discussion Section

The meaning that researchers give to the results plays an important role in reports. The discussion section is devoted to a thoughtful (and, it is hoped, insightful) analysis of the findings, leading to a discussion of their clinical and theoretical utility. A typical discussion section addresses the following questions: What were the main findings? What do the findings mean? What evidence is there that the results and the interpretations are valid? What limitations might threaten validity? How do the results compare with prior knowledge on the topic? What are the implications of the findings for future research? What are the implications for nursing practice?

TIP: The discussion is typically the most challenging section to write. It deserves your most intense intellectual effort—and careful review by peers. Peers should be asked to comment on how persuasive your arguments are, how well organized the section is, and whether it is too long, which is a common flaw.

Typically, the discussion section begins with a summary of key findings. The summary should be brief, however, because the focus of the discussion is on making sense of (and not merely repeating) the results.

Interpretation of results is a global process, encompassing the findings, methodologic strengths and limitations, sample characteristics, related research findings, clinical aspects, and theoretical issues. Researchers should justify their interpretations, explicitly stating why alternative explanations have been ruled out. Unsupported conclusions are among the most common problems in discussion sections. If the findings conflict with those of

earlier studies, tentative explanations should be offered. A discussion of the generalizability of study findings should also be included.

Implications of study findings are speculative and so should be couched in tentative terms, as in the following example: "The results *suggest* that nurses' communication about advanced directives is inconsistent, and that nurses' years of experience affect the nature and amount of communication." The interpretation is, in essence, a hypothesis that can be tested in another study. The discussion should include recommendations for research to test such hypotheses.

Finally, and importantly, implications of the findings for nursing practice need to be discussed. What aspects of the evidence are clinically significant, and how might the evidence be put to use by nurses? The importance of adequately addressing nursing implications has been discussed by the editors of several nursing journals (Becker, 2009; Gennaro, 2010).

Other Aspects of the Report

The materials covered in the four major IMRAD sections are found in some form in most quantitative research reports. In addition to these major divisions, other aspects of the report deserve mention.

Title. Every research report needs a title indicating the nature of the study. Insofar as possible, the dependent and independent variables (or central constructs under study) should be named in the title. It is also desirable to indicate the study population. Yet, the title should be brief (no more than about 15 words), so writers must balance clarity with brevity. The length of titles can often be reduced by omitting unnecessary terms such as "A Study of . . .," "Report of . . . ," or "An Investigation to Examine the Effects of . . . ," and so forth. The title should communicate concisely what was studied and stimulate interest in the research. A few journals, however, such as the *International Journal of Nursing Studies* (*IJNS*), request that the basic method or design be stated in the title, often indicated after a colon. For example, Mak and colleagues (2015) published a paper in *IJNS* entitled "Pressurised irrigation versus swabbing method in cleansing wounds healed by secondary intention: A randomised controlled trial with cost-effectiveness analysis." Thus, it is always important to review journal guidelines and requirements before finalizing a manuscript.

Abstract. Research reports usually include an abstract—brief descriptions of the problem, methods, and findings of the study, written so readers can decide whether to read the entire report. As noted in Chapter 3, journal abstracts are sometimes written as an unstructured paragraph of 100 to 200 words or in a structured form with subheadings. Weinert (2010) has offered tips on writing "strong, convincing" abstracts.

> **TIP:** Take the time to write a compelling abstract, which is your first main point of contact with reviewers and readers. It should demonstrate that your study is important clinically and that it was done with conceptual and methodologic rigor. It should also contain words that will help people find your paper if they search for articles on your topic.

Keywords. It is often necessary to include keywords that will be used in indexes to help others locate your study. Sometimes authors are given a list of keywords from which to choose (often Medical Subject Headings or MeSH terms), but additional keywords can often be added. Substantive, methodologic, and theoretical terms can be used as keywords.

References. Each report concludes with a list of references cited in the text, using a reference style specified in the journal's guidelines. References can be cumbersome to prepare, but software is available to facilitate the preparation of reference lists (e.g., EndNote, ProCite, Reference Manager, Format Ease).

Acknowledgments. People who helped with the research but whose contribution does not qualify them for authorship can be acknowledged in the report. This might include statistical consultants, data collectors, or people who reviewed the manuscript. Acknowledgments should also give credit to organizations that made the project possible, such as funding agencies or organizations that helped with subject recruitment.

Checklist. A few journals, such as the *International Journal of Nursing Studies*, require the completion of an author checklist that obliges authors to state their compliance with various conditions, such as total word count, declaration of keywords, and so on.

> **TIP:** Some specific advice about writing an article about pilot intervention studies is provided in the Supplement to this chapter on thePoint®.

Qualitative Research Reports

There is no single style for reporting qualitative findings, but qualitative research reports often follow the IMRAD format, or something akin to it. Thus, we present some issues of particular relevance for writing qualitative reports within the IMRAD structure.

Introduction

Qualitative reports usually begin with a problem statement, in a similar fashion to quantitative reports, but the focus is on the phenomenon under study. The way in which the problem is expressed and the types of questions the researchers sought to answer are usually tied to the research tradition underlying the study (e.g., grounded theory, ethnography), which is usually explicitly stated in the introduction. Prior research on the phenomenon under study may be summarized in the introduction but is sometimes described in the discussion section.

In many qualitative studies, but especially in ethnographic ones, it is critical to explain the study's cultural or social context. For studies with an ideologic orientation (e.g., critical theory or feminist research), it is also important to describe the sociopolitical context. For studies using phenomenologic or grounded theory designs, the philosophy of phenomenology or symbolic interaction, respectively, may be described.

As another aspect of explaining the study's background, qualitative researchers sometimes provide information about relevant personal experiences or qualifications. If a researcher who is studying decisions about long-term care placements is caring for two elderly parents and participates in a care-giver support group, this is relevant for readers' understanding of the study. In descriptive phenomenologic studies, researchers may discuss their personal experiences in relation to the phenomenon being studied to communicate what they bracketed.

The concluding paragraph of the introduction usually offers a summary of the purpose of the study or the research questions.

Method

Although the research tradition of the study is often noted in the introduction, the method section usually elaborates on specific methods used in conjunction with that tradition. Design features such as whether the study was longitudinal should also be noted.

The method section should provide a good description of the research setting, so that readers can assess transferability of findings. Study participants and methods by which they were selected should also be described. Even when samples are small, it is often useful to provide a table summarizing participants' key characteristics. If researchers have a personal connection to participants or to groups with which they are affiliated, this connection should be noted. At times, to disguise a group or institution, it may be necessary to omit or modify potentially identifying information.

Qualitative reports usually cannot provide much specific information about data collection, but some researchers provide a sample of questions, especially if a topic guide was used. The description of data collection methods should include how data were collected (e.g., interview or observation), who collected the data, how data collectors were trained, and what methods were used to record the data.

Information about quality and integrity is particularly important in qualitative studies. The more information included in the report about steps researchers took to ensure the trustworthiness of the data, the more confident readers can be that the findings are credible.

Quantitative reports typically have only brief descriptions of data analysis techniques because standard statistical procedures are widely understood.

By contrast, analytic procedures are often described in some detail in qualitative reports because readers need to understand how researchers organized, synthesized, and made sense of their data.

Results

In their results sections, qualitative researchers summarize their themes, categories, taxonomic structure, or the theory that emerged. The results section can be organized in a number of ways. For example, if a process is being described, results may be presented chronologically, corresponding to the unfolding of the process. Key themes, metaphors, or domains are often used as subheadings, organized in order of salience to participants or to a theory.

Example of Organization of Qualitative Results: Kirk and colleagues (2014) used feminist post-structuralism as the guiding framework in their study of the management of obesity. They found three themes in their analysis of data from 42 interviews with people with obesity and health care practitioners: (1) blame as a devastating relation of power, (2) tensions in obesity management and prevention, and (3) the prevailing medical management discourse. These themes were used as subheadings to organize the results section.

Sandelowski (1998) emphasized the importance of developing a story line before beginning to write the findings. Because of the richness of qualitative data, researchers have to decide which story, or how much of it, they want to tell. They must also decide how best to balance description and interpretation. The results section in a qualitative paper, unlike that in a quantitative one, intertwines data and interpretations of those data. It is important, however, to give sufficient emphasis to the voices, actions, and experiences of participants themselves so that readers can gain an appreciation of their lives and their worlds. Most often, this occurs through the inclusion of direct quotes to illustrate important points. Because of space constraints in journals, quotes cannot be extensive, and great care must be exercised in selecting the best possible exemplars. Gilgun (2005) offered guidance in writing up the results of qualitative research in a manner that has "grab."

TIP: Using quotes is not only a skill but also a complex process. When inserting quotes in the results section, pay attention to how the quote is introduced and how it is put in context. Quotes should not be used haphazardly or listed one after the other in a string.

Figures, diagrams, and word tables that organize concepts are often useful in summarizing an overall conceptualization of the phenomena under study. Grounded theory studies are especially likely to benefit from a schematic presentation of the basic social process. Ethnographers sometimes present taxonomies in tabular form.

Discussion

In qualitative studies, findings and interpretation are typically interwoven in the results section because the task of integrating qualitative materials is essentially interpretive. The discussion section of a qualitative report, therefore, is not so much designed to give meaning to the results but to summarize them, link them to other research, and suggest their implications for theory, research, or nursing practice.

Other Aspects of a Qualitative Report

Qualitative reports, like quantitative ones, include abstracts, keywords, references, and acknowledgments. Abstracts for journals that feature qualitative reports (e.g., *Qualitative Health Research*) tend to be the traditional (single-paragraph) type rather than structured abstracts.

The titles of qualitative reports usually state the central phenomenon under scrutiny. Phenomenologic studies often have titles that include such words as "the lived experience of . . . " or "the meaning of . . . " Grounded theory studies often indicate something about the *findings* in the title—for example, mentioning the core category or basic social process. Ethnographic titles usually indicate the culture being studied. Two-part titles are not uncommon, with substance and method, research tradition and findings, or theme and meaning separated by a colon. For example, Cognet and Coyer (2014) published a qualitative study with

this title: "Discharge practices for the intensive care patient: A qualitative exploration in the general ward setting."

TIP: Preparing a report for a mixed methods (MM) study has challenges of its own. Creswell and Plano Clark (2011) offer useful guidance for writing up integrated MM reports.

THE STYLE OF RESEARCH REPORTS

Research reports, especially for quantitative studies, are written in a distinctive style. Some style issues were discussed previously, but additional points are elaborated here.

A research report is not an essay. It is an account of how and why a problem was studied and what was discovered as a result. The report should not include overtly subjective statements, emotionally laden statements, or exaggerations. This is not to say that the research story should be told in a dreary manner. Indeed, in qualitative reports, there are ample opportunities to enliven the narration with rich description, direct quotes, and insightful interpretation. Authors of quantitative reports, although somewhat constrained by structure and the need to include numeric information, should strive to keep the presentation lively.

Quantitative researchers often avoid personal pronouns such as "I," "my," and "we" because impersonal pronouns, and use of the passive voice, may suggest greater impartiality. Qualitative reports, by contrast, are sometimes written in the first person and in an active voice. Even among quantitative researchers, however, there is a trend toward striking a greater balance between active and passive voice. If a direct presentation can be made without suggesting bias, a more readable product usually results.

It is not easy to write simply and clearly, but these are important goals of scientific writing. The use of technical jargon does little to enhance the communicative value of the report and should especially be avoided in conveying findings to practicing nurses. The style should be concise and straightforward.

If writers can add elegance to their reports without interfering with clarity and accuracy, so much the better, but the product is not expected to be a literary achievement.

A common flaw in reports of novice researchers is inadequate organization. The overall structure is fairly standard, but organization within sections and subsections also needs attention. Sequences should be in an orderly progression with appropriate transitions. Continuity and logical thematic development are critical to good communication.

It may seem a trivial point, but methods and results should be described in the past tense. For example, it is inappropriate to say, "Nurses who receive special training perform triage functions significantly better than those without training." In this sentence, "receive" and "perform" should be changed to "received" and "performed" to reflect the fact that the statement pertains only to a particular sample whose behavior was observed in the past.

TYPES OF RESEARCH REPORTS

This section describes features of several major kinds of research reports: theses and dissertations, traditional or online journal articles, and presentations at professional meetings. Reports for class projects are excluded—not because they are unimportant but rather because they so closely resemble theses on a smaller scale.

Theses and Dissertations

Most doctoral degrees, and some master's degrees, are granted on the successful completion of a research project. Most universities have a preferred format for their dissertations. Until recently, most schools used a traditional IMRAD format. The following organization for a traditional dissertation is typical:

- Front Matter: Title Page, Abstract, Copyright Page, Approval Page, Acknowledgment Page, Table of Contents, List of Tables, List of Figures, List of Appendices

- Main Body: Chapter I. Introduction, Chapter II. Review of the Literature, Chapter III. Methods, Chapter IV. Results, Chapter V. Discussion and Summary
- Supplementary Pages: Bibliography, Appendices, Curriculum Vitae

The **front matter** (preliminary pages) for dissertations are much the same as those for a scholarly book. The title page indicates such information as the title of the study, the author's name, the degree requirement being fulfilled, and the name of the university awarding the degree. The acknowledgment page gives writers the opportunity to thank those who contributed to the project. The table of contents outlines major sections and subsections of the report, indicating on which page readers will find sections of interest. The lists of tables and figures identify by number, title, and page the tabular and graphic material in the text.

The main body of a traditionally formatted dissertation incorporates the IMRAD sections described earlier. The literature review often is so extensive that a separate chapter may be devoted to it. When a short review is sufficient, the first two chapters may be combined. In some cases, a separate chapter may also be required to elaborate the study's conceptual framework.

> **➔ TIP:** In some traditional dissertations, the early chapters describe students' intellectual journey, including a description of the paths they took and decisions they made in selecting their final research question and methodology.

The supplementary pages include a bibliography or list of references used to prepare the report and one or more appendixes. An appendix contains materials relevant to the study that are either too lengthy or too tangential to be incorporated into the body of the report. Data collection instruments, scoring instructions, codebooks, cover letters, permission letters, IRB approval, category schemes, and peripheral statistical tables are examples of materials included in appendices. Some universities also require a *curriculum vitae* of the author.

A growing number of universities offer a new formatting option, what has been called the **paper format thesis** or **publication option** (Robinson & Dracup, 2008). In a typical paper format thesis, there is an introduction, two or more publishable papers, and then a conclusion. Such a format permits students to move directly from dissertation to journal submission but can be more demanding than the traditional format on both students and their advisers. Formats for the paper format thesis vary and are typically decided by the dissertation committee. Some universities require that a certain number of the publishable papers (e.g., two out of three) be data-based—that is, reports of original research. Other papers within the dissertation, however, might be publishable systematic reviews, concept analyses, or methodologic papers (e.g., describing the development of an instrument). Some universities require that the papers be under review or *in press* (i.e., accepted and awaiting publication), but other universities require that the papers be ready to submit.

If an academic institution does not accept paper format theses, students need to adapt their dissertations before submission to a journal. Several writers have provided guidance on converting a traditional dissertation into a manuscript, including Ahern (2012) and Heyman and Cronin (2005).

Journal Articles

Progress in evidence-based practice depends on researchers' efforts to share their work. Traditional dissertations, which are too lengthy for widespread use (and often difficult to access), are read only by a handful of people. Publication in a professional journal ensures broad circulation of research findings, and it is professionally advantageous—or even necessary—to publish. This section discusses issues relating to publication in journals.

> **TIP:** A valuable resource for nurse authors is the Nurse Author & Editor website at http://www.nurseauthoreditor.com/. This website offers helpful information for writing and publishing.

Traditional and Online (Open-Access) Journals

A major issue facing those preparing a manuscript concerns whether to publish in a traditional journal or an open-access journal. Traditional journals are typically available both in print and online, but access to the online versions is restricted to individuals and institutions that pay a subscription fee. **Open-access journals** are available online free of charge to those with access to the Internet.

A major benefit to authors is that open-access formats offer a worldwide audience of readers and hence can increase the visibility and impact of their research. Also, unlike traditional journals in which the journal publishers maintain the copyright for all publications, open-access journals usually allow authors to retain copyright. The legal basis for open access is the consent of the copyright holder, that is, the authors. In many cases, copyright holders demonstrate their consent to use open access by using something called the *Creative Commons licenses*. When authors consent to open-access, they are usually consenting up-front to unrestricted access, reading, downloading, copying, printing, and sharing of the work.

In most cases, an article accepted by an open-access journal gets published more quickly than is true for traditional print journals. Another advantage is that online journals are much less strict about page limitations. Qualitative researchers may benefit by this feature because it allows them to include more extensive verbatim quotes. Quantitative researchers can include more figures and tables than is true in traditional journal articles (although some journals publish online supplements that can be used to publish additional material).

> **TIP:** In selecting methodologic examples of nursing studies in this edition, we deliberately sought studies published as open-access articles, so that readers around the world would be able to obtain them. We have identified open-access articles in the chapter bibliographies, and links to the articles are provided in the Toolkit.

One potential drawback is that open-access journals often charge a fee to cover the cost of producing the journal. For example, in 2015, the open-access journal *BMC Nursing* charged authors US$2,145 (£1,370; €1,745) for an accepted article. However, many nurse authors are affiliated with institutions that are members of BioMed Central, in which case there is no fee—and in other cases, institutions pay publication fees for faculty members. (The fee for open-access journal publication is often waived for authors from low-income countries and is sometimes reduced for students.) Another drawback for nurse researchers is that, at the moment, few nursing journals are open-access, although that may change in the future. For example, the international open-access journal *Nursing-Plus Open* was launched by the publisher Elsevier in early 2015. The scarcity of open-access nursing journals has meant that a number of nurse researchers who seek open-access publication have opted to send their manuscripts to non-nursing journals.

⮕ TIP: The Directory of Open Access Journals (DOAJ) indexes and provides information for about 10,000 open-access journals, 56 of which were classified as having *nursing* as a subject code in early 2015 (http://doaj .org). Two examples include *Global Qualitative Nursing Research* and *Open Nursing Journal.* Many of the open-access nursing journals are ones subsidized by national governments (e.g., in Brazil and Iran).

As mentioned in Chapter 5, many traditional journals have moved to a hybrid model, in which authors can elect to have individual articles published as open-access—usually for an article-processing fee. However, many government agencies that fund health research (such as the National Institutes of Health [NIH] in the United States and Research Councils UK) now require that articles reporting government-funded studies be published as open-access. Some publishers deposit NIH-funded manuscripts directly into PubMed Central on behalf of the authors.

Also, some journals allow articles to be uploaded into *open-access repositories* such as ResearchGate or other institutional repositories. If open access is important but unaffordable, researchers should check a journal's policy about uploading to open-access repositories before submitting a manuscript—including whether or not there is a period of *embargo*. When there is an embargo, an article cannot be uploaded to the repository for a period after it first appears in print (e.g., 12 months). As noted by Griffiths (2014), editor of the journal *International Journal of Nursing Studies*, publishers and journals vary in their policies with regard to costs and embargos (or permission to upload at all), so authors "need to be wary to avoid breaking copyright laws" (p. 690).

When the open-access movement got underway, many expressed concerns that low-quality articles would increasingly find their way into publication. And, in fact, there are a number of so-called "predatory" open-access journals that charge fees without providing adequate review and editorial services. The names of publishers of such journals can be accessed at http://scholarlyoa.com/ publishers. However, there are many high-quality open-access journals that are fully peer-reviewed, and many have attained high prestige. All major open-access initiatives insist on the importance of high-quality scientific review of submitted articles.

Selecting a Journal

Hundreds of nursing journals exist and are indexed in CINAHL and in PubMed. In addition to variation in publication format, as just described, journals differ in focus, prestige, acceptance rates, word limits, and reference styles. Journals also vary in their goals, types of manuscript sought, review methods, and readership. These various factors need to be matched against personal ambitions and realistic assessments of the work. Writers should make efforts to develop a clear idea of the journal to which a manuscript will be submitted before writing begins.

All journals release goal statements as well as guidelines for preparing and submitting a manuscript. This information is published in journals themselves and on their websites.

Example of a Journal Goal Statement:
Qualitative Health Research is an international, interdisciplinary, refereed journal for the enhancement of health care and for furthering the development and understanding of qualitative research methods in health care settings. We welcome manuscripts in the following areas: the description and analysis of the illness experience, health and health-seeking behaviors, the experiences of caregivers, the sociocultural organization of health care, health care policy, and related topics. We also seek critical reviews and commentaries addressing conceptual, theoretical, methodologic, and ethical issues pertaining to qualitative inquiry.

Northam and colleagues (2010) reported information on the focus, word limit, reference style, and article review time for 63 nursing journals, although only a handful of the editors surveyed stated that research was their primary focus. The analysis revealed great variation for the journals across many dimensions, including article word limit (ranging from 1,200 to 9,000 words), number of issues (ranging from 2 to 26), and length of time from submission to acceptance or rejection decision (ranging from 3 to 45 weeks). Editors' reasons for rejection also varied, but among the research-focused articles, the primary reasons were poor writing and methodologic problems.

Many authors would like to know a journal's acceptance rate, but this information is not always available. Northam and colleagues (2000) conducted an earlier survey of journal editors and reported on the acceptance rate for 83 journals in nursing and related health fields. As might be expected, some journals were far more competitive than others. For example, *Nursing Research* accepted only 20% of submitted manuscripts, whereas the acceptance rates for many specialty journals were greater than 50%. Competition for journal publication likely became much keener in the years since that article was written.

➔ **TIP:** Some nursing journals do provide acceptance information on their websites. For example, the website for *Oncology Nursing Forum* stated in 2015 that the journal accepted 36% of manuscripts on first submission, and 52% after

revision. The website also noted that the peer review process took, on average, 6-8 weeks, and that the time to publication was 6-8 months.

Authors are often guided in their selection of a journal by the journal's *prestige*. Prestige is typically assessed in terms of a journal's **impact factor** (IF), which is a measure of citation frequency for an average article in a journal. Specifically, a journal's IF for, say, 2015 is the number of times in 2015 that articles published in the journal in the 2 prior years (2013 and 2014) were cited, divided by the number of the journal's articles in those 2 years that *could* have been cited (i.e., actual citations divided by potentially citable articles). As examples, the 2014 impact factor for *International Journal of Nursing Studies*, the highest ranking nursing journal in that year, was 2.90, while that for *Journal of Nursing Scholarship*, ranked 11th, was 1.64. Impact factor information can be found in *Journal Citation Reports* and also on the websites of most journals. Impact factor information for 2014 for several journals with a high concentration of research articles and impact factors of 1.20 or greater are shown in Table 30.2. Not all nursing journals are evaluated for impact factor, but the number included is now more than 100 and continues to grow (Polit & Northam, 2011).

➔ **TIP:** Only two journals in the nursing category of *Journal Citation Reports* in 2014 were open-access journal (*Revista da Escola de Enfermagem da USP*, ranked 105th and *Revista Latino-Americana de Enfermagem*, ranked 106th). *BMC Nursing* and *The Open Nursing Journal* have not been evaluated for their impact factors. By contrast, many open-access medical journals have high impact factors. *BMC Medicine* had a 2014 impact factor of 7.25, and *PLOS Medicine* had an impact factor of 14.43.

Query Letters

It is sometimes useful to send a **query letter** to a journal to ask the editor whether there is interest in a manuscript. The query letter should briefly describe the topic and methods, title, and a tentative

TABLE 30.2 • Impact Factor of Nursing Journals with High Concentration of Research Articles and a 2014 Impact Factor of 1.20 or Greater[a]

NAME OF JOURNAL	IMPACT FACTOR IN 2014[a]	JOURNAL RANK, 2014[b]
Advances in Skin & Wound Care	1.11	45
American Journal of Critical Care	2.12	21
Asian Nursing Research	1.00	54
Australian Critical Care	1.56	16
Australian Journal of Rural Health	1.23	37
Biological Research for Nursing	1.43	22
Birth	1.26	34
Cancer Nursing	1.97	7
Clinical Nursing Research	1.28	30
Critical Care Nurse	1.56	17
European Journal of Cancer Care	1.56	15
European Journal of Cardiovascular Nursing	1.88	9
European Journal of Oncology Nursing	1.43	23
Heart & Lung	1.29	29
International Journal of Mental Health Nursing	1.95	8
International Journal of Nursing Studies	2.90	1
Journal of Advanced Nursing	1.74	10
Journal of the Association of Nurses in AIDS Care	1.27	31
Journal of Cardiovascular Nursing	2.05	5
Journal of Clinical Nursing	1.26	35
Journal of Family Nursing	1.34	27
Journal of Human Lactation	1.99	6
Journal of Nursing Administration	1.27	32
Journal of Nursing Care Quality	1.39	24
Journal of Nursing Scholarship	1.64	11
Journal of Obstetric, Gynecologic, & Neonatal Nursing	1.02	50
Journal of Pediatric Health Care	1.44	20
Journal of Wound, Ostomy and Continence Nursing	1.18	39
Midwifery	1.57	13
Nurse Education Today	1.36	25
Nursing Outlook	1.59	12
Nursing Research	1.36	26
Oncology Nursing Forum	2.79	2
Pain Management Nursing	1.53	18
Qualitative Health Research	1.44	b
Research in Nursing & Health	1.27	33
Scandinavian Journal of Caring Sciences	1.20	b
Western Journal of Nursing Research	1.03	49
Women and Birth	1.57	14
Worldviews on Evidence-Based Nursing	2.38	3

[a]Impact factor information is from the *Journal Citation Reports* (JCR). Nursing journals are not listed if they are not primarily research-focused (e.g., *American Journal of Nursing*, impact factor = 1.30 in 2014), or if the 2014 impact factor was 1.20 or less (with the exception of a few journals with high research content). The median impact factor for the 110 journals in the Nursing category of the JCR Science Edition in 2014 was .97.
[b]Ranks are for rankings within the Nursing category of the JCR Science Edition. *Qualitative Health Research* was ranked 42nd in the Health Policy & Services category in 2014. The *Scandinavian Journal of Caring Sciences* is in the Nursing category of the Social Science Edition of JCR; it was ranked 35th in 2014.

submission date. Query letters are not essential if you have done a lot of homework about the journal's goals, but they might help to avoid impediments in some circumstances (e.g., if editors have recently accepted several papers on a similar topic and do not wish to consider another). Query letters can be submitted by e-mail using contact information provided on the journal's website. In Northam and colleagues' 2010 survey, editors had different views about the value of query letters, ranging from those who said they were not important (e.g., *Research in Nursing & Health*), somewhat important (*International Journal of Nursing Studies*), or very important (*Canadian Journal of Nursing Research*).

Query letters can be sent to multiple journals simultaneously, but ultimately, the manuscript can be submitted only to one—or rather to one at a time. If several editors express interest in reviewing a manuscript, journals can be prioritized according to criteria previously described. The priority list should be preserved because the manuscript can be resubmitted to the next journal on the list if the journal of first choice rejects it.

> **TIP:** A useful strategy in selecting a journal is to inspect your citation list. Journals that appear in your list have shown an interest in your topic and likely are strong candidates for publishing new studies on that topic.

Preparing the Manuscript

Once a journal has been selected, the information included in the journal's **Instructions to Authors** should be carefully reviewed. These instructions typically give authors such information as what the maximum page length is, what font and margins are permissible, what type of abstract is desired, what reference style should be used, and how to submit the manuscript online. It is important to adhere to the journal's guidelines to avoid rejection for a nonsubstantive reason. (The Toolkit section of the *Resource Manual* offers links to manuscript requirements for several nursing research journals.) In an informal survey of journal editors, Froman (2008) found that the most aggravating author behavior was "disregard for journal format or mission" (p. 399).

> **TIP:** Before you begin to write, it can be helpful to identify a research article to use as a model. Select a journal article on a topic similar to your own, or one that used similar methods, in the journal you have selected as first choice. When you have written a draft, a review by colleagues or advisers can be invaluable in improving its quality.

Typically, a manuscript for journals must be no more than 15 to 20 pages, double-spaced, not counting references and tables. The greatest amount of space usually should be allocated to methods and results. A frequent complaint of journal editors is that submitted manuscripts are too long (Northam et al., 2010).

Care should be taken in using and preparing citations. Some nursing journals suggest that there be not more than 15 references, or no more than three citations supporting a single point. In general, only published work can be cited (e.g., not papers presented at a conference nor manuscripts submitted but not accepted for publication). The reference style of the American Psychological Association (APA, 2010) is the style used by many nursing journals.

> **TIP:** There is a wealth of Internet resources to assist you with the APA style, including APA "crib sheets" and tutorials on the websites of university libraries. Several websites are listed in the Toolkit for you to click on directly. There is also software (e.g., StyleEase for APA and Chicago styles) that helps with formatting manuscripts.

Submission of a Manuscript

When the manuscript is ready for journal submission, a *cover letter* should be drafted. The cover letter should state the title of the paper and name and contact information of the **corresponding author** (the author with whom the journal communicates—usually, but not always, the lead author). The letter may include assurances that (1) the paper is original and has not been published or submitted elsewhere, (2) all authors have read and approved the manuscript, and (3) there are no conflicts of interest. Most traditional journals also require a signed *copyright transfer* form, which transfers all copyright ownership of the manuscript to the journal and warrants that all authors signing the form participated sufficiently in the research to justify authorship.

In submitting an article online, it is usually necessary to upload several files containing different parts of your manuscript. The title page, which has identifying information, should be in the first file. The next file usually contains the abstract, main text, and the reference list. Tables and figures are submitted separately, one file at a time. In other words, if there are two tables and one figure, these would be submitted in three files. At the end of the submission process, a pdf file that contains all the various elements is created for your review prior to submission. The entire process often takes a fair amount of time, but fortunately, it is usually possible to begin the process and return to it later if you need to track down information, such as the addresses of all coauthors.

> **TIP:** Nurses publish in many health-related journals, not just in nursing journals. Publishing opportunities for nurses in non-nursing journals have been discussed by Polit and Northam (2010).

Manuscript Review

Most nursing journals that include research reports—including those listed in Table 30.1—have a policy of independent **peer review** of manuscripts by two or more experts in the field. Reviewers are typically independent—they do not collaborate nor need they achieve consensus: The ultimate decision rests in the hands of journal editors. In most cases, peer review is a *blind review*, the idea being that greater candor is possible when there is anonymity. In a double-blind review, reviewers do not know the identity of the authors, and authors do not learn the identity of reviewers. (Relatively few nursing journals use a single-blind system in which only the referees' identities are hidden, but authors' are not.) Journals with peer reviewers are **refereed journals** and are in general more prestigious than

nonrefereed journals. When submitting a manuscript to a refereed journal, authors' names should not appear anywhere except on the title page.

Peer reviewers make recommendations to the editors about whether to accept the manuscript for publication, accept it contingent on revisions, or reject it. Relatively few manuscripts are accepted outright—both substantive and editorial revisions are the norm. Jennings (2010) has described how the review process works at *Research in Nursing & Health*.

> **Example of Reviewer Recommendation Categories:** The journal *Research in Nursing & Health* asks reviewers to make one of five recommendations: (1) Accept, (2) Minor revision, (3) Major revision, (4) Reject and resubmit, and (5) Reject.

Authors are sent information about the editors' decision, together with reviewers' comments. When resubmitting a revised manuscript to the same journal, each reviewer recommendation should be addressed, either by making the requested change, or by explaining in the cover letter accompanying the resubmission the rationale for not revising (Bearinger et al., 2010). Defending some aspect of a paper against a reviewer's recommendation often requires a strong supporting argument and citations. Typically, many months go by between submission of the original manuscript and the publication of a journal article, especially if there are revisions, as there usually are.

> **Example of Journal Timeline:** Beck et al. (2015) published a paper in the *Journal of Midwifery & Women's Health* entitled "A mixed methods study of secondary traumatic stress in certified nurse-midwives: Shaken belief in the birth process." The timeline for acceptance and publication of this manuscript, which was relatively fast, is as follows:

February 12, 2014	Manuscript submitted to *Journal of Midwifery & Women's Health* for review
March 29, 2014	Letter from editor informing of a provisional acceptance pending revisions
April 19, 2014	Revised manuscript resubmitted
May 24, 2014	Revised manuscript accepted for publication
February 2015	Publication in *Journal of Midwifery & Women's Health*

Many manuscripts, including many worthy and publishable ones, are rejected because of keen competition. If a manuscript is rejected, the reviewers' comments should be taken into consideration before submitting it to another journal. Manuscripts may need to be reviewed by several journals before final acceptance. Northam and colleagues (2010) offered this useful advice: "Resubmit to a different journal as soon as possible" (p. 35).

Presentations at Professional Conferences

Numerous international, national, and regional professional organizations sponsor meetings at which nursing studies are presented, either through an oral presentation or through visual display in a poster session. Professional conferences are particularly good forums for presenting results to clinical audiences. Researchers also can take advantage of meeting and talking with other conference attendees who are working on similar problems in different geographic regions.

The mechanism for submitting a presentation to a conference is simpler than for journal submission. The association sponsoring the conference ordinarily publishes an announcement or **Call for Abstracts** on its website or sends an e-mail to its members, 6 to 9 months before the meeting date. The notice indicates topics of interest, submission requirements, and deadlines for submitting a proposed paper or poster. Most universities and major health care agencies receive and post Call for Abstracts notices. Sigma Theta Tau International also posts a schedule of nursing conferences on its website (http://www.nursingsociety.org).

Oral Reports

Most conferences require prospective presenters to submit online abstracts of 250 to 1,000 words. Each conference has its own guidelines for abstract content and form. Abstracts are sometimes submitted to the organizer of a particular session; in other cases, conference sessions are organized after-the-fact, with related papers grouped together. Abstracts are evaluated based on the quality and originality of the research and the appropriateness of the paper for the conference audience. If abstracts are accepted, researchers are committed to appear at the conference to make a presentation.

Oral reports at meetings usually follow the IMRAD format. The time allotted for presentation usually is about 10 to 15 minutes, with 5 minutes or so for audience questions. Thus, only the most important aspects of the study, with emphasis on the results, can be included. It is especially challenging to condense a qualitative report to a brief oral summary without losing the rich, in-depth character of the data.

A handy rule of thumb is that a page of double-spaced text requires 2½ to 3 minutes to read aloud. Although presenters often prepare a written paper or a script, presentations are most effective if they are delivered informally or conversationally rather than if they are read verbatim. The presentation should be rehearsed to gain comfort with the script and to ensure that time limits are not exceeded.

➔ TIP: Most conferences presentations include visual materials, notably, PowerPoint slides. Visual materials should be kept simple for biggest impact. Tables are difficult to read on a slide but sometimes can be distributed to members of the audience in hard copy form. Make sure a sufficient number of copies is available.

The question-and-answer period can be a good opportunity to expand on aspects of the research and to get early feedback. Audience comments can be helpful in turning the conference presentation into a manuscript for journal submission.

Poster Presentations

Researchers sometimes present their findings or study protocols in **poster sessions**. Abstracts, often similar to those required for oral presentations, must be submitted to conference organizers according to specific guidelines. In poster sessions, several researchers simultaneously present visual displays summarizing study highlights, and conference attendees circulate around the exhibit area perusing displays. Those interested in a particular topic can devote time to discussing the study with the researcher and bypass posters dealing with topics of less interest. Poster sessions are efficient and encourage one-on-one discussions. Poster sessions are typically 1 to 2 hours in length. Researchers are expected to stand near their posters throughout the session to ensure effective communication and in some cases distribute handouts.

It is challenging to design an effective poster. The poster must convey essential information about the background, design, and results of a study in a format that can be perused in minutes. Bullet points, graphs, and photos are useful for communicating a lot of information quickly. Large, bold fonts are essential because posters are often read from a short distance. Posters must be sturdily constructed for transport to the conference site. It is important to follow conference guidelines in determining such matters as poster size, format, allowable display materials, and so on.

Several authors have offered advice on preparing for poster sessions (e.g., Hardicre et al., 2007; Miller, 2007; Nicol & Pexman, 2010; Shelledy, 2004). Russell and colleagues (1996) alerted qualitative researchers to the special challenges that await them in designing a poster. Software is available for producing posters (http://www.postersw.com). For those traveling long distances to conferences, it is worth noting that lightweight posters can now be created on fabric.

Electronic Dissemination

Computers and the Internet have changed forever how information of all types is disseminated. Earlier we discussed publishing in open-access online-only journals, but there are other ways to disseminate research findings on the Internet. For example, some researchers or research teams develop their own web page with information about their studies. When there are hyperlinks embedded in the websites, consumers can navigate between files and websites to retrieve relevant information on a topic of interest. Links to unpublished papers can also be uploaded on to the websites of individual researchers, their institutions, special interest organizations, and online repositories. The *International Journal of Advancements in Research & Technologies* (IJO-ART) provides some tips about online publication.

Such online dissemination avenues ensure timely distribution of information. One drawback of such dissemination opportunities, however, is that the papers are not subject to peer review. Researchers who want their evidence to have an impact on nursing practice should seek publication in outlets that subject manuscripts to external review.

CRITIQUING RESEARCH REPORTS

Although various aspects of study methodology can be evaluated using guidelines presented throughout this book, the manner in which study information is communicated in the research report can also be critiqued in a comprehensive critical appraisal. Box 30.2 summarizes major points to consider in evaluating the presentation of a research report.

An important issue is whether the report provided sufficient information for a thoughtful critique of other dimensions. When vital pieces of information are missing, researchers leave readers little choice but to assume the worst because this would lead to the most cautious interpretation of the results. For example, if there is no mention of blinding, then the safest conclusion is that blinding was not used.

Styles of writing differ for qualitative and quantitative reports, and it is unreasonable to apply the standards considered appropriate for one paradigm to the other. Regardless of style, however, you should, in critiquing a report, be alert to indications of overt biases, unwarranted exaggerations, or melodramatic language.

In summary, the research report is meant to be an account of how and why a problem was studied and what results were obtained. The report should be clearly written, cogent, and concise, and written in a manner that piques readers' interest.

SUMMARY POINTS

- In developing a dissemination plan, researchers select a communication outlet (e.g., journal article versus conference presentation), identify the audience whom they wish to reach, and decide on the content that can be effectively communicated.
- In the planning stage, researchers need to decide authorship credits (if there are multiple authors),

BOX 30.2 Guidelines for Critiquing the Presentation of a Research Report

1. Does the report include a sufficient amount of detail to permit a thorough critique of the study's purpose, conceptual framework, design and methods, handling of ethical issues, analysis of data, and interpretation?
2. Is the report well written and grammatical? Are pretentious words or jargon used when a simpler wording would have been possible?
3. Is the report well organized? Is there an orderly, logical presentation of ideas? Is the report characterized by continuity of thought and expression?
4. Does the report effectively combine text with tables or figures?
5. Does the report suggest overt biases, exaggerations, or distortions?
6. Is the report written using appropriately tentative language?
7. Is sexist or insensitive language avoided?
8. Does the title of the report adequately capture the key concepts and the population under investigation? Does the abstract (if any) adequately summarize the research problem, study methods, and important findings?

who the **lead author** and **corresponding author** will be, and in what order authors' names will be listed.

- Quantitative reports (and many qualitative reports) follow the **IMRAD format**, with the following sections: introduction, method, results, and discussion.
- The *introduction* acquaints readers with the research problem. It includes the problem statement and study purpose, the research hypotheses or questions, a brief literature review, and description of a framework. In qualitative reports, the introduction indicates the research tradition and, if relevant, the researchers' connection to the problem.
- The *method section* describes what researchers did to solve the research problem. It includes a description of the study design (or an elaboration of the research tradition), the sampling approach and a description of study participants, instruments and procedures used to collect and evaluate the data, and methods used to analyze the data.
- Standards for reporting methodologic elements now abound. Researchers reporting an RCT follow **CONSORT guidelines** (Consolidated Standards of Reporting Trials), which includes use of a flowchart to show the flow

of study participants. Other guidelines include **STROBE** for observational studies, and **COREQ** for certain qualitative studies.

- Guidelines for reporting aspects of an intervention include **CReDECI** and **TIDieR**.
- In the *results section*, findings from the analyses are summarized. Results sections in qualitative reports necessarily intertwine description and interpretation. Quotes from interview transcripts are essential for giving voice to study participants.
- Both qualitative and quantitative researchers include **figures** and **tables** that dramatize or succinctly summarize major findings or conceptual schema.
- The *discussion section* presents the interpretation of results, how the findings relate to earlier research, study limitations, and implications of the findings for nursing practice and future research.
- The major types of research reports are theses and dissertations, journal articles, and presentations at professional meetings.
- Theses and dissertations normally follow a standard IMRAD format, but some schools now accept **paper format theses**, which include an introduction, two or more publishable papers, and a conclusion.

- In selecting a journal for publication, researchers consider the journal's goals and audience, its prestige, and how often it publishes. Another major consideration is whether to publish in a traditional journal or in an online **open-access journal**. An advantage of open-access journals is speedy, worldwide dissemination.
- One proxy for a journal's prestige is its **impact factor**, the ratio between citations to a journal and recent citable items published. More than 100 nursing journals are now evaluated for their impact factors.
- Before beginning to prepare a **manuscript** for submission to a journal, researchers need to carefully review the journal's **Instructions to Authors**.
- Most nursing journals that publish research reports are **refereed journals** with a policy of basing publication decisions on **peer reviews** that are usually **double-blind reviews** (identities of authors and reviewers are not divulged).
- Nurse researchers can also present their research at professional conferences, either through a 10- to 15-minute oral report to a seated audience or in a **poster session** in which the "audience" moves around a room perusing information about the study on the posters. Sponsoring organizations usually issue a **Call for Abstracts** for the conference 6 to 9 months before it is held.

STUDY ACTIVITIES

Chapter 30 of the accompanying *Resource Manual for Nursing Research: Generating and Assessing Evidence for Nursing Practice*, *10th edition*, offers exercises and study suggestions for reinforcing the concepts presented in this chapter. In addition, the following questions can be addressed:

1. Skim a qualitative and a quantitative research report. Make a bullet-point list of differences in style and organization between the two.
2. Read a research report. Now, write a two- to three-page summary of the report that communicates the major points of the report to a clinical audience with minimal research skills.

STUDIES CITED IN CHAPTER 30

Ahern, K. (2012). How to create a journal article from a thesis. *Nurse Researchers, 19*, 21–25.

American Psychological Association. (2010). *Publication manual of the American Psychological Association* (6th ed.). Washington, DC: Author.

Baggs, J. G. (2008). Issues and rules for authors concerning authorship versus acknowledgements, dual publication, self-plagiarism, and salami publishing. *Research in Nursing & Health, 31*, 295–297.

Bearinger, L., Taliaferro, L., & Given, B. (2010). When R & R is not rest and recovery but revise and resubmit. *Research in Nursing & Health, 33*, 381–385.

Beck, C. T., LoGiudice, J., & Gable, R. K. (2015). A mixed methods study of secondary traumatic stress in certified nurse-midwives: Shaken belief in the birth process. *Journal of Midwifery & Women's Health, 60*, 16–23.

Becker, P. T. (2009). Thoughts on the end of the article: The implications for nursing practice. *Research in Nursing & Health, 32*, 241–242.

*Bossuyt, P., Reitsma, J., Bruns, D., Gatsonis, C., Glasziou, P., Irwiq, L., . . . de Vet, H. (2004). Towards complete and accurate reporting of studies of diagnostic accuracy: The STARD initiative. *Family Practice, 21*, 4–10.

Boutron, I., Moher, D., Altman, D., Schulz, K., & Ravaud, P. (2008). Extending the CONSORT statement to randomized trials of nonpharmacologic treatment: Explanation and elaboration. *Annals of Internal Medicine, 148*, 295–309.

*Campbell, M., Elbourne, D., & Altman, D. (2012). CONSORT 2010 statement: Extension to cluster randomised trials. *BMJ, 345*, e5661.

*Chan, A. W., Tetzlaff, J., Gotzsche, P., Altman, D., Mann, H., Berlin, J., . . . Moher, D. (2013). SPIRIT 2013 explanation and elaboration: Guidance for protocols of clinical trials. *BMJ, 346*, e7586.

Cognet, S., & Coyer, F. (2014). Discharge practices for the intensive care patient: A qualitative exploration in the general ward setting. *Intensive and Critical Care Nursing, 30*, 292–300.

Conn, V. S., Cooper, P., Ruppar, T., & Russell, C. (2008). Searching for the intervention in intervention research reports. *Journal of Nursing Scholarship, 40*, 52–59.

Conn, V. S., Ward, S., Herrick, L., Topp, R., Alexander, G., Anderson, C., . . . Georgesen, S. (2015). Managing opportunities and challenges of co-authorship. *Western Journal of Nursing Research, 37*, 134–163.

Creswell, J. W., & Plano Clark, V. L. (2011). *Designing and conducting mixed methods research* (2nd ed.). Thousand Oaks, CA: Sage.

*Des Jarlais, D., Lyles, C., & Crepaz, N. (2004). Improving the reporting quality of nonrandomized evaluations of behavioral and public health interventions: The TREND statement. *American Journal of Public Health, 94*, 361–366.

Dolgin, E. (2013). Publication checklist proposed to boost rigor of pilot trials. *Nature Medicine, 19*, 795–796.

Froman, R. (2008). Hitting the bull's eye rather than shooting yourself between the eyes. *Research in Nursing & Health, 31*, 399–401.

Gennaro, S. (2010). Closing the gap. *Journal of Nursing Scholarship, 42*, 357.

Gilgun, J. (2005). "Grab" and good science: Writing up the results of qualitative research. *Qualitative Health Research, 15*, 256–262.

*Glasziou, P., Meats, E., Heneghan, C., & Shepperd, S. (2008). What is missing from descriptions of treatment in trials and reviews? *BMJ, 336*, 1472–1474.

*Griffiths, P. (2014). Open access publication and the International Journal of Nursing Studies: All that glitters is not gold. *International Journal of Nursing Studies, 51*, 689–690.

Hardicre, J., Devitt, P., & Coad, J. (2007). Ten steps to successful poster presentation. *British Journal of Nursing, 16*, 398–401.

Heyman, B., & Cronin, P. (2005). Writing for publication: Adapting academic work into articles. *British Journal of Nursing, 14*, 400–403.

*Hoffmann, T. C., Glasziou, P. P., Boutron, I., Milne, R., Perara, R., Moher, D., . . . Michie, S. (2014). Better reporting of interventions: Template for intervention description and replication (TIDieR) checklist and guide. *BMJ, 348*, g1687.

*International Committee of Medical Journal Editors. (2013). *Recommendations for the conduct, reporting, editing, and publication of scholarly work in medical journals.* Retrieved from http://www.icmje.org

Jackson, D., Walter, G., Daly, J., & Cleary, M. (2014). Multiple outputs from single studies: Acceptable division of findings vs. "salami" slicing. *Journal of Clinical Nursing, 23*, 1–2.

Jennings, B. M. (2010). It takes a village to publish a manuscript in Research in Nursing & Health. *Research in Nursing & Health, 33*, 175–178.

Kearney, M. H. (2014). Be a responsible co-author. *Research in Nursing & Health, 37*, 1–2.

Kirk, S., Price, S., Penney, T., Rehman, L., Lyons, R., Piccinini-Vallis, H., . . . Aston, M. (2014). Blame, shame, and lack of support: A multilevel study of obesity management. *Qualitative Health Research, 24*, 790–800.

Kottner, J., Audigé, L., Brorson, S., Donner, A., Gajeweski, B., Hróbjartsson, A., . . . Streiner, D. (2011). Guidelines for reporting reliability and agreement studies (GRRAS). *International Journal of Nursing Studies, 48*, 661–671.

Lang, T. A. (2010). *How to write, publish, and present in the health sciences.* Washington, DC: American College of Physicians.

*Lang, T. A., & Altman, D. G. (2013). Basic statistical reporting for articles published in biomedical journals: The "Statistical Analyses and Methods in the Published Literature" or the SAMPL guidelines. In P. Smart, H. Maisonneuve, & A. Polderman (Eds), *Science editors' handbook.* Split, Croatia: European Association of Science Editors.

Mak, S. S., Lee, M., Cheung, J., Choi, K., Chung, T. Wong, T., . . . Lee, D. (2015). Pressurised irrigation versus swabbing method in cleansing wounds healed by secondary intention: A randomised controlled trial with cost-effectiveness analysis. *International Journal of Nursing Studies, 52*, 88–101.

*Mayo-Wilson, E., Grant, S., Hopewell, S., MacDonald, G., Moher, D., & Montegomery, P. (2013). Developing a reporting guideline for social and psychological intervention trials. *Trials, 14*, 242.

Michie, S., Richardson, M., Johnston, M., Abraham, C., Francis, J., Hardeman, W., . . . Wood, C. E. (2013). The behavior change technique taxonomy (v1) of 93 hierarchically clustered techniques: Building an international consensus for the reporting of behavior change interventions. *Annals of Behavioral Medicine, 46*, 81–95.

*Miller, J. E. (2007). Preparing and presenting effective research posters. *Health Services Research, 42*, 311–328.

*Moher, D., Hopewell, S., Schulz, K. F., Montori, V., Gotzsche, P., Devereaux, P., . . . Altman D. (2010). CONSORT 2010 explanation and elaboration: Updated guidelines for reporting parallel-group randomised trials. *BMJ, 340*, c869.

*Moher, D., Liberati, A., Tetzlaff, J., & Altman, D. (2009). Preferred reporting items for systematic reviews and meta-analyses: The PRISMA statement. *BMJ, 339*, b2535.

Möhler, R., Bartoszek, G., Köpke, S., & Meyer, G. (2012). Proposed criteria for reporting the development and evaluation of complex interventions in healthcare (CReDECI): Guideline development. *International Journal of Nursing Studies, 49*, 40–46.

Möhler, R., Köpke, S., & Meyer, G. (2015). Criteria for reporting the development and evaluation of complex interventions in healthcare: Revised guideline (CReDECI 2). *Trials, 16*, 204.

Nicol, A., & Pexman, P. (2010). *Displaying your findings: A practical guide for creating figures, posters, and presentations* (6th ed.). Washington, DC: American Psychological Association.

Northam, S., Trubenbach, M., & Bentov, L. (2000). Nursing journal survey: Information to help you publish. *Nurse Educator, 25*, 227–236.

Northam, S., Yarbrough, S., Haas, B., & Duke, G. (2010). Journal editor survey: Information to help authors publish. *Nurse Educator, 35*, 29–36.

Oermann, M., Galvin, E., Floyd, J., & Roop, J. (2006). Presenting research to clinicians: Strategies for writing about research findings. *Nurse Researcher, 13*, 66–74.

Oermann, M., & Hays, J. (2011). *Writing for publication* (2nd ed.). New York: Springer.

*Ogrinc, G., Mooney, S., Estrada, C., Foster, T., Goldmann, D., Hall, L., . . . Watts, B. (2008). The SQUIRE (Standards for QUality Improvement Reporting Excellence) guidelines for quality improvement reporting: Explanation and elaboration. *Quality & Safety in Health Care, 17*(Suppl. 1), 13–32.

Piaggio, G., Elbourne, D., Pocock, S., Evans S., & Altman, D. (2012). Reporting of noninferiority and equivalence randomized trials: Extension of the CONSORT 2010 statement. *Journal of the American Medical Association, 308,* 2594–2604.

Polit, D. F., & Gillespie, B. (2010). Intention-to-treat in randomized controlled trials: Recommendations for a total trial strategy. *Research in Nursing & Health, 33,* 355–368.

Polit, D. F., & Northam, S. (2010). Publication opportunities in nonnursing journals. *Nurse Educator, 35,* 237–242.

Polit, D. F., & Northam, S. (2011). Impact factors in nursing journals. *Nursing Outlook, 59,* 18–28.

Robinson, S., & Dracup, K. (2008). Innovative options for the doctoral dissertation in nursing. *Nursing Outlook, 56,* 174–178.

Russell, C. K., Gregory, D. M., & Gates, M. F. (1996). Aesthetics and substance in qualitative research posters. *Qualitative Health Research, 6,* 542–553.

Sandelowski, M. (1998). Writing a good read: Strategies for representing qualitative data. *Research in Nursing & Health, 21,* 375–382.

*Shelledy, D. C. (2004). How to make an effective poster. *Respiratory Care, 49,* 1213–1216.

Stroup, D., Berlin J., Morton, S., Olkin, I., Williamson, G., Rennie, D., . . . Thacker, S. (2000). Meta-analysis of observational studies in epidemiology: A proposal for reporting. Meta-analysis Of Observational Studies in Epidemiology (MOOSE). *Journal of the American Medical Association, 283,* 208–2012.

Strunk, W., Jr., & White, E. B. (2014). *The elements of style* (4th ed.). Essex, United Kingdom: Pearson Education.

*Tong, A., Flemming, K., McInnis, E., Oliver, S., & Craig, J. (2012). Enhancing transparency in reporting the synthesis of qualitative research. *BMC Medical Research Methodology, 12,* 181.

*Tong, A., Sainsbury, P., & Craig, J. (2007). Consolidated criteria for reporting qualitative research (COREQ): A 32-item checklist for interviews and focus groups. *International Journal for Quality in Health Care, 19,* 349–357.

*von Elm, E., Altman, D., Egger, M., Pocock, S., Gotzsche, P., & Vandenbroucke, J. (2014). The Strengthening the Reporting of Observational Studies in Epidemiology (STROBE) statement: Guidelines for reporting observational studies. *International Journal of Surgery, 12,* 1495–1499.

Wager, E. (2010). Getting *research published: An A-Z of publication strategy* (2nd ed.). London, United Kingdom: Radcliffe Books.

Weinert, C. (2010). Are all abstracts created equal? *Applied Nursing Research, 23,* 106–109.

Zinsser, W. (2006). On writing well: The classic guide to writing nonfiction (9th ed.). New York: Harper Collins.

*Zwarenstein, M., Treweek, S., Gagnier, J., Altman, D., Tunis, S., Haynes, B., . . . Moher, D. (2008). Improving reporting of pragmatic trials: Extensions of the CONSORT statement. *BMJ, 337,* 1–8.

A link to this open-access journal article is provided in the Toolkit for this chapter in the accompanying Resource Manual. ✪

31 | Writing Proposals to Generate Evidence

Research proposals communicate a research problem and proposed methods of solving it to an interested party. Research proposals are written both by students seeking faculty approval for studies and by researchers seeking financial support. In this chapter, we offer tips on how to improve the quality of research proposals and how to develop proficiency in **grantsmanship**—the set of skills involved in securing research funding.

OVERVIEW OF RESEARCH PROPOSALS

This section provides some general information regarding research proposals. Most of the information applies equally to dissertation proposals and grant applications.

Functions of a Proposal

Proposals are a means of opening communication between researchers and other parties. Those parties typically are either funding agencies or faculty advisers, whose job is to accept or reject the proposed plan or to request modifications. An accepted proposal is a two-way contract: Those accepting the proposal are effectively saying, "We are willing to offer our (professional or financial) support, for a study that proceeds as proposed," and those writing the proposal are saying, "If you offer support, then the study will be conducted as proposed."

Proposals often serve as the basis for negotiating with other parties as well. For example, a proposal may be shared with administrators when seeking institutional approval to conduct a study (e.g., for gaining access to participants). Proposals are often incorporated into submissions to human subjects committees or Institutional Review Boards.

Proposals help researchers to clarify their own thinking. By committing ideas to writing, ambiguities can be addressed at an early stage. Proposal reviewers also make suggestions for conceptual and methodologic improvements. When studies are undertaken collaboratively, proposals can help ensure that all researchers are "on the same page" about how the study is to proceed.

Proposal Content

Proposal reviewers want a clear idea of what the researcher plans to study, why the study is needed, what methods will be used to achieve study goals, how and when tasks will be accomplished, and whether the researcher has the skills to complete the project successfully. Proposals are evaluated on a number of criteria, including the importance of the question, the adequacy of the methods, and, if money is being requested, the reasonableness of the budget.

Proposal authors are usually given instructions about how to structure proposals. Funding agencies often supply an application kit that includes forms to be completed and specifies the format for organizing proposal content. Universities issue guidelines for dissertation proposals.

The content and organization of most proposals are broadly similar to that for a research report, but proposals are written in the future tense (i.e., indicating what the researcher *will* do) and obviously do not include results and conclusions.

Proposals for Qualitative Studies

Preparing proposals for qualitative research entails special challenges. Methodologic decisions typically evolve in the field, and therefore, it is seldom possible to provide detailed or in-depth information about such matters as sample size or data collection strategies. Sufficient detail needs to be provided, however, so that reviewers will have confidence that the researcher will assemble strong data and do justice to the data collected.

Qualitative researchers must persuade reviewers that the topic is important and worth studying, that they are sufficiently knowledgeable about the challenges of fieldwork and adequately skillful in eliciting rich data, and, in short, that the project would be a good risk. Knafl and Deatrick (2005) offered 10 tips for successful qualitative proposals. The first tip is to make the case for the *idea*, not the method. They also advised qualitative researchers to avoid methodologic tutorials, to use examples to clarify the research design, and to write for both experts and skeptics.

Resources are available to help qualitative researchers with proposal development. For example, an entire issue of the journal *Qualitative Health Research* was devoted to proposal writing—the July 2003 issue (volume 13, issue 6). Useful advice is also available in Carey and Swanson (2003), Padgett and Henwood (2009), and Sandelowski and colleagues (1989).

Proposals for Theses and Dissertations

Dissertation proposals are sometimes a bigger hurdle than dissertations themselves. Many doctoral candidates founder at the proposal development stage rather than when writing or defending the dissertation. Much of our advice—especially in our "Tips on Proposal Development" section later in this chapter—applies equally to proposals for theses and dissertations as for grant applications, but some additional advice might prove helpful.

The Dissertation Committee

Choosing the right adviser (if an adviser is chosen rather than appointed) is almost as important as choosing the right research topic. The ideal adviser is one who is a mentor, an expert with a strong reputation in the field, a good teacher, a patient and supportive coach and critic, and an advocate. The ideal adviser is also a person who has sufficient time and interest to devote to your research and who is likely to stick with your project until its completion. This means that it might matter whether the prospective adviser has plans for a sabbatical leave or is nearing retirement.

Dissertation committees often involve three or more members. If the adviser lacks certain "ideal" characteristics, those characteristics can be balanced across committee members by seeking people with complementary talents. Putting together a group who will work well together and who have no personal antagonism toward each other can, however, be tricky. Advisers can usually make good suggestions about other committee members.

Once a committee has been formed, it is important to develop a good working relationship with members and to learn about their viewpoints before and during the proposal development stage. This means, at a minimum, becoming familiar with their research and the methodologic strategies they have favored. It also means meeting with them and sounding them out with ideas about topics and methods. If the suggestions from two or more members are at odds, it is prudent to seek your adviser's counsel on how to resolve this.

TIP: When meeting with your adviser and committee members, take notes about their suggestions and write them out in more detail after the meeting while they are still fresh in your mind. The notes should be reviewed while developing the proposal.

Practices vary from one institution to another and from adviser to adviser, but some faculty require a prospectus before giving the go-ahead to prepare a full proposal. The prospectus is usually a three- to four-page paper outlining the research questions and proposed methods.

Content of Dissertation Proposals
Specific requirements regarding the length and format of dissertation proposals vary in different settings, and it is important to know at the outset what is expected. Typically, dissertation proposals are 20 to 40 pages in length. In some cases, however, committees prefer "mini-dissertations," that is, a document with fully developed sections that can be inserted with minor adaptation into the dissertation itself. For example, the review of the literature, theoretical framework, hypotheses, and the bibliography may be sufficiently refined at the proposal stage that they can be incorporated into the final product.

Literature reviews are often the most important section of a dissertation proposal (at least for quantitative studies). Committees may not desire lengthy literature reviews, but they want to be assured that students are in command of knowledge in their field of inquiry.

Dissertation proposals sometimes include elements not normally found in proposals to funding agencies. One such element may be table shells (see Chapter 19), which can demonstrate that the student knows how to analyze data and present results effectively. Another element is a table of contents for the dissertation. The table of contents serves as an outline for the final product and shows that the student knows how to organize material.

Several books provide additional advice on writing a dissertation proposal, including those by Locke et al. (2014), Roberts (2010), and Rudestam and Newton (2015).

FUNDING FOR RESEARCH PROPOSALS

Funding for research projects is becoming increasingly difficult to obtain because of keen and growing competition. Successful proposal writers need to have good research and proposal-writing skills, and they must also know from whom funding is available.

Federal Funding in the United States
The largest funder of research activities in the United States is the federal government. For health care researchers, National Institutes of Health (NIH) and the Agency for Healthcare Research and Quality (AHRQ) are leading agencies. Two major types of federal disbursements are grants and contracts. **Grants** are awarded for studies conceived by researchers themselves, whereas **contracts** are for studies desired by the government.

There are several mechanisms for NIH grants, which can be awarded to researchers in both domestic and foreign institutions. Most grant applications are unsolicited and reflect the research interests of individual researchers. Unsolicited applications should be consistent with the broad objectives of an NIH funding agency, such as the National Institute of Nursing Research (NINR). Investigator-initiated applications are submitted in response to **Parent Announcements**, which are covered under omnibus Funding Opportunity Announcements (FOAs).

NIH also issues periodic **Program Announcements** (PAs) that describe new, continuing, or expanded program interests. For example, in September 2014, NINR issued a program announcement entitled "Self-Management for Health in Chronic Conditions" (PA-14-344). The purpose of this PA, which expires in 2018, is "to support research in self-management focused across conditions . . . to reduce the burden of chronic illnesses/conditions."

Another grant mechanism allows federal agencies to identify a *specific* topic area in which they are interested in receiving proposals by a **Request for Applications (RFAs)**. RFAs are one-time opportunities with a single submission date. As an example, NINR issued an RFA entitled "Chronic Wounds: Advancing the Science from Prevention to Healing" in May 2014, with grant applications due in July 2014. The RFA states general guidelines and goals for the competition, but researchers can develop the specific research problem within the broad area of interest. A weekly electronic publication, the *NIH Guide for Grants and Contracts*, contains announcements about RFAs, PAs, and Parent Announcements.

In addition to grants, some government agencies award contracts to do *specific* studies. Contract offers are announced in a **Request for Proposals**

(RFP), which details the *exact* study that the government wants. Contracts, which are typically awarded to only one competitor, constrain researchers' activities and so most nurse researchers compete for grants rather than contracts. A summary of federal RFPs is published in the *Commerce Business Daily* (http://cbdnet.gpo.gov).

Government funding for nursing research is, of course, also available in many other countries. In Canada, for example, various types of health research are sponsored by the Canadian Institutes of Health Research (CIHR). Information about CIHR's program of grants, training awards, and other funding opportunities is available at its website (http://www.cihr.ca). In Australia, major government funding for health research comes from the National Health and Medical Research Council (NHMRC) (http://www.nhmrc.gov.au/grants/).

Private Funds

Health care research is supported by numerous philanthropic foundations, professional organizations, and corporations. Many researchers prefer private funding to government support because there is less "red tape" and fewer requirements.

Information about philanthropic foundations that support research is available through the Foundation Center (http://www.fdncenter.org). A comprehensive resource for identifying funding opportunities is the Center's *The Foundation Directory*, available online for a fee. The directory lists the purposes and activities of the foundations and information for contacting them. The Foundation Center also offers seminars and training on grant writing and funding opportunities in locations around the United States. Another resource for information on funding is the Community of Science, which maintains a database on funding opportunities (http://pivot.cos.com/).

Professional associations (e.g., the American Nurses Foundation, Sigma Theta Tau International) offer funds for conducting research. Health organizations, such as the American Heart Association and the American Cancer Society, also support research activities.

Finally, research funding is sometimes donated by private corporations, particularly those dealing with health care products. The Foundation Center publishes a directory of corporate grantmakers and provides links through its website to a number of corporate philanthropic programs. Additional information concerning corporate requirements and interests should be obtained either from the organization directly or from staff in the research administration offices of the institution with which you are affiliated.

GRANT APPLICATIONS TO NATIONAL INSTITUTES OF HEALTH

NIH funds many nursing studies through NINR and other institutes. Because of the importance of NINR as a funding source for nurse researchers, this section describes the process of proposal submission and review at NIH. AHRQ, which also funds nurse-initiated studies, uses the same application kit and similar procedures.

Types of National Institutes of Health Grants and Awards

NIH awards different types of research grants, and each has its own objectives and review criteria. The basic grant program—and the primary funding mechanism for independent research—is the traditional **Research Project Grant** (R01). The objective of R01 grants is to support specific research projects in areas reflecting the interests and competencies of a Principal Investigator (PI).

Beside the R01 grant program, three others that are available through NINR are worth noting. A special program (R15) has been established for researchers working in institutions that have not been major participants in NIH programs. These **Academic Research Enhancement Awards (AREA)** are designed to stimulate research in institutions that provide baccalaureate training for many individuals who go on to do health-related research. There is also a **Small Grant** Program (R03) that provides support for pilot, feasibility, and methodology development studies. R03 grants provide a maximum of $50,000 of direct support for up to 2 years. Finally, the R21 grant mechanism—the **Exploratory/Developmental Research Grant Award**—is intended to encourage new, exploratory and developmental research projects by providing support for early stages of research, such as for pilot or feasibility studies.

NIH and other agencies also offer individual and institutional predoctoral and postdoctoral fellowships as well as career development awards. Examples of individual fellowship mechanisms available through the National Research Service Award (NRSA) program within NINR include the following:

• F31, Ruth L. Kirschstein NRSA Individual Predoctoral Fellowships, support nurses in a supervised training leading to a doctoral degree in areas related to the NINR mission
• F32, Ruth L. Kirschstein NRSA Individual Postdoctoral Fellowships, support postdoctoral training to nurses to broaden their scientific background
• F33, Ruth L. Kirschstein NRSA Senior Fellowships, support doctorally trained researchers with at least 7 years of research in pursuing opportunities to change the direction of their research careers.

> **TIP:** Advice on developing a proposal for an NRSA fellowship has been offered in a paper by Parker and Steeves (2005).

Four important Career Development Awards offered through NINR are as follows:

• K01, Mentored Research Scientist Development Award, available to doctorally prepared scientists who would benefit from a mentored research experience with an expert sponsor
• K22, NINR's Career Transition Award, offers support to postdoctoral fellows in transition to a faculty position
• K23, Mentored Patient-Oriented Research Career Development Award, supports the career development of investigators who are committed to focusing their research on patient-oriented research
• K99, Pathway to Independence Award, provides for postdoctoral research activity leading to the submission of an independent research project application.

> **TIP:** If you have an idea for a study and are not sure which type of grant program is suitable—or you are unsure whether NINR or another NIH institute might be interested—you should contact NINR directly (Telephone number: 301-594-6906). NINR staff can provide feedback about whether your proposed study matches NINR's program interests. Information about NINR's ongoing priorities and areas of opportunity is available at http://www.ninr.nih.gov.

National Institutes of Health Forms and Schedule

In 2007, NIH transitioned from hard copy application submissions to electronic submissions for most competing applications using the SF424 (R&R) application through http://www.grants.gov. The SF424 is used for all the types of grants and awards described in the previous section, although there are supplemental components needed for some of them. Researchers use Adobe Reader to "fill in" and complete this application. There is abundant information online about the application process, and NIH offers training sessions on how to submit applications electronically. The application kit can be accessed from the NIH website at http://www.nih.gov under their "Grants & Funding" section.

New grant applications are usually processed in three cycles annually. Different deadlines apply to different types of grants, as shown in Table 31.1. For most new applications, except fellowships in the F series and AIDS-related research, the deadline for receipt is in February, June, and October. The scientific merit review dates are about 4-5 months after each submission date. For example, applications submitted for the February cycle are reviewed in June or July; the earliest project start date for applications funded in that cycle would be in September or December (depending on when the applications are reviewed by the NIH Advisory Council). Applicants should begin a registration process through the Electronic Research Administration (eRA) Commons at least 2 weeks prior to the submission date.

TABLE 31.1 • Schedule for Selected New Research Applications, National Institutes of Health

Application Due Date	MECHANISM OF SUPPORT (TYPE OF AWARD)				
	R01	**R03, R21**	**R15**	**K Series**	**F Series**
Cycle I[a]	February 5	February 16	February 25	February 12	April 8
Cycle II[b]	June 5	June 16	June 25	June 12	August 8
Cycle III[c]	October 5	October 16	October 25	October 12	December 8

AIDS-related applications are on a different schedule; consult the NIH website for information.
[a]Cycle I: Scientific Merit Review: June to July; earliest start date: September or December.
[b]Cycle II: Scientific Merit Review: October to November; earliest start date: April.
[c]Cycle III: Scientific Merit Review: February to March; earliest start date: July.

Preparing a Grant Application for National Institutes of Health

Although many substantive aspects of the NIH grant application have remained stable, the forms and procedures for NIH grant applications have been changing. It is crucial to carefully review up-to-date instructions for grant application submission rather than relying on information in this chapter.

Forms: Screens and Uploaded Attachments

The SF424 form set has numerous components. The "front matter" of SF424 consists of various forms that appear on a series of fillable screens. These forms help in processing the application and provide administrative information. Careful attention to detail with these forms is very important. Major forms include the following:

- *SF424 (R&R) Form.* On the cover form, researchers state a brief, descriptive title of the project (not to exceed 81 characters), the name and affiliation of the PI, and other administrative information.

TIP: The project title should be given careful thought. It is the first thing that reviewers see and should be crafted to create a good impression. The title should be concise and informative but should also be compelling.

- *Project/Performance Site Location Form.* The next screen requests information about the primary site where the work will be performed.
- *Other Project Information Form.* This screen is the mechanism for submitting key information. The form begins with questions about human subjects and the use of vertebrate animals. The last few items require attachments to be uploaded, including a project summary, a project narrative, bibliography, and facilities and equipment information. Attachments, which must be in PDF format, have strict size limitations. The *Project Summary* serves as a succinct description of aims and methods the proposed study and must be no longer than 30 lines. The *Project Narrative* is a brief (two to three sentences) description of the relevance of the research to public health. The *Bibliography* is a list of references cited in the research plan; any reference style is acceptable. The *Facilities* attachment is used to describe needed and available resources (e.g., laboratories). The *Equipment* attachment is used to list major items of equipment already available for the project.
- *Senior/Key Person Profile Form.* For each key or senior person, the form requests basic identifying information and calls for an attachment, a Biographical Sketch. The sketch should list education and training as well as the following: (a) a statement describing the qualifications

that make the person well suited for his or her role, (b) positions and honors, (c) selected peer-reviewed publications or manuscripts in press (no more than 15), and (d) selected completed and ongoing research support. A maximum of four pages is permitted for each person.

• *Budget Form.* For NIH applications, researchers must choose between two budget options—the R&R Budget Component or the PHS398 Modular Budget Component. Detailed R&R budgets showing specific projected expenses are required if annual direct project costs exceed $250,000, but for smaller projects, budget information is obtained in another section. (Modular budgets are appropriate only for R-type grants.)

➔ **TIP:** Cover letters to the funding agency are strongly encouraged. The cover letter should include such information as the application title; the name and number of the funding opportunity (PA or RFA); individuals who should not review the application and a rationale; disciplines involved, if multidisciplinary; and any request to be assigned to a particular review group.

For grant applications to NIH and other public health service agencies, additional forms referred to as PHS398 components are required and include the following:

• *PHS398 Cover Page Supplement Form.* This form supplements the SF424 cover page and requests mainly administrative information.

• *PHS398 Modular Budget Form.* **Modular budgets**, paid in modules of $25,000, are appropriate for R-series applications (e.g., R01s) requesting $250,000 or less per year of direct costs. (**Direct costs** include specific project-related costs such as staff and supplies; **indirect costs** are institutional **overhead** costs.) This form provides budget fields for annual summaries of projected costs for up to 5 years of support. There are also fields for cumulative summaries across all project years. A *budget justification* attachment, detailing primarily personnel costs, must be uploaded.

➔ **TIP:** Even though modular budget forms ask only for summaries of the funds needed to complete a study, you should prepare a more detailed budget to arrive at a reasonable projection of needed funds. Beginning researchers are likely to need the assistance of a research administrator or an experienced, funded researcher in developing their first budget. Higdon and Topp (2004) and Bliss (2005) have offered some advice on developing a budget.

• *PHS398 Research Plan Form.* The PHS398 Research Plan form asks about application type (e.g., new, resubmission) and then requires information, in the form of attachments, about the proposed study and the research plan. Research plan requirements are described in the next section.

➔ **TIP:** Examples of selected forms for SF424 are presented in the Toolkit of the *Resource Manual* in non-fillable form—that is, they are included simply as illustrations, not to be used for submitting a grant application.

The Research Plan Component

The research plan component consists of 14 items, not all of which are relevant to every application—for example, item 1 is for revised applications or resubmissions. Each item involves uploading a separate PDF attachment. In this section, we briefly describe guidelines for items 2 through 14, with emphasis on items 2 and 3. We also present some advice based on a study (Inouye & Fiellin, 2005) in which the researchers content analyzed the criticisms in the review sheets of 66 applications (R01s) submitted to a clinical research review group (not NINR). Thus, the advice relating to specific pitfalls is "evidence-based," that is, based on problems identified in actual applications.

➔ **TIP:** Based on their analysis, Inouye and Fiellin (2005) created a grant-writing checklist designed as a self-assessment tool for proposal developers. We have included an adapted and expanded checklist in the Toolkit in the accompanying *Resource Manual*.

Specific Aims (Item 2). In this section, which is restricted to a single page, researchers must provide a succinct summary of the research problem and the specific objectives of the study, including any hypotheses to be tested. The aims statement should indicate the scope and importance of the problem. Care should be taken to be precise and to identify a problem of manageable proportions.

Inouye and Fiellin (2005) found that the most frequent critique of the Specific Aims section was that the goals were overstated, overly ambitious, or unrealistic (18% of the review sheets). Other complaints were that the project was poorly conceptualized (15%) or that hypotheses were not clearly articulated (12%).

TIP: Some suggestions for describing the objectives of a pilot intervention study (see Chapter 29) are provided in the Supplement to this chapter on the**Point**°.

Research Strategy (Item 3). Unless otherwise specified in a Funding Opportunity Announcement (FOA), the Research Strategy section is restricted to 12 pages for R01 and R15 applications and to 6 pages for R03, R21, and F-series applications. For other funding mechanisms, page restrictions are specified in the FOA.

TIP: Career Development Awards (K-series) involve completion of a special form, requiring attachments that include a description of the applicant's background, a statement of career goals and objectives, career development or training activities during the award period, and training in the responsible conduct of research. The applicant's institution must also submit a letter describing its commitment to the candidate and to his or her development.

The Research Strategy section is organized into three subsections: Significance, Innovation, and Approach. In the Significance section, researchers must convince reviewers that the proposed study idea has clinical or theoretical relevance and that the study will make a contribution to scientific knowledge or clinical practice. Researchers describe the study context in this section through a brief analysis of existing knowledge and gaps on the topic. Researchers should demonstrate command of current knowledge in a field, but this section must be very tightly written. Inouye and Fiellin (2005) found that a frequent critique expressed by reviewers about this section was that the need for the study was not adequately justified (29%). In the Innovation section, researchers should describe how the proposed study challenges, refines, or improves current research or clinical practice paradigms.

The proposed design and methods for the study are described in the third subsection, Approach. This section, which is the heart of the application, should be written with extreme care and reviewed with a self-critical eye. The Approach section needs to be concise but with sufficient detail to persuade reviewers that methodologic decisions are sound and that the study will yield important and reliable evidence.

The Approach section typically describes the following: (1) the research design, including a discussion of comparison group strategies and methods of controlling confounding variables (for qualitative studies, the research tradition should be described); (2) the experimental intervention, if applicable, including a description of the treatment and control group conditions; (3) procedures, such as what equipment will be used, how participants will be assigned to groups, and what type of blinding, if any, will be achieved; (4) the sampling plan, including eligibility criteria and sample size; (5) data collection methods and information about the measurement properties of measures that will be used; and (6) data analysis strategies. The Approach should identify potential methodologic problems and intended strategies for handling such problems. In proposals for qualitative studies, steps that will be taken to enhance the integrity and trustworthiness of the study should be described.

Inouye and Fiellin (2005) found that *all* of the reviews they analyzed had one or more criticism of this section, the most general of which was that the description of methods was underdeveloped (15%). A few of the most persistent criticisms were as follows:

- Inadequate blinding for outcome assessment (36%)
- Sample was flawed—biased or unrepresentative (36%)
- Important confounding variables inadequately controlled (32%)
- Inadequate sample size or inadequate power calculations (26%)
- Insufficient description of the approach to data analysis (24%)
- Outcome measures inadequately specified or described (23%)

Although some of these concerns relate to clinical trials (e.g., blinding), many have broad relevance—small sample size, sample biases, and poorly described data collection and analysis plans can be problematic in any type of study.

The Approach section must also include information on Preliminary Studies. In new applications, researchers must describe the PI's preliminary or developmental studies and any experience pertinent to the application. This section must persuade reviewers that you have the skills and background needed to do the research. Any pilot work that has served as a foundation for the proposed project should be described. Inouye and Fiellin's (2005) analysis is especially illuminating with regard to Preliminary Studies. They found that the single biggest criticism across the 66 review sheets was that more pilot work was needed, mentioned in 41% of the reviews.

→ **TIP:** For applications submitted by an Early Stage Investigator (a person within 10 years of completing their terminal degree and who has not yet been awarded an RO1 grant), reviewers are instructed to place less emphasis on the applicant's Preliminary Studies.

Human Subjects Sections (Items 5-7). Researchers who plan to collect data from human beings must complete items relating to the protection of subjects. An entire section of the application kit ("Part II, Supplemental Instructions for Preparing the Human Subjects Section of the Research Plan") provides guidance on the attachments needed for these items. Applicants must either address the involvement of human subjects and describe protections from research risks or provide a justification for exemption with enough information that reviewers can determine the appropriateness of requests for exemption. If no exemption is sought, the section must address various issues, as outlined in the application kit. The application must also include various types of information regarding the inclusion of women, minorities, and children. For example, applicants must complete a Planned Enrollment Report and Cumulative Inclusion Enrollment Report, which ask for expectations for enrollment of subjects from various racial and ethnic categories, separately by gender. These sections often serve as the cornerstone of the document submitted to Institutional Review Boards.

Other Research Plan Sections (Items 8-13). Most remaining sections in the research plan are not relevant universally. These include such items as a description and justification of the use of vertebrate animals and a leadership plan if there are multiple principal investigators. One item, however, has relevance to many applications: Letters of Support (item 12). This item requires you to attach letters from individuals agreeing to provide services to the project, such as consultants and collaborators.

Appendix (Item 14). Grant applications often include appended materials. A maximum of 10 PDF attachments is allowed, and a summary sheet listing all appended items is encouraged. Examples of appended materials include data collection instruments, clinical protocols, detailed sample size calculations, complex statistical models, and other supplementary materials in support of the application. Researchers cannot submit publications, except under restricted circumstances (e.g., an accepted manuscript not yet published). Essential information should never be relegated to an appendix because only primary reviewers receive appendices. The guidelines warn that appendices should not be used to circumvent the page limitations of the Research Strategy section.

> ⮕ **TIP:** In terms of content, the research plan for NIH applications is similar to what is required in most research proposals—although emphases and page restrictions may vary, and supplementary information may be required.

The Review Process

Grant applications submitted to NIH are reviewed for completeness, relevance, and adherence to instructions by the NIH Center for Scientific Review. Acceptable applications are assigned to an appropriate Institute or Center and to a peer review group.

NIH uses a sequential, dual review system for informing decisions about its grant applications. The first level involves a panel of peer reviewers (not NIH employees), who evaluate applications for their scientific merit. These review panels are called **scientific review groups** (SRGs) or, more commonly, **study sections**. Each panel consists of about 20-25 researchers with backgrounds appropriate to the specific study section for which they have been selected and usually with a track record of NIH funding. Appointments to the review panels are for 4-year terms and are staggered so that about one fourth of each panel is new each year.

> ⮕ **TIP:** Applications by nurse researchers usually are assigned to the Nursing and Related Clinical Sciences Study Section (NRCS). However, applications by nurse researchers could be reviewed in several other study sections, such as Behavioral Medicine Interventions and Outcomes (BMIO) and Adult Psychopathology and Disorders of Aging (APDA).

The second level of review is by a National Advisory Council, which includes scientific and lay representatives. The Advisory Council considers not only the scientific merit of an application but also the relevance of the proposed study to the programs and priorities of the Center or Institute to which the application has been submitted as well as budgetary considerations.

During the first round of review in a study section, applications are assigned to primary and secondary (and sometimes a tertiary) reviewers for detailed analysis. Each assigned reviewer prepares comments and assigns scores according to five core review criteria.

1. *Significance*. Does this study address an important problem? If the aims of the application are achieved, how will scientific knowledge or clinical practice be advanced? What will be the effect of the study on the concepts or methods that drive this field?
2. *Investigator*. Is the investigator appropriately trained and well suited to carry out this work? Is the proposed work appropriate to the experience level of the PI and other researchers? Do Early Stage Investigators have appropriate training and experience?
3. *Innovation*. Does the project employ novel concepts, approaches, or methods? Are the aims original and innovative? Does the project challenge existing paradigms or develop new methods or technologies?
4. *Approach*. Are the overall strategy, design, methods, and analyses adequately developed and appropriate to the aims of the project? Does the applicant acknowledge potential problem areas and consider alternative tactics?
5. *Environment*. Does the scientific environment in which the work will be done contribute to the probability of success? Do the proposed experiments take advantage of unique features of the scientific environment or employ useful collaborative arrangements?

In addition to these five criteria, other factors are relevant in evaluating proposals, including the reasonableness of the proposed budget, the adequacy of protections for human or animal subjects, and the appropriateness of the sampling plan in terms of including women, minorities, and children as participants. These factors are not, however, formally scored.

Scoring of applications changed in 2010. In the current system, each of the five core criteria is scored on a scale from 1 (exceptional) to 9 (poor). Assigned reviewers score applications and submit their scores before attending a study section meeting and also submit a preliminary overall **impact score** (also called a **priority score**) on the same 1 to 9 scale. An impact score reflects a reviewer's

assessment of the extent to which the study will
exert a powerful influence in an area of research.
Based on preliminary impact scores, applications
with unfavorable scores (usually those in the lower
half) are not discussed or scored by the entire study
section in its meeting. This streamlined process was
instituted so that study section members could focus
their discussion on the most worthy applications.

For applications that *are* discussed in the meeting, each study section member (not just those who
were assigned as reviewers) designates an impact
score, based on their own critique of the application and the committee's discussion. Individual
impact scores from all committee members are
averaged, and the mean is then multiplied by 10
to arrive at a final score. Thus, final impact scores
for applications that are discussed can range from
10 (the best possible score) to 90 (the lowest possible score). Final scores tend to cluster in the 10
to 50 range, however, inasmuch as the least meritorious applications were previously screened out
and not scored by the full study section. Among the
scored applications, only those with the best priority scores actually obtain funding. Cutoff scores for
funding vary from institute to institute and year to
year, but a score of 20 or lower is usually needed to
secure funding.

➜ **TIP:** Some NIH institutes (but not NINR)
calculate and publish a *payline*—a percentile
rank for impact scores, up to which nearly all
RO1 applications are funded.

Within a few days after the study section meeting,
applicants are able to learn their priority score
and percentile ranking online via the NIH eRA
Commons (https://commons.era.nih.gov/commons).
Within about 30 days, applicants can access a
summary of the study section's evaluation. These
summary sheets include critiques written by the assigned reviewers, a summary of the study section's
discussion, study section recommendations, and
administrative notes of special consideration (e.g.,
human subjects issues). All applicants receive a summary sheet, even if their applications were unscored.
(Applicants of unscored applications also learn how
the assigned reviewers scored the five core criteria.)

➜ **TIP:** Unless an unfunded proposal is
criticized in some fundamental way (e.g., the
problem area was not judged to be significant),
applications often should be resubmitted, with
revisions that reflect the concerns of the peer
reviewers. When a proposal is resubmitted, the
next review panel members are given a copy of
the original application and the summary sheet
so that they can evaluate the degree to which
concerns have been addressed. Applications to
NIH can be resubmitted up to two times.

TIPS ON PROPOSAL DEVELOPMENT

Although it is impossible to tell you exactly what
steps to follow to produce a successful proposal, we
conclude this chapter with some advice that might
help to improve the process and the product. Many
of these tips are especially relevant for those preparing proposals for funding. Further suggestions for
writing effective grant applications may be found in
Grey (2000), Berg et al. (2007), Funk and Tornquist
(2015), and Inouye and Fiellin (2005).

Things to Do before Writing Begins

Advance planning is essential to the development
of a successful proposal. This section offers suggestions for things you can do to prepare for the
actual writing.

Start Early

Writing a proposal, and attending to all of the details
of a formal submission process, is time-consuming
and almost always takes longer than originally envisioned. Be sure to build in enough time that the
product can be reviewed and rereviewed by members of the team (including any faculty mentors)
and by willing colleagues. Build in adequate time
for administrative issues such as securing permissions and getting budgets approved.

Having a proposal timeline is a good way to impose discipline on the proposal development process. Figure 31.1 presents one example, but the list
of tasks is merely suggestive. Ask an experienced
person to review your timeline and try to adhere to
the timeline once you start.

Task	Timeline (Months Before Submission)												
	12+	12	11	10	9	8	7	6	5	4	3	2	1
Identify/conceptualize the problem	X												
Undertake a literature review	X												
Identify and approach possible data collection sites	X												
Initiate descriptive or pilot work	X												
Analyze pilot data, assess feasibility	X	X	X	X	X								
Develop a "brief," outlining significance & preliminary thoughts about overall study design		X	X										
Identify methodologic and content experts; solicit input and possible collaboration			X	X	X								
Begin building a team of co-investigators and consultants		X	X	X	X								
Identify and contact funder/program officer (as needed)		X	X										
Obtain all application forms and instructions		X	X										
Review funding agencies' priorities; review recently funded grants			X	X	X								
Develop research plan, identify instruments, etc.; consult with statisticians, psychometricians, etc., as needed				X	X	X	X	X	X	X			
Collect site data for describing site, staff, clients					X	X	X						
Obtain written letters of agreement and/or support from data collection sites					X	X	X						
Prepare an outline of the proposal; develop writing assignments						X	X						
Write draft of proposal							X	X	X	X	X	X	X
Draft a budget								X	X				
Draft other ancillary components (bio sketches, etc.)								X	X				
Internal review by team members									X	X	X		
Make revisions based on review										X	X	X	
External review by colleagues/experts										X	X	X	
Team review of comments, make final revisions											X	X	X
Write abstract/summary												X	X
Finalize budget and other ancillary components													X
Prepare all final documents, get needed signatures													X

FIGURE 31.1 Example of a grant-writing timeline.

TIP: It is advantageous to build pilot or preliminary work into your proposal development schedule, which may add many months to your timeline. As noted earlier, NIH reviewers frequently criticize the absence of adequate pilot work. Incremental knowledge building is attractive to reviewers. When you apply for funding, you are asking funders to make an *investment* in you; they will have the sense of being offered a better investment opportunity if some groundwork for a study has already been completed.

Select an Important Problem

A factor that is critical to the success of a proposal is selecting a problem that has clinical or theoretical significance. The proposal must make a persuasive argument that the research could make a noteworthy contribution to evidence on a topic that is important and appealing to those making judgments, that is, the reviewers.

Kuzel (2002), who shared some lessons about securing funding for a qualitative study, noted that researchers could profit by taking advantage of certain "hot topics" that have the special attention of the public and government officials. Proposals can sometimes be cast in a way that links them to topics of national concern, and such a linkage can contribute to a favorable review. Kuzel used as an example his funded study of quality of care and medical errors in primary care practices, with emphasis on patients' perspectives. The proposal was submitted at a time when the U.S. government was putting resources into research to enhance patient safety, and noted that "the reframing of 'quality' under the name of 'patient safety' has captured the stage and is likely to have an enduring effect on what work receives funding" (p. 141). Both qualitative and quantitative researchers should be sensitive to political realities.

Know Your Audience

Learn as much as possible about the audience for your proposal. For dissertations, this means getting to know your committee members and learning about their expectations, interests, and schedules. If you are writing a proposal for funding, you should obtain information about the funding organization's priorities. It is also wise to examine recently funded projects. Funding agencies often publish the criteria that reviewers use to make funding decisions—such as the ones we described for NIH—and these criteria should be studied carefully.

Grey (2000), in her tips on grantsmanship, urged researchers to "talk it up" (p. 91), that is, to call program staff in agencies and foundations, or to send letters of inquiry about possible interest in a project. Grey also noted the importance of *listening* to what these people say and following their recommendations.

Another aspect to "knowing your audience" concerns appreciating reviewers' perspective. Reviewers for funding agencies are busy professionals who are taking time away from their own work to consider the merits of proposed new studies. They are likely to be methodologically sophisticated and experts in *their* field—but they may have limited knowledge of your own area of research. It is therefore imperative to help time-pressured reviewers to grasp the merits of your proposed study, without relying on jargon or specialized terminology.

Review a Successful Proposal

Although there is no substitute for actually writing a proposal as a learning experience, novice proposal writers can profit by examining a successful proposal. It is likely that some of your colleagues or fellow students have written a proposal that has been accepted (either by a funding sponsor or by a dissertation committee), and many people are glad to share their successful efforts with others. Also, proposals funded by the government are usually in the public domain—that is, you can ask for a copy of funded proposals. To obtain a funded NIH project, for example, you can contact the NIH Freedom of Information Office Coordinator for the appropriate institute.

Several journals have published entire proposals, except for administrative and budgetary information. An early example was a proposal for a study of comprehensive discharge planning for the elderly (Naylor, 1990). More recently, a proposal for a qualitative study of adolescent fathers was published, together with reviewers' comments (Dallas et al., 2005a, 2005b).

➔ **TIP:** The accompanying *Resource Manual* includes the entire successful grant application to NINR by Deborah Dillon McDonald entitled "Older adults response to health care practitioner pain communication," together with reviewers' comments and McDonald's response.

Create a Strong Research Team

For funded research, it is important to think strategically in putting together a team because reviewers often give considerable weight to researchers' qualifications. It is not enough to have a team of competent people; it is necessary to have the right *mix* of competence. Gaps and weaknesses can often be compensated for by the judicious use of consultants.

Another shortcoming of some project teams is that there are too many researchers with small time commitments. It is unwise to propose a staff with five or more top-level professionals who are able to contribute only 5% to 10% of their time to the project. Such projects often run into management problems because no one is in control of the workflow. Although collaborative work is commendable, you should be able to justify the inclusion of every person.

Things to Do as You Write

If you have planned well and drafted a realistic schedule, the next step is to move forward with the development of the proposal. Some suggestions for the writing stage follow.

Build a Persuasive Case

In a proposal, whether or not funding is sought, you need to persuade reviewers that you are asking the right questions, that you are the right person to ask those questions, and that you will get valid and credible answers. You must also convince them that the answers will make a difference to nursing and its clients.

Beginning proposal writers sometimes forget that they are *selling* a product: themselves and their ideas. It is appropriate, therefore, to think of the proposal as a marketing opportunity. It is not enough to have a good idea and sound methods—you must have a persuasive presentation. When funding is at stake, the challenge is greater because *everyone is trying to persuade reviewers that their proposal is more meritorious than yours.*

Reviewers know that most applications they review will *not* get funded. For example, in fiscal year 2013, the *success rate* for all applications to NINR was 9.1% (53 applications with awards out of 581 applications reviewed). The success rate for R01s was slightly higher (16.4%), but that means that more than four out of five applications did not receive funding. The reviewers' job is to identify the most scientifically worthy applications. In writing the proposal, you must consciously include features that will put your application in a positive light. That is, you should think of ways to gain a competitive edge. Be sure to give thought to issues persistently identified as problematic by reviewers (Inouye & Fiellin, 2005) and use a well-conceived checklist to ensure that you have not missed an opportunity to strengthen your study design and your proposal.

The proposal should be written in a positive, confident tone. If you do not sound convinced that the proposed study is important and will be rigorously done, then reviewers will not be persuaded either. It is unwise to promise what cannot be achieved, but you should think about ways to put the proposed project in a positive light.

Justify Methodologic Decisions

Many proposals fail because they do not instill confidence that key decisions have a good rationale. Methodologic decisions should be made carefully, keeping in mind the benefits and drawbacks of alternatives, and a compelling—if brief—justification should be provided. To the extent possible, make your decisions evidence-based and *defend* the proposed methods with citations demonstrating their utility. Insufficient detail and scanty explanation of methodologic choices can be perilous, although page constraints often make full elaboration impossible.

Begin and End with a Flourish

The abstract or summary to the proposal should be crafted with extreme care. Because it is one of the first things that reviewers read, you need to be sure that it will create a favorable impression. (For NIH applications, non-assigned reviewers may read *only* the summary and not the entire application.) The ideal abstract is one that generates excitement and inspires confidence in the proposed study's rigor. Although abstracts appear at the beginning of a proposal, they are often written last.

Proposals typically conclude with material that is somewhat unexciting, such as a data analysis plan. A brief, upbeat concluding paragraph that summarizes the significance and innovativeness of the proposed project can help to remind reviewers of its potential to contribute to nursing practice and nursing science.

Adhere to Instructions

Funding agencies (and universities) provide instructions on what is required in a research proposal. It is crucial to read these instructions carefully and to follow them precisely. Proposals are sometimes rejected without review if they do not adhere to such guidelines as minimum font size or page limitations.

Pay Attention to Presentation

Reviewers are put in a better frame of mind if the proposals they read are attractive, well organized, grammatical, and easy to read. Glitzy figures are not needed, but the presentation should be professional and show respect for weary reviewers. In Inouye and Fiellin's (2005) study, 20% of the grant applications were criticized for such presentation issues as typographical or grammatical errors, poor layout, inconsistencies, and omitted tables.

well-chosen committee and adviser. Dissertation proposals are sometimes "mini-dissertations" that include sections that can be incorporated into the dissertation.

- The federal government is the largest source of research funds for health researchers in the United States. In addition to regular grants programs through **Parent Announcements**, federal agencies such as the National Institutes of Health (NIH) announce special opportunities in the form of **Program Announcements (PAs)** and **Requests for Applications (RFAs)** for **grants** and **Requests for Proposals (RFPs)** for **contracts**.

- Nurses can apply for a variety of grants from NIH, the most common being **Research Project Grants** (R01 grants), **AREA Grants** (R15), **Small Grants** (R03), or **Exploratory/Developmental Grants** (R21). NIH also awards training fellowships through the National Research Service Award (NRSA) program as F-series awards, and Career Development Awards (K-series awards).

- Grant applications to NIH are submitted online using the SF424, which has a series of special forms (fillable screens) that require uploaded PDF attachments.

- The heart of an NIH grant application is the **research plan component**, which includes two major sections: Specific Aims and Research Strategy. The latter, which is restricted to 12 pages for R01 applications, includes subsections called Significance, Innovation, and Approach.

- NIH grant applications also require budgets, which can be abbreviated **modular budgets** if requested funds for R01 grants do not exceed $250,000 in direct costs per year.

- Grant applications to NIH are reviewed three times a year in a dual review process. The first phase involves a review by a peer review panel (or **study section**) that evaluates each proposal's scientific merit; the second phase is a review by an Advisory Council.

- In NIH's review procedure, the study section assigns **priority (intensity) scores** only to applications judged to be in the top half of proposals based on a preliminary appraisal by

assigned reviewers. A final priority score of 10 by the study section is the most meritorious score, and 90 is the lowest possible score.

- All applicants for NIH grants are sent a summary statement, which offers a critique of the proposal. Applicants of scored proposals also receive information on the intensity score and percentile ranking.

- Some suggestions for writing a strong proposal include several for the planning stage (e.g., starting early, selecting an important topic, learning about the audience, reviewing a successful proposal, creating a strong team) and several for the writing stage (building a persuasive case, justifying methodologic decisions, beginning and ending with a flourish, adhering to proposal instructions, and having the draft proposal critiqued by reviewers).

STUDY ACTIVITIES

Chapter 31 of the accompanying *Resource Manual for Nursing Research: Generating and Assessing Evidence for Nursing Practice*, 10th edition, offers various exercises and study suggestions for reinforcing the concepts taught in this chapter. In addition, the following study questions can be addressed:

1. Suppose that you were planning to study the self-care behaviors of aging AIDS patients.
   a. Outline the methods you would recommend adopting.
   b. Develop a project timeline.
2. Suppose you were interested in studying separation anxiety in hospitalized children. Using references cited in this chapter, identify potential funding sources for your project.

STUDIES CITED IN CHAPTER 31

*Berg, K. M., Gill, T., Brown, A., Zerzan, J., Elmore, J., & Wilson, I. (2007). Demystifying the NIH grant application process. *Journal of General Internal Medicine, 22*, 1587–1595.

Bliss, D. Z. (2005). Writing a grant proposal: Part 6: The budget, budget justification, and resource environment. *Journal of Wound, Ostomy, and Continence Nursing, 32,* 365–367.

Carey, M. A., & Swanson, J. (2003). Funding for qualitative research. *Qualitative Health Research, 13,* 852–256.

Dallas, C., Norr, K., Dancy, B., Kavanaugh, K., & Cassata, L. (2005a). An example of a successful research proposal: Part I. *Western Journal of Nursing Research, 27,* 50–72.

Dallas, C., Norr, K., Dancy, B., Kavanaugh, K., & Cassata, L. (2005b). An example of a successful research proposal: Part II. *Western Journal of Nursing Research, 27,* 210–231.

Funk, S. G., & Tornquist, E. M. (2015). *Writing winning proposals for nurses and health care professionals.* New York: Springer.

Grey, M. (2000). Top 10 tips for successful grantsmanship. *Research in Nursing & Health, 23,* 91–92.

Higdon, J., & Topp, R. (2004). How to develop a budget for a research proposal. *Western Journal of Nursing Research, 26,* 922–929.

Inouye, S. K., & Fiellin, D. A. (2005). An evidence-based guide to writing grant proposals for clinical research. *Annals of Internal Medicine, 142,* 274–282.

Knafl, K., & Deatrick, J. (2005). Top 10 tips for successful qualitative grantsmanship. *Research in Nursing & Health, 28,* 441–443.

Kuzel, A. J. (2002). Some lessons from the story of a funded project. *Qualitative Health Research, 12,* 140–142.

Locke, L., Spirduso, W., & Silverman, S. (2014). *Proposals that work: A guide for planning dissertations and grant proposals* (6th ed.). Thousand Oaks, CA: Sage.

Naylor, M. D. (1990). An example of a research grant application: Comprehensive discharge planning for the elderly. *Research in Nursing & Health, 13,* 327–347.

Padgett, D., & Henwood, B. (2009). Obtaining large-scale funding for empowerment-oriented qualitative research: A report from personal experience. *Qualitative Health Research, 19,* 868–874.

Parker, B., & Steeves, R. (2005). The National Research Service Award: Strategies for developing a successful proposal. *Journal of Professional Nursing, 21,* 23–31.

Roberts, C. M. (2010). *The dissertation journey: A practical and comprehensive guide to planning, writing, and defending your dissertation.* Thousand Oaks, CA: Sage.

Rudestam, K., & Newton, R. (2015). *Surviving your dissertation: A comprehensive guide to content and process* (4th ed.). Thousand Oaks, CA: Sage.

Sandelowski, M., Davis, D., & Harris, B. (1989). Artful design: Writing the proposal for research in the naturalist paradigm. *Research in Nursing & Health, 12,* 77–84.

***A link to this open-access journal article is provided in the Toolkit for this chapter in the accompanying* Resource Manual.** ✶

Glossary

absolute risk (AR) The proportion of people in a group who experienced an undesirable outcome.

absolute risk reduction (ARR) The difference between the absolute risk in one group (e.g., those exposed to an intervention) and the absolute risk in another group (e.g., those not exposed); sometimes called the *risk difference* or *RD*.

abstract A brief description of a completed or proposed study, usually located at the beginning of a report or proposal.

accessible population The population of people available for a particular study; often a nonrandom subset of the target population.

acquiescence response set A bias in self-report instruments, especially in psychosocial scales, created when participants characteristically agree with statements ("yea-say"), independent of content.

adherence to treatment The degree to which those in an intervention group adhere to protocols or continue getting the treatment.

adjusted mean The group mean for an outcome variable after statistically removing the effect of covariates.

after-only design An experimental design in which data are collected from participants only after an intervention has been introduced.

AGREE instrument A widely used instrument (Appraisal of Guidelines Research and Evaluation) for systematically assessing clinical practice guidelines.

allocation concealment The process used to ensure that the people enrolling subjects into a clinical trial are unaware of upcoming assignments, that is, of the group to which new enrollees will be assigned.

alpha (α) (1) In tests of statistical significance, the significance criterion—the risk the researcher is willing to accept of making a Type I error; (2) in measurement, an index of internal consistency, that is, Cronbach's alpha.

alternative hypothesis In hypothesis testing, a hypothesis different from the one actually being tested—usually, an alternative to the null hypothesis.

analysis The organization and synthesis of data so as to answer research questions and test hypotheses.

analysis of covariance (ANCOVA) A statistical procedure used to test mean group differences on a dependent variable while controlling for one or more covariate.

analysis of variance (ANOVA) A statistical procedure for testing mean differences among three or more groups by contrasting variability between groups to variability within groups, yielding an *F*-ratio statistic.

analysis triangulation The use of two or more analytic approaches to analyze the same set of data.

analytic generalization One of three models of generalization, concerning researchers' efforts to generalize from particulars to broader conceptualizations and theories.

ancestry approach In literature searches, using citations from relevant studies to track down earlier research upon which the studies were based (the "ancestors").

anchor-based approach An approach to estimating a measure's responsiveness, and to developing a benchmark of importance for interpreting change scores, that relies on a "gold standard" or criterion as the anchor.

anonymity Protection of participants' confidentiality such that even the researcher cannot link individuals with the data they provided.

applied research Research designed to find a solution to an immediate practical problem.

area under the curve (AUC) In an ROC analysis, an index of the performance of a diagnostic or screening measure vis-à-vis diagnostic accuracy, summarized in a single value that typically ranges from .50 (no better than random classification) to 1.0 (perfect classification).

arm A particular treatment condition to which participants are allocated (e.g., the control *arm* or treatment *arm* of a controlled trial).

ascertainment bias Systematic differences between groups being compared in how outcome variables are measured, verified, or recorded when data collectors have not been blinded; also called *detection bias*.

assent The affirmative agreement of an individual (e.g., a child) to participate in a study, typically to supplement formal consent by a parent or guardian.

associative relationship An association between two variables that cannot be described as causal.

assumption A principle that is accepted as being true based on logic or reason, without proof.

asymmetric distribution A distribution of data values that is skewed, with two halves that are not mirror images of each other.

attention control group A control group that gets a similar amount of attention as those in the intervention group, without receiving the "active ingredients" of the treatment.

attrition The loss of participants over the course of a study, which can create bias by changing the composition of the sample initially drawn.

AUC See *area under the curve*.

audio-CASI (computer-assisted self-interview) An approach to collecting self-report data in which respondents listen through headphones to questions being read, and respond by entering information onto a computer.

audit trail The systematic documentation of material that allows an independent auditor of a qualitative study to draw conclusions about trustworthiness.

authenticity The extent to which qualitative researchers fairly and faithfully show a range of different realities in the collection, analysis, and interpretation of data.

auto-ethnography An ethnographic study in which researchers study their own culture or group.

axial coding The second level of coding in a grounded theory study using the Strauss and Corbin's approach, involving the process of categorizing, recategorizing, and condensing first-level codes by connecting a category and its subcategories.

back translation The translation of a translated text (from a forward translation) back into the original language, so that original and back-translated versions can be compared to assess semantic equivalence.

baseline data Data collected at an initial measurement (e.g., prior to an intervention), so that changes can be evaluated.

basic research Research designed to extend the base of knowledge in a discipline for the sake of knowledge production or theory construction rather than for solving an immediate problem.

basic social process (BSP) The central social process emerging through analysis of grounded theory data.

before–after design A design in which data are collected from participants both before and after the introduction of an intervention.

benchmark In measurement, a threshold value on a measure that corresponds to an important value, such as a threshold for interpreting whether a change in scores is meaningful or clinically significant.

beneficence An ethical principle that seeks to maximize benefits for study participants and prevent harm.

beta (β) (1) In multiple regression, the standardized coefficients indicating the relative weights of the predictor variables in the equation; (2) in statistical testing, the probability of a Type II error.

between-subjects design A research design in which separate groups of people are compared (e.g., smokers and nonsmokers; intervention and control group subjects).

bias Any influence that distorts the results of a study and undermines validity.

bibliographic database Data files containing bibliographic (reference) information that can be accessed electronically for the purpose of conducting a literature search.

bimodal distribution A distribution of data values with two peaks (high frequencies).

binomial distribution A statistical distribution with known properties describing the number of occurrences of an event in a series of observations; forms the basis for analyzing dichotomous data.

bivariate statistics Statistical analysis of two variables to assess the empirical relationship between them.

Bland-Altman plot A graphic depiction of the degree of agreement between two sets of scores, for people who have been measured twice on the same continuous measurement scale; the plot highlights random differences between the two measurements through the construction of a parameter called the *limits of agreement*.

blind review The review of a manuscript or proposal such that neither the author nor the reviewer is identified to the other party.

blinding The process of preventing those involved in a study (participants, intervention agents, data collectors, or health care providers) from having information that could lead to a bias, particularly information about which treatment group a participant is in; also called *masking*.

Bonferroni correction An adjustment made to establish a more conservative alpha level when multiple statistical tests are being run from the same data set; the correction is computed by dividing the desired α by the number of tests—for example, $.05 / 3 = .017$.

borrowed theory   A theory, borrowed from another discipline, that has utility for nursing practice or research.

bracketing   In phenomenologic inquiries, the process of identifying and holding in abeyance any preconceived beliefs and opinions about the phenomena under study.

bricolage   The tendency in qualitative research to derive a complex array of data from a variety of sources, using a variety of methods.

calendar question   A question used to obtain retrospective information about the chronology of events and activities in people's lives.

carry-over effect   The influence that one treatment (or measurement) can have on subsequent treatments (or measurements), notably in a crossover design or in test–retest reliability assessments.

case mean substitution   An approach to imputing missing values that involves substituting a missing value with the mean of other relevant variables from the case with the missing value (e.g., using the mean of 9 non-missing items on a scale to impute the value of the 10th item, which is missing).

case study   A method involving a thorough, in-depth analysis of an individual, group, or other social unit.

case-control design   A nonexperimental research design that compares "cases" (i.e., people with a specified condition, such as lung cancer) to matched controls (similar people without the condition).

categorical variable   A variable with discrete values (e.g., gender) rather than values along a continuum (e.g., weight).

category system   In studies involving observation, the prespecified plan for recording the behaviors and events under observation; in qualitative studies, the system used to sort and organize the data.

causal (cause-and-effect) relationship   A relationship between two variables wherein the presence or value of one variable (the "cause") determines the presence or value of the other (the "effect").

causal modeling   The development and statistical testing of an explanatory model of hypothesized causal relationships among phenomena.

cause-probing research   Research designed to illuminate the underlying causes of phenomena.

ceiling effect   The effect of having scores restricted at the upper end of a continuum, which limits discrimination at the upper end of the measurement, constrains true variability, and restricts the amount of upward change possible.

cell   (1) The intersection of a row and column in a table with two or more dimensions; (2) in an experimental design, the representation of an experimental condition in a schematic diagram.

census   A survey covering an entire population.

central category   The main category or pattern of behavior in grounded theory analysis; sometimes referred to as the *core category*.

central limit theorem   A statistical principle stipulating that the larger the sample, the more closely the sampling distribution of the mean will approximate a normal distribution, and that the mean of a sampling distribution equals the population mean.

central tendency   A statistical index of what is "typical" in a set of scores, derived from the center of the score distribution; indices of central tendency include the mode, median, and mean.

Certificate of Confidentiality   A certificate issued by the National Institutes of Health in the United States to protect researchers against forced disclosure of confidential research information.

change score   A person's score difference between two measurements on the same measure, calculated by subtracting the value at one point in time from the value at the second point.

chi-square test   A statistical test used in various contexts, most often to assess differences in proportions; symbolized as χ^2.

classical test theory (CTT)   A measurement theory that has traditionally been used in the development of multi-item scales; in CTT, any score on a measure is conceptualized as having a "true score" component and an error component, and the goal is to approximate the true score.

clinical practice guidelines   Practice guidelines that are evidence-based, combining a synthesis and appraisal of research evidence with specific recommendations for clinical decisions.

clinical relevance   The degree to which a study addresses a problem of significance to clinical practice.

clinical research   Research designed to generate knowledge to guide practice in health care fields.

clinical significance   The practical importance of research results in terms of whether they have genuine, palpable effects on the daily lives of patients or on the health care decisions made on their behalf.

clinical trial   A study designed to assess the safety, efficacy, and effectiveness of a new clinical intervention, sometimes involving several phases (e.g., Phase III typically is a *randomized controlled trial* using an experimental design).

clinimetrics   An approach to the quantitative measurement of clinical phenomena such as symptoms and signs; an alternative approach to psychometrics for health measurement.

closed-ended question   A question that offers respondents a set of specific response options; also referred to as a *fixed alternative question*.

cluster randomization   The random assignment of intact groups of subjects (e.g., hospitals), rather than individual subjects, to treatment conditions.

cluster sampling   A form of sampling in which large groupings ("clusters") are selected first (e.g., nursing schools), typically with successive subsampling of smaller units (e.g., nursing students) in a multistage approach.

Cochrane Collaboration   An international organization that aims to facilitate well-informed decisions about health care by preparing systematic reviews, primarily about the effects of health care interventions.

code of ethics   The fundamental ethical principles established by a discipline or institution to guide researchers' conduct in research with human (or animal) study participants.

codebook   A record documenting categorization and coding decisions.

coding   The process of transforming raw data into standardized form for data processing and analysis; in quantitative research, the process of attaching numbers to categories; in qualitative research, the process of identifying and indexing recurring words, themes, or concepts within the data.

coefficient alpha   The most widely used index of internal consistency that indicates the degree to which the items on a multi-item scale are measuring the same underlying construct; also referred to as *Cronbach's alpha*.

coercion   In a research context, the explicit or implicit use of threats (or excessive rewards) to gain people's cooperation in a study.

cognitive questioning   A method sometimes used in a pretest of an instrument in which respondents are asked to explain the process by which they answer questions; basic approaches include a *think-aloud* method and the use of targeted *probes*; also used in connection with content validity work.

cognitive test   A performance test designed to assess cognitive skills or cognitive functioning (e.g., an IQ test).

Cohen's *d*   An effect size index for comparing two group means, computed by subtracting one mean from the other and dividing by the pooled standard deviation; also called *standardized mean difference* or *SMD*.

Cohen's kappa   See *kappa*.

cohort design   A nonexperimental design in which a defined group of people (a cohort) is followed over time to study outcomes for the cohort; also called a *prospective design*.

comparison group   A group of study participants whose scores on a dependent variable are used to evaluate the outcomes of the group of primary interest (e.g., nonsmokers as a comparison group for smokers); term often used in lieu of control group when the study design is not a true experiment.

compensatory equalization   A potential threat to design-related construct validity that can occur if health care staff try to compensate for control group members' failure to receive a perceived beneficial treatment.

compensatory rivalry   A potential threat to design-related construct validity that can arise from the control group members' desire to demonstrate that they can do as well as those receiving a special treatment.

complex intervention   An intervention in which complexity exists along one or more dimensions, including number of components, number of targeted outcomes, and the time needed for the full intervention to be delivered.

composite scale   A measure of an attribute, involving the aggregation of information from multiple items into a single numerical value that places people on a continuum with respect to the attribute.

computer-assisted personal interviewing (CAPI)   In-person interviewing in which the interviewer reads questions from, and enters responses onto, a computer.

computer-assisted telephone interviewing (CATI)   Interviewing done over the telephone in which the interviewer reads questions from, and enters responses onto, a computer.

computerized adaptive testing (CAT)   An approach to measuring a latent trait in which computer algorithms are used to tailor a set of questions to individuals, usually using questions from an item bank created using item response theory; with CAT, highly precise measures of a trait typically can be secured with a small set of targeted items.

concealment   A tactic involving the unobtrusive collection of research data without participants' knowledge or consent, used to obtain an accurate view of naturalistic behavior when the known presence of an observer would distort the behavior of interest.

concept   An abstraction inferred from observation of behaviors, situations, or characteristics (e.g., stress, pain).

concept analysis A systematic process of analyzing a concept or construct, with the aim of identifying the boundaries, definitions, and dimensionality for that concept.

conceptual definition The abstract or theoretical meaning of a concept being studied.

conceptual equivalence The extent to which a construct of interest exists and is comparable in another culture; of relevance in the translation or cultural adaptation of an instrument.

conceptual file A manual method of organizing qualitative data, by creating file folders for each category in the coding scheme, and inserting relevant excerpts from the data.

conceptual map A schematic representation of a theory or conceptual model that graphically represents key concepts and linkages among them.

conceptual model Interrelated concepts or abstractions assembled in a rational and often explanatory scheme to illuminate relationships among them; sometimes called *conceptual framework*.

concurrent design A mixed methods study design in which the qualitative and quantitative strands of data collection occur simultaneously; symbolically designated with a plus sign, as in QUAL + QUAN.

concurrent validity The degree to which scores on an instrument are correlated with an external criterion, measured at the same time.

confidence interval (CI) The range of values within which a population parameter is estimated to lie, at a specified probability (e.g., 95% CI).

confidence limit The upper (or lower) boundary of a confidence interval.

confidentiality Protection of study participants so that data provided are never publicly divulged.

confirmability A criterion for trustworthiness in a qualitative inquiry, referring to the objectivity or neutrality of the data and interpretations.

confirmatory factor analysis (CFA) A factor analysis designed to confirm a hypothesized measurement model, using maximum likelihood estimation; used to provide evidence of structural validity.

confounding variable A variable that is extraneous to the research question and that confounds understanding of the relationship between the independent and dependent variables; confounding variables can be controlled in the research design or through statistical procedures.

consecutive sampling Involves recruiting *all* of the people from an accessible population who meet the eligibility criteria over a specific time interval, or for a specified sample size.

consent form A written agreement signed by a study participant and a researcher concerning the terms and conditions of voluntary participation in a study.

consistency check A procedure performed in cleaning a set of data to ensure that the data are internally consistent.

CONSORT guidelines Widely adopted guidelines (Consolidated Standards of Reporting Trials) for reporting information for a randomized controlled trial, including a checklist and flowchart for tracking participants through the trial, from recruitment through data analysis.

constant comparison A procedure used in a grounded theory analysis wherein newly collected data are compared in an ongoing fashion with data obtained earlier to refine theoretically relevant categories.

constitutive pattern In hermeneutic analysis, a pattern that expresses the relationships among relational themes and is present in all the interviews or texts.

construct An abstraction or concept that is invented (constructed) by researchers based on inferences from human behavior or human traits (e.g., health locus of control); sometimes referred to as a *latent trait*.

construct validity The degree to which evidence about study particulars supports inferences about the higher order constructs they are intended to represent; in measurement, the degree to which a measure truly captures the focal construct.

constructivist grounded theory An approach to grounded theory, developed by Charmaz, in which the grounded theory is constructed from shared experiences and relationships between the researcher and study participants and interpretive aspects are emphasized.

constructivist paradigm An alternative to the positivist paradigm that holds that there are multiple interpretations of reality and that the goal of research is to understand how individuals construct reality within their context; associated with qualitative research; also called *naturalistic paradigm*.

consumer An individual who reads, reviews, and critiques research findings and who attempts to use and apply the findings in his or her practice.

contact information Information obtained from study participants in longitudinal studies to facilitate locating them at a future date.

contamination The inadvertent, undesirable influence of one treatment condition on another treatment condition, as when members of the control group receive the intervention; sometimes called *treatment diffusion*.

content analysis The process of extracting, organizing, and synthesizing material from documents, often the narrative data from a qualitative study, according to key concepts and themes.

content validity The degree to which a multi-item instrument has an appropriate set of relevant items reflecting the full content of the construct domain being measured.

content validity index (CVI) An index summarizing the degree to which a panel of experts agrees on an instrument's content validity, that is, the relevance, comprehensiveness, and balance of items comprising a scale; both item content validity (I-CVI) and the overall scale content validity (S-CVI) can be assessed.

contingency table A two-dimensional table in which the frequencies of two categorical variables are cross-tabulated; also called a *crosstabs table*.

continuous variable A variable that can take on an infinite range of values along a specified continuum (e.g., height); less strictly, a variable measured on an interval or ratio scale.

control, research The process of holding constant confounding influences on the dependent variable under study.

control group Participants in an experimental study who do not receive the experimental treatment and whose performance provides a counterfactual, against which the effects of the treatment can be measured (see also *comparison group*).

controlled trial A trial that has a control group, with or without randomization.

convenience sampling Selection of the most readily available persons as participants in a study.

convergent design A concurrent, equal-priority mixed methods design in which different, but complementary data, qualitative and quantitative, are gathered about a central phenomenon under study; symbolized as QUAL + QUAN; sometimes called a *triangulation design*.

convergent validity A type of construct validity concerning the degree to which scores on a focal measure are correlated with scores on measures of constructs with which there is a hypothesized correlation (i.e., whether there is conceptual convergence).

core category (variable) In a grounded theory study, the central phenomenon that is used to integrate all categories of the data.

correlation An association or bond between variables, with variation in one variable systematically related to variation in another.

correlation coefficient An index summarizing the degree of relationship between variables, typically ranging from +1.00 (for a perfect positive relationship) through 0.0 (for no relationship) to −1.00 (for a perfect negative relationship).

correlation matrix A two-dimensional display showing the correlation coefficients between all pairs of variables in a set of several variables.

correlational research Research that explores the interrelationships among variables of interest without researcher intervention.

COSMIN The **Co**nsensus-based **S**tandards for the selection of health **M**easurement **In**struments, an initiative that developed an important measurement taxonomy and sought to standardize the definitions of measurement properties.

cost–benefit analysis An economic analysis in which both costs and outcomes of a program or intervention are expressed in monetary terms and compared.

cost-effectiveness analysis An economic analysis in which costs of an intervention are measured in monetary terms, but outcomes are expressed in natural units (e.g., the costs per added year of life).

cost–utility analysis An economic analysis that expresses the effects of an intervention as overall health improvement and describes costs for some additional utility gain—usually in relation to gains in quality-adjusted life years (QALY).

counterbalancing The process of systematically varying the order of presentation of stimuli or treatments to control for ordering effects, especially in a crossover design.

counterfactual The condition or group used as a basis of comparison in a trial, embodying what would have happened *to the same people* exposed to a causal factor if they *simultaneously* were *not* exposed to the causal factor.

covariate A variable that is statistically controlled (held constant) in ANCOVA, typically a confounding influence on, or a pre-intervention measure of, the dependent variable.

covert data collection The collection of information in a study without participants' knowledge.

Cox regression A regression analysis in which independent variables are used to model the risk (or hazard) of experiencing an event at a given point in time, given that one has not experienced the event before that time.

Cramér's V An index describing the magnitude of relationship between nominal-level data, used when the contingency table to which it is applied is larger than 2×2.

credibility A criterion for evaluating trustworthiness in qualitative studies, referring to confidence in the truth of the data; analogous to internal validity in quantitative research.

criterion sampling A purposive sampling approach used by qualitative researchers that involves selecting cases that meet a predetermined criterion of importance.

criterion validity The extent to which scores on a measure are an adequate reflection of (or predictor of) a criterion—that is, a "gold standard" measure.

critical case sampling A sampling approach used by qualitative researchers involving the purposeful selection of cases that are especially important or illustrative.

critical ethnography An ethnography that focuses on raising consciousness in the group or culture under study in the hope of effecting social change.

critical incidents technique A method of obtaining data from study participants by in-depth exploration of specific incidents and behaviors related to the topic under study.

critical region The area in the sampling distribution representing values that are "improbable" if the null hypothesis were true.

critical theory An approach to viewing the world that involves a critique of society, with the goal of envisioning new possibilities and effecting social change.

critique A critical appraisal that analyzes both weaknesses and strengths of a research report or proposal.

Cronbach's alpha A widely used index that estimates the internal consistency of a composite measure composed of several subparts; also called *coefficient alpha*.

cross-cultural validity The degree to which the items on a translated or culturally adapted scale perform adequately and equivalently, individually, and in the aggregate, in relation to their performance on the original instrument; an aspect of construct validity.

crossover design An experimental design in which one group of subjects is exposed to more than one condition or treatment, in random order.

cross-sectional design A study design in which data are collected at one point in time; sometimes used to infer change over time when data are collected from different age or developmental groups.

crosstabulation A calculation of frequencies for two variables considered simultaneously—for example, gender (male/female) crosstabulated with smoking status (smoker/nonsmoker).

cutpoint (cutoff point) The point in a distribution of scores used to classify or divide people into different groups, such as cases and noncases for a disease or health problem (e.g., the cutpoint for classifying newborns as being low birth weight is 5.5 pounds [2,500 grams]).

d A widely used effect size index for comparing two group means, computed by subtracting one mean from the other and dividing by the pooled standard deviation; also called *Cohen's d* or *standardized mean difference*.

data The pieces of information obtained in a study; the singular is *datum*.

data analysis The systematic organization and synthesis of research data and, in quantitative studies, the testing of hypotheses using those data.

data cleaning The preparation of data for analysis by performing checks to ensure that the data are consistent and accurate.

data collection The gathering of information to address a research problem.

data collection protocols The formal procedures researchers develop to guide the collection of data in a standardized fashion.

data entry The process of entering data onto an input medium for computer analysis.

data saturation See *saturation*.

data set The total collection of data on all variables for all study participants.

data transformation A step often undertaken before data analysis to put the data in a form that can be meaningfully analyzed (e.g., recoding of values).

data triangulation The use of multiple data sources for the purpose of validating conclusions.

debriefing Communication with study participants after participation is complete regarding aspects of the study.

deception The deliberate withholding of information, or the provision of false information, to study participants, usually to minimize potential biases.

deductive reasoning The process of developing specific predictions from general principles; see also *inductive reasoning*.

degrees of freedom (*df*) A statistical concept referring to the number of sample values free to vary (e.g., with a given sample mean, all but one value would be free to vary).

de-identified data Data or records from which identifying information is removed to protect the privacy of individuals.

delay of treatment design A design for an intervention study that involves putting control group members on a waiting list for the intervention until follow-up data are collected; also called a *wait-list design*.

Delphi survey A technique for obtaining judgments from an expert panel about an issue of concern; experts are questioned individually in several rounds, with a summary of the panel's views circulated between rounds, to achieve some consensus.

dependability A criterion for evaluating trustworthiness in qualitative studies, referring to the stability of data over time and over conditions; analogous to reliability in quantitative research.

dependent variable The variable hypothesized to depend on or be caused by another variable (the *independent variable*); the outcome variable of interest.

descendancy approach In literature searches, finding a pivotal early study and searching forward in citation indexes to find more recent studies ("descendants") that cited the key study.

descriptive research Research that typically has as its main objective the accurate portrayal of people's characteristics or circumstances and/or the frequency with which certain phenomena occur.

descriptive statistics Statistics used to describe and summarize data (e.g., means, percentages).

descriptive theory A broad characterization that thoroughly accounts for a phenomenon.

detection bias Systematic differences between groups being compared in how outcome variables are measured, verified, or recorded; a bias that can result when there is no blinding of data collectors.

determinism The belief that phenomena are not haphazard or random but rather have antecedent causes; an assumption in the positivist paradigm.

deviation score A score computed by subtracting an individual score from the mean of all scores.

diagnostic accuracy The degree to which a measure is accurate in diagnosing or predicting "caseness" and "noncaseness" for a condition, as established by a gold-standard criterion. See also *sensitivity, specificity*.

dichotomous variable A variable having only two values or categories (e.g., gender).

differential item functioning (DIF) The extent to which an item functions differently for one group than for another despite the groups being equivalent with respect to the underlying latent trait.

direct costs Specific project-related costs incurred during a study (e.g., for supplies, salaries).

directional hypothesis A hypothesis that makes a specific prediction about the direction of the relationship between two variables.

disconfirming case In qualitative research, a case that challenges the researchers' conceptualizations; sometimes used as part of a sampling strategy.

discourse analysis A qualitative tradition, from the discipline of sociolinguistics, that seeks to understand the rules, mechanisms, and structure of conversations.

discrete variable A variable with a finite number of values between two points.

discriminant validity See *divergent validity*.

discriminative validity See *known-groups validity*.

disproportionate sampling A sampling approach in which the researcher samples varying proportions of people from different population strata to ensure adequate representation from smaller strata.

distribution-based approach An approach to estimating a measure's responsiveness, and to developing a benchmark of importance for interpreting change scores, that relies on distributional properties of the data—often the distribution of change scores.

divergent validity An approach to construct validation that involves gathering evidence that the focal measure is not a measure of a different construct, distinct from the focal construct; also referred to as *discriminant validity*.

domain In ethnographic analysis, a unit or broad category of cultural knowledge.

domain analysis One of Spradley's levels of ethnographic analysis, focusing on the identification of domains, or units of cultural knowledge.

domain sampling model The model underpinning scale development in the classical test theory framework, which conceptually involves the random sampling of a homogeneous set of items from a hypothetical universe of items relating to the construct.

dose-response analysis An analysis to assess whether larger doses of an intervention are associated with greater benefits, usually in a quasi-experimental framework.

double-blind study A study (usually a clinical trial) in which two groups are blinded with respect to the group that a study participant is in; often a situation in which neither the subjects nor those who administer the treatment know who is in the experimental or control group.

dummy variable Dichotomous variables created for use in many multivariate statistical analyses, typically using codes of 0 and 1 (e.g., female = 1, male = 0).

ecologic momentary assessment (EMA) Repeated assessments of people's feelings, experiences, or behaviors in real time, within their natural environment, using contemporary technologies such as smartphones.

ecologic psychology A qualitative tradition that focuses on the environment's influence on human behavior and attempts to identify principles that explain the interdependence of humans and their environmental context.

economic analysis An analysis of the relationship between costs and outcomes of alternative health care interventions.

effect size (ES) In quantitative research, an index summarizing, in standardized units, the magnitude of change in a group or the amount of difference in two groups on a measure; for mean-difference situations, calculated by dividing the mean difference in two scores by an index of variability, usually the baseline *SD*; sometimes referred to as *Cohen's d* or the *standardized mean difference*; in metasynthesis, an index used to characterize the salience of a theme or category.

effectiveness study A clinical trial designed to shed light on effectiveness of an intervention under ordinary conditions, often with an intervention already found to be efficacious in an efficacy study.

efficacy study A tightly controlled trial designed to establish the efficacy of an intervention under ideal conditions, using a design that maximizes internal validity.

egocentric network analysis An ethnographic method that focuses on the pattern of relationships and networks of individuals; researchers develop lists of a person's network members (called *alters*) and seek to understand the scope and nature of interrelationships and social supports.

eigenvalue The value equal to the sum of the squared weights for a linear composite, such as a factor in a factor analysis, indicating how much variance in the solution is accounted for.

element The most basic unit of a population for sampling purposes, typically a human being.

eligibility criteria The criteria designating the specific attributes of the target population by which people are selected for inclusion in a study.

emergent design A design that unfolds in the course of a qualitative study as the researcher makes ongoing design decisions reflecting what has already been learned.

emergent fit A concept in grounded theory that involves comparing new data and new categories with previously existing conceptualizations.

emic perspective An ethnographic term referring to the way members of a culture themselves view their world; the "insider's view."

empirical evidence Evidence rooted in objective reality and gathered using one's senses as the basis for generating knowledge.

endogenous variable In a structural equations model or path analysis, a variable whose variation is determined by other variables within the model.

end point In a clinical trial, the target outcome of interest.

equivalence In the context of instrument translation, the degree to which the translated and original measures are comparable; many types of equivalence can be evaluated, including conceptual equivalence, content equivalence, semantic equivalence, technical equivalence, measurement equivalence, and factorial equivalence.

equivalence trial A trial designed to assess whether the outcomes of two or more treatments do *not* differ by a prespecified amount judged to be clinically unimportant.

error of measurement The deviation between hypothetical true scores and obtained scores of a measured characteristic.

error term The mathematic expression (e.g., in a regression analysis) that represents all unknown or unmeasurable attributes that can affect the dependent variable.

estimation procedures Statistical procedures that estimate population parameters based on sample statistics.

eta squared In ANOVA, a statistic calculated to indicate the proportion of variance in the dependent variable explained by the independent variables, analogous to R^2 in multiple regression.

ethics A system of moral values that is concerned with the degree to which research procedures adhere to professional, legal, and social obligations to study participants.

ethnography A branch of human inquiry, associated with anthropology, that focuses on the culture of a group of people, with an effort to understand the worldview and customs of those under study.

ethnomethodology A branch of human inquiry, associated with sociology, that focuses on the way in which people make sense of their everyday activities and come to behave in socially acceptable ways.

ethnonursing research The study of human cultures, with a focus on a group's beliefs and practices relating to nursing care and related health behaviors.

etic perspective In ethnography, the "outsider's" view of the experiences of a cultural group.

evaluation research Research that assesses how well a program, practice, or policy is working.

event history calendar A data collection matrix that plots time on one dimension and events or activities of interest on the other.

event sampling A sampling plan that involves the selection of integral behaviors or events to be observed.

evidence hierarchy A ranked arrangement of the strength of research evidence based on the rigor of the method that produced it; the traditional evidence hierarchy is appropriate primarily for cause-probing research.

evidence-based practice (EBP) A practice that involves making clinical decisions on the best available evidence, with an emphasis on evidence from disciplined research.

exclusion criteria The criteria specifying characteristics that a target population does *not* have.

exogenous variable In a structural equations model or path analysis, a variable whose determinants lie outside the model.

expectation bias The bias that can arise when study participants (or research staff) have expectations about treatment effectiveness in intervention research; the expectation can result in altered behavior or altered communication.

expectation maximization (EM) imputation A sophisticated single-imputation process that generates an estimated value for missing data in two steps (an expectation or E-step and a maximization or M-step), using maximum likelihood estimation.

experimental group The study participants who receive the experimental treatment or intervention.

experimental research A study using a design in which the researcher controls (manipulates) the independent variable by randomly assigning subjects to different treatment conditions; randomized controlled trials use experimental designs.

explanatory design A sequential mixed methods design in which quantitative data are collected in the first phase and qualitative data are collected in the second phase to build on or explain quantitative findings; symbolized as QUAN → qual or quan → QUAL.

exploratory design A sequential mixed methods design in which qualitative data are collected in the first phase and quantitative data are collected in the second phase based on the initial in-depth exploration; symbolized as QUAL → quan or qual → QUAN.

exploratory factor analysis (EFA) A factor analysis undertaken to explore the underlying dimensionality of a set of variables.

exploratory research A study that explores the dimensions of a phenomenon or that develops or refines hypotheses about relationships between phenomena.

external criticism In historical research, the systematic evaluation of the authenticity and genuineness of data.

external validity The degree to which study results can be generalized to settings or samples other than the one studied.

extraneous variable A variable that confounds the relationship between the independent and dependent variables and that needs to be controlled either in the research design or through statistical procedures; often called *confounding variable*.

extreme case sampling A sampling approach used by qualitative researchers that involves the purposeful selection of the most extreme or unusual cases.

extreme response bias A bias resulting from a respondent's consistent selection of extreme alternatives (e.g., *strongly agree* or *strongly disagree*) to scale items regardless of item content.

***F*-ratio** The statistic obtained in several statistical tests (e.g., ANOVA) in which variation attributable to different sources (e.g., between-group variation and within-group variation) is contrasted.

face validity The extent to which a measuring instrument looks as though it is measuring what it purports to measure.

factor analysis A statistical procedure for disentangling complex interrelationships among items and identifying the items that "go together" as a unified dimension.

factor extraction The first phase of a factor analysis, which involves the extraction of as much variance as possible through the successive creation of linear combinations of the variables or items in the data set.

factor loading In factor analysis, the weight associated with a variable or item on a given factor.

factor matrix In a factor analysis of scale items, a matrix with items on one dimension and factors on the other, with matrix entries being factor loadings of the items on the factors; factor matrices can be either *rotated* or *unrotated*.

factor rotation The second phase of factor analysis, during which the reference axes for the factors are pivoted to more clearly align items or variables with a single factor.

factorial design An experimental design in which two or more independent variables are simultaneously manipulated, permitting a separate analysis of the main effects of the independent variables and their interaction.

fail-safe number In meta-analysis, an estimate of the number of studies with nonsignificant results that would be needed to reverse the conclusion of a significant effect.

feasibility study Research completed prior to a main intervention study to test specific aspects of an emerging intervention or the anticipated trial (e.g., the intervention's acceptability).

feminist research   Research that seeks to understand, typically through qualitative approaches, how gender and a gendered social order shape women's lives and their consciousness.

field diary   A daily record of events and conversations in the field; also called a *log*.

field notes   The notes taken by researchers to record the unstructured observations made in the field and the interpretation of those observations.

field research   Research in which the data are collected "in the field" from people in their normal roles, with the aim of understanding the practices, behaviors, and beliefs of individuals or groups as they normally function in real life.

fieldwork   The activities undertaken by qualitative researchers to collect data out in the field, that is, in natural settings.

findings   The results of the analysis of research data.

Fisher's exact test   A statistical procedure used to test the significance of differences in proportions, used when the sample size is small or cells in the contingency table have no observations.

fit   An element in Glaserian grounded theory analysis in which the researcher develops categories of a substantive theory that fit the data.

fittingness   The degree of congruence between a sample of people in a qualitative study and another group or setting of interest, a concept often referred to as *transferability*.

fixed alternative question   A question that offers respondents a set of prespecified response options; also called a *closed-ended question*.

fixed effects model   In meta-analysis, a model in which studies are assumed to be measuring the same overall effect; a pooled effect estimate is calculated under the assumption that observed variation between studies is attributable to chance.

floor effect   The effect of having scores restricted at the lower end of a continuum, which limits the ability of the measure to discriminate at the lower end, constrains true variability, and limits the amount of downward change possible.

focus group interview   An interview with a small group of individuals assembled to provide feedback on a given topic, usually guided by a moderator using a semistructured topic guide.

focused interview   A loosely structured interview in which an interviewer guides the respondent through a set of questions using a topic guide.

follow-up study   A study undertaken to ascertain the outcomes of individuals who have a specified condition or who received a specified treatment.

forced-choice question   A question requiring respondents to choose between two statements that represent polar positions.

forest plot   A graphic representation of effects across studies in a meta-analysis, permitting a visual assessment of heterogeneity of effects.

formal grounded theory   A theory of a substantive grounded theory's core category that is extended by sampling other studies in a wide range of substantive areas.

formative evaluation   An ongoing assessment of a product or program as it is being developed to optimize its quality and effectiveness.

formative index   A multi-item measure whose items are viewed as "causing" or defining the construct of interest rather than being the effect of the construct; distinct from a *reflective scale*.

forward translation   The translation of an item (or any text, such as scale instructions) from an original source language into a target language. See also *back translation*.

framework   The conceptual underpinnings of a study— a *theoretical framework* in theory-based studies, or *conceptual framework* in studies based on a conceptual model.

frequency distribution   A systematic array of numeric values from the lowest to the highest, together with a count of the number of times each value was obtained.

frequency effect size   In a qualitative metasummary, the percentage of reports that contain a given thematic finding.

frequency polygon   Graphic display of a frequency distribution, in which dots connected by a straight line indicate the number of times score values occur in a data set.

Friedman test   A nonparametric analog of ANOVA, used with paired-groups or repeated measures situations.

full disclosure   The communication of complete, accurate information to potential study participants.

functional relationship   A relationship between two variables in which it cannot be assumed that one variable caused the other.

funnel plot   A graphical display that plots a measure of study precision (e.g., sample size) against effect size to explore the possibility of publication bias.

gaining entrée   The process of gaining access to study participants through the cooperation of key gatekeepers in the selected community or site.

general linear model (GLM)   A large class of statistical techniques (including regression analysis,

ANOVA, and correlational analysis) that describe the relationship between a dependent variable and one or more independent variables.

generalizability The degree to which the research methods justify the inference that the findings are true for a broader group than study participants; usually, the inference that the findings can be generalized from the sample to the population.

global rating scale (GRS) A single item designed to provide a summary measurement of a person's status on a construct, or his or her perception of change on a construct over a specified interval; also referred to as a *health transition rating*.

"going native" A pitfall in ethnographic research wherein a researcher becomes emotionally involved with participants and therefore loses the ability to observe objectively.

grand theory A broad theory aimed at describing large segments of the physical, social, or behavioral world; also called a *macrotheory*.

grand tour question A broad question asked in an unstructured interview to gain a general overview of a phenomenon on the basis of which more focused questions are subsequently asked.

grant A financial award made to a researcher to conduct a proposed study.

grantsmanship The combined set of skills and knowledge needed to secure financial support for a research idea.

graphic rating scale A scale in which respondents are asked to rate a concept along an ordered, numbered continuum, typically on a bipolar dimension (e.g., "excellent" to "very poor").

grey literature Unpublished, and thus less readily accessible, papers or research reports.

grounded theory An approach to collecting and analyzing qualitative data that aims to develop theories grounded in data from real-world observations.

handsearching The planned searching of a journal article by article (i.e., by hand) to identify relevant reports that might be missed by electronic searching.

Hawthorne effect The effect on the dependent variable resulting from people's awareness that they are participants under study.

health transition rating scale A single item, often on a 7-point scale, that asks people to rate the extent to which they have improved/deteriorated (e.g., slightly, moderately, greatly) or stayed the same with regard to a focal attribute.

hermeneutic circle In hermeneutics, a methodologic and interpretive process in which, to reach understanding, there is continual movement between the parts and the whole of the text that are being analyzed.

hermeneutics A qualitative research tradition, drawing on interpretive phenomenology, that focuses on the lived experiences of humans and on how they interpret those experiences.

heterogeneity The degree to which objects are dissimilar (i.e., characterized by variability) on some attribute.

hierarchical multiple regression A multiple regression analysis in which predictor variables are entered into the equation in a series of pre-specified steps.

histogram A graphic presentation of frequency distribution data.

historical comparison group A comparison group chosen from a group who were observed at some time in the past or for whom data are available through records.

historical research Systematic studies designed to discover facts and relationships about past events.

history threat The occurrence of events external to an intervention, but concurrent with it, that can affect the dependent variable and threaten the study's internal validity.

homogeneity The degree to which objects are similar (i.e., characterized by low variability).

homogeneous sampling A purposive sampling approach used by qualitative researchers involving the deliberate selection of cases with limited variation.

Hosmer-Lemeshow test A test used in logistic regression to evaluate the degree to which observed frequencies of predicted probabilities correspond to expected frequencies in an ideal model over the range of probability values; a good fit is indicated by lack of statistical significance.

hypothesis A prediction of outcomes, most often about predicted relationships between variables.

hypothesis-testing validity The extent to which it is possible to corroborate hypotheses regarding how scores on a measure function in relation to other variables; an important aspect of construct validity.

identical sampling An approach to sampling in mixed methods studies in which all of the participants are included in both the qualitative and quantitative strands of the study.

impact analysis An evaluation of the effects of a program or intervention on outcomes of interest, net of other factors influencing those outcomes.

impact factor An annual measure of citation frequency for an average article in a given journal over a 2-year period, that is, the ratio between citations and recent citable items published in the journal.

implementation analysis In evaluations, a descriptive analysis of the process by which a program or intervention was implemented in practice.

implementation potential The extent to which an innovation is amenable to implementation in a new setting, an assessment of which is usually made in an evidence-based practice project.

implied consent Consent to participate in a study that a researcher assumes has been given based on participants' actions, such as returning a completed questionnaire.

imputation methods A broad class of methods used to address missing values problems by estimating (imputing) the missing values.

IMRAD format The standard organization of a research report into four sections: the Introduction, Method, Results, and Discussion sections.

incidence rate The rate of new cases with a specified condition, computed by dividing the number of new cases over a given period of time by the number at risk of becoming a new case (i.e., free of the condition at the outset of the time period).

independent variable The variable that is believed to cause or influence the dependent variable; in experimental research, the manipulated (treatment) variable.

index A multi-item measure by convention differentiated from a *scale* in that the term *index* is used for a formative (rather than a reflective) measure.

indirect costs Administrative costs, over and above the specific (direct) costs of conducting the study; also called *overhead*.

inductive reasoning The process of reasoning from specific observations to more general rules (see also *deductive reasoning*).

inference In research, a conclusion drawn from the study evidence, taking into account the methods used to generate that evidence.

inference quality An overarching criterion for the integrity of mixed methods studies, referring to the believability and accuracy of inductively and deductively derived conclusions.

inferential statistics Statistics that permit inferences about whether results observed in a sample are likely to be reliable, that is, found in the population.

informant An individual who provides information to researchers about a phenomenon under study, usually in qualitative studies.

informed consent An ethical principle that requires researchers to obtain people's voluntary participation, after informing them of possible risks and benefits.

inquiry audit An independent scrutiny of qualitative data and relevant supporting documents by an external reviewer to evaluate the dependability and confirmability of qualitative data.

insider research Research on a group or culture—usually in an ethnography—by a member of the group or culture; in ethnographic research, an *autoethnography*.

Institutional Review Board (IRB) A term used primarily in the United States to refer to the institutional group that convenes to review proposed and ongoing studies with respect to ethical considerations.

instrument The device used to collect data (e.g., a questionnaire, test, observation schedule).

instrumentation threat The threat to the internal validity of the study that can arise if the researcher changes the measuring instrument between two points of data collection.

intensity effect size In a qualitative metasummary, the percentage of all thematic findings that are contained in any given report.

intensity sampling A sampling approach used by qualitative researchers involving the purposeful selection of intense (but not extreme) cases.

intention-to-treat A strategy for analyzing data in a randomized controlled trial that includes all randomized participants in the group to which they were assigned, whether or not they received or completed the treatment associated with the group, and whether or not their outcome data were missing.

interaction effect The effect of two or more independent variables acting in combination (interactively) on a dependent variable.

intercoder reliability The degree to which two coders, working independently, agree on coding decisions.

internal consistency The degree to which the subparts of a composite scale (i.e., the items) are interrelated and are all measuring the same attribute or dimension, usually as evaluated using coefficient alpha; a measurement property within the reliability domain.

internal criticism In historical research, an evaluation of the worth of the historical evidence.

internal validity The degree to which it can be inferred that an experimental intervention (independent variable), rather than confounding factors, caused the observed effects on the outcome.

interpretability In measurement, the degree to which it is possible to assign qualitative meaning to an instrument's scores or change scores.

interpretation The process of making sense of the results of a study and examining their implications.

interquartile range (*IQR*) A measure of variability, indicating the difference between Q_3 (the third quartile or 75th percentile) and Q_1 (the first quartile or 25th percentile).

interrater (interobserver) reliability   The degree to which two raters or observers, operating independently, assign the same ratings or score values for an attribute being measured.

interrupted time series design   See *time series design*.

interval estimation   A statistical estimation approach in which the researcher establishes a range of values that are likely, within a given level of confidence, to contain the true population parameter.

interval measurement   A measurement level in which an attribute or a variable is rank ordered on a scale that has equal distances between points on that scale (e.g., Fahrenheit degrees).

intervention   In experimental research (clinical trials), the treatment being tested.

intervention fidelity   The extent to which the implementation of a treatment is faithful to its plan.

intervention protocol   The specification of exactly what the intervention and alternative (or control) treatment conditions are and how they should be administered.

intervention research   Research involving the development, implementation, and testing of an intervention.

intervention theory   The conceptual underpinning of a health care intervention, which articulates the theoretical basis for what must be done to achieve desired outcomes.

interview   A data collection method in which an interviewer asks questions of a respondent, either face-to-face or by telephone.

interview schedule   The formal instrument that specifies the wording of all questions to be asked of respondents in structured self-report studies.

intraclass correlation coefficient (ICC)   The statistical index used to assess the reliability (e.g., test–retest reliability) of a measure; the ICC estimates the proportion of total variance in a set of scores that is attributable to true differences among the people or objects being measured.

intrarater reliability   The extent to which a rater or observer assigns the same score values for an attribute being observed on two separate occasions, as an index of self-consistency.

intuiting   The second step in descriptive phenomenology, which occurs when researchers remain open to the meaning attributed to the phenomenon by those who experienced it.

inverse relationship   A relationship characterized by the tendency of high values on one variable to be as-sociated with low values on the second variable; also called a *negative relationship*.

inverse variance method   In meta-analysis, a method that uses the inverse of the variance of the effect estimate (one divided by the square of its standard error) as the weight to calculate a weighted average of effects.

investigator triangulation   The use of two or more researchers to analyze and interpret a data set to enhance trustworthiness.

Iowa Model of Evidence-Based Practice   A widely used framework that can be used to guide the development and implementation of a project to promote evidence-based practice.

item   A single question on an instrument, or a single statement on a scale.

item analysis   A type of analysis used to assess whether items on a scale are tapping the same construct and are sufficiently discriminating.

item bank   A large collection of previously tested items, usually with the aim of using the items in computerized adaptive testing (e.g., the PROMIS® item bank established by NIH).

item characteristic curve (ICC)   In item response theory, a graphic representation of an item's performance that models the relationship between people's responses to the item and their level of the latent trait; typically an ICC is approximately S-shaped, and different parts of the curve yield information about different item parameters, such as difficulty and discrimination.

item discrimination   A parameter in item response theory models that indicates the degree to which an item can differentiate between people with different levels of the latent trait.

item location   A parameter in item response theory and Rasch models, indicating the amount of a latent trait a respondent must possess in order to "pass" (or endorse) an item; also referred to as *item difficulty*.

item response theory (IRT)   A "modern" measurement perspective, also referred to as *latent trait theory*, that is gaining favor in lieu of classical test theory in developing highly precise multi-item measures of latent traits; in IRT, the focus is on understanding item characteristics, independent of the people who complete the items.

joint interview   An interview where two or more people are interviewed simultaneously, typically using either a semistructured or unstructured interview.

jottings   Short notes jotted down quickly while engaged in fieldwork so as to not distract researchers from their observations or their role as participating members of a group.

journal article A report appearing in a professional journal such as *Nursing Research* or *International Journal of Nursing Studies*.

journal club A group that meets in clinical settings to discuss and critique research reports appearing in journals.

kappa A statistical index of chance-corrected agreement or consistency between two nominal (or ordinal) measurements, often used to assess interrater or intrarater reliability.

Kendall's tau A correlation coefficient used to indicate the magnitude of a relationship between ordinal-level variables.

key informant A person knowledgeable about a focal phenomenon and who is willing to share information and insights with the researcher (e.g., an ethnographer).

keyword An important term used to search for references on a topic in a bibliographic database and used by authors to enhance the likelihood that their report will be found.

knowledge translation (KT) The exchange, synthesis, and application of knowledge by relevant stakeholders within complex systems to accelerate the beneficial effects of research aimed at improving health care.

known-groups validity A type of construct validity that concerns the degree to which a measure is capable of discriminating between groups known or expected to differ with regard to the construct of interest; also called *discriminative validity*.

Kruskal-Wallis test A nonparametric test used to test the difference between three or more independent groups based on ranked scores.

last observation carried forward (LOCF) A method of imputing a missing outcome using the previous measurement of that same outcome.

latent trait An abstract human trait that is not directly observable or measurable but that can be inferred from people's behavior or their responses to a set of questions; term often used in the context of an item response theory analysis, confirmatory factor analysis, and structural equations modeling analysis; also referred to as a *latent variable*. See also *construct*.

latent trait scale A scale developed within an *item response theory* framework, an alternative psychometric theory to *classical test theory*.

least-squares estimation A method of statistical estimation in which the solution minimizes the sums of squares of error terms; also called *ordinary least squares* (*OLS*).

level of measurement A system of classifying measurements according to the nature of the measurement and the type of permissible mathematical operations; the levels are nominal, ordinal, interval, and ratio.

level of significance The risk of making a Type I error in a statistical analysis, with the criterion (alpha) established by the researcher beforehand (e.g., $\alpha = .05$).

life history A narrative self-report about a person's life experiences vis-à-vis a theme of interest.

likelihood ratio (LR) For a screening or diagnostic instrument, the relative likelihood that a given result is expected in a person with (as opposed to one without) the target attribute; LR indexes summarize the relationship between specificity and sensitivity in a single number.

likelihood ratio test A test for evaluating the overall model in logistic regression, or to test improvement between models when predictors are added.

Likert scale Traditionally, a type of scale to measure attitudes, involving the summation of scores on a set of items that respondents rate for their degree of agreement or disagreement; more loosely, the name attributed to many summated rating scales.

limits of agreement (LOA) An estimate of the range of differences in two sets of scores that could be considered random measurement error, typically with 95% confidence; graphically portrayed on Bland-Altman plots.

linear regression An analysis for predicting the value of a dependent variable from one or more predictors by determining a straight-line fit to the data that minimizes deviations from the line.

listwise deletion A method of dealing with missing values in a data set that involves the elimination of cases with missing data.

literature review A critical summary of research on a topic of interest, often prepared to put a research problem in context.

log In participant observation studies, the observer's daily record of events and conversations.

logical positivism The philosophy underlying the traditional scientific approach; see also *positivist paradigm*.

logistic regression A multivariate regression procedure that analyzes relationships between two or more independent variables and a categorical dependent variable.

logit The natural log of the odds used as the dependent variable in logistic regression; short for logistic probability unit.

longitudinal study A study designed to collect data at more than one point in time, in contrast to a cross-sectional study.

macrotheory A broad theory aimed at describing large segments of the physical, social, or behavioral world; also called a *grand theory*.

main effect In a study with multiple independent variables, the effect of a single independent variable on the dependent variable.

manifest variable An observed, measured variable that serves as an indicator of an underlying construct, that is, a latent trait; term used most often in a confirmatory factor analysis or structural equations analysis.

manipulation An intervention or treatment introduced by the researcher in an experimental or quasi-experimental study to assess its impact on the dependent variable.

manipulation check In experimental studies, a test to assess whether the manipulation was implemented or experienced as intended.

Mann-Whitney *U* test A nonparametric statistic used to test the difference between two independent groups, based on ranked scores.

MANOVA See *multivariate analysis of variance*.

masking See *blinding*.

matching The pairing of subjects in one group with those in another group based on their similarity on one or more dimension to enhance the comparability of groups.

maturation threat A threat to the internal validity of a study that results when changes to the outcome measure (dependent variable) result from the passage of time.

maximum likelihood estimation An estimation approach in which the estimators are ones that estimate the parameters most likely to have generated the observed measurements.

maximum variation sampling A sampling approach used by qualitative researchers involving the purposeful selection of cases with a wide range of variation.

McNemar test A statistical test for comparing differences in proportions when values are derived from paired (nonindependent) groups.

mean A measure of central tendency computed by summing all scores and dividing by the total number of cases.

mean substitution A relatively weak approach for addressing missing data problems that involves substituting missing values on a variable with the sample mean for that variable.

measure A device whose purpose is to obtain numeric information to quantify an attribute or construct.

measurement The process of assigning numbers to represent the amount of a construct or attribute that is present in a person (or object) according to specified rules.

measurement error The systematic and random error of a person's score on a measure, reflecting factors other than the construct being measured and resulting in an observed score that is different from a hypothetical true score; a measurement property within the reliability domain.

measurement model In structural equations modeling, the model that stipulates the hypothesized relationships among the manifest and latent variables.

measurement parameter A statistical index that estimates a measurement property of a measure within a population (e.g., Cronbach's alpha is a measurement parameter for the property of internal consistency).

measurement property A characteristic reflecting a distinct aspect of the measure's quality; properties include reliability, validity, reliability of change, and responsiveness.

median The point in a distribution of scores above and below which 50% of the values fall.

mediating variable A variable that mediates or acts like a "go between" in a causal chain linking two other variables; also called a *mediator*.

Medical Research Council framework A framework developed in the United Kingdom for developing and testing complex interventions.

member check A method of validating the credibility of qualitative data through debriefings and discussions with informants.

MeSH Medical Subject Headings, used to index articles in MEDLINE and also recommended by several nursing journals to help authors identify keywords for their articles.

meta-analysis A technique for quantitatively integrating the results of multiple similar studies addressing the same research question.

meta-inference A higher order inference that can be gleaned in a mixed methods study when findings from the two strands (qualitative and quantitative) are integrated and interpreted.

meta-matrix A device sometimes used in a mixed methods study that permits researchers to recognize important patterns and themes across data sources.

metaphor A figurative comparison used by some qualitative analysts to evoke a visual or symbolic analogy.

meta-regression In meta-analyses, an approach for statistically examining clinical, demographic, and methodologic factors contributing to heterogeneity of effects.

metasummary A type of qualitative research synthesis that uses quantitatively oriented methods to aggregate qualitative findings; it involves the development of a list of abstracted findings from primary studies and calculating manifest effect sizes (frequency and intensity effect size).

metasynthesis The grand narratives or interpretive translations produced from the integration or comparison of findings from multiple qualitative studies.

method triangulation The use of multiple methods of data collection about the same phenomenon to enhance rigor or validity.

methodologic notes In observational field studies, the researcher's notes about the methods used in collecting data.

methodologic study Research designed to develop or refine methods of obtaining, organizing, or analyzing data.

methods, research The steps, procedures, and strategies for gathering and analyzing data in a study.

middle-range theory A theory that focuses on only a piece of reality or human experience, involving a selected number of concepts (e.g., a theory of stress).

minimal important change (MIC) A benchmark for interpreting change scores that represents the smallest change that is important or meaningful to patients or clinicians.

minimal risk Anticipated risks that are no greater than those ordinarily encountered in daily life or during the performance of routine tests or procedures.

missing at random (MAR) Values that are missing from a data set in such a manner that missingness is unrelated to the value of the missing data after controlling for another variable; missingness is unrelated to the value of the missing data but *is* related to values of other variables.

missing completely at random (MCAR) Values that are missing from a data set in such a manner that missingness is unrelated to either the value of the missing data or the value of any other variable; the subsample with missing values is a totally random subset of the original sample.

missing not at random (MNAR) Values that are missing from a data set in such a manner that missingness *is* related to the value of the missing data and, usually, to values of other variables as well.

missing values Values missing for certain variables for some participants as a result of such factors as refusals, withdrawals from the study, failure to complete forms, or researcher error.

mixed design A design that lends itself to comparisons both within groups over time (within subjects) and between different groups of participants (between subjects).

mixed methods (MM) research Research in which both qualitative and quantitative data are collected and analyzed to address different but related questions.

mixed studies review A systematic review that integrates and synthesizes findings from qualitative, quantitative, and mixed methods studies on a topic.

modality A characteristic of a frequency distribution describing the number of peaks; that is, values with high frequencies.

mode A measure of central tendency; the value that occurs most frequently in a distribution of scores.

model A symbolic representation of concepts or variables, and interrelationships among them.

moderator variable A variable that affects (moderates) the strength or direction of a relationship between the independent and dependent variables.

MOOSE guidelines Guidelines for reporting meta-analyses of observational (nonexperimental) primary studies.

mortality threat A threat to the internal validity of a study, referring to differential attrition (loss of participants) from different groups.

multicollinearity A problem that can occur in multiple regression when predictor variables are too highly intercorrelated, which can lead to unstable estimates of the regression coefficients.

multilevel sampling An approach to sampling in mixed methods studies in which participants in the two strands are not the same and are drawn from different populations at different levels of a hierarchy (e.g., nurses, nurse administrators).

multimodal distribution A distribution of values with more than one peak (high frequency).

multiple comparison procedures Statistical tests, normally applied after an ANOVA indicates statistically significant group differences, that compare different pairs of groups; also called *post hoc tests*.

multiple correlation coefficient An index that summarizes the degree of relationship between two or more independent variables and a dependent variable; symbolized as R.

multiple imputation (MI) The gold standard approach for dealing with missing values, involving the imputation of multiple (m) estimates of the missing value, which are later pooled and averaged in estimating parameters.

multiple regression analysis A statistical procedure for understanding the effects of two or more independent (predictor) variables on a dependent variable.

multistage sampling A sampling strategy that proceeds through a set of stages from larger to smaller sampling units (e.g., from states, to census tracts, to households).

multitrait–multimethod matrix method A method of assessing an instrument's construct validity using multiple measures for a set of people; the target instrument is valid to the extent that there is a strong relationship between it and other measures of the same attribute (convergent validity) and a weak relationship between it and measures purporting to measure a different attribute (divergent validity).

multivariate analysis of variance (MANOVA) A statistical procedure used to test the significance of differences between the means of two or more groups on two or more dependent variables, considered simultaneously.

multivariate statistics Statistical procedures designed to analyze the relationships among three or more variables (e.g., multiple regression, ANCOVA).

N The symbol designating the total number of subjects (e.g., "The total *N* was 500").

n The symbol designating the number of subjects in a subgroup or cell of a study (e.g., "Each of the four groups had an *n* of 125, for a total *N* of 500").

Nagelkerke R^2 A pseudo R^2 statistic used as an overall effect size index in logistic regression, analogous to R^2 in least-squares multiple regression, but lacking the ability to truly capture the proportion of variance explained in the outcome variable.

narrative analysis A qualitative approach that focuses on the story as the object of the inquiry.

natural experiment A nonexperimental study that takes advantage of a naturally occurring event (e.g., an earthquake) that is explored for its effect on people's behavior or condition, typically by comparing people exposed to the event with those not exposed.

naturalistic paradigm See *constructivist paradigm*.

naturalistic setting A setting for the collection of research data that is natural to those being studied (e.g., homes, places of work, and so on).

nay-sayers bias A bias in self-report scales created when respondents characteristically disagree with statements ("nay-say"), independent of content.

needs assessment A study designed to describe the needs of a group, community, or organization, usually as a guide to policy planning and resource allocation.

negative case analysis The refinement of a theory or description in a qualitative study through the inclusion of cases that appear to disconfirm earlier hypotheses.

negative predictive value (NPV) A measure of the usefulness of a screening/diagnostic test that can be interpreted as the probability that a negative test result is correct; calculated by dividing the number with a negative test who do not have disease by the number with a negative test.

negative relationship A relationship between two variables in which there is a tendency for high values on one variable to be associated with low values on the other (e.g., as stress increases, emotional well-being decreases); also called an *inverse relationship*.

negative results Results that fail to support the researcher's hypotheses.

negative skew An asymmetric distribution of data values with a disproportionately high number of cases at the upper end; when displayed graphically, the tail points to the left.

nested sampling An approach to sampling in mixed methods studies in which some, but not all, of the participants from one strand are included in the sample for the other strand.

net effect The effect of an independent variable on a dependent variable after controlling for the effect of one or more covariates statistically (e.g., through multiple regression or ANCOVA).

network sampling The sampling of participants based on referrals from others already in the sample; also called *snowball sampling*.

nominal measurement The lowest level of measurement involving the assignment of numbers to categorical characteristics (e.g., males = 1; females = 2).

nondirectional hypothesis A research hypothesis that does not stipulate the expected direction of the relationship between variables.

nonequivalent control group design A quasi-experimental design involving a comparison group that was not created through random assignment.

nonexperimental research Studies in which the researcher collects data without introducing an intervention; also called *observational research*.

noninferiority trial A trial designed to assess whether the effect of a new treatment is not worse than a standard treatment by no more than a pre-specified, clinically important amount.

nonparametric statistics A class of statistical tests that do not involve stringent assumptions about the distribution of variables.

nonprobability sampling The selection of sampling units (e.g., participants) from a population using nonrandom procedures (e.g., convenience and quota sampling).

nonrecursive model A causal model that predicts reciprocal effects (i.e., a variable can be both the cause of and an effect of another variable).

nonresponse bias A bias that can result when a nonrandom subset of people invited to participate in a study fail to participate.

nonsignificant result The result of a statistical test indicating that group differences or an observed relationship could have occurred by chance, at a given probability level; sometimes abbreviated as NS.

normal distribution A theoretical distribution that is bell-shaped and symmetrical; also called a *normal curve* or a *Gaussian distribution.*

norms Performance standards based on test or scale score information from a large, representative sample.

novelty effect A potential threat to design-related construct validity that can occur when participants or research agents alter their behavior because an intervention is new or different, not because of its inherent qualities.

null hypothesis A hypothesis stating no relationship between the variables under study; used primarily in statistical testing as the hypothesis to be rejected.

number needed to treat (NNT) An estimate of how many people would need to receive an intervention to prevent one undesirable outcome, computed by dividing 1 by the value of the absolute risk reduction.

nursing research Systematic inquiry designed to develop knowledge about issues of importance to the nursing profession.

nursing sensitive outcome A patient outcome that improves if there is greater quantity or quality of nursing care.

objectivity The extent to which two independent researchers would arrive at similar judgments or conclusions (i.e., judgments not biased by personal values or beliefs).

oblique rotation In factor analysis, a rotation of factors such that the reference axes are allowed to move to acute or oblique angles, and hence, the factors are allowed to be correlated.

observation A method of collecting information and measuring constructs by directly watching and recording behaviors and characteristics.

observational notes An observer's in-depth descriptions about events and conversations observed in naturalistic settings.

observational research Studies that do not involve an experimental intervention—that is, nonexperimental research in which phenomena are merely observed.

observed (obtained) score The actual score or numerical value assigned to a person on a measure.

odds A way of expressing the chance of an event—the probability of an event occurring to the probability that it will not occur, calculated by dividing the number of people who experienced an event by the number for whom it did not occur.

odds ratio (OR) The ratio of one odds to another odds, for example, the ratio of the odds of an event in one group to the odds of an event in another group; an odds ratio of 1.0 indicates no difference between groups.

one-tailed test A statistical test in which only values in one tail of a distribution are considered in determining significance; sometimes used when the researcher states a directional hypothesis.

open coding The first level of coding in a grounded theory study, referring to the basic descriptive coding of the content of narrative materials.

open-access journal A journal that allows free online access to articles, without any user subscription costs (authors or their institutions typically pay publication costs); some traditional journals include articles that are open-access.

open-ended question A question in an interview or questionnaire that does not restrict respondents' answers to preestablished alternatives.

operational definition The definition of a concept or variable in terms of the procedures by which it is to be measured.

operationalization The process of translating research concepts into measurable phenomena.

opportunistic sampling An approach to sampling in qualitative studies that involves adding new cases based on changes in research circumstances or in response to new leads that develop in the field.

oral history An unstructured self-report technique used to gather personal recollections of events and their perceived causes and consequences.

ordinal measurement A measurement level that rank orders phenomena along some dimension.

ordinary least squares (OLS) regression Regression analysis that uses the least-squares criterion for estimating the parameters in the regression equation.

orthogonal rotation In factor analysis, a rotation of factors such that the reference axes are kept at right angles, and hence, the factors remain uncorrelated.

outcome analysis An evaluation of what happens to outcomes of interest after implementing a program or intervention, typically using a one group before–after design.

outcome variable A term often used to refer to the dependent variable, that is, a measure that captures the outcome (end point) of an intervention.

outcomes research Research designed to document the effectiveness of health care services and the end results of patient care.

outlier A value that lies outside the normal range of values on a measure, especially in relation to other cases in a data set.

p value In statistical testing, the probability that the obtained results are due to chance alone; the probability of a Type I error.

pair matching See *matching*.

pairwise deletion A method of dealing with missing values in a data set involving the deletion of cases with missing data selectively (i.e., on a variable by variable basis).

panel study A longitudinal survey study in which data are collected from the same people (*a panel*) at two or more points in time.

paradigm A way of looking at natural phenomena—a worldview—that encompasses a set of philosophical assumptions and that guides one's approach to inquiry.

paradigm case In a hermeneutic analysis following the precepts of Benner, a strong exemplar of the phenomenon under study, often used early in the analysis to gain understanding of the phenomenon.

parallel sampling An approach to sampling in mixed methods studies in which the participants in one strand are not included in the sample for the other strand, but sampling from both strands is from the same or a similar population.

parallel test reliability The extent to which scores for people who are administered two parallel tests are the same for both measures.

parameter A characteristic of a population (e.g., the mean age of all U.S. citizens).

parametric statistics A class of statistical tests that involve assumptions about the distribution of the variables and the estimation of a parameter.

partially randomized patient preference (PRPP) design A design that involves randomizing only patients without a strong preference for a treatment condition.

participant See *study participant*.

participant observation A method of collecting data through the participation in and observation of a group or culture.

participatory action research (PAR) A research approach based on the premise that the use and production of knowledge can be political and used to exert power.

path analysis A regression-based procedure for testing causal models, typically using correlational data.

path coefficient The weight representing the effect of one variable on another in a path analytic model.

path diagram A graphic representation of the hypothesized interrelationships and causal flow among variables.

patient acceptable symptom state (PASS) A threshold for interpreting "final state" scores on a measure, signifying a desirable or satisfactory outcome for a patient.

patient-centered intervention (PCI) An intervention tailored to meet individual needs or characteristics.

patient-reported outcome (PRO) A health outcome that is measured by directly asking the patient for information.

Pearson's r A correlation coefficient designating the magnitude of relationship between two variables measured on at least an interval scale; also called the *product–moment correlation*.

peer debriefing Sessions with peers to review and explore various aspects of a study; sometimes used to enhance trustworthiness in a qualitative study.

peer reviewer A researcher who reviews and critiques a research report or proposal of another researcher and who makes a recommendation about publishing or funding the research.

pentadic dramatism An approach for analyzing narratives, developed by Burke, that focus on five key elements of a story: act (what was done), scene (when and where it was done), agent (who did it), agency (how it was done), and purpose (why it was done).

per protocol analysis Analysis of data from a randomized controlled trial that excludes participants who did not obtain the protocol to which they were assigned (or who received an insufficient dose of the intervention); sometimes called an *on-protocol analysis*.

percentile A value indicating the percentage of people who score below a particular score value on a measure; the 50th percentile is the median for the distribution of scores.

perfect relationship A correlation between two variables such that the values of one variable permit perfect prediction of the values of the other; designated as 1.00 or -1.00.

performance bias In clinical trials, systematic differences in the care provided to (or care received by) members of different groups of participants, apart from the intervention that is the focus of the inquiry, which can occur when there is no blinding.

performance ethnography A scripted, staged reenactment of ethnographically derived findings that reflect an interpretation of the culture.

performance test A measure designed to assess a person's physical or cognitive abilities or achievements.

permuted block randomization Randomization that occurs for blocks of subjects (e.g., 6 or 8 at a time) to ensure a balanced allocation to groups within cohorts of participants; the size of the blocks is varied (permuted).

persistent observation A qualitative researcher's intense focus on the aspects of a situation that are relevant to the phenomena being studied.

person triangulation The collection of data from different levels of persons, with the aim of validating data through multiple perspectives on the phenomenon.

personal interview A face-to-face interview between an interviewer and a respondent.

personal notes In field studies, written comments about the observer's own feelings during the research process.

person-item map A graphic display of information from a Rasch analysis that shows the distribution of respondents on one side of a latent trait continuum or "ruler" and the distribution of items on the other side.

phenomenology A qualitative research tradition, with roots in philosophy and psychology, that focuses on the lived experience of humans.

phenomenon The abstract concept under study, often used by qualitative researchers in lieu of the term *variable*.

phi coefficient A statistical index describing the magnitude of relationship between two dichotomous variables.

photo elicitation An interview stimulated and guided by photographic images.

PICO framework A framework for asking well-worded questions and for searching for evidence, where P = population, I = intervention or influence, C = comparison, and O = outcome.

pilot study A small-scale version, or trial run, of a study done in preparation for a major study; designed to assess the feasibility of, and to support refinements of, the protocols, methods, and procedures to be used in a larger scale study, such as a clinical trial.

placebo A sham or pseudointervention, often used as a control group condition.

placebo effect Changes in the dependent variable attributable to the placebo condition.

plan-do-study-act A framework often used to guide quality improvement projects.

point estimation A statistical procedure in which information from a sample (a statistic) is used to estimate the single value that best represents the population parameter.

point prevalence rate The number of people with a condition or disease divided by the total number at risk, multiplied by the total number for whom the rate is being established (e.g., per 1,000 population).

population The entire set of individuals or objects having some common characteristics (e.g., all RNs in Canada); sometimes called *universe*.

positive predictive value (PPV) A measure of the usefulness of a screening/diagnostic test that can be interpreted as the probability that a positive test result is correct; calculated by dividing the number with a positive test who have the disease by the number with a positive test.

positive relationship A relationship between two variables in which high values on one variable tend to be associated with high values on the other (e.g., as physical activity increases, heart rate increases).

positive results Research results that are consistent with the researcher's hypotheses.

positive skew An asymmetric distribution of values with a disproportionately high number of cases at the lower end; when displayed graphically, the tail points to the right.

positivist paradigm The paradigm underlying the traditional scientific approach, which assumes that there is an orderly reality that can be objectively studied; often associated with quantitative research.

post hoc test A test for comparing all possible pairs of groups following a significant test of overall group differences (e.g., in an ANOVA).

poster session A session at a professional conference in which several researchers simultaneously present visual displays summarizing their studies while conference attendees circulate around the room perusing the displays.

posttest The collection of data after introducing an intervention.

posttest-only design An experimental design in which data are collected from participants only after the intervention has been introduced; also called an *after-only design*.

power The ability of a design or analysis strategy to detect true relationships that exist among variables.

power analysis A procedure used to estimate sample size requirements prior to undertaking a study or the likelihood of committing a Type II error.

practical (pragmatic) clinical trial Trials that address practical questions about the benefits, risks, and costs of an intervention as they would unfold in routine clinical practice, using designs that yield information needed for making clinical decisions.

pragmatism A paradigm on which mixed methods research is often said to be based, in that it acknowledges the practical imperative of the "dictatorship of the research question."

precision In measurement, the degree to which an obtained score (trait estimate) closely approximates a true score; precision corresponds to low errors of measurement and is usually expressed in terms of the width of the confidence interval.

prediction The use of empirical evidence to make forecasts about how variables will behave in a new setting and with a different sample.

predictive validity A type of criterion validity that concerns the degree to which a measure is correlated with a criterion measured at a future point in time.

pretest (1) The collection of data prior to the experimental intervention; sometimes called *baseline data*; (2) the trial administration of a newly developed measure to identify flaws or to gain better understanding of how the construct in question is conceptualized by respondents.

pretest–posttest design An experimental design in which data are collected from participants both before and after introducing an intervention; also called a *before–after design*.

prevalence The proportion of a population having a particular condition (e.g., multiple sclerosis) at a given point in time.

primary source First-hand reports of facts or findings; in research, the original report prepared by the investigator who conducted the study.

primary study In a systematic review, an original study whose findings are used as the data in the review.

principal components analysis (PCA) An analysis that some consider a type of factor analysis; PCA analyzes all variance in the observed variables, not just common factor variance, with 1s on the diagonal of the correlation matrix.

principal investigator (PI) The person who is the lead researcher and who will have primary responsibility for overseeing a study.

priority A key issue in mixed methods research, concerning which strand (qualitative or quantitative) will be given more emphasis; using symbols to represent a design, the dominant strand is in all capital letters, as QUAL or QUAN, and the nondominant strand is in lower case, as qual or quan.

PRISMA guidelines Guidelines for reporting meta-analyses of randomized controlled trials.

probability sampling The selection of sampling elements (e.g., participants) from a population using random procedures (e.g., simple random sampling).

probe A method used in interviews to get detailed and reflective information from a respondent; in cognitive interviews, a method used to obtain information about how a question was processed and answered.

problem statement The articulation of a dilemma or disturbing situation that needs investigation.

process analysis A descriptive analysis of the process by which a program or intervention gets implemented and used in practice.

process consent In a qualitative study, an ongoing, transactional process of negotiating consent with study participants, allowing them to play a collaborative role in decision making about their continued participation.

product–moment correlation coefficient (r) A correlation coefficient designating the magnitude of relationship between two variables measured on at least an interval scale; also called *Pearson's r*.

projective technique A data collection method designed to elicit information about a person's innermost feelings and emotions through the presentation of vague stimuli (e.g., the Rorschach inkblot test).

prolonged engagement In qualitative research, the investment of sufficient time during data collection to have an in-depth understanding of the group under study, thereby enhancing credibility.

propensity score A score that captures the conditional probability of exposure to a treatment, given various pre-intervention characteristics; can be used to match comparison groups or as a statistical control variable to enhance internal validity.

proportion of agreement In assessing agreement/consistency between two nominal or ordinal measurements, the proportion of cases for which there is total agreement.

proportional hazards model A model in which independent variables are used to predict the risk (hazard) of experiencing an event at a given point in time.

proportionate sampling A sample approach in which the researcher samples from different strata of the population in direct proportion to their representation in the population.

proposal A document for a proposed study that communicates a research problem, its significance, proposed procedures for solving the problem, and, when funding is sought, how much the study will cost.

prospective design A study design that begins with an examination of presumed causes (e.g., cigarette smoking) and then goes forward in time to observe presumed effects (e.g., lung cancer); also called a *cohort design*.

proximal similarity model A conceptualization relating to generalization that concerns the contexts that are more or less like the one in a study in terms of a *gradient of similarity* for people, settings, times, and contexts.

pseudo R^2 A type of statistic used to evaluate overall effect size in logistic regression, analogous to R^2 in least-squares multiple regression; the statistic does not, strictly speaking, indicate the proportion of variance explained in the outcome variable.

psychometric assessment An evaluation of the quality of an instrument in which its measurement properties (i.e., its reliability, validity, and responsiveness) are estimated.

psychometrics A field of inquiry concerned with the theory of measurement of abstract psychological constructs and the application of the theory in the development and testing of measures.

publication bias The bias resulting from the fact that published studies overrepresent statistically significant findings, reflecting the tendency of researchers, reviewers, and editors to not publish nonsignificant results; also called a *bias against the null hypothesis*.

purposive (purposeful) sampling A nonprobability sampling method in which the researcher selects participants based on personal judgment about which ones will be most informative.

Q sort A data collection method in which participants sort statements into a number of piles (usually 9 or 11) according to some bipolar dimension (e.g., most helpful/least helpful).

qualitative analysis The organization and interpretation of narrative data for the purpose of discovering important underlying themes, categories, and patterns of relationships.

qualitative data Information in narrative (nonnumeric) form, such as the information provided in an unstructured interview.

qualitative research The investigation of phenomena, typically in an in-depth and holistic fashion, through the collection of rich narrative materials using a flexible research design.

qualitizing The process of reading and interpreting quantitative data in a qualitative manner.

quality improvement (QI) Systematic efforts to improve practices and processes within a specific organization or patient group.

quantitative analysis The manipulation of numeric data through statistical procedures for the purpose of describing phenomena or assessing the magnitude and reliability of relationships among them.

quantitative data Information collected in a numeric (quantified) form.

quantitative research The investigation of phenomena that lend themselves to precise measurement and quantification, often involving a rigorous and controlled design.

quantitizing The process of coding and analyzing qualitative data quantitatively.

quasi-experiment A type of design for an intervention study in which participants are not randomly assigned to treatment conditions; also called a *nonrandomized trial* or a *controlled trial without randomization*.

quasi-statistics An "accounting" system used to assess the validity of conclusions derived from qualitative analysis.

query letter A letter written to a journal editor to ask whether there is interest in a proposed manuscript or to a funding source to ask if there is interest in a proposed study.

questionnaire A document used to gather self-report data via self-administration of questions.

quota sampling A nonrandom sampling method in which "quotas" for certain subgroups based on sample characteristics are established to increase the representativeness of the sample.

r The symbol for a bivariate correlation coefficient (*Pearson's r*), summarizing the magnitude and direction of a relationship between two variables measured on an interval or ratio scale.

R The symbol for the multiple correlation coefficient, indicating the magnitude (but not direction) of the relationship between a dependent variable and multiple independent (predictor) variables, taken together.

R^2 The squared multiple correlation coefficient, indicating the proportion of variance in the dependent variable explained by a group of independent variables.

random assignment The assignment of participants to treatment conditions in a random manner (i.e., in a manner determined by chance alone); also called *randomization*.

random effects model In meta-analysis, a model in which studies are not assumed to be measuring the same overall effect but rather a distribution of effects; often preferred to a fixed effect model when there is extensive heterogeneity of effects.

random number table A table displaying hundreds of digits (from 0 to 9) in random order; each number is equally likely to follow any other.

random sampling The selection of a sample such that each member of a population has an equal probability of being included.

randomization The assignment of subjects to treatment conditions in a random manner (i.e., in a manner determined by chance alone); also called *random assignment*.

randomized consent design An experimental design in which subjects are randomized prior to informed consent; also called a *Zelen design*.

randomized controlled trial (RCT) A full experimental test of an intervention, involving random assignment to treatment groups; sometimes, Phase III of a full clinical trial.

randomness An important concept in quantitative research, involving having certain features of the study established by chance rather than by design or personal preference.

range A measure of variability, computed by subtracting the lowest value from the highest value in a distribution of scores.

Rasch model A latent trait model, used to evaluate items for a scale or test, that estimates only item difficulty (location) parameters; mathematically similar to a one-parameter item response theory model.

rating scale A scale that requires ratings of an object or concept along a continuum.

ratio measurement A measurement level with equal distances between scores and a true meaningful zero point (e.g., weight).

raw data Data in the form in which they were collected, without being transformed or analyzed.

reactivity A measurement distortion arising from the study participant's awareness of being observed, or, more generally, from the effect of the measurement procedure itself.

readability The ease with which materials (e.g., a questionnaire) can be read by people with varying reading skills, often empirically evaluated through readability formulas.

RE-AIM framework (*Reach, Efficacy, Adoption, Implementation*, and *Maintenance*) A model for designing and evaluating intervention research that is strong on multiple forms of study validity, including external validity.

receiver operating characteristic curve (ROC curve) A statistical technique that involves plotting specificity against sensitivity for different scores on a measure and so can be used to determine the best cutoff score for "caseness"; also used to generate an index (the *area under the curve*) that has relevance for assessing validity and responsiveness in some situations.

rectangular matrix A matrix of data (variables × subjects) that is complete and contains no missing values.

recursive model A path model in which the causal flow is unidirectional, without any feedback loops; opposite of a nonrecursive model.

refereed journal A journal in which decisions about the acceptance of manuscripts are made based on recommendations from peer reviewers.

reflective scale A multi-item scale whose items are conceptualized as having been "caused" by the underlying trait that is being measured; items are viewed as the effects of an underlying construct; distinct from a *formative index*.

reflective notes Notes that document a qualitative researcher's personal experiences, reflections, and progress in the field.

reflexivity In qualitative studies, critical self-reflection about one's own biases, preferences, and preconceptions.

regression analysis A statistical procedure for predicting values of a dependent variable based on one or more independent variables.

relationship A bond or a connection between two or more variables.

relative risk (RR) An estimate of the risk of "caseness" in one group compared to another, computed by dividing the absolute risk for one group (e.g., an exposed group) by the absolute risk for another (e.g., the nonexposed); also called the *risk ratio*.

relative risk reduction (RRR) The estimated proportion of baseline (untreated) risk that is reduced through exposure to the intervention, computed by dividing the absolute risk reduction (ARR) by the absolute risk for the control group.

reliability The extent to which a measurement is free from measurement error; more broadly, the extent to which scores for people who have not changed are the same for repeated measurements; statistically, the proportion of total variance in a set of scores that is attributable to true differences among those being measured.

reliability coefficient A quantitative index, usually ranging in value from 0.00 to 1.00, that provides an estimate of how reliable an instrument is (e.g., the intraclass correlation coefficient).

reliable change index (RCI) An index (used especially in psychotherapy) that estimates the threshold for a "real" change in scores—that is, a change that, with 95% confidence, is beyond measurement error; similar in concept to the *smallest detectable change* but based on a different formula.

repeated measures design A design that involves the collection of data multiple points in time, to track changes in an outcome.

repeated-measures ANOVA An analysis of variance used when there are multiple measures of the dependent variable over time (e.g., in a crossover design).

replication The deliberate repetition of research procedures in a second investigation for the purpose of assessing whether earlier results can be confirmed.

representative sample A sample whose characteristics are comparable to those of the population from which it is drawn.

reputational case sampling A variant of purposive sampling used in qualitative studies that involves selecting cases based on a recommendation of an expert or key informant.

research Systematic inquiry that uses orderly, disciplined methods to answer questions or solve problems.

research control See *control, research.*

research design The overall plan for addressing a research question, including specifications for enhancing the study's integrity.

research hypothesis The actual hypothesis a researcher wishes to test (as opposed to the *null hypothesis*), stating the anticipated relationship between two or more variables.

research methods The techniques used to structure a study and to gather and analyze information in a systematic fashion.

research misconduct Fabrication, falsification, plagiarism, or other practices that seriously deviate from those that are commonly accepted within the scientific community for conducting or reporting research.

research problem An enigmatic or perplexing condition that can be investigated through disciplined inquiry.

research proposal A document for a proposed study that communicates a research problem, its significance, proposed procedures for solving the problem, and, when funding is sought, how much the study will cost.

research question A statement of the specific query the researcher wants to answer to address a research problem.

research report A document (often a journal article) summarizing the main features of a study, including the research question, the methods used to address it, the findings, and the interpretation of the findings.

research utilization The use of some aspect of a study in an application unrelated to the original research.

researcher credibility The faith that can be put in a researcher, based on his or her training, qualifications, and experiences.

residuals In multiple regression, the error term, that is, unexplained variance.

respondent In a self-report study, the person responding to questions posed by the researcher.

responder analysis An analysis that compares people who are *responders* to an intervention, based on their having reached a benchmark on a change score (e.g., the minimal important change), compared to people who are nonresponders (have not reached the benchmark).

response bias An influence that leads a person to select a response option that does not correspond to his or her hypothetical "true score" for an item.

response options The pre-specified list of possible answers to a closed-ended question or item; also called *response alternatives.*

response rate The rate of participation in a study, calculated by dividing the number of people participating by the number of people sampled.

response set bias The systematic bias resulting from the tendency of some individuals to respond to items in characteristic ways (e.g., always agreeing), independently of item content.

responsiveness The ability of a measure to detect change over time in a construct that has changed, commensurate with the amount of change that has occurred.

results The answers to research questions, obtained through an analysis of the collected data.

retrospective design A study design that begins with the manifestation of the dependent variable in the present (e.g., lung cancer), followed by a search for a presumed cause occurring in the past (e.g., cigarette smoking).

revelatory case sampling An approach to sampling in a case study that involves identifying and gaining access to a case representing a phenomenon that was previously inaccessible to research scrutiny.

risk ratio See *relative risk.*

risk/benefit ratio The relative costs and benefits, to an individual person and to society at large, of participation in a study; also the relative costs and benefits of implementing an innovation.

rival hypothesis An alternative explanation, competing with the researcher's hypothesis, for interpreting the results of a study.

ROC curve See *receiver operating characteristic curve.*

sample A subset of a population comprising those selected to participate in a study.

sample size The number of people who participate in a study; an important factor in the *power* of the analysis and in statistical conclusion validity.

sampling The process of selecting a portion of the population to represent the entire population.

sampling bias Distortions that arise when a sample is not representative of the population from which it was drawn.

sampling distribution A theoretical distribution of a statistic, using the values of the statistic (e.g., the means) computed from an infinite number of samples as the data points in the distribution.

sampling error The fluctuation of the value of a statistic from one sample to another drawn from the same population.

sampling frame A list of all the elements in the population from which the sample is selected.

sampling plan The formal plan specifying a sampling method, a sample size, and procedures for recruiting study participants.

saturation The collection of qualitative data to the point where a sense of closure is attained because new data yield redundant information.

scale Typically, a composite measure of an attribute or trait, involving the aggregation of information from multiple items into a single numerical value that places people on a continuum with respect to the trait. See also *reflective scale*.

scatter plot A graphic representation of the relationship between two continuous variables.

scientific merit The degree to which a study is methodologically and conceptually sound.

scientific method A set of orderly, systematic, controlled procedures for acquiring dependable, empirical—and typically quantitative—information; the methodologic approach associated with the positivist paradigm.

scoping review A preliminary review of research findings designed to refine the questions and protocols for a systematic review.

score A numerical value derived from a measurement that communicates *how much* of an attribute is present in a person or whether the attribute is present or absent.

screening instrument An instrument used to ascertain whether potential participants for a study meet eligibility criteria or for determining whether a person tests positive for a specified condition.

secondary analysis A form of research in which the data collected by one researcher are reanalyzed by another investigator to answer new questions.

secondary source Second-hand accounts of events or facts; in research, a description of a study prepared by someone other than the original researcher.

selection threat (self-selection) A threat to the internal validity of the study resulting from preexisting differences between groups under study; the differences affect the dependent variable in ways extraneous to the effect of the independent variable.

selective coding A level of coding in a grounded theory study that begins once the core category has been discovered and involves limiting coding to only those categories related to the core category.

selective deposit A bias that can result when records and documents that are stored are not a complete set of records but rather are selectively stored based on criteria that could bias the set.

selective survival A bias that can result when records and documents that are stored are not a complete set of records because of a nonrandom mechanism of maintaining them.

self-determination A person's right to voluntarily decide whether or not to participate in a study.

self-report A method of collecting data that involves a direct verbal report of information by the person who is being studied (e.g., by interview or questionnaire).

semantic differential A technique used to measure attitudes in which respondents rate concepts of interest on a series of bipolar rating scales.

semantic equivalence In a translation or adaptation of an instrument, the extent to which the meaning of an item is the same in the target culture after the item is translated as it was in the original.

semistructured interview An interview in which the researcher has a list of topics to cover rather than specific questions to ask.

sensitivity The ability of screening instruments to correctly identify a "case," that is, to correctly diagnose a condition.

sensitivity analysis An effort to test how sensitive the results of a statistical analysis are to changes in assumptions or in the way the analysis was done (e.g., in a meta-analysis, used to assess whether conclusions are sensitive to the quality of the studies included).

sequential clinical trial A trial in which data are continuously analyzed, and *stopping rules* are used to decide when the evidence about treatment efficacy is sufficiently strong that the trial can be stopped.

sequential design A mixed methods design in which one strand of data collection (qualitative or quantitative) occurs prior to the other, informing the second strand; symbolically shown with an arrow, as QUAL → QUAN.

setting The physical location and conditions in which data collection takes place in a study.

significance, clinical See *clinical significance*.

significance, statistical See *statistical significance*.

simple random sampling Basic probability sampling, involving the selection of sample members from a sampling frame through completely random procedures.

simultaneous multiple regression   A multiple regression analysis in which all predictor variables are entered into the equation simultaneously.

single-blind study   A study in which only one group (e.g., data collectors) do not know participants' status in terms of the group to which they have been assigned.

single-subject experiment   An intervention study that tests the effectiveness of an intervention with a single subject, typically using a time series design; sometimes called an *N-of-1 experiment*.

site   The overall location where a study is undertaken.

skewed distribution   The asymmetric distribution of a set of data values around a central point.

smallest detectable change (SDC)   An index that estimates the threshold for a "real" change in scores—that is, a change that, with 95% confidence, is beyond measurement error; the SDC is a change score that falls outside the limits of agreement on a Bland-Altman plot.

snowball sampling   The selection of participants through referrals from earlier participants; also called *network sampling*.

social desirability response bias   A bias in self-report instruments created when participants have a tendency to misrepresent their opinions in the direction of answers consistent with prevailing social norms.

space triangulation   The collection of data on the same phenomenon in multiple sites, to enhance the validity of the findings.

Spearman's rank-order correlation (Spearman's rho)   A correlation coefficient indicating the magnitude of a relationship between variables measured on the ordinal scale.

specificity   The ability of a screening or diagnostic instrument to correctly identify noncases.

standard deviation   The most frequently used statistic for measuring the degree of variability in a set of scores.

standard error   The standard deviation of a sampling distribution, such as the sampling distribution of the mean.

standard error of measurement (SEM)   An index that quantifies the amount of "typical" error on a measure and indicates the precision of individual scores.

standard score   A score expressed in terms of standard deviations from the mean, with raw scores typically transformed to have a mean of zero and a standard deviation of one; sometimes called a *z* score.

standardized mean difference (SMD)   In meta-analysis, the effect size index for comparing two group means, computed by subtracting one mean from the other and dividing by the pooled standard deviation; also called Cohen's *d*.

statement of purpose   A broad declarative statement of the overall goals of a study.

statistic   An estimate of a parameter, calculated from sample data.

statistical analysis   The organization and analysis of quantitative data using statistical procedures, including both descriptive and inferential statistics.

statistical conclusion validity   The degree to which inferences about relationships from a statistical analysis of the data are correct.

statistical control   The use of statistical procedures to control confounding influences on the dependent variable.

statistical heterogeneity   Diversity of effects across primary studies included in a meta-analysis.

statistical inference   An inference about the population based on information from a sample, using laws of probability.

statistical power   The ability of a research design and analytic strategy to detect true relationships among variables.

statistical process control (SPC)   A statistical method of monitoring a process unfolding over time; used originally to monitor quality in a manufacturing process, but SPC can be used to test hypotheses about changes over time (e.g., as the result of an intervention).

statistical significance   A term indicating that the results from an analysis of sample data are unlikely to have been the result of chance at a specified level of probability.

statistical test   An analytic tool that estimates the probability that results obtained from a sample reflect true population values.

stem   In an item for a scale, the portion of the item (either a question or declarative statement) designed to elicit a response.

stepwise multiple regression   A multiple regression analysis in which predictor variables are entered into the equation in steps, in the order in which the increment to R is greatest.

stipend   A monetary payment to individuals participating in a study, as an incentive for participation and/or to compensate for time and expenses.

strata   Subdivisions of the population according to some characteristic (e.g., males and females); singular is *stratum*.

stratification The division of a sample of a population into smaller units (e.g., males and females), typically to enhance representativeness or to explore results for subgroups of people; used in both sampling and in allocation to treatment groups.

stratified random sampling The random selection of study participants from two or more strata of the population independently.

STROBE guidelines Guidelines for reporting observational studies.

structural equations modeling (SEM) A statistical modeling procedures that involves equations representing the magnitude of hypothesized relations among sets of variables, typically used to test a model or theory in a path analysis and most often relying on maximum likelihood estimation.

structural validity The extent to which an instrument captures the hypothesized dimensionality of the broad construct; an aspect of construct validity.

structured data collection An approach to collecting data from participants, either through self-report or observations, in which categories of information (e.g., response options) are specified in advance.

study participant An individual who participates and provides information in a study.

study section Within the National Institutes of Health, a group of peer reviewers who evaluate grant applications in the first phase of a dual-review process.

subgroup effect The differential effect of the independent variable on the dependent variable for subsets of the sample.

subject An individual who participates and provides data in a study; term used primarily in quantitative research.

subscale A subset of items that measures one aspect or dimension of a multidimensional construct.

summated rating scale A composite scale consisting of multiple items that are added together to yield an overall, continuous measure of an attribute (e.g., a Likert scale).

superiority trial A trial in which the researchers hypothesize that the focal intervention is "superior to" (more effective than) the control condition; most clinical trials are superiority trials.

survey research Nonexperimental research that involves gathering information about people's activities, beliefs, preferences, and attitudes via direct questioning.

survival analysis A statistical procedure used when the dependent variable represents a time interval between an initial event (e.g., onset of a disease) and an end event (e.g., death).

symmetric distribution A distribution of values with two halves that are mirror images of the each other.

systematic review A rigorous synthesis of research findings on a particular research question, using systematic sampling and data collection procedures and a formal protocol.

systematic sampling The selection of sample members such that every *kth* (e.g., every tenth) person or element in a sampling frame is chosen.

table shell A table without any numeric values, prepared in advance of data analysis as a guide to the analyses to be performed.

tacit knowledge Information about a culture that is so deeply embedded that members do not talk about it or may not even be consciously aware of it.

target population The entire population in which a researcher is interested and to which he or she would like to generalize the study results.

taxonomy In an ethnographic analysis, a system of classifying and organizing terms and concepts, developed to illuminate the domain's internal organization and the relationship among the categories of the domain.

test statistic A statistic used to test for the reliability of relationships between variables (e.g., chi-squared, *t*); sampling distributions of test statistics are known for circumstances in which the null hypothesis is true.

testing threat A threat to a study's internal validity that occurs when the administration of a pretest or baseline measure of a dependent variable results in changes on the variable, apart from the effect of the independent variable.

test–retest reliability The type of reliability that concerns the extent to which scores for people who have not changed are the same when a measure is administered twice; an assessment of a measure's stability.

theme A recurring regularity emerging from an analysis of qualitative data.

theoretical notes In field studies, notes detailing the researcher's interpretations of observed behavior and events.

theoretical sampling In qualitative studies, especially in grounded theory studies, the selection of sample members based on emerging findings to ensure adequate representation of important theoretical categories.

theory An abstract generalization that presents a systematic explanation about the relationships among phenomena.

theory triangulation The use of competing theories or hypotheses in the analysis and interpretation of data.

thick description A rich and thorough description of the research context and findings in a qualitative study.

think aloud method A qualitative method used to collect data about cognitive processes (e.g., decision making), in which people's reflections on decisions or problem solving are captured as they are being made; sometimes used as part of a cognitive interview during the development of a new instrument.

threats to validity In research design, reasons that an inference about the effect of an independent variable (e.g., an intervention) on an outcome could be wrong.

time sampling In structured observations, the sampling of time periods during which observations will take place.

time series design A quasi-experimental design involving the collection of data over an extended time period, with multiple data collection points both prior to and after an intervention is introduced.

time triangulation The collection of data on the same phenomenon or about the same people at different points in time to enhance trustworthiness.

topic guide A list of broad question areas to be covered in a semistructured interview or focus group interview.

tracing Procedures used to relocate subjects to avoid attrition in a longitudinal study.

transferability The extent to which qualitative findings can be transferred to other settings or groups; analogous to generalizability.

translational research Research that focuses on how research findings can best be translated into practice.

treatment The intervention under study; the condition being manipulated.

treatment group The group receiving the intervention being tested; the experimental group.

TREND guidelines Guidelines (Transparent Reporting of Evaluations with Nonrandomized Designs) for reporting non-RCT intervention studies.

trend study A form of longitudinal study in which different samples from a population are studied over time with respect to some phenomenon (e.g., annual national polls on attitudes toward abortion).

triangulation The use of multiple methods to collect and interpret data about a phenomenon, so as to converge on an accurate representation of reality.

true score A hypothetical score that would be obtained if a measure were infallible.

trustworthiness The degree of confidence qualitative researchers have in their data and analyses, assessed using the criteria of credibility, transferability, dependability, confirmability, and authenticity.

***t*-test** A parametric statistical test for analyzing the difference between two means.

two-tailed tests Statistical tests in which both ends of the sampling distribution are used to determine improbable values.

Type I error An error created by rejecting the null hypothesis when it is true (i.e., the researcher concludes that a relationship exists when in fact it does not—a false positive).

Type II error An error created by accepting the null hypothesis when it is false (i.e., the researcher concludes that *no* relationship exists when in fact it does—a false negative).

underpowered A characteristic of a study that lacks sufficient statistical power to minimize the risk of a Type II error (i.e., the risk of concluding that a relationship does not exist when, in fact, it does).

unidimensional scale A scale that measures only one construct, or a unitary aspect or facet of a construct.

unimodal distribution A distribution of values with one peak (high frequency).

unit of analysis The basic unit or focus of a researcher's analysis—typically individual study participants.

univariate descriptive study A study that gathers information on the occurrence, frequency of occurrence, or average value of the variables of interest, one variable at a time, without focusing on interrelationships among variables.

univariate statistics Statistical analysis of a single variable for purposes of description (e.g., computing a mean).

unstructured interview An interview in which the researcher asks respondents questions without having a predetermined plan regarding the content or flow of information to be gathered.

unstructured observation The collection of descriptive data through direct observation that is not guided by a formal, prespecified plan for observing, enumerating, or recording the information.

urn randomization A method of randomizing participants to groups, in which group balance in monitored and the allocation probability is adjusted when imbalances occur.

validity A quality criterion referring to the degree to which inferences made in a study are accurate and well-founded; in measurement, the degree to which an instrument measures what it is intended to measure.

variability The degree to which values on a set of scores are dispersed.

variable An attribute that varies, that is, takes on different values (e.g., body temperature, heart rate).

variance A measure of variability or dispersion, equal to the standard deviation squared.

vignette A brief description of an event, person, or situation to which respondents are asked to express their reactions.

visual analog scale (VAS) A scaling procedure used to measure certain clinical symptoms (e.g., pain, fatigue) by having people indicate on a straight line the intensity of the symptom; usually measured on a 100 mm scale with values from 0 to 100.

vulnerable groups Special groups of people whose rights in studies need special protection because of their inability to provide meaningful informed consent or because their circumstances place them at higher than average risk of adverse effects (e.g., children, unconscious patients).

wait-list design A design for an intervention study that involves putting control group members on a waiting list for the intervention until follow-up data have been collected; also called a *delay of treatment design*.

Wald statistic A statistic, distributed as a chi-square, used to evaluate the significance of individual predictors in a logistic regression equation.

web-based survey A questionnaire delivered over the Internet on a dedicated survey website for self-administration.

weighting A procedure used to adjust estimated population values when a disproportionate sampling design has been used (or to give differential emphasis to different items on a scale).

Wilcoxon signed ranks test A nonparametric statistical test for comparing two paired groups, based on the relative ranking of values between the pairs.

wild code A coded value that is not legitimate within the coding scheme for that data set.

within-subjects design A research design in which a single group of participants is compared under different conditions or at different points in time (e.g., before and after surgery).

yea-sayers bias A bias in self-report scales created when respondents characteristically agree with statements ("yea-say"), independent of content.

z score A standard score, expressed in terms of standard deviations from the mean; raw scores are transformed such that the mean equals zero and the standard deviation equals 1.

Zelen design An experimental design in which subjects are randomized prior to informed consent; also called *randomized consent design*.

Appendix:

Statistical Tables of Theoretical Probability Distributions

TABLE A.1 • Critical Values for the *t* Distribution

df	α, 2-tailed test: α, 1-tailed test:	.10 .05	.05 .025	.02 .01	.01 .005	.001 .0005
1		6.314	12.706	31.821	63.657	636.619
2		2.920	4.303	6.965	9.925	31.598
3		2.353	3.182	4.541	5.841	12.941
4		2.132	2.776	3.747	4.604	8.610
5		2.015	2.571	3.376	4.032	6.859
6		1.953	2.447	3.143	3.707	5.959
7		1.895	2.365	2.998	3.449	5.405
8		1.860	2.306	2.896	3.355	5.041
9		1.833	2.262	2.821	3.250	4.781
10		1.812	2.228	2.765	3.169	4.587
11		1.796	2.201	2.718	3.106	4.437
12		1.782	2.179	2.681	3.055	4.318
13		1.771	2.160	2.650	3.012	4.221
14		1.761	2.145	2.624	2.977	4.140
15		1.753	2.131	2.602	2.947	4.073
16		1.746	2.120	2.583	2.921	4.015
17		1.740	2.110	2.567	2.898	3.965
18		1.734	2.101	2.552	2.878	3.922
19		1.729	2.093	2.539	2.861	3.883
20		1.725	2.086	2.528	2.845	3.850
21		1.721	2.080	2.518	2.831	3.819
22		1.717	2.074	2.508	2.819	3.792
23		1.714	2.069	2.500	2.807	3.767
24		1.711	2.064	2.492	2.797	3.745
25		1.708	2.060	2.485	2.787	3.725
26		1.706	2.056	2.479	2.779	3.707
27		1.703	2.052	2.473	2.771	3.690
28		1.701	2.048	2.467	2.763	3.674
29		1.699	2.045	2.462	2.756	3.659
30		1.697	2.042	2.457	2.750	3.646
40		1.684	2.021	2.423	2.704	3.551
60		1.671	2.000	2.390	2.660	3.460
120		1.658	1.980	2.358	2.617	3.373
∞		1.645	1.960	2.326	2.576	3.291

TABLE A.2 • Critical Values for the *F* Distribution
α = .05 (Two-Tailed)   α = .025 (One-Tailed)

df_W \ df_B	1	2	3	4	5	6	8	12	24	∞
1	161.4	199.5	215.7	224.6	230.2	234.0	238.9	243.9	249.0	254.3
2	18.51	19.00	19.16	19.25	19.30	19.33	19.37	19.41	19.45	19.50
3	10.13	9.55	9.28	9.12	9.01	8.94	8.84	8.74	8.64	8.53
4	7.71	6.94	6.59	6.39	6.26	6.16	6.04	5.91	5.77	5.63
5	6.61	5.79	5.41	5.19	5.05	4.95	4.82	4.68	4.53	4.36
6	5.99	5.14	4.76	4.53	4.39	4.28	4.15	4.00	3.84	3.67
7	5.59	4.74	4.35	4.12	3.97	3.87	3.73	3.57	3.41	3.23
8	5.32	4.46	4.07	3.84	3.69	3.58	3.44	3.28	3.12	2.93
9	5.12	4.26	3.86	3.63	3.48	3.37	3.23	3.07	2.90	2.71
10	4.96	4.10	3.71	3.48	3.33	3.22	3.07	2.91	2.74	2.54
11	4.84	3.98	3.59	3.36	3.20	3.09	2.95	2.79	2.61	2.40
12	4.75	3.88	3.49	3.26	3.11	3.00	2.85	2.69	2.50	2.30
13	4.67	3.80	3.41	3.18	3.02	2.92	2.77	2.60	2.42	2.21
14	4.60	3.74	3.34	3.11	2.96	2.85	2.70	2.53	2.35	2.13
15	4.54	3.68	3.29	3.06	2.90	2.79	2.64	2.48	2.29	2.07
16	4.49	3.63	3.24	3.01	2.85	2.74	2.59	2.42	2.24	2.01
17	4.45	3.59	3.20	2.96	2.81	2.70	2.55	2.38	2.19	1.96
18	4.41	3.55	3.16	2.93	2.77	2.66	2.51	2.34	2.15	1.92
19	4.38	3.52	3.13	2.90	2.74	2.63	2.48	2.31	2.11	1.88
20	4.35	3.49	3.10	2.87	2.71	2.60	2.45	2.28	2.08	1.84
21	4.32	3.47	3.07	2.84	2.68	2.57	2.42	2.25	2.05	1.81
22	4.30	3.44	3.05	2.82	2.66	2.55	2.40	2.23	2.03	1.78
23	4.28	3.42	3.03	2.80	2.64	2.53	2.38	2.20	2.00	1.76
24	4.26	3.40	3.01	2.78	2.62	2.51	2.36	2.18	1.98	1.73
25	4.24	3.38	2.99	2.76	2.60	2.49	2.34	2.16	1.96	1.71
26	4.22	3.37	2.98	2.74	2.59	2.47	2.32	2.15	1.95	1.69
27	4.21	3.35	2.96	2.73	2.57	2.46	2.30	2.13	1.93	1.67
28	4.20	3.34	2.95	2.71	2.56	2.44	2.29	2.12	1.91	1.65
29	4.18	3.33	2.93	2.70	2.54	2.43	2.28	2.10	1.90	1.64
30	4.17	3.32	2.92	2.69	2.53	2.42	2.27	2.09	1.89	1.62
40	4.08	3.23	2.84	2.61	2.45	2.34	2.18	2.00	1.79	1.51
60	4.00	3.15	2.76	2.52	2.37	2.25	2.10	1.92	1.70	1.39
120	3.92	3.07	2.68	2.45	2.29	2.17	2.02	1.83	1.61	1.25
∞	3.84	2.99	2.60	2.37	2.21	2.09	1.94	1.75	1.52	1.00

TABLE A.2 • Critical Values for the *F* Distribution (continued)

α = .01 (Two-Tailed)   α = .005 (One-Tailed)

df_B df_W	1	2	3	4	5	6	8	12	24	∞
1	4052	4999	5403	5625	5764	5859	5981	6106	6234	6366
2	98.49	99.00	99.17	99.25	99.30	99.33	99.36	99.42	99.46	99.50
3	34.12	30.81	29.46	28.71	28.24	27.91	27.49	27.05	26.60	26.12
4	21.20	18.00	16.69	15.98	15.52	15.21	14.80	14.37	13.93	13.46
5	16.26	13.27	12.06	11.39	10.97	10.67	10.29	9.89	9.47	9.02
6	13.74	10.92	9.78	9.15	8.75	8.47	8.10	7.72	7.31	6.88
7	12.25	9.55	8.45	7.85	7.46	7.19	6.84	6.47	6.07	5.65
8	11.26	8.65	7.59	7.01	6.63	6.37	6.03	5.67	5.28	4.86
9	10.56	8.02	6.99	6.42	6.06	5.80	5.47	5.11	4.73	4.31
10	10.04	7.56	6.55	5.99	5.64	5.39	5.06	4.71	4.33	3.91
11	9.65	7.20	6.22	5.67	5.32	5.07	4.74	4.40	4.02	3.60
12	9.33	6.93	5.95	5.41	5.06	4.82	4.50	4.16	3.78	3.36
13	9.07	6.70	5.74	5.20	4.86	4.62	4.30	3.96	3.59	3.16
14	8.86	6.51	5.56	5.03	4.69	4.46	4.14	3.80	3.43	3.00
15	8.68	6.36	5.42	4.89	4.56	4.32	4.00	3.67	3.29	2.87
16	8.53	6.23	5.29	4.77	4.44	4.20	3.89	3.55	3.18	2.75
17	8.40	6.11	5.18	4.67	4.34	4.10	3.78	3.45	3.08	2.65
18	8.28	6.01	5.09	4.58	4.29	4.01	3.71	3.37	3.00	2.57
19	8.18	5.93	5.01	4.50	4.17	3.94	3.63	3.30	2.92	2.49
20	8.10	5.85	4.94	4.43	4.10	3.87	3.56	3.23	2.86	2.42
21	8.02	5.78	4.87	4.37	4.04	3.81	3.51	3.17	2.80	2.36
22	7.94	5.72	4.82	4.31	3.99	3.76	3.45	3.12	2.75	2.31
23	7.88	5.66	4.76	4.26	3.94	3.71	3.41	3.07	2.70	2.26
24	7.82	5.61	4.72	4.22	3.90	3.67	3.36	3.03	2.66	2.21
25	7.77	5.57	4.68	4.18	3.86	3.63	3.32	2.99	2.62	2.17
26	7.72	5.53	4.64	4.14	3.82	3.59	3.29	2.96	2.58	2.13
27	7.68	5.49	4.60	4.11	3.78	3.56	3.26	2.93	2.55	2.10
28	7.64	5.45	4.57	4.07	3.75	3.53	3.23	2.90	2.52	2.06
29	7.60	5.42	4.54	4.04	3.73	3.50	3.20	2.87	2.49	2.03
30	7.56	5.39	4.51	4.02	3.70	3.47	3.17	2.84	2.47	2.01
40	7.31	5.18	4.31	3.83	3.51	3.29	2.99	2.66	2.29	1.80
60	7.08	4.98	4.13	3.65	3.34	3.12	2.82	2.50	2.12	1.60
120	6.85	4.79	3.95	3.48	3.17	2.96	2.66	2.34	1.95	1.38
∞	6.64	4.60	3.78	3.32	3.02	2.80	2.51	2.18	1.79	1.00

(continued)

TABLE A.2 • Critical Values for the F Distribution (continued)

α = .001 (Two-Tailed)   α = .0005 (One-Tailed)

df_B df_W	1	2	3	4	5	6	8	12	24	∞
1	405284	500000	540379	562500	576405	585937	598144	610667	623497	636619
2	998.5	999.0	999.2	999.2	999.3	999.3	999.4	999.4	999.5	999.5
3	167.5	148.5	141.1	137.1	134.6	132.8	130.6	128.3	125.9	123.5
4	74.14	61.25	56.18	53.44	51.71	50.53	49.00	47.41	45.77	44.05
5	47.04	36.61	33.20	31.09	29.75	28.84	27.64	26.42	25.14	23.78
6	35.51	27.00	23.70	21.90	20.81	20.03	19.03	17.99	16.89	15.75
7	29.22	21.69	18.77	17.19	16.21	15.52	14.63	13.71	12.73	11.69
8	25.42	18.49	15.83	14.39	13.49	12.86	17.04	11.19	10.30	9.34
9	22.86	16.39	13.90	12.56	11.71	11.13	10.37	9.57	8.72	7.81
10	21.04	14.91	12.55	11.28	10.48	9.92	9.20	8.45	7.64	6.76
11	19.69	13.81	11.56	10.35	9.58	9.05	8.35	7.63	6.85	6.00
12	18.64	12.97	10.80	9.63	8.89	8.38	7.71	7.00	6.25	5.42
13	17.81	12.31	10.21	9.07	8.35	7.86	7.21	6.52	5.78	4.97
14	17.14	11.78	9.73	8.62	7.92	7.43	6.80	6.13	5.41	4.60
15	16.59	11.34	9.34	8.25	7.57	7.09	6.47	5.81	5.10	4.31
16	16.12	10.97	9.00	7.94	7.27	6.81	6.19	5.55	4.85	4.06
17	15.72	10.66	8.73	7.68	7.02	6.56	5.96	5.32	4.63	3.85
18	15.38	10.39	8.49	7.46	6.81	6.35	5.76	5.13	4.45	3.67
19	15.08	10.16	8.28	7.26	6.61	6.18	5.59	4.97	4.29	3.52
20	14.82	9.95	8.10	7.10	6.46	6.02	5.44	4.82	4.15	3.38
21	14.59	9.77	7.94	6.95	6.32	5.88	5.31	4.70	4.03	3.26
22	14.38	9.61	7.80	6.81	6.19	5.76	5.19	4.58	3.92	3.15
23	14.19	9.47	7.67	6.69	6.08	5.65	5.09	4.48	3.82	3.05
24	14.03	9.34	7.55	6.59	5.98	5.55	4.99	4.39	3.74	2.97
25	13.88	9.22	7.45	6.49	5.88	5.46	4.91	4.31	3.66	2.89
26	13.74	9.12	7.36	6.41	5.80	5.38	4.83	4.24	3.59	2.82
27	13.61	9.02	7.27	6.33	5.73	5.31	4.76	4.17	3.52	2.75
28	13.50	8.93	7.19	6.25	5.66	5.24	4.69	4.11	3.46	2.70
29	13.39	8.85	7.12	6.19	5.59	5.18	4.64	4.05	3.41	2.64
30	13.29	8.77	7.05	6.12	5.53	5.12	4.58	4.00	3.36	2.59
40	12.61	8.25	6.60	5.70	5.13	4.73	4.21	3.64	3.01	2.23
60	11.97	7.76	6.17	5.31	4.76	4.37	3.87	3.31	2.69	1.90
120	11.38	7.31	5.79	4.95	4.42	4.04	3.55	3.02	2.40	1.56
∞	10.83	6.91	5.42	4.62	4.10	3.74	3.27	2.74	2.13	1.00

TABLE A.3 • Critical Values for the χ^2 Distribution

	LEVEL OF SIGNIFICANCE				
df	.10	.05	.02	.01	.001
1	2.71	3.84	5.41	6.63	10.83
2	4.61	5.99	7.82	9.21	13.82
3	6.25	7.82	9.84	11.34	16.27
4	7.78	9.49	11.67	13.28	18.46
5	9.24	11.07	13.39	15.09	20.52
6	10.64	12.59	15.03	16.81	22.46
7	12.02	14.07	16.62	18.48	24.32
8	13.36	15.51	18.17	20.09	26.12
9	14.68	16.92	19.68	21.67	27.88
10	15.99	18.31	21.16	23.21	29.59
11	17.28	19.68	22.62	24.72	31.26
12	18.55	21.03	24.05	26.22	32.91
13	19.81	22.36	25.47	27.69	34.53
14	21.06	23.68	26.87	29.14	36.12
15	22.31	25.00	28.26	30.58	37.70
16	23.54	26.30	29.63	32.00	39.25
17	24.77	27.59	31.00	33.41	40.79
18	25.99	28.87	32.35	34.81	42.31
19	27.20	30.14	33.69	36.19	43.82
20	28.41	31.41	35.02	37.57	45.32
21	29.62	32.67	36.34	38.93	46.80
22	30.81	33.92	37.66	40.29	48.27
23	32.01	35.17	38.97	41.64	49.73
24	33.20	36.42	40.27	42.98	51.18
25	34.38	37.65	41.57	44.31	52.62
26	35.56	38.89	42.86	45.64	54.05
27	36.74	40.11	44.14	46.96	55.48
28	37.92	41.34	45.42	48.28	56.89
29	39.09	42.56	46.69	49.59	58.30
30	40.26	43.77	47.96	50.89	59.70

TABLE A.4 • Critical Values of the *r* Distribution

	LEVEL OF SIGNIFICANCE FOR ONE-TAILED TEST				
	.05	.025	.01	.005	.0005
	LEVEL OF SIGNIFICANCE FOR TWO-TAILED TEST				
df	.10	.05	.02	.01	.001
1	.98769	.99692	.999507	.999877	.9999988
2	.90000	.95000	.98000	.990000	.99900
3	.8054	.8783	.93433	.95873	.99116
4	.7293	.8114	.8822	.91720	.97406
5	.6694	.7545	.8329	.8745	.95074
6	.6215	.7067	.7887	.8343	.92493
7	.5822	.6664	.7498	.7977	.8982
8	.5494	.6319	.7155	.7646	.8721
9	.5214	.6021	.6851	.7348	.8471
10	.4973	.5760	.6581	.7079	.8233
11	.4762	.5529	.6339	.6835	.8010
12	.4575	.5324	.6120	.6614	.7800
13	.4409	.5139	.5923	.5411	.7603
14	.4259	.4973	.5742	.6226	.7420
15	.4124	.4821	.5577	.6055	.7246
16	.4000	.4683	.5425	.5897	.7084
17	.3887	.4555	.5285	.5751	.6932
18	.3783	.4438	.5155	.5614	.5687
19	.3687	.4329	.5034	.5487	.6652
20	.3598	.4227	.4921	.5368	.6524
25	.3233	.3809	.4451	.5869	.5974
30	.2960	.3494	.4093	.4487	.5541
35	.2746	.3246	.3810	.4182	.5189
40	.2573	.3044	.3578	.3932	.4896
45	.2428	.2875	.3384	.3721	.4648
50	.2306	.2732	.3218	.3541	.4433
60	.2108	.2500	.2948	.3248	.4078
70	.1954	.2319	.2737	.3017	.3799
80	.1829	.2172	.2565	.2830	.3568
90	.1726	.2050	.2422	.2673	.3375
100	.1638	.1946	.2301	.2540	.3211

Index

Page numbers in bold type indicate glossary entries.
Entries in the chapter supplements are indicated by chapter number (e.g., an entry with Supp-1 is in the Chapter 1 Supplement).

This list contains some commonly used symbols in statistics. The list is in approximate alphabetical order, with English and Greek letters intermixed. Nonletter symbols have been placed at the end.

Symbol	Meaning
a	Regression constant, the intercept
α	Greek alpha; significance level in hypothesis testing, probability of Type I error; also, a reliability coefficient
b	Regression coefficient, slope of the line
β	Greek beta; probability of a Type II error; also, a standardized regression coefficient (beta weight)
χ^2	Greek chi squared, a test statistic for several statistical tests
CI	Confidence interval around estimate of a population parameter
d	An effect size index, a standardized mean difference
df	Degrees of freedom
η^2	Greek eta squared, index of variance accounted for in ANOVA context
f	Frequency (count) for a score value
F	Test statistic used in ANOVA, ANCOVA, and other tests
H_0	Null hypothesis
H_A	Alternative hypothesis; research hypothesis
λ	Greek lambda, a test statistic used in several multivariate analyses (Wilks' lambda)
μ	Greek mu, the population mean
M	Sample mean (alternative symbol for $\bar{X}$)
MS	Mean square, variance estimate in ANOVA
n	Number of cases in a subgroup of the sample
N	Total number of cases or sample members
NNT	Number needed to treat
OR	Odds ratio
p	Probability that observed data are consistent with null hypothesis
r	Pearson's product–moment correlation coefficient for a sample
r_s	Spearman's rank-order correlation coefficient
R	Multiple correlation coefficient
R^2	Coefficient of determination, proportion of variance in dependent variable attributable to independent variables
RR	Relative risk
ρ	Greek rho, population correlation coefficient
SD	Sample standard deviation
SEM	Standard error of the mean
σ	Greek sigma (lowercase), population standard deviation
Σ	Greek sigma (uppercase), sum of
SS	Sum of squares
t	Test statistics used in t-tests (sometimes called Student's t)
U	Test statistic for the Mann-Whitney U-test
$\bar{X}$	Sample mean
x	Deviation score
Y'	Predicted value of Y, dependent variable in regression analysis
z	Standard score in a normal distribution
$\|\ \|$	Absolute value
$\leq$	Less than or equal to
$\geq$	Greater than or equal to
$\neq$	Not equal to